SAUNDERS Review of
DENTAL
HYGIENE

SAUNDERS Review of DENTAL HYGIENE

Second Edition

Margaret J. Fehrenbach, RDH, MS
Dental Hygiene Educational Consultant
Dental Science Technical Writer
Seattle, Washington

Jane Weiner, RDH, BS Candidate
Owner, Jane Weiner, RDH, Board Reviews, Inc.
Faculty and Staff
Nova Southeastern University College of Dental Medicine
Fort Lauderdale, Florida

SAUNDERS

ELSEVIER

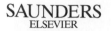

11830 Westline Industrial Drive
St. Louis, Missouri 63146

SAUNDERS REVIEW OF DENTAL HYGIENE, SECOND EDITION
Copyright © 2009, 2000 by Saunders, an imprint of Elsevier Inc.

ISBN: 978-1-4160-6255-4

Notice

Knowledge and best practice in this field are constantly changing. As new research and experience broaden our knowledge, changes in practice, treatment and drug therapy may become necessary or appropriate. Readers are advised to check the most current information provided (i) on procedures featured or (ii) by the manufacturer of each product to be administered, to verify the recommended dose or formula, the method and duration of administration, and contraindications. It is the responsibility of the practitioner, relying on their own experience and knowledge of the patient, to make diagnoses, to determine dosages and the best treatment for each individual patient, and to take all appropriate safety precautions. To the fullest extent of the law, neither the Publisher nor the Authors assume any liability for any injury and/or damage to persons or property arising out of or related to any use of the material contained in this book.

The Publisher

Library of Congress Cataloging-in-Publication Data
Fehrenbach, Margaret J.
Saunders review of dental hygiene / Margaret J. Fehrenbach, Jane Weiner. -- 2nd ed.
    p. ; cm.
  Rev. ed. of : Saunders review of dental hygiene / Debralee McKelvey Nelson. 1st ed. c2000.
  Includes bibliographical references and index.
   ISBN 978-1-4160-6255-4 (pbk. : alk. paper) 1. Dental hygiene. 2. Dental hygiene--Case studies.
3. Dental hygiene--Examinations, questions, etc. I. Weiner, Jane, 1944- II. Nelson, Debralee McKelvey.
Saunders review of dental hygiene. III. Title. IV. Title: Review of dental hygiene.
[DNLM: 1. Dental Prophylaxis--Case Reports. 2. Dental Prophylaxis--Examination Questions.
WU 18.2 F296w 2009]
RK60.7.N44 2009
617.6'01--dc22

2008034346

Vice President and Publisher: Linda Duncan
Senior Acquisitions Editor: John Dolan
Developmental Editor: Joslyn Dumas
Publishing Services Manager: Patricia Tannian
Design Direction: Jessica Williams

Printed in United States of America

Last digit is the print number: 9 8 7 6 5 4 3 2 1

To the student dental hygienists we have known who have gone on to become potent professionals and those we hope to meet, as well as their hardworking and devoted instructors, without whom learning would not be possible

Preface

ABOUT THE TEXT

Since its introduction 8 years ago, *Saunders Review of Dental Hygiene* has solidified its place in the market as one of the leading supplemental dental hygiene review books. Students often look for a supplemental text, in addition to their required texts, to help them prepare for exams. *Saunders Review of Dental Hygiene* has been that text for many students. The success of the first edition, as well as new guidelines in the areas of infection control and pharmacology, has made a second edition a necessity.

Examinations are designed to test and improve your intellect. They take both mental and physical stamina, and you should be well prepared for them as you enter your professional career. This text is a tool to help you prepare for the National Board of Dental Hygiene Exam (NBDHE), as well as to aid you in recognizing your strengths and weaknesses. The text will make obvious the areas you may need to review, strengthen your knowledge, and improve your test-taking abilities.

This **new** edition maintains many of the successful key features of the first edition, such as more than 60 clinical studies and over 1500 questions, while offering several exciting updates, including a CD-ROM. These elements will help you to better review the theories, skills, and conclusions you will be expected to know for the National Board Examination.

CD-ROM

The CD-ROM is an integral part of this text and offers another vehicle for reviewing. It includes a full-length computerized simulated exam that is divided into two sections, Component A and Component B. Component A consists of 200 randomly ordered questions with answers and rationales available. Component B includes 15 case studies with accompanying answers and rationales that test your ability to make case-based decisions. These cases are in the new format introduced by the American Dental Association.

You will be able to take the test in two formats. The first format will not be timed, and you will be able to move through the exam at your leisure. If an incorrect answer is chosen, you will be provided with the rationale for why that answer is incorrect. The second format will be timed, and you will have the same amount of time to complete the exam as you will when you actually take the NBDHE. At the end of the exam, the CD will score you and give you a breakdown of what answers you got correct and what answers were incorrect.

In addition to the computerized simulated exam, there are crossword puzzles and word searches to serve as study tools. These are available for each chapter and will aid you in memorizing terminology and recognizing anatomical structures. Key terms (in bold), references, weblinks, and other related articles are available for each chapter and provide additional resources for information to complement your school studies.

OTHER FEATURES

Updated case study format. The case studies on the CD-ROM have been created within the updated guidelines published by the ADA. This format allows you to consider other external factors that can have an effect on dental and general health. It also eliminates the use of names, removing any insinuation of ethnicity or nationality. The cases are designed to test your ability to make sound objective judgments when faced not only with dental but also with pharmacological and medical concerns. They are followed by test questions that focus on providing quality care to the patient. Within the computerized simulated exam on the CD-ROM, each case is presented with a patient history, dental charts, radiographs, and clinical photographs. In addition, throughout the text are clinical, community health, and professional practice studies in a "testlet" mode that combines a scenario with the case study format to further test your judgmental abilities.

Text written in an easy to read summary mode. The authors have remodeled the text into an easy to read summary format. This format provides a straightforward outline that makes vital material easier to retain. The format is consistent throughout the book, which gives the text a cohesive look and feel.

Fully modeled after specific NBDHE guidelines. The purpose of *Saunders Review of Dental Hygiene* is to provide you with a review text that will help you prepare for the NBDHE. Therefore it is essential that the NBDH format be followed as closely as possible. This allows you to get used to the testing conditions you will experience when you take the board exam. The full-length, computerized simulated exam on the CD-ROM is modeled directly after the NBDHE. The formats of each section, the amount of time you have, and the case studies are all representative of the NBDHE. Now you can take advantage of this invaluable resource to make the review process much easier.

The second edition of *Saunders Review of Dental Hygiene* will be a vital tool in helping you prepare for the NBDHE by both familiarizing you with the format you will see on the exam and improving your test-taking abilities. The benefit of this text is invaluable and will greatly reduce the anxiety associated with test-taking. All the elements of the text and CD package combine to deliver a review book that will carry you through the review process and aid in your success on the NBDHE.

Margaret J. Fehrenbach
Jane Weiner

Acknowledgments

We would like to thank Debralee McKelvey Nelson, RDH, MS, and her contributors from the first edition of this textbook. In addition, we would like to thank the editorial staff in Dentistry, Dental Assisting, Dental Hygiene at Elsevier, Inc., including John Dolan, Senior Editor, and Joslyn Dumas, Developmental Editor, as well as Patrica Tannian, Publishing Services Manager. We would also like to thank the following reviewers of this second edition:

Jorge Arenas, DMD
Department of Radiology
Nova Southeastern University, College of Dental
    Medicine
Fort Lauderdale, Florida
Radiology

Marge Bell, BS, RDH
Dental Hygiene Program Coordinator
Ozarks Technical Community College
Springfield, Missouri
Community Oral Health

Elizabeth L. Fehrenbach, BA
Student Nurse Practitioner, John Hopkins University
Baltimore, Maryland
*Anatomy, Biochemistry, and Physiology; Microbiology
    and Immunology*

Barbara G. Hammaker, RDH, BASDH
Adjunct Instructor
St. Petersburg College, St. Petersburg, Florida
Broward Community College, Davie, Florida
Pharmacology

Juli Kagan, RDH, MEd
Clinical Instructor and Lecturer, Department of
    Periodontology
Nova Southeastern University
College of Dental Medicine, Fort Lauderdale, Florida
Periodontology and Component B

Amy M. Nieves, RDH
Webmaster, amyrdh.com and www.amysrdhlist.com.
Preparing for the NBDHE

Michael A. Siegel, DDS, MS, FRCSEd
Professor and Chair, Department of Diagnostic Sciences
Nova Southeastern University College of Dental
    Medicine
Fort Lauderdale, Florida
House Staff, Department of Surgery, Division of Oral
    and Maxillofacial Surgery
Broward General Medical Center, Fort Lauderdale,
    Florida
*Dental and Medical Emergencies; Anatomy,
    Biochemistry, and Physiology*

Sharon Crane Siegel, DDS, MS
Chair and Associate Professor, Department of
    Prosthodontics
Nova Southeastern University, College of Dental
    Medicine
Fort Lauderdale, Florida
Clinical Associate Professor, Department of Restorative
    Dentistry
Baltimore College of Dental Surgery, University of
    Maryland
Baltimore, Maryland
Dental Biomaterials

Laura J. Webb, CDA, RDH, MS
Independent Consultant
Fallon, Nevada
Nutrition; Community Oral Health

Contents

SAUNDERS Review of
DENTAL
HYGIENE

CHAPTER 1

Preparing for the National Board Dental Hygiene Examination

NATIONAL BOARD DENTAL HYGIENE EXAMINATION

The National Board Dental Hygiene Examination (NBDHE) is developed and administered by the Joint Commission on National Dental Examinations of the American Dental Association. This examination fulfills or partially fulfills the examination requirement in all 50 states of the United States and the District of Columbia, Puerto Rico, and the Virgin Islands. Individual states determine the acceptance of the examination as a requirement, the period before expiration of results, and the percentage score accepted as passing. (See the WebLinks on the CD-ROM that accompanies the textbook for contact sites and candidate guidelines.)

The purpose of the NBDHE is to determine the professional competency of applicants for licensure. The examination assesses the candidate's ability to recall, analyze, and apply basic information and concepts typically taught in the dental hygiene curriculum.

The NBDHE is in English and consists overall of 350 multiple-choice questions. Of this total, approximately 200 questions are traditional (stand-alone) multiple-choice questions and the remaining 150 questions are based on approximately 12 to 15 dental hygiene treatment cases. The examination is comprehensive in that it covers topics taught to enable competency in performing dental hygiene care as determined by delegated functions of dental hygienists in the majority of the nation.

More specifically, Component A of the examination, the stand-alone multiple-choice section, has 176 independent items in the areas of basis for dental hygiene practice (~30%) and provision of clinical dental hygiene services (~60%) and 24 testlet-dependent items on community health or research principles (~10%).

Multiple-choice questions contain a question stem and four or five answer choices (see later discussion of question types, test-taking strategies, and test anxiety). Each question has only one CORRECT answer. It is important to note that some of the questions are ONLY for trial run to see if they will be included in future tests. Passage of the NBDHE requires a score of 75% or greater.

Component B of the examination contains 12 to 15 case-based problems with comprehensive scenarios (discussed later) that describe a specific situation and require you to demonstrate skill in the following areas:

- Assessing patient characteristics
- Obtaining and interpreting radiographs
- Planning and managing dental hygiene care
- Performing periodontal procedures
- Using preventive agents
- Providing supportive treatment service
- Professional responsibility

The case-based scenarios may include descriptions, photographs, illustrations, radiographs, dental and periodontal data, or other information necessary to present the case of both adult and child patients. Each case is followed by multiple-choice test items related to the scenario. Each examination includes at least one case regarding the following types of patients who may be encountered in dental practice: Geriatric, Adult-periodontal, Pediatric, Special Needs, and Medically Compromised; 80% of cases concern adult patients, and 20% children. Just as in a real dental setting, many distractions will be included!

USING *SAUNDERS REVIEW OF DENTAL HYGIENE*

The updated new second edition of this text has been prepared by well-respected dental hygiene educators who have researched the topics and concepts needed to succeed on the NBDHE. One author has been a member of the board examination basic science committee in the past and has textbooks on various dental science topics that are used in many dental hygiene programs in the United States and abroad. The other author owns her own NDHBE review company and conducts review courses for the board exam in venues across the United States. Both authors have worked hard to ensure that the text is to the point and easy to read and use as a study guide.

The material contained in the NBDHE is primarily applicable to dental hygiene practice. Success on the national board examination means that the test taker has an adequate understanding of the concepts and applications of the dental hygiene knowledge base. This updated edition of the textbook consists of 18 chapters. Its newly produced CD-ROM has a simulated NBDHE as well as other IMPORTANT and fun study features. The chapters provide a comprehensive review of basic knowledge of dental hygiene scientific subjects that are MORE likely to appear on the NBDHE, as well as complete discussion of each of the possible types of patients who may appear in the cases on the examination. The material provided is so much MORE than flash cards or dental study facts!

Each chapter in the new edition includes a short-form clinical study and/or testlet. It is a short-form case study, since it is without the photographs, illustrations, radiographs, and dental and periodontal data normally present for a complete clinical study. However, these are used to illustrate IMPORTANT application of content in the chapter and contain a scenario filled with common problems followed by a series of related open-ended questions with answers and rationale. Presenting clinical studies in this updated form FIRST is helpful in improving analytical and application skills. Even though testlets are used mainly with community health activity items on the NBDHE, a careful study of these short-form clinical studies and/or testlets with their discussions will help prepare you for more complex cases with closed-ended questions that appear on the NBDHE and for situations that arise in clinical practice.

Along with each clinical study is a comprehensive review of the subject with relevant material updated for this new edition. We recommend that you read each clinical study both before and after reviewing the chapter content related to it. After you study the entire chapter's content review and clinical studies, answer the review questions at the end of the chapter and compare the answers with those in the rationale section that follows. Questions included were specifically developed to be SIMILAR in format, content, and depth to those that appear on the NBDHE. The rationale with answer key is particularly useful because it contains discussion of why certain answers are correct or incorrect. Thus it can help you BETTER understand why one answer choice is better than another choice. In addition, the index in the text is a useful resource to look up information about a specific term or topic that comes up during your study for the examination.

CD-ROM with the Textbook

The CD-ROM accompanying the textbook has many sections useful in studying for the NDHBE.

The Computer-Simulated National Board Dental Hygiene Examination is comparable in length, format, and difficulty to the NBDHE. The computer-simulated examination can be taken as a timed examination or can be browsed through during initial studies.

The computer-simulated examination is broken down into two parts. Component A contains 200 randomly ordered, multiple-choice questions covering basic dental hygiene

science, provision of clinical dental hygiene services, and community health activities. Rationales for all questions are included.

Component B consists of 15 case-based studies developed to help you assess, plan, integrate, evaluate, and analyze clinical information. The case studies, selected to imitate situations a dental hygienist might encounter in practice, require you to carefully assess the information provided, including medical and dental data, photographs, and radiographs (enlarged slightly for learning purposes) to answer 150 case-specific questions. A thorough study of this section of the simulated examination will help you develop the knowledge and skills necessary to successfully manage the cases presented on the NBDHE and in clinical practice. Rationales for all questions are included.

Additional study resources on the CD-ROM include the following:
- Chapter Review Schedule
- Learning Strategies
- Mnemonic Study Tips
- Chapter Terms and Puzzles
- Study Programs
- Guidelines and Graphics
- Chapter WebLinks
- Textbook References

PREPARING FOR THE NDHBE

There is NO guaranteed method for a student dental hygienist to prepare for the NBDHE, but we would like to share some concepts with you as you prepare for the examination.
- Standardized testing attempts to assess knowledge and comprehension of specific subject matter, as well as the ability to analyze information and apply the knowledge in practical ways. Examination questions therefore run the gamut from easy (rote memory or recall) to difficult (analysis or case study). While memorization is adequate to answer simple questions, you MUST have a deeper understanding of concepts and theory to answer questions that assess higher level learning. However, you should NOT forget to include the fun hints and mnemonic devices that your instructors share with you (see Mnemonic Study Tips on the CD-ROM with the textbook).
- The BEST preparation for the NDHBE is thorough study throughout the course of the professional program. Also, attending a review course with your study group is invaluable and memorable, too! Review for the NBDHE and other professional examinations can refresh the memory and help clarify information NOT understood well previously.
- Proper preparation is essential for successful test taking. The MORE time you initially spend learning the material, the LESS time you will spend when reviewing material

for competency testing. Conversely, those who have NOT mastered a subject will need to spend MORE time reviewing for a competency examination, since they must "relearn" much of the material. (See Learning Strategies on the CD-ROM.)

- Becoming familiar with the NDHBE examination is vitally IMPORTANT in test taking. Take time to examine the testing materials and sample booklets that you can access through your program or online to gain a general knowledge of which topics are covered and in what depth, the type or style of questions on the examination and their depth and number, the sections or parts of the examination, the amount of time allowed to answer each question or section on the exam, common directions or instructions used, materials that can be used during the examination, and how the examination is scored. (See the WebLinks on the CD-ROM for candidate guidelines.)

- Schedule study time. Begin studying for national board examinations approximately 3 to 6 months in advance. Schedule study time into your weekly calendar, preferably setting aside the same period each week (for example, reserving Thursday mornings from 8 to 10 AM for review). In this way the review is organized, manageable, and NOT likely to be forgotten. Set up a schedule of study topics (use the Review Schedule on the CD-ROM). If inadequate time remains for a thorough review of all subject matter, select a few (three to five) of your *weakest* subjects or the subjects with *greater* coverage on the examination and learn them well. Trying to review the entire curriculum in too short a time will only frustrate you and seldom leads to much learning.

- Plan study time in 2- to 5-hour segments. Be sure to take scheduled, frequent breaks. The breaks should occur every 30 to 60 minutes and last less than 10 minutes. Set a timer to ring whenever a break is due. This technique is helpful for training you to concentrate on the task rather than on the clock. When a break arrives, use the time to visit the restroom, refill beverage containers, take a brisk walk, or exercise before sitting down to study again. Do NOT turn on the television, pick up a magazine, or do anything that might interfere with the resolve to study.

- Make it a rule to study the MOST difficult subject first, saving easier subjects for later in the study period. In this way you will avoid procrastination and achieve an immense sense of accomplishment. Use the Chapter Terms on the CD-ROM for clarification of each subject. If you are having difficulty with a particularly challenging subject, however, take on an easier one for a day and then go back to the harder one.

- Studying in groups or individually is a personal preference. For those who find it difficult to set a study schedule and follow through, group study may be the answer. While group study is MORE difficult to organize and somewhat MORE time consuming, it allows group members to learn from one another, is LESS boring, and sparks the discussion of topics. A *study group* should be limited to six or fewer members, have a set time and place for meeting, and require members to prepare for meetings.

  ▷ All members should be informed before the study period of what the topic of review is and how they should prepare for it. This can help bring members to a similar level of knowledge and will usually lead to a more meaningful discussion. Keeping members on the task of reviewing is the MOST difficult part of the group study. Keep discussion of children and pets to a minimum!

  ▷ Set a specific start and end time for each review session. This helps motivate you to stay on task. Planning the study period to end when a favorite television program or event begins can be a good incentive and reward. Using enjoyable means of learning is also helpful. (See Chapter Puzzles and Chapter WebLinks on the CD-ROM.)

  ▷ After every review session, check off the subject matter studied on the Review Schedule (on the CD-ROM) and plan the next review topic. Charting your progress on a form such as the Review Schedule provides the BEST sense of accomplishment and further incentive to continue reviewing.

  ▷ Studying individually also has its benefits and detriments. Individual study sessions are easier to organize, require less time, and allow the student to review at his or her own pace. This type of studying is BEST for the self-directed learner who is able to set a study schedule and follow through. Like study group sessions, individual study sessions should be held at specific times in specific locations.

- Getting enough rest is essential before a big examination. This is much easier to accomplish when you feel comfortably prepared for the examination. Not surprisingly, the ability to sleep well before a stressful event is much greater when you feel up to the task. It is MOST important that you not study the evening before a big examination. You should have completed all your preparation by noon the day before. Instead, do something relaxing to relieve anxiety—take a long walk, watch a favorite movie, prepare a nice meal, and go to bed at the usual time.

- Making sure to eat the CORRECT type of meals and knowing proper nutrition are essential while you are reviewing for the examination and before you take the exam. Your diet should be well balanced and provide enough calories for sustenance, as you have learned in your classes. Eating properly the day of the exam has been shown to affect exam results. Do NOT eat a heavy carbohydrate breakfast or lunch. Rather, eat a full breakfast that is *high* in protein and a light, *high*-protein lunch. This will help you stay alert throughout the exam day. See Chapter 7, Nutrition, for a good review of this information.

- After thorough preparation, attitude is probably the MOST important factor in successful test taking. Taking the exam with the attitude that you are prepared and capable of success is extremely important. Many people will attest that the pressure they put on themselves before an examination can adversely affect their performance. Think positively. Having a clear and relaxed mind is very important. A little anxiety is normal and can be beneficial during an examination (see later discussion of test-taking anxiety). After all, you have taken the CORRECT courses of study and have done well; now you are to be *tested on knowledge* that you already have in your head and for the most part will use in your new career!

- A thing you might find challenging on the exam day is time expediency. Do NOT panic if you think that you are taking too long to complete the test. That is why it is a timed exam. Some people will NOT require as much time as others, and that is OK. The important thing is NOT to change your answers and to answer every question, even questions on which you might need to "guesstimate." Once you answer, leave the answer as is. Usually when people randomly change an answer, that is when they get it wrong.

- Remember that this is what you want to do with your career, so be confident that the exam is one of the FIRST steps to reaching that first day in your profession. Smile and have fun with the dear friends you have made in your dental hygiene program; they will probably be your personal and professional friends for life!

Question Types on the NBDHE

Seven basic question formats are used on the NBDHE. These include the completion, question, negative, paired true-false, cause-and-effect, testlet, and case study question formats. Each question stem is followed by four or five answer choices.

Remember that you CANNOT learn everything and you CANNOT remember everything, but you can be familiar enough with the information that you will be able to make an educated decision and use critical thinking to identify the CORRECT answer out of four or five multiple-choice answers. Following are a brief description and example of each *type of question* (correct answers are marked with an asterisk).

Completion-type questions are simple and easy to read and understand. The question stem consists of a partial statement that the BEST answer completes.

Opsonins are
A. cytokines produced by B cells.
B. antigens that directly neutralize viruses.
C. antibodies deficient in the Fc region.
D. molecules that stimulate phagocytosis.*

Question-type questions are the simplest to read and understand. They ask a specific question for which there is one BEST answer.

Which one of the following collimator types can most effectively reduce scatter radiation to the patient?
A. Long round
B. Pointed plastic
C. Rectangular*
D. Short round

Negative-type (exception) questions ask the reader to determine which answer does NOT pertain to information in the question stem. They usually include the words "NOT," "LEAST LIKELY," or "EXCEPT."

Candida albicans is known or suspected to cause all of the following denture-related problems, EXCEPT one. Which one is the EXCEPTION?
A. Denture stomatitis
B. Thrush
C. Papillary hyperplasia*
D. Angular cheilitis

Paired true-false questions contain two statements about a related topic. You will be asked to determine if either *one* or *both* of the statements are TRUE. As with multiple-choice questions having four answer choices, you have a 25% chance of selecting the correct answer by guessing.

Gingival inflammation always precedes periodontal disease. Periodontal disease always follows gingival inflammation.
A. Both statements are true.
B. Both statements are false.
C. The first statement is true, the second is false.*
D. The first statement is false, the second is true.

Cause-and-effect questions are similar in format to paired true-false questions. They consist of a single statement that is divided into *cause*-and-*effect* portions. The two portions are separated by the word "because." You will be asked to determine if the statement and reason are CORRECT and related. As with multiple-choice questions having four or five answer choices, you have a 25% or 20% chance of selecting the correct answer by guessing.

Obesity is often associated with Type 1 diabetes mellitus because obesity affects insulin resistance.
A. Both the statement and reason are correct and related.*
B. Both the statement and reason are correct but NOT related.
C. The statement is correct, but the reason is NOT.
D. The statement is NOT correct, but the reason is correct.
E. NEITHER the statement NOR the reason is correct.

Testlet-type questions include a brief description of a situation or case study (usually one to two paragraphs in length) and a series of five or more situation-related questions. This type of question is commonly used on the NBDHE to test Community Health Activity items. (Refer to the Community Health Testlet on the simulated NBDHE on the CD-ROM that accompanies the textbook.) However, we expanded the use of this type of question format throughout the text in all areas of study, so you can become comfortable with its easy situational format and since it prepares you for the involved case-based-type queations.

Case-based-type questions contain patient information (medical and dental history, significant oral findings, radiographs, periodontal probe readings, photographs, etc.) followed by a series of 10 to 12 case-based questions. This type of question requires you to study the case information carefully, paying particular attention to its focus. You must identify and analyze information useful for answering the case questions. (Refer to the simulated NBDHE on the CD-ROM, discussed earlier.)

Test-Taking Strategies for a Multiple-Choice Style Test

Multiple-choice-style questions found on the NDHBE tend to be MORE time consuming than other questions. They require careful reading and analysis of the question stem for content and meaning. Following are some *standard guides* for taking multiple-choice-style tests.

1. You MUST read each question carefully for meaning.
   a. AVOID choices with the words "never," "always," and "all," since they are so restrictive that they seldom appear in the correct answer; nothing is ever a definite in science or health.
   b. When the question has the words "except," "not," or "but," the focus of the question changes and you MUST change your focus too.
   c. Look for answers that are different from the rest. If three answers say MAINLY the same thing but in different words, choose the answer that is more radically different than the others.
2. At the examination site, quickly preview each question in the examination *before* beginning to answer each of them.
   a. Try to answer each question *before* looking at the possible answer choices. Find an answer choice that parallels yours. If the correct answer cannot be determined easily, begin first by eliminating answer choices with the MOST obviously wrong answer. Once choices are limited to two or three, attempt to clarify the question by redefining or restating it or drawing on other knowledge.
   b. When unsure, choose the answer that was instinctively the FIRST choice.
3. Answer ALL questions while going through the examination and record the answers as indicated.

4. Remember that it does NOT matter if you are first or last to finish…take all the time you need and try NOT to be distracted as people leave the testing facility.

TEST-TAKING ANXIETY

Test anxiety has affected nearly everyone at some time. It is often described as an extreme anxiety that causes shaky legs, sick stomach, jittery hands, chaotic thinking, and outright panic. If unmanaged, it can result in wasted time and ineffective test taking. When you are prepared for an examination and have a *positive attitude* (confidence in your abilities) and a strategy to deal with the jitters, this allows you to take control of the anxiety and make test taking a success.

Mild anxiety is normal and is actually helpful because it increases alertness. When you are faced with the panicky feeling of high anxiety, however, your ability to concentrate is reduced. Following are several effective ways to prevent and control test anxiety (also see Learning Strategies on the CD-ROM).

- Careful preparation for an examination is essential in preventing test anxiety. Knowing the material on which you are being tested provides you with confidence to pass the exam. Procrastination and disorganized time management are usually the reasons for less than helpful exam preparation. Use the Review Schedule on the CD-ROM to plan study times and stick with them.
- Self-confidence is key to success. A positive attitude, along with careful exam preparation, is essential. The type of careful exam preparation that increases self-confidence includes a thorough review of exam subjects, adequate study time, familiarization with the exam format and instructions, and understanding of test scoring (e.g., whether wrong answers are penalized or not).
- Take the night off before the exam. Relax, eat properly, and get plenty of sleep. Be confident in your preparation; studying the evening before the exam increases anxiety.
- Plan to arrive at the exam site early with needed materials (identification, wristwatch, etc.) so that you have time to relax. Some of the hurdles you might find when taking the exam are extraneous noises (bring earplugs) or radiographs (remember your prescription or reading glasses).
- Relaxation techniques can help relieve anxiety. Practice deep breathing (breathe in deeply, hold breath a few seconds, then release) for at least 10 minutes whenever you feel muscle tension—when studying or during the examination. Visualization is another technique that can relieve tension. To visualize, close your eyes and sit comfortably. Use as many senses (hearing, vision, smell, taste, feel) as possible to relive a positive experience. Imagine floating on water in warm sunlight or hearing the sounds of nature on a hike in the woods.

CHAPTER 2

Embryology and Histology

EMBRYOLOGY

Embryology is the study of prenatal development (gestation period), which begins with fertilization and continues until birth. Divided into three periods: preimplantation, embryonic, fetal.

- See CD-ROM for Chapter Terms and WebLinks.
- See Chapters 9, Pharmacology: drugs and placental barrier; 11, Clinical Treatment: pregnant patient.

A. Preimplantation period (FIRST week):
1. Union of ovum and sperm undergoes **fertilization** to form egg (zygote) where final stages of **meiosis** occur in ovum:
   a. To allow formation of new individual, sperm and ovum when joined have CORRECT number of chromosomes (diploid number of 46).
   b. Ovum and sperm have to reduce by one half the normal number of chromosomes (to haploid number of 23).
   c. Thus zygote received half its chromosomes from female and half from male, with resultant genetic material a reflection of BOTH biological parents.
   d. Photographic analysis of person's chromosomes is done by orderly arrangement of pairs in a **karyotype.**
2. After fertilization, zygote undergoes **mitosis** (individual cell division); solid ball of cells is a morula; review of the stages and terms of mitosis is recommended (see CD-ROM WebLinks).
3. Because of ongoing process of mitosis and secretion of fluid by the cells within morula, zygote becomes a blastocyst (blastula), which undergoes successive cell divisions by mitosis:
   a. By end of first week, blastocyst stops traveling, undergoes implantation, and becomes embedded in prepared endometrium, which is the innermost layer of uterine lining.
   b. After 1 week of cleavage, blastocyst consists of trophoblast layer (layer of peripheral cells) and embryoblast layer (small inner mass of embryonic cells).

B. **Embryonic period** (weeks 2 through 8): implanted blastocyst becomes **embryo** after first week.
1. Second week:
   a. Increased number of cells creates embryonic cell layers (germ layers) and forms disc.
   b. *Bilaminar* disc (also known as disk); two-layered, flattened, essentially circular plate of cells with superior epiblast layer (high columnar cells) and inferior hypoblast layer (small cuboidal cells).
   c. Disc is suspended in uterus's endometrium between two fluid-filled cavities: amniotic cavity faces epiblast layer, and yolk sac faces hypoblast layer; BOTH serve as initial nourishment for embryonic disc.
   d. **Placenta:** prenatal organ that joins pregnant woman and developing embryo; permits selective exchange of soluble bloodborne substances (including drugs and nutrients) through the placental barrier.
2. Third week:
   a. Within the disc, primitive streak forms, which is a furrowed, rod-shaped thickening in the middle of the disc:
      (1) Cells from epiblast layer migrate *between* the two layers, becoming mesenchyme, embryonic connective tissue.
      (2) Mesenchyme layer has potential to proliferate and differentiate into IMPORTANT types of connective tissue-forming cells (e.g., fibroblasts, chondroblasts, osteoblasts).
   b. Differentiation of new embryonic layer within disc from mesenchyme, called **mesoderm:**
      (1) *Trilaminar* disc: three-layered disc with epiblast layer now ectoderm and hypoblast layer now endoderm.
         (a) Ectoderm: forms epidermis of skin, nervous system, other structures.
         (b) Mesoderm: forms muscle coats, connective tissues, vessels supplying tissues and organs, other tissues.
         (c) Endoderm: forms epithelial linings of respiratory passages and digestive tract, including some glandular organ cells.
   c. Disc now has a cephalic end (head) where oropharyngeal membrane (buccopharyngeal membrane, future mouth) forms and caudal end (tail) where cloacal membrane forms (future anus).
3. Fourth week:
   a. Central nervous system (CNS) begins to develop in embryo:

(1) Neuroectoderm differentiates from ectoderm, localized to neural plate.

(2) Neural plate is a band of cells that extends length of the embryo, from cephalic to caudal end.

(3) Plate undergoes further growth and thickening, which cause it to deepen and invaginate centrally, forming the neural groove.

(4) Neural groove deepens further and becomes surrounded by neural folds, which meet superior to neural groove, forming a neural tube.

(5) Neural tube undergoes fusion at its most superior portion, future spinal cord.

b. Neural crest cells develop from neuroectoderm, then migrate from neural folds and disperse within mesenchyme; they are IMPORTANT in development of head and neck structures such as branchial arches.

4. Embryo also undergoes folding, placing three types of tissues in proper positions; recognizably human at end of embryonic period (eighth week).

C. **Fetal period** (weeks 9 through birth): encompasses beginning of ninth week (third month) to ninth month; involves maturation of existing structures as embryo enlarges to become a **fetus.**

D. **Congenital malformations** (birth defects):

1. Developmental problems evident at birth (or before because of prenatal diagnostic tests): occur during BOTH preimplantation and embryonic periods, thus in first trimester of pregnancy. Examples:

a. Ectopic pregnancy: implantation that occurs outside the uterus.

b. Down syndrome (trisomy 21): extra chromosome present after meiotic division.

c. Ectodermal dysplasia: abnormal development of one or more ectodermal structures.

d. Spina bifida: neural tube defect.

2. Malformations: caused by genetic factors such as chromosome abnormalities, environmental agents, teratogens.

a. **Teratogens:** infections (e.g., rubella virus), drugs (e.g., fetal alcohol syndrome [FAS] causing serious physical and mental disorders, systemic tetracycline antibiotic therapy causing intrinsic dental staining), radiation.

b. Women of reproductive age should AVOID teratogens at time of first missed menstrual period and thereafter, to protect developing child.

E. **Amniocentesis:** sampling of amniotic fluid.

1. MOST common invasive prenatal diagnostic procedure.

2. Fluid sampled during fourteenth to sixteenth weeks after last missed menstrual period.

3. Performed in older age groups: one or both parents have chromosomal abnormality or neural tube defect, previous child was affected, or parents are carriers of inborn errors of metabolism, e.g., X-linked disorders such as hemophilia.

DEVELOPMENT OF FACE AND ORAL CAVITY ■■■

Face and structures of the oral cavity begin development early in embryonic period. ALL three embryonic layers are involved in facial development (layers are discussed earlier). Depends on five facial processes (prominences) that form during fourth week and surround stomodeum (primitive mouth): (1) single frontonasal process; (2 and 3) paired maxillary processes; and (4 and 5) paired mandibular processes (Figure 2-1). In the future, the stomodeum will form the oral cavity.

A. Facial processes are centers of growth for the face:

1. If an adult's face is divided into thirds, these portions roughly correspond to centers of facial growth:

a. Upper face: from frontonasal process.

b. Middle face (midface): from maxillary processes.

c. Lower face: from mandibular processes.

B. Overall growth of the face is in inferior and anterior direction in relation to cranial base:

1. Growth of upper face is MORE rapid, in keeping with association with developing brain; forehead ceases to grow much after age 12.

2. In contrast, middle and lower portions of the face grow MORE slowly over prolonged period of time:

a. Finally cease to grow late in puberty.

b. Eruption of permanent third molars at around 17 to 21 years marks end of major growth of lower two thirds of face.

C. Underlying facial bones also developing at this time depend on centers of bone formation by intramembranous ossification.

Stomodeum and Oral Cavity Formation

Before fourth week, stomodeum initially appears as a shallow depression in embryonic surface ectoderm at cephalic end, limited in depth by oropharyngeal membrane (Figure 2-1).

A. FIRST event during fourth week is disintegration of oropharyngeal membrane:

1. Stomodeum is increased in depth, enlarging it to become oral cavity.

2. Now there is access by way of stomodeum from internal primitive pharynx to outside fluids of amniotic cavity surrounding embryo.

B. Stomodeum will form oral cavity:

1. Lined by oral epithelium, which is derived from ectoderm, as a result of embryonic folding.

2. Oral epithelium and underlying tissues will form teeth and associated tissues.

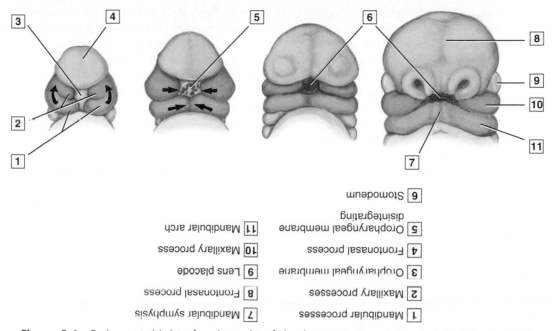

Figure 2-1 Embyro at third to fourth weeks of development. (From Bath-Balogh M, Fehrenbach MJ: *Illustrated dental embryology, histology, and anatomy, ed 2*, St. Louis, 2006, Saunders/Elsevier.)

1 Mandibular processes
2 Maxillary processes
3 Oropharyngeal membrane
4 Frontonasal process
5 Oropharyngeal membrane disintegrating
6 Stomodeum
7 Mandibular symphysis
8 Frontonasal process
9 Lens placode
10 Maxillary process
11 Mandibular arch

Mandibular Arch and Lower Face Formation

During fourth week, two bulges of tissue appear inferior to stomodeum; these paired mandibular processes are formed in part by neural crest cells that migrated to the facial region, covered externally by ectoderm and internally by endoderm (Figure 2-1).

A. Paired mandibular processes BOTH fuse at midline to form the mandibular arch (mandibular symphysis is indication):
   1. Mandibular arch and related tissues (also known as first branchial arch) are first portions of the face to form after creation of stomodeum.
   2. Directly forms lower face, including lower lip.
   3. Will also form mandible, mandibular teeth, associated tissues, as well as tongue.

B. Meckel's cartilage forms within each side of mandibular arch, IMPORTANT in alveolar bone development.
   1. Makes contribution to mandible, and portion of cartilage participates in formation of middle ear bones.
   2. Part of perichondrium surrounding Meckel's cartilage becomes ligaments of the jaws and middle ear.

C. Mesoderm of mandibular arch forms muscles of mastication, as well as some palatal muscles and suprahyoid muscles. Because these muscles are derived from mandibular arch, they are innervated by nerve of the first arch, fifth (V) cranial nerve (trigeminal).

Frontonasal Process and Upper Face Formation

During fourth week, frontonasal process is a bulge of tissue in upper facial area, at most cephalic end of embryo, which is also the cranial boundary of the stomodeum. In the future, frontonasal process will form upper face, which includes forehead, bridge of nose, primary palate, nasal septum, and all structures related to medial nasal processes (Figure 2-1).

A. Placodes become submerged, forming depression in center of each:
   1. Form nasal (olfactory) pits, which develop into nasal cavities.
   2. Deepening of nasal pits produces a nasal sac that grows internally toward developing brain; separated from the stomodeum by oronasal membrane.

B. On outer portion of nasal pits are two crescent-shaped swellings, lateral nasal processes that form the alae (sides of the nose).
   1. Middle portion of the tissue growing around nasal placodes appears as medial nasal processes.
   2. BOTH fuse together externally to form the middle portion of the nose from root to apex, center portion of upper lip, philtrum region.

C. BOTH paired medial nasal processes also fuse internally and grow inferiorly on inside of stomodeum:
   1. Form intermaxillary (premaxillary) segment, MOST anterior portion of the tissues.
   2. Involved in formation of maxillary incisor teeth and associated tissues, primary palate, nasal septum.

Maxillary Process and Midface Formation

During fourth week, adjacent swellings, the maxillary processes, form from increased growth of mandibular arch. Maxillary processes grow superiorly and anteriorly on each side of stomodeum (Figure 2-1).

A. Maxillary process will form the midface:
1. Includes sides of upper lip, cheeks, secondary palate.
2. Also posterior portion of maxilla, with maxillary canines and posteriors, associated tissues.
3. Also zygomatic bones and portions of temporal bones.

B. Each maxillary process fuses with each medial nasal process:
1. Contribute to sides of upper lip, and the two medial nasal processes contribute to middle of upper lip.
2. If the maxillary process on each side does NOT fuse with medial nasal process, cleft lip can result (discussed later).

Branchial Apparatus Formation

Branchial apparatus consists of the branchial arches, branchial grooves and membranes, pharyngeal pouches.

A. Arches are six pairs of U-shaped stacked bilateral swellings of tissue appearing inferior to the stomodeum and include the mandibular arch (FIRST branchial arch), which will form the lower face; each arch will form into different structures.
1. Each arch contains cartilaginous core, aortic arch, definite cranial nerve; each cranial nerve will supply the structures that develop from the mesenchyme of the arch.
2. Second (hyoid) arch enlarges and grows so that by the sixth week it will overlap the third, fourth, and sixth arches and cover them.
3. Tracts of epithelial cells can remain after development of the second pharyngeal arch; on occasion, a fistula opens to both the external surface and the pharynx, connecting these structures and becoming a complete branchial fistula.
4. However, a fistula can open externally on the anterolateral surface of the neck or internally to the pharynx by way of a ruptured pharyngeal membrane and become an incomplete branchial fistula.

B. Between neighboring branchial arches, branchial (pharyngeal) grooves are noted on each side of the embryo; FIRST groove forms the external auditory meatus and mesenchyme of first and second arches, which are located on either side of this pharyngeal groove, and will also give rise to the external ear.
1. Four well-defined pairs of pharyngeal pouches develop as endodermal evaginations form the lateral walls lining the pharynx and form different structures.
2. Space between the second arch and the other three arches is called the cervical sinus and is lined by ectoderm; sinus can undergo enlargement at a later time and form cervical cysts.

Palatal Development

Formation of the palate starts in the embryo during fifth week, takes place during several weeks of prenatal development, and is completed in twelfth week in the fetus (Figure 2-2). Formed from two separate embryonic structures, primary palate and secondary palate. Palate is developed in three consecutive stages: formation of primary palate, formation of secondary palate, completion of final (definitive) palate.

A. Intermaxillary segment forms primary (primitive) palate, a triangular mass:

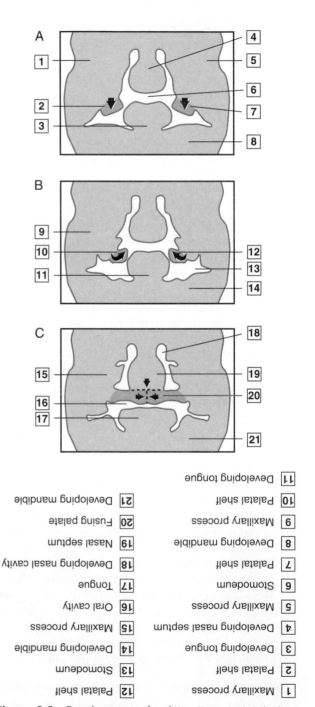

11 Developing tongue	
21 Developing mandible	10 Palatal shelf
20 Fusing palate	9 Maxillary process
19 Nasal septum	8 Developing mandible
18 Developing nasal cavity	7 Palatal shelf
17 Tongue	6 Stomodeum
16 Oral cavity	5 Maxillary process
15 Maxillary process	4 Developing nasal septum
14 Developing mandible	3 Developing tongue
13 Stomodeum	2 Palatal shelf
12 Palatal shelf	1 Maxillary process

Figure 2-2   Development of palate. (From Bath-Balogh M, Fehrenbach MJ: Illustrated dental embryology, histology, and anatomy, ed 2, St. Louis, 2006, Saunders/Elsevier.)

1. In the future, primary palate will form premaxillary portion of the maxilla, anterior one third of final (definitive) palate.
2. Consists of small portion of the hard palate, anterior to incisive foramen; contains maxillary incisor teeth.

B. During sixth week of prenatal development (within embryonic period), bilateral maxillary processes form two palatal shelves (lateral palatine processes), BOTH fusing together to form secondary palate (fusing from anterior to posterior):
1. Secondary palate will form MOST posterior two thirds of hard palate, contains maxillary canines and posteriors, posterior to incisive foramen as well as soft palate and its uvula (fusion line indicated by median palatine raphe).
2. If the palatal shelves do NOT fuse with the primary palate (or with each other), cleft palate can result, with varying degrees of disability (see next discussion).

Patient with Cleft Palate and/or Cleft Lip

Cleft palate and/or cleft lip are craniofacial deformities that occur during fourth to twelfth weeks of prenatal development. Etiology is unknown; may involve genetics and exposure to environmental factors such as drugs or toxins (tobacco use, retinoic acid analogues, alcohol, anticonvulsants) during early prenatal development. MOST common class of congenital malformations in United States.

A. **Cleft lip:** failure of fusion of maxillary processes with medial nasal process:
1. Located at side of upper lip; unilateral or bilateral; may range from LEAST severe case, notch in vermilion border of upper lip (incomplete cleft), to MORE severe cases (complete cleft) that extend into floor of the nostril and through alveolar process of maxilla.
2. Cleft lip, with or without cleft palate, occurs in about 1 in 1000 live births.
3. Cleft lip is MORE common and MORE severe in males and is MORE frequently unilateral, occurring on left side.

B. **Cleft palate:** failure of fusion of palatal shelves with primary palate (or with each other):
1. Cleft uvula (bifid uvula) is the LEAST severe form.
2. Occurs, with or without cleft lip, in 1 in 2500 live births.
3. Isolated forms are LESS common than cleft lip and are MORE common in females.

C. Surgical intervention:
1. Plastic surgery: lip closure (adhesion) is performed before third month of life; palatal closure is performed at 1 to 5 years of age.
2. Bone grafting, orthodontics, and speech and hearing evaluation and treatment occur at 6 to 15 years of age.
3. Final plastic surgical procedures and replacement of teeth occur after age of 15, when physical growth is complete.
4. Medical anomalies such as heart, ear, skeletal, and genitourinary tract deformities may also occur.

D. Oral signs: increased risk of oral infection (including periodontal disease, dental caries) from malpositioning of the teeth, wearing of a full or partial denture to replace teeth or use of an **obturator** (dental appliance covering clefted area), mouth breathing, associated oral deformities; all complications also make oral hygiene procedures MORE difficult.

E. Risk factors for oral health: upper respiratory and middle ear infections and inadequate nourishment (before completion of surgical procedures), since cleft complicates nursing and/or feeding.

F. Barriers to care:
1. Economic issues; multiple oral and facial surgeries and care by professionals from different disciplines are required to correct defect and associated conditions.
2. Difficult communication because of inadequate speech production, hearing loss related to defect, self consciousness.

G. Professional and homecare:
1. Frequent oral prophylaxis (every 3 or 4 months) to reduce risk of infection.
2. When premaxilla is unfixed or immediately after surgical procedures, fulcruming during instrumentation at the site SHOULD be avoided or limited.
3. Fluoride and calcium products to reduce incidence of caries.

H. Patient or caregiver education:
1. Supervision and/or performance of oral hygiene procedures, depending on age and abilities.
2. Care of dental appliance or prosthesis similar to care of denture; removal after meals to cleanse thoroughly and reduce halitosis (see Chapter 15, Dental Biomaterials).
3. Risk for infection and need for excellent daily homecare, frequent professional oral prophylaxis and examination; care to reduce periodontal disease or caries.

I. Commissural lip pits (dimple like) can occur at one or both commissures and are hereditary.

CLINICAL STUDY

Age	21 YRS	SCENARIO
Sex	☒ Male ☐ Female	Upon extraoral examination during an initial appointment, the dental hygienist notes that there is a notch in the upper lip on the left side of the patient. When asked about it, the patient says it has been there since he was born. Nothing else is noted.
Height	5'8"	
Weight	150 LBS	
BP	115/75	
Chief Complaint	None	
Medical History	Hay fever	
Current Medications	OTC allergy medications prn	
Social History	College student in engineering	

1. Why is there a notch noted the patient's upper lip?
2. How did this occur in the patient?
3. How will this affect the patient's treatment?

1. Notch in the vermilion border of upper lip may be an incomplete cleft of the lip.
2. Each maxillary process fuses with each medial nasal process to contribute to the sides of upper lip, and two medial nasal processes contribute to middle of upper lip. Failure of fusion of maxillary processes with medial nasal process can result in cleft lip. Clefts of the lip are located at one or both sides of upper lip; they are unilateral or bilateral and may range from notch in vermilion border of upper lip (incomplete cleft) to more severe cases (complete cleft) that extend into floor of nostril and through alveolar process of maxilla; sometimes associated with cleft palate. Cleft lip, with or without cleft palate, occurs in about 1 in 1000 live births.
3. Since it is only notch in the vermilion border of the lip, this will not affect treatment. However, the dental hygienist should ask if the patient has any surgical repair history or if any complications have resulted from the notch. Consideration should be given to the way the question is asked, since the patient may be sensitive about this facial difference. The dental hygienist may also ask if she can answer any questions about the disorder and note the presence of the notch in the chart. Cleft lip is more common and more severe in males, is more frequently unilateral, and occurs mostly on left side. If severe, it can complicate nursing and/or feeding, speech development, appearance, and oronasal infection levels. Treatment includes plastic surgery with dental intervention and speech and hearing therapy.

Tongue Development

Tongue develops during fourth to eighth weeks of prenatal development.

A. Develops from independent swellings located internally on floor of the primitive pharynx, formed by first four paired branchial arches:
   1. Body: develops from first paired branchial arches.
   2. Base: originates later from second, third, fourth paired branchial arches.
   3. Body and base fuse together; fusion demarcated by sulcus terminalis.
B. Ankyloglossia ("tongue tied"): short lingual frenum that extends to tongue apex:
   1. Restricts movement of tongue to varying degrees.
   2. Frenum usually stretches with time or myofunctional exercises; thus surgical correction may NOT be necessary.

TOOTH DEVELOPMENT

Child's primary (deciduous) dentition develops during prenatal period and consists of 20 teeth, which erupt and are later shed (lost). As primary teeth are shed and jaws grow and mature, permanent dentition, consisting of as many as 32 teeth, gradually erupts and replaces primary dentition (Figure 2-3). Primary dentition begins on average with eruption of the mandibular central incisor at 6 to 10 months and is completed with eruption of the maxillary second molar at 25 to 33 months. Permanent dentition begins on average with the eruption of the mandibular first molar or central incisor at 6 to 7 years and is completed with the eruption of the third molars at 17 to 21 years. Discussion of tooth development will center first on the primary dentition and then include the permanent dentition.
- See Chapters 4, Head, Neck, and Dental Anatomy: dentitions; 6, General and Oral Pathology: developmental dental disorders.
A. Initiation stage:
   1. FIRST stage for primary dentition begins between the sixth and seventh weeks (during embryonic period).

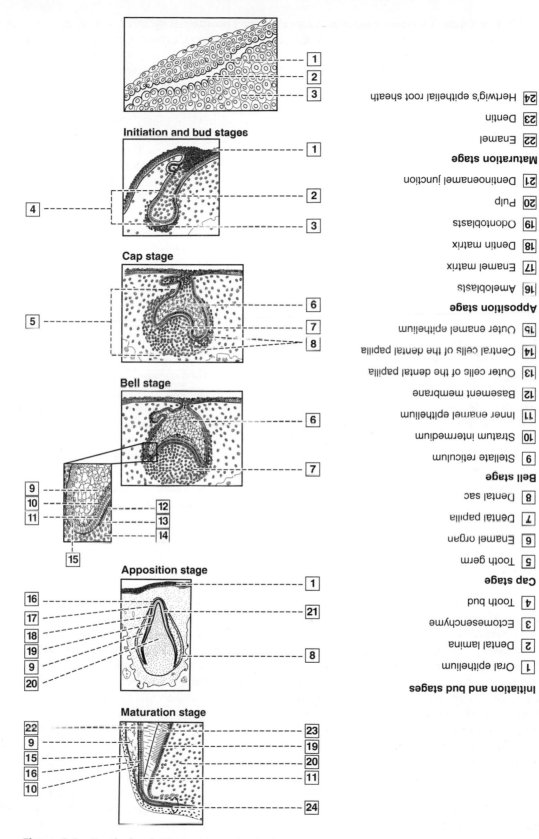

Figure 2-3   Tooth development. (From Fehrenbach MJ, ed: Dental anatomy coloring book, St. Louis, 2008, Saunders/Elsevier.)

2. Stomodeum (primitive mouth) is lined by ectoderm, with outer portion of ectoderm forming oral epithelium.

3. Deep to this is ectomesenchyme, influenced by neural crest cells; basement membrane separates the two tissues, future site of dentinoenamel junction (DEJ).

4. During seventh week, oral epithelium grows deeper into the ectomesenchyme and is induced to produce the dental lamina for the formation of the succedaneous teeth (all teeth EXCEPT permanent molars).

B. **Bud stage:**
   1. Second stage occurs at eighth week (during embryonic period).
   2. Growth of dental lamina into buds penetrating into ectomesenchyme; each will develop into a tooth germ.

C. **Cap stage:**
   1. Third stage occurs between ninth and tenth weeks (during fetal period).
   2. Differentiation of the tooth bud's dental lamina into the **enamel organ,** which will produce enamel, an ectodermal product, in the future.
      a. Enamel organ covers **dental papilla** from the ectomesenchyme.
      b. Dental papilla will produce future dentin and pulp tissue, which have mesenchymal origin.
      c. Remaining ectomesenchyme surrounding enamel organ (outside of the cap) forms into **dental sac** (follicle), which will produce periodontium, cementum, periodontal ligament (PDL), alveolar bone; all of mesenchymal origin.
   3. Together, enamel organ, dental papilla, and dental sac form the **tooth germ** (tooth primordium), giving the tooth bud its overall shape.
   4. Extension of dental lamina into ectomesenchyme lingual to developing primary tooth germs forms the **successional dental lamina** for the succedaneous permanent teeth; for nonsuccedaneous permanent molars, which have NO primary predecessors, these teeth will form from a posterior extension of the dental lamina.

D. **Bell stage:**
   1. Fourth stage occurs between eleventh and twelfth weeks (during fetal period).
   2. Stage marked by extensive proliferation, with differentiation of the enamel organ into four layers:
      a. Outer and inner enamel epithelium surrounds inner cells; inner cells become preameloblasts.
      b. Stellate reticulum and stratum intermedium are located *between* the two outer and inner layers; provide support for ameloblasts.

E. Apposition stage:
   1. Enamel, dentin, cementum are secreted in successive layers.
      a. Initially secreted as a matrix, extracellular substance that is partially calcified yet serves as a framework for later calcification:
         (1) Preameloblasts repolarize and differentiate into **ameloblasts** and then induce dental papilla cells to repolarize and become **odontoblasts.**
         (2) Thus odontoblasts produce predentin *before* ameloblasts produce enamel from Tomes' process.
      b. With enamel matrix in contact with predentin, mineralization of disintegrating basement membrane now occurs, forming DEJ.
   2. Structure responsible for root development is the cervical loop, most cervical portion of enamel organ:
      a. Bilayer rim consisting of ONLY inner and outer enamel epithelium.
      b. Grows deeper into the dental sac to become **Hertwig's epithelial root sheath** (HERS):
         (1) Function of HERS is to shape the root(s).
         (2) Also induces dentin formation in root area so that it is continuous with coronal dentin, as well as cementum on roots overlying the newly formed dentin.
      c. After the disintegration of HERS, its cells may become **epithelial rests of Malassez,** which are located in the mature PDL and may become cystic in the future (periapical cyst formation).
   3. Ectomesenchyme from dental sac (follicle) begins to form PDL, adjacent to newly formed cementum.
   4. After enamel apposition ceases in crown area, ameloblasts place an acellular dental cuticle on new enamel surface and the enamel organ is compressed, forming **reduced enamel epithelium** (REE).
   5. The REE fuses with oral epithelium lining the oral cavity to allow eruption process for both dentitions.
      a. Primary teeth act as guides for the developing permanent teeth; premature loss of primary teeth can have a serious effect on eruption of permanent teeth and their position in the dental arch.
      b. To allow removal of the primary for replacement by the permanent tooth, odontoclast resorption of primary teeth (MAINLY root, possibly crown) occurs.
      c. Succedaneous permanent tooth erupts into oral cavity in position lingual to roots of shed primary tooth, just as it will develop, EXCEPT permanent maxillary incisors, which move into a MORE facial position for eruption.
      d. After a permanent tooth erupts in the oral cavity, its root begins to form in the cervical area after

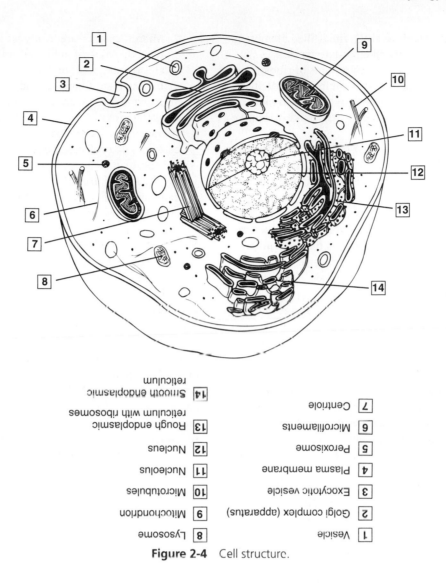

Figure 2-4   Cell structure.

1	Vesicle	8	Lysosome
2	Golgi complex (apparatus)	9	Mitochondrion
3	Exocytotic vesicle	10	Microtubules
4	Plasma membrane	11	Nucleolus
5	Peroxisome	12	Nucleus
6	Microfilaments	13	Rough endoplasmic reticulum with ribosomes
7	Centriole	14	Smooth endoplasmic reticulum

crown formation. Thus prevention of traumatic injury to the permanent teeth before they are fully anchored into the jaws is very important (see Chapter 11, Clinical Treatment).

   e. **Nasmyth's membrane:** residue of the eruption process that may form on newly erupted teeth of BOTH dentitions; leaves teeth with extrinsic green stain that is MAINLY removed by first brushing.

F. Maturation: reached when the dental tissues mineralize into their mature hard tissues.

GENERAL HISTOLOGY

Histology is the study of the structure, composition, and function of tissues that form organs and then into systems. **Tissues** consist of a group of similar cells that combine in a characteristic pattern and perform a specific function. In addition to cells, intercellular substance and tissue fluid tissues are found in tissues.

• See CD-ROM for Chapter Terms and WebLinks.

Cell Structure

A **cell** is the smallest unit of organization in the body. Cell structure includes cell components, such as **organelles,** plasma, and cytoskeletal elements. All are IMPORTANT in cell function (Figure 2-4).

• See Chapter 3, Anatomy, Biochemistry, and Physiology: cell physiology.

A. **Plasma membrane:** surrounds each cell; selectively allows movement of water and other substances into and out of cells and is involved in cell-to-cell recognition:

   1. Fluid mosaic model is the current working model of a membrane.

   2. Contains proteins that consist of channels, pumps, and transport systems; these regulate composition of the intracellular fluid.

   3. Components: phospholipids, which are polar and have charged heads; lipids, which are hydrophobic; cholesterol, which affects membrane fluidity; proteins, such as channels, enzymes, receptors, carbohydrates.

B. **Endoplasmic reticulum** (ER): fluid-filled membrane organelle found within cells; has two types:
 1. Rough ER: contains large amounts of ribosomes, involved in synthesis of proteins for cell structure and function, found in large amounts in growing cells and in cells that make digestive enzymes.
 2. Smooth ER: production of steroid hormones, detoxifies harmful substances, produces lysosomes, uses calcium in muscle cells for contraction and relaxation.

C. **Golgi apparatus** (complex): made up of layers of membranes and enclosed sacs, involved in processing substances made in the ER, directs finished products to intracellular or extracellular locations.

D. Vesicles: membrane-surrounded buds, formed from the Golgi apparatus:
 1. Coated vesicles contain chemicals for intracellular use; secretory vesicles are used for export **(exocytosis).**
 2. Also involved in trafficking substances into the cell from the environment (e.g., **endocytosis,** import; pinocytosis, absorption of fluids; **phagocytosis,** engulfing of solids).

E. **Lysosomes:** membrane-enclosed organelles derived from the Golgi apparatus, contain enzymes to digest unwanted debris and foreign matter, involved in apoptosis (tissue regression).

F. Peroxisomes: membrane-enclosed organelles that contain oxidative enzymes (e.g., catalase) for detoxifying chemicals.

G. **Mitochondria:** organelles with a folded inner membrane (containing cristae with respiratory enzymes) and outer membrane:
 1. Produce energy for cell in form of adenosine triphosphate (ATP), produce heat (e.g., in brown fat).
 2. Found in greater numbers within metabolically active cells such as cardiac and skeletal muscles.

H. **Ribosomes:** granules of RNA and proteins that are found on ER or are free in cytoplasm; involved in protein production.

I. **Nucleus:** contains DNA molecules that act as the genetic "blueprint" for the cell's protein production:
 1. Has inner and outer bilayers that make up **nuclear envelope;** pores for transporting substances across membranes.
 2. Has **nucleolus** that is involved in the assembly of ribosomes.
 3. Organelle MOST sensitive to radiation.

J. **Cytoskeleton:** three-dimensional system of support within the cell that includes microtubules, which are long, slender, hollow tubes involved in cell movement:
 1. Transport of vesicles within the cell, formation of mitotic spindles in cellular reproduction.

 2. Microfilaments are composed of helically intertwined chains of actin and myosin found in muscles (contraction) and microvilli.
 3. Intermediate filaments and rods are made of protein and form scaffolding (skeleton) of cell (cytoskeleton).

K. Extracellular fluid: interstitial fluid and plasma located outside cell; high in Na^+, Cl^-, Ca^{+2}; low in K^+; pH approximately 7.4.

L. **Cytoplasm** (intracellular fluid): located within the cell membrane, low in Na^+, Cl^-, Ca^{+2}; high in K^+; pH approximately 7.0.

Tissue Components and Types

Tissue components include cells, cell products (known as intercellular substance), and fluids derived from blood plasma (tissue fluid). Tissue cells vary considerably in size, shape, structure, and function. **Intercellular substance** consists of fibrous elements, such as collagen, and ground substance, known as mucopolysaccharides. Tissue fluid is a component of blood plasma that serves to carry nutrients to the cells of the tissue. **Tissues** may be grouped into four MAIN types: epithelial, connective, nerve, muscle. ALL types of tissues can be found in the oral cavity.

- See Chapters 3, Anatomy, Biochemistry, and Physiology: muscle tissue; 14, Pain Management: nerve tissue.

A. Epithelial tissues:
 1. Surface coverings (e.g., skin) lining tissues (e.g., mucous membranes, including oral mucosa in oral cavity) or specialized tissues (e.g., salivary glands and tooth enamel).
 2. Avascular (NO blood supply), rely on neighboring connective tissue for nutrients and removal of cell waste (via blood vessels in connective tissue).
 3. Classified according to type and arrangement of cells.
  a. Simple epithelium: single layer of squamous, cuboidal, or columnar cells.
  b. Pseudostratified epithelium: falsely appears stratified; ONLY one layer present.
  c. Stratified epithelium: consists of two or more layers of cells (discussed later); includes skin and oral mucosa of oral cavity.

B. Connective tissues:
 1. Contain fibers and cells: fibroblasts, macrophages, mast cells.
 2. Provide functions: transporting material (vascular tissue), providing structural support (cartilage and bone), forming ligaments, supporting and surrounding other tissues (located inferior to basement membrane of skin and mucous membranes, including oral cavity as the lamina propria and PDL).

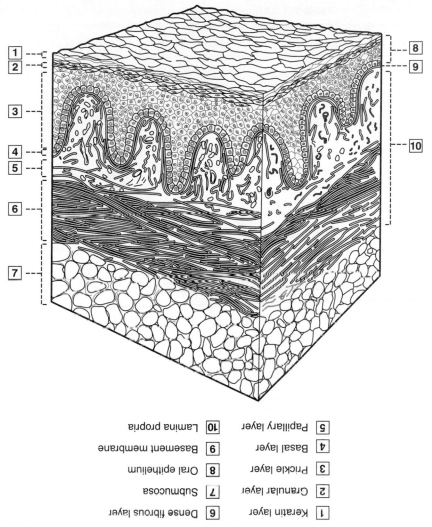

10	Lamina propria	5	Papillary layer
9	Basement membrane	4	Basal layer
8	Oral epithelium	3	Prickle layer
7	Submucosa	2	Granular layer
6	Dense fibrous layer	1	Keratin layer

Figure 2-5   Oral mucosa. (From Fehrenbach MJ, ed: Dental anatomy coloring book, St. Louis, 2008, Saunders/ Elsevier.)

3. Classified as loose, dense, cartilage; bone, or fluid (blood and lymph).

C. Muscle tissues:
   1. Specialized fibers that allow contraction.
   2. Classified as skeletal, smooth, or cardiac; considered involuntary (e.g., heart muscle, contracts in response to body controls) or voluntary (e.g., arm, leg, and trunk muscles).

D. Nerve tissue:
   1. Part of central nervous system (CNS: brain and spinal cord) and peripheral nervous system (PNS: associated with other body organs).

ORAL MUCOSA

Oral mucosa almost continuously lines the oral cavity. Composed of stratified squamous epithelium overlying lamina propria (connective tissue proper) (Figure 2-5). Three MAIN types of oral mucosa are found in the oral cavity: lining, masticatory, specialized mucosa; for regional differences associated with each type, see Table 2-1.

• See Chapter 6, General and Oral Pathology: oral mucosal hyperkeratinization.

A. **Lining mucosa:** buccal mucosa, labial mucosa, alveolar mucosa, floor of the mouth, ventral surface of the tongue, soft palate.
   1. *Nonkeratinized* squamous epithelium:
      a. Basal layer (stratum basale): innermost single layer of cuboidal epithelial cells, overlying basement membrane, superior to lamina propria.
         (1) Produces basal lamina of the basement membrane.
         (2) Mitosis (cell division) of epithelial cells occurs within, creating new cells for the tissue.
      b. Intermediate layer (stratum intermedium): superficial to the basal layer; composed of larger, stacked, polyhedral-shaped cells.
      c. Superficial layer (stratum superficiale): outermost layer; larger, similarly stacked, polyhedral epithelial cells; the MOST superficial flatten into squames, showing

Table 2-1   Regional differences in oral mucosa

Region/appearance	Epithelium	Lamina propria	Submucosa
LINING MUCOSA			
Labial mucosa and buccal mucosa: opaque pink, shiny, moist; with areas of melanin pigmentation and Fordyce's spots possible	Thick nonkeratinized	Irregular and blunt CT papillae, some elastic fibers, extensive vascular supply	Present with adipose and minor salivary glands, with firm attachment to muscle
Alveolar mucosa: reddish pink, shiny, moist, extremely mobile	Thin nonkeratinized	CT papillae sometimes absent, many elastic fibers, with extensive vascular supply	Present with minor salivary glands and many elastic fibers, with loose attachment to muscle or bone
Floor of the mouth and ventral tongue surface: reddish pink, moist, shiny, compressible, with vascular blue areas; mobility varies	Extremely thin nonkeratinized	Extensive vascular supply Floor: broad CT papillae Ventral tongue: numerous CT papillae, some elastic fibers, minor salivary glands	Present Floor: adipose with submandibular and sublingual glands, loosely attached to bone/muscles Ventral tongue: extremely thin and firmly attached to muscle
Soft palate: deep pink with a yellow hue and moist surface; compressible and extremely elastic	Thin nonkeratinized	Thick lamina propria with numerous CT papillae and distinct elastic layer	Extremely thin with adipose tissue and minor salivary glands, with a firm attachment to underlying muscle
MASTICATORY MUCOSA			
Attached gingiva: opaque pink, dull, firm, immobile; with areas of melanin pigmentation possible and varying amounts of slipping	Thick keratinized (mainly parakeratinized, some orthokeratinized)	Tall, narrow CT papillae, extensive vascular supply, and serves as a mucoperiosteum to bone	Not present
Hard palate: pink, immobile, and firm medial portion, with rugae and raphe; cushioned lateral portions	Thick orthokeratinized	Medial portion, rugae and raphe serve as a mucoperiosteum to bone	Present only in lateral portions, with anterior part having adipose and posterior part having minor salivary glands. Absent in medial portion.

CT, Connective tissue.

shedding or loss as they age and die during turnover of tissue.

B. **Masticatory mucosa:** attached gingiva, hard palate, dorsal surface of the tongue.
   1. *Keratinized* squamous epithelium:
      a. Deeper layers: same nonkeratinized squamous epithelium described above is present over basement membrane.
      b. Prickle layer (stratum spinosum): superficial to basal layer; cells look spiky when fixed.
      c. Granular layer (stratum granulosum): superficial to prickle layer; cells in this layer are flat and stacked and have keratohyaline granules in cytoplasm.
      d. Keratin layer (stratum corneum): MOST superficial, consists of squames filled with keratin;

two types of keratinization: *parakeratinized* (retained nuclei in cytoplasm) and *orthokeratinized* (NO nuclei); note that healthy skin does NOT show parakeratinization, which is normally found ONLY in oral cavity.
   2. **Lamina propria:** connective tissue *deep* to basement membrane for BOTH types of epithelium; has two layers:
      a. Papillary layer: MORE superficial; consists of loose connective tissue within connective tissue papillae.
      b. Dense layer: deepest dense connective tissue; large amount of fibers.
   3. Submucosa may or may NOT be present deep to lamina propria.

Table 2-2 Comparison of lingual papillae

Comparison	Filiform	Fungiform	Foliate	Circumvallate
Clinical appearance	Most common on body; fine-pointed cones give the tongue a velvety texture	Lesser numbers on body; mushroom-shaped small red dots	4 to 11 vertical ridges on the lateral surface of the posterior tongue	7 to 15 large raised mushroom-shaped structures anterior to the sulcus terminalis
Microscopic appearance	Pointed structure with a thick layer of keratinized epithelium, overlying a core of lamina propria; no taste buds.	Mushroom-shaped structure with a thin layer of keratinized epithelium overlying a core of lamina propria, with taste buds in the most superficial portion	Leaf-shaped structure of keratinized epithelium overlying a core of lamina propria, with taste buds superficial	Mushroom-shaped structure with similar histology to fungiform, that is, sunken deep to the tongue surface, taste buds in base, and surrounded by a trough, with von Ebner's minor salivary glands in the submucosa
Function	Possibly mechanical	Taste	Taste	Taste

C. **Specialized mucosa:** lingual papillae on dorsal and lateral surface of the tongue; consist of epithelium and lamina propria; see Table 2-2 for comparison of lingual papillae.

Gingival Tissues

Gingival tissues surround the teeth in the alveoli and cover the alveolar processes.

* See Chapters 6, General and Oral Pathology: gingival hyperplasia; 11, Clinical Treatment: periodontal evaluation and charting; 12, Instrumentation: probing; 13, Periodontology: gingival conditions or diseases.

A. **Marginal** (free) **gingiva:** located at gingival margin of each tooth:
1. Width is 0.5 to 1.5 mm (approximates level of base of gingival sulcus).
2. Continuous with attached gingiva; has SIMILAR features, with mainly parakeratinized epithelium.
3. Gingival margin (free gingival crest): MOST superficial portion of marginal gingiva.
4. Free gingival groove: shallow linear groove that demarcates marginal gingiva from attached gingiva.

B. **Attached gingiva:** composed of stratified, keratinized epithelial tissue firmly bound to underlying cementum and alveolar bone (masticatory mucosa); measured from free gingival margin to mucogingival junction; stippling can be present in health. Tissues can show orthokeratinization or (MAINLY) parakeratinization (retention of nuclei in superficial layers).
1. **Interdental papilla:** occupies interdental space between two adjacent teeth.

a. Tip and lateral borders are marginal tissue, continuous with the free gingiva.
b. Center of the papilla consists of attached gingiva; its shape is determined by amount of interproximal space created by contact point of adjacent teeth.
c. In healthy tissue is pointed in the anterior, then flatter and wider in the posterior.
2. **Col:** depression between lingual and facial papillae.
a. Shape conforms to interproximal space; consists of nonkeratinized tissue.
b. MORE susceptible to inflammation because of fragility; FIRST site of periodontal inflammation.
3. **Mucogingival junction:** scalloped line that marks connection between alveolar mucosa and attached gingiva.

C. **Alveolar mucosa:** movable tissue loosely attached to underlying bone; attached by frena (singular, frenum), band(s) of tissue that attaches MORE fixed tissue to MORE movable tissue; may pull (displace) tissue when attached gingival margin is narrow or missing.

D. Dentogingival junction tissues: ALL tissues that face the tooth; nonkeratinized epithelium, UNLIKE marginal and attached gingiva, with smooth interface between tissues and underlying lamina propria (Figure 2-6):
1. **Sulcular** (crevicular) **epithelium** (SE): stands away from the tooth, creating gingival sulcus, filled with **crevicular gingival fluid** (CGF) from blood vessels of lamina propria:
a. Depth of healthy gingival sulcus varies from 0.5 to 3 mm, with average of 1.8 mm.

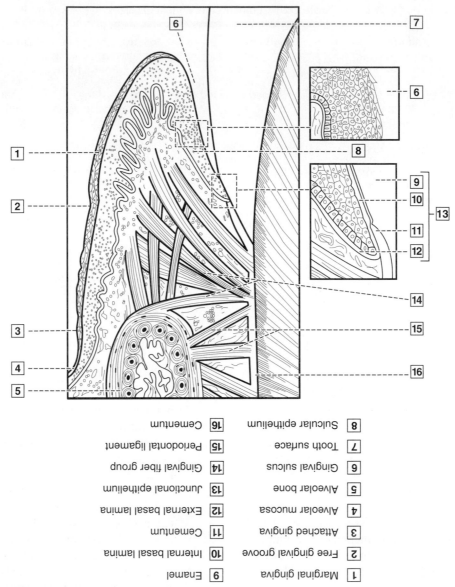

Figure 2-6 Dentogingival junction tissues. (From Fehrenbach MJ, ed: Dental anatomy coloring book, St. Louis, 2008, Saunders/Elsevier.)

16	Cementum	8	Sulcular epithelium
15	Periodontal ligament	7	Tooth surface
14	Gingival fiber group	6	Gingival sulcus
13	Junctional epithelium	5	Alveolar bone
12	External basal lamina	4	Alveolar mucosa
11	Cementum	3	Attached gingiva
10	Internal basal lamina	2	Free gingival groove
9	Enamel	1	Marginal gingiva

b. Normal gingival fluid flow rate of CGF is regular; however, amount in healthy state is minimal.

c. CGF seeps out between epithelial cells into the sulcus; includes white blood cells (WBCs); MAIN cells are polymorphonuclear leukocytes (PMNs, neutrophils) as well as IgG, IgM, serum IgA.

2. **Junctional epithelium** (JE): deeper extension of SE into sulcus:

a. Created during tooth eruption from fused tissues (REE) along tooth surface.

b. Continuous with SE of the gingival sulcus, lines floor of the gingival sulcus, attached to the tooth surface in a cufflike manner by way of **epithelial attachment** (EA):

(1) Thin tissue (15 to 30 cells thick), widest at its junction with the SE; superficial suprabasal epithelial cells provide hemidesmosomes and internal basal lamina that create EA (cell to noncellular intercellular junction type).

(2) Permeable tissue that allows emigration of large numbers of mobile WBCs from lamina propria's blood vessels into JE and then into GCF, even in healthy state to protect JE.

c. Basal layer of JE undergoes constant and rapid cell division:

(1) Cells do NOT mature UNLIKE other gingival tissues, but still migrate to surface and are lost in sulcus.

(2) Highest turnover time in entire oral cavity: 4 to 6 days.

3. Clinical probing depth of gingival sulcus is measured by calibrated periodontal probe; probe is gently inserted, slides by SE, and is stopped by EA in a healthy state, with NO bleeding on probing (BoP) noted; boundaries on probing gingival sulcus: (a) *inner:* tooth surface (enamel and/or cementum); (b) *outer:* SE; (c) *base:* JE lining sulcus, contacting EA.

DENTAL TISSUES

Tooth consists of enamel, dentin, cementum, and pulpal tissues. Hard tissues (enamel, dentin, cementum, as well as the surrounding bone) consist MAINLY of calcium hydroxyapatite with the chemical formula $Ca_{10}(PO_4)_6(OH)_2$. Soft tissues (pulp) are mesodermally derived connective tissues. See earlier discussion of the development of tissues.

- See Chapters 6, General and Oral Pathology: dental pathology; 11, Clinical Treatment: pulpal evaluation, dentinal hypersensitivity, enamel sealants; 15, Dental Biomaterials: endodontic therapy, whitening procedure.

A. **Enamel:** ~96% inorganic crystal (hardest calcified/mineralized tissue in the body):
  1. Covers dentin in crown; NOT found in the root; SAME calcium hydroxyapatite makeup.
  2. UNLIKE dentin, cementum, and bone, enamel does not contain collagen; instead, it is formed from two proteins, amelogenins and enamelins.
  3. Amelogenesis: process of enamel matrix formation during apposition stage:
     a. Ectodermal product from enamel organ, which is derived from the ectoderm.
     b. First formed in incisal or occlusal portion of future crown, near forming dentinoenamel junction (DEJ); then moves cervically to cementoenamel junction (CEJ).
  4. **Enamel rod** (prism): crystalline structural unit of enamel.
     a. **Tomes' process:** end portion of each ameloblast nearest the DEJ that dictates the specific shape of each rod; takes four ameloblasts to produce one enamel rod.
        (1) Each rod is cylindrical in longitudinal section; 4 micrometers (μm) in diameter.
        (2) Rods are stacked in rows; surrounding outer portion is interprismatic region (interrod enamel); each rod is oriented perpendicular to DEJ and outer surface (at angles from <90° to 60°).
        (3) MOST rods extend the width of the enamel from DEJ to outer surface; thus each rod varies in length because the width of enamel varies in different locations of crown area.
     b. Clinical ramifications of enamel rod structure:
        (1) Acid etch is briefly used to remove some of organic portions of enamel crystals and thus enable an enamel sealant or tooth-colored restoration to flow into newly created gaps; offers MORE surface area for better adherence (mechanical bonding).
        (2) Oxygen radicals from peroxide in the whitening (bleaching) agents contact stains in interprismatic spaces within enamel layer; when this occurs, the stains are removed (bleached).
  5. **Hunter-Schreger bands:** light or dark bands oriented perpendicular to DEJ, caused by curvature of rods.
  6. **Lines of Retzius:** dark incremental lines; in longitudinal sections appear as traverse rods; on transverse sections appear as concentric rings:
     a. **Perikymata:** raised imbrication lines (grooves) noted on nonmasticatory surfaces of some teeth in the oral cavity; wear away with attrition.
     b. **Neonatal line:** MOST accentuated incremental line; marks stress and/or trauma to ameloblasts during birth.
  7. Enamel spindles: short dentinal tubules near the DEJ; produced by odontoblasts that cross the basement membrane before it is mineralized into DEJ.
  8. Enamel tufts: small dark brushes with bases near DEJ.
  9. Enamel lamellae: partially calcified vertical sheets of enamel matrix that extend from the DEJ near the cervix to the outer occlusal surface.

B. **Dentin:** ~70% inorganic crystal (LESS hard than enamel; second hardest of dental tissues):
  1. Located in BOTH crown and root; covered by enamel in crown and cementum in root; encloses innermost pulp tissue.
  2. Makes up the bulk of tooth and protects the pulp.
  3. Dentinogenesis: process of dentin matrix formation during the apposition stage:
     a. **Predentin:** initial material laid down by odontoblasts; mesenchymal product; mantle dentin is first predentin.
        (1) Globular: areas where BOTH primary and secondary mineralization has occurred with complete crystalline fusion; appear as lighter rounded areas.
        (2) Interglobular: areas where ONLY primary mineralization occurred and globules did NOT fuse completely; appear as darker arclike areas.
     b. **Imbrication lines of von Ebner:** incremental lines (bands) that stain darkly, show daily production of 4-micrometer (μm) increment.

c. **Contour lines of Owen:** adjoining parallel imbrication lines; demonstrate disturbance in body metabolism that affects odontoblasts; neonatal line is MOST pronounced and occurs during trauma of birth.

4. **Tomes' granular layer:** peripheral portion of dentin beneath root's cementum, adjacent to dentinocemental junction (DCJ).

5. **Dentinal tubules:** long tubes in dentin that extend from DEJ in crown area or DCJ in root area to outer wall of pulp:

   a. **Dentinal fluid:** tissue fluid in tubule surrounding the cell membrane of the odontoblast, continuous from the cell body in the pulp; changes in flow are related to dental pain from the pulp (may cause dental hypersensitivity; see Chapter 11, Clinical Treatment).

   b. **Odontoblastic process:** long cellular extension located within dentinal tubule, still attached to cell body of odontoblast within pulp.

      (1) Avascular (NO blood supply); nutrition for odontoblasts comes from tissue fluid by way of tubule from blood vessels located in adjacent pulp.

      (2) Tubules become exposed as a result of caries, cavity preparation, recession, or attrition; open-ended dentinal tubules may be painful, causing dentinal hypersensitivity (see earlier discussion).

6. Types of dentin:

   a. Peritubular: creates wall of tubule; MOST mineralized; with age, diameter of tubule becomes narrower because of peritubular deposition.

   b. Intertubular: between tubules; LESS mineralized than peritubular.

   c. Circumpulpal: layer around outer pulpal wall.

   d. Primary: formed in a tooth *before* completion of apical foramen of the root, with regular pattern of tubules.

   e. Secondary: formed *after* the completion of the apical foramen and continues to form:

      (1) Formed MORE slowly than primary and LESS mineralized; fills in along the outer pulpal wall.

      (2) Made by the odontoblastic layer that lines the dentin-pulp interface, with a regular pattern of tubules.

   f. Tertiary (reparative, reactive): quickest type to form in localized regions in response to a localized trauma to exposed dentin:

      (1) MORE irregular course than in secondary.

      (2) Sclerotic: type of tertiary associated with chronic injury of caries and aging.

         (a) Has dead odontoblastic processes that leave tubules vacant but that become retrofilled, occluded by mineralized substance (calcium salts) similar to peritubular.

         (b) Noted with arrested caries; appears brown, smooth, shiny.

C. **Cementum:** ~65% inorganic (LESS hard than BOTH enamel and dentin; MORE similar to bone):

1. Covers the entire root, overlying Tomes' granular layer in dentin.

2. Thickest at apex and in interradicular areas of multirooted teeth; thinnest at CEJ at cervix (neck).

   a. Can form throughout life of the tooth; forms arrest lines (smooth lines formed by layered apposition).

   b. Repair of traumatic resorption involves apposition of cementum by cementoblasts in adjacent PDL, resulting in reversal lines (scalloped layers formed by absorption).

3. Part of periodontium that attaches the teeth to the alveolar bone by anchoring PDL:

   a. **Sharpey's fibers:** collagen fibers from PDL.

   b. "Brush ends" that are each partially inserted into outer cementum at 90°.

4. Formed from dental sac (follicle), formed on root after disintegration of HERS:

   a. **Cementoblasts** then disperse to cover the root dentin and undergo cementogenesis, laying down cementoid; many become entrapped, becoming **cementocytes.**

   b. Each cementocyte lies in lacuna (plural, lacunae), similar to pattern in bone, with canaliculi.

   c. All the canals are oriented toward PDL and contain cementocytic processes.

5. No innervation; avascular (NO blood supply), receiving nutrition by way of own cells from the surrounding PDL (reason for orientation of canals toward PDL).

6. CEJ exhibits varying patterns overall in each individual oral cavity and even on one tooth: (a) cementum overlaps enamel (MOST common at 60%; makes it hard to discern from calculus); (b) cementum and enamel meet end to end; (c) gap between cementum and enamel, leaving exposed dentin with increased risk of dentinal hypersensitivity.

D. **Pulp:** soft tissue; innermost tissue of tooth:

1. Formed from the central cells of the dental papilla (same derivation as dentin); mesenchymal product.

   a. Forms during odontogenesis, when dentin forms around dental papilla.

   b. Innermost tissue is considered pulp.

2. Anatomy:

   a. Pulp chamber: mass of pulp is contained within tooth.

   b. Coronal pulp: located in crown of tooth.

c. **Pulp horns:** smaller extensions of coronal pulp into the cusps of posteriors; MOST prominent under buccal cusp of premolar teeth and MB cusp of molar teeth and MOST primary teeth (care taken during restoration).

d. Radicular (root) pulp ("root canal") located in root:

 (1) **Apical foramen:** opening at the apex; surrounded by cementum; allows arteries, veins, lymphatics, nerves to enter and exit from PDL.

 (2) **Accessory** (lateral) **canals:** extra openings from pulp to PDL; NOT just laterally located.

3. Involved in support, maintenance, and continued formation of dentin because inner layer of the cell bodies of the odontoblasts remains along outer pulpal wall:

a. Fibroblasts: MOST common cells in the pulp; odontoblasts are second MOST common.

b. Fibers: mainly collagen fibers and some reticular fibers; NO elastic fibers.

c. Pulp has extensive vascular supply and rudimentary lymphatics; ALL sensation is transmitted as pain.

d. Pulp stones (denticles) are sometimes present; becomes MORE fibrotic with increased age and may make endodontic therapy MORE difficult.

4. With endodontic therapy, pulp is removed:

a. Tooth is NO longer vital; tooth may darken, become brittle, and fracture during mastication.

b. Full restorative coverage is recommended to protect tooth from fracture.

CLINICAL STUDY

Age	60 YRS		SCENARIO
Sex	☐ Male ☒ Female		A patient reports for new patient examination. Radiographs reveal endodontic therapy of tooth #30. The intraoral examination reveals that the distobuccal cusp of tooth #30 has fractured off.
Height	5'4"		
Weight	185 LBS		
BP	119/78		
Chief Complaint	"My tooth broke off, but there is no pain in any of my teeth."		
Medical History	Carpal tunnel surgery 5 years ago		
Current Medications	Scarlet fever and tonsillectomy as a child None except OTC vitamin E qd		
Social History	Grandmother and church organist		

1. Why is tooth #30 not painful?
2. Which cells are no longer active in tooth #30?
3. Discuss possible causes of the distobuccal cusp fracture on the tooth.

1. Although tooth exhibits a fractured cusp, patient feels no pain because nerve tissues within pulp were removed during endodontic therapy.
2. Cells associated with pulp tissue (odontoblasts, fibroblasts, histiocytes, undifferentiated mesenchymal cells) are not active, since they are no longer present after endodontic therapy; removed during therapy to control pulpal infection.
3. Endodontic therapy of tooth #30 has increased the likelihood that tooth will fracture in the future. Posteriors are often restored with full coverage such as a crown to reduce the chance of a tooth's fracturing after endodontic therapy. Age-related changes may also cause a tooth to become more brittle.

PERIODONTIUM

Periodontium includes alveolar bone and PDL, as well as gingival tissues and cementum (Figure 2-7). See also earlier discussion about development of the jaws and discussion of gingival tissues and cementum.

• See Chapters 2, Embryology and Histology: bone tissue; 11, Clinical Treatment: periodontal evaluation and charting.

A. **Alveolar bone:** ~60% inorganic (MORE similar to cementum than other dental tissues):

1. Part of the jaws that supports and protects teeth, attached to cementum of the tooth by way of PDL.

2. Formed from dental sac (similar to PDL); mesenchymal product.

3. Anatomy:

a. Basal bone is apical to roots, forms body of jaws.

b. Alveolar bone is the portion that contains the roots of the teeth.

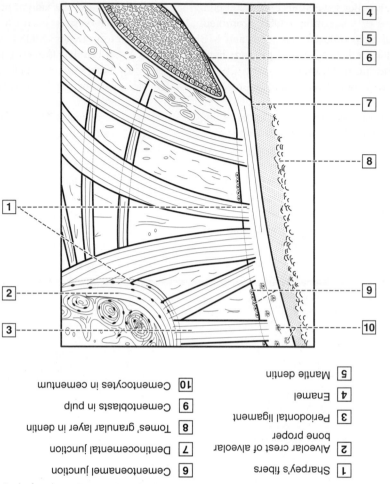

Figure 2-7 Periodontium. (From Fehrenbach MJ, ed: Dental anatomy coloring book, St. Louis, 2008, Saunders/Elsevier.)

1 Sharpey's fibers	6 Cementoenamel junction
2 Alveolar crest of alveolar bone proper	7 Dentinocemental junction
3 Periodontal ligament	8 Tomes' granular layer in dentin
4 Enamel	9 Cementoblasts in pulp
5 Mantle dentin	10 Cementocytes in cementum

(1) **Alveolar bone proper** (ABP) (cribriform plate, tooth socket): lining of alveolus (plural, alveoli).
  (a) Has Volkmann's canals, passing from alveolar bone into PDL, and Sharpey's fibers, portion of the fibers of PDL inserted here at 90°.
  (b) Consists of compact bone, noted on radiographs as **lamina dura,** a solid radiopacity surrounding radiolucency of PDL space.
  (c) Lamina propria of the attached gingiva serves as its mucoperiosteum.
  (d) **Alveolar crest:** MOST cervical rim of the ABP, apical to CEJ by approximately 1 to 2 mm.
c. Supporting alveolar bone: cortical plates and trabecular bone:
  (1) Cortical plates (bone): plates of compact bone on facial and lingual surfaces of alveolar bone.

(2) Trabecular bone: located between ABP and cortical plates; consists of cancellous (spongy) bone.
d. **Interdental septum:** alveolar bone between two neighboring teeth; consists of BOTH compact bone of ABP and cancellous bone of trabecular bone.
e. **Interradicular septum:** found ONLY on multirooted teeth; alveolar bone between the roots of the same tooth; consists of BOTH ABP and trabecular bone.
4. Ramifications of alveolar bone:
  a. Easily remodeled in comparison with cementum, thus allowing orthodontic tooth movement; shows arrest lines (smooth) and reversal (scalloped) lines:
    (1) On one side of tooth, compression zone in PDL leads to bone resorption.
    (2) At the same time, on opposite side of tooth and bone, tension zone develops in PDL and causes deposition of new bone.

b. Density of alveolar bone in an area also determines route that dental infection takes with abscess formation.

c. With the loss of teeth, patient becomes edentulous, either partially or completely, and alveolar bone undergoes resorption (loss); underlying basal bone and both the body of maxilla and mandible remain less affected.

B. **Periodontal ligament** (PDL): soft tissue that provides attachment of teeth to surrounding ABP by way of cementum; serves periosteum for these tissues:

1. Derived from the dental sac (similar to alveolar bone and cementum); mesenchymal product.

2. Organized fibrous connective tissue that maintains gingiva in proper relationship to the teeth.

3. Appears on radiographs as radiolucent **periodontal ligament space,** bordered by radiopaque lamina dura of ABP and then tooth root.

4. Transmits occlusal forces from the teeth to bone, allowing small amount of movement; nerve supply provides MOST efficient proprioceptive mechanism (as evidenced when biting on metal foil in candy wrappers—ewww!).

5. UNLIKE the pulp, transmits touch, pressure, and temperature sensations as well as pain.

6. Cells in tissue participate in formation and resorption of hard tissues of periodontium.

7. Has blood vessels that provide nutrition for its cells and surrounding cells of cementum and ABP.

8. Components:

a. Fibroblast is MOST common cell, with cementoblasts along cemental surface; osteoblasts are also present at the periphery of the ABP.

b. Osteoclasts, odontoclasts; also undifferentiated mesenchymal cells, which can differentiate into any of these cells if their cell populations are injured or lost.

c. Epithelial rests of Malassez become located in mature PDL after disintegration of HERS during formation of root; may become cystic.

d. Principal fiber groups of PDL (see Table 2-3 and Figure 2-8):

(1) Alveolodental group: largest of the five fiber groups of PDL; oblique fibers are MOST numerous.

(2) Approximately 5 mm in diameter; resist the forces exerted on tooth such as rotational, tilting, extrusive, or intrusive; some fibers resist a combination of forces.

(a) Sharpey's fibers: "brush ends" of the principal fibers are within ABP and cementum.

(b) Partially inserted into the hard tissues of periodontium (bone or cementum) at 90°.

Table 2-3   Fiber groups of the alveolodental ligament

Fiber group	Location	Function
Alveolar crest group	Originates in alveolar crest of ABP and fans out to insert into cervical cementum at various angles	To resist tilting, intrusive, extrusive, and rotational forces
Horizontal group	Originates in ABP apical to its alveolar crest and inserts into cementum in horizontal manner	To resist tilting forces and rotational forces
Oblique group	Originates in ABP and extends apically to insert more apically into cementum in oblique manner	To resist intrusive forces and rotational forces
Apical group	Radiates from apical region of cementum to insert into surrounding ABP	To resist extrusive forces and rotational forces.
Interradicular group (only on multirooted teeth)	Inserted on the cementum of one root to the cementum of the other root(s) superficial to the interradicular septum	To resist intrusive, extrusive, tilting, and rotational forces

ABP, Alveolar bone proper.

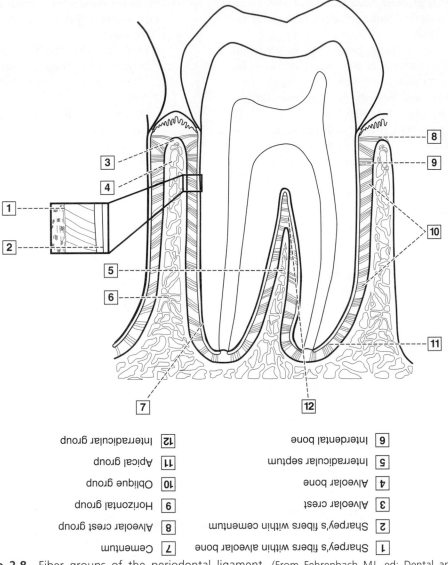

Figure 2-8 Fiber groups of the periodontal ligament. (From Fehrenbach MJ, ed: Dental anatomy coloring book, St. Louis, 2008, Saunders/Elsevier.)

12 Interradicular group	6 Interdental bone
11 Apical group	5 Interradicular septum
10 Oblique group	4 Alveolar bone
9 Horizontal group	3 Alveolar crest
8 Alveolar crest group	2 Sharpey's fibers within cementum
7 Cementum	1 Sharpey's fibers within alveolar bone

Review Questions

1 The midface and all structures of the oral cavity EXCEPT the posterior part of the tongue develop from the
A. frontal process and first branchial arch.
B. frontal process and second branchial arch.
C. stomodeum and buccopharyngeal membrane.
D. forebrain and tuberculum impar.

2 The formation of an ameloblast from cells of the inner enamel epithelium is an example of
A. histodifferentiation.
B. morphodifferentiation.
C. odontogenesis.
D. dentinogenesis.

3 Which structure becomes the dentinoenamel junction of the fully formed tooth?
A. Outer enamel epithelium
B. Stellate reticulum
C. Basement membrane
D. Dental papilla

4 Tooth development begins when a localized growth of cells on the jaw ridge produces a strand of epithelium. What is this strand called?
A. Tooth germ
B. Tooth bud
C. Dental lamina
D. Enamel organ

5 Which of the following develops into the posterior one third of the tongue?
   A. Meckel's cartilage
   B. Copula
   C. Tuberculum impar
   D. Lingual swellings

6 Which of the following determines the shape of the tooth root?
   A. Rests of Malassez
   B. Stellate reticulum
   C. Hertwig's sheath
   D. Dental lamina

7 Enamel contains which percentage of inorganic substance?
   A. 4%
   B. 38%
   C. 74%
   D. 96%

8 Which of the following is created with the changes in direction of developing enamel rods?
   A. Lines of Retzius
   B. Hunter-Schreger bands
   C. Perikymata lines
   D. Neonatal lines

9 Of what are perikymata an external manifestation?
   A. Lines of Retzius
   B. Hunter-Schreger bands
   C. Lines of Ebner and Owen
   D. Enamel spindles

10 An enamel pearl is
   A. located on the occlusal surface, causing discomfort during chewing.
   B. confused with calculus because of its location.
   C. present as an opacity ring on the facial surface of anterior teeth.
   D. located within the pulp chamber, obliterating the blood supply.

11 Where are odontoblast nuclei located in a tooth?
   A. Predentin
   B. Dentinal tubules
   C. Pulp tissue
   D. Periodontal ligament

12 Where is cellular cementum MOST likely to be found?
   A. At the apical portion of the tooth
   B. At the cementoenamel junction
   C. Equally throughout the root surface
   D. Closest to the dentin

13 A chronic inflammation of a tooth that causes a localized thickening of cementum is referred to as
   A. a cementicle.
   B. hypercementosis.
   C. cementogenesis.
   D. a cementoid.

14 Rank the following tissues from MOST to LEAST resistant to abrasion.
   A. Dentin, enamel, cementum
   B. Enamel, cementum, dentin
   C. Enamel, dentin, cementum
   D. Cementum, enamel, dentin

15 One of the following is NOT true as the pulp ages. Which one is the EXCEPTION?
   A. Vascularity decreases.
   B. Pulp chamber size decreases.
   C. Mineralization decreases.
   D. Sensitivity increases.

16 At which location does cementum have the greatest thickness?
   A. At the apex or furcation areas
   B. Closest to the cementoenamel junction
   C. At Sharpey's attachment sites
   D. At mesial root surfaces

17 Which cells are MOST active on the mesial side of a tooth being translated mesially during orthodontic treatment?
   A. Fibroblasts
   B. Osteoblasts
   C. Cementoblasts
   D. Osteoclasts

18 Which is the MOST common type of epithelium found in the oral cavity?
   A. Stratified squamous
   B. Cuboidal
   C. Transitional
   D. Simple squamous

19 One of the following lingual papillae is NOT considered a primary location for taste buds. Which one is the EXCEPTION?
   A. Circumvallate
   B. Fungiform
   C. Filiform
   D. Foliate

20 Epithelial rests of Malassez are associated with which of the following?
   A. Dental sac
   B. Dental papilla
   C. Enamel organ
   D. Lamina dura

21 Which of the following lingual papillae is MOST keratinized?
   A. Circumvallate
   B. Filiform
   C. Foliate
   D. Fungiform

22 Which of the following types of bone tissue increases in amount because of an increase in occlusal activity?
   A. Cortical
   B. Trabecular
   C. Circumferential
   D. Lamellar

23 The histological pocket depth is
   A. less than the clinical probing depth.
   B. equal to the clinical probing depth.
   C. greater than the clinical probing depth.
   D. lessened as periodontal disease increases.

24 One of the following is NOT true of sclerotic dentin. Which one is the EXCEPTION?

A. More rapid progression of caries than in normal dentin

B. Located in MOST older teeth

C. Located where odontoblasts have degenerated

D. Formed from calcium salts that have filled dentinal tubules

25 Corkscrew-shaped structures that lie among dentin are called

A. Tomes' fibers.

B. Korff's fibers.

C. enamel spindles.

D. dentinal tubules.

26 What is a commissural lip pit?

A. Cancerous lesion on the lips

B. Sunburned lips that are chapped

C. Dimplelike invaginations of the corner of the lips

D. Disturbance of lip development in utero

27 What is a bifid uvula?

A. Disruption in palatal fusion

B. Minor cleft of the posterior soft palate

C. Disturbance of lip development in utero

D. Dimplelike invaginations of the corner of the lips

28 How often does cleft lip occur?

A. 1 in 2500

B. 1 in 1000

C. 1 in 100

D. 1 in 50

29 Ankyloglossia is a short lingual frenum that extends to the tongue apex. Ankyloglossia restricts the movement of the tongue to varying degrees.

A. Both statements are true.

B. Both statements are false.

C. The first statement is true, the second is false.

D. The first statement is false, the second is true.

30 The secondary palate will form the posterior two thirds of the hard palate. The secondary palate contains the maxillary central and lateral incisors.

A. Both statements are true.

B. Both statements are false.

C. The first statement is true, the second is false.

D. The first statement is false, the second is true.

31 The branchial arches are six pairs of stacked bilateral swellings of tissue that appear inferior to the stomodeum. The branchial arches include the maxillary arch.

A. Both statements are true.

B. Both statements are false.

C. The first statement is true, the second is false.

D. The first statement is false, the second is true.

32 The tongue develops during the second to third weeks of prenatal development. The tongue develops from independent swellings located internally on the floor of the primitive pharynx.

A. Both statements are true.

B. Both statements are false.

C. The first statement is true, the second is false.

D. The first statement is false, the second is true.

33 The bell stage occurs between the eleventh and twelfth weeks of prenatal development. There is differentiation of the enamel organ into four layers during the bell stage.

A. Both statements are true.

B. Both statements are false.

C. The first statement is true, the second is false.

D. The first statement is false, the second is true.

34 Dentin is a crystalline material that is less hard than enamel because it is 70% inorganic.

A. Both the statement and reason are correct and related.

B. Both the statement and reason are correct but NOT related.

C. The statement is NOT correct, but the reason is correct.

D. NEITHER the statement NOR the reason is correct.

35 The lines of Retzius appear as incremental lines in dentin that stain brown. In transverse sections the lines of Retzius appear as concentric rings.

A. Both statements are true.

B. Both statements are false.

C. The first statement is true, the second is false.

D. The first statement is false, the second is true.

36 The hard tissues of the tooth consist mainly of calcium carbonate because it has the chemical formula $Ca_{10}(PO_4)_6(OH)_2$.

A. Both the statement and reason are correct and related.

B. Both the statement and reason are correct but NOT related.

C. The statement is NOT correct, but the reason is correct.

D. NEITHER the statement NOR the reason is correct.

37 With endodontic therapy the tooth may lighten because the tooth is no longer in occlusion.

A. Both the statement and reason are correct and related.

B. Both the statement and reason are correct but NOT related.

C. The statement is NOT correct, but the reason is correct.

D. NEITHER the statement NOR the reason is correct.

38 Enamel sealants must be placed in any of the pronounced occlusal fissures because the pulp horns are especially prominent under the mesiobuccal cusp of molar teeth.

A. Both the statement and reason are correct and related.

B. Both the statement and reason are correct but NOT related.

C. The statement is NOT correct, but the reason is correct.

D. NEITHER the statement NOR the reason is correct.

39 The alveolar crest is the MOST apical rim of the alveolar bone proper. The alveolar crest is apical to the cemento-enamel junction by approximately 1 to 2 mm.

A. Both statements are true.

B. Both statements are false.

C. The first statement is true, the second is false.

D. The first statement is false, the second is true.

40 The periodontal ligament provides a MOST efficient proprioceptive mechanism because the fibroblast is the MOST common cell in the ligament.

A. Both the statement and reason are correct and related.

B. Both the statement and reason are correct but NOT related.

C. The statement is NOT correct, but the reason is correct.

D. NEITHER the statement NOR the reason is correct.

41 The functions of the periodontium include all of the following, EXCEPT one. Which one is the EXCEPTION?
   A. Attaching the tooth to the bony socket
   B. Resisting forces generated by mastication and speech
   C. Defending against external noxious stimuli
   D. Protecting the tooth against cariogenic bacteria

42 Oral epithelium is classified as
   A. simple squamous epithelium.
   B. stratified squamous epithelium.
   C. pseudostratified columnar epithelium.
   D. simple cuboidal epithelium.

43 Sulcular or crevicular epithelium is
   A. keratinized.
   B. parakeratinized.
   C. pseudokeratinized.
   D. nonkeratinized.

44 Attached gingiva is found between the
   A. mucogingival junction and the free gingival groove.
   B. alveolar mucosa and the marginal gingiva.
   C. marginal gingiva and the free gingival groove.
   D. teeth of the dentition.

45 The connective tissue of the gingival tissues is called the
   A. lamina dura.
   B. lamina propria.
   C. lamina lucida.
   D. lamina densa.

46 One of the following descriptors does NOT pertain to the alveolar mucosa. Which is the EXCEPTION?
   A. Nonkeratinized
   B. Found beyond the mucogingival junction
   C. Flexible
   D. Component of gingiva

47 Brush ends of the fibers of the PDL that are embedded in both the cementum and alveolar bone are referred to as
   A. oblique fibers.
   B. Sharpey's fibers.
   C. principal fibers.
   D. transseptal fibers.

48 All of the following are terms given to the compact bone that surrounds the roots of the tooth and forms the lining of the tooth socket, EXCEPT one. Which is the EXCEPTION?
   A. Alveolar bone proper
   B. Cribriform plate
   C. Lamina dura
   D. Lamina propria

49 The supporting alveolar bone is made of
   A. compact and cancellous bone.
   B. cortical and spongy bone.
   C. cancellous and spongy bone.
   D. cortical, cancellous, and spongy bone.

50 Which of the following tissues lines the oral cavity?
   A. Simple squamous epithelium for diffusion of fluids
   B. Simple columnar epithelium for absorption
   C. Pseudostratified columnar epithelium with goblet cells for production of mucus
   D. Stratified squamous epithelium for protection from abrasion

Answer Key and Rationales

1 (A) Frontal process and first branchial arch are responsible for formation of the face and oral cavity, NOT including base of the tongue. Branchial arches II, III, and IV merge to form base of tongue. Stomodeum and buccopharyngeal (oropharyngeal) membranes are IMPORTANT in formation of primitive mouth. Tuberculum impar is IMPORTANT in formation of anterior portion of tongue.

2 (A) Formation of an ameloblast from cells of the inner enamel epithelium is an example of histodifferentiation, the formation of a MORE specialized cell from a primitive cell. Primitive cells are the cells of the inner enamel epithelium, and specialized cells are the ameloblasts. Morphodifferentiation is the development of a different form, such as occurs when cells of Hertwig's epithelial root sheath (HERS) align themselves to dictate the shape of the root. Odontogenesis refers to formation of teeth; dentinogenesis refers to formation of dentin.

3 (C) Basement membrane marks the junction where dentin and enamel will meet. Outer enamel epithelium and stellate reticulum are cell layers of the enamel organ. Dental papilla forms the pulp.

4 (C) Dental lamina is a strand of epithelial cells that marks the beginning of tooth formation and develops along jaw ridge. Primary dental lamina forms primary teeth, and secondary dental lamina is responsible for formation of permanent teeth. Tooth germ and tooth bud refer to later stages of tooth development. Enamel organ and dental papilla refer to tissues associated with tooth development after initial localized growth of cells.

5 (B) Copula is posterior swelling that forms the base of the tongue. Lingual swellings and tuberculum impar form the anterior two thirds of the tongue or body. First branchial arch is responsible for formation of the maxilla, mandible, and middle portion of the face. Meckel's cartilage is IMPORTANT in formation of alveolar bone.

6 (C) Shape of developing root is determined by HERS, which forms when outer and inner epithelial tissues join. Rests of Malassez are epithelial remnants of the sheath and are trapped in tissues of the periodontal ligament (PDL). Dental lamina and stellate reticulum are structures associated with the developing tooth and are NOT responsible for the shape of the root.

7 (D) Enamel is the hardest tissue in the body and contains *about* 96% inorganic (mineralized) material. Dentin contains *about* 70% inorganic material, and cementum, LIKE bone, contains *about* 65% inorganic material. When considering the inorganic percentage with each portion of the tooth (or alveolar bone), choose the *closest* one listed because the percentage can vary according to source.

8 (B) Light and dark bands of Hunter-Schreger are oriented perpendicular to the dentinoenamel junction (DEJ) and are caused by curvature of the developing enamel rods. Neonatal lines, lines of Retzius, and perikymata are also lines found in enamel.

9 (A) Perikymata are fine horizontal lines that may be visible on the enamel surface as a manifestation (or sign) of the lines of Retzius, seen microscopically as narrow lines that extend from dentinoenamel junction (DEJ) to cusp tips. Hunter-Schreger bands and enamel spindles are features of enamel that would NOT be visible on external enamel surface.

10 (B) Enamel pearl is often confused with calculus because of its location and shape. Enamel pearls often form near cementoenamel junction (CEJ) as rounded structures that protrude from the tooth surface. They are never found on the occlusal surface of teeth and are never seen as opacity rings on facial surfaces of anteriors. Denticles (pulp stones) are commonly found within pulp chamber, UNLIKE enamel pearls.

11 (C) Nuclei of odontoblasts, cells responsible for dentin formation, are found in pulp. Dentinal tubules may contain cytoplasmic extensions of odontoblast. Newly formed dentin (predentin) would NOT contain odontoblast nuclei.

12 (A) Apical and furcation areas are sites associated with cellular cementum. Cementocytes are NOT located equally throughout the root surface. Thin cervical cementum has few or no cementocytes. The region closest to dentin contains few cementocytes.

13 (B) Thickening of apical cementum is referred to as hypercementosis; it may be a result of persistent inflammation. Cementicle is a calcification found in PDL. Cementogenesis refers to normal formation of cementum. Cementoid is cementum MOST recently formed by cementoblasts.

14 (C) Enamel is the hardest and therefore MOST abrasion-resistant tissue, followed by dentin and cementum. Strength of enamel as the covering of the tooth is IMPORTANT in longevity of tooth structure.

15 (C) Mineralization of pulp increases as the tooth ages and has clinical significance when endodontic therapy is indicated. Both vascularity and pulp chamber size decrease as the result of aging. Increased occlusal function may cause pulp to fill completely with reparative dentin. As pulp shrinks, patients may note a decrease in tooth sensitivity.

16 (A) Apex and furcation areas are sites where cementum is thicker (>0.05 mm), while the cervical third is thinner (0.02 to 0.05 mm). Cementum is approximately 0.05 mm thick on remaining portions of the root surface.

17 (D) Cells would be MOST active on the mesial side of a tooth being moved mesially and would be cells responsible for bone removal and osteoclasts. Osteoblasts would become active on the distal side of mesially moved tooth. Fibroblasts and cementoblasts would NOT have a great change in activity.

18 (A) Stratified squamous epithelium is the MOST common type of soft tissue of the oral cavity. Cuboidal and simple squamous epithelial and transitional cells are NOT considered primary cell layers of oral cavity.

19 (C) Taste buds are NOT associated with filiform lingual papillae; they are associated with fungiform, foliate, and circumvallate lingual papillae.

20 (C) Epithelial rests are trapped epithelial cells associated with the inner and outer enamel epithelium that is associated with enamel organ. Dental sac and dental papilla are mesenchymal components of the tooth bud (germ) and would NOT be associated with trapped epithelial cells.

21 (B) Filiform lingual papillae are MORE keratinized than fungiform, foliate, and circumvallate lingual papillae.

22 (B) When tooth function increases, the amount of trabeculae also increases. Cortical, lamellar, and circumferential bone do NOT show significant changes as the result of increased occlusal forces.

23 (A) Histological depth is LESS than clinical probing depth. The probe will slightly penetrate junctional epithelium (JE), leading to greater clinical probing depth. As tissue health decreases as with periodontal disease, the probe penetrates MORE easily because of ulceration of the JE, so there is even greater clinical probing depth.

24 (A) Presence of sclerotic dentin may decrease the rate at which caries spreads. Sclerotic dentin is a site where odontoblasts have degenerated and may be noted in older teeth with arrested dentin. Dentinal tubules contain calcium salts.

25 (B) Korff's fibers are corkscrewlike collagen structures that lie among cytoplastic extensions of odontoblasts. Enamel spindles are extensions of the odontoblastic process into enamel. Dentinal tubules contain the odontoblastic process. Tomes' granular layer is an area of unmineralized regions in the peripheral portion of dentin beneath the root's cementum, adjacent to the dentinocemental junction (DCJ).

26 (C) Commissural lip pits are dimplelike invaginations of the corner (commissure) of lips. They may be unilateral or bilateral but generally occur on vermilion portion. Cleft lip is a disturbance of lip development in utero. Basal cell or squamous cell carcinoma is usually a cancerous lesion on the lips that presents as an ulcer.

27 **(B)** Bifid uvula (cleft uvula) is a minor cleft of the posterior soft palate. Cleft palate is a disruption in palatal fusion. Cleft lip is a disturbance of lip development in utero. Commissural lip pits are dimplelike invaginations of the corner of lips.

28 **(B)** Cleft lip, with or without cleft palate, occurs in about 1 in 1000 live births. Cleft palate, with or without cleft lip, occurs 1 in 2500 live births. Cleft palate is a disruption in palatal fusion. Cleft lip is a disturbance of lip development in utero.

29 **(A)** Both statements are true. Ankyloglossia is a short lingual frenum that extends to the tongue apex, restricting the movement of the tongue to varying degrees. Surgery may or may not be needed; if the condition is severe, therapy may help with speech problems.

30 **(C)** First statement is true, the second is false. The secondary palate will form posterior two thirds of the hard palate. However, the secondary palate contains maxillary canines and posteriors and NOT central and lateral incisors, which would be contained in the primary palate, the anterior one third of the hard palate.

31 **(C)** First statement is true, the second is false. Branchial arches are six pairs of stacked bilateral swellings of tissue that appear inferior to the stomodeum. However, branchial arches include the mandibular arch and NOT the maxillary arch.

32 **(D)** First statement is false, the second is true. The tongue develops from independent swellings located internally on floor of the primitive pharynx. However, the tongue develops during fourth to eighth weeks of prenatal development.

33 **(A)** Both statements are true. The bell stage occurs between the eleventh and twelfth weeks of prenatal development; there is differentiation of the enamel organ into four layers.

34 **(A)** Both the statement and the reason are correct and related. Dentin is a crystalline material that is LESS hard than enamel because it is 70% inorganic.

35 **(D)** First statement is false, the second is true. Lines of Retzius appear as incremental lines in enamel that stain brown and in transverse sections appear as concentric rings. Imbrication lines of von Ebner are incremental lines or bands that stain darkly in dentin.

36 **(C)** Statement is not correct, but the reason is correct. Hard tissues of the tooth consist mainly of calcium hydroxyapatite with the chemical formula $Ca_{10}(PO_4)_6(OH)_2$; they include enamel, dentin, and cementum.

37 **(D)** Neither the statement nor reason is correct. With endodontic therapy, tooth may darken because it is no longer vital. That is because the pulp that provided nutrients for the dentin has been removed. Teeth will lighten with the whitening (bleaching) process, whether vital or not. Oxygen radicals from peroxide in the whitening agents contact stains in interprismatic spaces within the enamel layer; when this occurs, stains will be bleached (whitened).

38 **(B)** Both the statement and reason are correct but not related. Pulp horns are MOST prominent under the MB cusp of molar teeth (and MOST primary teeth). Thus extra care MUST be taken when restorative treatment is performed. Enamel (pit and fissure) sealants are not invasive; however, they MUST be placed in any of pronounced occlusal fissures on molar teeth, even in adults, to prevent occlusal caries.

39 **(D)** First statement is false, the second is true. Alveolar crest is the MOST cervical, not apical, rim of alveolar bone proper, apical to the CEJ by approximately 1 to 2 mm.

40 **(B)** Both the statement and reason are correct but not related. The PDL does provides MOST efficient proprioceptive mechanism because of its innervation. However, fibroblast is MOST common cell in PDL and produces fibers for ligament.

41 **(D)** Protection against cariogenic bacteria has NOT been shown to be a function of periodontium. Functions of the periodontium include attaching tooth to its bony housing; providing resistance to forces of mastication, speech, and deglutition; maintaining body surface integrity by separating external and internal environments; defending against external noxious stimuli.

42 **(B)** Oral epithelium consists of keratinized (orthokeratinized or parakeratinized) stratified squamous epithelium. Simple epithelia, pseudostratified columnar epithelia, and simple cuboidal epithelia are found in other areas of the body but NOT in the oral mucosa lining the oral cavity.

43 **(D)** Sulcular and crevicular epithelium is nonkeratinized. ONLY masticatory mucosa, such as the attached gingiva and hard palate, is keratinized (orthokeratinized or parakeratinized). No areas of the mouth are considered pseudokeratinized.

44 **(A)** Attached gingiva is portion that is firmly bound to underlying bone and is located between free gingival groove and mucogingival junction. Free gingival groove demarcates part of the tissues that are marginal (free) and NOT attached to the tooth. Alveolar mucosa is loose and movable. Connective tissue of PDL is ONLY tissue that attaches to tooth.

45 **(B)** Lamina propria is the connective tissue of the gingival tissues that contains collagen fibers, fibroblasts, undifferentiated cells, macrophages. Lamina dura is the radiographic term for alveolar bone proper (ABP), which surrounds tooth root. Lamina lucida and lamina densa are BOTH components of basement membrane between lamina propria and the attached gingiva.

46 **(D)** Alveolar mucosa is nonkeratinized, flexible, located beyond mucogingival junction. However, it is a separate part of oral mucosa and is NOT classified as gingiva.

47 **(B)** Brush ends of principal fibers of the PDL that are embedded in both cementum and alveolar bone are referred to as Sharpey's fibers. Transseptal and the rest of the principal fibers span across entire PDL space; do NOT refer to just embedded portions of the fibers.

48 **(C)** Lamina propria is the oral connective tissue. Alveolar bone proper (ABP) is compact bone that forms housing of the root and tooth socket. Referred to histologically as cribriform plate, anatomically as bundle bone, and radiographically as lamina dura.

49 **(C)** Supporting alveolar bone contains BOTH compact and cancellous bone. Facial and lingual cortical plates are compact, and spongy bone between these plates is cancellous.

50 **(C)** Diffusion and absorption do NOT occur across tissue that lines the oral cavity. Mucus in oral cavity is a component of the saliva produced by salivary glands. Lining of oral cavity is subject to abrasion by food during mastication; therefore the lining consists of many layers of cells, primarily stratified squamous epithelium, to provide protection from abrasive action.

CHAPTER 3

Anatomy, Biochemistry, and Physiology

GENERAL ANATOMY

Anatomy is the study of structure; **physiology** is the study of function; **gross anatomy** is the study of the body's structure that is visible with the naked eye; and **microanatomy** (histology) examines the cellular composition of tissues. Structures and associated functions are organized in interacting hierarchy from simple to complex (i.e., chemicals, cells, tissues, organs, body systems, total organism).

Organs of the body include integumentary, skeletal, muscular, nervous (including special sense organs), endocrine, cardiovascular, lymphatic, respiratory, digestive, urinary, and reproductive. Knowing these systems can help you to understand a medical term. A term related to each of these systems might be augmented with roots, prefixes, and suffixes (see CD-ROM for commonly encountered ones), filling out the other two thirds of the term. If you know those, plus the name of the body system, you are well on your way to understanding another third or more of a term. In addition, **anatomical nomenclature** includes directional terms that describe relative position of body parts in **anatomical position** (see CD-ROM).

- See CD-ROM for Chapter Terms and WebLinks.
- See Chapter 2, Embryology and Histology: cell structure.

Integumentary System

Integumentary system consists of skin (cutaneous membrane), including glands, hair, and nails (adnexa). Skin has *outermost* epidermis and *innermost* dermis anchored to underlying tissues by hypodermis or subcutaneous tissue; it is the largest external organ.

A. **Epidermis:** stratified squamous epithelium, five layers in thicker areas or four layers in thinner areas (Figure 3-1):
  1. Stratum corneum: outermost layer of dead cells, continually sloughed off, replaced by cells from deeper layers; contains keratin.
  2. Stratum lucidum: thin, clear layer just beneath stratum corneum; not in thinner areas.
  3. Stratum granulosum: appears granular because organelles are shrinking, with intracellular keratin (keratin granules) being deposited.
  4. Stratum spinosum: located next to stratum basale; undergoes limited mitosis and adds strength to the skin owing to intracellular bridging.

  5. Stratum basale: innermost layer and closest to blood supply; active mitotic layer; contains melanocytes (produce dark pigment, melanin) and immune cells (Langerhans' cells); tissue color depends on melanocytic activity, amount of carotene (yellow pigment), dermal blood supply.
B. Basement membrane: where epidermis and dermis interface; derives components from both layers.
C. **Dermis** (stratum corium): superior papillary layer of fibrous connective tissue; contains vessels, nerves, embedded accessory structures; lower reticular layer is meshwork of collagen and elastic fibers.
D. Hypodermis (subcutaneous tissue): deep to dermis and serves to anchor skin to underlying organs; composed of loose connective tissue and adipose tissues; acts as cushion and insulates body from heat and cold.
E. Accessory structures (e.g., glands, hair, nails): derived by mitosis in stratum basale of epidermis:
  1. Sweat glands: merocrine (MORE numerous, widely distributed) and apocrine (larger, LESS numerous); sebaceous glands are oil glands associated with hair follicles.
  2. Hair: divided into visible shaft and root, embedded in skin and surrounded by a follicle; central core: medulla, surrounded by cortex, cuticle, arrector pili muscles (contract in response to cold or fear to make hair stand on end).
  3. Nails: thin plates of hardened stratum corneum; each has free edge, nail body, root, eponychium, nail bed, nail matrix, lunula.

Skeletal System

Skeletal system (206 bones) includes axial skeleton (80), forming axis of the body, and appendicular skeleton (126), consisting of appendages and attachments. System functions to provide support, protect soft body parts, produce movement with muscles, store minerals (calcium), form blood cells.

- See Chapter 4, Head, Neck, and Dental Anatomy: skull, hyoid bone.
A. Osseous tissue: **osteons** (Haversian systems) (Figure 3-2):
  1. Compact bone: MORE dense; osteons are packed closely together.

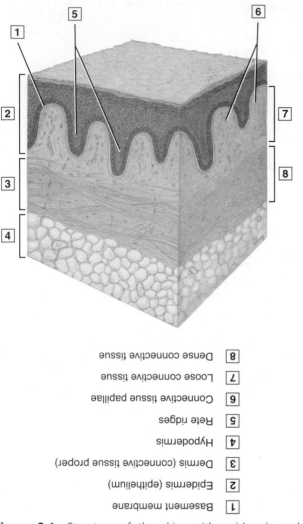

8 Dense connective tissue
7 Loose connective tissue
6 Connective tissue papillae
5 Rete ridges
4 Hypodermis
3 Dermis (connective tissue proper)
2 Epidermis (epithelium)
1 Basement membrane

Figure 3-1 Structure of the skin, with epidermis and dermis. (From Bath-Balogh M, Fehrenbach MJ: Illustrated dental embryology, histology, and anatomy, ed 2, St. Louis, 2006, Saunders/Elsevier.)

2. Spongy bone: LESS dense; consists of bony plates called trabeculae around irregular spaces that contain red bone marrow.
B. Long bones, such as femur, humerus, phalanges:
    1. Diaphysis: located around medullary cavity, with epiphysis at each end.
    2. Epiphysis: covered with articular cartilage; remainder of the bone is covered with periosteum.
C. Surface markings (elevations and depression) on bones: allow articulation, muscle attachment; openings: allowed for vessels.
D. **Axial skeleton:** skull, hyoid, vertebral column, thoracic cage:
    1. Skull: 28 bones:
        a. Cranium: 8 bones (frontal, occipital, 2 parietal, 2 temporal, ethmoid, sphenoid).

b. Facial: 14 bones (2 maxillae, 2 zygomatic, 2 nasal, 2 inferior nasal conchae, 2 lacrimal, 2 palatine, 1 mandible, 1 vomer).
        c. Auditory ossicles (malleus, incus, stapes in each ear): 6 bones.
    2. **Hyoid bone:** midline body and two pairs of projections, greater and lesser cornu:
        a. Forms base of the tongue and larynx; suspended in the neck, mobile, LACKS other bony articulations but is attached to many muscles.
        b. Superior and anterior to thyroid cartilage of the larynx (voice box).
    3. Vertebral column (26): separated by intervertebral discs (7 cervical, 12 thoracic, 5 lumbar, 1 sacrum, 1 coccyx):
        a. Atlas (C1): allows back-and-forth movement of skull.
        b. Axis (C2): allows side-to-side movement of skull (contains dens, pivoting fulcrum for atlas).
    4. Thoracic cage (25): 1 sternum and 24 ribs (12 pairs).
E. **Appendicular skeleton:** upper and lower extremities, pectoral and pelvic girdles, attaching extremities to axial skeleton (Figure 3-3):
    1. Upper extremities (60): each extremity consists of 30 bones (1 humerus in arm, 1 lateral radius and 1 medial ulna in forearm, 8 carpals in wrist, 5 metacarpals in hand, and 14 phalanges in fingers).
    2. Pectoral girdle (4): clavicle (collar bone) and scapula (shoulder blade) on each side.
    3. Lower extremities (60): 30 bones in each extremity (1 femur in the thigh, 1 medial tibia and 1 lateral fibula in the leg, 7 tarsals in the ankle and instep, 5 metatarsals in the foot, 14 phalanges in the toes, and 1 patella [kneecap]).
    4. Pelvic girdle (2): os coxae (innominate bones); each is formed from ilium, ischium, pubis, fused together; acetabulum, a large depression, provides socket for head of femur.
F. Articulations (joints): bones are held together by fibrous joint capsule lined with synovial membrane; secretes synovial fluid for lubrication and protection:
    1. Synarthrosis: immovable fibrous joint, e.g., suture in skull.
    2. Amphiarthrosis: slightly movable joint; bones are connected by hyaline cartilage or fibrocartilage; e.g., symphysis pubis, intervertebral discs.
    3. Diarthrosis (synovial joint): freely movable joint; motion limited ONLY by surrounding tendons, ligaments, bones; joint movement includes gliding, condyloid, hinge, saddle, pivot, ball-and-socket; e.g., temporomandibular, hip, knee, shoulder, elbow, wrist.

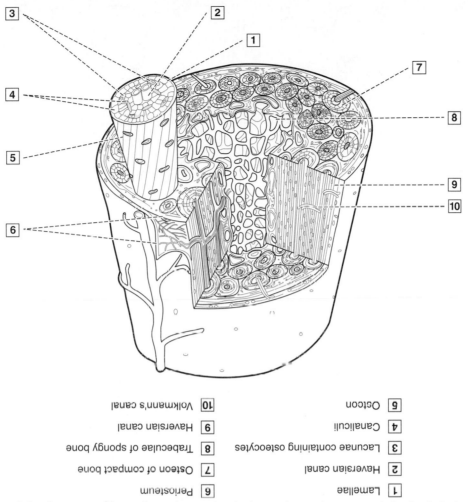

Volkmann's canal **10**

Haversian canal **9**

Trabeculae of spongy bone **8**

Osteon of compact bone **7**

Periosteum **6**

Osteon **5**

Canaliculi **4**

Lacunae containing osteocytes **3**

Haversian canal **2**

Lamellae **1**

Figure 3-2　Structure of bone tissue. (From Fehrenbach MJ, ed: Dental anatomy coloring book, St. Louis, 2008, Saunders/Elsevier.)

Muscular System

Muscular system includes skeletal muscle tissue that can be controlled voluntarily. Functions include moving the skeleton, maintaining posture, supporting soft tissues, producing heat to maintain body temperature.

- See Chapter 4, Head, Neck, and Dental Anatomy: muscles.

A.　Structure of **skeletal muscle** (Figure 3-4):

　1.　Muscles and muscle fibers are surrounded by connective tissue coverings, extend beyond muscle to form tendons; endomysium surrounds individual muscle fibers; perimysium surrounds each fasciculus (functional muscle fiber group); epimysium covers entire muscle.

　2.　Each skeletal muscle fiber represents single muscle cell: sarcolemma, sarcoplasm, sarcoplasmic reticulum, mitochondria, and myofibrils composed of myofilaments actin and myosin, organized in repeating sarcomeres; arrangement is responsible for striations in skeletal muscle fibers.

B.　Attachments and actions: muscles are attached to bones by tendons:

　1.　**Origin** is the LESS movable attachment; **insertion** is the MORE movable attachment.

　2.　In function, insertion moves *toward* origin.

C.　Major axial muscles (according to site of action):

　1.　Head and neck: facial expression, mastication, cervical.

　2.　Spine: erector spinae, forming a mass on either side of vertebral column.

　3.　Trunk: thoracic wall (external and internal intercostals), abdominal wall (external and internal oblique, transversus abdominis, rectus abdominis), diaphragm.

　4.　Pelvic floor: superficial (bulbospongiosus, ischiocavernosus, transversus perinei) and deep (levator ani, coccygeus).

D.　Major appendicular (Figure 3-5):

　1.　Shoulder (trapezius, serratus anterior); arm (pectoralis major, latissimus dorsi, deltoid, rotator cuff).

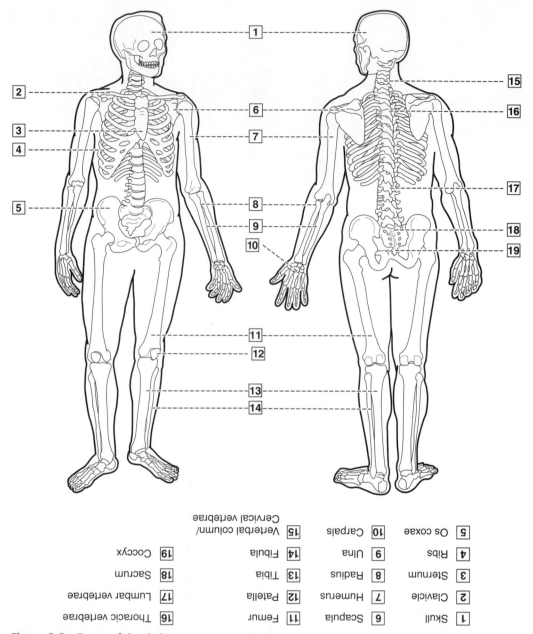

Figure 3-3 Bones of the skeleton. (From Fehrenbach MJ, ed: Dental anatomy coloring book, St. Louis, 2008, Saunders/Elsevier.)

1	Skull	6	Scapula	11	Femur	16	Thoracic vertebrae
2	Clavicle	7	Humerus	12	Patella	17	Lumbar vertebrae
3	Sternum	8	Radius	13	Tibia	18	Sacrum
4	Ribs	9	Ulna	14	Fibula	19	Coccyx
5	Os coxae	10	Carpals	15	Vertebal column/ Cervical vertebrae		

2. Forearm (triceps brachii, biceps brachii, brachialis, brachioradialis); hand (extensors on posterior surface of forearm, flexors on anterior surface, pronator, supinator).

3. Thigh: abduct ("move away") and rotate (gluteus maximus, gluteus medius, gluteus minimus, tensor fasciae latae), adduct ("move toward") (adductor longus, adductor brevis, adductor magnus, gracilis), flex (iliopsoas).

4. Leg: extensors are the quadriceps femoris in anterior compartment (vastus lateralis, vastus medialis, vastus intermedius, rectus femoris); flexors are

hamstrings in posterior compartment (semimembranosus, semitendinosus, biceps femoris).

5. Ankle and foot: dorsiflexion (tibialis anterior in anterior compartment), plantar flexion (gastrocnemius and soleus in posterior compartment), eversion (peroneus in lateral compartment).

Nervous System

Nervous system includes all neural tissue (neurons and neuroglia). The synapse is in the region of communication between neurons; communication occurs through the effects of neurotransmitters. **Sensory nerves**

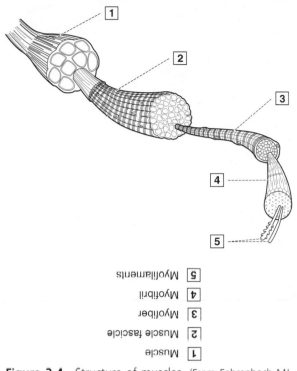

5 Myofilaments
4 Myofibril
3 Myofiber
2 Muscle fascicle
1 Muscle

Figure 3-4 Structure of muscles. (From Fehrenbach MJ, ed: Dental anatomy coloring book, St. Louis, 2008, Saunders/Elsevier.)

(dorsal root) transmit information to the brain and spinal cord. **Motor nerves** (ventral root) transmit information from the brain and spinal cord to effectors, such as muscles and glands. Integrative functions interpret the sensory information and act by stimulating motor pathways. Divided into **central nervous system** (CNS) and **peripheral nervous system** (PNS), which function together to integrate and coordinate body activities, assimilate experiences, and assist in memory and learning.

- See Chapters 6, General and Oral Pathology: nervous system pathology; 9, Pharmacology: drugs and nervous system; 14, Pain Management: nerve anatomy and physiology.

A. CNS: composed of the brain and spinal cord (Figures 3-6 and 3-7):
  1. Within the brain, covered by meninges: outermost layer (dura mater), middle layer (arachnoid), and innermost layer (pia mater); subarachnoid space between arachnoid and pia mater contains blood vessels and cerebrospinal fluid.
  2. Components of the brain:
    a. Cerebrum: largest portion, divided into two hemispheres by longitudinal fissure; connected by band of white fibers, corpus callosum, responsible for higher level thought processes (i.e., what we need to channel during the case study portions of NDHBE):

(1) Outer surface is cerebral cortex, composed of gray matter and marked by gyri (raised folds) and sulci (grooves, furrows).
(2) Each hemisphere has frontal, parietal, occipital, temporal lobe, insula; primary somatosensory area is in parietal, primary somatomotor area is in frontal, visual cortex is in occipital, auditory and olfactory areas are in temporal, taste is in parietal.
  b. Diencephalon: surrounded by cerebrum; includes thalamus, hypothalamus, pituitary gland:
    (1) Thalamus: serves as relay station for sensory impulses that travel to cerebral cortex; hypothalamus plays MAIN role in maintaining homeostasis (body's thermostat).
    (2) Brainstem: between diencephalon and spinal cord; consists of midbrain, pons, medulla oblongata; midbrain: contains voluntary motor tracts and visual and auditory reflex centers; pons: contains the pneumotaxic and apneustic areas that help regulate breathing movements; medulla oblongata: contains ascending and descending tracts and vital cardiac, vasomotor, and respiratory centers.
  c. Cerebellum: second largest portion; motor area that coordinates skeletal muscle activity; maintains muscle tone, posture, balance.
  3. Spinal cord: continuation of medulla oblongata and extends from foramen magnum to first lumbar vertebra; acts as conduction pathway and reflex center:
    a. Ascending tracts: conduct sensory impulses *to* brain.
    b. Descending tracts: carry motor impulses *from* brain *to* effectors.
B. PNS includes all cranial and spinal nerves:
  1. Consists of afferent (sensory) division and efferent (motor) division; efferent division includes somatic nervous system (SNS), which enables voluntary control over skeletal muscle contraction, and autonomic nervous system (ANS), which regulates smooth and cardiac muscle contraction and glandular activity.
  2. Components: bundles of nerve fibers (axons and dendrites), 12 pairs of cranial nerves that emerge from inferior surface (caudal) of brain (see next section).
  3. Spinal nerves contain both sensory and motor fibers; 31 pairs emerge from spinal cord and are grouped according to origin; in all but thoracic region, MAIN portions of nerves form complex networks called plexuses (cervical, brachial, lumbar, sacral); nerves emerge from plexuses to supply specific regions.

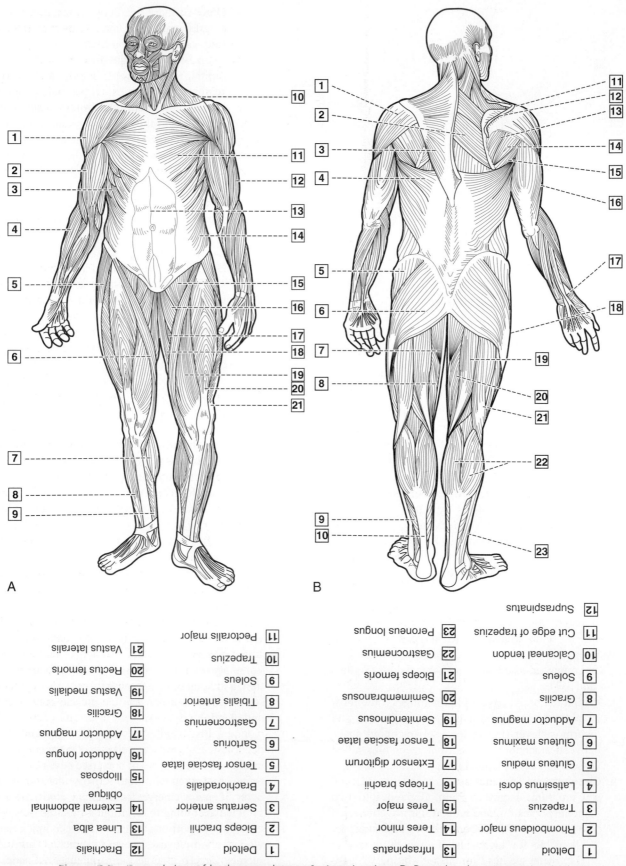

A

B

Figure 3-5 General view of body musculature. **A,** Anterior view. **B,** Posterior view. (From Fehrenbach MJ, ed: Dental anatomy coloring book, St. Louis, 2008, Saunders/Elsevier.)

11	Pectoralis major
21	Vastus lateralis	10	Trapezius
20	Rectus femoris	9	Soleus
19	Vastus medialis	8	Tibialis anterior
18	Gracilis	7	Gastrocnemius
17	Adductor magnus	6	Sartorius
16	Adductor longus	5	Tensor fasciae latae
15	Iliopsoas	4	Brachioradialis
14	External abdominal oblique	3	Serratus anterior
13	Linea alba	2	Biceps brachii
12	Brachialis	1	Deltoid

23	Peroneus longus	12	Supraspinatus
22	Gastrocnemius	11	Cut edge of trapezius
21	Biceps femoris	10	Calcaneal tendon
20	Semimembranosus	9	Soleus
19	Semitendinosus	8	Gracilis
18	Tensor fasciae latae	7	Adductor magnus
17	Extensor digitorum	6	Gluteus maximus
16	Triceps brachii	5	Gluteus medius
15	Teres major	4	Latissimus dorsi
14	Teres minor	3	Trapezius
13	Infraspinatus	2	Rhomboideus major
		1	Deltoid

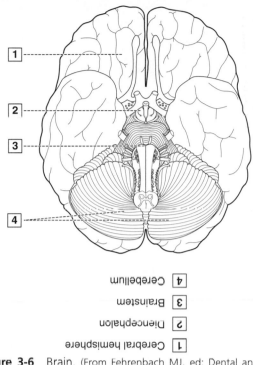

1. Cerebral hemisphere
2. Diencephalon
3. Brainstem
4. Cerebellum

Figure 3-6 Brain. (From Fehrenbach MJ, ed: Dental anatomy coloring book, St. Louis, 2008, Saunders/Elsevier.)

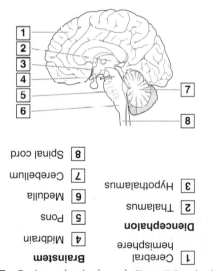

Diencephalon
1. Cerebral hemisphere
2. Thalamus
3. Hypothalamus

Brainstem
4. Midbrain
5. Pons
6. Medulla
7. Cerebellum
8. Spinal cord

Figure 3-7 Brain and spinal cord. (From Fehrenbach MJ, ed: Dental anatomy coloring book, St. Louis, 2008, Saunders/Elsevier.)

4. **Autonomic nervous system** (ANS) is a visceral efferent system part of PNS; innervates smooth muscle, cardiac muscle, and glands; has two divisions, with MOST organs being innervated by BOTH to maintain homeostasis:
   a. **Sympathetic division** (thoracolumbar division) (SANS) is energy-expending system that is MOST active when body is in emergencies or stressful conditions; MOST postganglionic neurons release norepinephrine.
   b. **Parasympathetic division** (craniosacral division) (PANS) is energy-conserving system that is MOST active when the body is in normal relaxed condition; MOST postganglionic neurons release acetylcholine.

Cranial Nerves

Cranial nerves are part of the PNS; designated by both number and Roman numerals I through XII, as well as specific name (Figure 3-8). Include 12 pairs that are connected to the brain at its base and pass through the skull by way of fissures and foramina; may be either *afferent* or *efferent* or have both types.

- See Chapters 4, Head, Neck, and Dental Anatomy: fifth (trigeminal) and seventh (facial); 6, General and Oral Pathology, and 16, Special Needs Patient Care: neurological disorders.
A. First (I) (olfactory): *afferent* for smell from the nasal mucosa to the brain, enters skull through perforations in cribriform plate of ethmoid to join olfactory bulb in brain.
B. Second (II) (optic): *afferent* for vision from retina to brain, enters skull through optic canal of sphenoid, where right and left optic nerves join at the optic chasm and where many fibers cross to the opposite side before continuing into the brain as optic tracts. Glaucoma results from damage to this nerve.
C. Third (III) (oculomotor): *efferent* to eye muscles, carries preganglionic parasympathetic fibers to ciliary ganglion near the eyeball and postganglionic fibers innervate muscles inside the eyeball; located in lateral wall of cavernous sinus and then exits skull through superior orbital fissure on its way to the orbit; strabismus (lack of eye coordination, "cross-eyed") can occur with damage.
D. Fourth (IV) (trochlear): *efferent* to one eye muscle (superior oblique) for proprioception; runs in lateral wall of cavernous sinus and exits skull through the superior orbital fissure on its way to the orbit.
E. Fifth (V) (trigeminal): *efferent* for muscles of mastication and for other cranial muscles; *afferent* for ALL of oral cavity, including teeth and portions of tongue, and for MOST of facial skin; trigeminal neuralgia is a neural lesion involving afferent nerves to the face.
   1. Trigeminal ganglion (semilunar, gasserian) is on anterior surface of petrous portion of temporal bone; largest cranial nerve; has two roots: sensory and motor:
      a. Sensory root has three divisions: ophthalmic, maxillary, mandibular; each enters skull in different location in sphenoid:

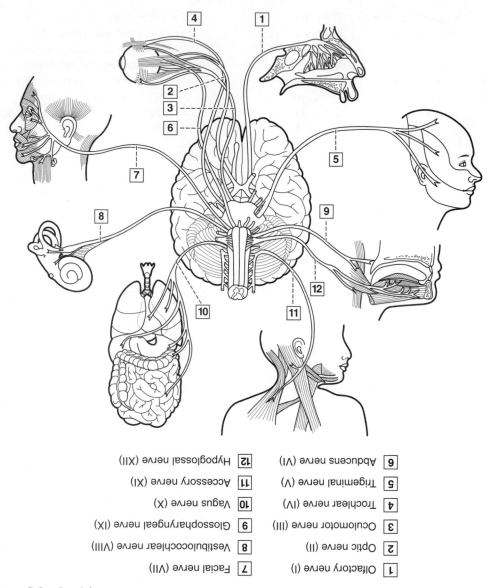

Figure 3-8   Cranial nerves. (From Fehrenbach MJ, ed: Dental anatomy coloring book, St. Louis, 2008, Saunders/Elsevier.)

1 Olfactory nerve (I)	**7** Facial nerve (VII)
2 Optic nerve (II)	**8** Vestibulocochlear nerve (VIII)
3 Oculomotor nerve (III)	**9** Glossopharyngeal nerve (IX)
4 Trochlear nerve (IV)	**10** Vagus nerve (X)
5 Trigeminal nerve (V)	**11** Accessory nerve (XI)
6 Abducens nerve (VI)	**12** Hypoglossal nerve (XII)

(1) Ophthalmic division: provides sensation for upper face and scalp; enters through superior orbital fissure (SOF).

(2) Maxillary division: provides sensation for middle face; enters by way of foramen rotundum.

(3) Mandibular division: provides sensation for lower face and sensory for anterior one third of tongue; enters by way of foramen ovale.

b. Motor root accompanies mandibular division of the sensory root and also exits skull through foramen ovale.

F. Sixth (VI) (abducens): *efferent* to one of the eyeball muscles (lateral rectus); exits skull through superior orbital fissure on its way to the orbit; runs through cavernous sinus; often is FIRST nerve affected by sinus infection.

G. Seventh (VII) (facial): *efferent* for muscles of facial expression, for preganglionic parasympathetic innervation of lacrimal, and for submandibular and sublingual; *afferent* for skin behind the ear, for taste sensation, and for the body of the tongue:

1. Leaves cranial cavity by passing through internal acoustic meatus; leads to facial canal inside temporal bone; exits the skull by way of stylomastoid foramen.

2. Nerve lesions include permanent or transient facial paralysis, loss of movement of muscles of facial expression caused by injury to nerve or Bell's palsy (BOTH motor and sensory deficit).

H. Eighth (VIII) (vestibulocochlear): *afferent* for hearing and balance; enters cranial cavity through internal acoustic meatus.

I. Ninth (IX) (glossopharyngeal): *efferent* for pharyngeal muscle (stylopharyngeal) and preganglionic parasympathetic innervation for parotid; *afferent* for pharynx (swallowing), taste, and general sensation from base of tongue (posterior one third of tongue).
   1. Passes through skull by way of jugular foramen and tympanic branch; has sensory fibers for middle ear and preganglionic parasympathetic fibers for parotid; arises within the gland and reenters the skull.
   2. After supplying ear, parasympathetic fibers leave skull through foramen ovale as lesser petrosal nerve; these preganglionic fibers then end in otic ganglion, located near mandibular division of trigeminal.

J. Tenth (X) (vagus): longest nerve in body; *efferent* for muscles of soft palate, pharynx, and larynx and for parasympathetic fibers to many major body organs, including thymus, heart, stomach; *afferent* for skin around ear and for taste sensation of the epiglottis; passes through skull by way of the jugular foramen; originates in brainstem and terminates in transverse colon.

K. Eleventh (XI) (accessory): *efferent* for trapezius and sternocleidomastoid, as well as muscles of soft palate and pharynx; ONLY partly a cranial nerve; consists of two roots: one arising from brain and one from spinal cord; exits skull through jugular foramen.

L. Twelfth (XII) (hypoglossal): *efferent* for intrinsic and extrinsic muscles of tongue; exits skull through hypoglossal canal; tongue is ONLY organ in the body with own cranial nerve; damage, such as by cerebrovascular accident (CVA, stroke), can result in deviation of tongue to one side.

Sense Organs

Sense organs include the widely distributed general senses and localized special senses of taste, smell, vision, hearing, equilibrium.

• See Chapter 4, Head, Neck, and Dental Anatomy: lacrimal gland.

A. General senses: widely distributed in the body; include touch, pressure, proprioception, thermoreception, pain:
   1. Touch and pressure: free nerve endings, Meissner's corpuscles, pacinian corpuscles.
   2. Proprioception (sense of position or orientation): Golgi tendon organs and muscle spindles.
   3. Thermoreception (temperature changes): thermoreceptors are free nerve endings; some are sensitive to heat, others to cold; extremes in temperature stimulate pain receptors.
   4. Pain (nociceptors): free nerve endings that are stimulated by tissue damage.

B. Gustatory (taste) and olfactory (smell) are localized special senses, closely related, complementary:
   1. Taste buds are located on the lingual papillae on the dorsal surface of tongue; salty, sweet, sour, bitter are four taste sensations (possibly savory is another) (see Chapter 4, Head, Neck, and Dental Anatomy).
   2. Seventh cranial nerve (facial): transmits taste impulses from *anterior two thirds* of tongue's body, and ninth cranial nerve (glossopharyngeal) transmits impulses from *posterior one third* of tongue's root; impulses are interpreted in parietal lobe of brain.
   3. Receptors for smell: located in olfactory epithelium of nasal cavity; first cranial nerve (olfactory) transmits impulses from olfactory epithelium; impulses are perceived as odors in temporal lobe of brain.

C. Visual sense is a localized special sense:
   1. Protective features of eye: eyebrows, eyelids, and eyelashes (cilia) protect from foreign particles and irritants; lacrimal glands produce antibacterial tears that moisten, cleanse, protect.
   2. Structure of eyeball: sclera (white) and cornea (clear): outermost fibrous layer; iris: middle vascular layer that regulates pupil size; retina: innermost neural layer and contains visual receptors (Figure 3-9).
   3. Refraction (bending of light rays): necessary to focus light rays on retina; in normal relaxed eye, refractive media are sufficient to focus light rays from 20 or more feet on retina; closer objects require accommodation to focus, which involves change in shape of lens, convergence of eyes, constriction of pupil.
   4. Photoreceptors are rods for vision in dim light and cones for color and acuity in bright light; cones are concentrated in fovea centralis and rods are located peripherally in retina; visual pathway begins with impulses that are triggered by chemical reactions in rods and cones that are transmitted to second cranial nerve (optic).
   5. There is 25% crossover of visual fields between right (o.d.) and left eye (o.s.).

D. Auditory sense is a localized special sense (Figure 3-10):
   1. Regions of ear include outer ear (auricle and external auditory meatus), ending at tympanic membrane; middle ear, containing auditory ossicles (malleus, incus, stapes); inner ear, containing vestibule, semicircular canals, cochlea.
   2. Receptors for hearing: located in organ of Corti in cochlea.
   3. Sound waves cause tympanic membrane vibrations, which are transmitted to inner ear by

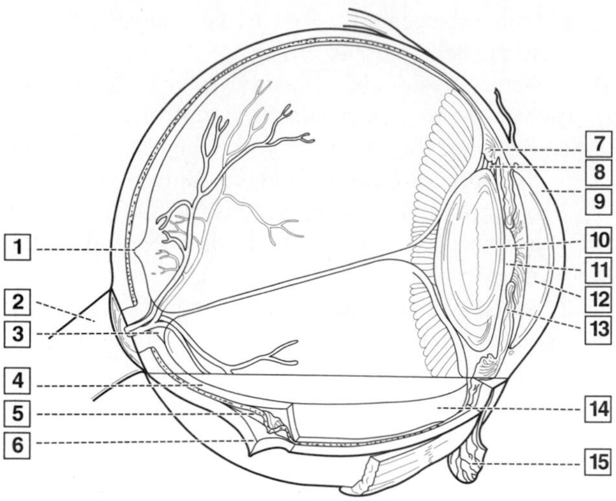

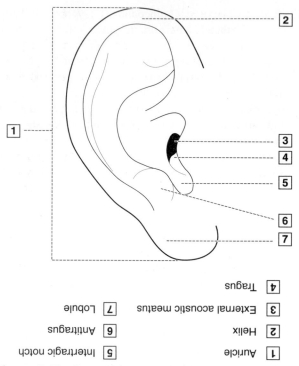

Figure 3-9, eye labels (shown inverted/rotated):

8 Suspensory ligament	
15 Conjunctiva	7 Ciliary body
14 Vitreous humor	6 Sclera
13 Iris	5 Choroid
12 Anterior cavity filled with aqueous humor	4 Retina
11 Pupil	3 Optic disk
10 Lens	2 Optic nerve
9 Cornea	1 Fovea centralis

Figure 3-9 Anatomy of the eye. (From Fehrenbach MJ, ed: Dental anatomy coloring book, St. Louis, 2008, Saunders/Elsevier.)

Figure 3-10, ear labels (shown inverted):

		4 Tragus
7 Lobule	3 External acoustic meatus	
6 Antitragus	2 Helix	
5 Intertragic notch	1 Auricle	

Figure 3-10 External ear. (From Fehrenbach MJ, ed: Dental anatomy coloring book, St. Louis, 2008, Saunders/Elsevier.)

ossicles; organ of Corti moves and hairs bend, triggering impulses transmitted by eighth cranial nerve (vestibulocochlear) to brain, where impulses are interpreted as sound.

E. Sense of equilibrium is a localized special sense:
  1. Receptors are located in vestibule and semicircular canals of inner ear.
  2. As fluids in inner ear move relative to gravity, hairs bend, triggering impulses transmitted to eighth cranial nerve (vestibulocochlear); brain interprets impulses in terms of acceleration and position.

CLINICAL STUDY

Age	68 YRS	SCENARIO
Sex	☐ Male ☒ Female	The dental hygienist calls to remind the patient that she is due for her 3-month recall appointment. The patient says that she has just been diagnosed with an eye disease that has permanently narrowed her field of vision. She does not like the drops prescribed and wonders why she should take them.
Height	5'5"	
Weight	145 LBS	
BP	118/74	
Chief Complaint	"How am I going to get to the appointment?"	
Medical History	Osteoarthritis in both hands and neck Removal of gallstones Basal cell carcinoma of the lip Past history of smoking	
Current Medications	Ibuprofen p.r.n.	
Social History	Retired grade school teacher	

1. What has happened to the patient's eyesight? What is the reason for it?
2. How does this affect her eyesight? To what drug is she referring, and should she take it?
3. What type of test did she have? How often should persons at risk have the test?
4. What factors would reduce the effectiveness of oral care in the dental office for this patient?

1. The patient probably has glaucoma, a group of eye diseases of second (II) cranial nerve (optic), which involves loss of retinal ganglion cells in characteristic pattern of optic neuropathy. Raised intraocular pressure (ocular hypertension) is significant risk factor, as well as female gender, age, family history, race (African-American or Asian), diabetes mellitus (DM). Unstable ocular blood flow could be involved in pathogenesis; may be related to hypertension (high blood pressure). This information should be added to patient's health history.
2. Involves loss of visual field that often occurs gradually and may not be recognized until advanced. Once lost, the visual field can never be recovered. Glaucoma is second leading cause of blindness in United States. If increased intraocular pressure (above 20 mm Hg) is present, can be lowered with drugs, usually eye drops, or surgery if severe. Major reason for vision loss is poor compliance with drugs and follow-up visits. One type of drop medication is pilocarpine, a nonselective muscarinic receptor agonist in the parasympathetic nervous system, which relieves the symptoms by decreasing intraocular pressure (also available in weekly time-released inserts). This drug is also given in intraoral form (Salagen) for non-drug-induced xerostomia. Any new medications should be added to patient's drug history.
3. The patient had a dilated eye examination to check nerve. Includes measurements of intraocular pressure via tonometry, changes in size or shape of eye, and retinal examination of nerve to look for visible damage; if damage is suspected, formal visual field test is performed. Those at risk are advised to have the test at least once a year.
4. For visually impaired, not being able to see objects in path or to view instructions or procedures being done.

Endocrine System

Endocrine system consists of endocrine glands (release product into bloodstream) and hormones produced (Figure 3-11). Acts with nervous system to regulate body activities to maintain homeostasis. Nervous system acts through electrical impulses and uses a **neurotransmitter,** and effects are MORE localized and of LESS duration; endocrine system acts through a chemical messenger

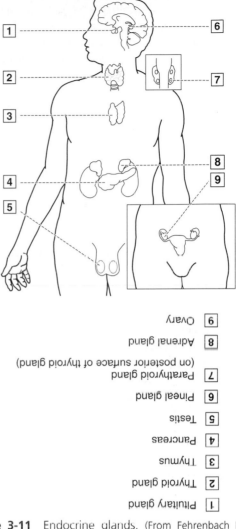

9	Ovary
8	Adrenal gland
7	Parathyroid gland (on posterior surface of thyroid gland)
6	Pineal gland
5	Testis
4	Pancreas
3	Thymus
2	Thyroid gland
1	Pituitary gland

Figure 3-11 Endocrine glands. (From Fehrenbach MJ, ed: Dental anatomy coloring book, St. Louis, 2008, Saunders/Elsevier.)

called a **hormone,** and effects are MORE generalized and of MORE duration.

Endocrine glands are ductless; secretions flow directly into blood, which carries the hormones to appropriate region (exocrine glands release product to the body surface). Exert effects on specific target organs by attaching to receptor sites, causing some type of reaction in organ.

A. Chemical classes of hormones:
1. Proteins and polypeptides: long chains of amino acids; class includes MOST of hormones NOT listed below.
2. Amines: derivatives of amino acids; class includes epinephrine, norepinephrine, thyroxine.
3. Steroids: derivatives of cholesterol, lipid; class includes sex hormones and adrenal cortex hormones.

B. Mechanism of hormone action: react with specific receptor sites on or in cells; cells with appropriate receptors make up the target tissues.
  1. Protein hormones react with receptors on the cell membrane; amines and steroids react with receptors in the cytoplasm or nucleus.
  2. MOST action is regulated by negative feedback, with some positive feedback; stimulus may be other hormones, substances in the blood, or direct neural stimulation.
C. Endocrine glands and related hormones:
  1. Anterior pituitary (adenohypophysis): growth hormone (GH), adrenocorticotropic hormone (ACTH), thyroid-stimulating hormone (TSH), follicle-stimulating hormone (FSH), luteinizing hormone (LH), prolactin.
  2. Intermediate pituitary (pars intermedius): melanocyte-stimulating hormone (MSH).
  3. Posterior pituitary (neurohypophysis): antidiuretic hormone (ADH) and oxytocin.
  4. Thyroid gland: thyroxine, triiodothyronine (iodinated amino acids), calcitonin; parathyroid gland: parathyroid (PTH) (see Chapter 4, Head, Neck, and Dental Anatomy).
  5. Adrenal (suprarenal) cortex: mineralocorticoids (aldosterone), glucocorticoids (cortisol), sex steroids; adrenal (suprarenal) medulla: epinephrine and norepinephrine.
  6. Pancreas (islets of Langerhans): insulin and glucagon.
  7. Testes: androgens (testosterone); ovaries: estrogen and progesterone.

Cardiovascular System

Cardiovascular system (CVS) includes blood, heart, and blood vessels.
- See Chapters 8, Microbiology and Immunology: immunology of the blood; 9, Pharmacology: drugs that affect CVS.
A. Blood (liquid connective tissue):
  1. Composition: MOSTLY plasma at ~55% of blood volume; formed elements compose ~45% of volume.
  2. Plasma: MAINLY water; also contains plasma proteins, nutrients, gases, electrolytes, nitrogenous waste compounds.
  3. Formed elements in blood:
    a. **Erythrocytes** (red blood cells [RBCs]): biconcave disks without nuclei that contain hemoglobin, transport oxygen (O_2) and carbon dioxide (CO_2).
    b. **Leukocytes** (white blood cells [WBCs]): have nuclei and do NOT have hemoglobin; five types include neutrophils (polymorphonuclear leukocytes [PMNs], MOST numerous), monocytes, lymphocytes, eosinophils, basophils;

provide defense against disease, mediate inflammatory reactions. See Table 3-1 for more information.
    (1) Lymphocytes: second MOST common leukocytes; three types: B cells, T cells, NK (natural killer) cells.
      (a) B cells: mature in bone marrow and gut-associated lymphoid tissue such as lymph nodes.
      (b) T cells: mature in thymus.
      (c) NK cells: mature in bone marrow, large cells involved in first line of defense against tumor cells or virally infected cells by killing them; thus are NOT considered part of immune response.
    (2) **Cytokines:** chemical mediators of immune response; produced by B and T cells.
    (3) B cells divide during immune response to form plasma cells:
      (a) **Plasma cell:** round cell with a single round nucleus (cartwheel appearance).
      (b) Once mature, plasma cells produce **antibody** (immunoglobulin [Ig]).
      (c) Five distinct classes of antibodies (Igs): IgA, IgE, IgD, IgG, IgM (Table 3-2).
      (d) Two types of IgA: serum and secretory.
      (e) Thrombocytes (platelets), small fragments of cells, aid in blood clotting.
  4. Blood types (ABO and Rh):
    a. ABO blood types are based on agglutinogens (antigens) and agglutinins (antibodies).
    b. In **transfusion reactions,** recipient's agglutinins react with donor's agglutinogens; type AB is *universal recipient;* type O is *universal donor*.
    c. Example: people with Rh+ blood have Rh agglutinogens; those with Rh− blood do NOT; neither type has anti-Rh agglutinins; exposure to Rh+ blood causes an Rh− individual to develop anti-Rh agglutinins, and subsequent exposures may result in transfusion reaction.
B. Heart: muscle that pumps the blood, with two thirds on the left of the sternum; enclosed in fibrous pericardial sac lined with serous membrane (Figure 3-12):
  1. Heart wall: outermost layer of epicardium; thickest middle layer of myocardium composed of cardiac muscle; innermost layer of endocardium.
  2. Four chambers: atria are thin-walled receiving chambers (superior); ventricles are thick-walled pumping chambers (inferior).
  3. Right atrium: receives O_2-poor blood from systemic circulation through inferior and superior venae cavae; left atrium receives O_2-rich blood from lungs through pulmonary veins; the ONLY veins that carry oxygenated blood.

Table 3-1 Blood cells and related tissue cells

Cells	Microscopic appearance	Description	Functions
Neutrophil or polymorphonuclear leukocyte (PMN)		Multilobulated nucleus with granules	Inflammatory response: phagocytosis
Lymphocyte		Round eccentric nucleus without granules, B, T, and NK types	B and T types of cells: immune response: humoral and cell-mediated; also NK cell: defense against tumor cells and virally infected cells
Plasma cell		Round nucleus derived from B-cell lymphocytes	Humoral immune response: produces immunoglobulins
Monocyte (blood) or macrophage (tissue)		Bean-shaped nucleus with poorly staining granules	Inflammatory and immune response: phagocytosis as well as process and present immunogens
Eosinophil		Double-lobed nucleus with red granules	Immune response
Basophil		Irregularly shaped double-lobulated nucleus with blue granules	Immune response
Mast cell (tissue eosinophil)		Irregularly shaped double-lobulated nucleus with red granules	Immune response

From Bath-Balogh M, Fehrenbach MJ: Illustrated dental embryology, histology, and anatomy, ed 2, St. Louis, 2006, Saunders/Elsevier.

4. Right ventricle: pumps blood *to* lungs through pulmonary trunk; left ventricle pumps blood *to* systemic circulation through aorta.
5. Four heart valves: maintain unidirectional flow of blood by opening and closing depending on the difference in pressure on each side.
   a. Atrioventricular valves: between atria and ventricles; tricuspid valve is on right and bicuspid (mitral) valve is on left.
   b. Semilunar valves: at exits from heart; pulmonary semilunar valve regulates flow from right ventricle into pulmonary trunk; aortic semilunar valve is between left ventricle and ascending aorta.

6. Purkinje fibers: in inner ventricular walls; conduct electrical impulse that enables heart to contract in coordinated fashion; work with sinoatrial node (SA node, has inherent rhythmicity) and atrioventricular node (AV node, bundle of His) to control heart rate.
C. Blood vessels:
   1. Arteries: carry blood away from heart; thicker muscular walls than veins:
      a. Radial artery, located on thumb side of wrist, palpated by two fingers of clinician to obtain radial pulse so as to measure heart rate in conscious adults; in unconscious adults, common

Table 3-2 Known immunoglobulins (antibodies)

Immunoglobulin	Description
IgA	Has two subgroups: serous in blood and secretory in saliva and other secretions; aids in defense against proliferation of microorganisms in body fluids
IgE	Involved in hypersensitivity reactions, since can bind to mast cells and basophils and bring about release of bioactive substances such as histamine
IgD	Functions in activation of B-cell lymphocytes.
IgG	Major antibody in blood serum; can pass placental barrier and forms first passive immunity for newborn
IgM	Involved in early immune responses owing to involvement with IgD in activation of B-cell lymphocytes

carotid artery in neck palpated on ONLY one side by emergency personnel.

   b. Arterioles: small arteries that branch off larger artery; connect with capillary beds.

   c. Capillary beds: form connection between arteries and veins; site for exchange of materials between blood and cells.

  2. Veins: carry blood toward heart; walls are thinner and have valves to prevent backflow of blood (EXCEPT for emissary veins of face):

   a. Veins are BEST point of access to bloodstream, permitting withdrawal of blood specimens (venipuncture) for testing purposes and intravenous (IV) delivery of fluid, electrolytes, nutrition, drugs by needle or catheter.

   b. Venules: smaller veins; drain the capillaries of a tissue area and then join larger veins.

   c. Venous sinuses: blood-filled spaces between two layers of tissue.

  3. Anastomosis: communication (joining) of one blood vessel with another by connecting channel.

  4. Plexus: network of blood vessels (usually veins).

  5. Pressure of circulating blood decreases as blood moves through arteries, arterioles, capillaries, venules, veins; blood pressure refers to arterial pressure in larger arteries.

D. Circulatory pathways (Figure 3-13):

  1. Pulmonary circulation: transports O_2-poor blood from right ventricle through pulmonary arteries to lungs, where blood picks up new O_2 supply; then pulmonary veins return O_2-rich blood to left atrium.

  2. Systemic circulation: carries O_2-rich blood from left ventricle through systemic arteries to capillaries in the tissues of the body for O_2 and CO_2 exchange; systemic veins transport O_2-poor blood containing CO_2 from capillaries to superior and inferior venae cavae and then into right atrium.

  3. Hepatic portal circulation: carries venous blood from digestive system to liver, filters through sinusoids, and then enters hepatic veins to inferior vena cava (IVC).

Lymphatic System

Lymphatic system is composed of lymph, lymphatic organs, lymphatic vessels. Functions to return excess interstitial fluid to the blood, absorb fats and fat-soluble vitamins from digestive system, provide defense against invading microorganisms and disease. Lymph is interstitial fluid that has entered lymph vessels.

- See Chapters 4, Head, Neck, and Dental Anatomy: nodes, tonsils; 6, General and Oral Pathology: lymphadenopathy.

A. Lymphatic organs include lymph nodes, tonsils, spleen, thymus (Figure 3-14):

  1. **Lymph nodes:** dense mass of lymphocytes separated by spaces called sinuses; filters and cleanses lymph before enters blood; periphery of node contains B cells, and germinal center contains T cells:

   a. Nodes cluster in three areas: inguinal nodes cluster in groin, axillary nodes in armpit, and cervical nodes in neck; NO nodes exist in CNS; must be enlarged (lymphadenopathy) to be palpated.

   b. **Tonsil:** aggregate of lymphatic tissue that provides protection against pathogens that enter through nose, mouth, and throat; pharyngeal (adenoids) are located in nasopharynx; palatine are located in oropharynx; lingual are located at posterior portion of tongue.

  2. **Spleen:** large masses of lymphocytes and macrophages supported by reticular fibrous framework; SIMILAR to lymph node but is larger and filters blood instead of lymph, also acts as reservoir for blood; contains red and white pulp.

  3. **Thymus:** processes and matures T-cell lymphocytes, involved in defense against pathogens; also produces hormone thymosin; involutes (shrinks) with aging.

B. Lymphatic vessels carry fluid from interstitial spaces and return it to subclavian veins, where it becomes part of blood plasma:

  1. Vessels have thin walls and valves; small lymphatic vessels merge to form larger ones until there

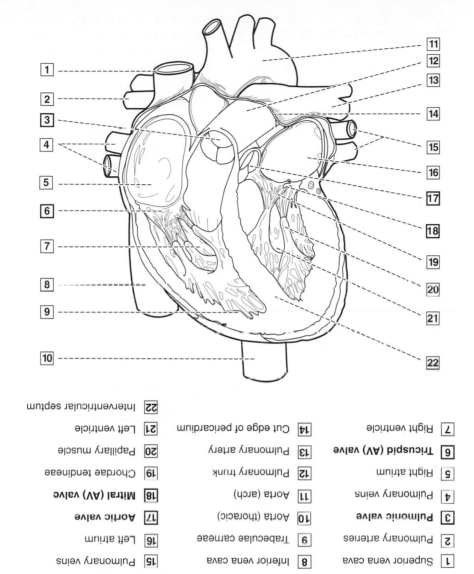

22	Interventricular septum				
21	Left ventricle	14	Cut edge of pericardium	7	Right ventricle
20	Papillary muscle	13	Pulmonary artery	6	**Tricuspid (AV) valve**
19	Chordae tendineae	12	Pulmonary trunk	5	Right atrium
18	**Mitral (AV) valve**	11	Aorta (arch)	4	Pulmonary veins
17	**Aortic valve**	10	Aorta (thoracic)	3	**Pulmonic valve**
16	Left atrium	9	Trabeculae carneae	2	Pulmonary arteries
15	Pulmonary veins	8	Inferior vena cava	1	Superior vena cava

Figure 3-12   Internal view of the heart. (From Fehrenbach MJ, ed: Dental anatomy coloring book, St. Louis, 2008, Saunders/Elsevier.)

are two MAIN ducts that empty into subclavian veins.

2. *Afferent* lymph flows into node; *efferent* lymph flows out (area of hilum).

3. Lymphatic ducts: larger lymphatic vessels; drain smaller vessels, then empty into venous system; right lymphatic duct drains upper right quadrant of body, and thoracic duct drains remainder of body.

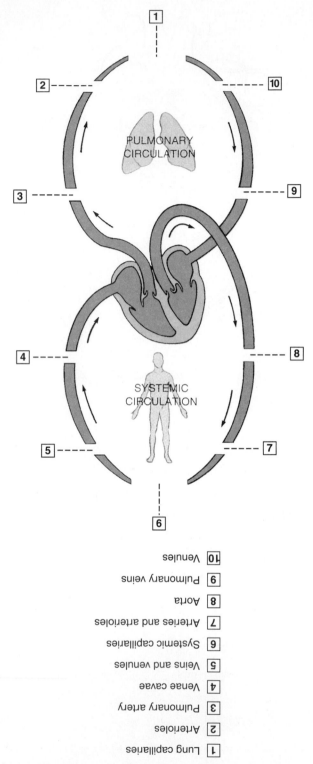

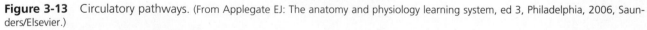

Figure 3-13 Circulatory pathways. (From Applegate EJ: The anatomy and physiology learning system, ed 3, Philadelphia, 2006, Saunders/Elsevier.)

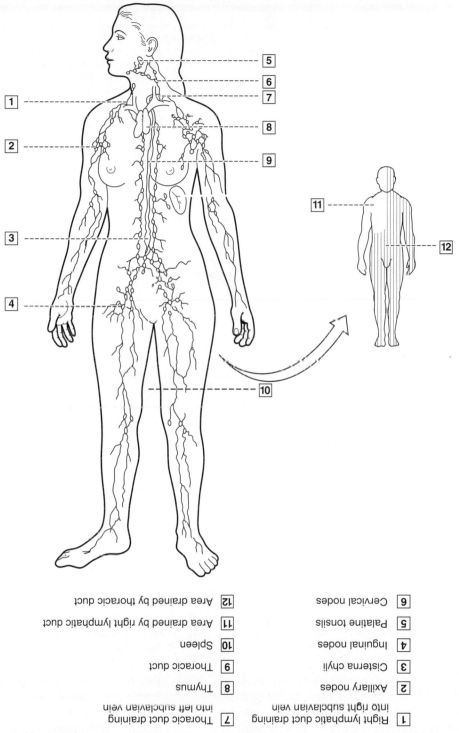

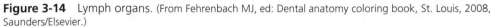

12	Area drained by thoracic duct	6	Cervical nodes
11	Area drained by right lymphatic duct	5	Palatine tonsils
10	Spleen	4	Inguinal nodes
9	Thoracic duct	3	Cisterna chyli
8	Thymus	2	Axillary nodes
7	Thoracic duct draining into left subclavian vein	1	Right lymphatic duct draining into right subclavian vein

Figure 3-14   Lymph organs. (From Fehrenbach MJ, ed: Dental anatomy coloring book, St. Louis, 2008, Saunders/Elsevier.)

CLINICAL STUDY ▬▬▬▬▬▬▬▬▬▬▬▬▬▬▬▬▬▬

		SCENARIO
Age	23 YRS	During an extraoral examination, a hard fixed mass, approximately 6 mm wide by 36 mm long by 6 mm deep, is noted on the right side of the neck; enlargement is clearly visible but no discomfort is noted when it is palpated. Other enlarged areas have been detected by the patient in his armpit and groin areas on same side. He states that he feels fine, although he tires easily. Intraoral exam shows poor oral hygiene and moderate gingivitis but no evidence of caries, only decalcification.
Sex	☒ Male ☐ Female	
Height	6′2″	
Weight	185 LBS	
BP	112/69	
Chief Complaint	"There is a swelling on my neck that has been there for 6 months and is getting larger."	
Medical History	Broken kneecap at age 8	
Current Medications	None	
Social History	Real estate lawyer Drinks diet colas to keep awake	

1. What could the enlargement along the right side of the patient's neck possibly be?
2. What would cause such a severe enlargement on his neck?
3. Identify the treatment planning procedures that should be completed.

1. Enlargement along right side of neck is most likely either a tumor or an enlarged cervical lymph node (lymphadenopathy) along sternocleidomastoid (SCM) muscle of right side.
2. If involving the lymph nodes, such severe enlargement is indicative of severe infection (local or systemic) or malignancy (cancer). Severe infection should be painful; lack of pain is prognostically threatening and points to its being an early malignancy.
3. Treatment planning procedures should include thorough intraoral examination for possible causes of swelling (e.g., pulpal infection, periodontal infection) and panoramic radiograph (shows entire jaw areas). If no evidence suggests dental causative factors, oral prophylaxis should be rescheduled until patient has seen his physician. Imperative that he seek immediate medical consult. (Later, Hodgkin's lymphoma, a cancer of lymph nodes, was diagnosed in this patient.)

Respiratory System

Respiratory system includes the upper and lower respiratory tracts and the lungs (Figure 3-15). It functions to move gases to and from exchange surfaces, where diffusion can occur. Defends body against pathogens, permits speech, helps regulate acid-base balance in body.

A. Upper respiratory tract:
   1. Nose (nasal cavity): warms, moistens, and filters air; opens to outside through external nares and in to pharynx through internal nares; separated from oral cavity by palate.
   2. **Pharynx** (throat): passageway for air; divided into nasopharynx, oropharynx, laryngopharynx; opening from oral cavity into oropharynx is the fauces.
   3. Larynx (voice box): formed by nine cartilages that are connected by muscles and ligaments:
      a. Three largest cartilages are thyroid, cricoid, epiglottis.
      b. Vocal folds (cords): present in central region; air passing through vibrates vocal folds to produce sound. Hoarseness indicates inflammation or possibly cancer if chronic.
B. Lower respiratory tract:
   1. Trachea (windpipe): framework supported by cartilage; divides into right and left primary bronchi.
   2. Bronchial tree:
      a. Bronchi enter lungs and subdivide; branching pattern continues into smaller passages until terminates in alveoli with alveolar sac; permits rapid diffusion of oxygen and CO_2.
   3. Lungs: formed by bronchial tree and alveoli.
      a. Right lung: three lobes; shorter, broader, and has greater volume than left lung.
      b. Left lung: two lobes and indentation (cardiac notch) to accommodate apex of heart.
      c. Air flows *into* and *out of* lungs through conducting passages because of pressure differences between atmosphere and gases inside alveoli. This gas exchange is passed onto the rich vascular network within the lung interstitium.

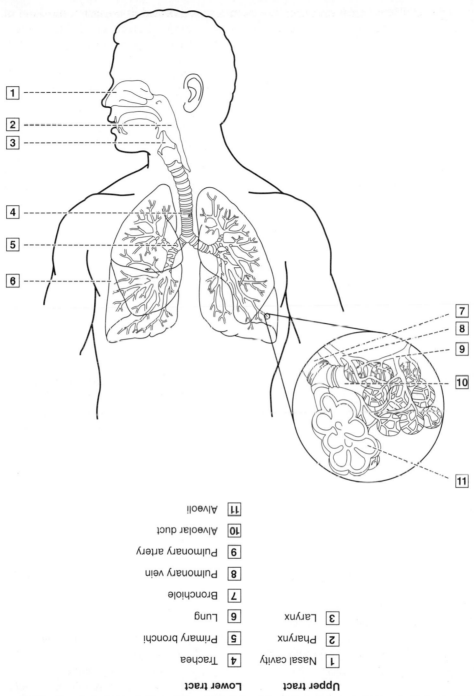

Figure 3-15 Respiratory tract. (From Fehrenbach MJ, ed: Dental anatomy coloring book, St. Louis, 2008, Saunders/Elsevier.)

Upper tract		Lower tract	
1 Nasal cavity		**4** Trachea	
2 Pharynx		**5** Primary bronchi	
3 Larynx		**6** Lung	
		7 Bronchiole	
		8 Pulmonary vein	
		9 Pulmonary artery	
		10 Alveolar duct	
		11 Alveoli	

Digestive System

Digestive system includes gastrointestinal (alimentary) tract (GIT; includes oral cavity, pharynx, esophagus, stomach, small intestine, large intestine, rectum, anus) and accessory organs (liver, gallbladder, pancreas) (Figure 3-16). Embryologically and physiologically, the mouth is the beginning of GIT. Functions include ingestion, mechanical digestion, chemical digestion, secretion, mixing and propelling movements, absorption, elimination of waste products, immunological functions (e.g., secretory IgA).

- See Chapter 4, Head, Neck, and Dental Anatomy: oral cavity structure.
- A. Pharynx (throat): muscles in wall contract during deglutition (swallowing) to propel food along passageway into esophagus, then into stomach.
- B. **Esophagus:** carries liquids and solids *from* pharynx *to* stomach:

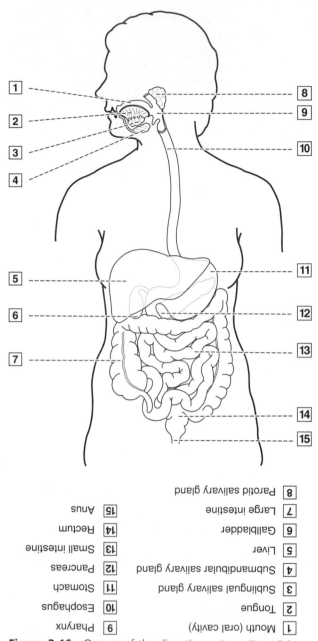

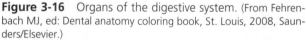

8	Parotid salivary gland
15	Anus
14	Rectum
13	Small intestine
12	Pancreas
11	Stomach
10	Esophagus
9	Pharynx

7	Large intestine
6	Gallbladder
5	Liver
4	Submandibular salivary gland
3	Sublingual salivary gland
2	Tongue
1	Mouth (oral cavity)

Figure 3-16 Organs of the digestive system. (From Fehrenbach MJ, ed: Dental anatomy coloring book, St. Louis, 2008, Saunders/Elsevier.)

1. Located posterior to trachea and anterior to vertebral column; passes through diaphragm, enters cardiac region of stomach.
2. Lower esophageal (cardiac) sphincter: controls passage of food from esophagus into stomach.

C. **Stomach:** involved in temporary storage of ingested food, maceration and mixing of ingested materials, secretion of enzymes that begin breaking chemical bonds (digestion), production of intrinsic factor, absorption of fluoride (IMPORTANT with toxicity):

1. Located in upper left quadrant of abdomen, anterior to spleen; divided into fundus, cardiac region, body, pyloric region.
2. Mucosal lining has folds (wrinkles) called rugae, which increase surface area for absorption, and glandular cells; parietal cells secrete hormone gastrin that stimulates gastric acid production (hydrochloric acid) and intrinsic factor (necessary for the absorption of vitamin B_{12}); also causes chief cells to secrete pepsinogen, which then is converted to pepsin by acids.
3. Chyme: semifluid mixture of ingested food, liquids, and gastric juice that passes through pyloric sphincter into small intestine; pH of contents as low as 2.

D. **Small intestine:** extends from pyloric sphincter to ileocecal valve; materials require ~5 hours to pass through and into the large intestine; divided into duodenum (MOST enzymes), jejunum, ileum:

1. Glandular cells in mucosa produce peptidase, which acts on proteins; maltase, sucrose, and lactase, which act on disaccharides; lipase, which acts on neutral fats.
2. Produces two hormones, secretin and cholecystokinin; secretin stimulates pancreas to produce fluid rich in bicarbonates; cholecystokinin stimulates gallbladder to secrete bile and stimulates pancreas to secrete digestive enzymes.

E. **Large intestine:** divided into cecum, colon, rectum, anal canal; MAIN functions are to absorb water, electrolytes, and vitamins; compact feces; and store fecal material before defecation:

1. Cecum: short region inferior to ileocecal valve; vermiform appendix is attached to cecum.
2. Rectum and anal canal: terminal portions of digestive system.

F. Accessory organs:

1. **Pancreas:** extends from duodenum to spleen:
   a. Composed MAINLY of exocrine cells, which produce enzymes amylase, trypsin, peptidase, lipase; pancreatic enzymes are carried to duodenum by pancreatic duct (of Wirsung).
   b. Endocrine cells (islets of Langerhans) produce insulin and glucagon.

2. **Liver:** largest visceral organ; located in upper right quadrant of abdomen:
   a. Lobule consists of hepatocytes arranged like spokes of a wheel around central vein and separated by sinusoids.
   b. Blood is brought to liver by portal vein and hepatic artery, flows through sinusoids into central vein and then into hepatic veins.
   c. Functions include production of bile (yellow color from bilirubin, breakdown of hemoglobin), production of plasma proteins, detoxification of harmful substances, filtering of blood, nutrient metabolism, immunological response via Kupffer cells.

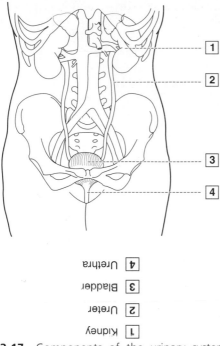

1. Kidney
2. Ureter
3. Bladder
4. Urethra

Figure 3-17 Components of the urinary system. (From Fehrenbach MJ, ed: Dental anatomy coloring book, St. Louis, 2008, Saunders/Elsevier.)

3. **Gallbladder:** attached to visceral surface of liver by cystic duct; joins hepatic duct to form common bile duct; empties into duodenum; functions to store, concentrate, secrete bile produced by liver. Contracts in response to cholecystokinin, hormone secreted by duodenum.

Urinary System

Urinary system consists of kidneys, ureters, urinary bladder, urethra (Figure 3-17). Functions to rid wastes, regulate fluid volume, maintain electrolyte concentrations, control blood pH, secrete renin and erythropoietin responsible for long-term maintenance of blood pressure.

A. **Kidney:** one of a pair that are located behind peritoneum (retroperitoneal) between twelfth thoracic and third lumbar vertebrae:
   1. Enclosed by capsule; blood vessels enter at ureter and leave at hilum.
   2. Peripheral region is cortex; inner region is medulla; left kidney higher than right one.
   3. **Nephron:** functional unit of kidney; consists of corpuscle and tubule.
      a. Corpuscle in cortex includes glomerulus and Bowman's capsule; blood filtration occurs in glomerulus and filtrate passes into capsule (Figure 3-18).
      b. Reabsorption of water and electrolytes to adjust volume and content of urine occurs in tubule;

straight portions in medulla, convoluted portions in cortex.
      c. Juxtaglomerular apparatus associated with nephron secretes renin, which becomes angiotensin and increases blood pressure.
      d. Kidneys excrete fluoride.
B. Ureters: enter urinary bladder; urine is formed in kidney, leaves kidney through ureters, is transported to urinary bladder; bladder is posterior to symphysis pubis in pelvic cavity and stores urine until micturition.
C. Urethra: transports urine from urinary bladder to exterior.
D. Urine: fluid produced by nephrons of kidney, usually 1 to 2 L per 24 hours.
E. Blockages (renal calculi, kidney stones) along any of these structures result in increased pressure, may damage kidneys.

Reproductive System

Reproductive system consists of the gonads (testes), ducts, accessory glands, penis in the male and gonads (ovaries), uterine tubes, uterus, vagina, external genitalia, mammary glands in the female.

A. Female (Figure 3-19):
   1. Ovaries: located in pelvic cavity on each side of uterus; ovum production occurs monthly in ovarian follicles as part of ovarian cycle; follicle cells produce estrogen.
   2. Uterine tubes (fallopian tubes, oviducts): extend laterally from uterus; site for fertilization.
   3. Uterus: consists of a fundus, body, and cervix; superficial layer is sloughed off during menstruation.
   4. Vagina: muscular tube that extends from cervix to exterior.
   5. Mammary glands located in breast; consist of lobules of glandular units that produce milk; estrogen and progesterone stimulate breast development; prolactin stimulates milk production; oxytocin causes ejection (let-down) of milk.
B. Male (Figure 3-20):
   1. Testes: begin development in abdominal cavity and then descend into scrotum shortly before birth; physically outside of the body because body temperature impairs sperm production.
   2. Testes: composed of seminiferous tubules, which produce sperm, and interstitial cells, which produce testosterone.

BIOCHEMISTRY

Biochemistry is the study of living matter or organisms at a molecular level. Requires understanding of how molecules are structured, bonding to form MORE complex structures and thus affect living matter. Hydrocarbons

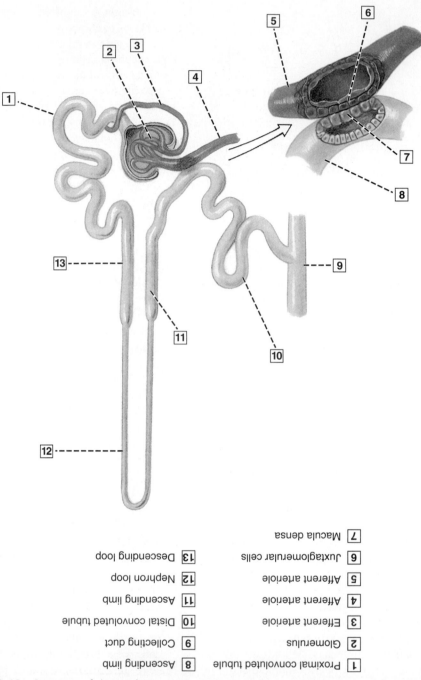

Figure 3-18   Structure of the nephron. (From Applegate EJ: The anatomy and physiology learning system, ed 3, Philadelphia, 2006, Saunders/Elsevier).

1	Proximal convoluted tubule	8	Ascending limb
2	Glomerulus	9	Collecting duct
3	Efferent arteriole	10	Distal convoluted tubule
4	Afferent arteriole	11	Ascending limb
5	Afferent arteriole	12	Nephron loop
6	Juxtaglomerular cells	13	Descending loop
7	Macula densa		

are carbon- and hydrogen-based molecules that exist in several different forms and have various properties. Found within several products used daily (including in the dental office) and also form major components of the body.

- See CD-ROM for Chapter Terms and WebLinks.

A. Parent hydrocarbons have chemical characteristics that can be greatly influenced by replacement of hydrogen atoms with one or MORE functional groups:

1. Alcohols: components of several natural products, including menthol (throat lozenges).

2. Ethers: used as general anesthetics.

3. Aldehydes: variety of uses, e.g., formaldehyde used for preservation of biological samples.

4. Ketones: include progesterone and testosterone (sex hormones); produced in uncontrolled DM.

5. Carboxyl groups (salicylic acid, constituent of aspirin).

6. Organohalogens: several uses; found in insecticides and BEST for treatment of brain cancer.

7. Amines: treatment of several ailments, including migraine headaches, hypertension, inflammation.

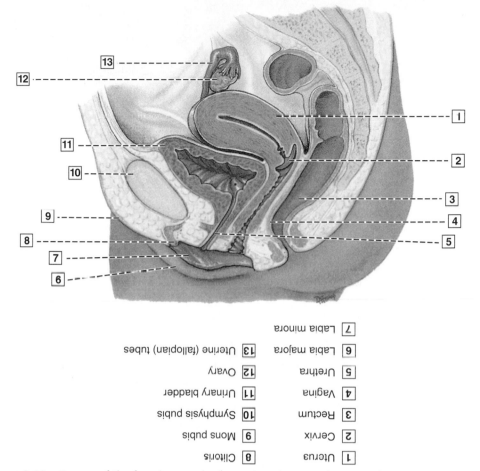

Figure 3-19 Organs of the female reproductive system. (From Applegate EJ: The anatomy and physiology learning system, ed 3, Philadelphia, 2006, Saunders/Elsevier).

1 Uterus	8 Clitoris
2 Cervix	9 Mons pubis
3 Rectum	10 Symphysis pubis
4 Vagina	11 Urinary bladder
5 Urethra	12 Ovary
6 Labia majora	13 Uterine (fallopian) tubes
7 Labia minora	

8. Esters: used MAINLY topically; NO longer used as injected local anesthetics; frequent allergies to ester agents (e.g., PABA) have stopped use as injectables.
9. Amides: used MAINLY as injected local anesthetic agents or topically (but at lower levels than topical esters); LESS allergenic than esters.

B. Saturated hydrocarbons:
1. Molecules that contain hydrogen atoms and carbon atoms connected by single bonds.
2. Can be straight chain, branched, or cyclic; straight chain hydrocarbons have higher boiling points than branched hydrocarbons because MORE surface contact is allowed between straight chain hydrocarbons.

C. Unsaturated hydrocarbons: carbon- and hydrogen-based molecules that contain at least one double or triple bond between carbon atoms (e.g., vitamin A).

Biomolecules

Biomolecules are found in living organisms and are classified as belonging to one of four major groups: carbohydrates, lipids, proteins, nucleic acids.

• See Chapter 7, Nutrition: biomolecules.

A. **Carbohydrates:** transport, energy, and structure of the cell:
1. Monosaccharides: basic units of complex carbohydrates (e.g., glucose, provides energy to brain).
2. Disaccharides: two monosaccharides (e.g., lactose, milk sugar).
3. Oligosaccharides: consists of 2 to 10 monosaccharides (e.g., sucrose-6 monosaccharides); GREATEST effect on caries process.
4. Polysaccharides: many monosaccharides (e.g., starch); LEAST effect on caries process.

B. **Lipid** (fat): energy and structure of the cell:
1. Fatty acids: carboxylic acids with hydrocarbon side chains; exist as major component of other naturally existing lipids.
2. Triacylglycerols: three fatty acids that are esterified to a glycerol molecule; exist as a form of energy storage.
3. Structural lipids: found in biological membranes and also work in transport of other lipids in the circulatory system.

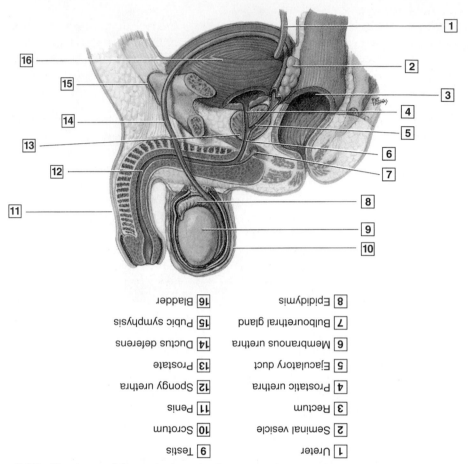

16 Bladder	8 Epididymis
15 Pubic symphysis	7 Bulbourethral gland
14 Ductus deferens	6 Membranous urethra
13 Prostate	5 Ejaculatory duct
12 Spongy urethra	4 Prostatic urethra
11 Penis	3 Rectum
10 Scrotum	2 Seminal vesicle
9 Testis	1 Ureter

Figure 3-20 Structures of the male reproductive system. (From Applegate EJ: The anatomy and physiology learning system, ed 3, Philadelphia, 2006, Saunders/Elsevier).

4. Steroids, prostaglandins, leukotrienes: involved in regulation of body functions.

5. High-density lipoproteins (HDL): carry fatty acids and cholesterol from tissues to the liver ("good" cholesterol).

6. Low-density lipoprotein (LDL): transports cholesterol and triglycerides from liver to tissues and regulates cholesterol synthesis at sites ("bad" cholesterol).

C. Amino acids, peptides, and proteins: components in the development of molecules used by the body for forming cell structure, catalyzing reactions, and transmitting signals.

1. **Amino acids:** building blocks (chemical structures) of peptides and proteins; thus proteins are degraded into amino acids when denatured.

2. Peptides: molecules that consist of more than one amino acid linked by peptide bond.

3. **Proteins:** functional molecules that consist of one or more peptide molecules present in the cells of all living organisms; important components in chemical and physical cell functioning.

4. **Nucleic acids:** encode genetic information and are the molecular basis of heredity; made up of nucleotides, which consist of nitrogenous base, sugar, phosphate; allow cellular reproduction:

a. Adenosine monophosphate (AMP).

b. Guanosine monophosphate (GMP).

c. Cytosine monophosphate (CMP).

d. Thymidine monophosphate (TMP); found ONLY in **deoxyribonucleic acid** (DNA).

e. Uridine monophosphate (UMP); found ONLY in **ribonucleic acid** (RNA).

5. Include RNA and DNA; located in nucleus (DNA and RNA) and in cytoplasm (RNA):

a. Structure and replication of DNA is a double helix with two strands of DNA that run complementary (antiparallel) to each other:

(1) The two strands are held together by formation of hydrogen bonds between nucleotide on one strand of DNA and nucleotide on other strand of DNA.

(2) Deoxy AMP forms base pair by forming two hydrogen bonds with deoxy TMP.

(3) Deoxy GMP forms base pair by forming three hydrogen bonds with deoxy CMP.

(4) Semiconservative replication:

(a) During replication, two complementary strands of DNA are separated.

(b) Separation allows protein DNA polymerase to synthesize new strand of DNA complementary to each original strand of DNA.

(c) Replication of one double-stranded DNA molecule results in two double-stranded molecules of DNA, identical to original molecule of DNA.

(d) Process of DNA replication is necessary for cell division; when cell divides into two, each daughter cell receives one of DNA molecules.

b. Structure and function of RNA:

(1) RNA is similar to DNA in structure EXCEPT that:

(a) RNA contains ribose sugar instead of deoxyribose sugar.

(b) RNA contains UMP instead of TMP.

(c) RNA is a single-stranded rather than a double-stranded molecule.

(2) Overall function of mRNA, tRNA, rRNA is the synthesis of proteins.

c. **Transcription:** transfer of genetic information from DNA to messenger RNA (mRNA) transcript; genetic information from an mRNA transcript is used as a guide for protein synthesis.

d. **Translation:** transferring genetic information from mRNA to synthesis of proteins.

e. **Mutagenesis:** alteration in the DNA that changes the encoded genetic information; chemicals, viruses, radiation are three classes of agents that cause mutation.

f. Gene expression: regulated by a number of proteins called transcription factors, regulated by other internal and external stimuli.

g. Genetic engineering: using specific techniques for manipulating genetic information; e.g., gene for human insulin can be placed in bacteria, allowing expression of large quantity of human insulin (protein can then be purified from bacteria and used for diabetic therapy).

h. Gene therapy: type of genetic engineering; involves compensating for damaged gene responsible for causing illness by expressing foreign gene in affected cells.

Metabolism

Metabolism is the process of producing and using energy and includes BOTH catabolism and anabolism.

A. Catabolism:

1. Process of breaking down large complex molecules into *simpler* molecules.

2. Produces energy for physical activity; helps maintain body temperature and elimination of body waste.

B. Anabolism:

1. Process of building larger, more *complex* molecules from smaller, simpler units.

2. Important in new cell development and in older cell maintenance.

C. Enzymes (most): functional proteins involved in catalyzing specific reactions.

D. Adenosine triphosphate (ATP): main form of energy storage:

1. Energy released from exothermic reactions can be stored in the form of ATP by addition of inorganic phosphate (P_i) to molecule of ADP.

2. Energy stored in the form of ATP can be donated to an endothermic reaction by hydrolysis of the inorganic phosphate (P_i) from the ATP molecule, resulting in a molecule of ADP.

3. Glycolysis: pathway for catabolism of the simple sugar glucose.

4. Pyruvate dehydrogenase: enzyme that catalyzes conversion of molecule of pyruvate into acetyl CoA, which can be used in the tricarboxylic acid cycle (TCA cycle) for further production of energy.

5. Tricarboxylic acid cycle: pathway for further catabolism of glucose to produce energy.

6. Electron transport and oxidative phosphorylation: pathway by which electrons proceed down the electron transport chain and result in the reduction of O_2 to H_2O and eventually the production of ATP.

7. Overall goal of these metabolic pathways: use food taken into the body for production of ATP, enabling body to store energy for later use.

PHYSIOLOGY

Physiology is the study of function of organ systems. Lends meaning to anatomical structure; conversely, anatomy is what makes physiology possible. **Homeostasis** refers to the relative constancy or equilibrium of the internal environment. Maintained by negative feedback mechanisms, under regulation from nervous and endocrine systems. When lacking, results in illness or disease.

• See CD-ROM for Chapter Terms and WebLinks.

Cell Physiology

Cell physiology is study of general and specific functions of cells and requires understanding of cell structure and environment.

• See Chapter 2, Embryology and Histology: cell structure.

A. Physiological functions of cell:
   1. Response to environment:
      a. Production of substances (e.g., mucus in response to tobacco smoke).
      b. Movement (e.g., of cell part, such as cilia, or entire cell, such as lymphocyte).
      c. Ingestion of substances (e.g., nutrients or bacteria).
      d. Generation of electrical impulses (e.g., action potential).
   2. Synthesis of proteins for structural and functional requirements.
   3. Use of membrane transport for:
      a. Separation of internal and external cell environments.
      b. Communication between cells.
      c. Intracellular communication.
      d. Fluid volume regulation.
   4. Duplication for:
      a. Growth (mitosis).
      b. Reproduction (meiosis).
   5. Differentiation and specialization as:
      a. Muscle cells (skeletal, smooth, and cardiac).
      b. Nervous cells (neurons).
      c. Epithelial cells (lining of organs and tissues).
      d. Connective tissue cells (fibroblasts, WBCs).
B. Specific cell functions:
   1. Transport of substances across the plasma membrane:
      a. Permeability: ability of substance to move across membrane.
         (1) Completely permeable: anything can cross.
         (2) Impermeable: nothing can cross.
         (3) Semipermeable: ONLY some substances can cross.
   2. Diffusion mechanism of transport:
      a. Random movement of molecules from a higher to a lower concentration gradient; once concentrations differences are eliminated, NO net movement occurs.
      b. Following factors affect the diffusion rate:
         (1) Higher the temperature, greater the diffusion.
         (2) Smaller the molecule, faster it diffuses.
         (3) Shorter the distance across the membrane, faster the rate of diffusion.
         (4) Greater the available surface area for diffusion, higher the rate of diffusion.
         (5) MORE lipid soluble the substance, MORE readily it moves across the membrane.
      c. Movement of ions depends on their charge (different charges attract, similar ones repel) and their concentration gradients.
      d. **Osmosis:** net movement of water down its concentration gradient.
         (1) Amount of water that moves depends on concentration of water relative to solute and relative permeability of membrane to solute.
         (2) Isotonic solution has same osmotic characteristics on both sides of the membrane; no net movement of water occurs.
         (3) Hypotonic solution contains MORE water outside the cell than inside the cell; water moves into the cell and exerts a pressure; with increased volume, cell may burst.
         (4) Hypertonic solution contains LESS water outside than inside cell; movement of water out of cell makes it shrink (crenation).
   3. Carrier-mediated transport:
      a. Uses molecules to move substances across plasma membrane.
      b. Exhibits selectivity for a substance, saturation, or a transport maximum (limit to how much can be moved); competition for transporting substances that are closely related chemically.
      c. Types of carrier-mediated transport:
         (1) Facilitated diffusion for molecules, like glucose, moves down a concentration gradient; uses no energy.
         (2) Primary active transport: moves substances against their concentration gradients; uses energy in the form of ATP (e.g., Na^+, K^+ transmembrane ATPase pumps).
         (3) Secondary active transport (more than one molecule is moved); uses energy:
            (a) Moves molecules against their concentration gradients.
            (b) Creates gradient to move second substance with the energy used to move one ion (e.g., coupled transport of sodium with amino acids in the intestine).
C. Cell communication:
   1. Examples of communication *between* cells:
      a. Hormones: made by one cell type are transported in blood and affect cells at distant site.
      b. Neurotransmitters: chemicals produced by one neuron that affect neurons or muscle cells.
      c. Paracrine secretion: involves one cell secreting a chemical (e.g., neurotransmitter, cytokine, gas such as nitrous oxide) that affects nearby cell.
      d. Tight (nexus) junctions: specialized connections between cells that restrict movement of substances between cells.
   2. Examples of communication from the *outside* of a cell to *its interior*:
      a. Channels: allow fluxes of ions (e.g., Na^+, Cl^-, K^+) or water into or out of a cell.
      b. Receptors:
         (1) Bind chemicals from outside of the cell that couple to membrane-bound enzymes

(e.g., adenosine cyclase), affect intracellular second messenger systems (e.g., elevate calcium levels).

    (2) Large intracellular response occurs (amplification) when ONLY a small number of membrane receptors are activated.

D. Membrane potential:

  1. Occurs when there is a difference in the numbers and charges of ions across plasma membrane.

  2. Does NOT exist when the number and charge characteristics of ions are the same on either side of the membrane.

  3. Increases as both the concentration gradient and difference in charge across the membrane increase.

  4. Affected by the permeability of a membrane for an ion:

    a. Membranes are "leaky" for K^+ but "tight" for Na^+.

    b. Proteins have a negative charge and are trapped *within* the cell; K^+ that leaves the cell because of "leakiness" results in a relative negative charge inside the cell compared with *outside* the cell.

Neurophysiology

Neurophysiology is the study of the nervous system; includes central (CNS) and peripheral nervous systems (PNS). Systems are responsible for sensing and responding to both external and internal stimuli. For more on organization of nervous system, see earlier discussion.

• See Chapters 14, Pain Management: nerve anatomy and physiology; 9, Pharmacology: products involved in nervous systems; 16, Special Needs Patient Care: neural disease.

Skeletal Muscle Physiology

Skeletal muscles are relatively large cells and are involved in locomotion, work, heat production. See earlier discussion on muscular system.

• See Chapter 16, Special Needs Patient Care: muscle diseases.

A. Basic structural components of skeletal muscle (Figure 3-21):

  1. Connective tissue surrounds muscles, fascicles (functional unit of the muscle), and fibers:

    a. Muscles are surrounded by epimysium.

    b. Each muscle consists of fascicles surrounded by perimysium.

    c. Muscle fibers are surrounded by endomysium.

  2. Individual muscle cells or fibers are surrounded by sarcolemma, which invaginates into cell, forming "T" tubules:

    a. Muscle cells are large, multinucleated.

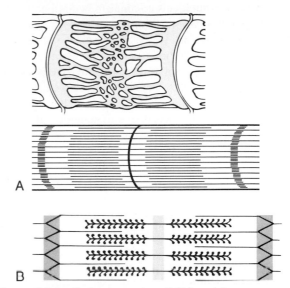

Figure 3-21 Skeletal muscle cell **(A)** and its components and the sarcomere **(B)**, the contractile unit.

    b. Endoplasmic reticulum (ER), involved in energy generation, is well developed; actin and myosin filaments make up myofibrils.

  3. Contractile unit of the muscle is the sarcomere:

    a. "A" band: myosin (thick filaments composed of heads and tails) and actin (thin filaments); "M" line: ONLY myosin.

    b. Actin filaments: surrounded by tropomyosin, to which troponins are attached; these molecules interact with calcium ions and allow actin to bind to myosin heads; also allow filaments to slide (causing contraction of the muscle).

    c. The "I" band: contains actin filaments and other proteins linked to "Z" line; the "H" zone contains ONLY myosin filaments.

B. Skeletal muscle function:

  1. Neuromuscular junction and excitation-contraction coupling:

    a. Motoneurons release acetylcholine, which binds to receptors on muscle endplate.

    b. Receptors form channels that respond to binding of acetylcholine by allowing influx of cations into muscle cell, resulting in action potential that travels along and into muscle fiber by means of the "T" tubules.

    c. Action potential causes release of calcium from sarcoplasmic reticulum (SR); calcium binds to troponin and results in a conformational change of tropomyosin, allowing actin to bind to myosin heads activated with ATP.

    d. Interaction of actin and myosin results in SR shorting (contraction); actin and myosin filaments require ATP to separate.

e. If calcium levels continue to be high within the cell, *contraction* continues; if NOT, *relaxation* occurs because of calcium reuptake in SR.

2. Factors involved in muscle contraction:
   a. Active tension develops from interaction of actin and myosin against connective tissue outside and proteins within muscle fibers.
   b. Motor unit consists of a motoneuron and all of the muscle fibers it innervates.
   c. Types of fatigue:
      (1) Muscle fatigue:
         (a) Inability of a muscle to continue to work at a given level.
         (b) May be caused by increases of waste products (lactic acid), lower energy stores (phosphates), muscle disease (muscular dystrophy).
      (2) Neuromuscular junction fatigue: inability to manufacture enough acetylcholine presynaptically.
      (3) Central fatigue: inability of the CNS to drive muscles; may occur in response to muscle fatigue.
      (4) General fatigue at end of day (or at the end of this chapter!): may be due to iron deficiency (hypochromic anemia).
      (5) Chronic fatigue syndrome (CFS): unknown etiology; associated with fibromyalgia (widespread pain of unknown origin).

Endocrinology

Endocrinology is the study of endocrine glands, the hormones secreted, and effects on body. See earlier discussion of endocrine system.

- See Chapters 6, General and Oral Pathology: hormonal pathology; 9, Pharmacology: hormones.

A. Endocrine system: slower control system compared with CNS; allows for ability to "fine tune":
   1. Produces some hormones in periphery and some in CNS, but functions differ in each location.
   2. Produces hormones in rhythmic manner (e.g., circadian, monthly).

B. Chemical categories of hormones:
   1. Peptide and protein:
      a. Hydrophilic (water-soluble); transported as free hormones.
      b. Produced in hypothalamus, pineal, pancreas, parathyroid, gastrointestinal tract, kidneys, liver, thyroid, heart, and other organs.
   2. Amines (tyrosine derivatives):
      a. Catecholamines (hydrophilic), produced in adrenal medulla.
      b. Thyroid hormones (iodinated tyrosine derivatives), lipophilic (lipid soluble), act at genomic level to produce new proteins.

c. Bind to plasma proteins.
   3. Steroid (cholesterol derivatives):
      a. Lipophilic and easily enter cells; bind to both membrane and intracellular receptors.
      b. Can activate genes to initiate protein synthesis and may activate second messengers.
      c. Produced in adrenal cortex, gonads (testes and ovaries), placenta.

C. Hormones produced by CNS:
   1. Pineal produces **melatonin:**
      a. Induces sleep; involved in modulation of body rhythms.
      b. Affects reproduction: increased levels lead to decreased reproduction.
      c. Acts as antioxidant; enhances immune system.
   2. Hypothalamus stimulates release:
      a. Thyrotropin-releasing (TRH): **thyroid-stimulating hormone** (TSH) from anterior pituitary, regulates production of thyroid hormones.
      b. Corticotropin-releasing (CRH): **adrenocorticotropin** (ACTH), acts on adrenal cortex to increase cortisol in response to stress.
      c. Gonadotropin-releasing (GnRH): follicle-stimulating (FSH) and luteinizing (LH) from anterior pituitary.
         (1) FSH in females: growth of ovarian follicles, production of estrogen.
         (2) FSH in males: sperm development in testes.
         (3) LH in females: formation of corpus luteum, production of estrogen and progesterone.
         (4) LH in males: production of testosterone in testes.
   3. Pituitary stimulates release:
      a. Growth hormone–releasing hormone (GH-RH) stimulates release:
         (1) **Growth hormone** (GH) by anterior pituitary.
         (2) GH acts directly or through production of somatomedins:
            (a) Increases protein synthesis, influx of amino acids into cells.
            (b) Decreases cellular uptake of glucose, promotes blood glucose levels.
            (c) Stimulates insulin secretion and cartilage and bone growth.
      b. Somatostatin inhibits release of GH.
      c. Prolactin-releasing factor (PRF) stimulates anterior pituitary to release prolactin, affects development of breast and milk production.
      d. **Antidiuretic hormone** (ADH, vasopressin) and oxytocin are produced by hypothalamus but stored in and released from posterior pituitary:
         (1) ADH: decreases water excretion from the kidney, involved in stress responses; contracts blood vessels (EXCEPT in lungs).

(2) Oxytocin: promotes uterine contractions and aids in milk ejection (let-down) by breast with nursing.

D. Hormones produced by PNS:

1. Thyroid hormones:
   a. Produced and stored in thyroid gland, transported in blood bound to plasma proteins.
   b. Include BOTH **thyroxine** (T_4, tetraiodothyronine) and triiodothyronine (T_3):
      (1) T_4 can be converted to T_3 by deiodinase in brain, kidneys, liver, brown fat.
      (2) Major systemic source of T_3 is derived by conversion from T_4 in liver and kidneys.
      (3) Production is regulated in negative feedback manner by TSH (Figure 3-22).
   c. Major functions: normal is considered euthyroid.
      (1) Regulation of metabolic rate, heat production, body temperature.
      (2) Increases number of catecholaminergic receptors on cells, heart rate, force of heart muscle contraction.
      (3) Intermediary metabolism of carbohydrates and fats.
      (4) Stimulates growth, teeth eruption, CNS development by interaction with GH.
   d. Thyroid hormone disorders:
      (1) Consequences are dictated by severity of disorder, duration, time of onset.
      (2) Hypothyroidism (decreased hormones) and hyperthyroidism (increased hormones).

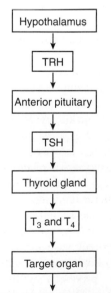

Figure 3-22 Negative feedback in the endocrine system. *TRH,* Thyroid-releasing hormone; *TSH,* thyroid-stimulating hormone; T_3, triiodothyronine; T_4, thyroxine.

(3) Goiter: enlarged thyroid (can occur with EITHER hypothyroidism or hyperthyroidism).

2. Hormones that affect calcium metabolism:
   a. Calcium levels in plasma are tightly regulated; the active form is free (1.3 mmol/L), NOT bound to plasma proteins; largest store of calcium is in bone calcium and is also stored and released at the SR.
   b. Deviations from normal range of calcium levels can affect:
      (1) Neuromuscular excitability; low levels (hypocalcemia) result in contraction and twitching of skeletal muscles; excitation-contraction coupling in cardiac and smooth muscles.
      (2) CNS excitability; stimulus-secretion coupling of hormones and neurotransmitters.
      (3) Maintenance of tight junctions between epithelial cells.
      (4) Clotting of blood.
   c. **Parathyroid hormone** (PTH): regulates calcium, produced in parathyroid glands (within thyroid) along with phosphorus and magnesium; vitamin D (cholecalciferol) produced by the skin is necessary for absorption of calcium as well as phosphorus:
      (1) Decreased plasma calcium levels stimulate release of PTH.
      (2) PTH stimulates kidneys to conserve calcium and phosphate.
      (3) In conjunction with vitamin D, PTH increases intestinal reabsorption of calcium and phosphate and increases bone reabsorption.
      (4) LOW levels of PTH can affect tooth development and may result in delayed tooth eruption along with defects in matrix, enamel mineralization, and dentin production.
   d. **Calcitonin:** affects BOTH calcium and phosphate handling; produced by thyroid C (interfollicular) cells (within thyroid):
      (1) Increased levels of calcium increase release of calcitonin.
         (a) Calcitonin (short-term increase): decreases movement of calcium from bone into plasma.
         (b) Calcitonin (long-term increase): decreases bone reabsorption by inhibiting osteoclasts, thereby decreasing plasma calcium and phosphate levels.

3. Hormones of pancreas: BOTH exocrine and endocrine functions:
   a. Exocrine glands (acini): secrete enzymes (proteases, amylase, lipases) and aqueous bicarbonate-rich fluid into intestine.

b. Cells in the isles of Langerhans: produce insulin, glucagon, somatostatin, pancreas polypeptide:

  (1) **Insulin:** produced in beta cells: decreases blood glucose, fatty acid, amino acid levels; increases storage of these nutrients as glycogen, triglycerides, and protein; increases uptake of glucose:

    (a) Release is stimulated MAINLY by elevations in blood glucose levels.

    (b) Release also occurs with increased blood amino acid levels and PNS stimulation.

  (2) **Glucagon:** produced in alpha cells; counteracts many of the effects of insulin; increases breakdown of glycogen to glucose; produces ketone bodies from breakdown of fatty acids; inhibits liver protein synthesis and increases protein degradation; excess glucagon increases effect of insulin deficiencies (e.g., DM).

4. Hormones of adrenal glands: cortical and medullary regions have different endocrine functions:

  a. Hormones secreted by adrenal cortex:

    (1) **Mineralocorticoids** (MAINLY aldosterone): produced in zona glomerulosa; increases sodium retention and potassium elimination by the kidneys, thus involved in long-term regulation of blood volume and pressure; secretion is stimulated by renin-angiotensin system; decreases plasma sodium levels; increases potassium levels.

    (2) **Glucocorticoids:** produced in zona fasciculata; include cortisol, regulated by ACTH, which increases gluconeogenesis, increases protein degradation in muscle (wasting), facilitates lipolysis; have permissive effect on actions of catecholamines; exert antiinflammatory and immunosuppressive effects.

    (3) Sex steroid hormones (discussed later): produced in zona reticularis; dehydroepiandrosterone (DHEA) is MOST important form of androgen; production peaks at 25 to 30 years and then decreases.

  b. Medulla secretes MAINLY epinephrine and some norepinephrine; control of medullary secretion is through the SNS.

5. Testicular hormones:

  a. Testosterone: produced in the testes under the stimulation of LH, in conjunction with FSH:

    (1) Increases production of RBCs.

    (2) Increases production of sperm; involved in growth and maturation of male reproductive organs at puberty; induces development of secondary male sexual characteristics.

    (3) Increases production in muscles; increases long bone growth.

  b. Inhibin: produced by Sertoli cells; inhibits FSH production.

6. Ovarian hormones and the menstrual cycle (see birth control pills and hormone replacement therapy in Chapter 9, Pharmacology):

  a. Hormones involved in female health:

    (1) Estrogens (estradiol [MOST important], estrone, estriol):

      (a) Essential for follicular (egg) maturation and release; stimulate development and maintenance of the female reproductive tract; induce production of progesterone and oxytocin receptors.

      (b) Increase fat deposition, which then decreases blood cholesterol levels.

      (c) Close epiphyseal plates and increase bone density.

      (d) Act as antioxidants and increase vasodilation.

    (2) Inhibin inhibits production of FSH during menstrual cycle.

    (3) Progesterone: prepares uterus for developing fetus; inhibits GnRH production; stimulates alveolar development in breasts and inhibits milk-secreting action of prolactin; stimulates ventilation.

  b. Hormonal changes during menstrual cycle: ovarian cycles begin at puberty (~12 years, "menarche") and continue until menopause (~50 years), with possible breaks during pregnancy and lactation.

  c. Hormones involved in fluid volume and blood pressure regulation:

    (1) Renin: produced by the kidney and stimulated by:

      (a) Low plasma sodium levels, decreased extracellular fluid volume.

      (b) Decrease in blood pressure as sensed by the kidney; SNS stimulation.

    (2) Angiotensin I and II:

      (a) Renin is converted via enzyme angiotensinogen (made in the liver, released into plasma) into angiotensin I (AI).

      (b) In the lungs, angiotensin-converting enzyme (ACE) converts AI to angiotensin II (AII).

      (c) Potent vasoconstrictors; also increase production of aldosterone.

    (3) ADH produced by hypothalamus in the CNS, NOT peripherally:

      (a) Stimuli for its release include AII, decrease in extracellular fluid volume, stress, increase in extracellular fluid osmolarity.

(b) ADH increases water retention by the kidney and is a potent vasoconstrictor.

(4) Atrial natriuretic peptide is produced in the right heart chamber and in the lungs:

   (a) Production is influenced by increase in extracellular fluid volume.

   (b) Increases water excretion (diuretic); increases sodium excretion (natriuretic).

   (c) Increased plasma levels are found in patients with congestive heart failure (CHF).

d. Hormones that regulate satiety (feeling of fullness, disappearance of hunger):

   (1) Leptin is produced peripherally by white adipose cells:

      (a) Transported in the blood across the blood-brain barrier by selective carriers; in brain acts on receptors located in the hypothalamus and brainstem regions to affect a number of physiological functions.

      (b) Also regulates reproductive behaviors and sleep.

   (2) Other neuromodulators and neurotransmitters associated with feeding include opioids, galanin, neuropeptide.

Respiratory Physiology

Respiratory physiology is the study of the respiratory system, which controls gas exchange, acid-base balance, and vocalization and enhances venous return. See earlier discussion on the respiratory system.

- See Chapters 6, General and Oral Pathology: respiratory disorders; 16, Special Needs Patient Care: respiratory disabilities; 14, Pain Management: nitrous oxide administration.

A. Functions of the respiratory system:

1. Gas exchange of oxygen (O_2) and carbon dioxide (CO_2):

   a. Exchange with environment in the lungs (ventilation).

   b. Exchange between lungs, circulatory system, and cells (diffusion and transport).

   c. Exchange in cells involves use of O_2 and production of CO_2 (respiration).

2. Acid-base balance with maintenance of blood pH at ~7.4:

   a. Rapid response system that alters plasma levels of CO_2.

   b. Works in conjunction with other buffering systems, including blood, kidneys, bones, other cells.

3. Regulation of airflow involved in vocalization.

4. Metabolism and elimination of substances via the pulmonary circulation (e.g., conversion of AI to AII).

5. Defense against inhaled particles (airways and nose) and emboli (pulmonary circulation).

6. Means for drug delivery because of the lung's large surface area and ready access to circulatory system.

7. Enhancement of venous return.

B. Specific functions of the respiratory system:

1. Process of ventilation:

   a. **Tidal volume** (TV, minimum flow rate): volume of breath that depends on force of respiratory muscle contractions and elasticity of lung; IMPORTANT during administration of gases such as nitrous oxide during dental treatment.

      (1) Part of breath goes to alveolar sacs for gas exchange.

      (2) Part of breath remains in conducting branches of lung, forming "dead space" volume.

      (3) During inspiration, alveolar pressures are *below* atmospheric pressure and suck air into lung.

      (4) During expiration, alveolar pressures are *above* atmospheric pressures and push air out of lungs.

      (5) Frequency of breathing in adults is between 14 and 20 breaths/min.

      (6) Minute ventilation is product of TV and frequency of breaths per minute.

   b. Multiple factors drive ventilation: elevated levels of CO_2 in plasma are sensed MAINLY by neurons within ventral medulla of brain:

      (1) Decreased levels of O_2 are sensed by carotid bodies.

      (2) Increased levels of hydrogen ions are sensed by carotid bodies.

      (3) Within airways and lung, receptors are sensitive to stretch, congestion (e.g., pneumonia, pulmonary emboli), irritation (e.g., smoke).

   c. Ventilation *increases* with:

      (1) Increased metabolic demands, e.g., exercise.

      (2) Use of stimulants, e.g., caffeine and progesterone.

      (3) Decreased levels of O_2 found at high altitudes and with cardiopulmonary disease (COPD).

      (4) Acidosis with uncontrolled DM, results in ketone body formation.

   d. Ventilation *decreases* with:

      (1) Metabolic alkalosis.

      (2) Overdose of some drugs (e.g., morphine, heroin).

      (3) Respiratory muscle failure.

      (4) Use of supplemental O_2 by patients with COPD; low levels of O_2 provide ONLY chemical drive to breathing, whereas in

healthy people the major drive is elevations in CO_2 levels.

2. Lung mechanics and volumes:
   a. **Compliance:** measure of distensibility of lung.
      (1) Increases in emphysema (type of COPD) because of destruction of connective tissue.
      (2) Decreases in pneumonia (increased lung water) and in diseases that decrease levels of lung surfactant (e.g., adult respiratory distress syndrome [ARDS] and cystic fibrosis [CF]).
   b. **Resistance:** measure of the ease with which air moves in or out of the lung, related to radius of airways; *small* decreases in radius have *large* effects on airway resistance:
      (1) Decreased by excess mucus (bronchitis), airway edema, tumors within or around airways.
      (2) Increased by agents that cause contraction of airway smooth muscles (e.g., acetylcholine, histamine, leukotrienes).
      (3) Changes in mechanics, such as decreased compliance (lung fibrosis with emphysema or lung cancer) or increased resistance (asthma), can increase the work of breathing, resulting in breathlessness even when performing minor tasks.
      (4) Lung volumes: influenced by lung and chest wall mechanics (Figure 3-23):
         (a) Smaller: pulmonary fibrosis (possibly an aftereffect of infection, with added factors such as smoking, environmental pollutants).
         (b) Larger: hyperinflation caused by emphysema.

3. Handling of O_2 and CO_2 by the body:
   a. MAJOR sources of O_2 are lungs and blood (~8 L), transported in dissolved state, bound to hemoglobin or myoglobin.
   b. The CO_2 is produced by aerobic metabolism, transported in blood, some dissolved, with MAJORITY transported as bicarbonate; at level of the lung, this reaction is reversed and CO_2 is released by lungs.

4. Diffusion of gases across lungs:
   a. Occurs in areas that both are ventilated and perfuse with blood.
   b. Depends on solubility of gas in plasma membranes; CO_2 is 20 times MORE soluble than O_2.
      (1) Arterial blood: partial pressure ("P," tension) of O_2 is 100 mm Hg; of CO_2 is 40 mm Hg.
      (2) Mixed venous blood: pCO_2 45 mm Hg; pO_2 40 mm Hg.

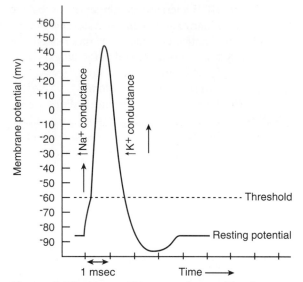

Figure 3-23 Lung volumes and capacities in a normal adult. Residual volume and any capacities containing residual volume cannot be determined using a spirometer.

   c. Affected by thickness of alveolar-capillary barrier; increases during lung edema.

5. Regulation of acid-base balance by lungs occurs by increasing or decreasing ventilation of CO_2:
   a. If amount of CO_2 produced by body is *equal* to ventilation, pH remains *constant* (7.4).
   b. If amount of CO_2 produced by body is *greater* than ventilation, pH *decreases* and acidosis results (pH <7.35).
   c. If ventilation is *greater* than amount of CO_2 produced by body, pH *increases* and alkalosis results (pH >7.45).
   d. Hydrogen ions are produced by metabolism and during periods of low O_2 and buffered by bicarbonate ions (HCO_3^-) produced from reaction of CO_2 and H_2O (see above).
   e. Resulting decrease in bicarbonate ions can be addressed by the kidneys ONLY.

6. Decreased delivery to or use of O_2 occurs when:
   a. Alveolar pO_2 is decreased (hypoxic hypoxia).
      (1) In high altitudes (decreased barometric pressure).
      (2) During lung disease and respiratory failure.
   b. Amount of functional hemoglobin decreases (anemic hypoxia):
      (1) In anemia caused by decreased RBC production, abnormal forms of hemoglobin (sickle cell anemia), or blood loss.
      (2) In carbon monoxide (CO) poisoning, prevents hemoglobin from binding to O_2 (CO binds to hemoglobin 150 times greater than does O_2).

c. Poisoning of enzymes involved in using O_2 to form ATP (histotoxic hypoxia):
  (1) CO.
  (2) Cyanide.

d. Blood flow to the tissues decreases (ischemia or stagnant hypoxia) as a result of:
  (1) Arteriosclerosis.
  (2) Congestive heart failure (CHF).
  (3) Stroke (cerebrovascular accident [CVA]).
  (4) Effect of DM on blood vessels.

CLINICAL STUDY

Age	14 YRS	SCENARIO
Sex	☒ Male ☐ Female	Patient's mother is calling to cancel his recall appointment. He has developed an upper respiratory infection (URI) with symptoms of cough, sore throat, fever, and dyspnea (difficulty breathing). Now she says that his end tidal pCO_2 has increased from 45 to 55 mm Hg. His maximal inspiratory pressure (MIP) and maximal expiratory pressures (MEP) dropped from 30 cm H_2O to 10 cm H_2O; vital capacity also dropped. He has had this situation before, and they anticipate that it should clear up in 2 weeks' time.
Height	4'3"	
Weight	80 LBS	
Chief Complaint	"He can't make his dental appointment since he is so sick today."	
Medical History	Duchenne muscular dystrophy (MD) Slight cognitive disability Wheelchair bound	
Current Medications	prednisone (Deltasone) 15 mg qd deflazacort (Calcort) 6 mg qd	
Social History	Grade school student at a special school	

1. Why would the pCO_2 increase in the patient?
2. What could be the reason for decreased respiratory muscle strength exemplified by decrease in MIP, MEP, and vital capacity?
3. The decrements in lung function were reversible. What does this say about the effects of the URI in the patient?
4. What lymph nodes can be affected by his sore throat? Which organ is responsible for his fever, and what does it mean?
5. What type of MD is this? How wide does the entry to the dental operatory have to be for him to get his wheelchair through when he is again able to visit the dental office?

1. Increase in pCO_2 indicates alveolar hypoventilation, which may be associated with marked respiratory weakness (normal values of MIP and MEP would be more than double the pre-URI values in this case) and increased airway resistance (decreased airway diameter) caused by inflammation and edema. Increased pCO_2 may also occur because of increased metabolism (fever) and an inability of the weakened ventilatory muscles to compensate.
2. Marked decrease in respiratory muscle strength during URI may be caused by release of cytokines, muscle injury from free radical production, or anorexia; all affect respiratory muscle performance.

3. Resolution of increased pCO_2 and decreased respiratory muscle strength occurs as URI clears up and factors mentioned above disappear.
4. Superior cervical nodes would be involved because of drainage from infection of pharynx (throat), especially jugulodigastric (tonsillar or sentinel node), below posterior belly of digastric muscle. Hypothalamus is body's thermostat and regulates temperature; can produce a fever, in which body temperature is elevated by at least full degree; occurs with infection, acute inflammation, shock, and/or changes in temperature exposure.
5. Duchenne MD is a form characterized by decreasing muscle mass and progressive loss of muscle function in male children; caused by a mutation in a specific gene within the X chromosome. The patient takes the corticosteroid medications to increase energy and strength and defer severity of some symptoms. Minimum 32-inch door opening is needed to enter the dental operatory, with at least 18 inches of clear wall space on pull side of door next to handle. The door handle must be no higher than 48 inches above the floor and of a lever type that can be operated with a closed fist.

Renal Physiology

Renal physiology is the study of the urinary system; consists of kidneys, ureter, bladder, urethra. Kidneys selectively excrete substances, reabsorb nutrients (via active

transport) and water, affect blood pressure, influence acid-base balance. See earlier discussion on the urinary system.
- See Chapter 14, Pain Management: metabolism of drugs in kidneys.

A. Major functions of the kidneys:
1. Conservation of water, electrolytes (especially sodium), and nutrients.
2. Regulation of acid-base balance in conjunction with other systems (lungs, blood, bone).
3. Secretion of erythropoietin (hormone that stimulates production of RBCs).
4. Elimination of waste and foreign products (including excretion of local anesthetic agents, fluoride).
5. Regulation of plasma volume, which affects blood pressure.
6. Secretion of renin, enzyme that produces AI from angiotensinogen, resulting in peripheral vasoconstriction.
7. Production of active form of vitamin D involved in calcium handling by body.

B. Nephron is functional unit of kidney: shorter nephrons are called cortical nephrons; longer nephrons involved in concentrating urine are juxtamedullary nephrons.
1. Basic components of nephrons (structures listed in series):
   a. Vascular components:
      (1) Afferent arteriole: delivers blood to nephron.
      (2) Glomerulus: dense capillary bed formed from arteriole that acts to filter plasma, allowing ALL substances in the blood EXCEPT proteins and cells to enter nephron.
      (3) Efferent arteriole: carries blood from glomerulus.
      (4) Peritubular capillaries: formed from efferent arteriole and supply blood to rest of nephron.
      (5) Juxtamedullary apparatus (JMA): vascular and nephron tubular components, macula densa, juxtaglomerular cells of afferent arteriole; produces chemicals that affect blood flow to kidneys.
   b. Tubular components:
      (1) Bowman's capsule: composed of two epithelial layers (visceral and parietal) that enable filtration of plasma. Filtered plasma enters here.
      (2) Proximal convoluted tubule (PCT): reabsorbs MOST filtered constituents; secretion of H^+ and organic ions may occur.
      (3) Loop of Henle: concentrates urine in conjunction with distal convoluted tubule (DCT) and collecting duct; loops are especially long in medullary nephrons.
      (4) DCT and collecting duct: variable control (by means of hormones such as aldosterone, ADH, atrial natriuretic peptide) of sodium, potassium, hydrogen ions, water.

2. Processes performed by nephron:
   a. Glomerular filtration rate (GFR) involves indiscriminate filtration of plasma; depends on:
      (1) Blood pressure. See later discussion.
      (2) Leakiness of glomerular (fenestrated) capillaries and Bowman's capsule.
      (3) *Afferent* versus *efferent* vasoconstriction: afferent leads to decreased GFR and decreased perfusion of the rest of nephron; efferent leads to increased GFR and increased perfusion of the rest of nephron.
      (4) Tubular reabsorption: selective, high-volume process dependent on:
         (a) Energy: Na^+ reabsorption (water and Cl^- follow passively; glucose, phosphate, amino acids are transported secondarily).
         (b) Concentration of substances: normally higher in proximal tubule than in peritubular vessels.
         (c) Hormones: aldosterone (for sodium), ADH (for water), atrial natriuretic peptide (for both sodium and water).
         (d) Tubular maximum for the substance: once this is reached, substance is "dumped" into urine (e.g., higher plasma glucose levels in DM result in glucose in urine; ALL glucose in nephron is reabsorbed back into the blood).
      (5) Tubular secretion results in movement of substances from peritubular capillaries into nephron for excretion.
         (a) Secretion of hydrogen and bicarbonate ions depends on acid-base status.
         (b) Potassium secretion is dependent on amount of aldosterone present.
         (c) Organic ions and cations (especially some drugs and endogenous substances such as histamine, epinephrine, creatinine) are secreted.
      (6) Plasma clearance and urinary excretion:
         (a) **Clearance** of substance by kidneys refers to volume of plasma that is completely cleared of substance per unit of time.
         (b) Inulin is filtered, NOT reabsorbed or secreted; completely cleared by kidney, measured clinically to determine GFR.
         (c) Glucose in healthy person is filtered but completely reabsorbed; therefore NO glucose is cleared by the kidneys.

3. Excretion is the measure of the amount of urine output per unit of time:
   a. Difference between what is filtered and what is reabsorbed plus what is secreted; normal excretion rates are 1 mL/min.

b. Excretion rates depend on the concentration of the urine, modulated by osmolarity of plasma and hormonal status; rates decreased during dehydration, decreased blood pressure, renal disease.

c. Acid-base handling by the kidney involves reabsorption or secretion of H^+ and HCO_3^-; if disturbance is caused by kidney or metabolic source, respiratory system tries to compensate:
   (1) Healthy: metabolically produced acids are buffered by HCO_3^-, replaced by the kidneys.
   (2) Metabolic acidosis: H^+ is secreted and HCO_3^- is reabsorbed; increase in ventilation eliminates CO_2 produced by combining the excess H^+ with HCO_3^-.
   (3) Respiratory acidosis (hypoventilation): HCO_3^- and H^+ are generated from CO_2 and H_2O; H^+ is secreted and HCO_3^- is reabsorbed.
   (4) Respiratory alkalosis (hyperventilation): excess HCO_3^- is secreted by the kidneys and H^+ is retained; CO_2 levels in blood are LOWER.
   (5) Metabolic alkalosis: handled by the kidney in a similar manner to respiratory alkalosis, but metabolic alkalosis depresses ventilation and CO_2 builds up in the plasma to compensate.

Blood Pressure

Blood pressure is the force that drives blood through vessels to carry nutrients and oxygen to tissues and waste products and metabolized substances away from tissues. **Mean arterial pressure** (MAP) is a term used to describe an *average* blood pressure.

• See Chapters 6, General and Oral Pathology: high blood pressure; 11, Medical and Dental Emergencies: blood pressure readings, classifications, related emergencies.

A. MAP (cardiac output [CO] × total peripheral resistance of blood vessels [TPR]).

B. Blood pressure medications act on one of these three variables; factors that affect MAP:
  1. The CO is the amount of blood pumped by the heart per minute:
     a. Equal to the heart rate (HR) multiplied by the stroke volume (SV) (CO = HR × SV).
     b. The HR is the number of beats per minute and the SV is the volume pumped per beat (e.g., 70 beats per minute [HR], 70 mL blood is ejected with each beat [SR]).
     c. The HR:
        (1) Increased by sympathetic division (SANS) stimulation and release of norepinephrine and epinephrine.
        (2) Decreased by parasympathetic division (PANS) stimulation.
     d. The SV is influenced by:
        (1) Amount of blood returning to the heart (venous return), increased by an increase in blood volume, decreased right atrial pressure, skeletal muscle contractions, increasing venous tone.
        (2) Contractility of heart muscle is increased by the SAME factors that increase HR.
        (3) Condition of the heart; as heart fails, CO decreases.
  2. The TPR is influenced by:
     a. Diameter of blood vessels, especially "resistance" vessels and arterioles that have large amount of smooth muscle; diameter is affected by:
        (1) SANS stimulation, leads to constriction.
        (2) Local conditions, e.g., decreased O_2 and increased metabolites, cytokines, adenosine, and histamine increase dilation.
        (3) Circulating hormones, ADH and angiotensin, are constrictors and atrial natriuretic peptide is a dilator.
     b. Blood viscosity affected by:
        (1) Dehydration; leads to increased viscosity and resistance.
        (2) Number of RBCs; viscosity is increased in polycythemia (increased RBCs) and decreased in anemia (decreased RBCs).
        (3) Pancytopenia: decreased number of total circulating blood cells.

C. *Short-term* regulation of blood pressure:
  1. The CNS regulates blood pressure for the short term.
     a. Pressure and volume sensors are located in:
        (1) Carotid sinus and aortic arch (pressure).
        (2) Right atrium and lungs (volume).
  2. Afferent pathways to the CNS include medulla oblongata, hypothalamus, cortex.
  3. CNS responses to decreased blood pressure include:
     a. Increased SANS outflow.
     b. Release of hormones such as ADH from the pituitary.
     c. Stimulation of renin release by the kidneys.
  4. Systemic consequences include:
     a. Increased CO.
     b. Increased TPR.
     c. Production of AII and aldosterone.

D. *Long-term* regulation of blood pressure:
  1. Influenced by the kidneys; retain and/or excrete sodium and water.
  2. Involves measurement of MAP by means of:
     a. Direct use of indwelling catheter (thank goodness we do not have to do this to our patients!).
     b. Indirect use of pressure cuff, sphygmomanometer, stethoscope:

(1) Systolic: 120 mm Hg in a resting, healthy adult.
(2) Diastolic: 80 mm Hg in a resting, health adult.
(3) MAP = DP + ⅓ (SP − DP).

E. Blood pressure abnormalities according to the Joint National Committee 7 on Prevention, Detection, Evaluation, and Treatment of High Blood Pressure (see CD-ROM for guidelines):
1. Prehypertension: 120/80 to 139/89 mm Hg; lifestyle changes are needed to prevent hypertension.
2. **Hypertension** (high blood pressure [HBP]): with systolic/diastolic of >140/>90 mm Hg; can involve systolic and/or diastolic.
3. May be caused or increased by:
   a. Excess fluid retention cause by hormonal abnormalities (e.g., increased levels of aldosterone).
   b. Stress and obesity.
   c. Renal disease and DM.
   d. Aging (may instead lead to hypotension).

4. Consequences of HBP include:
   a. Increased work by the heart; may lead to cardiac failure and then heart attack (myocardial infarction [MI]).
   b. Stresses on blood vessels; may lead to atherosclerosis and then stroke (cerebrovascular accident [CVA]).
5. **Hypotension** (low blood pressure) caused by:
   a. Cardiovascular disease (CVD) that leads to decreased CO.
   b. Decreased SANS function or β-adrenergic receptor blockade (drugs, such as propranolol [Inderal]).
   c. Shock related to:
      (1) Blood loss (such as by hemorrhage [excessive bleeding]), termed hypovolemic shock.
      (2) Septic (bacterial) infections.
      (3) Neurogenic causes (fainting [syncope]).
      (4) Anaphylactic reactions (e.g., allergy to bee stings results in the release of mediators such as histamine from mast cells).

CLINICAL STUDY

Age	66 YRS	SCENARIO
Sex	☒ Male ☐ Female	The patient was admitted to the hospital while visiting his dental office. The dental staff sent him by ambulance, since he had a sudden onset of pain affecting his left arm right before his dental appointment. Patient had stopped taking his prescribed daily medication, since he did not like the side effect of coughing.
Height	5′11″	
Weight	260 LBS	
BP	210/120	
Chief Complaint	"My wife could not get me out of bed this morning."	
Medical History	Essential hypertension Angina pectoris	
Current Medications	nitroglycerin, sl prn captopril (Capoten) 25 mg bid	
Social History	Retired bar owner who used to smoke	

1. What does a blood pressure reading mean? What is MAP? What organ maintains the long-term regulation of blood pressure?
2. What level of high blood pressure is the patient experiencing?
3. What may be happening to the patient because of his high blood pressure? Did the dental office need to have him sent to the hospital?

1. Blood pressure is force that drives blood through vessels to carry nutrients and oxygen to tissues, and waste products and metabolized substances away from tissues. Mean arterial pressure (MAP) is a term used to describe an average blood pressure (heart rate × stroke volume × total peripheral resistance), with a systolic pressure of <120 mm Hg and a diastolic pressure of <80 mm Hg in a resting, healthy adult. Long-term regulation of blood pressure is influenced by the kidneys, which either retain or excrete sodium and water.
2. Patient has a history of hypertension (high blood pressure [HBP]), with past readings of systolic/diastolic >140/90 mm Hg. With this latest reading, he is at stage 2, severe HBP (≥180/≥110 mm Hg), so the dental office needs to activate the emergency medical services (EMS) system and treat as emergency.
3. Patient could again be having angina pectoris, chest pain caused by decreased oxygen flow to the heart,

or could be having an MI, since pain can spread from chest to other areas. The pain is of greater intensity and duration than angina pectoris, and the pain he is feeling in left arm could be an indicator of MI. Considering the symptoms, the dental office acted correctly by sending him to hospital by ambulance for emergency care. A delay of 4 to 6 weeks after this cardiac episode, as well as follow-up medical consult, will be needed before dental care (either emergency or elective), and patient must meet the 4 METs to determine his FC levels to reduce future cardiac risk during dental treatment.

Gastrointestinal Tract Physiology

Gastrointestinal (alimentary) tract (GIT) consists of the oral cavity, esophagus, stomach, small and large intestines. MAINLY responsible for the digestion of food into MORE usable forms of nutrients for the cells of the body. See earlier discussion about GIT.

- See Chapter 4, Head, Neck, and Dental Anatomy: oral cavity structure.

A. Functions of GIT:

1. Digestion of food into nutrients that can be absorbed and used by cells for energy, growth, repair, heat production, differentiation:
   a. **Motility:** movement and mixing of food along GIT.
   b. **Secretion:** production and release of enzymes, hormones, fluids, mucus, or electrolytes that aid in digestion.
   c. **Digestion:** breakdown of ingested food into nutrients that may be used by the body.
   d. **Absorption:** uptake of digested materials across GIT into blood and lymphatics for delivery to cells.

2. Defense against ingested substances that may be harmful to the body.

B. Anatomical structures and functions of digestion:

1. Oral cavity is the site for the ingestion of foods:
   a. Tongue mixes food with saliva and contains taste buds; fluid in saliva helps dissolve foods to be "tasted."
   b. Teeth chew food into more manageable pieces, allowing better mixing of food with saliva, which acts as a lubricant.

2. Salivary glands and accessory digestive glands produce secretions:
   a. Saliva (fluid, mucus, lysozyme, bicarbonate):
      (1) Production is tonically stimulated by the PANS, by smell or sight of food or anticipatory reflex.
      (2) Fluid and lysozymes have antibacterial actions, as well as helping to reduce acids to help prevent caries.
      (3) Contains sIgA (secretory), which provides immune resistance against bacteria, food residues, fungi, parasites, viruses (also in tears, sweat, gut fluid).
      (4) Histatins function as antifungal.
   b. **Salivary amylase:** enzyme that begins to digest starches in the oral cavity (such as carbohydrates; see earlier discussion) to dextran and maltose (disaccharide).

3. Pharynx allows movement of gases into the lungs and chewed food into esophagus; during swallowing, glottis closes to prevent foodstuff from entering lungs.

4. Esophagus is tubelike and consists of both smooth and skeletal muscle:
   a. Moves chewed food from the mouth toward the stomach by peristaltic contractions.
   b. Mucus produced by cells lining the lumen is protective and helps movement of food.
   c. After the gastroesophageal sphincter relaxes, food enters the stomach.

5. Stomach functions:
   a. Storage of ingested food until it is emptied into the small intestine.
   b. Secretion of HCl and enzymes that initiate digestion.
   c. Pulverization and mixing of food to produce chyme (thick liquid mixture).
   d. Major secretions of stomach (and locations):
      (1) Oxyntic mucosa (fundus and body):
         (a) Mucous neck cells produce thin mucus.
         (b) Gastrin secreted by the duodenum initiates gastric acid production.
         (c) Chief cells produce pepsinogen, which can be converted to enzyme pepsin under influence of chloride to initiate protein digestion.
         (d) Parietal (oxyntic) cells produce HCl and intrinsic factor, which help absorb vitamin B_{12} in ileum.
         (e) Epithelial cells secrete thick mucus to protect stomach from autodigestion.
      (2) Pyloric area contains G cells that secret gastrin, hormone that stimulates parietal and chief cells.
   e. Emptying of chyme from stomach:
      (1) Depends on volume and fluidity of chyme; initiates gastrin production and reflexes (by way of vagus nerve and intrinsic nervous system) that stimulate antrum contraction, leading to stomach emptying.
      (2) Presence of acid and/or fat in duodenum initiates enterogastric reflex and release of secretin, cholecystokinin, and gastric inhibitory peptides that prevent emptying.
      (3) Vomiting (emesis) is caused by active contraction of respiratory muscles that act on stomach emptying.

f. Gastric secretion is stimulated during phases:
  (1) Cephalic phase: smell or thought of food leads to secretion of HCl, gastrin, pepsinogen.
  (2) Gastric phase: large volume of food, caffeine, or alcohol leads to gastrin and HCl secretion.
  (3) Intestinal phase: chyme enters duodenum, leading to decreased gastrin and HCl secretion.
g. Stomach absorbs fluoride at about 86% to 97%.

6. Functions of pancreas and liver (accessory organs):
  a. Pancreas:
    (1) Produces enzymes (e.g., trypsin [activated by enterokinase], chymotrypsin, amylase, lipase) and an alkaline watery solution, secreted into small intestine; lipase acts on fats to become fatty acids and glycerol.
    (2) Endocrine organ that produces insulin, glucagon, somatostatin (see section on endocrinology).
  b. Liver produces bile, cholesterol, lecithin, which facilitate absorption of fats; bile produced by the liver is stored in gallbladder.
  c. Additional functions of liver NOT associated with digestion include:
    (1) Detoxification of waste products and foreign substances.
    (2) Storage of glycogen.
    (3) Production of fibrinogen and prothrombin, involved in blood clotting.
    (4) Synthesis of amino acids and proteins.
    (5) Production of RBCs in fetus and destruction of RBCs in adult.
    (6) Immune surveillance via Kupffer cells (reticuloendothelial cells).
  d. All blood that leaves the gut passes through liver by way of portal vein, allowing additional processing of nutrients and blood detoxification.

7. Role of small intestine in digestion and absorption:
  a. Segmentation, results in mixing and moving of chyme:
    (1) Initiated by pacemaker cells in GIT.
    (2) Responds to presence of chyme in stomach and production of gastrin by duodenum.
    (3) Stimulated by PANS and inhibited by SANS.
  b. Digestion of chyme occurs by:
    (1) Pancreatic enzymes released into the small intestine.
    (2) Intracellular enzymes.
    (3) Crypts of Lieberkühn (between villi), which secrete water and electrolytes, constantly replace epithelial cells that secrete mucus.
  c. Small intestine has large surface area for absorption (presence of villi and microvilli):
    (1) MOST occurs in duodenum and jejunum.

  (2) Absorption of vitamin B_{12} and bile salts occurs in terminal ileum.
  (3) Absorption of calcium and iron depends on body's needs.
8. Processing of substances NOT absorbed in small intestine by large intestine (colon, cecum, appendix, rectum) includes electrolytes and water.

Review Questions

1 Some cells that line the respiratory tract produce mucus, which traps inhaled particles and subsequently is propelled upward for expectoration. This upward movement is produced by the action of
A. ribosomes.
B. cilia.
C. flagella.
D. centrioles.

2 One of the following is NOT a type of connective tissue. Which one is the EXCEPTION?
A. Blood
B. Bone
C. Cartilage
D. Muscle

3 Which of the following describes the type of membrane lining the respiratory tract?
A. Mucous
B. Cutaneous
C. Serous
D. Parietal

4 An abrasion on the surface of the skin heals when new cells form to replace the damaged cells. The layer of skin that produces the replacement cells is the stratum
A. lucidum.
B. corneum.
C. granulosum.
D. basale.

5 A fracture of the radius is also a fracture of the
A. axial skeleton.
B. medial side of the forearm.
C. brachium or arm.
D. lateral side of the forearm.

6 Diarthrotic joints (diarthroses)
A. have a synovial membrane lining the fibrous joint capsule.
B. are immovable joints.
C. include the intervertebral discs.
D. are fibrous joints.

7 One of the following muscles is NOT associated with the lower extremity. Which one is the EXCEPTION?
A. Adductor longus
B. Sternocleidomastoid
C. Biceps femoris
D. Gastrocnemius

8 One of the following is NOT a part of the central nervous system. Which one is the EXCEPTION?
A. Cranial nerves
B. Cerebrum
C. Cerebellum
D. Spinal cord

9 Which of the following statements is related to the function of the cerebellum?
A. Contains centers that help regulate breathing movements
B. Regulates heart rate and blood pressure
C. Is important in maintaining posture and equilibrium
D. Contains centers for hearing and vision

10 The afferent division of the peripheral nervous system
A. consists entirely of cranial nerves.
B. consists entirely of spinal nerves.
C. carries sensory impulses to the central nervous system.
D. carries motor impulses from the central nervous system to the effectors.

11 One of the following descriptors is NOT true about the autonomic nervous system. Which one is the EXCEPTION?
A. Visceral efferent system
B. Divided into sympathetic and parasympathetic divisions
C. System effectors are skeletal muscles
D. Part of the peripheral nervous system

12 Which of the following is CORRECT about taste and smell?
A. General senses
B. Localized and closely related
C. Type of proprioception
D. Detected by Meissner's and pacinian corpuscles

13 Where are the rods and cones of the eye located?
A. Innermost eye layer
B. Cornea
C. Ciliary body
D. Lens

14 The organ of Corti
A. is located in the middle ear.
B. contains the malleus, incus, and stapes.
C. functions to provide equilibrium.
D. contains the receptors for hearing.

15 Which of the following describes the hormone aldosterone?
A. Reacts with receptors on cell membrane surface
B. Considered sex hormones in the body
C. Produced by the adenohypophysis
D. Derivative of cholesterol

16 Which of the formed elements of the blood contain hemoglobin and transport oxygen?
A. Thrombocytes
B. Leukocytes
C. Monocytes
D. Erythrocytes

17 Which of the following transfusions can be given to a person with type A blood?
A. Type A or type AB
B. Type A or type O
C. Type B or type AB
D. Type AB or type O

18 During which of the following situations can an Rh factor reaction occur?
A. Anti-Rh agglutinins of the fetus come in contact with agglutinogens from an Rh– mother.
B. Rh+ agglutinogens of the fetus come into contact with anti-Rh agglutinins from an Rh– mother.
C. Rh+ agglutinogens of the fetus come into contact with Rh– agglutinogens from an Rh– mother.
D. Anti-Rh agglutinins of the fetus come into contact with anti-Rh agglutinins from an Rh– mother.

19 Which of the following describes the blood in the hepatic portal vein?
A. Lower oxygen content than blood in the hepatic artery
B. Higher oxygen content than blood in the descending aorta
C. Higher oxygen content than blood in the left atrium
D. Lower glucose content than blood in the hepatic artery

20 Into where does the lymph from the right inguinal lymph nodes flow?
A. Thoracic duct, then into the right subclavian vein
B. Thoracic duct, then into the left subclavian vein
C. Right lymphatic duct, then into the right subclavian vein
D. Right lymphatic duct, then into the left subclavian vein

21 The MOST diffusion of oxygen and carbon dioxide occurs across the walls of the
A. trachea.
B. bronchi.
C. alveoli.
D. hypopharynx.

22 Which of the following is one of the differences between the right lung and the left lung?
A. Left lung has a greater volume because it is longer than the right lung.
B. Right lung is covered by a serous membrane but the left lung is not.
C. Right lung has an indentation for the base of the heart but the left lung does not.
D. Right lung has three lobes but the left lung has two.

23 One of the following is NOT secreted by the mucosal cells of the stomach. Which one is the EXCEPTION?
A. Hydrochloric acid
B. Gastrin
C. Pepsinogen
D. Amylase

24 Cells of the small intestine secrete both enzymes and hormones. Secretin is a hormone produced by the small intestine that stimulates
A. contraction of the gallbladder.
B. production of pancreatic enzymes.
C. secretion of an alkaline fluid from the pancreas.
D. secretion of hydrochloric acid from the stomach.

25 One of the following statements is NOT true about the liver. Which one is the EXCEPTION?
A. Blood is drained from the liver by the hepatic portal vein.
B. Liver produces bile for digestion.
C. Liver is located in the upper right quadrant of the abdomen.
D. Oxygenated blood is brought to the liver by the hepatic artery.

26 Which of the following sequences BEST describes the directional flow of urine to outside the body?
   A. Urinary bladder, urethra, ureter, kidney
   B. Kidney, urethra, urinary bladder, ureter
   C. Kidney, ureter, urinary bladder, urethra
   D. Urinary bladder, ureter, urethra, kidney

27 If a male has had mumps, what side effect is possible?
   A. Emesis
   B. Orchitis
   C. Inflamed prostate gland
   D. Fluid from the penis

28 What is the basic structure of the helix of DNA?
   A. Single
   B. Double
   C. Triple
   D. Quadratic

29 All the following are ways that RNA is dissimilar to DNA, EXCEPT one. Which one is the EXCEPTION?
   A. Formed as single stranded
   B. Contains uridine monophosphate
   C. Assists in protein translation
   D. Involved in transcription

30 What is the process of breaking large, complex molecules into smaller, simpler units called?
   A. Anabolism
   B. Catabolism
   C. Electron transport
   D. Oxidative phosphorylation

31 The products of aerobic metabolism include all of the following, EXCEPT one. Which one is the EXCEPTION?
   A. H_2O
   B. Heat
   C. Lactic acid
   D. ATP
   E. CO_2

32 According to Fick's law of diffusion, the greatest net movement of a substance across a membrane will occur if the
   A. concentration gradient is small.
   B. thickness of the membrane is great.
   C. temperature is low.
   D. available surface area is large.
   E. membrane permeability for a substance is low.

33 Which of the following statements can describe the process of osmosis?
   A. Associated with movement of H_2O across a membrane
   B. Unrelated to membrane permeability
   C. Associated primarily with movement of solutes across a membrane
   D. Unrelated to the concentration gradient

34 All are characteristics of carrier-mediated transport EXCEPT one. Which one is the EXCEPTION?
   A. Movement of substances across membrane
   B. Specificity
   C. Saturation or transport maximum
   D. Competition
   E. Requirement of energy (ATP)

35 Which of the following can be used to describe the autonomic nervous system?
   A. Not part of the peripheral nervous system
   B. Innervates only smooth and cardiac muscles
   C. Consists of the sympathetic and parasympathetic nervous systems
   D. Innervates skeletal muscles
   E. Uses the neurotransmitter glutamate

36 All of the following are true of skeletal muscles, EXCEPT one. Which one is the EXCEPTION?
   A. Contain actin and myosin microfilaments
   B. Require external Ca^{+2} for contraction
   C. Use acetylcholine as the neurotransmitter
   D. Contain an extensive sarcoplasmic reticulum
   E. Need energy for both contraction and relaxation

37 Which of the following statements is CORRECT concerning cardiac muscles?
   A. Need no external Ca^{+2} for contraction
   B. Have action potentials that last more than 200 msec
   C. Contain few mitochondria
   D. Contract in response to acetylcholine
   E. Exhibit summation

38 How can hormones be divided into classes of chemicals?
   A. Amines, peptides, and steroids
   B. Free fatty acids, peptides, and amines
   C. Steroids, free fatty acids, and phospholipids
   D. Amines, phospholipids, and steroids

39 Which of the following is related to the role of parathyroid hormone in the body?
   A. Decreases Ca^{+2} plasma levels in response to hypocalcemia
   B. Acts on the kidney to conserve Ca^{+2}
   C. Acts with vitamin D to decrease intestinal absorption of Ca^{+2}
   D. Affects only phosphate metabolism in muscle

40 Which of the following is the role of the pancreas in the body?
   A. Only an endocrine gland within the body
   B. Produces glucagon, which decreases glucose levels
   C. Produces insulin, which promotes cellular uptake of plasma glucose
   D. Secretes hormones that break down carbohydrates and proteins

41 Which of the following describes the hormone aldosterone?
   A. Produced in the adrenal medulla
   B. Stimulated by increased Na^+ plasma levels
   C. Regulation of blood volume by means of effects on the kidneys
   D. Stimulated by a rise in blood pressure or a fall in K^+ plasma levels
   E. Stimulated by high estrogen levels only

42 Glucocorticoids such as cortisol have all of the following characteristics, EXCEPT one. Which one is the EXCEPTION?
   A. Promote muscle breakdown
   B. Promote gluconeogenesis
   C. Involved in stress responses
   D. Stimulate the immune system
   E. Are regulated by ACTH

43 Which of the following statements describes the role of testosterone in the body?
A. Produced by Leydig cells in testes
B. Stimulates production of sperm in Sertoli cells
C. Decreases red blood cell production
D. Decreases protein production in muscles

44 Estrogen is a hormone that
A. induces production of testosterone receptors in the uterus.
B. is essential for follicular maturation.
C. promotes oxygen production.
D. decreases bone density.

45 Hormones involved in fluid volume regulation include all the following, EXCEPT one. Which one is the EXCEPTION?
A. Angiotensin II
B. Aldosterone
C. Antidiuretic hormone
D. Inhibin
E. Atrial natriuretic peptide

46 How does gas exchange occur across the lung?
A. Depends on alveoli that are ventilated and perfused by blood
B. Is similar for oxygen and carbon dioxide
C. Occurs in the bronchi
D. Depends on a large pressure gradient for CO_2
E. Occurs primarily in the pulmonary artery

47 Which of the following statements can be used to describe the pleural space?
A. Normally contains a large amount of fluid
B. Contains positive (above atmospheric) pressure
C. Helps attach the chest wall and lung for ventilation
D. Produces surfactant

48 Which of the following is a factor related to ventilation of the lungs?
A. Determined by the product of tidal volume and frequency of breathing
B. Little influenced by the body's O_2 demands
C. Stimulated by high levels of CO_2
D. Stimulated by anoxia

49 How is MOST of the carbon dioxide (CO_2) transported in blood?
A. In the form of bicarbonate ions
B. Dissolved in the blood
C. Bound to plasma proteins
D. Bound to hemoglobin
E. In the form of H_2CO_3

50 Decreased access to oxygen by cells of the body can occur in all of the following conditions, EXCEPT one. Which one is the EXCEPTION?
A. Inhalation of carbon monoxide
B. Decreased hemoglobin levels
C. High altitude
D. Increased blood flow to the cells
E. Cyanide poisoning

51 What is the role of alveolar hyperventilation in the body?
A. Decreases O_2 levels in blood
B. Increases CO_2 levels in blood
C. Decreases the pH of blood
D. Decreases H^+ in blood

52 Secretions produced by the stomach include all of the following, EXCEPT one. Which one is the EXCEPTION?
A. Mucus
B. Hydrochloric acid (HCl)
C. Intrinsic factor
D. Vitamin B_{12}
E. Pepsinogen

53 Which of the following is considered a function of the liver?
A. Detoxification of wastes
B. Production of red blood cells in adults
C. Synthesis of steroid hormones
D. Production of vitamin A
E. Synthesis of fats

54 Functions of the small intestine include all of the following, EXCEPT one. Which one is the EXCEPTION?
A. Absorption of digested foodstuff
B. Production of fluids and electrolytes
C. Production of enzymes released into the intestine
D. Movement of chyme through the intestine
E. Absorption of vitamin B_{12} and bile salts

55 Which of the following is a function of the large intestine?
A. Absorbs food
B. Produces water and electrolytes
C. Produces mucus for protection and lubrication
D. Absorbs hormones
E. Produces intrinsic factor

56 Major functions of the kidneys include all of the following, EXCEPT one. Which one is the EXCEPTION?
A. Production of erythropoietin
B. Production of renin
C. Production of angiotensin II
D. Regulation of blood volume
E. Acid-base regulation

57 What can occur with a blockage of the ureter?
A. More pressure within kidney
B. Increased urine excretion
C. Increased overall size of nephrons
D. Formation of prostatic hypertrophy

58 Components of a nephron include all of the following, EXCEPT one. Which one is the EXCEPTION?
A. Glomerulus
B. Juxtaglomerular apparatus
C. Bowman's capsule
D. Urethra
E. Loop of Henle

59 Which of the following statements is CORRECT concerning the glomerular filtration rate?
A. Increased by an increase of blood pressure
B. Decreased by constriction of the efferent arteriole
C. Decreased by increasing the leakiness of the Bowman's capsule
D. Increased by constriction of the afferent arteriole

60 Which of the following occurs during respiratory acidosis?
A. Kidneys play no role.
B. Kidneys compensate by producing chloride.
C. Kidneys compensate by reabsorbing HCO_3^-.
D. Kidneys compensate by reabsorbing H^+.

61 Which of the following can cause a change in cardiac output?
A. Increased by an increase in contractility of the heart
B. Increased when the heart rate decreases
C. Decreased by an increase in venous return
D. Decreased by an increase in stroke volume

62 Which of the following can occur with changes in total peripheral resistance?
A. Increased as the diameter of blood vessels decreases
B. Decreased by angiotensin II
C. Independent of blood viscosity
D. Increased by increased production of metabolites
E. Decreased with dehydration

63 Blood pressure or volume is sensed by receptors in all of these locations, EXCEPT one. Which one is the EXCEPTION?
A. Right atrium
B. Carotid sinus
C. Carotid body
D. Aortic sinus

64 Which of the following can happen when there is a decrease in blood pressure?
A. Release of acetylcholine
B. Increased sympathetic nervous system discharge
C. Decreased heart rate
D. Decreased cardiac output

65 Which of the following statements is CORRECT concerning hypertension?
A. Decreases the work of the heart
B. Contributes to the formation of atherosclerotic plaques
C. Affects only the pulmonary circulation
D. Is age independent
E. Is lower in obese people

66 Hypotension may occur in all the following situations, EXCEPT one. Which one is the EXCEPTION?
A. Heart failure occurs.
B. Rapid release of epinephrine occurs.
C. Blood is lost.
D. Septic shock occurs.
E. Sympathetic nervous system–blocking drugs are taken.

67 Functions of the plasma membrane include all of the following, EXCEPT one. Which one is the EXCEPTION?
A. Selectively allows movement of substances into the cell interior
B. Contains receptors that allow communication between cells
C. Synthesizes proteins
D. Is involved in cell division
E. Forms vesicles for endocytosis

68 Which of the following organelles produces ATP?
A. Mitochondria
B. Golgi apparatus
C. Peroxisomes
D. Lysosomes
E. Vesicles

69 Loss of the sense of smell could result from injury to which of the following cranial nerves?
A. I
B. III
C. V
D. VII
E. IX

70 What is the largest visceral organ of the body?
A. Skin
B. Liver
C. Stomach
D. Gallbladder

71 Which of the following provides energy to the brain?
A. Glucagon
B. Glucose
C. Glycogen
D. Glycolic acid

72 Alpha and beta cells are found in which of the following organs?
A. Pancreas
B. Liver
C. Kidney
D. Adrenal glands

73 What is the primary form of carbohydrate storage?
A. Glucose
B. Sucrose
C. Glycogen
D. Starch

74 Starch digestion is initiated in the
A. oral cavity.
B. stomach.
C. small intestine.
D. large intestine.

75 Which of the following cranial nerves is also designated as the trigeminal nerve?
A. V
B. VII
C. X
D. XII

Answer Key And Rationales

1 **(B)** Both cilia and flagella are involved in movement; flagella move cells and cilia move substances across cell surface, and ciliary action moves mucus with trapped particles upward for subsequent removal from the body. Ribosomes are involved in protein synthesis, and centrioles function in cell division.

2 **(D)** Four main categories of tissue are epithelial, connective, muscle, and nervous. Blood, bone, cartilage, along with areolar tissue, adipose tissue, tendons, and ligaments, are examples of connective tissue.

3 **(A)** Serous membranes line body cavities that do NOT open to the outside and consist of parietal and visceral layers. Cutaneous membrane is the skin. Mucous membranes line body cavities that open to

the exterior, such as the respiratory and digestive tracts.

4 (D) Stratum basale is the actively mitotic layer that produces new cells. Other layers consist of dead or dying cells and have no mitotic ability, with EXCEPTION of stratum spinosum, which has limited mitotic ability.

5 (D) Radius is bone of appendicular skeleton and is located on lateral side of forearm. Humerus is bone in brachium or arm.

6 (A) Diarthrotic joints are freely movable joints whose range of motion is limited by adjacent muscles, bones, and ligaments. Joint has a fibrous joint capsule lined with a synovial membrane that secretes synovial fluid into the joint cavity for lubrication. Immovable joints are synarthroses. Intervertebral discs are located between vertebral bodies to form slightly movable joints or amphiarthroses.

7 (B) Adductor longus, biceps femoris, and gastrocnemius are associated with the lower extremity. Adductor longus adducts thigh at hip joint; biceps femoris is one of the hamstrings on posterior side of the thigh and flexes the knee; gastrocnemius is located on posterior leg and plantar flexes the foot. Sternocleidomastoid (SCM) is a neck muscle.

8 (A) Central nervous system (CNS) includes brain and spinal cord; cerebrum and cerebellum are parts of brain. Peripheral nervous system (PNS) consists of 12 pairs of cranial nerves and 31 pairs of spinal nerves.

9 (C) Pons in the brainstem contains apneustic and pneumotaxic centers, which regulate rate and depth of breathing. Heart rate and blood pressure are established by vital centers in the medulla oblongata. Auditory cortex is in temporal lobe, and visual cortex is in occipital lobe; both are in cerebrum. Cerebellum is motor area that coordinates skeletal muscle activity and is important in maintaining muscle tone, posture, and equilibrium.

10 (C) Afferent division of peripheral nervous system (PNS) carries sensory impulses to the central nervous system, and the efferent division carries motor impulses from central nervous system (CNS) to muscles and glands (effectors). Some, but NOT all, cranial nerves are sensory; some are motor, and others have BOTH sensory and motor components. All spinal nerves have BOTH sensory and motor components.

11 (C) Autonomic nervous system (ANS) is the visceral efferent portion of peripheral nervous system (PNS). Includes sympathetic (SANS) and parasympathetic (PANS) divisions, and its effectors are cardiac muscle, smooth muscle, and glands.

12 (B) General senses are widely distributed in the body. Proprioception is a general sense of position

or orientation, detected by Golgi tendon organs and muscle spindles. Meissner's and pacinian corpuscles are receptors that detect the general senses of touch and pressure. Taste and smell are special senses that are localized and closely related.

13 (A) Rods and cones are visual receptors (photoreceptors) located in the retina, the innermost layer of the eye. Cornea is the clear portion of outermost fibrous layer. Ciliary body changes shape of the lens to focus light rays on visual receptors of the retina.

14 (D) Middle ear contains malleus, incus, and stapes, three ossicles that transmit sound waves to inner ear. Receptors for hearing are located in organ of Corti, part of cochlea of the inner ear. Receptors for equilibrium are located in vestibule and semicircular canals of inner ear.

15 (D) Aldosterone is a steroid hormone that helps regulate fluid and electrolyte balance and is produced by adrenal cortex. Steroids are derivatives of cholesterol and react with receptors inside the cell. Protein hormones react with receptors on cell membrane.

16 (D) Monocytes are a type of leukocytes, cells that do NOT contain hemoglobin. Thrombocytes or platelets are fragments of cells and function in blood clotting. Erythrocytes are red blood cells (RBCs), which contain hemoglobin and transport oxygen.

17 (B) Blood types are determined by the agglutinogens on the surface of the RBC (red blood cell). Type A blood has A agglutinogens and anti-B agglutinins. In transfusion reactions the recipient's agglutinins react with the agglutinogens of the donor. The anti-B agglutinins of the type A blood (recipient) will react with type B agglutinogens found in type B and type AB blood; therefore these two blood types CANNOT be used as donors. Type O blood has no agglutinogens on the RBC surface and is considered the universal donor.

18 (B) Under normal conditions, no anti-Rh agglutinins are present in either Rh+ or Rh− blood on the red blood cells (RBCs). An Rh− person who comes into contact with Rh+ blood, however, develops these agglutinins. If such a woman becomes pregnant with an Rh+ fetus, some of her anti-Rh agglutinins may cross the placenta and react with the Rh+ agglutinogens of the fetus. Reaction may cause breakdown of the fetal RBCs, resulting in hemolytic disease of the newborn (erythroblastosis fetalis).

19 (A) Descending aorta and left atrium contain blood that has been freshly oxygenated in the lungs. Venous blood, such as that in the hepatic portal vein, has lower oxygen content. Hepatic portal vein receives blood from digestive system and has higher nutrient (glucose) content than other vessels.

20 (B) Right lymphatic duct collects lymph from upper right quadrant, which then drains into the right subclavian vein. Lymph from the remaining three quarters, including inguinal lymph nodes, enters the thoracic duct, which carries it to the left subclavian vein.

21 (C) Pharynx, trachea, and bronchi are conducting passages for air. Diffusion of gases, oxygen, and carbon dioxide occurs across the simple squamous epithelial walls of the alveoli.

22 (D) Right lung is shorter and wider and has a greater volume than the left. BOTH lungs are covered by the pleura, a serous membrane. Left lung is divided into two lobes and has an indentation for the apex of the heart. Right lung is divided into three lobes by oblique and horizontal fissures.

23 (D) Amylase is an enzyme that hydrolyzes starches into disaccharides. It is produced by both salivary glands and the pancreas but NOT by the stomach. Hydrochloric acid, gastrin, and pepsinogen are all produced by stomach mucosa.

24 (C) Cholecystokinin (pancreozymin) stimulates contraction of the gallbladder and production of pancreatic enzymes. Gastrin is a hormone that increases stomach activity. Secretin is a hormone produced by the small intestine that stimulates the pancreas to secrete a fluid that is rich in bicarbonate ions. Alkalinity of the bicarbonate ions neutralizes the acid chyme from the stomach so that pancreatic enzymes can function.

25 (A) Oxygenated blood is transported to the liver by hepatic artery. Hepatic portal vein delivers nutrient-rich blood from the digestive tract to the liver. Venous blood is drained from the liver by the hepatic vein. Bile (gall) is yellow-green alkaline fluid secreted by hepatocytes (cells) from the liver.

26 (C) Urine is produced in the kidney, flows into the ureter, and transports urine to the bladder for storage. During micturition, urine flows from the bladder through the urethra to the exterior.

27 (B) Orchitis is an acute inflammatory reaction of the testis caused by infection. MOST cases are associated with a viral infection like mumps. Emesis is vomiting. Prostate becomes enlarged as a result of infection and/or cancer. No glandular cells in the penis contribute to the seminal fluid.

28 (B) Basic structure of the helix of DNA is a double helix with two strands of DNA running antiparallel to each other. RNA is a single-stranded molecule.

29 (D) Both RNA and DNA are involved in transcription, the process of transferring genetic information from DNA to mRNA. RNA is dissimilar to DNA in that it is single stranded, contains uridine monophosphate, and is involved in translation of protein.

30 (B) Process of breaking large complex molecules into smaller, simpler units is called catabolism. Anabolism is a process of building large complex molecules from smaller molecules. Electron transport and oxidative phosphorylation constitute the pathway by which electrons are donated from NADH and $FADH_2$ to a series of proteins, which results in production of ATP.

31 (C) Lactic acid is a product of anaerobic metabolism. Constantly produced from pyruvate by way of enzyme lactate dehydrogenase (LDH), in process of fermentation during normal metabolism and exercise. Does NOT increase in concentration until the rate of lactate production exceeds the rate of lactate removal; this is governed by a number of factors, including monocarboxylate transporters, concentration and isoform of LDH, and oxidative capacity of tissues. Concentration of blood can rise during intense exertion.

32 (D) According to Fick's law of diffusion, the greatest net movement of a substance across a membrane will occur if the available surface area is large. If the concentration gradient was great, the thickness of the membrane was small, the temperature was increased, and the permeability was high, such conditions would ALL facilitate diffusion.

33 (A) Osmosis is associated with water movement across a membrane. Membrane permeability may affect solute movement, which in turn drags water with it, affecting osmosis. Osmosis is IMPORTANT in biological systems, since many biological membranes are semipermeable. These membranes are impermeable to organic solutes with large molecules, such as polysaccharides, while permeable to water and small, uncharged solutes. Others are NOT true of osmosis.

34 (E) Facilitated diffusion does NOT require ATP. Facilitated diffusion (facilitated transport) is a process of diffusion, a form of passive transport facilitated by transport proteins. Facilitated diffusion may occur either across biological membranes or through aqueous compartments of organism.

35 (C) Autonomic nervous system (ANS) is part of the peripheral nervous system (PNS) and innervates NOT only smooth and cardiac muscles, but also glands. Major neurotransmitters include acetylcholine (parasympathetic) and norepinephrine (sympathetic).

36 (B) NO external Ca^{+2} is needed for contraction. ALL Ca^+ release is regulated by sarcoplasmic reticulum.

37 (B) Unlike skeletal muscles, which have contraction times of 60 msec, cardiac muscles have greater contraction times of 200 msec. This length of time ensures that this muscle will NOT exhibit summation. Cardiac muscles contain MORE mitochondria and contract in response to norepinephrine but NOT acetylcholine.

38 (A) Three chemical classes of hormones are amines, peptides, and steroids. Hormone is a chemical messenger that carries a signal from one cell (or group of cells) to another via the blood. Regulates function of target cells, i.e., cells that express a receptor. Action (net effect) of hormones is determined by a number of factors, including pattern of secretion and response of the receiving tissue (signal transduction response). Endocrine molecules are secreted (released) directly into the bloodstream, whereas exocrine molecules are secreted directly into the duct and from the duct flow either into the bloodstream or from cell to cell by diffusion.

39 **(A)** Parathyroid hormone decreases Ca^{+2} plasma levels in response to hypercalcemia. Acts with vitamin D to increase intestinal absorption of Ca^{+2}. It may influence phosphate handling, but NOT metabolism, by kidneys.

40 **(C)** Pancreas is BOTH endocrine and exocrine gland. Produces glucagon, elevates plasma glucose levels. Exocrine function results in secretion of enzymes (NOT hormones) that break down carbohydrates and proteins.

41 **(C)** Aldosterone is produced by the adrenal cortex, and its secretion is stimulated by LOW plasma levels of Na^+ and high levels of K^+. Low blood pressure through the renin-angiotensin system also stimulates its production.

42 **(D)** Glucocorticoids suppress the immune system. Class of steroid hormones characterized by an ability to bind with the cortisol receptor and trigger similar effects. Distinguished from mineralocorticoids and sex steroids by the specific receptors, target cells, and effects. Corticosteroid refers to BOTH glucocorticoids and mineralocorticoids but is often used as synonym for glucocorticoid. Cortisol (hydrocortisone) is MOST important. Essential for life, and regulates or supports a variety of important cardiovascular, metabolic, immunological, homeostatic functions.

43 **(B)** Testosterone production is stimulated by luteinizing hormone, stimulates protein production, and increases red blood cell production, resulting in higher hematocrit values (number of RBCs in blood) in men compared with those in women. Testosterone is a steroid hormone from the androgen group. Testosterone is secreted MAINLY in the testes of males and the ovaries of females, although small amounts are also secreted by the adrenal glands. MAIN male sex hormone and anabolic steroid.

44 **(B)** Estrogen induces the production of progesterone receptors in the uterus, acts as antioxidant, and increases bone density. Estrogens are a group of steroid compounds, named for importance in the estrous cycle, and functioning as the MAIN female sex hormone. Estrogens are used as part of some oral contraceptives (birth control pills [BCP]), in estrogen replacement therapy of postmenopausal women, and

in hormone therapy for transsexual women. Like all steroid hormones, estrogens readily diffuse across the cell membrane; inside the cell, they interact with estrogen receptors.

45 **(D)** Inhibin is a peptide that inhibits production of follicle-stimulating hormone. Thus it participates in the regulation of the menstrual cycle. Produced in gonads, pituitary gland, placenta, other organs.

46 **(A)** Alveolar perfusion by blood is a major factor associated with normal gas exchange. Because of differences in solubilities for CO_2 and O_2 (GREATER for CO_2 than O_2), gas exchange for oxygen is MORE limited than CO_2 movement. Thus gradient for O_2 is 60 mm Hg and gradient for CO_2 is 5 mm Hg. No gas exchange occurs in bronchi or pulmonary artery.

47 **(C)** Pleural space normally contains ONLY a small amount of fluid. Pressure within is negative (below atmospheric) because of opposing forces of lung and chest wall and fluid movements out of the space. Surfactant is produced by type II cells in lungs.

48 **(A)** Metabolism generally is coupled with ventilation; thus as O_2 demands increase, ventilation increases. Ventilation is depressed by high levels of CO_2 and by anoxia.

49 **(A)** Bicarbonate ions are ~72% of the CO_2 that is transported.

50 **(D)** Increased blood flow to the cells is the ONLY listed condition that would increase O_2 transport or access. Inhalation of carbon monoxide would decrease the amount of O_2 bound to hemoglobin; decreased hemoglobin levels would decrease the amount of hemoglobin available; high altitudes would decrease the alveolar and arterial pO_2 and cyanide poisons enzymes that use O_2 to make ATP.

51 **(D)** Hyperventilation results in the "blowing off" of CO_2 and also causes a decrease in H^+ and increase in level of O_2. State of breathing faster and/or deeper than necessary thereby reduces CO_2 concentration of blood below normal. Can cause such symptoms as numbness or tingling in hands, feet, and lips, lightheadedness, dizziness, headache, chest pain, slurred speech, and sometimes fainting, particularly when accompanied by the Valsalva maneuver.

52 **(D)** Intrinsic factor is essential to absorption of vitamin B_{12}. Stomach does NOT produce vitamin B_{12}, but parietal cells of stomach produce glycoprotein, which is necessary for absorption of vitamin B_{12} later in the terminal ileum. Upon entry into stomach, vitamin B_{12} becomes bound to one of two B_{12}-binding proteins present in gastric juice. In the LESS acidic environment of small intestine, these proteins dissociate from vitamin, enabling it to bind to intrinsic factor and enter portal circulation through a receptor in ileal mucosa specific for the B_{12}–intrinsic factor complex.

53 (A) Liver produces red blood cells in the embryo and fetus. Synthesizes factors needed for clotting and amino acids. Also stores glycogen, iron, copper, and vitamins A and D. Steroid hormones are synthesized MAINLY in gonads and in adrenal cortex.

54 (C) Enzymes that digest chyme in the lumen are produced by the pancreas. Small intestine produces ONLY intracellular enzymes.

55 (C) Neither food NOR hormones are absorbed by large intestine. Major functions include reabsorption of water and electrolytes. Intrinsic factor is produced in the stomach.

56 (C) Angiotensin II is produced by endothelial cells in lung. Angiotensin is an oligopeptide in blood that causes vasoconstriction, increased blood pressure, release of aldosterone from adrenal cortex. Powerful dipsogen. Derived from precursor molecule angiotensinogen, serum globulin produced in liver. Plays IMPORTANT role in renin-angiotensin system. Angiotensin I is converted to angiotensin II through removal of two terminal residues by the enzyme angiotensin-converting enzyme (ACE, kinase), found MAINLY in capillaries of lung. Angiotensin II acts as endocrine or autocrine, paracrine, or intracrine hormone. Angiotensin II is degraded to angiotensin III by angiotensinases that are located in red blood cells and vascular beds of MOST tissues. Has a half-life of around 30 seconds in circulation but as long as 15 to 30 minutes in tissue. Angiotensin II thus increases blood pressure; ACE inhibitor drugs are major drugs against hypertension (high blood pressure).

57 (A) Blockage of ureter increases pressures within kidney and decreases urine excretion. Ureters are ducts that carry urine from kidneys to the urinary bladder. They are muscular tubes that can propel urine along by motions of peristalsis.

58 (D) Urethra is a part of urinary system but is NOT part of nephron. Others are parts of nephron. Urethra is tube that connects bladder to the outside of body. Has excretory function in both genders to pass urine to outside, and also reproductive function in the male, as passage for sperm.

59 (A) Efferent arteriole constriction increases GFR. Increase in the leakiness of the Bowman's capsule also increases GFR. Constriction of afferent arteriole decreases GFR.

60 (C) During respiratory acidosis, kidneys retain HCO_3^- and excrete H^+. Respiratory acidosis is acidosis (abnormal acidity of the blood) caused by decreased ventilation of pulmonary alveoli, leading to elevated arterial carbon dioxide concentration (Pa_{CO_2}). Clinical disturbance that is due to alveolar hypoventilation. Production of CO_2 occurs rapidly, and failure of ventilation promptly increases level of Pa_{CO_2}.

61 (A) Cardiac output (CO) is increased by increase in contractility of heart. Other factors that increase cardiac output are increased heart rate, venous return, stroke volume. The CO is volume of blood being pumped by heart, in particular by a ventricle in a minute.

62 (A) Factors that influence total peripheral resistance include diameter or radius of blood vessels (where R = ¼) and viscosity (increased viscosity leads to increased resistance). Thus as diameter of blood vessels decreases, total peripheral resistance increases. Radii of blood vessels are increased by production of metabolites, cytokines, histamine. Viscosity is increased during dehydration.

63 (C) Chemoreceptor for O_2, CO_2, pH; all others sense pressure or volume changes. Sensory receptor that transduces a chemical signal into an action potential. Detects certain chemical stimuli in the environment.

64 (B) Decreased blood pressure causes increased SNS discharge.

65 (B) Hypertension contributes to formation of atherosclerotic plaques. Also increases work of heart; tends to increase with BOTH age and obesity.

66 (B) All of these situations, EXCEPT when epinephrine is released rapidly, result in decrease in blood pressure.

67 (C) Ribosomes that produce protein are located on rough endoplasmic reticulum (RER) or in cytoplasm, NOT plasma membrane.

68 (A) Mitochondria produce ATP. Others are involved in metabolic handling of internally produced chemicals (Golgi apparatus) and/or externally produced chemicals (peroxisomes and lysosomes) but do NOT produce ATP.

69 (A) First (I) cranial nerve (olfactory) is FIRST of 12 cranial nerves. Specialized olfactory receptor neurons of the olfactory nerve are located in the olfactory mucosa of the upper parts of the nasal cavity. Nerve consists of collection of sensory nerve fibers that extend from olfactory epithelium to the olfactory bulb, passing through many openings of cribriform plate, sievelike structure. Sense of smell (olfaction) arises from stimulation of olfactory receptors by activation from gas molecules that pass by nose during respiration. Resulting electrical activity is transduced into olfactory bulb, which then transmits electrical activity to other parts of olfactory system and rest of central nervous system by way of olfactory tract.

70 (B) Liver is LARGEST visceral organ (internal organ of the body); skin is LARGEST external organ.

71 (B) Glucose provides energy to brain. Monosaccharide (simple sugar) is an important carbohydrate. Insulin reaction and other mechanisms regulate concentration of glucose in blood; high fasting blood sugar level is indication of prediabetic and diabetic conditions.

72 **(A)** Pancreas has both alpha and beta cells. Alpha cells release glucagon, and beta cells produce insulin.

73 **(C)** Glycogen provides a food storage system for all forms of animal life. One area of storage is in liver, which assists in regulating blood sugar. Glycogen storage also occurs in the muscle, where glycogen serves as an energy source for muscle contraction.

74 **(A)** Initiation of starch digestion begins in the oral cavity during chewing. Enzyme salivary amylase begins to break starch into disaccharides such as maltose. Stomach acids hydrolyze maltose and sucrose, but ONLY to a small extent. Digestion continues in the small intestine; there, enzyme pancreatic amylase (from the pancreas) breaks down the remaining disaccharides into monosaccharides.

75 **(A)** Trigeminal is also designated as fifth (V) cranial nerve (V). Seventh (VII) cranial nerve is the facial. Tenth (X) cranial nerve is the vagus. Twelfth (XII) cranial nerve is the hypoglossal. However, others innervate important structures of the oral cavity. Facial nerve is responsible for sensation in the face. Sensory information from the face and body is processed by parallel pathways in the central nervous system. Trigeminal is MAINLY a sensory nerve from the oral cavity, but it also has certain motor functions (biting, chewing, swallowing), such as innervating muscles of mastication.

CHAPTER 4

Head, Neck, and Dental Anatomy

REGIONS OF THE HEAD

Regions of the head include frontal, parietal, occipital, temporal, orbital, nasal, infraorbital, zygomatic, buccal, oral, mental regions. Specific landmarks are noted for each region.

- See CD-ROM for Chapter Terms and WebLinks.
- See Chapter 3, Anatomy, Biochemistry, and Physiology: general anatomy.

A. Frontal region: supraorbital ridge under each eyebrow; frontal eminence forms the prominence of the forehead.

B. Parietal and occipital regions: covered by scalp, which may be covered by hair.

C. Temporal region and external ear: include auricle and external acoustic meatus (EAM):
   1. Helix: superior and posterior free margin of auricle, ends inferiorly at lobule (earlobe).
   2. Tragus: part of auricle anterior to external acoustic meatus; antitragus: flap of tissue opposite tragus (radiographic landmarks).

D. Orbital region: includes eyeball and supporting structures within orbit (bony socket):
   1. Lateral canthus: outer corner where upper and lower eyelids meet; medial canthus: inner corner of eye.
   2. Upper and lower eyelids: cover and protect each eyeball; lacrimal gland: located behind each upper eyelid and within orbit and produces lacrimal fluid (tears).
   3. Sclera: white area of eyeball; iris: circular central area of color; pupil: central opening in iris.
   4. Conjunctiva: membrane that lines inside of eyelids and front of eyeball.

E. Nasal region and external nose: root of nose is located between eyes:
   1. Nasion: midpoint landmark; bridge of nose is inferior.
   2. Nares (nostrils): separated by midline nasal septum, bounded laterally by alae.
   3. Apex of nose: tip.

F. Infraorbital region: inferior to orbital region and lateral to nasal region; zygomatic region overlies cheekbone; buccal region is composed of soft tissues of cheek:
   1. Zygomatic arch: extends from just below lateral margin of eye to upper part of ear.
   2. Temporomandibular joint (TMJ): inferior to zygomatic arch and just anterior to ear, where upper skull forms a joint with lower jaw.
   3. Cheek: forms the side of face between nose, mouth, and ear; composed MAINLY of fat (buccal fat pad) and muscles, including masseter muscle; angle of mandible, sharp angle of lower jaw that is inferior to earlobe.

G. Oral region: includes lips, oral cavity, palate, tongue, floor of mouth, parts of pharynx:
   1. Nasolabial sulcus: groove running upward between labial commissure and ala of nose; labiomental groove: horizontal groove to which lower lip extends and which separates lower lip from chin in mental region.
   2. Vermilion zone: darker portion of lips than surrounding skin; vermilion border: outlines lips from surrounding skin, transition zone.
   3. Philtrum: vertical groove on midline of upper lip, extending downward from nasal septum; tubercle of upper lip: thicker area where philtrum terminates; labial commissure: where upper and lower lips meet at each corner of mouth.

H. Mental region: chin's mental protuberance (prominence), with possible midline depression (dimple) that marks underlying bony fusion of lower jaw.

Oral Cavity

Oral cavity is the inside of the mouth and includes jaws, palate, tongue, floor of the mouth, pharynx, and all associated oral mucosal tissues.

- See Chapters 2, Embryology and Histology: oral cavity histology; 3, Anatomy, Biochemistry, and Physiology: pharynx, digestion.

A. Structures labeled according to location: (1) lingual, if closest to tongue; (2) palatal, if closest to palate; (3) facial, if closest to facial surface; (4) buccal, if closest to inner cheek; (5) labial, if closest to lips.

B. Mucous membranes (oral mucosa): line inner oral cavity; parts of the lips are lined by labial mucosa; buccal mucosa lines inner cheek, covers buccal fat pad, including parotid papilla, and contains a duct opening from parotid salivary gland.

C. Maxillary and mandibular bones (jaws): lie beneath the respective lips and contain primary and/or permanent teeth, including incisors, canines, premolars, molars, depending on dentition present.

1. Maxillary and mandibular vestibules: upper and lower spaces between cheeks, lips, and gingival tissues.
2. Alveolar mucosa: lines each vestibule and meets labial or buccal mucosa at the mucobuccal fold (depth or height is location for local anesthetic nerve injections given into soft tissue).
3. Labial frenum: fold of tissue located at the midline between the labial mucosa and alveolar mucosa of the maxilla and mandible.
4. Gingival tissues (discussed later): surround maxillary and mandibular teeth.

D. Palate (roof of mouth):
1. Anterior part: hard palate and includes median palatine raphe (median palatal suture), incisive papilla, and palatine rugae, which are irregular ridges of tissue directly posterior to the incisive papilla; posterior part: soft palate and includes uvula.
2. Pterygomandibular fold: extends from junction of the hard and soft palates down to mandible, just posterior to the most distal mandibular tooth; separates cheek from pharynx; retromolar pad is located just distal to last tooth of the mandible.

E. Tongue (Figure 4-1):
1. Body: *anterior two thirds* and includes the tip (apex).
2. Base: *posterior one third*, which attaches to floor of the mouth; does NOT lie within the oral cavity but rather in the oral part of pharynx.
3. Lateral surfaces: located on each side; dorsal surface is located on top and includes median lingual sulcus; ventral surface (underside) has visible deep lingual veins (varicosities in elderly) and plicae fimbriatae, with fringelike projections.
4. Lingual papillae: elevated structures of specialized mucosa on tongue surface, some of which are associated with taste buds (see Chapters 2, Embryology and Histology; 3, Anatomy, Biochemistry, and Physiology: lingual papillae, taste sensation).
5. Sulcus terminalis: V-shaped groove located posteriorly on dorsal surface that separates base from body.
6. Foramen cecum: pitlike depression in center of sulcus terminalis; point of attachment of thyroglossal duct, embryological connection for development of thyroid gland.
7. Lingual tonsil: irregular mass of tonsillar tissue located more posteriorly than sulcus terminalis on the dorsal surface.

F. Floor of the mouth: located inferior to ventral surface of tongue (Figure 4-2):
1. Lingual frenum: midline fold of tissue between ventral surface of tongue and floor of mouth.

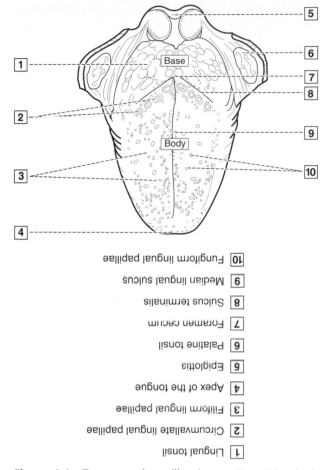

Figure 4-1 Tongue and tonsillar tissues. (From Fehrenbach MJ, ed: Dental anatomy coloring book, St. Louis, 2008, Saunders/Elsevier.)

1	Lingual tonsil
2	Circumvallate lingual papillae
3	Filiform lingual papillae
4	Apex of the tongue
5	Epiglottis
6	Palatine tonsil
7	Foramen cecum
8	Sulcus terminalis
9	Median lingual sulcus
10	Fungiform lingual papillae

2. Sublingual fold: V-shaped ridge of tissue on floor of mouth; contains duct openings from sublingual salivary gland.
3. Sublingual caruncle: small papilla at anterior end of each sublingual fold; contains duct openings from BOTH submandibular and sublingual salivary glands.

G. Pharynx (throat): muscular tube that serves BOTH respiratory and digestive systems, divided into nasopharynx, oropharynx, laryngopharynx.

REGIONS OF THE NECK

Neck is divided by the cervical muscle, **sternocleidomastoid muscle** (SCM), diagonally each side into anterior cervical and posterior cervical triangles.

A. Anterior region: corresponds to two anterior cervical triangles, separated by midline, and subdivided into submandibular and midline submental triangle by digastric muscle (Figure 4-3).
B. Posterior cervical triangle: considered lateral region and is posterior to the SCM on each side.

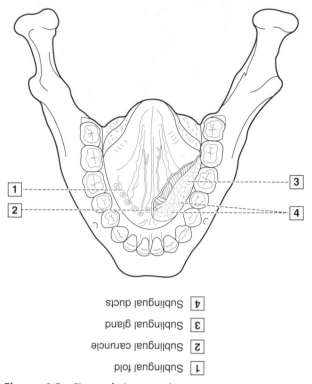

4 Sublingual ducts

3 Sublingual gland

2 Sublingual caruncle

1 Sublingual fold

Figure 4-2 Floor of the mouth. (From Fehrenbach MJ, ed: Dental anatomy coloring book, St. Louis, 2008, Saunders/Elsevier.)

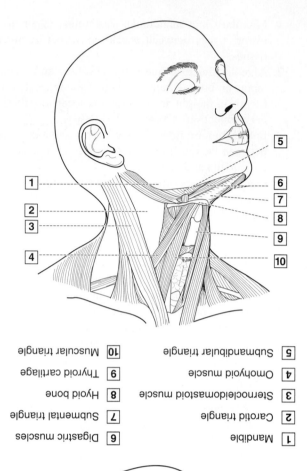

10 Muscular triangle	5 Submandibular triangle
9 Thyroid cartilage	4 Omohyoid muscle
8 Hyoid bone	3 Sternocleidomastoid muscle
7 Submental triangle	2 Carotid triangle
6 Digastric muscles	1 Mandible

C. Thyroid cartilage: prominence of larynx at anterior midline; vocal cords (ligaments) are attached to posterior surface.

D. Hyoid bone: suspended in anterior midline; superior to thyroid cartilage, attached to many muscles; controls position of base of tongue (see Chapter 3, Anatomy, Biochemistry, and Physiology).

SKULL

Skeletal system serves as a base during palpation of soft tissues and as a marker during location of soft tissue lesions, administration of local anesthesia, radiographic procedures. Bones may be a factor in spread of dental infection and may undergo a disease process themselves.

Skull (22 bones), with single and paired bones. Immovable, with EXCEPTION of mandible and temporomandibular joint (TMJ). Has movable articulation with bony vertebral column in neck area. Contains bony openings for important nerves and blood vessels (Table 4-1). Has paranasal sinuses within that serve to lighten bony mass. Has many associated processes that are involved in important structures. To study its landmarks, important to view from superior, lateral, inferior, anterior. Its bones are divided into three categories: cranial, facial, hyoid, which are noted on each view; each category is discussed separately next.

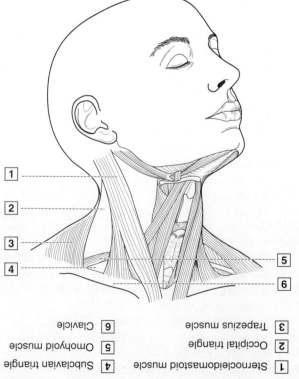

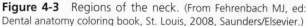

6 Clavicle	3 Trapezius muscle
5 Omohyoid muscle	2 Occipital triangle
4 Subclavian triangle	1 Sternocleidomastoid muscle

Figure 4-3 Regions of the neck. (From Fehrenbach MJ, ed: Dental anatomy coloring book, St. Louis, 2008, Saunders/Elsevier.)

Table 4-1 Bony openings in the skull and their associated nerves and blood vessels

Bony opening	Bony location	Nerves and vessels
Carotid canal	Temporal	Internal carotid artery
Cribriform plate with foramina	Ethmoid	Olfactory nerves
External acoustic meatus	Temporal	(Opening to tympanic cavity)
Foramen lacerum	Sphenoid, occipital, temporal	(Cartilage)
Foramen magnum	Occipital	Spinal cord, vertebral arteries, eleventh cranial nerve
Foramen ovale	Sphenoid	Mandibular division of fifth cranial nerve
Foramen rotundum	Sphenoid	Fifth cranial nerve
Foramen spinosum	Sphenoid	Middle meningeal artery
Greater palatine foramen	Palatine	Greater palatine nerve and vessels
Hypoglossal canal	Occipital	Ninth cranial nerve
Incisive foramen	Maxilla	Nasopalatine nerve and branches of sphenopalatine artery
Inferior orbital fissure	Sphenoid and maxilla	Infraorbital and zygomatic nerves, infraorbital artery, ophthalmic vein
Infraorbital foramen and canal	Maxilla	Infraorbital nerve and vessels
Internal acoustic meatus	Temporal	Seventh and eighth cranial nerves
Jugular foramen	Occipital and temporal	Internal jugular vein and ninth, tenth, eleventh cranial nerves
Lesser palatine foramen	Palatine	Lesser palatine nerve and vessels
Mandibular foramen	Mandible	Inferior alveolar nerve and vessels
Mental foramen	Mandible	Mental nerve and vessels
Optic canal and foramen	Sphenoid	Optic nerve and ophthalmic artery
Petrotympanic fissure	Temporal	Chorda tympani nerve
Pterygoid canal	Sphenoid	Area nerves and vessels
Stylomastoid foramen	Temporal	Seventh cranial nerve
Superior orbital fissure	Sphenoid	Third, fourth, sixth cranial nerves and ophthalmic nerve and vein

From Fehrenbach MJ, Herring SW: Illustrated anatomy of the head and neck, ed 3, St. Louis, 2007, Saunders/Elsevier.

- See Chapter 3, Anatomy, Biochemistry, and Physiology: skeletal system.
A. Superior view of skull: major bones and sutures (joints between bones of the skull are immovable; fontanelles ["soft spots"] on an infant's head).
    1. Coronal suture: frontal and parietal bones.
    2. Sagittal suture: paired parietal bones.
    3. Lambdoidal suture: single occipital bone and paired parietal bones.
B. Anterior view of skull: orbits and nasal cavity (Figure 4-4):

1. Orbits: contain and protect eyeballs:
    a. Orbital walls: orbital plates of frontal, ethmoid, lacrimal; orbital surfaces of maxilla; zygomatic bone; and orbital surface of greater wing of sphenoid.
    b. Orbital apex: lesser wing of sphenoid and palatine bones; optic canal is opening in orbital apex.
    c. Superior orbital fissure (SOF): located between the greater and lesser wings of sphenoid and connects orbit and cranial cavities; carries oculomotor, trochlear, abducens, ophthalmic vessels.

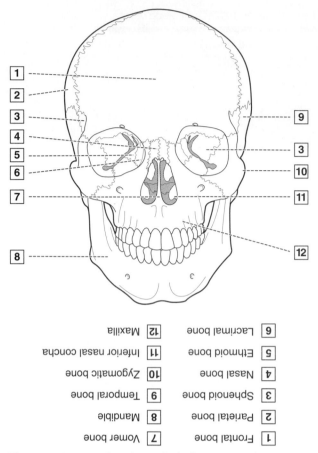

12	Maxilla	6	Lacrimal bone
11	Inferior nasal concha	5	Ethmoid bone
10	Zygomatic bone	4	Nasal bone
9	Temporal bone	3	Sphenoid bone
8	Mandible	2	Parietal bone
7	Vomer bone	1	Frontal bone

Figure 4-4 Anterior view of skull. (From Fehrenbach MJ, ed: Dental anatomy coloring book, St. Louis, 2008, Saunders/Elsevier.)

d. Inferior orbital fissure (IOF): located between greater wing of sphenoid and maxilla; connects orbit with infratemporal and pterygopalatine fossae; carries infraorbital and zygomatic nerves, branches of maxillary, infraorbital, and inferior ophthalmic vessels.

2. Nasal cavity: has piriform aperture for anterior opening; lateral boundaries are formed by maxillae:
   a. Nasal septum: divides nasal cavity into two parts; formed by nasal septal cartilages, perpendicular plate of ethmoid bone, vomer.
   b. Nasal conchae: located on each lateral wall; superior nasal concha and middle nasal concha are formed from ethmoid bone; inferior nasal concha is separate facial bone.
   c. Nasal meatus: grooves beneath each concha, have openings through which paranasal sinuses and nasolacrimal duct communicate with nasal cavity.

C. Lateral view of skull (Figure 4-5):
   1. Superior temporal line: superior ridge; inferior temporal line: superior boundary of temporal fossa; squamosal suture is between temporal and parietal bones.

2. Temporal fossa: formed by several bones of skull, contains body of temporalis; infratemporal fossa: inferior to temporal fossa; pterygopalatine fossa: deep to infratemporal fossa.
3. Zygomatic arch: formed by union of temporal process of zygomatic bone and zygomatic process of temporal bone.
4. TMJ: ONLY freely movable joint in the head, between temporal bone and mandible.

D. Inferior view of external surface of skull (Figure 4-6):
   1. Hard palate: forms floor of nasal cavity and roof of mouth at anterior section; formed by palatine processes of maxilla and horizontal plates of palatine bones; bordered by alveolar process of maxilla and maxillary teeth (Figure 4-7).
   2. Median palatine suture: midline articulation between palatine processes of maxillae anteriorly as well as horizontal plates of palatine bones posteriorly, noted clinically as the median palatal raphe, MORE prominent and thicker in the soft palate region; transverse palatine suture articulates with palatine processes of maxillae and horizontal plates of palatine bones.
   3. Jugular foramen: opening through which internal jugular vein and glossopharyngeal, vagus, accessory nerves pass; foramen lacerum is large, irregularly shaped, filled with cartilage.

E. Superior view of internal surface of skull (Figure 4-8).

Cranial Bones

Cranial bones (8) form cranium and include occipital, frontal, parietal, temporal, sphenoid, ethmoid. See earlier views of skull.

A. Occipital: *single* that is located in MOST posterior part of skull:
   1. Foramen magnum on external surface: largest skull opening; carries spinal cord, vertebral arteries, accessory nerve.
   2. Occipital condyles: pair located lateral and anterior to foramen magnum; movable articulation with atlas.
   3. Basilar part: four-sided plate; pharyngeal tubercle is midline projection anterior to foramen magnum, with paired hypoglossal canals that carry hypoglossal nerve.

B. Frontal: *single* that forms forehead and superior part of orbits:
   1. Frontal sinuses: pair contained within, superior to nasal cavity; each sinus communicates with and drains into nasal cavity by means of frontonasal duct to middle nasal meatus.
   2. Supraorbital ridges: elevations over superior part of orbit, and supraorbital notch is located on medial part of the supraorbital ridge; lacrimal fossa is located just inside lateral part of supraorbital ridge and contains lacrimal gland, which produces lacrimal fluid.

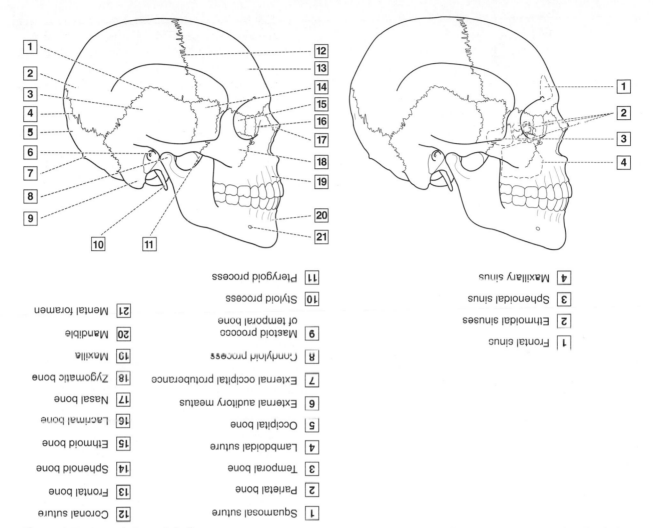

1	Squamosal suture	12	Coronal suture
2	Parietal bone	13	Frontal bone
3	Temporal bone	14	Sphenoid bone
4	Lambdoidal suture	15	Ethmoid bone
5	Occipital bone	16	Lacrimal bone
6	External auditory meatus	17	Nasal bone
7	External occipital protuberance	18	Zygomatic bone
8	Condyloid process	19	Maxilla
9	Mastoid process of temporal bone	20	Mandible
10	Styloid process	21	Mental foramen
11	Pterygoid process		

1	Frontal sinus
2	Ethmoidal sinuses
3	Sphenoidal sinus
4	Maxillary sinus

Figure 4-5   Lateral view of skull. (From Fehrenbach MJ, ed: Dental anatomy coloring book, St. Louis, 2008, Saunders/Elsevier.)

C. Parietal bones: *paired* and BOTH articulate with each other at sagittal suture.
D. Temporal bones: *paired* and form lateral walls of skull:
   1. Tympanic part: forms MOST of external acoustic meatus; petrous part contains mastoid process and carotid canal, which carries internal carotid artery; mastoid notch is medial to mastoid process; styloid process is bony projection.
   2. Stylomastoid foramen: carries seventh cranial nerve (facial), located between styloid process and mastoid process; internal acoustic meatus is on intracranial surface, carries vestibulocochlear nerve and seventh cranial nerve (facial).
E. Sphenoid ("butterfly"): *single* in midline; MOST complex; articulates with frontal, parietal, ethmoid, temporal, zygomatic, palatine, occipital bones, maxillae, vomer:
   1. Foramen ovale: oval opening that carries mandibular division of fifth cranial nerve (trigeminal); foramen rotundum: round opening that carries maxillary division of the same nerve; foramen spinosum: near spine and carries middle meningeal artery into cranial cavity.
   2. Body: middle position; contains sphenoidal sinus, which communicates with and drains into nasal cavity through opening superior to each superior nasal concha:
      a. Lesser wing of sphenoid: anterior and forms base of orbital apex; greater wing of sphenoid bone: posterolateral process with spine at each corner, divided by infratemporal crest.
      b. Pterygoid process: inferior and consists of lateral and medial plates, between which is pterygoid fossa; hamulus: inferior termination of medial pterygoid plate.
F. Ethmoid: *single* in midline and adjoins vomer:
   1. Two unpaired plates that cross each other, with perpendicular plate midline and vertical, cribriform plate horizontal, perforated by foramina to allow passage of olfactory nerves.

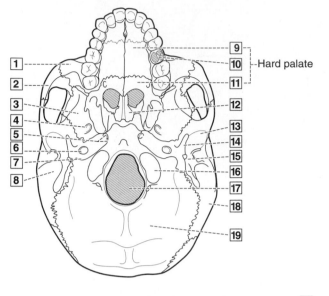

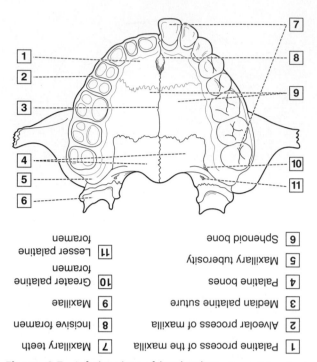

9	Palatine bone (horizontal plate)
10	Alveolar process
9	Maxilla (palatine process)
8	Mastoid process
7	Jugular foramen
6	Carotid canal
5	Foramen lacerum
4	Foramen ovale
3	Sphenoid bone
2	Zygomatic bone
1	Zygomatic process of maxilla

19	Occipital bone
18	Temporal bone
17	Foramen magnum
16	Occipital condyle
15	Stylomastoid foramen
14	Styloid process
13	Mandibular fossa
12	Vomer bone

Figure 4-6 Inferior view of external surface of skull. (From Fehrenbach MJ, ed: Dental anatomy coloring book, St. Louis, 2008, Saunders/Elsevier.)

2. Crista galli: vertical midline continuation of perpendicular plate into cranial cavity; ethmoidal sinuses: in the lateral masses, which open into superior and middle meatus of nasal cavity, forms superior and middle nasal conchae in nasal cavity.

Facial Bones

Facial bones (14) create facial features and serve as base for the dentition. Include vomer, lacrimal, zygomatic, palatine, maxilla, mandible. See earlier skull views. Many landmarks of the facial bones are used for local anesthetic delivery.
- See Chapter 5, Radiology: radiographic descriptions of bones.
A. Vomer: *single* that forms posterior part of nasal septum; located in midsagittal plane, inside nasal cavity; has free posteroinferior border.
B. Smaller bones (but they do just fine unless they participate in any bar fights!):

11	Lesser palatine foramen	6	Sphenoid bone
10	Greater palatine foramen	5	Maxillary tuberosity
9	Maxillae	4	Palatine bones
8	Incisive foramen	3	Median palatine suture
7	Maxillary teeth	2	Alveolar process of maxilla
		1	Palatine process of the maxilla

Figure 4-7 Inferior view of hard palate. (From Fehrenbach MJ, ed: Dental anatomy coloring book, St. Louis, 2008, Saunders/Elsevier.)

1. Lacrimal: *paired* that form small part of anterior medial wall of orbit; nasolacrimal duct is formed at junction of lacrimal and maxillary bones; lacrimal fluid from gland drains into inferior nasal meatus.
2. Nasal: *paired* that form bridge of nose and articulate with each other in the midline above piriform aperture; paired inferior nasal conchae project off maxilla to form part of lateral walls of nasal cavity.
3. Inferior nasal conchae: project off maxilla to form part of lateral walls of nasal cavity.
C. Zygomatic: *paired* that form cheek bones (malar surfaces), each composed of frontal, temporal, maxillary processes:
1. Orbital surface of frontal process forms anterior lateral orbital wall; temporal process of zygomatic bone joins zygomatic process of temporal bone to form zygomatic arch; orbital surface of maxillary process forms part of lateral orbital wall.
D. Palatine: *paired* that consist of horizontal and vertical plates; articulate with each other and with maxillae and sphenoid:
1. Horizontal plates: form posterior part of hard palate, also floor of nasal cavity; posterior part of median palatine suture is located at articulation of two horizontal plates; vertical plates: form part of lateral walls of nasal cavity; BOTH plates contribute to orbital apex.
2. Greater palatine foramen: located in posterolateral region of each of the palatine bones, distal to maxillary third molar, carries greater palatine nerve and

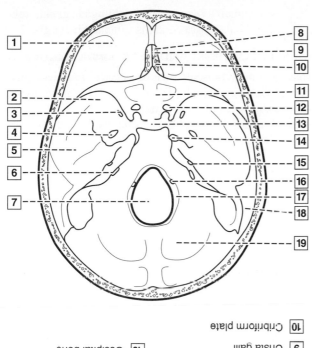

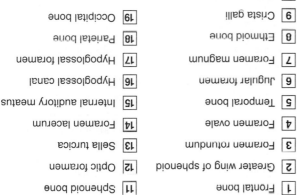

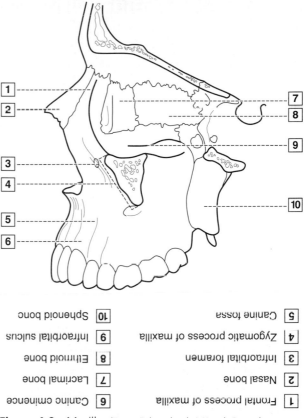

10	Cribriform plate
9	Crista galli
8	Ethmoid bone
7	Foramen magnum
6	Jugular foramen
5	Temporal bone
4	Foramen ovale
3	Foramen rotundum
2	Greater wing of sphenoid
1	Frontal bone

19	Occipital bone
18	Parietal bone
17	Hypoglossal foramen
16	Hypoglossal canal
15	Internal auditory meatus
14	Foramen lacerum
13	Sella turcica
12	Optic foramen
11	Sphenoid bone

Figure 4-8 Superior view of internal surface of skull. (From Fehrenbach MJ, ed: Dental anatomy coloring book, St. Louis, 2008, Saunders/Elsevier.)

10	Sphenoid bone
9	Infraorbital sulcus
8	Ethmoid bone
7	Lacrimal bone
6	Canine eminence

5	Canine fossa
4	Zygomatic process of maxilla
3	Infraorbital foramen
2	Nasal bone
1	Frontal process of maxilla

Figure 4-9 Maxilla. (From Fehrenbach MJ, ed: Dental anatomy coloring book, St. Louis, 2008, Saunders/Elsevier.)

blood vessels; lesser palatine foramen: nearby to carry own vessel to soft palate and tonsils.

E. **Maxilla:** upper jaw, consists of *two* maxillary bones (maxillae) fused together; articulates with frontal, lacrimal, nasal, inferior nasal concha, sphenoid, ethmoid, palatine, zygomatic bones, vomer (Figure 4-9); each maxilla has a body and frontal, zygomatic, palatine, alveolar processes:

1. Body of maxilla contains maxillary sinus located just posterior to maxillary canine and premolars; largest sinus; drains into middle meatus.
2. Inferior orbital fissure: separates each orbital surface from sphenoid; carries infraorbital and zygomatic nerves, infraorbital artery, inferior ophthalmic vein.
3. Infraorbital sulcus groove in floor of orbital surface: becomes infraorbital canal, then terminates as infraorbital foramen; carries infraorbital vessels.

4. Canine fossa: depression posterosuperior to maxillary canine roots; canine eminence is facial ridge over maxillary canine.
5. Lateral wall of nasal cavity: made up mainly of maxilla; floor of nasal cavity is formed by palatine process of maxilla anteriorly, also anterior part of hard palate.
6. Anterior part of median palatine suture: articulation of two fused maxillae (two palatine processes); incisive foramen in anterior midline part of palatine process, just posterior to maxillary central incisors; carries branches of BOTH right and left nasopalatine vessels.
7. **Alveolar process:** contains roots of maxillary teeth; maxillary tuberosity on posterior part is perforated by posterior superior alveolar foramina, allowing entry for posterior superior alveolar vessels.

F. **Mandible:** lower jaw, *single,* ONLY freely movable bone of skull; articulates with temporal bones at each TMJ (Figure 4-10):
1. Mental protuberance: prominence of chin; mandibular symphysis is ridge where bone was formed by fusion.
2. Mental foramen: on outer (lateral) surface of mandible, between apices of mandibular premolars; allows entrance of mental nerve and blood vessels into mandibular canal.

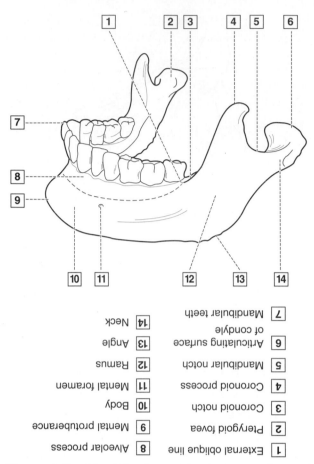

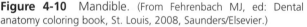

14 Neck		**7**	Mandibular teeth
13 Angle		**6**	Articulating surface of condyle
12 Ramus		**5**	Mandibular notch
11 Mental foramen		**4**	Coronoid process
10 Body		**3**	Coronoid notch
9 Mental protuberance		**2**	Pterygoid fovea
8 Alveolar process		**1**	External oblique line

Figure 4-10 Mandible. (From Fehrenbach MJ, ed: Dental anatomy coloring book, St. Louis, 2008, Saunders/Elsevier.)

3. Mandibular foramen: on inner (medial) surface of ramus, from which inferior alveolar vessels exit mandible after traveling in mandibular canal.
4. Lingula: sharp spine that overhangs mandibular foramen and gives attachment to the sphenomandibular ligament; at its lower and back part is a notch from which the mylohyoid groove runs obliquely downward and forward and lodges the mylohyoid vessels and nerve.
5. Alveolar process: contains roots of the mandibular teeth; ramus extends upward and backward from the body on each side and terminates in coronoid process and coronoid notch.
6. Body: inferior to alveolar process.
7. External oblique line (ridge): outer crest where ramus joins the body; ramus extends from angle to condyle and articulates with TMJ; mandibular notch is located between coronoid process and condyle.
8. Genial tubercles: midline of medial surface; retromolar triangle is at lateral end of each alveolar process.
9. Internal oblique (mylohyoid) line (ridge): extends posteriorly and superiorly on inner surface;

sublingual fossa contains sublingual gland; submandibular fossa contains submandibular gland.

MUSCLES OF HEAD AND NECK

Head and neck muscles include cervical muscles, muscles of facial expression, muscles of mastication, hyoid muscles, muscles of the tongue.
• See Chapter 3, Anatomy, Biochemistry, and Physiology: skeletal muscles.

Cervical Muscles

Cervical muscles include SCM and trapezius.
A. The SCM: *paired* that serves as MAIN muscular landmark, divides neck region into anterior and posterior cervical triangles (Figure 4-3):
   1. Originates from clavicle and sternum, inserts on mastoid process of temporal bone.
   2. If ONLY one SCM contracts, the head and neck bend to the same side and the face and front of the neck rotate to the opposite side; if BOTH SCMs contract, head flexes at the neck and extends at the junction between the neck and skull; innervated by accessory nerve.
B. Trapezius: *paired* that covers the lateral and posterior surfaces of the neck:
   1. Originates from occipital bone and posterior midline of the cervical and thoracic regions; inserts on clavicle's lateral third and parts of scapula.
   2. Acts to lift clavicle and scapula; innervated by accessory nerve and third and fourth cervical nerves.

MUSCLES OF FACIAL EXPRESSION

Muscles of facial expression act in various combinations to alter appearance of face; innervated by the facial nerve, seventh (VII) cranial nerve (Figure 4-11).
A. Epicranial muscle (epicranius), located in scalp region, with frontal and occipital bellies, which are separated by a scalp tendon, epicranial aponeurosis; raises eyebrows and scalp to express surprise.
B. Orbicularis oculi encircles eye, closes eyelid; orbicularis oris encircles mouth, closes lips.
C. Corrugator supercilii is deep to superior part of orbicularis oculi muscle; originates on frontal bone and inserts into skin tissue of eyebrow; causes vertical wrinkles in forehead (frowning).
D. Buccinator forms anterior part of cheek; originates from alveolar processes of maxilla, mandible, and pterygomandibular raphe (ligament that extends from hamulus and attaches to mylohyoid line); pulls angle of mouth laterally and shortens cheek BOTH vertically and horizontally; keeps food in CORRECT position during chewing.
E. Risorius originates from fascia superficial to masseter and inserts in skin tissue at angle of mouth; widens mouth to stretch lips.

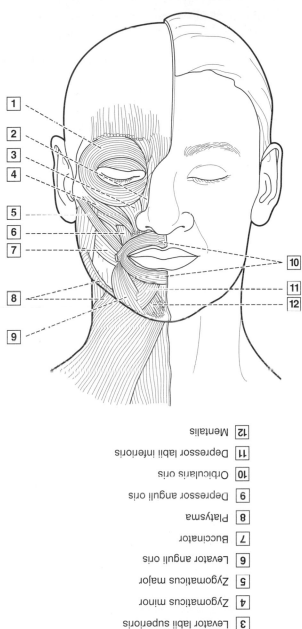

1. Orbicularis oculi
2. Levator labii superioris alaeque nasi
3. Levator labii superioris
4. Zygomaticus minor
5. Zygomaticus major
6. Levator anguli oris
7. Buccinator
8. Platysma
9. Depressor anguli oris
10. Orbicularis oris
11. Depressor labii inferioris
12. Mentalis

Figure 4-11 Muscles of facial expression. (From Fehrenbach MJ, ed: Dental anatomy coloring book, St. Louis, 2008, Saunders/Elsevier.)

F. Levator labii superioris originates from infraorbital region of maxilla and inserts in skin tissue of upper lip; raises upper lip.

G. Levator labii superioris alaeque nasi originates from frontal process of maxilla and inserts into skin tissue of ala of nose and upper lip; raises upper lip and dilates ala of nose for sneering.

H. Zygomaticus major originates from zygomatic bone and inserts in skin tissue at angle of mouth; raises angle of upper lip and pulls it laterally; zygomaticus minor originates on zygomatic bone and inserts in skin tissue of upper lip; raises upper lip for smiling.

I. Levator anguli oris originates superior to root of maxillary canine teeth and inserts in skin tissues at angle of mouth; raises angle of mouth; depressor anguli oris originates on mandible and inserts in skin tissue at angle of mouth; lowers angle of mouth for smiling and then frowning.

J. Depressor labii inferioris originates from mandible and inserts in skin tissues of lower lip; lowers lower lip.

K. Mentalis originates near mandible midline and inserts in skin tissue of chin; raises chin, causing lower lip protrusion and narrowing of oral vestibule.

L. Platysma runs from the neck to the mouth, covering anterior cervical triangle; originates in skin tissue superficial to the clavicle and shoulder and inserts on mandible and muscles surrounding mouth; raises skin of the neck and pulls down the corner of mouth (making anyone a Mr. Grimace, so *stretch* it out now as you study anatomy).

Muscles of Mastication

Muscles of mastication are *paired* muscles that attach to mandible and work with TMJ to accomplish movements of mandible: depression, elevation, protrusion, retraction, lateral deviation (Figures 4-12 and 4-13). Innervated by mandibular division of fifth (V) cranial nerve (trigeminal). Include masseter, temporalis, medial pterygoid, lateral pterygoid. Involved in temporomandibular joint disorder (TMD). See later discussion on occlusion in regard to masseter.

• See Chapter 6, General and Oral Pathology: TMD discussion.

A. **Masseter:** MOST superficially located and one of strongest muscles; located anterior to parotid gland:
   1. Two heads, superficial and deep, originate from different areas of zygomatic arch and insert on mandible (two heads are better than one).
   2. Superficial head inserts on lateral surface of angle; deep head inserts on ramus.
   3. When bilateral contraction occurs during closing of jaws, mandible raised.
   4. Can become increased in size (enlarged) with clenching and/or grinding (bruxism) of teeth.

B. Temporalis: originates from entire temporal fossa, inserts on coronoid process of mandible:
   1. When entire muscle contracts during closing of jaws, mandible raised.
   2. When only posterior part contracts, muscle moves mandible backward, causing retraction of jaw (usually during jaw closing).

C. Medial pterygoid: SIMILAR to but *deeper* to masseter:
   1. Originates from pterygoid fossa, on medial surface of lateral pterygoid plate; inserts on medial surface of angle of mandible.

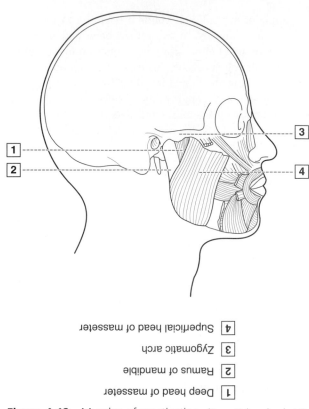

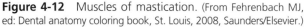

Figure 4-12 Muscles of mastication. (From Fehrenbach MJ, ed: Dental anatomy coloring book, St. Louis, 2008, Saunders/Elsevier.)

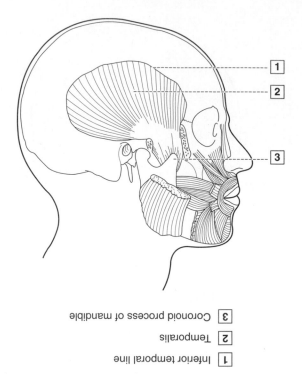

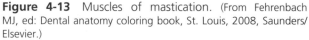

Figure 4-13 Muscles of mastication. (From Fehrenbach MJ, ed: Dental anatomy coloring book, St. Louis, 2008, Saunders/Elsevier.)

2. Raises mandible during closing of jaws.

D. Lateral pterygoid: two separate heads of origin, superior and inferior, separated by slight interval anteriorly; heads fuse posteriorly, within infratemporal fossa, deep to temporalis:

1. Superior head originates from greater wing of sphenoid; inferior head originates from lateral pterygoid plate; BOTH heads unite and insert on mandibular condyle.

2. Has tendency to lower mandible during opening of jaws; when BOTH muscles contract, serve to bring mandible forward, causing protrusion of mandible (during opening); when ONLY one is contracted, mandible shifts to opposite side, causing lateral deviation of mandible.

Hyoid Muscles

Hyoid muscles are located superficially in neck tissues, attached to hyoid. Assist in the actions of mastication and swallowing (Figure 4-14).

• See Chapter 3, Anatomy, Biochemistry, and Physiology: hyoid.

A. Suprahyoids: *paired* that are located superior to hyoid:

1. Act to raise hyoid and larynx by contraction of muscles of mastication when mandible is stabilized, which occurs during swallowing.

2. Contraction of anterior muscles causes mandible to lower and jaws to open when hyoid is stabilized by contraction of both posterior suprahyoid and infrahyoid muscles.

3. Categorized according to anterior or posterior position relative to hyoid:

a. Digastric: anterior and posterior bellies (separate); *anterior* belly is part of anterior suprahyoids; *posterior* belly is part of posterior suprahyoids:

(1) Each muscle demarcates superior part of anterior cervical triangle, forming (with the mandible) submandibular triangle on each side of neck.

(2) Right and left anterior bellies form midline submental triangle; anterior belly arises from intermediate tendon and inserts close to symphysis on inner surface of mandible, and posterior belly arises from mastoid process and inserts on intermediate tendon; anterior belly innervated by mylohyoid nerve; posterior belly innervated by posterior digastric nerve.

b. Mylohyoid: located *deep* to the digastric; its fibers run transversely between the two sides of mandible, where it originates from mylohyoid line (on inner surface of mandible):

(1) Unite medially, forming floor of mouth, and most posterior fibers insert on body of hyoid.

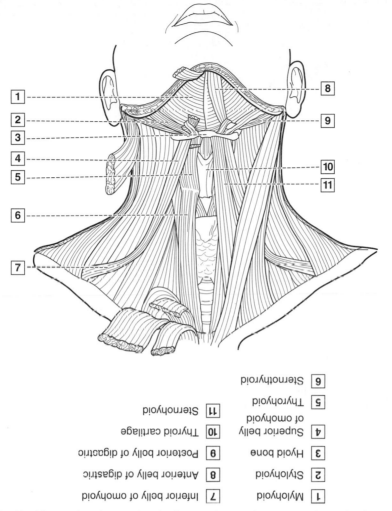

The following labels appear inverted below the figure:

9 Sternothyroid	
5 Thyrohyoid	
11 Sternohyoid	**4** Superior belly of omohyoid
10 Thyroid cartilage	**3** Hyoid bone
9 Posterior belly of digastric	**2** Stylohyoid
8 Anterior belly of digastric	**1** Mylohyoid
7 Inferior belly of omohyoid	

Figure 4-14 Hyoid muscles. (From Fehrenbach MJ, ed: Dental anatomy coloring book, St. Louis, 2008, Saunders/Elsevier.)

(2) Helps raise tongue; also raises hyoid bone or lowers mandible; innervated by mylohyoid nerve.

c. Stylohyoid: anterior and superficial to posterior belly of digastric:
  (1) Originates from styloid process of temporal bone and inserts on body of hyoid.
  (2) Innervated by stylohyoid nerve.

d. Geniohyoid: originates from medial surface of mandible:
  (1) Inserts near the symphysis at genial tubercles.
  (2) Innervated by first cervical nerve by way of twelfth (XII) cranial nerve (hypoglossal).

B. Infrahyoids: *paired* that are located *inferior* to hyoid; innervated by second and third cervical nerves; generally act to lower hyoid unless indicated:
  1. Sternothyroid: superficial to thyroid gland, deep and medial to sternohyoid; originates from sternum and inserts on thyroid cartilage and lowers thyroid cartilage and larynx; does NOT directly lower hyoid.
  2. Sternohyoid: superficial to sternothyroid, thyroid, cartilage; originates from sternum and inserts on hyoid.
  3. Omohyoid: lateral to BOTH sternothyroid and thyrohyoid; has superior and inferior bellies:
    a. Inferior belly: originates from scapula and passes beneath SCM, where it attaches by short tendon to superior belly.
    b. Superior belly: originates from short tendon attached to inferior belly and inserts on hyoid.
  4. Thyrohyoid: covered by omohyoid and sternohyoid; originates from thyroid cartilage and inserts on hyoid; appears as a continuation of sternothyroid; raises thyroid cartilage and larynx in addition to lowering hyoid.

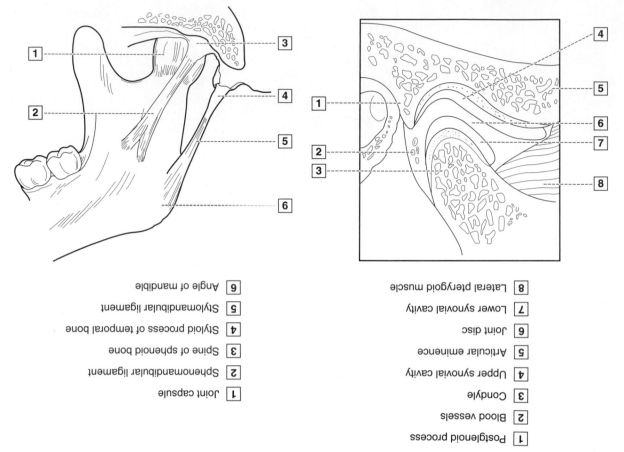

Figure 4-15 Temporomandibular joint. (From Fehrenbach MJ, ed: Dental anatomy coloring book, St. Louis, 2008, Saunders/Elsevier.)

6 Angle of mandible	8 Lateral pterygoid muscle
5 Stylomandibular ligament	7 Lower synovial cavity
4 Styloid process of temporal bone	6 Joint disc
3 Spine of sphenoid bone	5 Articular eminence
2 Sphenomandibular ligament	4 Upper synovial cavity
1 Joint capsule	3 Condyle
	2 Blood vessels
	1 Postglenoid process

Muscles of the Tongue

Tongue performs complex movements during mastication, speaking, and swallowing as a result of combined action of muscles. Muscles of the tongue are divided into intrinsic and extrinsic. Muscles innervated by twelfth (XII) cranial nerve (hypoglossal).

A. Intrinsic: located mainly inside the tongue; change shape of tongue:
 1. Named according to their orientation.
 2. Include superior longitudinal, transverse, vertical, inferior longitudinal.
B. Extrinsic: originate *outside* the tongue, yet insert *inside* tongue:
 1. Move the tongue while suspending and anchoring tongue to mandible, styloid process, hyoid.
 2. Include genioglossus, styloglossus, hyoglossus.

TEMPOROMANDIBULAR JOINT

Temporomandibular joint (TMJ) is located on each side of the head and allows movement of the mandible for speech and mastication (Figure 4-15). Innervated by mandibular division of fifth cranial nerve (trigeminal) and blood supply from the external carotid artery.

Patients may experience a temporomandibular joint disorder (TMD) of one or BOTH of these joints. Bones of the TMJ are discussed in skeletal system section.

A. Joint capsule: completely encloses TMJ; membranes that line inside of joint capsule secrete synovial fluid, which helps lubricate joint.
B. Disc: located between temporal bone and condyle, completely divides the TMJ into two synovial cavities, upper and lower, filled with synovial fluid:
 1. Attached to mandibular condyle anteriorly and NOT to temporal bone, except indirectly through capsule.
 2. Divided posteriorly into two areas where it blends with capsule: upper division is attached to postglenoid process, lower division is attached to condyle.
 3. Nerves and blood vessels enter joint in posterior area of attachment to capsule.
C. Ligaments associated with TMJ:
 1. TMJ ligament: on lateral side of each joint and reinforced capsule; prevents excessive retraction of mandible.
 2. Stylomandibular: variable ligament that is formed by thickened cervical fascia; runs from styloid

process of temporal bone to angle of mandible; becomes taut when mandible protrudes.
3. Sphenomandibular: NOT considered a part of TMJ; on medial side of mandible, some distance

from joint; runs from angular spine of sphenoid to lingula; becomes taut when mandible protrudes and can prevent diffusion of local anesthetic agent during inferior alveolar nerve block.

CLINICAL STUDY

Age	58 YRS	**SCENARIO**
Sex	☐ Male ☒ Female	The first afternoon patient has not had a dental examination since her last dentist retired 2 years ago. An initial extraoral examination indicates that her zygomatic region is firm and enlarged; she currently has no pain or discomfort in the jaw area. She does admit to frequently grinding her teeth at night.
Height	5'6"	
Weight	75 LBS	
BP	115/68	
Chief Complaint	"My jaws really ache when I wake up."	
Medical History	Hysterectomy 5 years ago Hypothyroidism (no goiter formation)	
Current Medications	levothyroxine sodium (Synthroid) 1 mg qd	
Social History	Internal revenue investigator Likes hockey	

1. What caused the patient's firmly enlarged zygomatic region? Why is there no jaw discomfort except in the morning?
2. Does the condition of cheek firmness and enlargement require treatment? If so, what may be recommended?

1. Patient's firm zygomatic region and enlarged cheeks are caused by an overuse of masseter muscle with grinding during sleep. The muscle underwent hypertrophy (enlargement by increase in size of cells, not number of cells). Jaw discomfort that is a dull ache only upon awakening is indicative of nighttime bruxism (grinding) and/or clenching habit. That is why there is no pain, since now she is at an afternoon appointment.
2. Her teeth should be checked for the presence of occlusal wear (attrition) and cusp fracture. The condition may require noninvasive treatment initially with a flat-plane splint (mouthguard), which prevents full closure and allows the masseter muscle to relax. It also helps distribute forces and prevent further wear to the occlusal surfaces of the teeth.

ARTERIAL BLOOD SUPPLY OF THE HEAD AND NECK

MAJOR arteries that supply the head and neck are the subclavian and the common carotid. Their paths from the heart to the head and neck are different, depending

on side of the body; other arteries of the head and neck are symmetrically located on each side of body. Vascular system supplies tissues with nutrients. May become compromised by disease process or during dental procedure.
• See Chapter 3, Anatomy, Biochemistry, and Physiology: vascular system.
A. Subclavian:
1. Located lateral to the common carotid artery.
2. Has branches that supply BOTH cranial structures.
B. Common carotid:
1. Branchless and travels up the neck, lateral to the trachea and larynx, then to thyroid cartilage.
2. Contained in a sheath beneath the SCM, along with the internal jugular vein and vagus nerve, until it ends by dividing into internal and external carotid arteries at level of larynx.
3. Bifurcates just past location of carotid sinus, a swelling (dilation); provides MOST reliable arterial pulse (used during emergencies by trained personnel).
C. Internal carotid:
1. After leaving common carotid, is hidden by the SCM; has no branches in neck but continues adjacent to internal jugular vein within carotid sheath to the skull base, where enters cranium to supply intracranial structures.
2. Source of ophthalmic artery, which supplies the eye, orbit, lacrimal gland.

D. External carotid:
  1. Arises from common carotid; supplies extracranial tissues, including oral cavity.
  2. Has anterior, medial, posterior, terminal branches.
  3. Anterior branches of external carotid:
     a. Superior thyroid branches into infrahyoid, sternocleidomastoid, superior laryngeal, and superior and inferior thyroid arteries, which supply tissues inferior to hyoid, including infrahyoid muscles, SCM, muscles of larynx, thyroid gland.
     b. Lingual arises above superior thyroid, at level of hyoid; travels anteriorly to tongue apex; supplies tissues superior to hyoid, including suprahyoid muscles and floor of mouth by the dorsal lingual, deep lingual, sublingual, suprahyoid branches; also supplies tongue.
     c. Sublingual supplies mylohyoid muscle, sublingual gland, floor of mouth; suprahyoid branch supplies suprahyoid muscles.
     d. Facial arises slightly superior to lingual as it branches off anteriorly and has a complicated path; supplies the face in the oral, buccal, zygomatic, nasal, infraorbital, orbital regions with its major branches, including ascending palatine, submandibular and submental, inferior labial, superior labial, angular (may share common trunk with lingual).
  4. Medial branch of external carotid includes ascending pharyngeal artery and pharyngeal and meningeal branches.
  5. Posterior branches of external carotid:
     a. Occipital includes muscular, SCM, auricular, meningeal branches.
     b. Posterior auricular arises superior to the occipital branch and stylohyoid muscle, level with the tip of the styloid process.
  6. Terminal branches of external carotid:
     a. Superficial temporal arises within parotid gland and may be clinically visible in temporal region; transverse facial branch supplies parotid; middle temporal branch supplies temporalis; frontal and parietal branches supply scalp.
     b. Maxillary gives off many branches within infratemporal and pterygopalatine fossae, such as middle meningeal and inferior alveolar arteries, and has branches near the muscles supplied, including deep temporal, pterygoid, masseteric artery, and buccal muscles, then branches into inferior alveolar (IA), posterior superior alveolar (PSA), infraorbital (IO), greater (GP) and lesser palatine (LP) (Figure 4-16).
     c. The IA arises from maxillary artery in infratemporal fossa, turns inferiorly to enter mandibular foramen, then enters mandibular canal and IA, branches into mylohyoid before it enters the

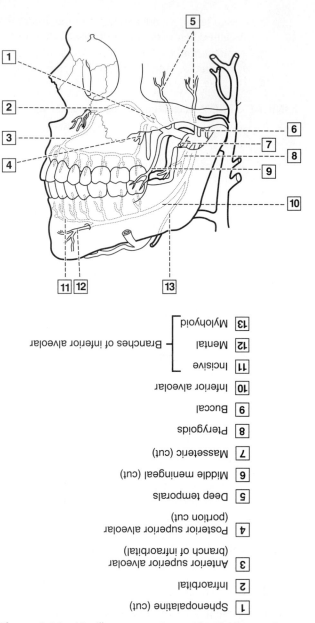

Figure 4-16 Maxillary artery. (From Fehrenbach MJ, ed: Dental anatomy coloring book, St. Louis, 2008, Saunders/Elsevier.)

1	Sphenopalatine (cut)
2	Infraorbital
3	Anterior superior alveolar (branch of infraorbital)
4	Posterior superior alveolar (portion cut)
5	Deep temporals
6	Middle meningeal (cut)
7	Masseteric (cut)
8	Pterygoids
9	Buccal
10	Inferior alveolar
11	Incisive
12	Mental	Branches of inferior alveolar
13	Mylohyoid

canal; in canal, branches into mandibular posterior and alveolar (dental) branches to supply teeth, periodontium, and associated gingiva.
     d. Mylohyoid arises before main artery enters mandibular canal by way of mandibular foramen and travels in the mylohyoid groove to supply floor of mouth and mylohyoid.
     e. Mental arises from main artery and then exits mandibular canal by way of mental foramen to supply the chin tissues; anastomoses with inferior labial artery.
     f. Incisive branches off main artery and remains in mandibular canal, divides into dental branches

to supply mandibular anteriors and alveolar branches to supply periodontium; anastomoses with alveolar branches of incisive artery on other side of mouth.

g. The PSA artery is given off just as maxillary artery leaves infratemporal fossa and enters pterygopalatine fossa, enters PSA foramina, and gives off dental branches (to supply the maxillary posteriors) and alveolar branches (to supply periodontium and maxillary sinus); anastomoses with anterior superior alveolar artery.

h. The IO artery branches from the maxillary in the pterygopalatine fossa and may share common trunk with the PSA artery; enters orbit through the inferior orbital fissure and travels through the IO canal; gives off orbital branches to the orbit; gives off anterior superior alveolar (ASA).

i. The ASA arises from IO artery and gives off dental branches to supply the maxillary anteriors and alveolar branches to supply periodontium; anastomoses with the PSA; after giving off these branches in infraorbital canal orbit, emerges onto the face from IO foramen to IO region of face; anastomoses with facial.

j. The GP and LP arteries arise from maxillary in the pterygopalatine fossa, which travels to the palate through the pterygopalatine canal and GP and LP foramina to supply hard and soft palate, respectively.

k. Maxillary artery ends by becoming sphenopalatine, which supplies nasal cavity and gives rise to posterior lateral nasal branches and septal branches, including nasopalatine branch that accompanies nasopalatine nerve through incisive foramen.

VENOUS DRAINAGE OF THE HEAD AND NECK

Veins are symmetrically located but have greater variability in location than do arteries. Veins anastomose freely and generally are larger and MORE numerous than arteries in same tissue. Internal jugular drains brain and other tissue; external jugular drains only some extracranial tissues, with many anastomoses between them. Internal and external jugular are major venous drainage vessels of head and neck (Figure 4-17). Leaving the head near the base of neck, veins become larger. Vascular system is capable of spreading infection or cancerous cells in head and neck area because valveless veins control direction of blood flow.

A. Facial: includes superior labial, inferior labial, submental, lingual; drains into internal jugular:
   1. Begins at medial canthus, at junction of supratrochlear and supraorbital, which anastomoses with ophthalmic that drains orbit tissues and provides communication with cavernous venous sinus.

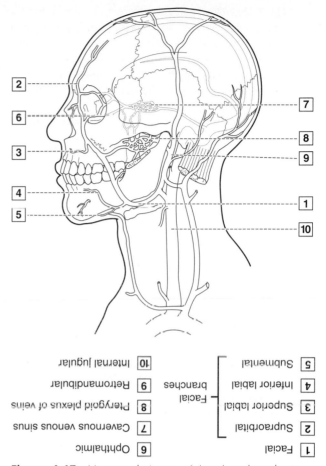

Figure 4-17 Venous drainage of head and neck. (From Fehrenbach MJ, ed: Dental anatomy coloring book, St. Louis, 2008, Saunders/Elsevier.)

1	Facial
2	Supraorbital
3	Superior labial
4	Inferior labial
5	Submental
6	Ophthalmic
7	Cavernous venous sinus
8	Pterygoid plexus of veins
9	Retromandibular
10	Internal jugular

2. Receives branches from same facial areas supplied by facial artery and anastomoses with deep veins, such as the pterygoid plexus in infratemporal fossa and retromandibular vein, before joining internal jugular vein at level of hyoid.
3. Has oral tributaries:
   a. Superior labial, drains upper lip; inferior labial, drains lower lip.
   b. Submental, drains chin tissues and submandibular region.
   c. Lingual, including dorsal lingual, which drains dorsal surface of tongue; deep lingual veins, which drain ventral surface; and sublingual veins, which drain floor of the mouth; may join to form a single vessel or may empty into larger vessels separately, either indirectly into facial or directly into internal jugular.
B. Retromandibular:
   1. Formed by union of superficial temporal and maxillary; emerges from parotid; drains areas similar to those supplied by superficial temporal and maxillary arteries.

2. Divides below parotid; anterior division joins facial, and posterior division continues and is then joined by posterior auricular vein, which drains scalp behind ear and becomes external jugular:
   a. Superficial temporal drains lateral scalp; drains into and forms retromandibular, along with maxillary.
   b. Maxillary:
      (1) Begins in infratemporal fossa; drains pterygoid plexus near maxillary artery and receives middle meningeal, posterior superior alveolar, inferior alveolar, and other veins, such as those from nose and palate (areas served by maxillary artery).
      (2) Merges with superficial temporal to drain into and form retromandibular.
      (3) Can be pierced during PSA block, causing hematoma, when needle overreaches target of apices of maxillary posteriors.

C. **Pterygoid plexus of veins:**
   1. Collection of small anastomosing vessels around pterygoid muscles and surrounding maxillary artery, protecting it from compression in infratemporal fossa; drains blood from maxillary and middle meningeal veins, which drain blood from meninges and deep facial parts.
   2. Anastomoses with BOTH facial and retromandibular veins; may be involved in spread of infection to cavernous venous sinus (needletrack infections); also drains PSA vein, formed by union of dental branches of maxillary teeth and alveolar branches of periodontium.
   3. Also drains inferior alveolar (IA) vein, which is formed by union of dental branches of mandibular teeth, alveolar branches of periodontium, and mental branches that enter mental foramen after draining chin area, where they anastomose with branches of facial vein.
   4. Can be pierced during PSA block, causing hematoma, when needle overreaches target of apices of maxillary posteriors; can also involve serious infection if needle-track infection is involved (causing cavernous sinus thrombosis).

GLANDULAR TISSUE

Glandular tissues include the lacrimal, salivary, thyroid, parathyroid, thymus glands.
- See Chapters 6, General and Oral Pathology: glandular diseases or conditions; 9, Pharmacology: secretions.
A. Lacrimal glands:
   1. Paired exocrine glands that secrete lacrimal fluid (tears) for lubrication of conjunctiva, which leaves gland through tubules.
   2. After passing over eyeball, drained through a hole in each eyelid, gland terminates in nasolacrimal sac, structure behind medial canthus.

B. **Salivary glands** (Figure 4-18):
   1. Produce saliva, which lubricates and cleanses oral cavity and aids digestion; include BOTH major and minor glands, defined by their size; exocrine glands with ducts that drain saliva directly into oral cavity where it is used; controlled by ANS.
   2. With connective tissue of gland divided into capsule, which surrounds outer part, and septa (plural of septum), each septum helps divide inner part of the gland into larger lobes and smaller lobules.
   3. Major glands are large paired glands; ducts are named after them; include parotid, submandibular, sublingual.
   4. Parotid:
      a. Largest encapsulated gland; provides only 25% of total volume; has purely serous secretion; divided into two lobes: superficial and deep.
      b. Parotid duct (Stensen's), which emerges from anterior border of gland, pierces buccinator, then opens into oral cavity at parotid papilla; occupies parotid fascial space, posterior to ramus, anterior and inferior to the ear; extends irregularly from zygomatic arch to angle of mandible.
      c. Innervated by parasympathetic nerves of the otic ganglion of ninth cranial nerve (glossopharyngeal), as well as afferent nerves from auriculotemporal branch of the fifth cranial nerve (trigeminal); drains into deep parotid nodes; supplied by branches of external carotid artery.
      d. Becomes enlarged and tender with mumps (unilateral or bilateral parotitis, inflammation of gland), viral disease that because of introduction of a vaccine is NOT a common childhood disease; the salivary gland MOST commonly involved in tumorous growth, which can change consistency and cause unilateral facial pain on involved side (seventh [VII] cranial nerve [facial] travels through gland).
      e. Trauma can also occur to nerve from accidental overreaching of needle during inferior alveolar nerve block, causing unilateral transient facial paralysis, temporary loss of movement of muscles of facial expression on affected side; patient CANNOT close one eye, smiles asymmetrically, has drooping lip on that side.
   5. Submandibular:
      a. Second largest encapsulated gland; provides 60% to 65% of total volume with mixed secretion.
      b. Submandibular duct (Wharton's), which arises from deep lobe and remains inside mylohyoid, travels along anterior floor of the mouth

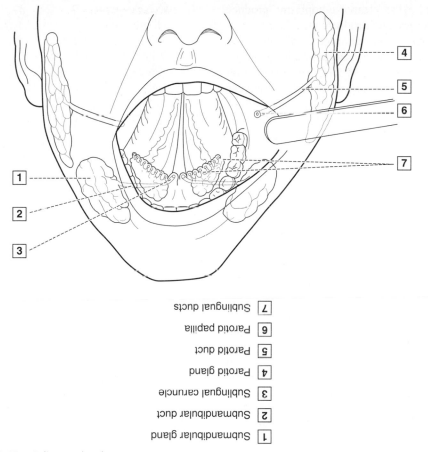

7 [Sublingual ducts

6 [Parotid papilla

5 [Parotid duct

4 [Parotid gland

3 [Sublingual caruncle

2 [Submandibular duct

1 [Submandibular gland

Figure 4-18 Salivary glands. (From Fehrenbach MJ, ed: Dental anatomy coloring book, St. Louis, 2008, Saunders/Elsevier.)

and then opens into oral cavity at the sublingual caruncle; tortuous travel may be reason that it is gland MOST often involved in stone formation.

c. Occupies submandibular fossa in submandibular fascial space, mostly superficial to the mylohyoid; deep lobe wraps around the posterior part and is posterior to the sublingual.

d. Innervated by parasympathetic fibers of chorda tympani and submandibular ganglion of seventh (VII) cranial nerve (facial); drains into submandibular nodes; supplied by branches of facial and lingual arteries.

6. Sublingual:

a. Smallest and ONLY unencapsulated gland; provides only 10% of total volume with mixed secretion.

b. NOT just one major duct; sublingual ducts (Bartholin's) open directly into oral cavity through gland and have other ducts that open along the sublingual fold; located in sublingual fossa in sublingual fascial space at the floor of the mouth; superior to mylohyoid, medial to body of mandible, anterior to submandibular.

c. Innervated by parasympathetic fibers of chorda tympani and submandibular ganglion of seventh (VII) cranial nerve (facial); drains into submandibularnodes; supplied by sublingual and submental arteries.

7. Minor salivary glands:

a. Smaller than major glands but MORE numerous, exocrine glands with unnamed ducts that are shorter than major glands; scattered in buccal, labial, and lingual mucosa, soft palate, lateral parts of hard palate, floor of the mouth; include von Ebner's glands (associated with circumvallate lingual papillae).

b. Secrete MAINLY mucous saliva, EXCEPT von Ebner's glands, which secrete only serous secretions.

c. Innervated by seventh (VII) cranial nerve (facial); drain into various lymph nodes; supplied by various arteries.

8. Histology of salivary glands:

a. Secretory cells: produce saliva; two types of epithelial cells in glands:

(1) Mucous cells: cloudier-looking cytoplasm; produce mucous secretory product.

(2) Serous cells: clearer cytoplasm; produce serous secretory product.

   b. Acinus: single layer of cuboidal epithelial cells surrounding lumen, where saliva is deposited after being produced; MOST acini match with type of cell, but mucoserous acini have mucous cells surrounding lumen, with serous demilune located superficially.

   c. Myoepithelial cells: on surface of some acini to help flow of saliva (squeeze play).

   d. Duct system: intercalated duct is associated with acinus, connected to striated duct, then excretory duct.

C. **Thyroid gland** (Figure 4-19):

   1. Located in anterior and lateral regions of neck, inferior to thyroid cartilage, at junction between larynx and trachea.

   2. Produces thyroxine, secreted directly into blood, stimulating metabolic rate.

   3. LARGEST endocrine gland; has NO ducts but is encapsulated; consists of two lateral lobes, right and left, connected anteriorly by isthmus.

   4. Innervated by sympathetic nerves through cervical ganglia; drains into superior deep cervical nodes; supplied by superior and inferior thyroid arteries.

   5. May become enlarged during disease process, producing goiter.

D. **Parathyroid glands** (Figure 4-19):

   1. Located close to or inside thyroid on posterior surface; consist of four endocrine glands, two on each side, with NO ducts; produce parathyroid hormone secreted directly into blood to regulate calcium and phosphorus levels.

   2. Innervated by sympathetic nerves through cervical ganglia; drain into superior deep cervical nodes; supplied MAINLY by inferior thyroid arteries

   3. May alter thyroid if involved in disease process.

E. **Thymus gland:**

   1. Ductless endocrine gland located in thorax and anterior region of base of neck, inferior to thyroid, deep to sternum; its muscles, superficial and lateral to trachea, consist of two lateral lobes in close contact at midline.

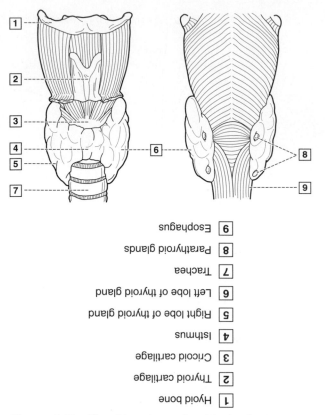

Figure 4-19	Label
1	Hyoid bone
2	Thyroid cartilage
3	Cricoid cartilage
4	Isthmus
5	Right lobe of thyroid gland
6	Left lobe of thyroid gland
7	Trachea
8	Parathyroid glands
9	Esophagus

Figure 4-19 Thyroid and parathyroid glands. (From Fehrenbach MJ, ed: Dental anatomy coloring book, St. Louis, 2008, Saunders/Elsevier.)

   2. Part of immune system and fights disease process; T-cell lymphocytes mature in gland in response to stimulation by thymus hormones.

   3. Innervated by branches of tenth cranial nerve (vagus) and cervical nerves, with lymphatics that arise within the substance of gland and terminate in internal jugular vein; supplied by inferior thyroid and internal thoracic arteries.

   4. Grows in size from birth *to* puberty, then stops growing and starts to shrink; thyroid cancer may develop as a result of mistaken past radiation therapy to shrink gland.

CLINICAL STUDY

Age	49 YRS	SCENARIO
Sex	☒ Male ☐ Female	The intraoral examination of the patient reveals a number of carious lesions, and the oral mucosa appears quite dry.
Height	6'5"	
Weight	175 LBS	
BP	112/62	
Chief Complaint	"My mouth is so sore when I eat!"	
Medical History	Recent radiation therapy for low-grade adenoid cystic carcinoma of the submandibular gland after surgical removal	
Current Medications	None	
Social History	Basketball coach at high school Past history of spit tobacco use	

1. What is the cause of the patient's dry mouth? What type of tumor is this? Why is the patient not taking any medications?
2. What are recommendations for treatment of dryness?
3. What types of cells were most damaged during radiation treatment provided?

1. Primary cause of xerostomia is radiation treatment the patient received for tumor. Radiation treatment causes glandular tissue fibrosis or atrophy, resulting in partial or total loss of secretory function of the submandibular salivary gland (hypofunction). Submandibular is the second largest encapsulated gland; provides 60% to 65% of total saliva volume with mixed secretion, thus most of the volume of saliva. Discomfort and difficulty speaking and swallowing are common complaints of those suffering from inadequate saliva production. Adenoid cystic carcinoma (ACC) is uncommon except in salivary glands, is usually a painless, slow-growing mass, and often appears to be a low-grade tumor; hard to get rid of completely and very often comes back after surgery. There is no effective medication or chemotherapy for this type of tumor.
2. Patient may use salivary substitute throughout the day to provide moisture for the mouth when speaking and swallowing. Sipping water frequently, sucking on sugar-free lozenges, and humidifying air in the home have also been found to be beneficial. Daily use of mineralizing fluoride and calcium product helps prevent formation of caries.
3. Secretory cells that make up submandibular glands are serous and mucous cells, since it is a mixed gland, and both types of cells can be damaged by radiation treatment. Gland occupies submandibular fossa in submandibular fascial space, mostly superficial to the mylohyoid; deep lobe wraps around the posterior part and is posterior to the sublingual.

TRIGEMINAL NERVE AND SENSORY ROOT

Trigeminal nerve (fifth cranial nerve [V]) is formed by ophthalmic, maxillary, mandibular branches.
- See Chapters 3, Anatomy, Biochemistry, and Physiology, and 14, Pain Management: nervous system, oral cavity nerves; 6, General and Oral Pathology: trigeminal neuralgia.
A. Ophthalmic division (ophthalmic nerve, V_1) is FIRST and smallest division, carried by way of superior orbital fissure; includes frontal, lacrimal, nasociliary.
B. Maxillary division (maxillary nerve, V_2) of fifth cranial nerve (trigeminal) (Figure 4-20):
   1. Second division of trigeminal, with nerve trunk formed in pterygopalatine fossa by convergence of MANY nerves; enters skull through foramen rotundum; contains branches: zygomatic, infraorbital (IO), anterior superior alveolar (ASA), middle superior alveolar (MSA), posterior superior alveolar (PSA), greater palatine (GP), lesser palatine (LP), nasopalatine (NP).
   2. Zygomatic: union of zygomaticofacial and zygomaticotemporal in orbit and is *afferent;* conveys postganglionic parasympathetic fibers to lacrimal gland; courses posteriorly along lateral orbit floor, enters pterygopalatine fossa through inferior orbital fissure, then joins maxillary.
   3. The IO: passes into IO foramen; then travels through IO canal, along with infraorbital blood vessels; then joined by ASA, which is *afferent* and is formed by a union of cutaneous branches from the upper lip, medial part of cheek, lower eyelid,

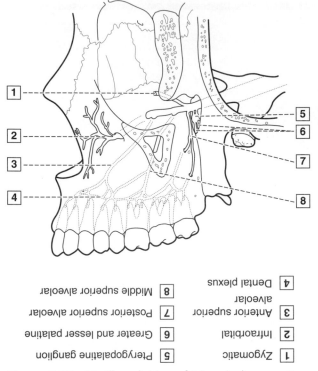

8 Middle superior alveolar	4 Dental plexus
7 Posterior superior alveolar	3 Anterior superior alveolar
6 Greater and lesser palatine	2 Infraorbital
5 Pterygopalatine ganglion	1 Zygomatic

Figure 4-20 Maxillary division of trigeminal nerve. (From Fehrenbach MJ, ed: Dental anatomy coloring book, St. Louis, 2008, Saunders/Elsevier.)

side of nose; then passes from IO canal and groove into pterygopalatine fossa through inferior orbital fissure; after leaving IO groove, and within pterygopalatine fossa, receives PSA.

4. The ASA: ascends along anterior wall of maxillary sinus to join IO in IO canal; *afferent* for maxillary anteriors by way of dental and interdental branches; forms dental plexus and innervates overlying facial gingiva; crossover can occur over midline.

5. The MSA: *afferent* for maxillary premolar teeth and possibly mesial buccal (MB) root of maxillary first molar; originates from dental, interdental, interradicular branches, forming dental plexus; then ascends to join IO by running in lateral wall of maxillary sinus and communicates with BOTH the ASA and PSA; may or may not be present; if NOT present, area is innervated by BOTH the ASA and PSA, but MAINLY the ASA.

6. The PSA joins IO (or maxillary directly) in the pterygopalatine fossa; *afferent* for most parts of maxillary molar teeth (possibly NOT MB root of maxillary first molars) and maxillary sinus:
   a. Some branches remain external to posterior surface of maxilla and provide innervation for buccal gingiva overlying maxillary molars; others originate from dental, interdental,

and interradicular branches, forming dental plexus; all internal branches exit from PSA foramina.
   b. BOTH external and internal branches ascend along maxillary tuberosity, which forms in posterolateral wall of maxillary sinus, to join IO or maxillary.

7. Greater palatine (GP, anterior palatine): located between mucoperiosteum and bone of anterior hard palate; communicates with terminal fibers of nasopalatine (NP):
   a. Enters GP foramen in palatine bone to travel in pterygopalatine canal, along with GP blood vessels and lesser palatine (LP) and blood vessels, ascends through pterygopalatine canal, toward maxillary nerve in pterygopalatine fossa; *afferent* for posterior hard palate and posterior lingual gingiva.
   b. The LP (posterior palatine): *afferent* for soft palate and palatine tonsillar tissues; enters LP foramen in the palatine bone, along with LP blood vessels; then joins GP nerve and blood vessels in pterygopalatine canal; then ascends through pterygopalatine canal toward maxillary nerve in pterygopalatine fossa.

8. The NP: originates in the mucosa of anterior hard palate; *afferent* for anterior hard palate, lingual gingiva of maxillary anteriors, nasal septal tissues; communicates with GP; has right and left nerves; BOTH enter incisive canal by way of incisive foramen; then travel along nasal septum.

C. Mandibular division (mandibular nerve, V₃) of fifth cranial nerve (trigeminal) (Figure 4-21):
   1. Largest of three divisions that form trigeminal and innervates ALL muscles of mastication:
      a. Has meningeal and muscular branches, which arise from trunk before separation into two trunks; main trunk is formed by union of anterior and posterior trunks in infratemporal fossa, before passing through foramen ovale; muscular branches arise from motor root of trigeminal; have deep temporal nerves that are *efferent* for temporalis and include masseteric nerve, which is *efferent* for masseter, and sensory branch to TMJ and lateral pterygoid nerve, which is *efferent* for lateral pterygoid.
      b. Anterior trunk formed by union of buccal nerve and muscular branches; posterior formed by union of auriculotemporal, lingual, inferior alveolar (IA); mandibular division joins ophthalmic and maxillary to form trigeminal ganglion; includes buccal, muscular, lingual, IA, mental, incisive, mylohyoid, and auriculotemporal, which is *efferent* for the external ear and scalp; then joins posterior trunk.

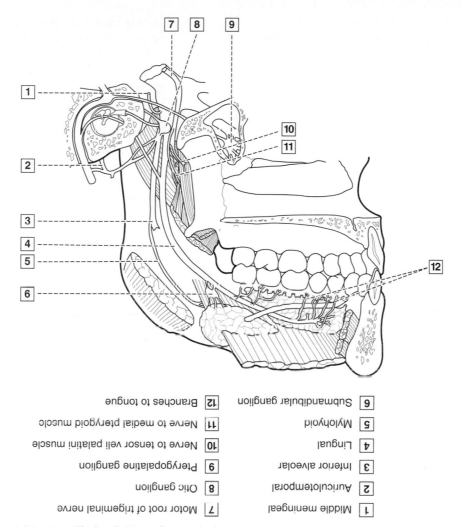

Figure 4-21 Mandibular division of trigeminal nerve (From Fehrenbach MJ, ed: Dental anatomy coloring book, St. Louis, 2008, Saunders/Elsevier.)

1 Middle meningeal	**7** Motor root of trigeminal nerve
2 Auriculotemporal	**8** Otic ganglion
3 Inferior alveolar	**9** Pterygopalatine ganglion
4 Lingual	**10** Nerve to tensor veli palatini muscle
5 Mylohyoid	**11** Nerve to medial pterygoid muscle
6 Submandibular ganglion	**12** Branches to tongue

2. Buccal (long buccal): not to be confused with buccal nerve that serves the buccinator muscle of the cheek:
   a. Located on surface of buccinator and travels posteriorly in cheek, deep to masseter, then crosses in front of the anterior border of the ramus, between two heads of lateral pterygoid, to join anterior trunk.
   b. *Afferent* for skin of cheek, buccal mucous membranes, buccal gingiva of mandibular posteriors.
3. Mental: external branches that are *afferent* for chin, lower lip, and labial mucosa near mandibular anteriors; then enters mental foramen to merge with incisive to form IA in mandibular canal.
4. Incisive: *afferent;* composed of dental branches from the mandibular anteriors and interdental branches, which form dental plexus; then merges with mental, just posterior to mental foramen, to form the IA in mandibular canal; crossover can occur over midline.

5. Lingual:
   a. Formed from afferent branches from the body of tongue that travel along its lateral surface; *afferent* for general sensation of body of tongue, floor of the mouth, lingual gingiva of mandibular teeth.
   b. Then passes posteriorly from medial to the lateral side of submandibular gland and communicates with submandibular ganglion located superior to deep lobe of submandibular gland, which is part of the parasympathetic efferent innervation for sublingual and submandibular glands (chorda tympani travels along with lingual nerve).
   c. At the base of tongue, ascends and runs between medial pterygoid and mandible, anterior and slightly medial to IA, then continues to travel upward to join posterior trunk.

6. The IA:
  a. *Afferent* for mandibular posteriors, formed from union of mental and incisive, then continues to travel posteriorly through mandibular canal, along with IA blood vessels.
  b. Joined by dental, interdental, and interradicular branches from the mandibular posteriors, forming a dental plexus; then exits mandible through mandibular foramen, where it is joined by mylohyoid nerve; then travels lateral to medial pterygoid, between sphenomandibular ligament and ramus and within pterygomandibular space, posterior and slightly lateral to lingual; then joins posterior trunk.

7. Mylohyoid: branch of IA nerve after it exits mandibular foramen, then pierces sphenomandibular ligament; runs in mylohyoid groove and then onto lower surface of the mylohyoid; *efferent* for mylohyoid and anterior belly of digastric.

CLINICAL STUDY

Age	25 YRS	SCENARIO
Sex	☒ Male ☐ Female	The dental hygienist previously performed a localized scaling of #14 and #15, with local anesthesia. Since the area continued to be sore at the patient's next appointment 2 weeks later, the supervising dentist referred him to an oral surgeon, with tooth #16 circled on the referral form. However, after extraction 1 week ago, he is now presenting with a fever and swollen lymph nodes and poor oral hygiene at extraction site. Antibiotics have been prescribed.
Height	5'8"	
Weight	190 LBS	
BP	118/78	
Chief Complaint	"My upper left jaw is still really sore."	
Medical History	Laser eye surgery 2 years ago Broken nose as child	
Current Medications	None	
Social History	Computer graphics engineer	

1. What three local anesthesia blocks would have to have been done to make the patient completely anesthetized for his localized scaling?
2. Which tooth was extracted by oral surgeon? Which nerves should be anesthetized to extract tooth #16 comfortably?
3. What types of roots might oral surgeon encounter when extracting tooth #16? From which bone and its process did the extraction of #16 take place?
4. Which blood vessels supply the area of extraction site?
5. Which primary and secondary lymph nodes might be involved in infection of tooth #16?

1. For the patient to be completely anesthetized on #14 and #15, the following nerve blocks would be needed: posterior superior alveolar (PSA) and middle superior alveolar (MSA) (both used for anesthesia of tooth and its pulp, associated periodontium, overlying buccal gingiva), as well as greater palatine (GP) (for overlying anesthesia of lingual gingiva). All nerves anesthetized are branches of maxillary nerve (maxillary division, V_2) of fifth (V) cranial nerve (trigeminal).

2. Tooth #16 (wisdom tooth, maxillary left third molar) was extracted. Crown has no standard form; smallest molar and most variable in shape in permanent dentition. Occlusal table with heart-shaped occlusal outline is most common; similar to maxillary second molar but with more supplemental grooves; has only three cusps (MB, DB, and ML). With rhomboid occlusal outline, has four cusps; no oblique ridge on small DL cusp. Both PSA and GP nerves must be anesthetized to extract tooth #16.

3. Tooth #16 was extracted from alveolar process of maxilla, the tooth-bearing part of upper jaw where each alveolus (tooth socket) is located. Posterior superior alveolar artery (branch off maxillary artery) and vein (begins as maxillary vein) supply tooth #16 and area.

4. Roots of #16, as third molar, may be partially or fully fused, poorly developed, and/or curved distally; may have accessory root. May even have dilaceration, a curvature of the root that is developmental anomaly and may be caused by trauma during tooth development; this presents the greatest challenge to the oral surgeon.

5. Primary lymph nodes that directly drain tooth #16 are superior deep cervical nodes, located deep beneath sternocleidomastoid muscle (SCM), superior to where

omohyoid muscle crosses internal jugular vein. Drain posterior nasal cavity, posterior part of hard palate, soft palate, base of tongue, maxillary third molars, esophagus, trachea, thyroid gland. Then drain into secondary nodes, inferior deep cervical nodes, or can drain directly into jugular trunk.

FACIAL NERVE

Facial nerve (seventh cranial [VII]) innervates muscles of facial expression. Carries BOTH efferent and afferent nerves. Branches include greater petrosal, chorda tympani, posterior auricular, stylohyoid, posterior digastric.

- See Chapters 6, General and Oral Pathology: Bell's palsy, CVA; 14, Pain Management: transient facial paralysis.
A. Facial: emerges from brain and enters internal acoustic meatus; gives off *efferent* branches to middle ear muscle and greater petrosal and chorda tympani nerves, which carry parasympathetic fibers.
B. Main trunk then emerges from skull through stylomastoid foramen, gives off posterior auricular nerve and branch to posterior belly of digastric and stylohyoid muscles, then passes into parotid gland and forms numerous branches to supply ALL muscles of facial expression (but NOT to the parotid):
  1. Greater petrosal: branches off facial before exiting skull; has efferent fibers that are preganglionic parasympathetic fibers to pterygopalatine ganglion in pterygopalatine fossa.
  2. Has postganglionic fibers that arise in pterygopalatine ganglion, then join with branches of maxillary division of trigeminal, carried to lacrimal gland (by way of zygomatic and lacrimal nerves), nasal cavity, minor salivary glands of hard and soft palate; *afferent* for taste sensation in palate.
  3. Chorda tympani: branch of facial and is parasympathetic; *efferent* for submandibular and sublingual glands and *afferent* for taste sensation for body of tongue:
    a. After branching off facial, within petrous part of temporal bone, crosses tympanic membrane (eardrum); exits skull by way of petrotympanic fissure, which is located immediately posterior to TMJ.
    b. Then travels with lingual along floor of the mouth in same nerve bundle; in submandibular triangle, appears alongside of lingual nerve and has communication with submandibular ganglion.
  4. Posterior auricular, stylohyoid, posterior digastric nerves: given off by facial nerve after it exits stylomastoid foramen; are all efferent; posterior auricular nerve supplies occipital belly of epicranial

muscle, and other two nerves supply stylohyoid muscle and posterior belly of the digastric, respectively.
  5. Branches to muscles of facial expression are efferent branches of facial, which originate in parotid gland and pass to the muscles innervated; include temporal, zygomatic, buccal, (marginal) mandibular, cervical; RARELY seen as five independent nerves; vary in number and connect irregularly.

LYMPH NODES OF HEAD AND NECK

Lymph nodes are part of immune system and help to fight disease. Network of lymphatic vessels that link lymph nodes throughout MOST of body. NOT palpable unless involved in a disease state.

- See Chapters 3, Anatomy, Biochemistry, and Physiology: lymphatics; 11, Clinical Treatment: extraoral examination.
A. Lymph nodes of head are either superficial or deep:
  1. Superficial nodes of head (Figure 4-22):
    a. Occipital: bilaterally in occipital region; drain part of scalp, then empty into inferior deep cervical nodes.
    b. Retroauricular (mastoid, posterior auricular): posterior to ears; drain surrounding area, then empty into superior deep cervical nodes.
    c. Anterior auricular: anterior to each ear; drain surrounding area, then empty into superior deep cervical nodes.
    d. Superficial parotid (paraparotid): superficial to parotids; drain surrounding area, then empty into superior deep cervical nodes (anterior auricular and superficial parotid may be grouped).
    e. Facial: along length of facial vein to drain area with descending subgroups: malar (infraorbital), nasolabial, buccal, mandibular; drain into each other, then into submandibular nodes.
  2. Deep nodes of head (too deep to palpate):
    a. Deep parotid: deep in gland; drain middle ear, auditory tube, gland, then empty into superior deep cervical nodes.
    b. Retropharyngeal: near deep parotid; drain pharynx, palate, paranasal sinuses, nasal cavity; then empty into superior deep cervical nodes.
B. Cervical nodes: in neck, divided into superficial and deep.
  1. Superficial cervical nodes (Figure 4-23):
    a. Submental: inferior to chin in submental fascial space, superficial to the mylohyoid, near midline; drain BOTH sides of chin, lower lip, floor of the mouth, apex of tongue, mandibular incisors, then empty into submandibular or deep cervical nodes.

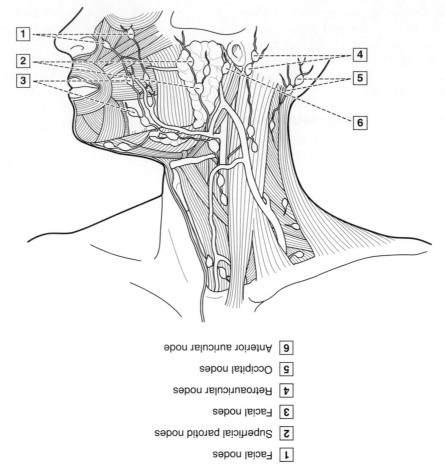

Anterior auricular node **6**

Occipital nodes **5**

Retroauricular nodes **4**

Facial nodes **3**

Superficial parotid nodes **2**

Facial nodes **1**

Figure 4-22   Superficial nodes of the head. (From Fehrenbach MJ, ed: Dental anatomy coloring book, St. Louis, 2008, Saunders/Elsevier.)

b. Submandibular: inferior border of the ramus, superficial to submandibular gland and within submandibular fascial space; drain the cheeks, upper lip, body of tongue, anterior part of hard palate, and ALL teeth (EXCEPT mandibular incisors and maxillary third molars); may be secondary nodes for the submental and facial regions because they also drain sublingual and submandibular glands and then empty into superior deep cervical nodes.

c. External jugular (superficial lateral cervical): on side of the neck along external jugular vein, superficial to SCM; may be secondary nodes for the occipital, retroauricular, anterior auricular, superficial parotid; then empty into the superior or inferior deep cervical nodes.

d. Anterior jugular (superficial anterior cervical): on side of the neck, along the length of the anterior jugular vein, anterior to SCM; drain infrahyoid region of neck, then empty into inferior deep cervical nodes.

2. Deep cervical nodes (Figure 4-24):
   a. Superior deep cervical: deep beneath SCM, superior to omohyoid muscle crosses internal jugular vein; drain posterior nasal cavity, posterior part of hard palate, soft palate, base of tongue, maxillary third molars, esophagus, trachea, thyroid gland:
      (1) May be secondary nodes for ALL other nodes of head and neck (EXCEPT occipital and inferior deep cervical nodes), then empty into inferior deep cervical nodes or directly into jugular trunk.
      (2) Jugulodigastric (tonsillar or sentinel node): below posterior belly of digastric; EASILY becomes palpable when palatine tonsils and pharynx are inflamed.
   b. Inferior deep cervical: continuation of superior deep cervicals, located deep to SCM, at level where omohyoid crosses internal jugular vein or inferior to this point; extend inferiorly into supraclavicular fossa, superior to each clavicle.

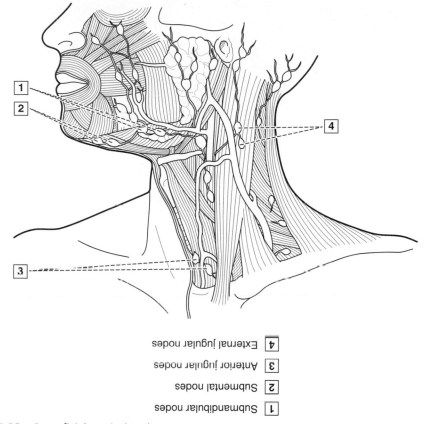

Figure 4-23   Superficial cervical nodes. (From Fehrenbach MJ, ed: Dental anatomy coloring book, St. Louis, 2008, Saunders/Elsevier.)

The following legend appears upside-down in the image:

4	External jugular nodes
3	Anterior jugular nodes
2	Submental nodes
1	Submandibular nodes

(1) Drain posterior part of scalp and neck, superficial pectoral region, part of arm; may be secondary nodes for occipital and superior deep cervical.

(2) Jugulo-omohyoid: located at crossing of omohyoid and internal jugular vein; drains tongue and submental region.

3. Accessory: along accessory nerve; drain scalp and neck, then empty into supraclavicular nodes.

4. Supraclavicular (transverse cervical): located along clavicle; drain lateral cervical triangles, then empty into either one of jugular trunks or into right lymphatic or thoracic duct; communicate with axillary lymph nodes that drain breast region (may be enlarged and hard if involved with breast cancer).

C. Efferent vessels form jugular trunk, one of tributaries of right lymphatic duct (on right side) and thoracic duct (on left).

Tonsillar Tissue

Tonsils are masses of lymphoid tissue that drain into the superior deep cervical nodes, especially jugulodigastric (tonsillar or sentinel) lymph node. Includes palatine, lingual, pharyngeal, tubal tonsils. Enlargement (lymphadenopathy) occurs in disease states.

A. Palatine tonsils: two rounded masses of variable size, between anterior and posterior tonsillar pillars (Figure 4-1).

B. Lingual tonsil: indistinct layer of lymphoid tissue located on base of dorsal surface of tongue (Figure 4-1).

C. Pharyngeal tonsils (adenoids): on posterior wall of nasopharynx; normally temporarily enlarged in children.

D. Tubal tonsils: in nasopharynx, posterior to openings of eustachian (auditory) tubes.

CLINICAL STUDY

Scenario: An intraoral examination of the 12-year-old patient reveals a 6-mm circular vesicle on the hard palate, near his maxillary anteriors. Bilaterally enlarged tonsils, near the throat, are also noted. He has a cold and is on cough medicine.

1. Which nerves are involved in the patient's discomfort from the blister?

2. Which bone underlies the tissue in the sore area?

3. Identify the unique intraoral landmark located near or within the sore area.

4. Which tonsils are involved in the enlargement? Which primary lymph nodes would one expect to find enlarged during the extraoral examination?

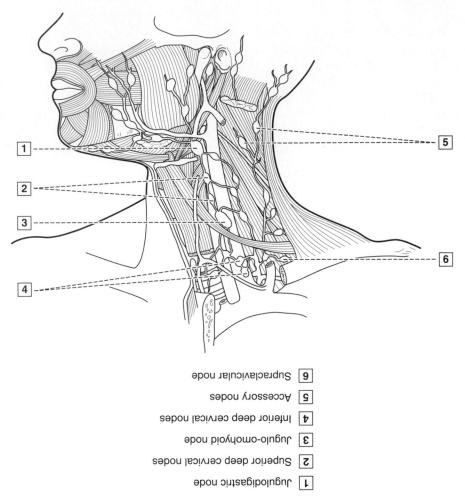

6	Supraclavicular node
5	Accessory nodes
4	Inferior deep cervical nodes
3	Jugulo-omohyoid node
2	Superior deep cervical nodes
1	Jugulodigastric node

Figure 4-24 Deep cervical nodes. (From Fehrenbach MJ, ed: Dental anatomy coloring book, St. Louis, 2008, Saunders/Elsevier.)

1. Nasopalatine nerve is involved in patient's discomfort from vesicle (blister) from the thermal burn.
2. Maxillary bone underlies soft tissues in burn area.
3. Unique intraoral landmark located near or within burn area is incisive papilla, centrally located on the hard palate, around 10 mm posterior to the maxillary central incisors.
4. Palatine tonsils are enlarged between anterior and posterior tonsillar pillars. Palpation of neck would reveal enlargement (lymphadenopathy) of primary nodes for the region, superior deep cervical lymph nodes, especially the jugulodigastric (tonsillar or sentinel node), below posterior belly of digastric.

Dental Anatomy and Dentitions

The **dentition** consists of the natural teeth in the jaw bones and includes BOTH primary and permanent dentitions. It is understood that the teeth being discussed on examinations are *permanent* unless otherwise designated (as on NBDHE).

- See CD-ROM for Chapter Terms and WebLinks.

- See Chapters 6, General and Oral Pathology: dental disorders; 11, Clinical Treatment: dental charting.
A. Primary (deciduous) dentition is the FIRST dentition; consists of 20 teeth (8 incisors, 4 canines, and 8 molars).
   1. Are exfoliated (shed) and replaced by permanent dentition (Figure 4-25).
   2. Begins on average with eruption of the mandibular central incisor at 6 to 10 months and is completed with the eruption of the maxillary second molar at 25 to 33 months.
B. Permanent (adult) dentition is the second dentition; replaces primary dentition; consists of 32 teeth (8 incisors, 4 canines, 8 premolars, and 12 molars).
   1. Anterior and premolar teeth are succedaneous (have primary predecessors); molars are nonsuccedaneous (do NOT have primary predecessors) (Figure 4-26).
   2. Begins on average with the eruption of the mandibular first molar or central incisor at 6 to 7 years and is completed with the eruption of the third molars at 17 to 21 years.

Tooth Types

Tooth types with their specific anatomy are related to masticatory function of the tooth and to its role in speech and esthetics (Figure 4-26). Form and function of each type are somewhat similar for BOTH primary and permanent dentitions. Types include incisors, canines, premolars, and molars; premolars (bicuspids) ONLY in permanent dentition.

A. Incisors: bite and cut food because of triangular proximal form.
B. Canines (cuspids): pierce or tear food because of prominent cusp and tapered shape.
C. Premolars (bicuspids): assist molars in grinding food because of broad occlusal surface and prominent cusps and assist canines in piercing and tearing food with their cusps.
D. Molars: grind food, assisted by premolars, because of broad occlusal surfaces and prominent cusps.

Tooth Surfaces

Includes **facial** (buccal), **lingual,** occlusal, and interproximal surfaces. Interproximal surfaces are complex (as is the care of the area).

A. **Contact point:** point on the proximal surface where two adjacent teeth actually touch each other (if not present, may have an open contact).
B. **Interproximal space:** area between two teeth.
   1. Part of the interproximal space is occupied by the interdental papilla.
   2. Part of the interproximal space not occupied is called the embrasure.
C. **Embrasure:** area bordered by interdental papilla, proximal surfaces of the two adjacent teeth, and contact point.
   1. If there is no contact point between the teeth, the area between is a diastema instead of an embrasure.

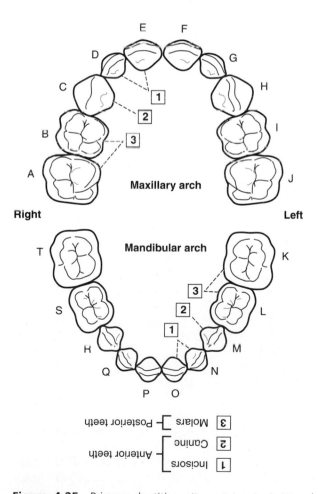

Figure 4-25 Primary dentition. (From Fehrenbach MJ, ed: Dental anatomy coloring book, St. Louis, 2008, Saunders/Elsevier.)

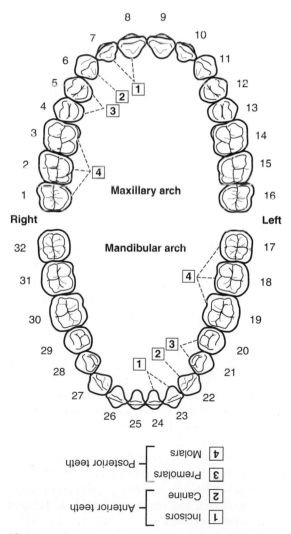

Figure 4-26 Permanent dentition. (From Fehrenbach MJ, ed: Dental anatomy coloring book, St. Louis, 2008, Saunders/Elsevier.)

D. **Height of contour** (crest of curvature):
1. Located on the mesial and distal surfaces at the contact area (also greatest elevation of the tooth either incisocervically or occlusocervically on a specific surface of the crown).
2. Also located on the facial and lingual surfaces as is easily seen when viewing the tooth's profile from the proximal.

Tooth Designation

Two systems of tooth designation are widely used. These systems offer standardized method of identifying teeth for purposes of treatment, identification, documentation. Palmer method is older method used by orthodontists and uses quadrant and position within it in numbering.
A. **Universal Tooth Designation System:** used in the United States; adaptable to electronic data transfer (used on the NDHBE):
1. Primary teeth are designated by the capital letters A through T, consecutively, starting with the maxillary right second molar, moving in a clockwise fashion, and ending with the mandibular right second molar (Figure 4-25).
2. Permanent teeth are designated by numbers #1 through #32, consecutively, starting with the maxillary right third molar, moving in a clockwise fashion, and ending with the mandibular right third molar (Figure 4-26).
B. **International Standards Organization Designation System** (ISO System) by the World Health Organization: used internationally; adaptable to electronic data transfer; teeth are designated by a two-digit code; first digit indicates quadrant, second indicates the tooth in quadrant.

Dentition Periods and Eruption Timetable

Dentition present may be within three periods: primary, mixed, permanent.
• See Chapter 2, Embryology and Histology: dental developmental.
A. Dentition periods:
1. Primary dentition period:
a. Begins with eruption of primary mandibular central incisor.
b. Occurs approximately from 6 months to 6 years; ends when first permanent tooth, mandibular first molar, erupts.
2. Mixed dentition period:
a. Follows primary dentition period; occurs approximately from 6 to 12 years.
b. Begins with eruption of first permanent tooth (mandibular first molar); ends with shedding of last primary tooth.
3. Permanent dentition period:
a. Begins with shedding of last primary tooth.

b. Occurs just after 12 years and includes eruption of all permanent teeth.
B. Eruption sequence: see Tables 4-2 and 4-3 for *approximate* eruption times and Figure 4-27 for favorable sequence of eruption for permanent teeth.
C. Premature eruption: early loss of primary tooth and premature eruption of permanent, can be caused by:
1. Not enough root for stability in primary tooth.
2. Gross caries in primary molars, resulting in early loss.
3. Bone resorption beneath primary tooth resulting from abscess.
D. Variables thought to influence permanent tooth eruption:
1. Genetic: familial, race, sex (females slightly earlier than males).
2. Environmental:
a. Low-birth-weight babies have delayed eruption, especially primary dentition.
b. Nutrition has little or no effect on eruption.
c. Systemic factors:
(1) Delayed: hypopituitarism, hypothyroidism, low levels of growth hormone.
(2) Premature exfoliation: hyperpituitarism, hyperthyroidism, cherubism, localized aggressive periodontitis, Papillon-Lefèvre syndrome, leukemia, cyclic neutropenia.

PERMANENT TEETH

Permanent dentition makes up the second dentition. Replaces primary dentition; some are **succedaneous** (having primary predecessor), others **nonsuccedaneous.**
A. There are 32 permanent teeth, 16 per dental arch:

Table 4-2 *Approximate* eruption and shedding ages for primary teeth

Tooth	Eruption (months)	Shedding (years)
MAXILLARY		
Central incisor	8-12	6-7
Lateral incisor	9-13	7-8
Canine	16-22	10-12
First molar	13-19	9-11
Second molar	25-33	10-12
MANDIBULAR		
Central incisor	6-10	6-7
Lateral incisor	10-16	7-8
Canine	14-18	9-12
First molar	17-23	9-11
Second molar	23-31	10-12

From Bath-Balogh M, Fehrenbach MJ: Illustrated dental embryology and anatomy, ed 2, Philadelphia, 2006, Saunders/Elsevier.

Table 4-3 *Approximate* eruption and root completion ages for permanent teeth (in years)

Tooth	Eruption	Root completion
MAXILLARY		
Central incisor	7-8	10
Lateral incisor	8-9	11
Canine	11-12	13-15
First premolar	10-11	12-13
Second premolar	10-12	12-14
First molar	6-7	9-10
Second molar	10-12	14-16
Third molar	17-21	18-25
MANDIBULAR		
Central incisor	6-7	9
Lateral incisor	7-8	10
Canine	9-10	12-14
First premolar	10-12	12-13
Second premolar	11-12	13-14
First molar	6-7	9-10
Second molar	11-13	14-15
Third molar	17-21	18-25

From Bath-Balogh M, Fehrenbach MJ: Illustrated dental embryology and anatomy, ed 2, Philadelphia, 2006, Saunders/Elsevier.

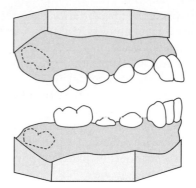

Figure 4-27 Favorable sequence of eruption per arch of the permanent dentition. (From Bath-Balogh M, Fehrenbach MJ: Illustrated dental embryology and anatomy, ed 2, Philadelphia, 2006, Saunders/Elsevier.)

1. Include anterior teeth: 4 incisors and 4 canines, and posterior teeth: 8 premolars and 8 molars; labeled in Universal Tooth Designation System by numbers, #1 to #32.
2. Eruption of the FIRST permanent tooth is the mandibular first molar at 6 years of age (NOT usually noticed, since it appears similar to the primary second molar anterior to it); completed at 17 to 25 years, after third molars have erupted.
3. By the age of 13, ALL primary teeth have been replaced; takes ~3½ years for primary to lose its roots and be replaced by permanent tooth.
B. Larger and with yellower enamel than primary teeth; jaws grow in size to accommodate difference.

Permanent Anteriors

Anteriors include incisors and canines. Composed of four developmental lobes, three labial and one lingual, and two vertical labial developmental depressions. Succedaneous teeth replace primary teeth of same type.
A. Crown: long with incisal masticatory surface:
    1. Outline is trapezoidal from labial and lingual and triangular from its proximal; compared with posteriors, anteriors are wider mesiodistally than labiolingually.
    2. Height of contour for the labial and lingual surfaces is in cervical third.

B. Proximal: contact areas are centered labiolingually on proximal surfaces, have smaller area than contact areas of posteriors but greater cementoenamel junction (CEJ) curvature than posteriors.
C. Lingual: cingulum with raised, rounded area on cervical third, in varying degrees of development; ridges are bordered mesially and distally by marginal ridges.
    1. May have a fossa, which is a shallow, wide depression; also may have pits located in deepest part of fossa.
    2. May have developmental groove, which marks junction among developmental lobes, and supplemental groove, which is MORE shallow and irregular.
D. Root: one.

Permanent Incisors

Incisors are of two types, central and lateral (Figure 4-28). When newly erupted, may contain three mamelons (rounded enamel extensions) on the incisal ridge, which are extensions from labial developmental lobes. The two incisal angles are formed from the incisal ridge on each proximal surface. Incisal ridge is flattened and becomes an incisal edge through attrition. Cingulum, lingual fossa, and marginal ridges are located on lingual surface at different levels, depending on type of incisor.
A. Maxillary incisors: maxillary central and lateral incisors resemble each other MORE than resemble similar type of incisors of opposing arch; maxillary central is larger than lateral incisor but has SIMILAR form; BOTH are wider mesiodistally than labiolingually.
    1. Crown: larger in ALL dimensions, especially mesiodistally, compared with mandibular incisors; labial surfaces are more rounded from incisal aspect, with tooth tapering toward lingual.
    2. Lingual: MORE prominent features than on the mandibular; incisal edge is just labial to long axis of root from either proximal; shovel-shaped form has greater prominence of marginal ridges, deeper

fossa; pit susceptible to caries, and presence of radicular lingual groove (RLG) can increase risk of periodontal disease.

3. Roots: SHORT compared with other maxillary teeth; do NOT have concavities.

B. Maxillary central incisors (#8, #9): largest incisors.

1. Crown: widest of any anterior, and outline when viewed from labial or lingual is trapezoidal, with lingual surface narrower overall than labial.

2. Lingual: horizontally placed groove; may have linguogingival groove or pit.

3. Proximal: CEJ curvature on mesial is deep incisally and has greatest depth of curvature of any tooth surface in permanent dentition; largest height of contour for BOTH labial and lingual surfaces.

4. Root: conical shape, which is smooth and slightly straight; narrows through middle to blunt apex.

    a. Approximately same length or shorter but wider than lateral of same arch and triangular in cervical cross section because wider on labial.

    b. Pulp cavity has only one canal and large chamber, three sharp horns.

C. Maxillary lateral incisor (#7, #10):

1. Crown: greater variation in form than any other permanent, EXCEPT for third molars.

    a. Resembles maxillary central incisor but has smaller and slightly more rounded crown; is frequently confused with small mandibular canine, yet has NO depressions on proximal surface as is common on mandibular canine.

    b. Outline is more rounded or oval from incisal, NOT triangular as central; mesiodistal measurement is wider than labiolingual measurement; labial surface is more rounded than central.

2. Lingual: horizontal groove is more common and better developed than on central, with pit common.

3. Root: conical in shape, relatively smooth and straight, yet may curve slightly to the distal.

    a. Same length or longer than central, yet thinner; apex is NOT rounded like central but rather is sharp.

    b. Pulp cavity is simple in form; one canal.

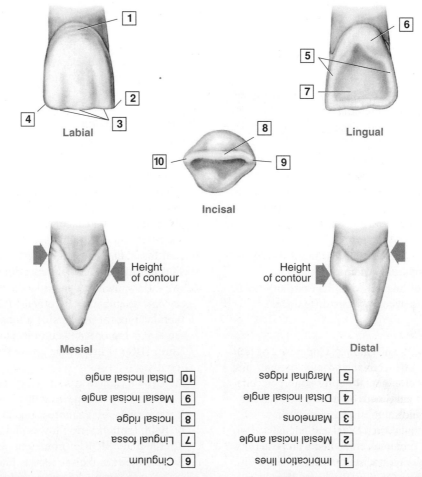

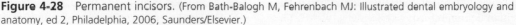

Figure 4-28 Permanent incisors. (From Bath-Balogh M, Fehrenbach MJ: Illustrated dental embryology and anatomy, ed 2, Philadelphia, 2006, Saunders/Elsevier.)

4. MOST common for partial microdontia (peg lateral) and MOST common for partial anodontia (congenitally missing).

D. Mandibular incisors: smallest and MOST symmetrical, uniform teeth.
   1. Crown: may have attrition to incisal edge, changing symmetrical form.
   2. Root: elliptical on cervical cross section; narrow on labial and lingual; wide on BOTH proximal surfaces; proximal concavities are also present and, if deep enough, give double-rooted appearance.

E. Mandibular central incisor (#24, #25):
   1. Crown: difficult to distinguish between right and left.
   2. Root has pronounced proximal root concavities and pulp cavity is simple; one canal and three horns.

F. Mandibular lateral incisor (#23, #26): NOT as symmetrical as that of central; from BOTH labial and lingual appears tilted or twisted distally in comparison with the long axis.
   1. Crown: slightly larger than central, yet resembles it.
   2. Root: pronounced proximal concavities, especially on distal surface, varying in BOTH length and depth; pulp cavity is simple; one canal, three horns.

CLINICAL STUDY

Age	20 YRS		SCENARIO
Sex	☐ Male ☒ Female		The patient comes into the office without an appointment because of concern about her teeth. During the intraoral examination, she says her palate feels sore and her face seems to be changing too, with some "downy" hair on it. However, the photographers like her more round face and square jaw.
Height	6'2"		
Weight	125 LBS		
BP	90/54		
Chief Complaint	"My teeth look thinner and transparent and even more gray in my recent photographs! How can I fix them?"		
Medical History	Breast augmentation 2 years ago Liposuction 1 year ago		
Current Medications	Laxatives for constipation		
Social History	Model		

1. What has happened to the patient's teeth? What teeth are involved and why just them? Why is her palate sore?
2. What could be the barriers to care for her now and later?
3. After working past any denial problems, what should her patient education emphasize?

1. Patient may have bulimia, a compulsive disorder that involves periods of starvation and bingeing and perceived lack of control over eating behavior; affected individuals engage in an average of two episodes a week (see Chapter 7, Nutrition). Cause is unknown but is likely to be stress related, affecting young women. Enamel erosion (perimolysis) occurs because of stomach acids from vomiting on maxillary anteriors, with dishing of lingual surfaces. This would involve the lingual surfaces of her maxillary lateral and central on both sides of her mouth (teeth #7, #8, #9, #10), since that is where the vomit always contacts. It would make the teeth thinner, thus appearing grayer. There is also salivary gland enlargement caused by the bulimia, with change in shape of face (round) and jaw (square) and with "downy" hair occurring on her face. Her palate is sore from forced vomiting (by fingers, knuckles, or other objects).

2. Initially, lack of communication could be a barrier to oral care because of denial, guilt, fear of gaining weight, and lack of compliance; also results from an inability to gain trust and confidence. She really needs to be referred to her physician to deal with her disorder. Economic barriers may come into play later because of cost of repairing oral damage.

3. Discussion of oral and medical problems associated with purging, diuretics, and laxative use. Also, she needs to neutralize vomit acid by rinsing with tap water, or possibly mix of water and sodium bicarbonate or magnesium hydroxide, as well as to avoid toothbrushing and flossing immediately after vomiting to reduce abrasion. Use of saliva substitutes or sugarless gums (possibly with xylitol) to increase salivary flow and daily use of mineralizing fluoride and calcium

products should be explained. Nutritional concerns may enter into discussion.

Permanent Canines

Maxillary and mandibular canines (cuspids) are similar (Figures 4-29 and 4-30). Have LARGER cingulum and marginal ridges on their lingual surfaces, which are narrower than the labial surfaces, and crowns that taper lingually. Longest teeth; each has a long, thick root, externally manifested by canine eminence on maxillary arch. Proximal root concavities are on BOTH proximal root surfaces and are ovoid on cervical cross section, with wide facial and proximal surfaces that show increased convergence to narrow lingual surface.

A. Maxillary canines (#6, #11):
   1. Crown: similar in length to or even shorter than maxillary central incisor.
      a. Outline is asymmetrical from incisal; distal part appears thinner than mesial and gives impression of being "stretched" to make contact with first premolar.
      b. Arch space is often partially closed and may erupt labially or lingually to surrounding teeth or may NOT erupt and remain impacted.

   2. Root: longest in maxillary arch; with blunt apex and developmental depressions on BOTH proximal surfaces, especially on the distal; one canal and large chamber, with only one horn.
B. Mandibular canines (#22, #27):
   1. Crown: can be as long as or even longer than maxillary canine; rarely has lingual pits or grooves.
   2. Root: may be as long as that of maxillary canine but is somewhat shorter; longest mandibular root, with slight mesial inclination.
      a. More pronounced and often deeper mesial developmental depression than in the maxillary canine.
      b. Distal developmental depression similar to mesial, giving double-rooted appearance.
      c. Pulp cavity resembles that of maxillary canine, with only one horn; may have two separate canals (one labially and one lingually), may join at the apex or have separate apical foramina.

Permanent Posteriors

Posteriors include premolars and molars.
A. Crowns: trapezoidal from the buccal and lingual.

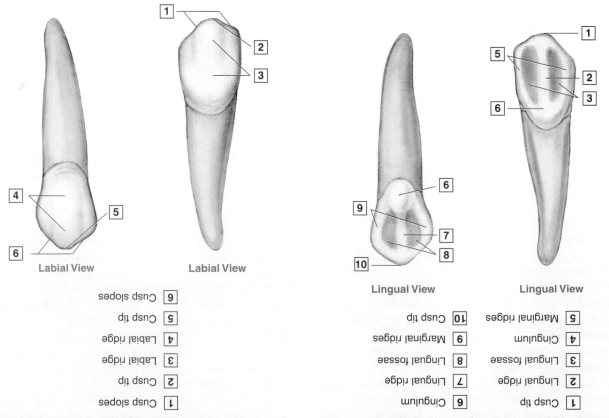

Labial View   Labial View

9	Cusp slopes
5	Cusp tip
4	Labial ridge
3	Labial ridge
2	Cusp tip
1	Cusp slopes

Figure 4-29 Labial view of permanent right canines. *Left,* Maxillary; *right,* mandibular. (From Bath-Balogh M, Fehrenbach MJ: Illustrated dental embryology and anatomy, ed 2, Philadelphia, 2006, Saunders/Elsevier.)

Lingual View   Lingual View

10	Cusp tip	5	Marginal ridges
9	Marginal ridges	4	Cingulum
8	Lingual fossae	3	Lingual fossae
7	Lingual ridge	2	Lingual ridge
6	Cingulum	1	Cusp tip

Figure 4-30 Lingual view of permanent right canines. *Left,* Maxillary; *right,* mandibular. (From Bath-Balogh M, Fehrenbach MJ: Illustrated dental embryology and anatomy, ed 2, Philadelphia, 2006, Saunders/Elsevier.)

1. Height of contour for the buccal surface is in cervical third and for lingual surface is in middle or occlusal third.
2. Wider labiolingually than mesiodistally, except for mandibular molars, when compared with anteriors.

B. Proximal:
   1. Contact areas are wider for posteriors than those of anteriors and are located to the buccal of center; also are closer to same level on each side.
   2. CEJ curvature is less pronounced on posteriors than on anteriors, may be quite straight.

C. Occlusal table: bordered by raised marginal ridges located on the distal and mesial and have two or more cusps (see Figures 4-32 to 4-39 for comparison to anterior teeth).
   1. With four cusp ridges descending from each cusp tip and inclined cuspal planes between them, triangular cusp ridges descend from cusp tips toward central part.
   2. May have a transverse ridge that occurs with the joining of two triangular ridges that cross occlusal table transversely or from the labial to lingual outline.
   3. Shallow and wide fossae; central fossae are located at converging of cusp ridges in central point, where there is junction of grooves and triangular fossa that appears to have triangular shape at convergence of cusp ridges, associated with termination of triangular grooves.
   4. Developmental grooves or primary grooves are sharp, deep, with V-shaped linear depressions; MOST prominent is central groove, which travels mesiodistally and separates occlusal table buccolingually.
   5. Marginal grooves cross marginal ridges, and triangular grooves separate marginal ridge from triangular ridge of a cusp, forming triangular fossa at termination.
   6. Supplemental grooves or secondary grooves are shallower, more irregular linear depressions.
   7. Developmental pits, where two or more grooves meet; can be located in deepest parts of fossa, making it susceptible to caries.

Permanent Premolars: First and Second

Premolars (bicuspids) are succedaneous and replace primary first and second molars; they are found ONLY in permanent dentition. May be extracted in each quadrant for orthodontic purposes to improve dental arch spacing (first premolar). Shorter crown than anteriors and buccal surface is rounded, with prominent buccal ridge and buccal developmental depressions. Height of contour labially is in cervical third, similar to anteriors, and lingually is in middle third. MOST have one root, except for maxillary first, which has two roots. Have proximal

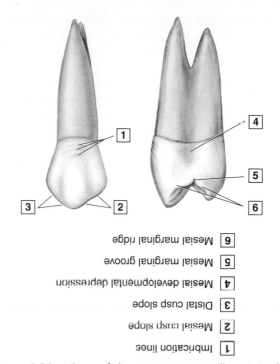

1 Imbrication lines
2 Mesial cusp slope
3 Distal cusp slope
4 Mesial developmental depression
5 Mesial marginal groove
6 Mesial marginal ridge

Figure 4-31 Views of the permanent maxillary right first premolar. (From Bath-Balogh M, Fehrenbach MJ: Illustrated dental embryology and anatomy, ed 2, Philadelphia, 2006, Saunders/Elsevier.)

root concavities. MOST susceptible to abfraction and labial cervical recession and enamel breakage caused by oral habits.

A. Maxillary premolars: BOTH types resemble each other MORE than mandibular premolar; first is larger than second.
   1. Crown: two cusps of almost equal size, centered over long axis of tooth from proximal.
      a. Shorter occlusocervically than maxillary canines, yet slightly longer than molars.
      b. Unlike crowns of mandibular premolars, centered over root and show no lingual inclination.
      c. Greater buccolingual than mesiodistal width compared with mandibular premolars.
   2. Proximal: trapezoidal.
   3. Occlusal table: somewhat hexagonal.
   4. Roots: shorter than maxillary canines and same length as molars.
      a. Show a slight lingual and distal inclination.
      b. On cervical cross section, appear elliptical; appearance may be slightly altered by proximal concavities.
      c. May penetrate maxillary sinus during accidental trauma or during tooth extraction because of close proximity; discomfort from sinusitis may be confused with tooth-related discomfort or vice-versa.

B. Maxillary first premolars (#5, #12) (Figure 4-31):
   1. Crown: widest mesiodistally of all premolars; wide at the level of contact areas and more narrow at CEJ. Occlusal table: transverse ridge perpendicular to central groove, mesial and distal pits.
   2. Roots: ONLY premolar with two roots, two branches or bifurcated in apical third; one buccal and one lingual or palatal; may be fused or laminated.
      a. DISTINCT mesial concavity is present on trunk, extending from contact area to bifurcation; increases periodontal risk, since allows increased deposit level.
      b. Pulp cavity shows two horns (one for each cusp) and two canals (one for each root).
C. Maxillary second premolar (#4, #13):
   1. Crown: less angular and more rounded in shape than the maxillary first, with more variations.
   2. Occlusal table: numerous supplemental grooves radiating from a central groove.
   3. Roots: has one; may have two, however; less pronounced greater length of second mesial concavity; pulp cavity has one canal and two horns.
D. Mandibular premolars: do NOT resemble each other as much as those of maxillary premolars; first smaller than second.
   1. Crowns: buccal outline shows strong lingual inclination proximally; occlusally, appears almost round, with strong buccal ridge; may have more than two cusps; lingual are always smaller than buccal.
   2. Proximal: outlines are rhomboidal, with lingual incline; contact areas are nearly on same level and have similar CEJs.
   3. Root: has one, with a slight distal inclination; in cervical cross section is either ovoid or elliptical; may be slightly altered by proximal concavities, MOST frequently found on mesial surface.
E. Mandibular first premolar (#21, #28): shows transition in dental arch from canine to molarlike second premolar.
   1. Crown: resembles mandibular canine in many more ways than it does mandibular second premolar, smaller overall than canine.
   2. Occlusal table: lingual cusp is very small, no more than half height of buccal, with four lingual cusp ridges, four lingual inclined cuspal planes, and lingual triangular ridge.
   3. Root: smaller and shorter than mandibular second premolar.
      a. May have deep groove on distal.
      b. Pulp cavity consists of one canal and two horns; each horn is located within cusp; buccal horn more pronounced.
F. Mandibular second premolars (#20, #29) (Figure 4-32):

   1. Crown has two types, three-cusp and two-cusp crowns.
      a. The three-cusp (tricuspidate) develops from three lobes:
         (1) MOST common; one large buccal cusp and two smaller lingual cusps.
         (2) Grooves form distinctive Y-shaped pattern on the occlusal table, resembling a small molar.
      b. The two-cusp (bicuspidate) develops from two lobes.
         (1) Similar to that of mandibular first premolars, one larger buccal cusp and one smaller lingual cusp;
         (2) Central groove is crescent or U shaped, appears rounded from occlusal.
   2. Root: larger and longer than first premolar, yet shorter than maxillary premolars.
      a. Pronounced proximal concavities.
      b. Pulp cavity for three-cusp type has three pointed horns; two-cusp type has two horns.

Permanent Molars: First, Second, and Third

Molars are nonsuccedaneous and do NOT replace primary teeth (Figures 4-33 and 4-34). They show evidence of developmental lobe separation in developmental grooves on occlusal table; do NOT exhibit buccal developmental depressions. Have large crowns in comparison with rest of the permanent dentition and are shorter occlusocervically than teeth anterior to them.

A. Crown: three or more cusps, of which at least two are buccal cusps, and its buccal surface has a prominent cervical ridge running mesiodistally in cervical one third.
B. Occlusal table: bordered by cusp ridges and marginal ridges.
   1. MORE complicated than premolars because there are more developmental grooves, supplemental grooves, occlusal developmental pits.
   2. Grooves (fissures) and pits are located on occlusal and lingual surfaces of maxillary and on occlusal and buccal surfaces of mandibular molars (Figure 4-35).
C. Roots: multirooted; maxillary molars usually have three branches; mandibular usually have two.
   1. Cervical cross section of trunk follows form of crown but then divides into number of branches.
   2. Furcations lie between two or more of these branches before dividing from trunk; furcation crotches are the spaces between roots at furcation and concavities are found on many branches and furcal surfaces.
   3. With the loss of periodontal tissue support from advanced periodontal disease, furcations, furcation crotches, and concavities of the molars may lose their bony coverage in varying degrees and

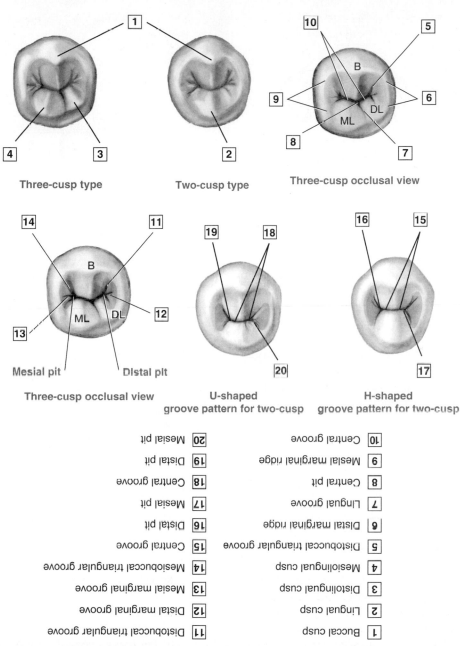

Three-cusp type   Two-cusp type   Three-cusp occlusal view

Three-cusp occlusal view   U-shaped groove pattern for two-cusp   H-shaped groove pattern for two-cusp

20	Mesial pit	10	Central groove
19	Distal pit	9	Mesial marginal ridge
18	Central groove	8	Central pit
17	Mesial pit	7	Lingual groove
16	Distal pit	6	Distal marginal ridge
15	Central groove	5	Distobuccal triangular groove
14	Mesiobuccal triangular groove	4	Mesiolingual cusp
13	Mesial marginal groove	3	Distolingual cusp
12	Distal marginal groove	2	Lingual cusp
11	Distobuccal triangular groove	1	Buccal cusp

Figure 4-32 Occlusal view of the two types of permanent mandibular right second premolars: three-cusp and two-cusp. Occlusal table, Y-shaped groove pattern, fossae, and U- and H-shaped groove patterns shown. (From Bath-Balogh M, Fehrenbach MJ: Illustrated dental embryology and anatomy, ed 2, Philadelphia, 2006, Saunders/Elsevier.)

present a challenge during instrumentation and performance of oral hygiene.
D. Localized enamel hypoplasia from congenital syphilis can result in mulberry molars, when molars have one or more tubercles or accessory cusps; dilaceration can also occur, making extraction and endodontic treatment difficult.
E. Maxillary molars:
　1. Crown: shorter occlusocervically than teeth anterior to them, but larger in all other measurements than other maxillary teeth.
　　a. Wider buccolingually than mesiodistally; from occlusal, outline is rhomboidal, and from proximal, trapezoidal.
　　b. Possible lingual pit that is susceptible to caries.
　2. Occlusal table:
　　a. Has four major cusps, with two cusps on buccal and two on lingual (Figure 4-36).
　　b. ONLY teeth with oblique ridge, transverse ridge formed by union of triangular ridge of DB cusp and the distal cusp ridge of ML cusp.

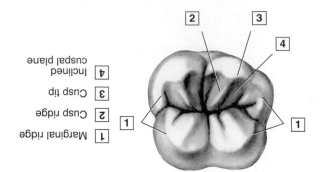

Inclined 4 cuspal plane

Cusp tip 3

Cusp ridge 2

Marginal ridge 1

Figure 4-33 Example of occlusal surface of permanent molar. (From Bath-Balogh M, Fehrenbach MJ: Illustrated dental embryology and anatomy, ed 2, Philadelphia, 2006, Saunders/Elsevier.)

3. Roots: ONLY teeth with three roots, trifurcated into three branches (MB, DB, and lingual [palatal]).
    a. Lingual branch is largest and longest; when located farther (distally) in the maxillary arch, have shorter and more varied roots in size, shape, and curvature but are less divergent.
    b. Show great lingual and moderate distal inclination and have three furcations, located on the mesial, buccal, and distal surfaces, that begin near the junction of the cervical and middle thirds.
    c. May have concavities on the mesial surface of MB root, on lingual surface of lingual root, and on all three furcal surfaces.
    d. May penetrate the maxillary sinus, from accidental trauma or during tooth extraction owing to close proximity, MOST commonly associated with discomfort from sinusitis.
    e. Teeth MOST commonly involved in concrescence in permanent dentition.
F. Maxillary first molars (#3, #14): five developmental lobes: two buccal and three lingual.
    1. Crown: largest among those of the permanent dentition; more complex form than nearby maxillary premolars; LEAST variable form among maxillary molars.
    2. Occlusal table:
        a. ML cusp is largest cusp, with rounded cusp tip (Figure 4-37).
        b. May have minor (fifth) cusp of Carabelli, with its groove; smallest cusp.
        c. Has three triangular grooves (MB, ML, D) and oblique ridge.
    3. Roots: larger and more divergent than those of second molar, more complex in form than roots of maxillary premolars.
        a. Twice as long as crown; thus furcations are well removed from cervical area.
        b. Pulp cavity has one horn for each major cusp; roots have three main pulp canals.
G. Maxillary second molars (#2, #15):
    1. Crown: two outline types, either rhomboid or heart shaped.

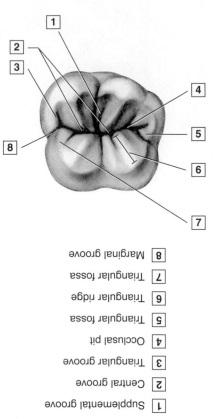

Marginal groove 8

Triangular fossa 7

Triangular ridge 6

Triangular fossa 5

Occlusal pit 4

Triangular groove 3

Central groove 2

Supplemental groove 1

Figure 4-34 Example of occlusal table on permanent molar. (From Bath-Balogh M, Fehrenbach MJ: Illustrated dental embryology and anatomy, ed 2, Philadelphia, 2006, Saunders/Elsevier.)

    2. Occlusal table:
        a. Rhomboid type: cusps similar to major cusps of maxillary first molar.
        b. Heart-shaped type: has DL cusp that is small, sometimes absent.
    3. Roots: show furcation notches that are narrower than first molar.
        a. Greater chance of fusion, especially of buccal roots or all three roots.
        b. Pulp cavity consists of chamber, three main canals, four horns.
H. Maxillary third molars (#1, #16) (wisdom tooth):
    1. Crown: no standard form; smallest molar and MOST variable in shape in permanent dentition.
    2. Occlusal table: two outline forms, heart shaped or rhomboidal.
        a. Heart shaped: MOST common; similar to maxillary second molar but with more supplemental grooves; only three cusps (MB, DB, ML).
        b. Rhomboid occlusal: four cusps; no oblique ridge on small DL cusp.
    3. Roots: trifurcated and fused, either partially or fully.
        a. Poorly developed and shorter than second molar, curved distally; may have accessory root.

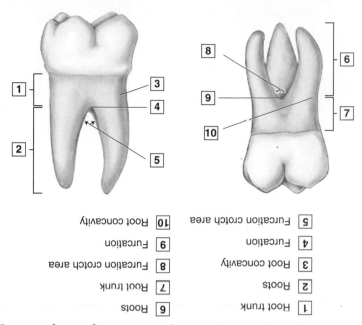

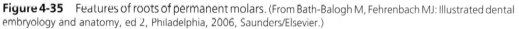

10	Root concavity		5	Furcation crotch area
9	Furcation		4	Furcation
8	Furcation crotch area		3	Root concavity
7	Root trunk		2	Roots
6	Roots		1	Root trunk

Figure 4-35 Features of roots of permanent molars. (From Bath-Balogh M, Fehrenbach MJ: Illustrated dental embryology and anatomy, ed 2, Philadelphia, 2006, Saunders/Elsevier.)

b. Pulp cavity may have a chamber and three canals; number of horns varies, depending on the number of cusps present.

4. May show partial microdontia (peg third molar) or partial anodontia (congenitally missing) or may fail to erupt and remain impacted.

I. Mandibular molars:

1. Crown: wider mesiodistally than buccolingually, similar to anteriors.

a. From occlusal, have an outline that is rectangular or pentagonal; buccal view shows strong lingual inclination proximally (like nearby premolars) and is rhomboidal.

b. Have four or five major cusps; always with two lingual cusps of approximately same width.

2. Roots: two roots or bifurcated, with mesial and distal; show distal inclination.

a. Have two furcations located on buccal and lingual surfaces, midway between proximal surfaces.

b. Concavities on mesial surface of mesial root and on furcal surfaces of BOTH mesial and distal roots; concavities on mesial root are especially prominent if this root also has two canals.

J. Mandibular first molars (#19, #30):

1. Crown: widest mesiodistally of any permanent tooth because of fifth major cusp; has three buccal and two lingual cusps.

2. Occlusal table: MOST complex groove pattern of all mandibular molars: Y-shaped groove pattern

by cusps and MB, DB, lingual grooves; NO transverse ridges (Figure 4-38).

3. Roots: widely separated buccally; trunk is shorter than second and pulp cavity has three canals and five horns.

K. Mandibular second molars (#18, #31):

1. Crown: smaller than first molar and rectangular occlusally.

2. Occlusal table: cross-shaped groove pattern formed by well-defined grooves that divide into four parts, with four nearly equal-sized cusps (Figure 4-39).

3. Roots: smaller, shorter, less divergent, and closer together than in first molar, and pulp cavity can have two canals (one for each root).

L. Mandibular third molars (#17 and #32) (wisdom tooth):

1. Crown: NO standard form; often has oval occlusal outline; can be smaller or same size as first molar of same arch.

2. Occlusal table: two mesial cusps, larger than two distal cusps; irregular groove pattern, with numerous supplemental grooves and occlusal pits.

3. Roots: two roots OFTEN are fused, irregularly curved, shorter than mandibular second molar; pulp cavity is similar to second molars, with four horns and two or three canals.

4. May fail to erupt and remain impacted or partially erupted; may exhibit partial anodontia (congenitally missing).

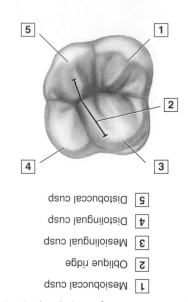

Figure 4-36 labels (shown inverted):

5 Distobuccal cusp
4 Distolingual cusp
3 Mesiolingual cusp
2 Oblique ridge
1 Mesiobuccal cusp

Figure 4-36 Occlusal view of permanent maxillary molar. (From Bath-Balogh M, Fehrenbach MJ: Illustrated dental embryology and anatomy, ed 2, Philadelphia, 2006, Saunders/Elsevier.)

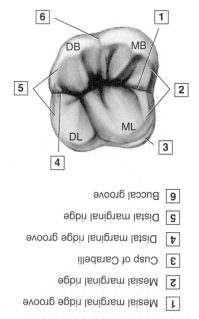

Figure 4-37 labels (shown inverted):

6 Buccal groove
5 Distal marginal ridge
4 Distal marginal ridge groove
3 Cusp of Carabelli
2 Mesial marginal ridge
1 Mesial marginal ridge groove

Figure 4-37 Occlusal table of permanent maxillary right first molar. (From Bath-Balogh M, Fehrenbach MJ: Illustrated dental embryology and anatomy, ed 2, Philadelphia, 2006, Saunders/Elsevier.)

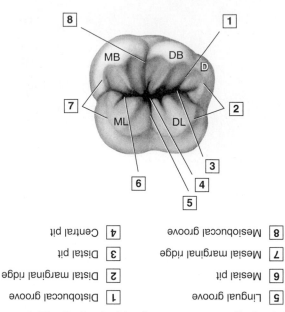

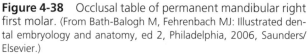

Figure 4-38 labels (shown inverted):

8 Mesiobuccal groove	4 Central pit
7 Mesial marginal ridge	3 Distal pit
6 Mesial pit	2 Distal marginal ridge
5 Lingual groove	1 Distobuccal groove

Figure 4-38 Occlusal table of permanent mandibular right first molar. (From Bath-Balogh M, Fehrenbach MJ: Illustrated dental embryology and anatomy, ed 2, Philadelphia, 2006, Saunders/Elsevier.)

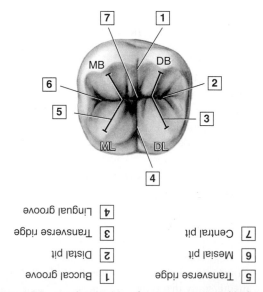

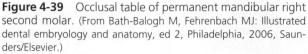

Figure 4-39 labels (shown inverted):

7 Central pit	4 Lingual groove
6 Mesial pit	3 Transverse ridge
5 Transverse ridge	2 Distal pit
	1 Buccal groove

Figure 4-39 Occlusal table of permanent mandibular right second molar. (From Bath-Balogh M, Fehrenbach MJ: Illustrated dental embryology and anatomy, ed 2, Philadelphia, 2006, Saunders/Elsevier.)

PRIMARY TEETH

Primary teeth make up first dentition. Exfoliated (shed) and replaced by permanent dentition (Figure 4-40).

A. There are 20 primary teeth, 10 per dental arch.
   1. Include 4 incisors, 4 canines, and 8 molars; labeled in Universal Tooth Designation System by capital letters, A through T.
   2. Begin calcification at 13 to 16 weeks' gestation; by 18 to 20 weeks' gestation have started to calcify.
   3. Eruption of primary mandibular central incisor occurs FIRST at average age of 8 months; thus NO primary teeth are visible at birth.
   4. Root formation takes from 2 to 3 years to be completed, including completion of roots of maxillary second molar; 6-month delay or acceleration is considered normal (see earlier discussion).

B. Smaller and whiter enamel than permanents (parents can be so jealous); may demonstrate extensive extrinsic green staining because of Nasmyth's membrane.

C. Crowns:
1. Shorter relative to the total length and MORE constricted (narrower) at the CEJ, which makes them appear bulbous.
2. Cervical ridges on BOTH labial and lingual surfaces of anteriors and buccal surfaces of molars; masticatory surfaces may show high levels of attrition.

D. Roots:
1. Narrower and longer when compared with overall crown length and may show partial resorption.
2. Hold eruption space for succedaneous permanent teeth; early assessment for appropriate preventive orthodontic intervention is important; supervising adults and child patients sometimes discount the importance of these teeth.

E. Pulp cavity:
1. Relatively large in proportion to the permanent dentition, especially larger mesial horns of the molars, increases risk of exposure during cavity preparation.
2. Thinner enamel and dentin than permanent teeth; risk of endodontic complications is greater.

Primary Incisors

Primary incisors include primary maxillary and mandibular central and lateral.

A. Primary maxillary central incisor (E, F):
1. Crown: wider mesiodistally than incisocervically (opposite of permanent successor).
   a. Appears thick even at incisal third (can be altered by attrition); incisal edge is nearly straight; no mamelons and no lingual pits, unlike its permanent successors.
   b. Cingulum and marginal ridges are more prominent and lingual fossae are deeper than in permanents.
2. Proximal: the CEJ curves distinctly toward incisal, but not as much as on permanent successor.
3. Root: one; is round and tapers evenly to apex.
B. Primary maxillary lateral incisor (D, G):
1. Crown: similar to central incisor but is much smaller; longer incisocervically than mesiodistally and incisal angles that also are more rounded than those of the central incisor.
2. Root: is also similar to that of central incisor, but apex is sharper.
C. Primary mandibular central incisor (O, P):
1. Crown: more like that of primary mandibular lateral incisor than permanent successor or any other primary maxillary incisor.
   a. Symmetrical tooth, similar to permanent successor, with incisal edge centered over root;

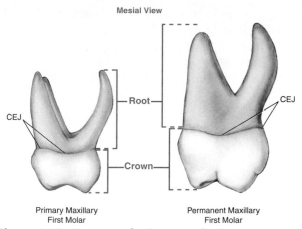

Figure 4-40 Features of primary teeth. (From Bath-Balogh M, Fehrenbach MJ: Illustrated dental embryology and anatomy, ed 2, Philadelphia, 2006, Saunders/Elsevier.)

NOT as constricted at CEJ as primary maxillary central.
   b. Labially, appears wide in comparison with permanent successor; has mesial and distal outlines that taper evenly from the contacts.
   c. Lingual appears smooth and tapers toward prominent cingulum, which has less pronounced marginal ridges and shallow lingual fossa.
   d. Mesially, much wider labiolingually than permanent successor.
2. Root: one, long and slender; labial and lingual are rounded, yet proximals are slightly flattened.
D. Primary mandibular lateral incisor (Q and N):
1. Crown: similar in form of mandibular central incisor, wider and longer than central, but NOT as symmetrical.
   a. Cingulum more developed; offset toward distal.
   b. Deeper lingual fossa than central; incisal edge slopes distally; distoincisal angle more rounded.
2. Root: may have distal curvature in apical third and distal longitudinal groove.

CLINICAL STUDY

Scenario: During an emergency dental appointment for a 2-year-old, the patient's mother tells how he slipped in the bathtub and hit his upper front teeth. He is bleeding profusely, and his upper lip is severely swollen. Both primary maxillary central incisors are intruded into the maxilla. "My son's front teeth are pushed into the gums!"

1. How many teeth can the patient have at present, and what dentition period is present?
2. At 2 years of age, which teeth should be fully erupted?
3. Identify the blood and nerve vessels that are most likely to be injured in this situation.
4. What effect might this trauma have on the patient's oral development?

1. He is in the primary (deciduous) dentition period in which 20 teeth are usually present.
2. At 2 years, primary maxillary and mandibular central and lateral incisors, canines, first molars are fully erupted. Primary second molars erupt at 27 to 29 months, depending on arch.
3. Infraorbital (IO) artery supplies upper lip, and anterior superior alveolar (ASA) nerve innervates maxillary anterior teeth and bone.
4. Intrusion injury occurs when the tooth root is forcibly compressed into alveolar bone. This severe injury caused damage to primary maxillary central incisor roots and alveolar bone. When injury occurs in primary dentition, displacement of tooth can also cause injury to adjacent developing permanent maxillary teeth. Enamel development of the permanent maxillary central and lateral incisors begins 3 to 4 months after birth and continues to age 5; therefore permanent maxillary central incisors may possibly exhibit slight to moderate enamel defects (hypoplasia and/or hypocalcification).

Primary Canines

Primary canines include primary maxillary and mandibular canines.
A. Primary maxillary canine (C, H):
   1. Crown: relatively longer, with sharper cusp than permanent successor, when first erupts.
      a. Rounder mesial and distal outlines that greatly overhang cervical line; mesial cusp slope is longer than distal.
      b. Cingulum, lingual ridge, and marginal ridges are well developed; tubercle often present on cingulum.
      c. Lingual ridge divides lingual into shallow ML and DL fossae.
      d. Incisally, diamond shaped; cusp tip offset distally.
   2. Root: twice as long as crown, more slender than permanent successor, inclined distally.
B. Primary mandibular canine (M, R):
   1. Crown: resembles primary maxillary canine.
      a. Smaller labiolingually; incisal edge straight and centered labiolingually.
      b. Distal cusp slope longer than the mesial and lingual is smoother than maxillary canine, with shallow lingual fossa.
   2. Root: long, narrow, almost twice crown length; shorter and more tapered than maxillary canine.

Primary Molars

Primary molars include primary maxillary and mandibular first and second molars.
A. Crown:
   1. Does NOT resemble any other tooth in either dentition; primary second in BOTH arches does resemble permanent first molars that will erupt distal to them (may make it hard to see permanent's eruption, so that there is failure of oral homecare and dental care).
   2. Shorter occlusocervically than mesiodistally.
B. Occlusal table:
   1. More constricted buccolingually than permanent molars, with buccal and lingual surfaces flatter occlusal to CEJ.
   2. Anatomy of cusps NOT as pronounced as on permanent successors.
C. Roots:
   1. Have a short trunk, creating more space for developing permanent premolar crowns.
   2. Flare beyond crown outlines; widely separated to create additional space between roots for developing permanent premolar crowns.
   3. Greater spread of roots, along with narrow shape and lack of trunk, making it easier to fracture during extraction procedures.
D. Primary maxillary first molar (B, I):
   1. Crown: does NOT resemble other crowns of either dentition.
      a. From buccal, mesial and distal outlines are rounded and constricted at CEJ, and on mesial half of buccal surface curves around prominent buccal cervical ridge.
      b. Height of contour on buccal is at cervical one third and for lingual is at middle one third.
   2. Occlusal table: can have four cusps (MB, ML, DB, DL).
      a. Mesial cusps are largest and distal cusps are very small; frequently has only three cusps; DL cusp may be absent.
      b. Has prominent transverse ridge and oblique ridge running between ML cusp and DB cusp, although NOT as prominent as on permanent counterpart.
      c. Has H-shaped groove pattern and central, mesial triangular, and distal triangular fossae, with central groove connecting the central, mesial, and distal pits; buccal groove separates MB and DB cusps, and distal triangular fossa contains disto-occlusal groove.
   3. Roots: SAME number and position as those of permanent dentition.
      a. Short trunk, with three branches that are thinner and have greater flare than on permanent molar.
      b. The MB root is wider buccolingually than DB root; lingual root is longest and MOST divergent.
E. Primary maxillary second molar (A, J):
   1. Crown and occlusal table: MOST closely resembles the permanent maxillary first molar.
      a. Yet is smaller in all dimensions.
      b. Has cusp of Carabelli, minor fifth cusp.

F. Primary mandibular first molar (L, S):
   1. Crown: unlike any other tooth of either dentition.
      a. Has prominent buccal cervical ridge on mesial half of buccal.
      b. Height of contour on the buccal is at cervical one third and for lingual is in middle one third.
      c. The ML line angle is rounder than any other.
   2. Occlusal table: four cusps; mesial cusps are larger; ML cusp is long, pointed, and angled; transverse ridge runs between MB and ML cusps.
   3. Roots: BOTH positioned similarly to other primary and permanent mandibular molars.
G. Primary mandibular second molar (K, T):
   1. Crown: larger than primary mandibular first molar; MOST closely resembles form of permanent mandibular first molar that erupts distal to it (may make it hard to notice permanent's eruption, so that there is failure of oral homecare and/or dental care).
   2. Occlusal table: five cusps; three buccal cusps of nearly equal size, with overall oval occlusal shape.
   3. Roots: positioned similarly to those of other primary and permanent mandibular molars.

OCCLUSION

Occlusion is the contact relationship between the maxillary and mandibular teeth when the jaws are in a fully closed position. Also refers to the relationship between teeth in the same arch. Occlusion develops as the primary teeth erupt. Involves interrelated factors in development, such as associated musculature, neuromuscular patterns, temporomandibular joint functioning.
- See Chapter 13, Periodontology: occlusal trauma.
A. **Mandibular rest position:** physiological rest position of mandible when relaxed; 2 to 3 mm of interocclusal clearance between arches; failure may mean parafunctional habits, which may be involved in occlusal problems.
B. **Occlusal plane:** maxillary and mandibular teeth in centric occlusion along BOTH anteroposterior and lateral curves (noted by the linea alba).
   1. Arches do NOT conform to flat planes but are curves; maxillary arch is convex occlusally, and mandibular arch is concave:
      a. **Curve of Spee:** anteroposterior concave curve of the occlusal plane produced by the alignment of the posteriors.
         (1) Noted when viewing posteriors from the buccal.
         (2) Beginning at the tip of the mandibular canine, following the buccal cusps of the natural premolars and molars, and continuing to the anterior border of the ramus.

         (3) MOST important when mounting radiographs.
      b. **Curve of Wilson:** lateral concave curve of the occlusal plane produced by the alignment of the posteriors.
         (1) Noted when a frontal section is taken through each set of both maxillary and mandibular molars: the firsts, seconds, and then thirds.
         (2) Formed by the lingual inclination of the posteriors because the lingual cusps are lower than the buccal cusps.
C. **Centric occlusion** (CO) (habitual occlusion):
   1. Voluntary position of dentition that allows maximum contact when teeth occlude, equalizing forces of impact; serves as basis for reference.
   2. In CO, relation of permanent maxillary first molar to mandibular arch is established when ML cusp interdigitates with the central fossa of mandibular first molar (see following discussion of occlusal evaluation).

Occlusal Evaluation

Normal occlusion is an ideal occlusion. However, it rarely exists; the concept provides a basis for treatment. Occlusal disharmony may lead to occlusal trauma, which could be an adverse factor in periodontal disease development; must be considered during dental treatment; occlusal adjustment involving removal of restorative, prosthetic, or natural tooth material may be needed.
A. American Association of Orthodontists (AAO) recommends that all children have orthodontic evaluation no later than age 7.
   1. Posterior occlusion is established when the first molars erupt; evaluation of the anteroposterior and transverse occlusal relationships can be performed and any functional shifts discovered.
   2. Incisors have begun to erupt, and problems such as crowding, habits, deep bites, open bites, some facial asymmetries can be detected.
   3. Early intervention and/or early treatment presents the opportunity to:
      a. Influence jaw growth in a positive manner and harmonize width of the dental arches.
      b. Improve eruption patterns and lower risk of trauma to protruded maxillary incisors.
      c. Correct harmful oral habits and improve esthetics and self-esteem.
      d. Simplify and/or shorten treatment time for later corrective orthodontics and reduce likelihood of impacted permanent teeth.
      e. Improve some speech problems and preserve or gain space for erupting permanent teeth.
B. **Malocclusions:** misalignment of teeth and jaws; can be a factor in oral health and hygiene; crowding is MOST common type (Figure 4-41):

1. **Overbite:** vertical overlap between maxillary and mandibular anterior teeth, normal overbite is only 2 to 3 mm or one third overlap.
   a. Measure vertical overlap with a periodontal probe and record in millimeters; described as slight (in the incisal one third), moderate (in the middle one third), or severe (in the gingival one third).
   b. Over closed, deep bite, or severe overbite: maxillary incisors overlap into gingival one third of the mandibular incisors.
2. **Overjet:** horizontal distance between maxillary and mandibular incisors; normal overjet is only 2 to 3 mm.
   a. Measured as horizontal distance between linguals of maxillary anterior teeth and facials of mandibular anterior teeth with a periodontal probe and recorded in millimeters.
   b. Excessive overjet is second MOST common form of malocclusion.
3. **Openbite:** lack of incisal or occlusal contact or overlap between maxillary and mandibular teeth; usually canines, laterals, centrals.
4. **Edge-to-edge bite** (end to end): NOT any vertical overlap between the arches (incisal edge of maxillary teeth meets incisal edge of mandibular teeth); occurs with anteriors and/or posteriors.
5. **Anterior crossbite:** maxillary incisors are lingual to mandibular incisors.
6. **Posterior crossbite:** maxillary posteriors are lingual or facial to ideal position (buccal or lingual to maxillary arch).
7. Labioversion: tooth lies labial to normal position; linguoversion: tooth lies lingual to normal position.

C. Angle's classification of malocclusion: serves to initially address malocclusion (Table 4-4).
D. Malposed dentition factors:
   1. Oral musculature force (tongue thrusting, cheek or lip biting, mouth breathing, abnormal tongue position) and tooth loss:
      a. Tongue exerts *outward* pressure, lips and cheeks provide balancing *inward* force.
      b. Strong forward thrust of tongue can force teeth out of position, also happens when adult continues swallowing patterns of childhood.
   2. Foreign object-to-tooth parafunctional habits (holding pin or pipe between teeth, nail biting, finger and/or thumb sucking).
      a. *Outward* pressure of a finger-sucking habit pushes maxillary anterior and jaw forward and out of alignment.
   3. Tooth-to-tooth parafunctional habits (clenching and/or bruxism [grinding]).
   4. Teeth that are in contact with opposing teeth (occlusal antagonist) in opposing jaw undergo super-eruption (increased eruption) that can decrease alveolar bone support and thus increase mobility.
   5. Iatrogenic factors: poorly contoured restorations, improper fit of removable appliance.
E. Primary dentition occlusal evaluation: tooth eruption usually begins at 6 to 10 months of age and is completed at 2½ to 3 years of age; MOST variability in eruption for dentitions.
   1. **Primate spaces:** normal developmental spaces, usually located between maxillary lateral incisors and canines and between mandibular canines and first molars; necessary for proper alignment of future permanents.

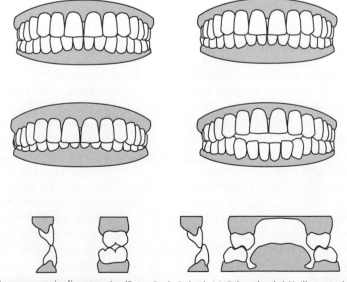

Figure 4-41 Common misalignments. (From Bath-Balogh M, Fehrenbach MI: Illustrated dental embryology and anatomy, ed 2, Philadelphia, 2006, Saunders/Elsevier.)

Table 4-4   Angle's classification of malocclusion*

Class	Model	Arch relationships	Descriptions
Class I		Molar: MC cusp of the maxillary first occluding with the MB groove of the mandibular first Canines: maxillary occluding with the distal half of the mandibular canine and the mesial half of the mandibular first premolar	Dental malalignment(s) present (see text), such as crowding or spacing; mesognathic profile; facial profile is flat with chin in same plane as forehead
Class II	Division I Division II	Molar: MB cusp of the maxillary first occluding (by more than the width of a premolar) mesial to the MB groove of the mandibular first Canines: distal surface of the mandibular canine distal to the mesial surface of the maxillary canine by at least the width of a premolar	Division I: maxillary anteriors protruding facially from the mandibular anteriors, with deep overbite; retrognathic profile Division II: maxillary central incisors either upright or retruded, and lateral incisors either tipped labially or overlapping the central incisors with deep overbite; mesognathic profile. Facial profile is convex with chin retruded
Class III		Molar: MB cusp of the maxillary first occluding (by more than the width of a premolar) distal to the MB groove of the mandibular first Canines: distal surface of the mandibular mesial to the mesial surface of the maxillary by at least the width of a premolar	Mandibular incisors in complete crossbite; prognathic profile; facial profile is concave with chin protruded

From Bath-Balogh M, Fehrenbach MJ: Illustrated dental embryology and anatomy, ed 2, Philadelphia, 2006, Saunders/Elsevier.
MB, Mesiobuccal.
*Note that this system deals with the classification of the permanent dentition.

2. **Terminal plane:** permanent first molars are guided by distal surface of primary second molars into preferred positioning.
   a. Mesial step: mandibular second molar is mesial to maxillary molar; ideal molar relationship will occur.
   b. Flush terminal plane: maxillary second molars lie end to end with mandibular second primary molars; ideal molar relationship may occur.
3. Distal step: mandibular second molar is distal to maxillary second molar, NOT type of terminal plane relationship; ideal molar relationship does NOT usually occur.
4. Slight to moderate amounts of attrition owing to bruxism; BOTH deep overbite and overjet are often present.
F. Mixed dentition occlusal evaluation: BOTH primary and permanent teeth are present (around 6 to 12 years):

1. Succedaneous (successional) replace primary teeth; nonsuccedaneous (accessional) erupt distal in the arch and do NOT replace any primary teeth.
2. Leeway space: sum width of MD widths of primary canines through primary second molars.
   a. Enhances development of a normal occlusion in permanent dentition.
   b. Usually greater on the maxillary arch, usually greater than the space needed for successional teeth.
   c. If primary is lost (caries or trauma) before permanent is ready to replace it, space maintainer (fixed or removable) can keep leeway space open.
G. Permanent dentition occlusal evaluation: eruption of all permanents (except third molars) is usually completed by age of 12:
   1. **Centric occlusion** (CO): maximum intercuspation when jaws are fully closed (discussed earlier).

2. **Centric relation** (CR): MOST retruded (unstrained) relationship of mandible to the maxilla and MOST reproducible relationship; position from which lateral excursions are made.
3. Contact areas: protect interdental gingiva and stabilize each tooth in arch; open contact allows food impaction and reduces mesiodistal stability.
4. Centric stops: occur in three places: (1) between the two arches where the teeth contact; (2) at the height of cusp contour of supporting cusps; (3) at marginal ridges and central fossae.
5. Centric prematurity: occlusal factor that is determined when guiding the mandible into centric relation closure.
6. Protrusive excursion: forward movement of lower jaw until mandibular anterior incisors meet the maxillary incisors edge to edge.
7. Lateral excursion: movement of the mandible from centric occlusion to the right or left until canines on the same side meet cusp tip to cusp tip.

Review Questions

1 How many erupted primary teeth does a 4-year-old child have?
A. 10
B. 12
C. 16
D. 18
E. 20

2 Which of the following are considered functions of the incisors?
A. Biting and tearing
B. Grinding and cutting
C. Biting and cutting
D. Tearing and grinding

3 Which of the following structures or features are found in numbers of four in the oral cavity only during the permanent dentition period?
A. Molars
B. Dental arches
C. Canine cusp slopes
D. Maxillary premolars
E. Quadrants

4 When viewed proximally, the crown of the mandibular first molar is inclined
A. buccally.
B. lingually.
C. mesially.
D. distally.

5 Which of the following BEST describes the groove pattern on the occlusal table of the mandibular second molar?
A. Linear
B. Snake eyes
C. Crescent
D. Cross

6 Which of the following teeth is considered succedaneous?
A. #13
B. #14
C. #18
D. #19

7 Which of the following features is located on the lateral surface of the mandible?
A. Lingula
B. Submandibular fossa
C. Genial tubercles
D. External oblique line
E. Mental foramen

8 Which of the following bones of the skull is paired?
A. Sphenoid
B. Ethmoid
C. Occipital
D. Vomer
E. Parietal

9 Which of the following bones of the skull is considered a facial bone?
A. Occipital
B. Parietal
C. Sphenoid
D. Zygomatic
E. Frontal

10 Which of the following landmarks of the temporomandibular joint is located on the mandible?
A. Articular eminence
B. Coronoid process
C. Articular fossa
D. Postglenoid process

11 Which of the following lymph nodes are initially affected in a patient who develops an infection in the lower lip after trauma from an accident?
A. Submandibular
B. Deep cervical
C. Submental
D. Buccal
E. Malar

12 Which of the following nerves serves the parotid salivary gland and can be affected by medication, thus causing xerostomia?
A. Facial
B. Trigeminal
C. Glossopharyngeal
D. Chorda tympani

13 Which of the following arteries of the head and neck provides the MOST reliable arterial pulse of the body?
A. Internal carotid
B. Common carotid
C. Lingual
D. Facial
E. Superior thyroid

14 Which muscle can become enlarged in the presence of the parafunctional habit of bruxism?
   A. Mentalis
   B. Masseter
   C. Orbicularis oris
   D. Risorius
   E. Epicranial

15 Which of the following muscles is palpated during an extra-oral examination of the posterior cervical triangle?
   A. Suprahyoid
   B. Infrahyoid
   C. Sternocleidomastoid
   D. Temporalis

16 Which teeth may cause sensations that suggest a carious and/or endodontic situation when only a sinus infection is diagnosed?
   A. Maxillary anteriors
   B. Maxillary posteriors
   C. Mandibular anteriors
   D. Mandibular posteriors

17 Which of the following salivary glands is MOST commonly involved in stone formation?
   A. Parotid
   B. Submandibular
   C. Sublingual
   D. Submandibular and sublingual

18 Which of the following structures divides the tongue into the body and the base?
   A. Circumvallate lingual papilla
   B. Sulcus terminalis
   C. Foramen cecum
   D. Median lingual sulcus
   E. Lingual tonsil

19 One of the following situations present in a primary dentition will NOT allow the efficient eruption of a normal permanent dentition. Which one is the EXCEPTION?
   A. Presence of primate spaces
   B. Mesial step
   C. Distal step
   D. Flush terminal plane

20 Which of the following terms is used to describe the maxillary incisors overlapping the mandibular incisors in centric occlusion?
   A. Overbite
   B. Crossbite
   C. Overjet
   D. End to end

21 Which of the following nerves or branches of a nerve causes discomfort during disorders of the temporomandibular joint?
   A. Lingual
   B. Auriculotemporal
   C. Inferior alveolar
   D. Buccal

22 Which pair of bones forms the floor of the nasal cavity?
   A. Frontal and ethmoid
   B. Ethmoid and lacrimal
   C. Lacrimal and maxillary
   D. Maxillary and palatine
   E. Zygomatic and palatine

23 Which of the following methods is MOST commonly used in the United States for the designation of teeth?
   A. Universal Tooth Designation System
   B. Palmer Method for Tooth Designation
   C. International Standards Organization Designation System
   D. World Health Organization system

24 Which of the following statements is CORRECT concerning the pterygoid plexus of veins?
   A. Located around the infrahyoid muscles
   B. Protects the superficial temporal artery
   C. Contains valves to prevent the backflow of blood
   D. Injury can lead to hematoma

25 Which of the following teeth has an oblique ridge?
   A. Mandibular second molar
   B. Maxillary first molar
   C. Mandibular third molar
   D. Maxillary third molar

26 Which tooth has a buccal pit that is susceptible to caries?
   A. Mandibular first molar
   B. Maxillary first molar
   C. Mandibular second molar
   D. Maxillary second molar

27 Which of the following structures is located just posterior to the MOST distal molar of the mandibular dentition?
   A. Maxillary tuberosity
   B. Median palatine suture
   C. Incisive foramen
   D. Greater palatine foramen
   E. Retromolar triangle

28 The mandibular third molar, compared with the mandibular second molar, is
   A. larger in the crown.
   B. less smooth on its occlusal surface.
   C. less variable in form.
   D. longer in the roots.

29 Which of the following nerves supplies the muscles of mastication?
   A. Hypoglossal
   B. Vagus
   C. Facial
   D. Chorda tympani
   E. Trigeminal

30 The submandibular duct opens into the oral cavity
   A. opposite the maxillary second molar.
   B. on the sublingual caruncle.
   C. on the buccal mucosa.
   D. at the base of the mandibular labial frenum.

31 Which of the following teeth has two roots?
   A. Maxillary first molar
   B. Maxillary second premolar
   C. Maxillary first premolar
   D. Maxillary third molar

32 Which of the following teeth has two pulp canals?
   A. Maxillary first premolar
   B. Mandibular first premolar
   C. Maxillary first molar
   D. Mandibular first molar

33 Which of the following muscles, when fully contracted, helps close the jaws?
   A. Lateral pterygoid
   B. Platysma
   C. Mentalis
   D. Buccinator
   E. Temporalis

34 Accumulation of food in the left vestibule might suggest malfunction of which of the following muscles?
   A. Buccinator
   B. Risorius
   C. Orbicularis oris
   D. Medial pterygoid
   E. Levator anguli oris

35 Damage to the facial nerve within the parotid salivary gland with local anesthesia may cause
   A. drooping of the lips.
   B. spasm of the muscles of mastication.
   C. temporary facial paralysis on the affected side.
   D. deviation of the tongue to the affected side.

36 Which of the following structures are found in the pterygomandibular space?
   (1) Inferior alveolar nerve
   (2) Lingual artery
   (3) Hypoglossal nerve
   (4) Inferior alveolar artery
   (5) Sphenomandibular ligament
   A. (1), (2), and (3)
   B. (1), (2), and (4)
   C. (1), (4), and (5)
   D. (2), (3), and (4)
   E. (2), (3), and (5)

37 Which of the following are contained within the sheath of the lingual nerve as it passes medial to the mandible, anterior to the mandibular foramen?
   A. Sensory fibers to the lip
   B. Motor fibers to the masseter muscle
   C. Parasympathetic motor secretory fibers to the submandibular gland
   D. Special sense fibers to the anterior two thirds of the tongue
   E. Somatic sensory fibers to the posterior one third of the tongue

38 The floor of the mouth and the tongue both receive their blood supply by way of which of the following arteries?
   A. Facial
   B. Lingual
   C. Mylohyoid
   D. Maxillary

39 Which of the following nerves exits the cranium through the foramen ovale?
   A. Facial
   B. Maxillary
   C. Ophthalmic
   D. Mandibular
   E. Glossopharyngeal

40 Which of the following arteries is a branch of the maxillary artery?
   A. Facial
   B. Lingual
   C. Superior thyroid
   D. Inferior alveolar
   E. Ascending pharyngeal

41 Which of the following lymph nodes receives lymphatic drainage from maxillary teeth?
   A. Buccal
   B. Submental
   C. Infraorbital
   D. Submandibular

42 Which of the following nerves innervates the mandibular posterior teeth?
   A. Mental
   B. Buccal
   C. Incisive
   D. Inferior alveolar

43 Which nerve listed is affected if a patient complains of being unable to experience touch, pain, hot, cold, or pressure on the anterior two thirds of the tongue?
   A. Vagus
   B. Lingual
   C. Hypoglossal
   D. Chorda tympani
   E. Glossopharyngeal

44 The nasopalatine nerve enters the oral cavity by way of which of the following foramina?
   A. Mental
   B. Incisive
   C. Pterygopalatine
   D. Lesser palatine
   E. Greater palatine

45 Which of the following is supplied by the hypoglossal nerve?
   A. Sublingual salivary gland
   B. Muscles of the tongue
   C. Mucous membrane of the floor of the oral cavity
   D. Muscles of facial expression

46 The rest position of the temporomandibular joint is NOT with the teeth biting together because during mastication of food the mandible returns to the center.
   A. Both the statement and reason are correct and related.
   B. Both the statement and reason are correct but NOT related.
   C. The statement is correct, but the reason is NOT.
   D. The statement is NOT correct, but the reason is correct.
   E. NEITHER the statement NOR the reason is correct.

47 Which of the following nerves or branches of a nerve contains pain fibers affected by disturbances of the temporomandibular joint?
   A. Chorda tympani
   B. Auriculotemporal
   C. Zygomaticotemporal
   D. Temporal branch of the facial nerve

48 The parotid duct pierces which of the following muscles before entry into the oral cavity?
A. Masseter
B. Mylohyoid
C. Buccinator
D. Medial pterygoid

49 The lateral pterygoid muscle inserts into the
A. coronoid process.
B. articular eminence.
C. mandibular condyle.
D. angle of the mandible.
E. internal oblique line.

50 Pain impulses from the periodontal ligament are carried by which of the following cranial nerves?
A. I
B. II
C. V
D. VII
E. IX

51 Mandibular teeth are vascularized by branches of which of the following arteries?
A. Facial
B. Labial
C. Lingual
D. Maxillary

52 During instrumentation, longitudinal developmental grooves would probably be noted on which of the following root surfaces of a maxillary first premolar?
A. Lingual
B. Mesial
C. Facial
D. Palatal

53 The roots of which of the following premolars present the greatest difficulty in endodontic therapy?
A. Maxillary first
B. Maxillary second
C. Mandibular first
D. Mandibular second

54 Which of the following occlusal factors is determined when guiding the mandible into centric relation closure?
A. Canine rise
B. Degree of overbite
C. Centric prematurity
D. Working interference
E. Balancing interference

55 Which of the following is a normal pattern for eruption of primary teeth?
A. Maxillary central incisors erupt before mandibular central incisors.
B. Maxillary canines erupt before maxillary lateral incisors.
C. Maxillary first molars erupt before maxillary canines.
D. Mandibular canines erupt before mandibular first molars.
E. Mandibular second molars erupt before mandibular first molars.

56 Which of the following premolars often has three cusps?
A. Maxillary first
B. Maxillary second
C. Mandibular first
D. Mandibular second

57 The tooth that has the longest crown is the
A. maxillary lateral incisor.
B. maxillary central incisor.
C. mandibular canine.
D. maxillary first molar.

58 Blood vessels are more numerous than lymphatic vessels in the head and neck; however, the venous vessels mainly parallel the lymphatic vessels in location.
A. Both statements are true.
B. Both statements are false.
C. The first is true, the second is false.
D. The first is false, the second is true.

59 Which of the following premolars frequently lacks a transverse ridge?
A. Maxillary first
B. Maxillary second
C. Mandibular first
D. Mandibular second

60 How does the mandibular second molar differ in related numbers from the mandibular first molar?
A. Cusps
B. Roots
C. Lingual grooves
D. Marginal ridges

61 Where is the cingulum normally located on the teeth indicated?
A. Incisal third of the lingual surface of anterior teeth
B. Middle third of the lingual surface of posterior teeth
C. Cervical third of the lingual surface of anterior teeth
D. Occlusal third of the lingual surface of posterior teeth

62 In centric occlusion the normal relation of the maxillary first molar to the mandibular arch is established when the
A. maxillary first molar occludes with the mandibular second premolar and first molar.
B. distal surface of the maxillary first molar is in the same plane as the distal surface of the mandibular first molar.
C. distofacial cusp of the maxillary first molar falls in the same plane as the distal surface of the mandibular first molar.
D. mesiolingual cusp of the maxillary first molar falls in the central fossa of the mandibular first molar.

63 Where is the height of contour of the buccal surface of the mandibular first molar located?
A. Junction of the occlusal and middle thirds
B. Center of tooth surface
C. Junction of the cervical and middle thirds
D. Lingual of tooth surface

64 The pulp horns MOST likely to be exposed accidentally in the preparation of a Class II cavity in the maxillary first molar are the
A. mesiobuccal and mesiolingual.
B. mesiolingual and distolingual.
C. distolingual and distobuccal.
D. distobuccal and mesiobuccal.

65 What does the vermilion border consist of?
A. Internal lining of the lip
B. Inner epithelial lining of the cheeks
C. Junction of the lip with the skin
D. Formed by palatopharyngeus muscle

66 Where is the soft palate located?
   A. Dorsal aspect of the oral cavity
   B. Just posterior to the hard palate
   C. Center of the hard palate
   D. Within the pillars

67 Where is the median palatine raphe more prominent?
   A. Hard palate
   B. Soft palate
   C. Tonsillar pillars
   D. Near oropharynx

68 Where is the lingual tonsil located?
   A. Posterior to the circumvallate lingual papillae
   B. Posterolateral border of the tongue
   C. Along the sulcus terminalis on the tongue
   D. Lateral border and anterior tip of the tongue

69 The thyroid gland produces thyroxine, which it secretes directly into the blood. Thyroxine is a hormone that stimulates the metabolic rate.
   A. Both statements are true.
   B. Both statements are false.
   C. The first statement is true, the second is false.
   D. The first statement is false, the second is true.

70 Which of the following glands is unencapsulated?
   A. Submandibular
   B. Thyroid
   C. Parotid
   D. Sublingual

71 The temporal bone and the mandible come together to form the temporomandibular joint because a joint is defined as a junction or union between two or more bones.
   A. Both the statement and reason are correct and related.
   B. Both the statement and reason are correct but NOT related.
   C. The statement is correct, but the reason is NOT.
   D. The statement is NOT correct, but the reason is correct.
   E. NEITHER the statement NOR the reason is correct.

72 The lymphatics of the right side of the head and the neck converge by way of the right jugular trunk. Then these lymphatics join the lymphatics from the right arm and thorax to form the thoracic duct.
   A. Both statements are true.
   B. Both statements are false.
   C. The first is true, the second is false.
   D. The first is false, the second is true.

73 The superior and posterior free margin of the auricle, known as the helix, ends inferiorly at the lobule. The lobule is a small flap of tissue, which is the part of the auricle anterior to the external acoustic meatus.
   A. Both statements are true.
   B. Both statements are false.
   C. The first is true, the second is false.
   D. The first is false, the second is true.

74 During the extraoral examination, feeling inferior to and medial to the angles of the mandible is important because this will allow the dental hygienist to effectively palpate the hyoid bone.
   A. Both the statement and reason are correct and related.
   B. Both the statement and reason are correct but NOT related.
   C. The statement is correct, but the reason is NOT.
   D. The statement is NOT correct, but the reason is correct.
   E. NEITHER the statement NOR the reason is correct.

75 The lymphatics are a portion of the immune system, and they help fight disease processes. Another component of the lymphatic system is the thymus gland because it works within the immune system.
   A. Both statements are true.
   B. Both statements are false.
   C. The first is true, and the second is false.
   D. The first is false, and the second is true.

76 The dental professional must be thoroughly familiar with the surface anatomy of the head and neck to examine patients because features of the surface provide essential landmarks for many deeper anatomical structures.
   A. Both the statement and reason are correct and related.
   B. Both the statement and reason are correct but NOT related.
   C. The statement is correct, but the reason is NOT.
   D. The statement is NOT correct, but the reason is correct.
   E. NEITHER the statement NOR the reason is correct.

77 An extrinsic tongue muscle that retracts the tongue is the
   A. palatoglossus muscle.
   B. inferior longitudinal muscle.
   C. styloglossus muscle.
   D. genioglossus muscle.

78 Occlusal evaluation defines the contact relationship between the maxillary and mandibular teeth when the
   A. anterior teeth are contacting end to end.
   B. teeth are fully closed.
   C. mandibular teeth are in the most protruded position.
   D. maxillary and mandibular first molar interproximal spaces coincide.
   E. contact occurs only on posterior teeth.

79 Overbite presents with which of the following situations?
   A. Vertical overlap between maxillary and mandibular anterior teeth
   B. Horizontal overlap between maxillary and mandibular anterior teeth
   C. Vertical overlap of the first molars when the anterior teeth are missing
   D. Horizontal overlap of the first molars when the anterior teeth are missing

80 In the primary dentition, when the maxillary second molars occlude end to end with the mandibular second molars, it is referred to as which of the following?
   A. Mesial step
   B. Distal step
   C. Flush terminal plane
   D. End-to-end occlusion
   E. Class I occlusion

Answer Key and Rationales

1 (E) All of 4-year-old child's primary teeth would have erupted into oral cavity because average age for primary (deciduous) dentition completion is approximately age 3. There are 20 teeth in the primary dentition.

2 (C) Incisors function as instruments for biting and cutting food during mastication because of incisal ridge, triangular proximal form, and arch position. There are eight incisors, two of each type, central and lateral.

3 (D) Only during permanent dentition period are four maxillary premolars (bicuspids) present, two of each type, first and second. The two types of molars, first and second molars, are found during primary dentition period. The three types of molars are found during permanent dentition period. Only two arches are found in BOTH primary and permanent dentition periods. Only two canine cusp slopes per tooth are found during BOTH periods. There are four quadrants, present during BOTH primary and permanent dentition periods.

4 (B) ALL permanent mandibular molars, including first molar, show strong lingual inclination when viewed proximally. This inclines crown lingually on root base, bringing cusps into proper occlusion with maxillary antagonists and the distribution of forces along the long axis.

5 (D) Cross-shaped groove pattern is formed on occlusal table of permanent mandibular second molar when the well-defined central groove is crossed by buccal groove and lingual groove, dividing the occlusal table into four parts that are NEARLY equal.

6 (A) Tooth #13 (permanent second premolar) is succedaneous for primary second molar. ALL others are permanent molars, and ALL molars are nonsuccedaneous because they do NOT have primary predecessors and erupt distal to primary second molar.

7 (E) Mental foramen is located on lateral surface of mandible. ALL others are located on internal (medial) surface of the mandible.

8 (C) Occipital bone is the ONLY *paired* bone of skull. Others are *single* bones of skull.

9 (D) Zygomatic bone is considered a facial bone because it helps create facial features and serves as base for the dentition. Vomer, lacrimal, palatine, maxilla, mandible are also facial bones. ALL others are considered cranial bones because they form cranium. Cranial bones form cranium and include occipital, frontal, parietal, temporal, sphenoid, ethmoid bones.

10 (B) Coronoid process is located on mandible and is part of TMJ. ALL others are part of joint but are located on temporal bone. Coronoid process is a thin, triangular eminence, flattened from side to side.

11 (C) Lower lip drains directly into submental lymph nodes, which serve as *primary* nodes during an infection. Submandibular and cervical nodes would serve as *secondary* nodes if infection progressed. Buccal and malar nodes drain upper and middle cheek.

12 (C) Parotid gland is supplied by ninth cranial nerve (glossopharyngeal, IX) (with preganglionic parasympathetic innervation). Even though seventh cranial nerve (facial, VII) travels through parotid, does NOT supply it. Chorda tympani supplies submandibular and sublingual salivary glands, which may also be affected by drugs to produce xerostomia (dry mouth). Trigeminal (fifth cranial nerve [V]) serves many other oral cavity structures but NOT the parotid.

13 (B) Common carotid artery provides MOST reliable carotid pulse from carotid sinus, the swelling of the common carotid before it bifurcates into internal and external carotid arteries. Others are branches from internal carotid artery after bifurcation. Carotid pulse is used in emergencies ONLY by emergency personnel, and radial pulse is used when taking vital sign of a baseline pulse at other times.

14 (B) Masseter muscle can become enlarged (hypertrophied) in a patient who habitually grinds (bruxism) or clenches the teeth. Action of masseter muscle during bilateral contraction of the entire muscle is to raise or elevate the mandible, thus raising the lower jaw. Elevation of the mandible occurs during closing of the jaws or grinding of the teeth. ALL others are of facial expression and NOT of mastication.

15 (C) Sternocleidomastoid muscle (SCM) divides each side of the neck into the anterior and posterior cervical triangle. Posterior cervical triangle is located on side of the neck, and the anterior cervical triangle corresponds to the anterior region of the neck that contains both the suprahyoid and infrahyoid muscles. Temporalis is located in the temporal region on the lateral surface of the skull.

16 (B) Discomfort from sinusitis can be confused with tooth-related discomfort from the maxillary posteriors because the roots are in close proximity to maxillary sinus. Others are NOT near maxillary sinus, the sinus MOST commonly involved in sinus infections.

17 (B) Duct for submandibular gland is the submandibular duct (Wharton's duct); long duct travels along the anterior floor of the mouth. Its tortuous upward travel for a considerable distance during its course may be the reason that the gland is MOST commonly involved in salivary stone formation.

18 (B) Sulcus terminalis divides tongue into posterior base and anterior body. Dorsum (top) surface is convex and marked by sulcus terminalis; this sulcus ends behind, about 2.5 cm from the root of the tongue, in a depression, foramen cecum, from which a shallow groove, terminal sulcus, runs lateralward and forward on either side to the margin of tongue. Others are also on dorsal surface.

19 **(C)** Distal step will NOT allow efficient eruption of a normal permanent dentition. Distal step occurs when primary mandibular second molar is distal to maxillary second molar and thus is NOT in a terminal plane relationship. Mesial step and flush terminal plane are BOTH types of terminal plane relationships that allow efficient eruption, along with primate spaces. Flush terminal plane occurs when primary maxillary and mandibular second molars are in an end-to-end relationship; mesial step occurs when primary mandibular second molar is mesial to maxillary molar. If primate spacing exists in primary mandibular arch after eruption of permanent first molar, this tooth will put pressure on primary second and first molars, causing forward movement of primary mandibular canine and first molar.

20 **(A)** In centric occlusion, maxillary incisors overlap mandibular incisors, causing an overbite. When maxillary dental arch naturally "overhangs" the mandibular arch facially, an overjet is caused. Crossbite occurs when mandibular tooth or teeth are placed facially to maxillary teeth. End-to-end bite occurs when teeth occlude WITHOUT maxillary teeth overlapping mandibular teeth.

21 **(B)** Auriculotemporal nerve serves as an *afferent* nerve for the external ear and scalp near TMJ. Auriculotemporal nerve is a branch of mandibular nerve that runs with the superficial temporal artery and vein and provides sensory innervation to various regions on the side of head. ALL others are *afferent* for oral structures.

22 **(D)** Horizontal plates of palatine bones and the palatine process of maxilla together form floor of nasal cavity. Also forms the anterior portion of hard palate (roof) of the oral cavity. ALL others form orbital walls.

23 **(A)** Universal Tooth Designation System is the MOST used system in United States for the designation of BOTH dentitions because it is adaptable to electronic data transfer. Palmer Method for Tooth Designation is used in orthodontic offices. International Standards Organization Designation System is used MAINLY internationally by World Health Organization (WHO) system.

24 **(D)** Pterygoid plexus of veins is around pterygoid muscles and surrounds maxillary artery on each side of the face in infratemporal fossa. Protects maxillary artery from being compressed during mastication and may be involved in the spread of infection to the cavernous venous sinus because it does NOT have valves.

When it is pierced, small amount of blood escapes and enters the tissues, causing a hematoma. Can be pierced when posterior superior alveolar (PSA) block is administered and needle overreaches for target of apices of maxillary posteriors.

25 **(B)** Maxillary first molar has an oblique ridge that is formed by union of triangular ridge of the DB cusp and distal cusp ridge of the ML cusp, crossing occlusal table obliquely. All others do NOT have oblique ridges.

26 **(A)** Mandibular first molar's MB groove almost always ends in the buccal pit, susceptible to caries because of increased dental biofilm retention and because of the thin enamel that forms the walls of the pit. Enamel sealants can be placed in buccal pit to protect the tooth from caries. All others do NOT have buccal pits.

27 **(E)** Retromolar triangle is located just posterior to MOST distal molar of mandibular dentition. ALL others are found on maxilla, near maxillary dentition.

28 **(B)** Generally, the MORE posterior the tooth, the MORE supplemental grooves are present, such that occlusal table appears more "wrinkled." Thus mandibular third molar is LESS smooth on its occlusal surface than third molar of same arch. Others refer to second molar and NOT the third molar.

29 **(E)** Muscles of mastication are four *paired* muscles attached to the mandible; include masseter, temporalis, medial pterygoid, lateral pterygoid. Mandibular division of fifth (V) cranial nerve, trigeminal, innervates ALL muscles of mastication. Seventh (VII) cranial nerve is the facial. Tenth (X) cranial nerve is the vagus. Twelfth (XII) cranial nerve is the hypoglossal. Chorda tympani is a branch of the facial nerve (seventh [VII] cranial nerve). However, others innervate important structures of the oral cavity.

30 **(B)** Submandibular duct opens up into the oral cavity on the sublingual caruncle, on the floor of the mouth. Parotid duct opens opposite maxillary second molar on buccal mucosa. Mandibular labial frenum has ONLY minor salivary gland ducts nearby in labial mucosa.

31 **(C)** Maxillary first premolar has two roots. ALL maxillary molars have three roots (trifurcated); however, sometimes the roots of the third molar are so close together that they are fused roots, either partially or fully, giving appearance of one root. Maxillary second premolar has one root and only occasionally has two roots (bifurcated).

32 **(A)** Pulp cavity for maxillary first premolar has two pulp canals, even if there is ONLY one undivided root. Mandibular first premolar has one canal. BOTH maxillary and mandibular first molars MOSTLY have three canals.

33 **(E)** BOTH lateral pterygoid and temporalis are muscles of mastication that affect the movement of the jaws. If the entire temporalis muscle contracts, its MAIN action is to elevate the mandible, thus raising the lower jaw. Elevation of the mandible occurs during the closing of the jaws. MAIN action when BOTH lateral pterygoid muscles contract is to bring the lower jaw forward, thus causing the protrusion of the mandible. Protrusion of the mandible often occurs during the opening of the jaws. If ONLY one lateral pterygoid muscle is contracted, the lower jaw shifts to the opposite side, causing a lateral deviation of the mandible. ALL other muscles listed are muscles of facial expression.

34 (A) Buccinator muscle is the muscle of the cheek and aids in the cleaning of food from the oral vestibule. Because the buccinator is innervated by the buccal branch of the facial nerve (seventh cranial nerve [VII]), injury to nerve will affect the action of the muscle (e.g., Bell's palsy).

35 (C) Damage to facial nerve (seventh cranial nerve [VII]) within the parotid gland may cause unilateral transient facial paralysis of the facial muscles on the affected side. Temporary situation can occur when a local anesthetic agent is injected by overreaching the needle during a inferior alveolar block into the parotid gland, since it contains the facial nerve; nerve serves the muscles of facial expression on each side. Thus patient will have a drooping lip on one side but NOT both sides. Contacting medial surface of the ramus of the mandibular bone during the injection prevents this from occurring.

36 (C) Following structures are found in pterygomandibular space: inferior alveolar (IA) nerve, IA artery, sphenomandibular ligament. Injection site for IA nerve block. Lingual artery will be superficial to this site. Hypoglossal (twelfth cranial nerve [XII]) is found in the hypoglossal canals of occipital bone.

37 (D) Special sense fibers to anterior two thirds of the tongue are contained within the sheath of lingual nerve as it passes medial to the mandible (and inferior alveolar nerve), anterior to mandibular foramen. Tongue thus becomes anesthetized as the local anesthetic agent diffuses to lingual nerve FIRST during the IA nerve block. Lingual nerve shock can also occur when the needle touches lingual nerve during the injection.

38 (B) Floor of the mouth and tongue receive blood supply by way of lingual artery. Facial artery with its major branches supplies the face in the oral, buccal, zygomatic, nasal, infraorbital, and orbital regions. Mylohyoid artery supplies the floor of the mouth and the mylohyoid muscle. Maxillary artery has branches near the muscles supplied.

39 (D) Mandibular nerve is the third of the three divisions of the fifth (V) cranial nerve (trigeminal). First division (ophthalmic, V_1) exits through superior orbital fissure, second division (maxillary, V_2) through foramen rotundum (round shaped), and the third (mandibular, V_3) through foramen ovale (oval shaped). Fissure and foramen are located in the sphenoid. Fissure also caries third, fourth, sixth cranial nerves and ophthalmic vein.

40 (D) Maxillary artery is one of the two terminal branches of the external carotid artery. Branches supply teeth and supporting structures of BOTH arches. Blood supply to mandibular teeth and supporting structures is MAINLY from inferior alveolar branch of the maxillary artery.

41 (D) Submandibular lymph node receives lymphatic drainage from maxillary teeth. Facial nodes are positioned along the length of the facial vein to drain the area and include the buccal and infraorbital. However, do drain *into* each other and then into the submandibular nodes. Submental nodes drain BOTH sides of the chin, lower lip, floor of the mouth, apex of the tongue, mandibular incisors, then empty into submandibular nodes or deep cervical nodes.

42 (D) Inferior alveolar (IA) nerve innervates the mandibular posteriors. Buccal (long buccal) nerve is *afferent* for the skin of the cheek, buccal mucous membranes, buccal gingiva of mandibular posteriors. Mental nerve is composed of external branches that are *afferent* for the chin, lower lip, and labial mucosa near the mandibular anteriors.

43 (B) Lingual nerve is affected if a patient complains of being unable to experience touch, pain, hot, cold, or pressure on the *anterior* two thirds of the tongue, which is a branch of the mandibular nerve from fifth (V) cranial nerve (trigeminal). Ninth (IX) cranial nerve (glossopharyngeal nerve) covers the general sensation from the base of the tongue. Tenth (X) cranial nerve (vagus nerve) is *efferent* for muscles of the soft palate, pharynx, and larynx. Chorda tympani is a branch of the facial nerve (seventh cranial nerve [VII]) and *afferent* for taste sensation for the body of the tongue.

44 (B) Nasopalatine (NP) nerve enters the oral cavity by way of incisive foramen on hard palate. Lesser palatine (LP, posterior palatine) nerve enters LP foramen in the palatine bone. Mental nerve enters mental foramen. Greater palatine (GP, anterior palatine) nerve enters the GP foramen in the palatine bone.

45 (B) Muscles of the tongue are supplied by hypoglossal (twelfth cranial nerve [XII]), which is *efferent* for intrinsic and extrinsic muscles of the tongue and exits the skull through the hypoglossal canal. Facial (seventh cranial nerve [VII]) serves muscles of facial expression. Lingual nerve serves floor of the mouth, as well as submandibular gland (parasympathetic efferent innervation) and branch off mandibular nerve.

46 (B) Both statements are true but are not related. Statement describes the rest position of the temporomandibular joint (TMJ), while the reason describes the power stroke, which occurs during mastication. Teeth are NOT occluding or biting together when the TMJ is at rest. Mandible is brought back to the center during mastication owing to the power stroke or the teeth crunching the food.

47 **(B)** Auriculotemporal nerve contains pain fibers affected by disturbances of the temporomandibular joint (TMJ). Also serves as an *afferent* nerve for the external ear and scalp near the TMJ. Chorda tympani is a branch of the facial nerve (seventh cranial nerve [VII]) and *afferent* for taste sensation for the body of the tongue. Zygomatic nerve is composed of the union of zygomaticofacial and zygomaticotemporal in orbit and is afferent; conveys postganglionic parasympathetic fibers to the lacrimal.

48 **(C)** Buccinator muscle is pierced by parotid duct before entry into the oral cavity, after it emerges from the anterior border of the gland. Parotid duct (Stensen's) serves the gland; it opens up into the oral cavity at the parotid papilla on the buccal mucosa, opposite maxillary first molar.

49 **(C)** Lateral pterygoid inserts into the mandibular condyle; this includes BOTH heads. Superior head originates from greater wing of the sphenoid; inferior head originates from lateral pterygoid plate. Temporalis inserts on the coronoid process of mandible. Masseter inserts on the lateral surface of the angle. Medial pterygoid inserts on medial surface of the angle of the mandible. ALL are muscles of mastication.

50 **(C)** Fifth (V) cranial nerve (trigeminal) carries pain impulses from the periodontal ligament (PDL) of ALL the teeth to the brain by its two MAJOR nerve branches, maxillary and mandibular nerves, which serve (respectively) the maxillary and mandibular teeth.

51 **(D)** Mandibular teeth are vascularized by branches of the maxillary arteries, by way of inferior alveolar (IA) artery, as well as the maxillary teeth. The IA arises from the maxillary artery in infratemporal fossa, turns inferiorly to enter the mandibular foramen, and then enters the mandibular canal and the inferior alveolar nerve; it branches into mylohyoid before it enters the canal. In the canal it branches into mandibular posterior and alveolar (dental) branches to supply the teeth and periodontium of these teeth, and also associated gingiva.

52 **(B)** Longitudinal developmental grooves (root concavity) would probably be noted on mesial root surfaces of maxillary first premolar (#5, #12). Because of its depth, there may be increased deposits in this area that may require instrumentation.

53 **(A)** Roots of the maxillary first premolar (#5, #12) present GREATEST difficulty in endodontic therapy as compared with all the other premolars, whether first or second or even mandibular, because of its two roots; has one buccal and one lingual (palatal) root. May be fused or laminated. In addition, crown is widest mesiodistally of all premolars.

54 **(C)** Centric prematurity is an occlusal factor that is determined when guiding mandible into centric relation closure. Centric stops occur in three places between the two arches where the teeth contact: at the height of cusp contour of supporting cusps, at the marginal ridges, and at the central fossae. With canine rise, the tooth should be the only tooth in function during lateral occlusion. Overbite occurs as the maxillary incisors overlap the mandibular incisors to allow maximum contact of the posteriors. Overjet occurs when the maxillary dental arch naturally overhangs the mandibular arch facially. BOTH are measured in millimeters with a probe. Evaluation of lateral occlusion is made by moving the mandible laterally left until the canines on that side are in a cusp-to-cusp relationship. Side to which the mandible has been moved is the working side; opposite side is the balancing side.

55 **(C)** Primary maxillary first molars (B, I) erupt at 13 to 19 months, before maxillary canines (C, H) (16 to 22 months), which is a normal pattern for eruption of primary (deciduous) teeth. Unless designated otherwise, the teeth in the exam SHOULD be considered a part of the permanent (adult) dentition.

56 **(D)** Mandibular second premolar (#20, #29) has three cusps in one of its two types. Its tricuspidate form has one large buccal cusp and two smaller lingual cusps; grooves form a distinctive Y-shaped pattern on the occlusal table; resembles small molar. Other premolars have two cusps.

57 **(C)** Mandibular canine (#22, #27) has longest crown in the permanent dentition; can be as long as or even LONGER than maxillary canine.

58 **(D)** First statement is false: blood vessels are LESS numerous than lymphatic vessels. Second statement is true: venous vessels MAINLY parallel lymphatic vessels in location.

59 **(B)** Mandibular second premolar (#20, #29) has either two or three cusps. The two-cusp type has a transverse ridge, the MORE common three-cusp type does NOT. Bicuspidate form is similar to that of the mandibular first premolars; has one larger buccal cusp and one smaller lingual cusp; central groove is crescent or U shaped; appears rounded from occlusal.

60 **(A)** Mandibular second premolar (#20, #29) differs from the mandibular first molar (#19, #30) by the number of cusps; has either two or three cusps. Molar has five cusps. BOTH teeth have two roots and two marginal ridges, and BOTH have a lingual groove that cuts the occlusal outline on the lingual surface, if the premolar has the bicuspid form.

61 **(C)** Cingulum is normally located in cervical third of the lingual surface of anteriors. Includes incisors and canines, BOTH maxillary and mandibular teeth. Raised, rounded area; varying degrees of development.

62 (D) In centric occlusion the normal relation of the permanent maxillary first molar to the mandibular arch is established when the mesiolingual cusp of the maxillary first molar falls in the central fossa of the mandibular first molar.

63 (C) Height of contour of the buccal surface of the mandibular first molar (#19, #30) is located at the junction of the cervical and middle thirds. Height of contour is the greatest elevation of tooth, either incisocervically or occlusocervically, on a specific surface of the crown.

64 (A) Pulp horns MOST likely to be exposed accidentally in the preparation of a Class II cavity in the maxillary first molar are the MB and ML. Cavity preparation would involve the occlusal surface of the tooth. Tooth has three horns, one for each major cusp. The ML and MB are BOTH very large horns, and the MB is large on all molars and can be exposed more easily during cavity preparation than the other horns.

65 (C) Vermilion border is smooth, well-delineated, and slightly raised junction of the lip with the skin. Internal lining of the lip is the labial mucosa. Inner epithelial lining of the cheeks is the buccal mucosa. Posterior tonsillar pillar is formed by palatopharyngeus muscle.

66 (B) Soft palate is just posterior to the hard palate. Location of the hard palate is on the dorsal aspect of the oral cavity. Median palatal raphe is in the center of the hard palate. Tonsils (palatal), which are lymphoid tissue, lie between the tonsillar pillars. Soft palate is the soft tissue constituting the back of the roof of the mouth; distinguished from the hard palate at the front of the mouth in that it does NOT contain bone.

67 (B) Median palatal raphe is MORE prominent and thicker in the center of soft palate, clinical evidence of the median palatine suture line showing the fusion of the palatal processes from the maxillary process during the development of the secondary palate. Median palatal cyst is a rare cyst that may occur anywhere along the median palatal raphe; may produce a swelling because of infection, treated by excision or surgical removal. Soft palate is located in the posterior part of the palate (roof) of the oral cavity; soft tissue constituting the back of the roof of mouth; distinguished from hard palate at the front of mouth in that it does NOT contain bone.

68 (A) Lingual tonsil is located on dorsal lateral aspect of the tongue, posterior to circumvallate lingual papillae. Lingual tonsil is an irregular mass of tonsillar tissue. Location for the foliate is on the posterolateral border of the tongue. Location of circumvallate is along the sulcus terminalis on the tongue. Fungiform papillae are mostly located on the lateral border and anterior apex (tip) of the tongue.

69 (A) Both statements are true. Thyroxine (T_4) is the MAJOR hormone secreted by the follicular cells of the thyroid gland. T_4 is transported in blood. T_4 is involved in controlling the rate of metabolic processes in the body and influencing physical development. Increases rate of chemical reactions in cells and helps control growth and development. Thyroxin is version manufactured in the laboratory; used to treat thyroid disorders.

70 (D) Sublingual gland is NOT capsulated; others (submandibular, thyroid, parotid) are encapsulated. Gland is located in the sublingual fossa in sublingual fascial space at the floor of the mouth. Superior to mylohyoid, medial to the body of mandible, and anterior to submandibular gland.

71 (A) Statement is correct: temporomandibular joint (TMJ) is a junction between temporal bone and mandible. Reason is also correct: joint is defined as union between two or more bones. Thus both statement and reason are related.

72 (C) First statement is true: lymphatics of right side of head and neck converge by way of right jugular trunk. Second statement is false: lymphatics on right side of head and neck converge by way of right jugular trunk to join lymphatics from right arm and thorax to form right lymphatic duct, which drains into venous system at junction of right subclavian and right internal jugular veins. Lymphatic vessels of left side of head and neck converge into left jugular trunk, a short vessel, and then into thoracic duct.

73 (C) First statement is true: superior and posterior free margin of the auricle, known as the helix, ends inferiorly at lobule. Second statement is false; this is the definition of the tragus, NOT the lobule. Thus tragus is a small flap of tissue, which is the part of auricle anterior to external acoustic meatus.

74 (A) Both the statement and the reason are correct and related: hyoid bone is located in anterior midline, superior to thyroid cartilage, where the angles of the mandible are located. Angle of mandible is also the landmark used to locate the hyoid bone. Palpation of angles of mandible is also part of extraoral examination.

75 (C) First statement is true: lymphatics are a portion of the immune system and help fight disease processes. Second statement is false: thymus gland is NOT a component of lymphatic system even though it works within the immune system.

76 (A) Both the statement and reason are correct and are related. Dental professionals must have knowledge of normal or healthy structures to identify and locate deeper anatomical landmarks, which are needed to perform certain dental procedures such as administration of local anesthetic or radiographic exposures.

77 (C) Styloglossus muscle moves the tongue superiorly and posteriorly. Palatoglossus elevates the tongue against the soft palate during swallowing. Inferior longitudinals are intrinsic tongue muscles, and the genioglossus acts to protrude the tongue.

78 (B) Teeth have to be fully closed for evaluation of occlusion.

79 (A) Vertical overlap between maxillary and mandibular anterior teeth is called overbite. Overjet is the horizontal overlap between maxillary and mandibular anterior teeth.

80 (C) Flush terminal plane occurs in the primary dentition when the maxillary second molars occlude end to end with the mandibular second molars; ideal molar relationship may occur. Mesial step occurs when mandibular second molar is mesial to maxillary molar; ideal molar relationship will occur. Distal step is when mandibular second molar is distal to maxillary second molar, NOT type of terminal plane relationship; ideal molar relationship will rarely occur. An end-to-end occlusion occurs when the buccal cusps of maxillary and mandibular molars occlude with one another. A Class I occlusion applies to the permanent dentition.

CHAPTER 5

Radiology

FUNDAMENTAL RADIATION PHYSICS

Understanding radiation physics requires a basic knowledge of atomic structure, radiation types, properties of radiation.
- See CD-ROM for Chapter Terms and WebLinks.
A. Atomic structure: nucleus and electrons in orbiting shells of an atom function in state of equilibrium until ionization occurs (Figure 5-1):
1. Nucleus:
   a. Contains protons, with positive charge.
   b. Contains neutrons, with NO electrical charge.
2. Orbiting shells:
   a. Contain electrons, with negative charge, and circle the nucleus in shells.
   b. Have binding energy, which keeps electrons in their shells as a result of centripetal force and attraction of opposites.
3. Ionization:
   a. Occurs when an atom loses an electron from one of its shells and becomes part of **ion pair** (not unlike the celebrity world with its changing pairs); this process elicits chemical changes in matter.
   b. Ion pair is created when an x-ray photon ejects a negative electron from its shell and neutral atom becomes positive.
   c. **Ionizing radiation** is any radiation that is capable of producing ions.
B. Types of radiation: particulate and electromagnetic radiation are types of ionizing radiation:
1. Particulate (corpuscular) radiation:
   a. Involves mass and particles that travel in straight lines at high speeds.
   b. Four types:
      (1) Electrons: originate from radioactive atoms; called beta particles.
      (2) Protons: heavily charged particles (namely, hydrogen nuclei).
      (3) Neutrons: have mass but NO electrical charge.
      (4) Alpha particles: large and emitted from nucleus of heavy metals; usually unable to penetrate tissue.
2. Electromagnetic radiation:
   a. Comprises electric and magnetic fields of energy that move through space in wavelike motion.

b. Some forms are ionizing and others are not, depending on their energy (wavelengths) (e.g., x-rays have short wavelengths and are ionizing).
c. Arranged in a **spectrum** according to its energies, which is demonstrated by its wavelengths and frequencies; wave concept suggests that electromagnetic radiation is much like waves or ripples of water and involves wave frequency and length.
   (1) **Wavelength:**
      (a) Distance between the peaks or crests of a wave.
      (b) Determines energy of radiation; longer the distance, LESS energetic the radiation, LESS ability it has to penetrate objects.
      (c) Measured according to distance between peaks; longer wavelengths are measured in meters; shorter wavelengths are measured in nanometers (0.01 to 0.05 nm).
   (2) Frequency:
      (a) Number of peaks or crests that occur in a given amount of time.
      (b) Frequency of the peaks determines energy of the wavelength; MORE frequent the peaks, shorter and MORE energetic the radiation.
C. Properties of x-rays:
1. **X-rays** are ionizing forms of radiation that have unique properties.
2. Bundles of pure energy (short wavelengths) that have NO electrical charge.
3. Travel at speed of light (3×10^8 m/sec) *(The Flash!)*.
4. Invisible, weightless, undetectable by any of the senses.
5. Absorbed by matter according to atomic structure of material that is exposed.
6. Cause ionization, which produces biological change in interaction with matter.

X-Ray Machine and Components

X-ray machine has basic operable components and internal components that are important for safe operation and functioning.

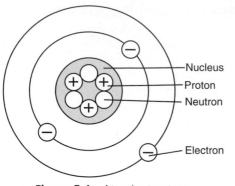

Figure 5-1 Atomic structure.

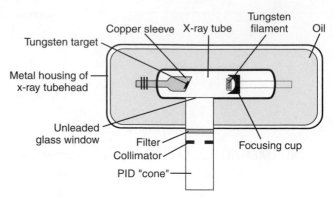

Figure 5-2 Components of x-ray machine.

A. Basic operable components: include control panel, tubehead, position-indicating device (PID):
1. Control panel:
   a. Operated by visible on-off switches, exposure button, indicator light.
   b. Controls milliamperage, time, kilovoltage settings by dials on panel.
2. **Tubehead** (Figure 5-2):
   a. Heavy metal housing for transformers and x-ray tube that serves as attachment for PID, filter, collimator.
   b. Contains insulating oil, which surrounds x-ray tube and transformers to prevent overheating.
3. **Position-indicating device** (PID):
   a. Attaches to the tubehead.
   b. Lead-lined, open-ended cylinder or rectangle that directs **x-ray beam** to object and film.
B. Internal components: include x-ray tube, power supply, circuit, transformer:
1. X-ray tube:
   a. Lead glass vacuum tube that is 1 inch by several inches long.
   b. Contains two types of electrodes:
      (1) **Cathode** (negative) electrode:
         (a) Has tungsten **filament,** which is a wire that is source of electrons when heated.
         (b) Has molybdenum cup, semicircular in shape, to focus direction of electrons toward anode.
         (c) Contains milliamperage (mA) control.
      (2) **Anode** (positive) electrode:
         (a) Has tungsten plate (or target) that electrons hit (when they leave the cathode) to produce x-rays and heat.
         (b) Has copper stem with an anode embedded in it to dissipate excessive amount of heat produced.
         (c) Has focal spot, hit by the electrons leaving cathode.
         (d) Contains kVp control

2. Power supply:
   a. Electricity that provides energy to unit to produce x-rays and is described by its current, amperage, voltage.
   b. Electric current (or flow) of electrons through a wire in a given point of time:
      (1) When a direct current (DC), electrons flow in one direction.
      (2) When an alternating current (AC), electrons flow in one direction and then change to flow in another direction.
   c. Usually measured in amperes; however, in dentistry, milliampere ($\frac{1}{1000}$ of ampere) is used.
   d. Uses voltage as the unit of force between two points; measured in kilovolts (1000 volts).
3. Circuit:
   a. Route the electrical current takes.
   b. Filament and high-voltage are two types of circuits:
      (1) Filament circuit:
         (a) Adjusts flow through a low-voltage circuit.
         (b) Controls the heating of a filament and quantity of available electrons.
         (c) Controlled by milliamperage (mA) setting.
      (2) High-voltage circuit, uses 65,000 to 100,000 volts to provide high voltage necessary to propel electrons and produce x-rays.
4. **Transformer:**
   a. Mechanism used in electrical circuit to increase or decrease the voltage.
   b. May be a step-up, step-down, or autotransformer type:
      (1) Step-down transformer:
         (a) Needed to produce electrons by heating the tungsten filament in a cathode.
         (b) Decreases incoming line voltage (110 to 220) to required 3 to 5 volts.

(c) Has MORE wires in primary coil (input coil) than in secondary coil (output coil).

(2) Step-up transformer:

(a) Provides energy needed to propel electrons from the negative pole to positive pole to produce x-rays.

(b) Increases incoming line voltage (110 to 220) to required 65,000 to 100,000 volts.

(c) Has MORE wires in secondary coil than in primary coil.

c. Autotransformer: changes voltage input into primary coil of step-up transformer.

Generation of X-Rays

X-rays are produced in x-ray tube through complex process that involves negative and positive poles and differing types of x-rays produced.

A. X-ray process: involves use of both cathode and anode:

1. Cathode: negative pole in x-ray tube:

a. Contains tungsten filament that is heated by filament circuit and generates electrons:

(1) Heating temperature is controlled by milliamperage.

(2) Available electrons are "boiled off" from filament by process called thermionic emission.

b. Includes focusing cup, made of molybdenum; cup surrounds filament and directs electrons to focal spot on anode.

2. Anode: positive pole in x-ray tube:

a. Has copper stem that serves as thermal conductor and dissipates heat away from the anode.

b. Includes target made of tungsten, embedded in the copper stem:

(1) Target's purpose is to convert the electrons from cathode into x-rays.

(2) Process results in generation of x-rays (1%) and heat (99%).

B. X-ray production:

1. Produced in an x-ray tube when kinetic energy from electrons hits the target in the anode.

2. Types include Bremsstrahlung and characteristic radiation:

a. **Bremsstrahlung radiation:**

(1) Means "braking action" in German; MAJOR source of x-rays produced in dentistry.

(2) Results when high-energy electrons come close to the nuclei of tungsten atoms but are slowed down by the positive pull of the nuclei.

(3) X-ray production results from the slowing down of the electrons, which releases energy.

b. **Characteristic radiation:**

(1) NOT generated frequently; involves electrons dislodging electrons from the K/L shell of tungsten atom.

(2) Requires filling of a vacancy by lower energy shell electron, resulting in an x-ray that comprises the binding energy between these two different shell electrons.

Interaction of X-Rays with Matter

An X-ray weakens whenever reacts with matter. When x-rays pass through atoms of tissue but do NOT react with the tissue, NO interaction occurs.

A. **Photoelectric effect:**

1. Ionization that occurs when x-ray photon interacts with inner shell electron.

2. When photons are absorbed and electrons are ejected, effect ceases to exist (NO penetrating power).

3. Responsible for ~30% of all interactions in dental x-rays.

B. **Compton scatter (effect):**

1. Ionization that occurs when x-ray photon interacts with an outer shell electron.

2. Occurs when electron is ejected and x-ray photon scatters in a different direction.

3. Responsible for ~62% of all scatter in dental x-rays.

C. **Thompson (coherent) scatter:**

1. Results without the occurrence of ionization.

2. Occurs when low-energy photon reacts with an outer shell electron and NO loss of energy occurs.

3. X-ray photon scatters in a different direction.

Units of Radiation Measurement

Two units of radiation were established to measure exposure, dose, and dose equivalent by the International Commission on Radiation Units and Measurements. Two systems are used for each unit: Standard and Système International (SI).

A. Exposure:

1. Radiation quantity that measures ionization in air; described in roentgens or SI units.

a. Intensity measured by the **roentgen** (R).

b. In other SI units, equivalent to coulombs per kilogram (C/kg).

B. Dose:

1. Amount of radiation energy absorbed by tissue:

a. Rate is amount of radiation absorbed per unit of time.

b. Often identified with **radiation absorbed dose (RAD):**

(1) Traditional unit of dose.

(2) The SI equivalent is the gray (Gy) or J/kg.

(3) Conversion:
    (a) 1 Gy = 100 rad
    (b) 1 rad = 0.01 Gy
    (c) 1 J/kg = 100 rad

C. Dose equivalent:
1. Has differing biological effects when compared with different types of radiation.
2. Quality factor is a specific number, according to exposure effect, that is given to each type of radiation.
3. Roentgen-equivalent-man (REM):
    a. Traditional unit of absorbed dose.
    b. The SI equivalent is the sievert (Sv).
    c. Conversion:
        (1) 1 Sv = 100 rem
        (2) 1 rem = 0.01 Sv

Mechanisms of Radiation Injury

Two theories attempt to explain biological effects of radiation that result in injury to living tissues, and dose-response curve is a graphic means of showing those effects.

A. Direct theory:
1. Radiation damage to tissues is caused by a direct hit on the DNA molecule of a cell, which causes cell death.
2. Seldom causes radiation injury.
B. Indirect theory:
1. Radiation damage to tissues involves the formation of free radicals.
2. Applies when x-ray photon is absorbed in a cell, which creates toxins (free radicals) and damages the cell.
3. Indirect injuries are common because of the reaction with water (70% to 80%) in cells (i.e., formation of hydrogen peroxide).
C. **Dose-response curve:**
1. Graphic means of plotting biological response (damage) to radiation exposure (dose) to determine acceptable levels of radiation exposure.
2. For low doses of radiation, very little information is available about acceptable levels.
3. Graphically, linear nonthreshold curve occurs, which indicates that response is seen at any dose.
4. Results indicate that there is *NO* true safe level of radiation exposure.

Factors That Determine Radiation Injury

Several factors determine amount of injury that occurs from radiation: total dose, amount of area exposed, types of cells exposed, cell sensitivity.

A. **Total dose:** amount of radiation absorbed in the tissue that determines effect.
1. Acute exposure: ionizing radiation given in shorter amount of time; results in MORE dramatic biological effects.
2. Chronic exposure: small amounts of ionizing radiation given over longer period; results in less effect on tissue.
3. Latent period: time (hours, days, or months) between radiation exposure and observed clinical effect.
B. **Exposure area:** amount of the body exposed to radiation, also determines biological effect of radiation on the tissues.
1. Whole-body exposure: exposure of entire body, results in MORE severe biological effects; can be acute or chronic.
    a. Acute: occurs in nuclear warfare and with occupational hazards; can result in such symptoms as nausea, vomiting, bleeding, diarrhea.
    b. Chronic: exposure to natural background radiation; largest single cause is cosmic rays.
2. Limited-area exposure: irradiation to specific body area; can be acute or chronic.
    a. Acute: to higher doses directed at specific area, such as occurs during radiation therapy (see effects on cells and organs listed below).
    b. Chronic: to lower doses, such as occurs during dental radiography.
C. Cell types: effects of radiation are determined by cell maturity and cell type:
1. **Law of Bergonié and Tribondeau** states that the greatest radiation effects occur in cells that are immature, are NOT highly specialized, and frequently divide.
    a. Cell maturity:
        (1) Immature cells are nonspecialized; experience rapid cell division.
        (2) Mature cells are specialized in function; divide at slower rate or do NOT divide at all.
    b. Cell types:
        (1) Somatic tissue cells are NOT inherited and NOT involved in reproduction (e.g., skin, kidney cells).
        (2) Genetic tissue cells are reproductive tissue cells (e.g., ovaries in woman and testes in man).
D. **Radiosensitivity:** human tissue cells have different sensitivities to radiation:
1. Radiosensitive tissues and cells are highly sensitive to radiation (e.g., bone marrow, reproductive, small lymphocyte).
2. Radioresistant tissues and cells are MORE resistant to radiation (e.g., salivary glands, lungs, kidneys, muscle).
3. In order of MOST sensitive to least sensitive: blood-forming and reproductive cells, gastrointestinal tract, immature bone, epithelial (glandular) and muscle tissues, adult bone and nerve tissue; blood type does NOT affect sensitivity.

E. Critical organs and radiation:
  1. When sensitive organs and tissues are exposed to radiation during dental irradiation, significant decrease in quality of person's life may occur.
  2. Include skin, eye lens, thyroid, bone marrow (hematopoietic):
     a. Skin irradiation may lead to erythema: FIRST clinical sign of overexposure (250 rad in 14-day period).
     b. Eye irradiation can lead to cataract formation if exposure to eyes is 200,000 mrad.
     c. Thyroid irradiation can result in increased cancer risk, particularly when radiation exposure of 6000 mrad or more occurs.
     d. Bone marrow irradiation poses increased cancer risk (particularly leukemia) at exposures of 5000 mrad or more of radiation.
     e. Organs MOST affected by continued low doses of radiation in order from MOST sensitive to least sensitive are thyroid, skin, brain.

Radiation Exposure and Risks

Exposure and risks associated with radiation include those from environment (background) and those associated with direct irradiation of organs. (See the WebLink on the CD-ROM for the ADA and FDA Guide to Patient Selection for Dental Radiographs.)

A. Background radiation: GREATEST contribution to radiation is from naturally occurring sources in environment:
  1. External radiation: from cosmic and terrestrial sources, comprises ~15% of the radiation exposure to the population.
  2. Internal radiation: from exposure to radionuclides through inhalation and ingestion; comprises ~67% of radiation exposure; radon is the LARGEST single contributor to natural radiation.
B. Artificial radiation: includes such sources as medical and dental radiation:
  1. Comprises ~17% of radiation exposure.
  2. Exposure is equivalent to few days' worth of background radiation or environmental radiation exposure, or similar to dose received during cross-country airplane flight.

Radiation Protection

Proper use of equipment, patient and clinician positioning, and technique can provide acceptable limits to incidental radiation exposure. Advances in dental radiograph technology have reduced scatter radiation, the reason for protective boxes; lead-lined radiograph storage boxes are thus unnecessary and should be discarded, since they contaminated the film. There is controversy over need for lead (or lead equivalent) aprons for patient protection. Note that term "clinician" is used for operator.

A. Patient: patient exposure to radiation MUST BE reduced by using filtration, collimation, positioning, shielding:
  1. Filtration involves filtering-out of nonproductive x-rays; inherent filtration plus added filtration equals total filtration for the machine:
     a. Inherent filtration is inside tubehead (i.e., oil, glass window, tubehead seal).
     b. Added filtration includes aluminum disc (disk) placed around seal of machine:
        (1) Used to filter out longer, nonproductive wavelengths, resulting in primary beam with MORE energy.
        (2) Federal and state laws dictate thickness of total filtration according to kilovolt peak (kVp) setting of the machine ($\leq$70 kVp = 1.5-mm thickness of aluminum; $\geq$70 kVp = 2.5-mm thickness).
  2. Collimation restricts size and shape of x-ray beam (reducing film fog) and therefore restricts patient exposure (scatter exposure):
     a. **Collimator:** lead diaphragm placed over opening of tubehead.
     b. Exposure reduction is possible by limiting size of x-ray beam at end of PID to no more than 2.75 inches in diameter, using rectangular PID, and placing tubehead 1½ to 2 inches from patient.
  3. The PID (beam-indicating device [BID]): aiming device that is used to direct the x-ray beam:
     a. Cone-shaped PID: closed, pointed, plastic device that increases scatter radiation and should NOT be used.
     b. Round PID: open ended, circular, and lead lined; standard lengths are 8 inches and 16 inches; 16 inches is MAINLY used because provides MORE parallel rays.
     c. Rectangular lead-lined PID: highly recommended because offers MOST reduction in radiation exposure to the patient; standard lengths are 8 inches and 16 inches.
  4. Lead aprons or lead equivalent (contains 0.25 to 0.3 mm of lead thickness) shields; aprons worn by patients to protect tissues from scatter radiation; mandated by law in many states; should be used in conjunction with thyroid collar for intraoral films (questionable use now).
  5. Fast film: one of the MOST effective means of reducing patient exposure; F-speed film is fastest and is MORE than twice as fast as D-speed film; F-speed film needs 60% LESS exposure time and E-speed film needs 50% LESS exposure time than D-speed film; thus E- and F-speed films recommended.
  6. Film-holding devices: method necessary to stabilize film and ultimately reduce additional exposure to patient.

B. Clinician: measures MUST be taken to protect clinician from unnecessary radiation; include proper positioning, use of monitors, attention to proper methods of taking radiographs:
1. Positioning:
   a. Involves awareness of distance; remaining at least 6 feet from the source of radiation and in a safe quadrant (at right angles to the primary beam) is one of the MOST effective ways to eliminate unnecessary clinician exposure.
   b. Clinician SHOULD never hold the tubehead or film in patient's mouth during exposure.
   c. Clinician should stand behind lead shield or barrier whenever possible (cinderblock or 2½ inches of drywall provides adequate protection).
2. Monitoring:
   a. Involves using personnel monitoring devices and following national guidelines when measuring occupational radiation exposure; **film badges** that measure exposure to low doses of radiation should be worn at waist level; two types of monitoring available.
      (1) Metal filters: located inside badge, measure amount of radiation but can be worn for ONLY 1 month; hard radiation shows faint shadow; soft radiation casts pronounced shadow.
      (2) Thermoluminescent **dosimeter** (TLD): device that contains lithium fluoride crystals that absorb x-ray energy; MORE sensitive and can be worn for 3 months but is MORE expensive.
   b. **Maximum permissible dose** (MPD): developed by National Council on Radiation Protection (NCRP):
      (1) Relates to amount of radiation exposure that is permissible through occupational exposure.
      (2) Considered to be maximum dose that does NOT produce significant injury in a lifetime.
      (3) Formula represents whole-body dose equivalent of ionizing and electromagnetic radiations and is expressed in sieverts.
      (4) The MPD for occupationally exposed persons:
         (a) Per year = 50 mSv (5 rem, 5000 mrem).
         (b) Per month = 4 mSv (400 mrem).
         (c) Per week = 1 mSv (100 mrem).
      (5) The MPD for nonoccupational (whole-body) exposure: 10% of that for worker, or 5 mSv (500 mrem) per year.
      (6) Maximum accumulated dose = 5 rem × N −18 (N = age).
   c. The ALARA concept: As Low As Reasonably Achievable.
      (1) Philosophy of radiation protection that is currently practiced by all radiation workers.
      (2) Implies that every effort will be made to keep radiation exposure, whether occupational or nonoccupational, as LOW as possible (see later discussion of guidelines for patient radiographic examination).

Digital Imaging

With digital imaging, nonfilm sensor is placed inside the mouth; electronically attached to computer, immediately producing image on monitor.
A. Principles:
   1. Requires conventional equipment to generate x-rays; see earlier discussion.
   2. Image captured is SIMILAR to conventional film.
   3. When sensor is exposed to radiation, electronic chart is produced on its surface.
   4. Direct or indirect (scanned):
      a. Direct: sensor in rigid case, either charge-coupled device (CCD) or complementary metal-oxide semiconductor (CMOS), is used; immediate image and immediate reuse.
      b. Indirect: photostimulable phosphor (PSP) plate is used to store image, which is then scanned, read, and erased; conventional films can also be scanned and converted to digital.
B. Advantages:
   1. Images can be stored, retained as a hard copy, or sent to a different site.
   2. Images can be displayed immediately, which is useful for intraoperative procedures such as endodontic treatment; eliminates darkroom procedures.
   3. Provides less radiation exposure to the patient but poorer resolution, costs MORE, large sensors, manipulated films, MORE exposures because of small sensor size.
   4. Associated software using a database can analyze changes in radiographic density to identify demineralized areas and determine probability that caries is present.
C. Disadvantages: initial cost, uncomfortable sensors, infection control of sensors by plastic sleeves and NOT heat sterilization.

CLINICAL STUDY

Age	42 YRS	SCENARIO
Sex	☐ Male ☒ Female	The new patient's intraoral examination reveals several suspect areas and fractured restorations on the maxillary arch. It has been at least 6 or 7 years since patient has had radiographs taken. The dental hygienist recommends a full-mouth series (FMX). However, the patient is reluctant because of what she has heard about the dangers and misuse of radiation.
Height	5'4"	
Weight	170 LBS	
BP	118/76	
Chief Complaint	"Boy, the fillings in my upper back teeth are so sensitive! They feel like they are moving when I bite down."	
Medical History	Has had a bad cold for 2 weeks with postnasal drip Mother died of breast cancer Has mammograms every 6 months because of high risk	
Current Medications	None	
Social History	Bus driver Single mom with two children Likes bowling	

1. What is the most probable diagnosis of the patient's condition? Identify all possible causes for her symptoms. What other information should be gathered to determine the cause of the sensitivity?
2. What issue must be addressed to provide this patient with the best treatment?
3. What procedures are used to protect the patient from unnecessary radiation?

1. Sinus infection *and* carious lesions are present. Sensitivity of maxillary teeth could be related to the closeness of the roots of maxillary teeth to enlarged, inflamed sinuses; such sensitivity should dissipate as sinusitis clears up. Movement of restorations is more serious in nature and is indicative of fractured restorations. Ill-fitting restorations often have marginal leakage and/or recurrent caries. Other information can be gained by asking: "What are the teeth sensitive to (e.g., temperature, pressure, sweets)?", "How long have they been sensitive?", and "Does anything seem to exacerbate or alleviate the discomfort?"
2. Benefit versus risk of having radiographs taken should be discussed with patient. Clinical examinations warrant FMX radiographs to confirm exact diagnosis and direction of proper treatment. Although minimal amount of radiation exposure occurs, benefit of diagnosis far outweighs risk of allowing carious lesions to continue without diagnosis and then treatment.

3. Devices on x-ray machine such as filter, collimator, lead-lined PID reduce radiation exposure to patient. Using lead apron or lead equivalent with thyroid collar and film-holding devices with fast-speed film (F-speed film is fastest) keeps patient exposure to minimum while providing excellent-quality diagnostic radiographs.

CHARACTERISTICS OF RADIATION IMAGES

Radiation images are characterized by their quantity, quality, intensity, clarity.

A. Quantity: number of x-rays that are produced; measured in amperes, milliampere-seconds, density of the radiographs.
   1. Ampere: number of electrons that flow through a filament:
      a. **Milliampere** (mA) is equal to $\frac{1}{1000}$ of an ampere.
      b. Milliamperage controls temperature of the cathode filament.
   2. Milliampere-seconds (mA-s): combination of milliamperes and seconds:
      a. Milliamperes have a direct effect on the number of electrons produced.
      b. Seconds have the same effect on the quantity of electrons produced.
      c. To maintain similar density:
         (1) Increased seconds, milliamperage MUST be decreased.
         (2) Decreased seconds, milliamperage MUST be increased.

3. Density: overall darkness of radiograph:
    a. Affected by milliamperage and by quantity of electrons produced.
        (1) Increased mA, film will be darker.
        (2) Decreased mA, film will be lighter.
B. Quality: energy and penetrating power of the beam; measured in kilovolts; affects image contrasts:
    1. **Kilovolt** (kV): equal to 1000 volts and is measurement used to determine energy in a tubehead:
        a. **Kilovoltage peak** (kVp) represents peak or maximum voltage; determines speed and ultimately energy of electrons.
        b. With increased kVp, primary beam will have MORE energy and density will increase.
    2. Contrast: difference between lighter and darker shades (grays) on radiograph:
        a. Increased kVp (≥90) results in many shades of gray on the film (long-scale contrast); BEST for detecting bone abnormalities.
        b. Decreased kVp (65 to 70) results in MORE black and white areas on a radiograph (short-scale contrast); BEST for detecting caries.
C. Beam intensity: affected by mA, kVp, exposure time, distance:
    1. The mA affects intensity by controlling the number of electrons produced; higher the mA, MORE intense the beam.
    2. The kVp controls energy of electrons traveling from the cathode to the anode; higher the kVp, MORE intense the beam.
    3. Exposure time affects the intensity in the same manner as mA; increase in time = MORE intense beam.
    4. Distance also affects beam intensity; as beam travels longer distance to film or tooth, becomes LESS intense:
        a. Inverse square law states that "intensity of radiation is inversely proportional to square of the distance from the source of radiation"; explains how the beam loses its intensity as it travels farther from the source.
        b. Half-value layer describes the reduction in beam intensity by one half with the use of aluminum filters; filters remove LESS penetrating, longer wavelengths in the beam.
D. Accurate image (geometric) formation: BEST produced by controlling image sharpness, magnification, distortion:
    1. Sharpness (detail, definition): umbra is increased clarity or distinctness of outlines of object; penumbra is fuzziness or LACK of sharpness in image.
        a. Influenced by focal spot size; tungsten target of anode should be small to increase sharpness.
        b. Associated with film composition; size of crystals on film determines sharpness; larger the crystals, LESS sharp the image.
        c. MAINLY influenced by patient and tubehead movement; either will reduce image sharpness.
    2. Magnification: enlargement of actual image:
        a. Influenced by target-film distance; increased distance from target in the x-ray tube to film allows MORE parallel rays to hit film, LESS magnification.
        b. Affected by object-film distance; closer the tooth to film, LESS the magnification.
    3. Distortion: disfigurement of the shape and size of an image:
        a. Affected by the object-film alignment; film and long axis of the tooth MUST be parallel to each other (so that rays will hit at a right angle) to decrease distortion.
        b. Influenced by beam direction; beam MUST be directed perpendicular to both the film and the tooth to record accurate, distortion-free image.
    4. Pneumatization: with free airspace in a structure or tissue, one area is MORE radiolucent than another area (frequently seen when maxillary sinus has dropped).

RADIOGRAPHIC EXAMINATION

Radiographic examination involves intraoral, extraoral, and special imaging techniques to produce high-quality radiographs for use in examination, interpretation, diagnosis of dental conditions and diseases. (See the CD-ROM for WebLink to the ADA/FDA Guide to Patient Selection for Dental Radiographs, which includes the chart Guidelines for Prescribing Dental Radiographs.) These guidelines will allow for ALARA concept, although each case is subject to clinical judgment.

Intraoral Radiographic Views

Views include **periapical** (PA), **bitewing** (BW), **occlusal, full-mouth series** (FMX).
A. The PA view: captures from cementoenamel junction (CEJ) to root on the film; included in FMX; uses size 1 to 2 films:
    1. Used for diagnosis of a pathological changes in a specific tooth by its root and surrounding bone.
    2. Especially if there is a need for endodontic therapy (late finding).
B. The BW view: visualizes crowns, contacts, height of alveolar bone in relation to CEJ; included in FMX; uses size 1 to 2 films:
    1. Used for diagnosis of a series of teeth as they contact on the occlusal.
    2. Used for diagnosis of dental caries (ONLY interproximal early, with occlusal and root late) and periodontal disease (ONLY bone loss on interproximal alveolar crest is shown, NOT facial or lingual plates).
    3. Can be either horizontal or vertical in placement; vertical used to evaluate alveolar bone loss.

C. Occlusal view: reveals bone surrounding tooth, floor of the mouth, or presence of sialolith (stone) in parotid (Stensen's) duct; NOT included in FMX; uses size 4 films.
D. FMX: complete set of intraoral radiographs: number depends on size of films:
   1. Use size 1 for anteriors and size 2 for others: 20 films, 4 BWs and 16 PAs.
   2. Use only size 2: 20 films, 4 BWs and 14 PAs.

Intraoral Techniques

Intraoral radiography includes bisecting, paralleling, and occlusal techniques.

A. **Bisecting** (angle) **technique** (Figure 5-3):
   1. Based on rule of isometry: two triangles are equal if they have equal angles and share common side.
   2. Requires bisection of the angle, forms two equal triangles; angle formed by plane of film and plane of long axis of tooth.
   3. If technique is strictly followed, directs primary beam 90° to bisected line, resulting in accurate image.
   4. MORE distortion than paralleling technique because of position of the palate.
B. **Paralleling technique:**
   1. Based on geometric figures of parallelism.
   2. Requires that film be placed parallel to long axis of the tooth.
   3. Requires film holder for proper film placement.
   4. Directs primary beam perpendicular to film and long axis of the tooth.
C. **Occlusal technique:**
   1. For anterior topographical mandibular occlusal:
      a. Head tilted backward, using negative 55° vertical angle.
      b. Central ray directed through point of the chin.
   2. For anterior topographical maxillary occlusal:
      a. Sagittal plane perpendicular to floor; occlusal plane parallel to floor.
      b. Positive vertical angle of 65°; central ray is directed just superior to tip of nose.
   3. For cross-sectional maxillary occlusal:
      a. Sagittal plane perpendicular to floor; occlusal plane parallel to floor.
      b. Central ray directed to film at 90°, with PID centered between the eyebrows.
   4. For cross-sectional mandibular occlusal:
      a. Head tilted backward until ala-tragus line is almost perpendicular to floor.
      b. A 90° vertical angle, central ray directed 3 cm inferior to the chin.
D. **Buccal object** (SLOB: <u>S</u>ame <u>L</u>ingual, <u>O</u>pposite <u>B</u>uccal) **rule:** shows whether artifact or object is lingual or buccal; in second radiograph, if central ray is moved and object moves in same direction, then lingual, if it moves in opposite direction, buccal; used mainly in endodontics, since on PAs, roots are often superimposed on one another and require separation for proper identification so as to visualize lengths and anatomy.

Intraoral Technique Errors

Proper recognition of errors can help clinician correct a technique problem before it is repeated, possibly subjecting patient to unnecessary radiation and producing nondiagnostic radiographs.

A. Overlap (Figure 5-4):
   1. Adjacent tooth structures superimposed on each other.
   2. Corrected by redirecting primary beam *through* contacts (change in horizontal angulation).
B. Foreshortening (Figure 5-5):
   1. Teeth shorter than actual size because of excessive vertical angulation.
   2. Corrected by decreasing the vertical angulation.

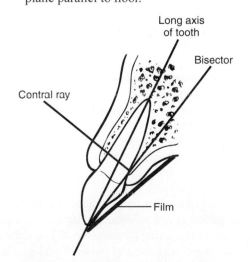

Figure 5-3   Bisecting (angle) technique.

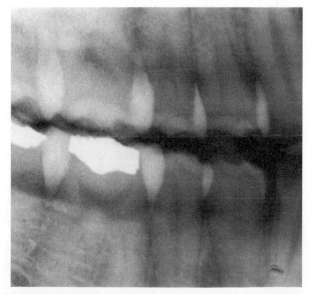

Figure 5-4   Overlapping of tooth structures caused by faulty horizontal angulation.

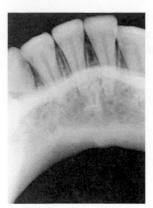

Figure 5-5 Foreshortening from excessive vertical angulation.

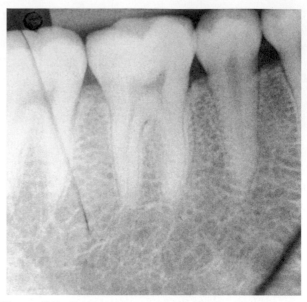

Figure 5-7 Radiolucent mark associated with creased or bent film.

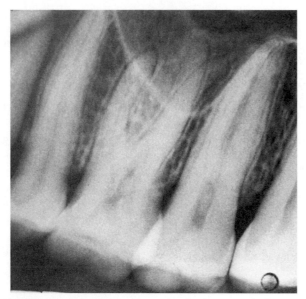

Figure 5-6 Elongation from inadequate vertical angulation.

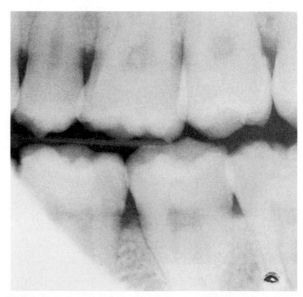

Figure 5-8 Cone cut caused by inadequate position-indicating device (PID) coverage of the film.

C. Elongation (Figure 5-6):
 1. Teeth distorted and larger than actual size because of insufficient vertical angulation, and apices of the teeth are NOT included.
 2. Corrected by increasing the vertical angulation.
D. Bent film (Figure 5-7):
 1. Radiolucent mark across film; caused by creasing or improperly placing film.
 2. Corrected by NOT creasing film corners and by positioning film to keep the surface of film in the same plane.
E. Cone cut (Figure 5-8):
 1. Radiopaque area with circular or rectangular border; caused because PID did NOT cover entire surface of film.
 2. Corrected by redirecting the PID to cover the surface of the film.

F. Backward placement (Figure 5-9):
 1. Film appears much lighter, with a herringbone or waffle patterned effect on both sides; caused by backward placement of the film in the mouth, with lead foil in the packet closest to (facing) tooth and x-ray source.
 2. Corrected by placing the film with the *smooth* side next to the tooth (*pebble* side away).
G. Movement (Figure 5-10):
 1. Blurred or unclear image; caused by movement of the patient and/or tubehead during exposure of film.
 2. Corrected by giving the patient MORE specific directions about NOT moving and by checking to be sure the tubehead is stabilized before exposing the film.

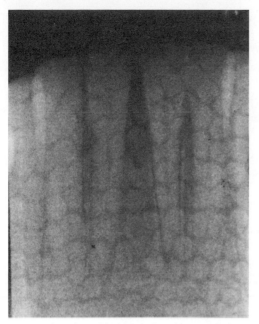

Figure 5-9 Film placed backward in the mouth has a waffle or herringbone appearance.

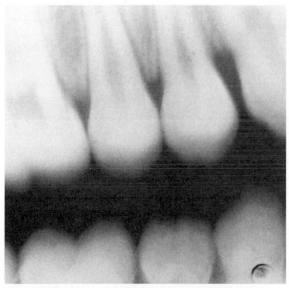

Figure 5-10 Blurred image is caused by movement of either patient or tubehead during film exposure.

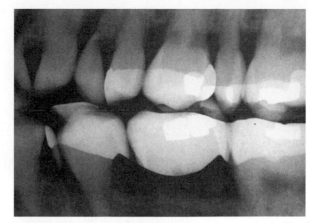

Figure 5-11 Double exposure occurs when a single film is exposed to radiation twice.

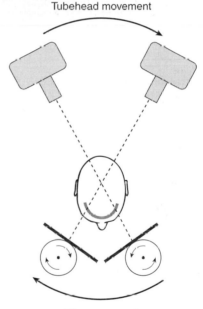

Tubehead movement

Film movement

Figure 5-12 Focal trough used in panoramic imaging.

H. Double exposure (Figure 5-11):
   1. Darker film with distinct outlines of many teeth; caused by NOT organizing film order during exposure or by exposing a single film twice.
   2. Corrected by keeping film in order of exposure and by keeping exposed film in a different place.

Extraoral Techniques

During extraoral techniques, film is placed outside of the mouth during exposure; MOST of these require use of screen film (if NOT using digital method). Includes panoramic imaging, lateral jaw exposures, cephalometry, Waters projection techniques. (See the Chapter 5 Extras on the CD-ROM for discussion of panoramic imaging.)

A. **Panoramic imaging:** movement of film cassette and radiation source around the head (Figure 5-12).
   1. Uses focal trough or plane of acceptable focus in shape of the dental arches.
   2. Any images inside this trough are *clearer;* images outside the trough are *blurred;* thus CORRECT patient positioning is crucial.
   3. Evaluates impacted teeth, eruption patterns, growth; used to detect diseases, conditions of the jaw, trauma.
   4. Errors in panoramic technique are common:
      a. Lip and tongue placement: IMPORTANT in quality of film.

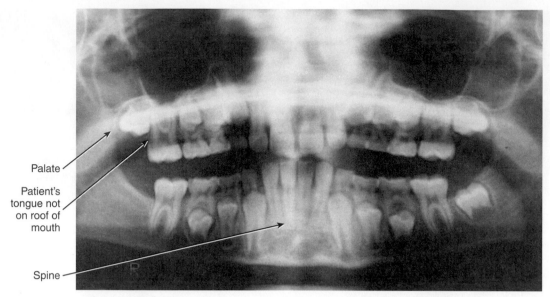

Figure 5-13 Panoramic film demonstrating improper tongue placement.

(1) NOT closing lips; lips must be closed to prevent appearance of dark shadow on anteriors.

(2) Tongue NOT on palate; tongue must be placed on the palate to prevent appearance of radiolucent areas over apices of maxillary teeth (Figure 5-13).

b. Chin placement: MUST be parallel to floor.

(1) If chin is tipped up, "frown" results, with blurring and magnification of maxillary teeth.

(2) If chin is tipped down, "exaggerated smile" results, with blurring and magnification of mandibular incisors.

(3) Shadow of chin rest.

c. Placement of anterior teeth: MUST be placed correctly in focal trough.

(1) If anterior teeth are placed forward to the focal trough (notch in the bite-block), will appear thinner.

(2) If anterior teeth are placed behind the focal trough (notch in the bite-block), will appear thicker and wider.

B. **Lateral jaw exposure:** film cassette placed laterally to jaw during exposure (Figure 5-14):

1. Used to examine posterior portion of mandible or for those who CANNOT open the mouth because of swelling or possible fractures.

2. Also, lateral areas of the mandible are too large for PA film.

C. **Lateral cephalometric projection:** film cassette placed on the side of head to image outline of face; evaluates trauma, facial growth and development, developmental abnormalities (Figure 5-15).

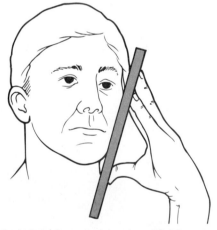

Figure 5-14 Lateral jaw exposure is useful for examining traumatic injury to the posterior jaw.

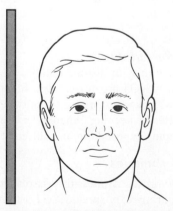

Figure 5-15 Lateral cephalometric projection is often used to detect developmental or traumatic disturbances.

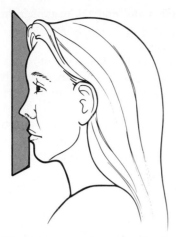

Figure 5-16 Posteroanterior projection is used to evaluate the frontal and ethmoidal sinuses, the eye orbits, and the nasal cavity.

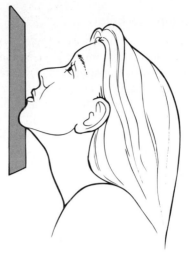

Figure 5-17 Waters projection is useful for examining maxillary sinuses.

D. **Posteroanterior projection:** film cassette placed on face, with forehead and nose touching it; shows frontal and ethmoidal sinuses, orbits, nasal cavity (Figure 5-16).

E. **Waters projection:** film cassette placed on face, with chin touching it, with head tipped back so that tip of the nose is 1 inch from it; specifically evaluates maxillary sinus area (Figure 5-17).

CLINICAL STUDY

Age	8 YRS	SCENARIO
Sex	☒ Male ☐ Female	At his first dental appointment, the patient demonstrates nervousness and a short attention span.
Chief Complaint	His guardian asks, "My foster child often has bad breath. Is it due to cavities?"	
Medical History	Fetal alcohol syndrome (FAS) Moderate cognitive disability	
Current Medications	None because of cost factors at this time	
Social History	Does not attend school at the present time because of mother's recent incarceration	

1. What is FAS and what are the oral manifestations of this disorder?
2. What radiographs are recommended and why?
3. A double image appeared on one of the two films. What caused this?

1. FAS is caused by maternal ingestion of alcohol during pregnancy. Alcohol ingestion during the early stages of pregnancy often leads to intellectual disability (mental retardation) and other developmental disabilities in the child. Hyperactivity and attention deficit disorder (ADD) often accompany the syndrome, as they do in this case. Oral manifestations may include flattened nose or extremely wide bridge, cleft lip with or without cleft palate, underdeveloped maxilla, micrognathia.

2. Panoramic radiograph with accompanying BWs is recommended because of the FAS and lack of drugs for ADD or hyperactivity, since he will have trouble sitting still for a long period needed for any other radiographs. In addition, his small jaw size would make numerous intraoral films difficult to obtain.

3. Blurred image on a film is caused by movement of either tubehead or patient during exposure. In this situation, most likely it is caused by patient movement because this patient is not taking any drugs for hyperactivity that accompanies FAS.

Special Imaging Techniques

Magnetic resonance imaging, computed tomography, sialography are specialized imaging techniques.

A. Magnetic resonance imaging (MRI): derives energy from powerful magnetic field:
   1. Hydrogen nuclei in the body are realigned by radiofrequency pulses, received by the sensor and transmitted to computer to generate mage.
   2. BEST for imaging soft tissue, especially within temporomandibular joint.
B. Computed tomography (CT scanning, CAT scan): computer generated; uses ionizing radiation as energy source:
   1. MUST be performed in special CT unit in the hospital; special software is required.
   2. Allows multiple images to be fed into a computer, resulting in image on monitor or film.
   3. Useful in dentistry for implant planning and soft tissue lesions, especially in salivary glands.
C. **Cone beam computed tomography** (CBCT): computer-generated imaging of hard tissues of maxillofacial region, providing three-dimensional representation of skeleton with minimal distortion; high diagnostic quality of resolution, with short scanning time and radiation dosages lower than CT scans; highly recommended for implant placement, preoperative and postoperative endodontic procedures with cracked teeth and missing canals, and apical surgery.
D. **Sialography:** used ONLY for radiographic examination of ductal system of salivary glands by use of contrast agent to check for salivary stones and other blockage.

Image Production

Producing a good image requires knowledge of proper film processing and darkroom techniques, processing problems and solutions, film reproduction methods, infection control practices.

A. Film processing: transformation of latent image into visible image by means of chemical processing; can be manual or automatic:
   1. Manual processing (time-temperature method) involves, in order: manual developing, washing, fixing, washing, drying.
      a. BEST developing takes ~5 minutes at 68° F; reduces exposed silver halide crystals into black metallic silver through four ingredients in solution:
         (1) Hydroquinone (gives contrast) or elon (gives detail): developing agent that converts energized crystals into metallic silver.
         (2) Sodium sulfite: preservative that prevents rapid oxidation of developer.
         (3) Sodium carbonate: softens film emulsion and speeds up action of developing agents.
         (4) Potassium bromide: restrainer that inhibits development of unexposed silver halide crystals.
      b. Fixing takes ~10 minutes, or TWICE developing time; clears all unexposed silver halide crystals from film emulsion by means of four ingredients in solution:
         (1) Sodium thiosulfate: clears unexposed silver halide crystals from emulsion.
         (2) Sodium sulfite: prevents the breakdown of sodium thiosulfate.
         (3) Potassium alum: shrinks and hardens emulsion.
         (4) Acetic acid: acidifier that keeps medium acidic and stops additional development.
   2. Automatic processing: automatically processes film; roller transport system moves film through solutions in order: developer, fixer, water, drying chamber.
      a. Developing and fixing solutions are different from those used in manual processing.
         (1) Developing solution works at higher temperature and MORE rapidly.
         (2) Fixing solution has a hardening agent to keep the film sturdy as it continues through the rollers.
      b. Rollers MUST be clean, or radiolucent bands will appear on films.
   3. Rapid (hot) processing method: concentrated or higher temperature solutions process in 1 minute or less; BEST for endodontic therapy or emergency procedures; quality of film is less than with standard methods.
B. Darkroom lighting: important in film processing:
   1. Without any light leaks to prevent fogging of the film.
   2. Filter that removes blue-green wavelengths; red both intraoral and extraoral, orange intraoral ONLY.
   3. Safelights (direct illumination) must be spaced at least 4 feet from working surface with low-wattage bulb (7½/15 watts).
   4. LED safelights: replace conventional filtered lights; offer MORE efficient light.
C. Film duplication: copying or reproducing a second film or set of films without reexposing the patient to radiation:
   1. Requires special duplicating film that must be used under safelight conditions.
      a. Duplicating film is coated on ONLY one side.
      b. Duplicating film is direct positive film:
         (1) Darker film requires LESS exposure time.
         (2) Conversely, lighter film requires MORE exposure time.
   2. Used for third-party payment, patient transfer, referral, litigation.

3. Procedure requires placing original film next to the light source, placing duplicate film on top of it, and exposing the films to the light source for specified amount of time.

D. Film mounting: processed radiographs are organized and placed in a frame for ease of reading, to protect films from wear, to reduce interpretation errors:
   1. Depending on the teaching method, radiographs are mounted either "dots-in" or "dots-out."
      a. Dots-in or lingual method (as if inside the mouth looking out): films are mounted with the patient's left side films on left side of the mount and right side films on right side of the mount; less common method.
      b. Dots-out or labial method (as if outside the mouth looking in): films are mounted with the patient's right side films on the left side of the mount and the left side films on the right side of the mount; MORE common method.
   2. Mounting procedure: once films are dry, placed on clean viewbox surface with dots up; use of magnifying viewer is helpful.
      a. Films are initially separated into maxillary, mandibular, BW sections:
         (1) BWs are mounted FIRST, using curve of Spee so that the "smile" is directed up and distally, to guide placement of posterior PA films; maxillary molars have three roots and mandibular molars have two roots.
         (2) Posterior films with most posterior structures are placed in molar areas; subsequently, posterior films with least posterior structures are placed in premolar areas.
         (3) Anterior films with both central incisors are placed in appropriate maxillary and mandibular central anterior sections.
         (4) Remaining right- and left-of-central anterior films are placed in appropriate sections to either side of the central films.
      b. Films are then arranged by the anatomical landmarks as if facing the dental arches: maxillary posterior right, posterior left, and anterior; mandibular posterior right, posterior left, anterior.

E. Quality assurance program: systematic procedure used to guarantee that high-quality radiographs are produced with minimal exposure to the patient:
   1. X-ray equipment:
      a. Evaluated annually as recommended by American Academy of Oral and Maxillofacial Radiology (AAOMR).
      b. Inspected by specifically trained inspectors who check kVp, mA output, half-value layer, timer, collimation, beam alignment, tubehead stability.

   2. Radiographer expertise: ONLY individuals skilled in radiographic procedures and techniques should expose patients to x-rays.
   3. Processing solutions (manual and automatic):
      a. Mixed and replenished according to the manufacturer's recommendations and dated.
      b. Changed as needed according to degree of use and dated.
      c. Can be evaluated by:
         (1) Stepwedge (constructed of aluminum layers) to provide standard radiograph for evaluating density on daily basis.
         (2) Dental radiographic normalizing device (DRND) to compare density of film and monitor strength of the solution.
   4. Darkroom:
      a. Safelight is evaluated every 6 months (see earlier discussion).
      b. Evaluated for light leaks around doors and vents by means of coin test.
   5. Cassette intensifying screens: inspected and cleaned monthly.

F. Administration:
   1. Assign duties to appropriate personnel; write descriptions of the plan and its expectations.
   2. Maintain records for equipment; create forms to keep records of monitoring procedures.
   3. Document all monitoring procedures.

Processing Problems and Solutions

Many problems occur when processing technique and procedure errors are made even with automatic processing.

A. Overdeveloped film too dark (Figure 5-18):
   1. Overdevelopment (excessive development time).
   2. Developing solution at a temperature that is too high.
   3. Developing solution that was incorrectly mixed or too concentrated.

B. Underdeveloped film too light (Figure 5-19):
   1. Underdevelopment (inadequate development time).
   2. Developing solution at a temperature that is too low.
   3. Exhausted (overused) developing solution.

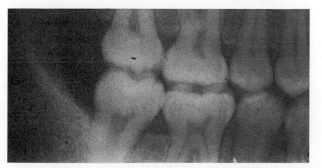

Figure 5-18 Overdeveloped film appears too dark.

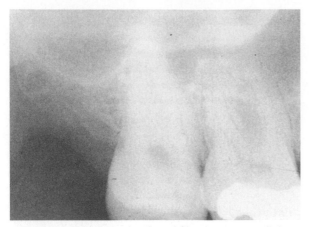

Figure 5-19 Underdeveloped film appears too light.

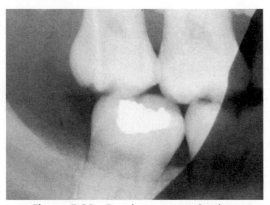

Figure 5-20 Developer contamination.

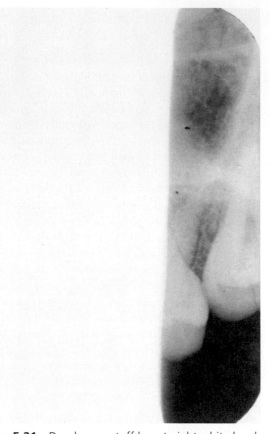

Figure 5-21 Developer cutoff has straight white border.

C. Reticulation: cracked emulsion; caused by sudden temperature change between developer and fixer solution.
D. Contamination from chemicals:
1. Developer contamination: darker areas; caused when developing solution comes into contact with film before processing procedure (Figure 5-20).
2. Fixer contamination: lighter areas; caused when fixer solution comes into contact with film before processing procedure.
E. Other errors:
1. Exhausted solutions or insufficient time in solutions: yellow-brown stains.
2. Developer cutoff: straight white border; caused by a low level of solution (Figure 5-21).
3. Fixer cutoff: straight black border; caused by incomplete immersion of film into fixer solution (Figure 5-22).
4. Overlapped films: white and dark areas in the shape of outline border of another film; caused when films contact each other in solutions (Figure 5-23).

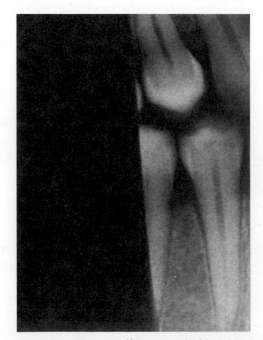

Figure 5-22 Fixer cutoff has straight black border.

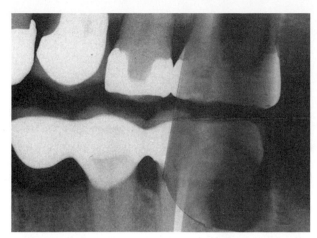

Figure 5-23 Overlapped films have an outline shape of a second film.

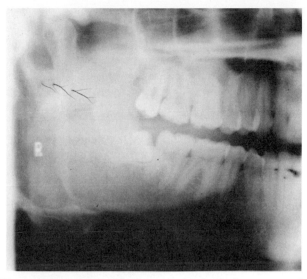

Figure 5-24 Static electricity on this half of a panoramic film caused a black, branchlike image.

5. Air bubbles: white spots; caused by air that is trapped on surface of film during processing.
6. Static electricity: thin, black, branchlike lines; caused by low humidity and opening film packet too quickly (Figure 5-24).

7. Scratched films: white lines; caused by removal of emulsion during processing process.
8. Fogged films: gray hue; caused by improper safelighting, outdated film, or light leaking into darkroom.

CLINICAL STUDY

Age	85 YRS	**SCENARIO**
Sex	☒ Male ☐ Female	The patient fell while getting dressed yesterday and hit his head on the headboard of his bed. Visual examination at his winter dental office during the emergency appointment reveals a large bruise on the right side of his face along the lower jaw line. Teeth #30 and #31 are missing their anatomical crowns.
Height	5'10"	
Weight	178 LBS	
BP	110/69	
Chief Complaint	"My jaw is sore and I can't open my mouth!"	
Medical History	Shielded pacemaker placed 10 years ago	
Current Medications	warfarin (Coumadin) 10 mg qd to prevent blood clots from forming	
Social History	Retired fireman Travels to Arizona during the winter months	

1. Which type of radiograph would provide the best assessment of this patient's jaw and teeth? What information should be obtained from the radiograph? Describe the appearance of such information.
2. After the film is processed, a 9-mm semicircular radiopaque mark is found on the lower right corner of the radiographs. What is the mark, and what caused it?

3. During examination of the processed film, a pyramid-shaped radiopacity is observed in the center of the panoramic image. What is it, and how was it caused?
4. "Branch-out" radiolucent marks appear on several areas of the film. What are they, and what caused them?

1. Panoramic radiograph should be taken to allow assessment of a larger area of the jaws and teeth; also is easier for patient, given that he has difficulty opening his mouth. Indications of jaw fracture (vertical radiolucent line) should be looked for on right side; possible tooth discoloration, noncontinuous lamina dura, and infected retained root tips on right side.
2. The 9-mm semicircular radiopaque mark located on the lower edge of film is most likely a fingernail scratch mark caused by improper handling of film during processing. Scratching of emulsion caused the radiopaque artifact on processed film.
3. Pyramid-shaped opacity is a ghost image of spine caused by slumped position of patient during exposure. Patient should be required to stand erect so that spinal column is not superimposed on the film.
4. These "treelike" marks are artifacts caused by static electricity; usually occur because of low humidity, as is the case in Arizona.

Radiology Infection Control

Disinfection and sterilization of equipment and clinical areas involve proper attention to infection control procedures and standards.

- See Chapter 8, Microbiology and Immunology: standard precautions.
A. Equipment and supplies:
   1. Chair, headrest, tubehead, PID SHOULD be covered with disposable barrier material such as plastic bag.
   2. Controls on the machine, including activating switch, SHOULD be covered with clear wrap or a disposable item.
   3. Lead apron or shielding equivalent SHOULD be sanitized by misting with disinfectant and wiping surface; should NOT be contaminated during procedure.
   4. Surface of the work area SHOULD be covered with disposable barrier material.
   5. Film holders SHOULD be sterilized, and film should have protective coverings or be contained in disposable cup to prevent contamination of other surfaces.
   6. If lead barrier is used, barrier SHOULD have protective coverings on all handled areas.
B. Clinician preparation (includes personal protective equipment [PPE]):
   1. Hands SHOULD be washed and gloved; mask and eyewear are optional.
   2. Clinician SHOULD wear a gown or protective outerwear.
C. Exposure procedures:
   1. Contaminated items (e.g., paper cups, BW tabs, cotton rolls) SHOULD be carefully discarded.
   2. All uncovered surfaces (e.g., armrests, chair, countertops) that might be contaminated SHOULD be disinfected with EPA-registered disinfectant; clinician SHOULD wear utility gloves.

Normal Anatomical Landmarks

Familiarity with normal anatomical landmarks of the oral cavity is essential for the development of proper radiographic technique, assessment, diagnosis. **Radiopaque** or **radiolucent** appearance of image helps determine specific landmarks; however, NOT all landmarks are seen on every FMX. When a lesion is suspect, appropriate landmarks for that site should be ruled out.

- See Chapter 4, Head, Neck, and Dental Anatomy: normal landmarks.
A. Tooth tissues and periodontium (in order of density or mineralization; lighter [highly mineralized] to darker [nonmineralized]): enamel, dentin, cementum, bone (first cortical bone as lamina dura, then supporting bone as spongy), periodontal ligament (PDL space), pulp.
B. Maxillary films have 11 common intraoral landmarks:
   1. Incisive foramen (Figure 5-25):
      a. Passageway for nasopalatine nerves and vessels in middle of hard palate, posterior to central incisors.
      b. Centrally located radiolucent oval-shaped object between roots of central incisors.
   2. Median palatal suture (intermaxillary suture) (Figure 5-25):
      a. Radiolucent thin line between roots of central incisors, with thin lines of cortical bone on each side.
      b. Runs vertically from alveolar crest to hard palate.
   3. Nasal fossae (Figure 5-25):
      a. Centrally located air-filled spaces.
      b. Radiolucent oval shapes superior to central incisors, outlined by radiopaque bone.
   4. Nasal septum (Figure 5-25):
      a. Thin wall that divides two spaces, formed by ethmoid and vomer bones and cartilage.
      b. Centrally located radiopaque vertical strip that separates the nasal fossae.
   5. Anterior nasal spine (Figure 5-25):
      a. Pointed projection of bone anterior and inferior to nasal cavity, between central incisors.
      b. Radiopaque triangular shape at median palatal suture where nasal septum and fossae meet.
   6. Maxillary sinus (Figure 5-26):
      a. Hollow spaces in bone superior to molar and premolar apices.
      b. Large, oval radiolucent areas (multilocular structure) outlined with thin lines of cortical bone.

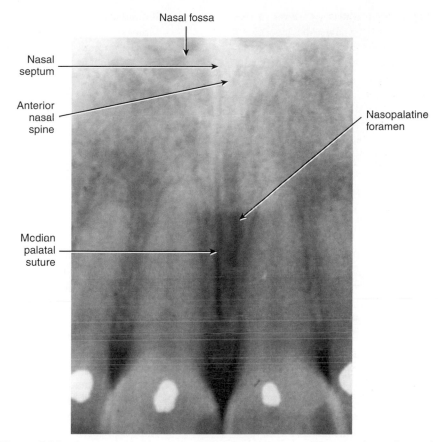

Nasal fossa

Nasal
septum

Anterior
nasal
spine

Nasopalatine
foramen

Mcdian
palatal
suture

Figure 5-25   Anatomical structures commonly seen on maxillary anterior radiographs.

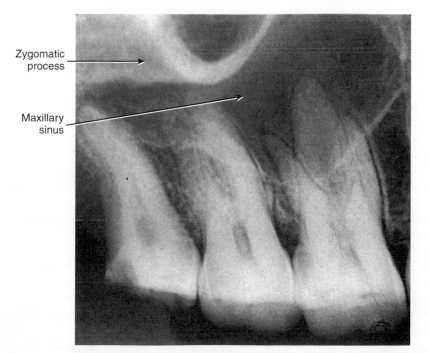

Zygomatic
process

Maxillary
sinus

Figure 5-26   Maxillary sinus and zygomatic process commonly appear on maxillary posterior radiographs.

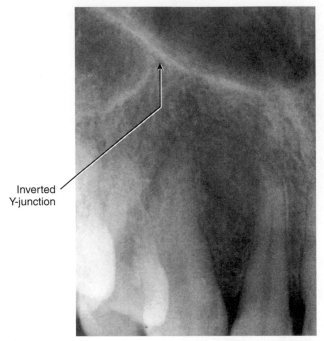

Figure 5-27   Inverted Y-junction is the meeting point of the nasal fossa and maxillary sinus.

7. Inverted Y-junction of two anatomical landmarks (Figure 5-27) (Let's all go to the YMCA!)
    a. Point where nasal fossa and maxillary sinus meet.
    b. Two oval radiolucent areas outlined by thin line of cortical bone, superior to canine apices.
8. Maxillary tuberosity (Figure 5-28):
    a. MOST distal portion of alveolar process.
    b. Rounded, radiopaque elevation distal to third molar region.
9. Hamulus (Figure 5-29):
    a. Extension of medial pterygoid plate of sphenoid bone.
    b. Radiopaque, hooklike protrusion posterior to maxillary tuberosity.
10. Zygomatic process (Figure 5-26):
    a. Together with zygomatic bone forms zygomatic arch.
    b. Starts as U-shaped band superior to molar apices, extends posteriorly continuing as a radiopaque band.
11. Coronoid process of mandible (Figure 5-28):
    a. Anterior portion of ramus.
    b. Radiopaque triangular projection, usually superimposed over maxillary tuberosity.
C. Mandibular films have eight common intraoral landmarks:
    1. Genial tubercles (Figure 5-30):
        a. Four bony spines used for muscle attachment for genioglossus and geniohyoid muscles.

b. Circular radiopacities inferior to central incisor apices.
2. Lingual foramen (Figure 5-30):
    a. Exit for incisive vessel branches.
    b. Radiolucent circle inside opaque genial tubercles.
3. Mental ridge (Figure 5-31):
    a. Ridge of bone located on anterior surface of mandible.
    b. Bilateral radiopaque lines, starting inferior to premolar apices, extending anterior to midline.
4. Mental foramen (Figure 5-32):
    a. Opening for mental nerve and vessels inferior to premolar apices.
    b. Round radiolucent area that can be mistaken for periapical disease or condition.
5. External oblique line (ridge) (Figure 5-33):
    a. Raised superior linear area of bone on external surface of mandible.
    b. Radiopaque line running anterior from ramus across molars.
6. Internal oblique (mylohyoid) line (ridge) (Figure 5-33):
    a. Raised inferior linear area of bone on internal surface of mandible.
    b. Radiopaque line running anterior along the premolar and molar apices, from anterior part of ramus to anterior part of alveolar process.
7. Mandibular canal (Figure 5-34):
    a. Canal for incisive and then inferior alveolar nerves and vessels; its posterior opening is the mandibular foramen (NOT visible on radiographs), and its anterior opening is the mental foramen (visible).
    b. Radiolucent band; outlined with a thin line of cortical bone inferior to premolar and molar apices.
8. Submandibular fossa (Figure 5-34):
    a. Thin, depressed area of bone on internal surface of mandible that contains submandibular salivary gland.
    b. Radiolucent band inferior to internal oblique (mylohyoid) line (ridge) and premolar and molar apices.
9. Nutrient canals: parallel radiolucent bands between the teeth; may be mistaken for bone fractures.

RADIOGRAPHIC INTERPRETATION

Radiographic interpretation involves the explanation and clarification of what is seen on dental radiograph. Teeth appear lighter (see earlier discussion) than MOST pathological conditions because LESS radiation penetrates them to reach the film; dental caries and other pathological conditions, such as changes in the bone density and the periodontal ligament, appear darker because x-rays readily penetrate these LESS dense structures.

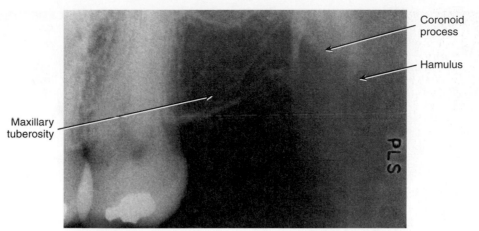

Coronoid
process

Hamulus

Maxillary
tuberosity

PLS

Figure 5-28   Coronoid process appears superimposed over the maxillary tuberosity.

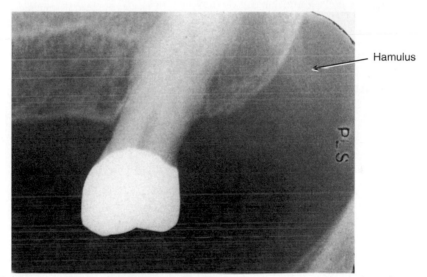

Hamulus

PLS

Figure 5-29   Hamulus is a radiopaque protrusion posterior to the maxillary tuberosity.

- See Chapters 6, General and Oral Pathology: diagnostic procedure, developmental presentations; 11, Clinical Treatment: diagnosis of caries; 13, Periodontology: diagnosis of periodontal disease; 15, Dental Biomaterials: restorations.

A. Dental caries: loss of tooth structure caused by acid by way of diet or microorganisms; radiolucent. Only about 50% to 75% sensitive on detection, NOT "gold standard"; MUST be accompanied by clinical detection.

  1. Interproximal caries located on mesial and distal surfaces (Figure 5-35):
     a. May progress from incipient to advanced, depending on length of time.
     b. Radiolucencies that advance as caries becomes larger.

  2. Occlusal caries: located on biting surfaces of posterior teeth:

     a. Radiolucent shadows under enamel as progression occurs.
     b. NOT apparent on radiographs until large.
     c. MORE effectively diagnosed by clinical examination.

  3. Root surface caries: exposed roots, preceded by bone loss and gingival recession; increased levels in older adults (Figure 5-36):
     a. Ditched-out radiolucent area or dot on the root.
     b. NOT apparent on radiographs until large.
     c. MORE effectively diagnosed by clinical examination.

B. Restorations and associated materials:

  1. CANNOT determine if material used is gold, silver, or metal alloy (amalgam); can be determined ONLY by size and contour of restoration.

  2. CANNOT determine surface of the tooth the restoration is on; image of one can be superimposed on

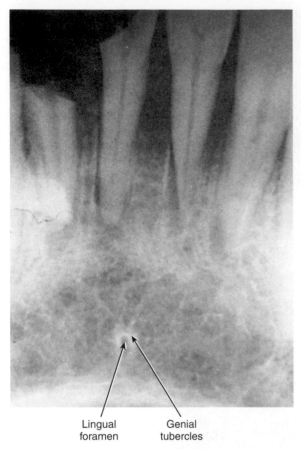

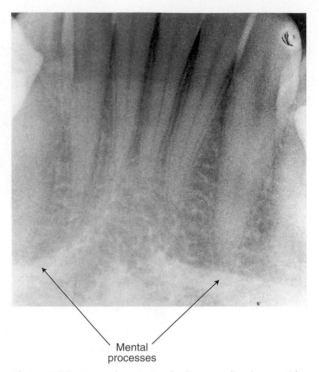

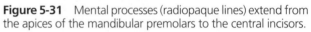

Mental
processes

Figure 5-31 Mental processes (radiopaque lines) extend from
the apices of the mandibular premolars to the central incisors.

Lingual   Genial
foramen   tubercles

Figure 5-30 Lingual foramen (radiolucent) is surrounded
by the genial tubercles (radiopaque).

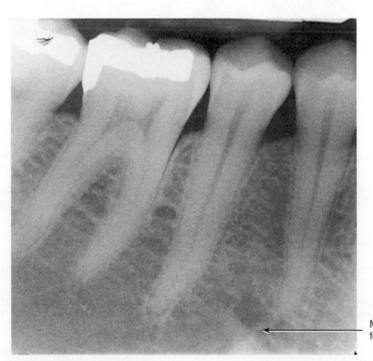

Mental
foramen

Figure 5-32 Mental foramen, located inferior to mandibular premolar apices, may be mistaken for
periapical pathological condition.

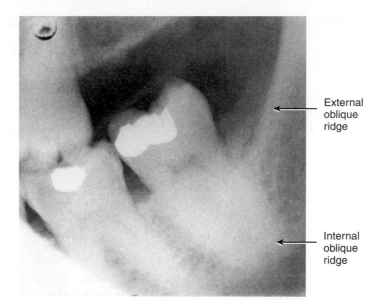

Figure 5-33   Internal and external oblique ridges are radiopaque structures that run from the ramus through the molar region (external) or to the anterior region (internal).

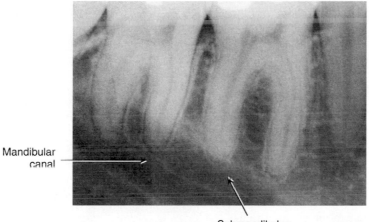

Figure 5-34   Mandibular canal and submandibular fossa are located inferior to apices of the mandibular molars and premolars.

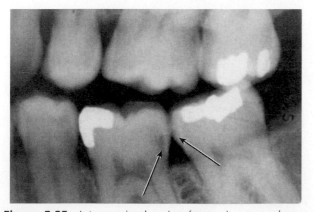

Figure 5-35   Interproximal caries *(arrows)* commonly appears as radiolucencies at the contact areas between adjacent teeth.

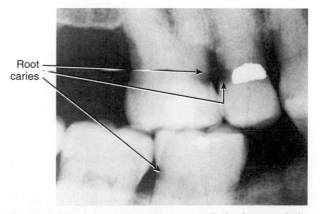

Figure 5-36   Root caries appears as ditched-out radiolucent areas located at the cervical third of the exposed root surface.

another restoration, giving appearance of ONLY one instead of two.

3. May appear lighter (radiopaque) or darker (radiolucent) depending on density of material.
   a. Radiopaque (lighter):
      (1) Retention pins appear as short rods near larger radiopaque casting restorations of gold, silver, or alloy (amalgam).
      (2) Whereas first-generation tooth-colored (composite) restorations were radiolucent, second-generation materials feature high level of radiopaque fillers.
      (3) Some restorative cements can be differentiated ONLY by location and degree of radiopacity; these include zinc phosphate, ZOE, calcium hydroxide cements.
      (4) Amalgam tattoo results from amalgam particles embedded into tissues during restorative procedures.
      (5) Gutta-percha and silver pins appear as rods within pulp canals.
      (6) Implant(s) with varying degrees of surrounding osteointegration opacity depending on length of time of placement in jaws (Figure 5-37).
   b. Radiolucent (darker):
      (1) Glass ionomers appear MORE radiolucent than surrounding teeth.
      (2) Porcelain, acrylic resins, sealants, older composites.

4. Distinguishing cement-retained single-unit implant restoration from natural tooth is often difficult without accompanying radiograph.

C. Torus (plural, tori): slow-growing bone mass on mandibular alveolar process, unilateral or bilateral radiopacity superimposed superior to or inferior to apices on mandible on PAs; palatal, central radiopacity on occlusal films of palate.

D. Periodontal disease: affects periodontium (supporting structures of teeth) (Figure 5-38).
   1. Gingivitis: inflammation that affects marginal gingiva.
      a. NOT apparent on radiographs.
      b. Diagnosed ONLY by clinical examination.
   2. Periodontitis (chronic): inflammation that involves alveolar bone loss.
      a. Appears as radiolucency (but ONLY in two dimensions):
         (1) FIRST noted as fuzzy or ditched-out area where destruction of cortical alveolar crest of bone occurs.
         (2) In MORE advanced stages as horizontal or vertical bone loss (Figure 5-39):
            (a) Horizontal bone loss appears radiographically *parallel* to CEJ of adjacent teeth.

(b) Vertical bone loss appears along one side of a tooth in *angular* form; NOT parallel to CEJ of adjacent teeth.
            (3) Bone loss is NOT the only diagnostic factor; also evaluated are calculus, overhanging margins of restorations, caries, root resorption, as well as periapical and pathological lesions.
      b. Radiographic appearance is NOT the only diagnostic factor; clinical examination is also used for diagnosis:
         (1) Does NOT show loss on facial and lingual places, ONLY on interproximal alveolar crest.
         (2) When becomes apparent, as much as 20% of bone may have already been lost.

E. Traumatic lesions, injuries caused by external forces:
   1. Occlusal forces:
      a. Trauma: widening of radiolucent PDL space surrounding root, outlined by radiopaque lamina

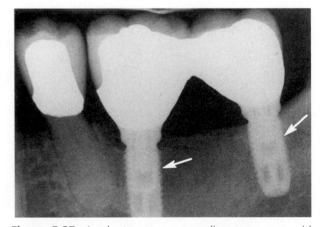

Figure 5-37 Implants appear as radiopaque areas with varying degrees of osseous integration opacity *(arrows)*. (From Bath-Balogh M, Fehrenbach MJ: Illustrated dental embryology and anatomy, ed 2, St. Louis, 2006, Saunders/Elsevier.)

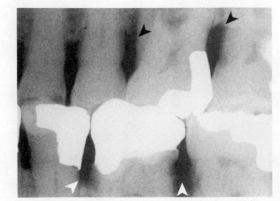

Figure 5-38 Periodontal disease is typified on radiographs by fuzzy appearance of alveolar crest bone; arrows indicate areas of advanced bone loss.

dura, possibly excess opaque cementum at apex of root(s) (hypercementosis).

   b. Lack of occlusal contact: narrowed radiolucent PDL space (may also have extrusion or hyper-eruption).

2. Tooth fractures:
   a. Crown fracture usually involves anteriors and results from fall or blows to face or mouth; space from missing structure appears radiolucent on radiograph.
   b. Root fracture occurs MOST frequently in anteriors; appears as radiolucent horizontal line on root.

3. Resorption: loss of tooth structure with NO resultant clinical recognition; either internal or external:
   a. External resorption, which starts FIRST on the root surface with loss and a flat rather than conical appearance radiographically; bone and lamina dura appear normal; can result from orthodontic therapy when teeth have been moved TOO rapidly (Figure 5-40).
   b. Internal resorption, which appears as asymptomatic radiolucency; results from trauma or pulp capping; begins in pulp and travels into dentin.

4. Enamel pearl: round, radiopaque calcifications MOST commonly seen externally on multirooted teeth in furcation area or at CEJ.

5. Cementicle: round, radiopaque calcifications on the root surface within the PDL space.

6. Extraction: radiolucent space in bone that fills in with time.

7. Avulsion: complete accidental removal of the tooth from the bone; radiolucent space in bone.

F. Pulpal lesions: commonly seen on radiographs:
   1. Pulp stones: round, radiopaque calcifications MOST commonly seen in molars (Figure 5-41).
   2. Pulp erasure: disappearance of usually radiolucent canal because of cavity trauma caused by caries, abrasion, or abnormal forces; appears radiopaque because of secondary dentin.
   3. Periapical lesions: usually located around apex but can be at ANY point around root because of lateral canals; ONLY a late finding on radiograph; clinical examination used to detect early lesions.
      a. Periapical abscess: radiolucent area located at end of apex of symptomatic tooth with infected pulp; appears as widening of PDL space and obliteration of lamina dura.
      b. Periapical granuloma: radiolucent area at the apex of nonvital, usually asymptomatic tooth (caused by pulp death or necrosis).
      c. Periodontal abscess: radiolucent area located at end or lateral part of root; may be result of

instrumentation and debris that irritate sulcus area, something left in sulcus after initial periodontal scaling, or primary tooth's root portion left after shedding.

   d. Condensing osteitis (chronic focal sclerosing osteomyelitis): radiopaque area attached to apex of a nonvital tooth with a low-grade infection (Figure 5-42).
   e. Sclerotic bone (osteosclerosis): radiopaque, defined area around apices of asymptomatic, noncarious, nonvital tooth; MOST likely associated with inflammation (Figure 5-43).

G. Malignancy (cancer): destructive radiolucency usually centrally in mandible (molar or premolar), occasionally apex of tooth.

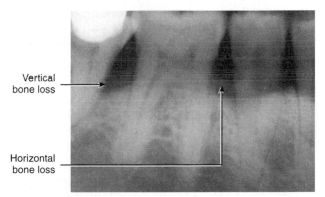
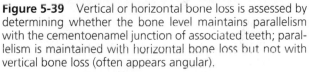

Vertical bone loss

Horizontal bone loss

Figure 5-39 Vertical or horizontal bone loss is assessed by determining whether the bone level maintains parallelism with the cementoenamel junction of associated teeth; parallelism is maintained with horizontal bone loss but not with vertical bone loss (often appears angular).

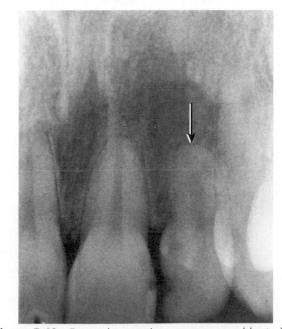

Figure 5-40 External resorption appears as a blunted or flat appearance of the apices.

Pulp stones

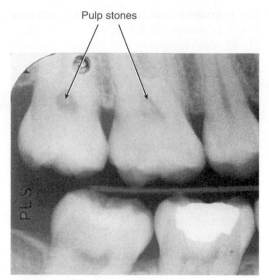

Figure 5-41 Pulp stone calcifications in the pulps of molars.

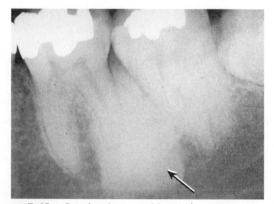

Figure 5-42 Condensing osteitis at the root apex of a nonvital tooth.

1. **Diffuse** "moth-eaten," "ratty"; NO corticated outline; adjacent teeth being displaced, loosened, and/or absorbed; certain breast and prostate metastases may be radiopaque owing to osteogenic qualities of tumor, with areas of bone production and sclerosis.
2. Primary: squamous cell carcinoma; secondary: from breast, bronchus, prostate, kidney, or thyroid cancers metastasized to jaws.

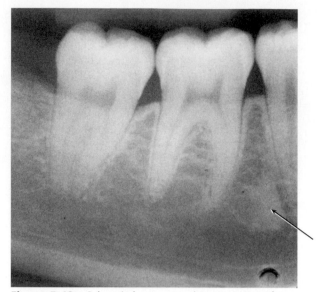

Figure 5-43 Sclerotic bone near the root apex of asymptomatic vital tooth.

3. CANNOT determine whether it is a primary or secondary tumor from radiographic presentation alone.
H. Other pathological lesions with radiographic presentations (see also Chapter 6, General and Oral Pathology):
1. Ameloblastoma: aggressive benign tumor with **multilocular** radiolucent bone destruction having "soap bubble" appearance.
2. Cherubism (familial fibrous dysplasis): disorder with bilateral, symmetrical, well-defined, well-corticated multilocular radiolucency in posterior mandible and displacement of teeth.
3. Fibrous dysplasia: disorder with **unilocular** or multilocular radiolucency having "ground glass" appearance because of the many C-shaped trabeculae.
4. Multiple myeloma: cancer that on a skull radiograph shows radiolucent "punched-out" lesions.
5. Osteoradionecrosis: postradiation complication that shows wide spectrum of presentations from normal to osteolysis (dissolution or degeneration of bone tissue); does NOT always correlate with severity or detect presence.
6. Paget's disease: disorder with an enlarged maxilla, overall loss of lamina dura, "cotton-wool" appearance of bone, patchy opacities.

CLINICAL STUDY

Age	32 YRS	SCENARIO
Sex	☐ Male ☒ Female	The patient recently had her orthodontic bands removed. Visual intraoral examination reveals a large restoration on tooth #30, recession on the right side of her mouth, and no apparent caries or other restorations. During examination of her past radiographs, well-defined radiopacity is seen apical to tooth #30. Also, the apices of teeth #27 and #28 appear blunted and roots appear shorter than normal.
Height	5'2"	
Weight	130 LBS	
BP	119/78	
Chief Complaint	"My lower right back teeth are sensitive when I eat."	
Medical History	Second month of pregnancy No complications except morning sickness	
Current Medications	Folic acid and prenatal vitamins qd	
Social History	Stay at home mom with twin 4-year-old boys	

1. What is (are) the most likely reason(s) for the patient's sensitive teeth? What homecare recommendations can be made?
2. Given the patient's history, what types of radiographs are recommended?
3. What is the radiopacity noted with #30, and how does it relate to her sensitivity?
4. What does the condition noted with #27 and #28 most likely indicate?

1. The patient's sensitivity may be caused by gingival recession, recent removal of orthodontic bands, or erosion associated with morning sickness. Further information must be gathered to determine cause. Because patient did not present clinically with caries and has only one restoration, the best approach is to provide oral hygiene instructions on toothbrushing technique (modified Stillman's method) to reduce incidence of recession and encourage use of mineralizing fluoride and calcium products (for sensitivity). She should be examined in 1 month to evaluate effectiveness of homecare procedures in reducing sensitivity.
2. Because the patient is pregnant and has no obvious signs of decay, radiographs can be postponed until after pregnancy unless sensitivity does not abate after practice of homecare recommendations. Although use of a lead apron or lead equivalent with a thyroid collar reduces chance of radiation reaching developing fetus, most dental practitioners prefer to take only those radiographs that are believed to be absolutely necessary to the safety and health of the pregnant patient. If the tooth discomfort continues at the 1-month visit, specific areas of sensitivity must be identified and appropriate radiographs must be exposed.
3. Radiopaque area most likely indicates condensing osteitis (chronic focal sclerosing osteomyelitis), which results from a low-grade infection or mild irritation. Tooth is most likely nonvital; teeth that contain large restorations are the most frequently affected. Condensing osteitis most commonly occurs in mandibular first molars in adults. Because this condition is asymptomatic, no treatment is necessary. Pulp testing is also indicated.
4. This most likely indicates external resorption of apices of teeth #27 and #28 from mechanical forces placed on them by orthodontic movement. This type of resorption does not have any signs or symptoms and cannot be detected clinically. No treatment for external resorption is needed.

Review Questions

1 Which one of the following energies in the electromagnetic spectrum is considered ionizing radiation?
   A. Radar rays
   B. Radio waves
   C. Infrared rays
   D. Gamma rays
2 What is the source of electrons used for x-ray production?
   A. Tungsten filament
   B. Molybdenum cup
   C. Tungsten target
   D. Copper stem
3 What part of the circuit provides the energy to propel the electrons and produce x-rays?
   A. Filament circuit
   B. High-voltage circuit
   C. Step-down transformer
   D. Milliampere

4 Where does the generation of x-rays in the x-ray tube actually occur?
A. Tungsten filament
B. Focusing cup
C. Copper stem
D. Tungsten target

5 When x-rays interact with an outer shell electron of an atom, causing ionization and scattering in a different direction, it is called
A. the photoelectric effect.
B. Thompson scatter.
C. Compton scatter.
D. no interaction.

6 Which theory BEST describes the free radical formation that is so injurious to living tissue?
A. Direct theory
B. Indirect theory
C. Dose-response curve
D. Buccal object rule

7 What unit of radiation represents the amount of radiation energy absorbed by the tissue?
A. Roentgen
B. Sievert
C. Dose rate
D. Gray

8 What factor is MOST important in a consideration of the biological effects of radiation used in dentistry?
A. Whole-body exposure
B. Limited area exposure
C. Acute exposure (limited area)
D. Latent period

9 Which one of the following cell types is MOST sensitive to radiation?
A. Highly specialized cells
B. Mature cells
C. Slowly dividing cells
D. Immature cells

10 All of the following reduce patient exposure to radiation, EXCEPT one. Which one is the EXCEPTION?
A. Filtration
B. Collimation
C. Positioning
D. Lead apron

11 Which one of the following reduces operator exposure to radiation?
A. Fast film
B. Distance
C. PID
D. Film-holding device

12 Which radiographic technique has LESS distortion and magnification and creates a MORE accurate image on film?
A. Bisecting-angle
B. Occlusal
C. Paralleling
D. Panoramic

13 Which one of these extraoral techniques is used specifically to evaluate the maxillary sinuses?
A. Waters
B. Lateral cephalometric
C. Panoramic
D. Lateral jaw

14 Which one of the following is used to restrict the size of the x-ray beam?
A. Filtration
B. Collimation
C. Film-holding device
D. Fast film

15 If the source-to-film distance is changed from 8 to 24 inches, the intensity of the beam becomes
A. three times as intense.
B. nine times as intense.
C. one-ninth as intense.
D. one-third as intense.

16 Magnification occurs when there is a
A. long object-film distance.
B. small focal spot.
C. parallel object and film.
D. short target-film distance.

17 Which one of these film-processing ingredients converts energized crystals into metallic silver?
A. Sodium carbonate
B. Sodium thiosulfate
C. Potassium alum
D. Hydroquinone

18 What is the processing order that films undergo in an automatic film processor?
A. Water, developer, water, fixer, dry
B. Developer, water, fixer, dry
C. Developer, fixer, water, dry
D. Developer, water, fixer, water, dry

19 Which of the following is LEAST likely to cause fogged film?
A. Improper safelighting
B. Developer spots
C. Outdated film
D. Light leakage

20 Which radiopaque maxillary anatomical landmark is MOST likely to be seen on a maxillary incisor periapical radiograph?
A. Nasal septum
B. Median palatal suture
C. Zygomatic process
D. Genial tubercles

21 Which radiolucent mandibular anatomical landmark is MOST likely to be seen on a mandibular molar periapical radiograph?
A. Lingual foramen
B. External oblique line
C. Submandibular fossa
D. Mental foramen

22 Which is the FIRST step in the radiograph mounting process?
A. Organizing films by anatomical area
B. Separating maxillary from mandibular films
C. Placing films dot-side up
D. Mounting premolar films first

23 Root caries of a tooth is
A. typically located at the middle third of the root.
B. identified as well-circumscribed radiopacity.
C. associated with bone loss and gingival recession.
D. found more often in adolescents.

24 If partially formed third molars are noted on a panoramic radiograph, how old is the patient?
A. 6 to 10 years of age
B. 11 to 15 years of age
C. 16 to 20 years of age
D. 21 to 25 years of age

25 Overlap on a left molar bitewing radiograph is caused by improper
A. exposure time.
B. horizontal angulation.
C. film placement.
D. patient movement.

26 When placed backward, a film exposed in the mouth will exhibit
A. fogginess.
B. no image.
C. waffle pattern.
D. cone cut.

27 A patient of record complains of temperature sensitivity in the maxillary right second molar region of the mouth. A full-mouth series of radiographs was taken 2 years previously. Which radiographs should be prescribed?
A. Panoramic
B. Horizontal bitewings
C. Vertical bitewing
D. Periapical

28 The "coin test" is a method of assessing
A. film freshness.
B. proper kVp settings.
C. contamination by developer.
D. proper safelighting.

29 If films were properly exposed at 6 mA for 4 seconds, films exposed for 3 seconds would have an mA of
A. 2.
B. 8.
C. 16.
D. 24.

30 Which of the following situations created the error of a radiolucent shadow that obscures the apices of the maxillary dentition on a panoramic film?
A. Lips were not closed.
B. Midsagittal plane was not perpendicular to the floor.
C. Tongue was not touching the palate.
D. Teeth were not in the focal trough.

31 If the x-ray machine is operating at 70 kVp, what thickness of filtration is necessary?
A. 1.5 mm
B. 2.0 mm
C. 2.5 mm
D. 3.0 mm

32 The lead diaphragm in the tubehead is referred to as the
A. target.
B. filament.
C. filter.
D. collimator.

33 Developing solution splashed on the film before processing will result in
A. white spots.
B. dark spots.
C. brown stain.
D. yellow stain.

34 Which of the following situations increases penumbra?
A. Increased object-to-film distance
B. Reduced focal spot size
C. Faster-speed film
D. Movement of film

35 The lingual foramen should be evident on the
A. maxillary posterior film.
B. maxillary anterior film.
C. mandibular posterior film.
D. mandibular anterior film.

36 On a mandibular molar film the MOST superior radiopaque anatomical landmark is the
A. external oblique ridge.
B. coronoid process.
C. internal oblique line.
D. mental process.

37 Exposure of a radiograph for ⅗ of a second is equal to how many impulses?
A. 3
B. 15
C. 22
D. 36

38 A white area with a right-angle-shaped border on a film is caused by
A. rectangular PID.
B. cylindrical PID.
C. fixer cutoff.
D. developer cutoff.

39 What is the inverted Y-junction in a radiograph?
A. Triangular shape at median palatal suture where nasal septum and fossa meet
B. Rounded, radiopaque elevation distal to the third molar region
C. Radiopaque, hooklike protrusion posterior to the maxillary tuberosity
D. Point where the nasal fossa and maxillary sinus meet

40 Which of the following diseases has a "ground glass" appearance on radiographs?
A. Osteoradionecrosis
B. Multiple myeloma
C. Fibrous dysplasia
D. Cherubism

41 Root fracture occurs MOST frequently in the anterior portion of the mouth. Root fracture appears as a radiopaque horizontal line on the root.
A. Both statements are true.
B. Both statements are false.
C. The first statement is true, the second is false.
D. The first statement is false, the second is true.

42 Film duplication is the process of copying or reproducing a second film or set of films. With film duplication, there is no need to reexpose the patient to radiation.
A. Both statements are true.
B. Both statements are false.
C. The first statement is true, the second is false.
D. The first statement is false, the second is true.

43 Contrast is the difference between lighter and darker shades (grays) on the radiograph. Decreased kVp (90 or higher) results in many shades of gray on the film.
   A. Both statements are true.
   B. Both statements are false.
   C. The first statement is true, the second is false.
   D. The first statement is false, the second is true.

44 Optimum developing takes approximately 10 minutes at 50° F. Developing reduces exposed silver halide crystals into black metallic silver through one ingredient in solution.
   A. Both statements are true.
   B. Both statements are false.
   C. The first statement is true, the second is false.
   D. The first statement is false, the second is true.

45 The bitewing view visualizes crowns, contacts, and height of alveolar bone. The bitewing view is not included in a full-mouth series.
   A. Both statements are true.
   B. Both statements are false.
   C. The first statement is true, the second is false.
   D. The first statement is false, the second is true.

46 Overdeveloped film that is too dark may occur because developing solution is at too high a temperature.
   A. Both the statement and reason are correct and related.
   B. Both the statement and reason are correct but NOT related.
   C. The statement is correct, but the reason is NOT.
   D. The statement is NOT correct, but the reason is correct.
   E. NEITHER the statement NOR the reason is correct.

47 Fogged films with white streaks may occur because there is improper safelighting in the darkroom.
   A. Both the statement and reason are correct and related.
   B. Both the statement and reason are correct but NOT related.
   C. The statement is correct, but the reason is NOT.
   D. The statement is NOT correct, but the reason is correct.
   E. NEITHER the statement NOR the reason is correct.

48 Genial tubercles are an exit for incisive vessel branches. Genial tubercles appear as radiolucent circle inside opaque lingual foramen tubercles.
   A. Both statements are true.
   B. Both statements are false.
   C. The first statement is true, the second is false.
   D. The first statement is false, the second is true.

49 Lateral cephalometric projection evaluates
   A. posterior portion of mandible only.
   B. lateral areas of mandible that are too large for periapical film.
   C. trauma and facial growth and development.
   D. frontal and ethmoidal sinuses only.

50 Compton scatter
   A. is ionization that occurs when x-ray photon interacts with an inner shell electron.
   B. occurs when electron is ejected and x-ray photon scatters in a different direction.
   C. is responsible for approximately 10% of all scatter in dental x-rays.
   D. is a result without any occurrence of ionization.

Answer Key and Rationales

1 (D) Gamma rays are ionizing forms of radiation in electromagnetic spectrum. Radar rays and infrared rays are NOT high-energy forms of radiation and thus do NOT cause ionization. Radio waves have long wavelengths and therefore CANNOT cause ionization.

2 (A) Heating tungsten filament is necessary to provide a source of electrons for generation of x-rays. Molybdenum cup directs the electrons to the tungsten target in the anode. Tungsten target is the spot in anode that electrons hit to produce x-rays. Copper stem in the anode dissipates the heat that is produced.

3 (B) High-voltage circuit provides the voltage necessary to propel electrons to the anode. Filament circuit controls the heating of the filament and quantity of available electrons. Step-down transformer is necessary to decrease incoming voltage to heat the filament. Milliampere is $\frac{1}{1000}$ of an ampere and determines quantity of electrons produced.

4 (D) Electrons hit tungsten target and convert kinetic energy into heat and x-rays. Tungsten filament has to be heated to provide electrons for x-ray production. Focusing cup in cathode surrounds filament and directs electrons to target. Target is embedded in copper stem, helping keep target cool.

5 (C) Compton scatter occurs when an outer shell electron is removed and scatters in a different direction. Photoelectric effect occurs when an inner shell electron is removed and is absorbed so that it ceases to exist. Coherent or Thompson scatter occurs when an outer shell electron scatters in a different direction but no ionization takes place. No interaction occurs when x-rays pass through the atoms of tissue but NEVER react with them.

6 (B) Indirect theory explains tissue damage by positing that x-ray photons are absorbed into cells, causing the production of free radicals (toxins); this damage is believed to be caused by the water content in cells. Direct theory explains damage as occurring from direct hit to the target within a cell; this damage seldom occurs. Dose-response curve graphically demonstrates that any level of radiation exposure causes a response from the tissue. Buccal object (SLOB) rule is whether artifact or object is lingual or buccal: in second radiograph, if central ray is moved and object moves in same direction, then object is lingual, if it moves in the opposite direction, buccal.

7 (D) Gray is (SI) unit that represents amount of energy absorbed by tissue. Roentgen is standard unit for measuring the quantity of ionization in air. Sievert is SI unit for dose equivalent and is used to compare different types of radiation. Dose rate is amount of radiation absorbed per unit of time.

8 **(B)** Limited area exposure refers to radiation in small area, such as occurs in dental radiation. Whole-body exposure is MORE extensive but is NOT used in dentistry. Acute exposure (limited area) refers to exposure to high doses of radiation in a specific area. Latent period is the time between exposure and the observable effect.

9 **(D)** Immature cells divide rapidly and therefore are the MOST sensitive to radiation. Highly specialized cells are MORE radioresistant to radiation. Mature cells do NOT change; because they are MORE specialized in function, they are LESS sensitive to radiation. Cells that divide at a slow rate have LESS cell activity and LESS reaction to radiation.

10 **(C)** Positioning patient reduces risk of exposure to operator but NOT to patient. Filtration reduces radiation by filtering out the nonproductive x-rays. Collimation reduces radiation exposure by restricting size of the beam directed at the patient's face. Lead apron or equivalent protects patient from unnecessary nonproductive scatter radiation.

11 **(B)** Distance of at least 6 feet from the primary beam is essential for reducing operator exposure. Faster film reduces exposure to the patient. The position-indicating device (PID) should be lead lined and rectangular to reduce patient exposure. Film-holding devices reduce exposure to the patient's hand.

12 **(C)** Paralleling technique is BEST and provides a MORE accurate image because the primary beam is at right angles to the tooth and the film. Bisecting (angle) technique is NOT as accurate because the use of bisecting line allows MORE errors. Occlusal technique results in a large amount of distortion, which is caused by the dramatic angles used and the need for greater coverage. Panoramic technique leads to greater distortion because the need for a larger survey leads to blurred images outside the focal trough.

13 **(A)** Waters projection specifically shows maxillary sinus area. Lateral cephalometric technique shows trauma, facial growth, and development. Panoramic projection is used to evaluate impactions, diseases, growths of the jaw. Lateral jaw exposure shows posterior part of the mandible and is used for patients who are unable to open their mouths.

14 **(B)** Collimation is a lead diaphragm that restricts size of the x-ray beam directed at the patient's face to 2.75 inches. Filtration uses aluminum disc to filter out the nonproductive, longer wavelengths from primary beam. Film-holding device is used to hold the film in place but does NOT restrict the size of the primary beam. Fast film (F-speed film is fastest) reduces radiation exposure to the patient but does NOT restrict the size of the beam.

15 **(C)** According to the inverse square law, intensity decreases as distance from the source increases; this would be adding the same amount of distance each time when it really should be squared. Intensity of the beam does NOT increase as this suggests, but decreases; because distance is three times the original, intensity CANNOT be one-third the original.

16 **(A)** Increased target-film distance allows MORE parallel rays to hit the film; thus less magnification occurs. Small focal spot size in the x-ray tube increases sharpness. If the object and film are parallel to each other, distortion is decreased. Short target-film distance increases magnification because fewer parallel rays hit the film.

17 **(D)** Hydroquinone (or elon) in developing solution converts energized crystals into metallic silver. Sodium carbonate softens emulsion and speeds up action of developing agents. Sodium thiosulfate, in fixer solution, clears unexposed silver halide crystals from the emulsion. Potassium alum, in fixer, shrinks and hardens emulsion.

18 **(C)** Processing order in which films go through the automatic processor is "developer-fixer-water-dry." In automatic processing, a reduced number of water baths and the addition of hardeners in the developer and fixer solutions allow film emulsion to remain firm throughout the automated procedure. Film exposed to too much moisture will become soft and prone to stick to the machine roller. In manual processing, water baths between developing and fixing are necessary and film softness is NOT an issue because the chemical concentrations and temperatures used are NOT as high as those used in automatic processing.

19 **(B)** Developer spots occur when the developing solution contacts the film before processing procedures begin. Proper safelighting is necessary. safelights (direct illumination) MUST be spaced at least 4 feet from working surface with low-wattage bulb (7½/15 watts). The expiration date on the film SHOULD be checked, and the film SHOULD be stored in a cool, dry environment. Because film is sensitive to white light, the darkroom should be "white-light tight."

20 **(B)** The nasal septum is a vertical opaque strip that separates the nasal fossae. The median palatine suture is a thin radiolucent line between the maxillary central incisors. The zygomatic process is a radiopaque U-shaped band located superior to the apices of the maxillary molars. Genial tubercles are four radiolucent bony spines located inferior to the apices of the mandibular central incisors.

21 **(C)** Submandibular fossa is a radiolucent band that runs inferior to mylohyoid and apices of molars. Lingual foramen is a radiolucent circle inside the genial tubercles, inferior to apices of mandibular central incisors. External oblique line is a radiopaque line that runs anterior from ramus across mandibular molars. Mental foramen is a radiolucent oval inferior to apices of premolars.

22 **(C)** Films should be placed dot-side up on a lighted viewbox first. Next, films should be organized by anatomical area, separated into maxillary and mandibular groups, and subsequently mounted in the appropriate area. Premolar films are mounted after the molar films are in place.

23 **(A)** Root caries is associated with bone loss and gingival recession, is located on exposed root surfaces (often in cervical areas), and is identified as a ditched-out radiolucency; found MORE often in older adults (who experience MORE root exposure and are at risk of medication-induced xerostomia).

24 **(B)** Partially formed third molars on a panoramic radiograph indicate that the patient is MOST likely to be 11 to 15 years old. Roots of third molars develop approximately 6 years before their expected eruption at age 18 to 21. Third molars may NOT be present in individuals 6 to 10 years old. Individuals 16 years and older should show well-formed third molars.

25 **(B)** Overlap on left molar bitewing radiograph is caused by improper horizontal angulation. Improper exposure time affects the darkness and lightness of film; poor film placement affects which teeth are exposed or how well film is centered; patient movement results in blurring.

26 **(C)** Film that is exposed when placed backward in the mouth will have a waffle or herringbone pattern. Fogginess is associated with old film; no image indicates lack of exposure; cone cut is associated with cone placement.

27 **(D)** For a patient of record with a specific complaint (temperature sensitivity in the maxillary right second molar region of the mouth) and a recent FMX, a periapical (PA) radiograph is the BEST choice. Temperature sensitivity is often associated with pulpal pathology, and PA provides coverage of the entire tooth structure and the bone surrounding the apex of the specific site. Panoramic film is NOT recommended because it may NOT provide the clarity required to detect pulpal pathological or other site-specific conditions and it requires exposure to greater amounts of radiation than a PA film. Horizontal and vertical bitewing films do NOT provide coverage of apices (root apex) and surrounding bone and thus are NOT as helpful.

28 **(D)** The "coin test" is a method of assessing improper safelighting caused by excessive bulb wattage, improper distance, or inadequate filtration. Film freshness is confirmed by the expiration date and by the absence of film fogginess. Proper kVp settings affect film quality as determined by the gray, black, white tones of a film. Contamination by developer solution is identified by dark spots on the film.

29 **(B)** Multiplying milliamperage and time gives total number of x-rays produced (mA × seconds = mAs). Total number of x-rays produced affects film density; therefore increase in one (mA/time) requires decrease in the other (time/mA) to maintain a similar density.

30 **(C)** Patient's tongue must be touching the palate or the resulting airspace will appear as a radiolucent line, obscuring apices of the anterior teeth. Open lips result in a radiolucent shadow that obscures anterior teeth. Improper midsagittal alignment results in unequal magnification of ramus and posterior teeth. Distortion of anterior teeth (wide and thin appearance) occurs if the teeth are outside the focal trough.

31 **(C)** According to federal and state regulations, filtration (thickness of aluminum) for machines operating below 70 kVp is 1.5 mm. Machines operating at 70 kVp and above are required to have filtration thickness of 2.5 mm.

32 **(D)** Collimator, located in tubehead, is a lead doughnut or diaphragm. Target refers to tungsten target in anode. Filament is the tungsten filament in the cathode. Filter refers to aluminum filter that is used to eliminate longer wavelengths from beam.

33 **(B)** Recontamination of film with developing solution results in an overdevelopment of the affected areas and causes dark spots. Recontamination with fixer solution clears film of silver halide in emulsion, resulting in white spots. Insufficient washing of films after fixing results in brown and yellow stains.

34 **(B)** Reducing the focal spot size increases penumbra (fuzziness, less sharpness); film movement and increase in the object-to-film distance or film speed decrease penumbra.

35 **(D)** Because the lingual foramen is located inferior to apices of the mandibular anterior incisors at the midline, it can be seen ONLY on mandibular anterior film.

36 **(A)** External oblique ridge is the MOST superior radiopaque anatomical landmark on mandibular molar film. Coronoid process appears ONLY on maxillary molar films. Internal oblique line is the inferior radiopaque landmark on a mandibular film, and the mental process is a radiopaque landmark located inferior to mandibular incisors.

37 **(D)** Converting seconds to impulses requires cross-multiplication. It is necessary to know that each impulse equals $\frac{1}{60}$ of a second (3/5 = x/60; 5x = 180; x = 36). Therefore $\frac{3}{5}$ of a second equals 36 impulses.

38 **(A)** Right-angle shape is the border of a rectangular PID. Circular border is caused by a cylindrical PID. Fixer cutoff has a straight black border, developer cutoff has a straight white border.

39 **(D)** Inverted Y-junction in a radiograph is a point where the nasal fossa and maxillary sinus meet. Rounded, radiopaque elevation distal to the third molar region is the retromolar pad. Radiopaque, hooklike protrusion posterior to the maxillary tuberosity is the hamulus, extension of medial pterygoid plate of the sphenoid bone. Anterior nasal spine is the triangular shape at the median palatal suture where nasal septum and fossa meet.

40 **(C)** Fibrous dysplasia shows unilocular or multilocular radiolucency with "ground glass" appearance caused by many trabeculae. Osteoradionecrosis demonstrates wide spectrum of presentations from normal to osteolysis. Skull radiograph of multiple myeloma shows "punched-out lesions." Cherubism shows well-defined, well-corticated, multilocular, radiolucent, bilateral, symmetrical lesions in posterior mandible.

41 **(C)** First statement is true, second is false. Root fracture occurs MOST frequently in anterior portion of mouth, appearing as radiolucent horizontal line on root.

42 **(A)** Both statements are true. Film duplication is process of copying or reproducing second film or set of films without reexposing patient to radiation.

43 **(C)** First statement is true, second is false. Contrast is the difference between lighter and darker shades (grays) on radiograph. Increased kVp (≥ 90) results in many shades of gray on the film.

44 **(B)** Both statements are false. Optimum developing takes approximately 5 minutes at 68° F. Developing reduces exposed silver halide crystals into black metallic silver through four ingredients in solution.

45 **(C)** First statement is true, second is false. Bitewing (BW) view visualizes crowns, contacts, and height of alveolar bone, included in a full-mouth series (FMX).

46 **(A)** Both statement and reason are correct and related. Overdeveloped film that is too dark may be caused by developing solution at too high a temperature. It could also be due to excessive development time.

47 **(D)** Statement is not correct, but reason is correct. Fogged films with a gray hue may occur because there is improper safelighting in the darkroom.

48 **(B)** Both statements are false. Genial tubercles are four bony spines used for muscle attachment. They appear as circular radiopacities inferior to apices of central incisors. Lingual foramen is an exit for incisive vessel branches and appears as radiolucent circle inside opaque genial tubercles.

49 **(C)** Lateral cephalometric projection is used to evaluate trauma and facial growth and development. Posteroanterior projection is used to evaluate frontal and ethmoidal sinuses, as well as orbits and nasal cavity. Lateral jaw exposure is used to evaluate posterior portion of the mandible or lateral areas that are too large for periapical film.

50 **(B)** Compton scatter is ionization that results when x-ray photon interacts with outer shell electron. Occurs when electron is ejected and x-ray photon scatters in a different direction. Responsible for approximately 62% of all scatter in dental x-rays. Thompson (coherent) scatter results without the occurrence of any ionization.

CHAPTER 6

General and Oral Pathology

PATHOLOGY

General pathology includes the study of the destruction and repair of bodily tissues. Oral pathology is the study of the destructive conditions associated with the mouth, head, neck. Can be either primary or secondary (follows and results from an earlier disease), or there can be comorbidity, with more than one pathological condition present. MOST conditions and diseases go through periods of exacerbation (relapse, attack, flare-up), with an increase in the severity of a disease or its symptoms, as well as periods of remission (absence of disease activity).

In many cases **etiology** (cause) of disease is unknown. **Pathogenesis** is the course of a disease or how it progresses. Even if etiology and pathogenesis are known, many conditions and diseases still can be treated ONLY by palliative methods, care concentrated on reducing severity of symptoms (see following discussion). Risk factors for NOT achieving oral health are listed so that the medically compromised patient will receive correct dental hygiene care.

- See CD-ROM for Chapter Terms and WebLinks.
- See Chapters 9, Pharmacology: specific usage; 10, Medical and Dental Emergencies: emergencies in the dental setting; 11, Clinical Treatment, and 16, Special Needs Patient Care: related medical disabilities.

INJURY, INFLAMMATION, AND REPAIR

Disease causes various injuries to the body. ALL diseases include processes of inflammation and repair. Inflammation is always FIRST response to injury; it can be BOTH protective and destructive process. Repair occurs in response to inflammation; involves BOTH regenerative and reparative processes.

A. Injury can have various causes:
  1. **Hypoxia** (lack of oxygen): from chemical, physical, or microbial agents, e.g., heart attack (myocardial infarction).
  2. Immunological factors: such as anaphylactic reactions and reactions to self-antigens, e.g., asthma.
  3. Genetic defects: result in pathological changes, e.g., sickle cell anemia.
  4. Nutritional imbalances: including lack of sufficient proteins or other nutrients and dietary excesses, e.g., high intake of animal fats.
  5. Mechanisms of injury:
    a. Type, duration, severity of injury.
    b. Type of cell injured; different types of cells have variable responses to injury.
    c. Biochemical considerations, including integrity of cell membranes, adenosine triphosphate (ATP) production systems, protein synthesis mechanisms, genetic apparatus.
B. Response to injury: inflammation:
  1. (Cardinal) signs: heat, redness, swelling, pain, loss of function.
  2. Pathogenesis involves circulatory changes, alterations in blood vessel permeability, leukocyte response, chemical mediators.
  3. Types:
    a. Acute: immediate response to injury, with increased blood flow, increased vessel permeability, movement of leukocytes into the tissue (MAINLY neutrophils [polymorphonucleocytes, PMNs], FIRST at site of injury).
    b. Chronic: low-grade inflammation that lasts weeks to years, during which inflammation, injury, healing occur all at once, with migration of phagocytes (monocytes, macrophages), plasma cells, lymphocytes.
  4. Functions:
    a. Neutralize, destroy, isolate, remove injurious agent.
    b. Remove necrotic debris.
    c. Initiate repair and regeneration.
C. Response to injury:
  1. Regeneration: replacement of injured cells with cells of same type, dependent on cell type.
  2. Repair: restoration of cell function and morphology (form) after injury:
    a. Response to severe or persistent injury; repair CANNOT be accomplished by regeneration alone.
    b. Usually accomplished by fibrous connective tissue (scar).
  3. Factors:
    a. Angiogenesis: proliferation of new blood vessels.
    b. Remodeling: secretion of collagen-degrading enzymes.
    c. Fibrosis: repair by excessive fibrous connective tissue.

D. **Latent period:** time elapsed between exposure to injury and first appearance of symptoms and signs.

Diagnostic Process

Diagnosis is translation of data gathered by clinical and radiographic examination into organized, classified definition of conditions or diseases present. Preliminary diagnosis may be made with one or more components of diagnostic process. Differential diagnosis requires use of diagnostic components to rule out other possibilities. **Dental hygiene diagnosis** involves interpreting data into coherent description of condition or disease in terms that can be addressed by dental hygienist.

- See Chapter 11, Clinical Treatment: standards for clinical dental hygiene practice, contraindications, treatment planning.
A. Patient history: medical, dental, lesion histories.
B. Clinical assessment: identification of lesion color, size, shape, location.
   1. **Sign:** objective evidence of disease that can be discerned by clinician and/or patient
   2. **Symptoms:** subjective information about disease by patient.
C. Lab assessment: includes microscopic analysis, blood tests, biopsy, radiographs (BEST for osseous and periapical pathological conditions).
D. Surgical assessment: visual examination of surgical site; therapeutic trial uses effective treatment to assist in diagnostic process.

Prognosis, Treatment, and Care

Prognosis is prediction of how condition or disease will progress and whether there is chance of recovery or cure with treatment. However, treatment does NOT always involve cure of condition or disease. **Palliative care** is any form of medical care or treatment that concentrates on reducing severity of disease symptoms, *rather* than providing a cure; prevents and relieves suffering and improves quality of life for serious, complex illness. Nonhospice palliative care is NOT dependent on prognosis and is offered in conjunction with curative and all other appropriate forms of medical treatment. Hospice care delivers palliative care to those at the end of life.

Inflammatory Diseases

Inflammatory diseases include several common forms of dermatitis, acute or chronic inflammation of skin. Etiology can involve chemicals (drugs), radiation, trauma, metabolic and immunological factors. Types include eczema (nonspecific lesions and itching), seborrheic dermatitis (inflammation of sebaceous glands, redness, itching, scaling), and psoriasis (raised **papules** or patches with silvery scales and thickened skin on extremities).

Infectious Diseases

Infectious diseases may be bacterial, viral, or fungal. Note that hepatitis is also discussed under metabolic disorders.

- See Chapters 8, Microbiology and Immunology: infectious diseases and microorganisms; 9, Pharmacology: drug usage for infections.
A. Bacterial infections (include common diseases and infective agents):
   1. Acne: multiple facial lesions because of plugged sebaceous glands and hair follicles.
      a. MOST common in adolescence.
      b. Involves heredity and hormonal factors; aggravated by stress and drugs.
   2. **Abscess:** raised pocket of necrotic tissue and purulent exudate.
      a. MOST are around trauma sites or associated with obstructed skin appendage on skin.
      b. Also called boil (furuncle) on the skin (tooth-associated discussed later).
   3. Impetigo: infectious **pustules** with itchy, yellow scabs.
      a. MOST are around mouth and face.
      b. Highly contagious; can be either staphylococcal or streptococcal infection.
B. Viral infections (include common diseases and infective agents):
   1. Localized viral diseases: include warts, caused by strains of human papillomavirus (HPV).
   2. Involve discrete proliferation of squamous epithelium; may disappear spontaneously.

Metabolic Disorders

Metabolic disorders often manifest themselves as overproduction or underproduction of secretions. **Hypersecretion** (overproduction) occurs because of a tumor of gland; **hyposecretion** (underproduction) occurs because of agenesis (failure of an organ to develop), atrophy (partial or complete wasting away), or destruction of secretory cells. Treatment for hypersecretion is removal or destruction of all or part of gland; hormone supplementation is prescribed for hyposecretion. Clinician will need a medical consult regarding metabolic disorder or its history before dental care.

- See Chapters 3, Anatomy, Biochemistry, and Physiology: physiological processes; 8, Microbiology and Immunology: infectious agents involved in hepatitis; 9, Pharmacology: hormones and replacement therapy; 9, Pharmacology, and 11, Clinical Treatment: alcoholic patient, hyposecretion of salivary gland with geriatric patient.
A. Endocrine gland disorders:
   1. Pituitary:
      a. Hyperpituitarism: gigantism and acromegaly from overproduction of growth hormone (GH), caused primarily by pituitary adenoma; oral

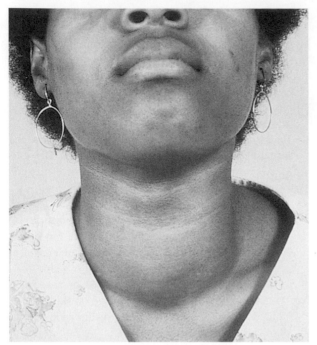

Figure 6-1 Goiter formation from thyroid gland disorder. (From Fehrenbach MJ, Herring SW: Illustrated anatomy of the head and neck, ed 3, St. Louis, 2008, Saunders/Elsevier.)

signs: macroglossia and mandibular prognathism (enlarged jaw to continued bone growth).

b. Hypopituitarism and panhypopituitarism: associated with diabetes insipidus (sometimes mistakenly confused with diabetes mellitus); urine production is copious because of lack of antidiuretic hormone (ADH) from pituitary.

2. Thyroid:

a. BOTH disorders can lead to **goiter** formation, thyroid gland enlargement (Figure 6-1).

b. Hyperthyroidism: MAINLY associated with Graves' disease, autoimmune hypertrophy of gland, with hypersecretion of thyroxine; causes exophthalmos (protruding eyes), tachycardia (increased pulse rate), severe weight loss, sweating, tremors, heat intolerance, frequent bowel movements:

(1) In children: premature primary exfoliation, early eruption of permanents.

(2) In adults: aggressive periodontal disease, dental caries, osteoporosis of jaws, burning tongue, increased salivation.

(3) Treatment: radioactive iodine (MOST common) or antithyroids, such as methimazole (Tapazole) or propylthiouracil (PTU); possibly partial surgical gland removal.

(4) Risk factors: thyroid storm (thyrotoxicosis) if undiagnosed or uncontrolled; emergency with fever, elevated blood pressure, heart dysrhythmia, tachycardia, hypermetabolism, can result in death; vasoconstrictors should NOT be used.

(5) No barriers to care; professional care and homecare: thorough extraoral and intraoral examination for increases in thyroid gland and lymph node size; home and professional fluoride to reduce incidence of caries as well as calcium products; frequent examination and oral prophylaxis to manage bone loss, caries, periodontal infection.

(6) Patient or caregiver education: instruction in dental biofilm removal methods to prevent periodontitis; adequate diet to reduce risk of osteoporosis; mineralizing fluoride and calcium products.

c. Hypothyroidism:

(1) Associated with hyposecretion of thyroxine; MOST common is Hashimoto's thyroiditis, autoimmune disorder that attacks gland; LESS common are secondary forms (iodine therapy, thyroid surgery, developmental disturbances, iodine deficiency [uncommon in United States, where salt is iodized], pituitary disease).

(2) Also associated with cretinism, congenital lack of thyroxine; causes dwarfism with stocky stature, protruding abdomen, underdeveloped sex organs, misshapen face.

(3) In children: delayed development (physical and mental).

(4) In adults: symmetrically enlarged thyroid gland, may have **nodules;** signs and symptoms include myxedema (fatigue and weight gain from slow metabolism), skin dryness, hair coarseness, face puffiness, intolerance to cold temperatures, constipation, muscle cramping, mental slowness, low blood pressure, slow pulse; sometimes confused with Sjögren's syndrome.

(5) Oral signs:

(a) In children: both enlarged tongue and lips, with delayed tooth eruption and possible enamel hypoplasia.

(b) In adults: enlarged tongue; chronic, severe periodontal disease; slow, hoarse speech; possibly gingival hyperplasia.

(6) Treatment: thyroid hormone supplementation (e.g., with levothyroxine [Synthroid, Levoxyl, Levothroid, Unithroid]).

(7) No significant risk factors; professional care and homecare: thorough extraoral and intraoral inspection for increases in thyroid gland or lymph node size, frequent oral examination and recare.

(8) Patient or caregiver education: instruction in thorough dental biofilm control and need

for frequent recare to reduce incidence of periodontal destruction.

3. Adrenal:
   a. Hyperadrenalism: Cushing's syndrome with hypersecretion of glucocorticoid hormones; causes obesity, striae, easy bruising, red face, pathological fractures, hyperglycemia, hypertension; drug therapy (corticosteroids), which can result in "moon face," "buffalo hump," and osteoporosis.
   b. Hypoadrenalism: Addison's disease with hyposecretion of adrenal cortex (NOT medulla) hormones; causes dehydration, electrolyte imbalances, hypotension (low blood pressure), weight loss, pigmented skin and oral mucosa; orthostatic hypotension risk.

4. Parathyroid: hyperparathyroidism that causes radiolucencies in mandible and mobile teeth.

B. Liver disorders:
   1. Cirrhosis: chronic destruction of liver cells with fibrous, nodular regeneration.
      a. Etiology: drugs, alcohol, viral infections; may be unknown.
      b. Systemic signs: jaundice (yellow skin, sclera), puffy eyes, facial redness, hepatic encephalopathy, ascites, splenomegaly, bleeding.
      c. Oral signs: xerostomia, reduced ability to taste, glossitis, increased risk of caries, periodontal disease, oral cancer, alcohol breath, enlargement of parotid gland, facial and dental trauma from falls and injuries.
      d. Treatment for alcoholics: alcohol abstinence; occasionally involves surgical operations to relieve portal circulatory disruptions.
      e. Risk factors: nutritional deficiencies, infections, trauma, oral cancer (especially if tobacco is also used); relative contraindication when administering amide local anesthetics (lowering amount) and nitrous oxide sedation (metabolism difficulties).
      f. Barriers to care:
         (1) Communication difficulties; may not appear for appointments when actively drinking.
         (2) Transportation problems, if the alcoholic does not drive or has lost driving privileges and must rely on others.
         (3) Economic problems, if unable to hold a job or on a fixed income.
      g. Professional care and homecare:
         (1) Need for frequent oral cancer evaluations.
         (2) Nonalcoholic mouthrinses (Rembrandt, Biotene).
         (3) Possible bleeding problems from damaged liver, need INR (international normalized ratio) number.
         (4) Daily fluoride and calcium product supplementation as needed.
         (5) Dealing with possible intoxication and difficulty in keeping appointments.
      h. Patient or caregiver education: need for frequent recall, fluoride and calcium supplementation, saliva substitutes, good homecare practices because of risk of infection.

   2. Viral hepatitis: caused by several viruses known as hepatitis A, B, C, D, or E (see Chapter 8, Microbiology: related discussion).
      a. MOST prevalent liver disease in world; vaccines for hepatitis A and B.
      b. Systemic signs: anorexia, malaise, jaundice, enlarged liver, high levels of aspartate aminotransferase (AST, enzyme released into blood after liver injury), dark urine (contains bilirubin).
      c. Types and pathogenesis:
         (1) Hepatitis A (HAV):
            (a) Transmission: fecal-oral route (contaminated food and water and sewage), includes shellfish.
            (b) Incubation period: 15 to 50 days, with short-lived, slight flulike symptoms, rapid recovery, NO long-term consequences.
         (2) Hepatitis B (HB): dental healthcare personnel (DHCP) are at highest risk for contracting.
            (a) Transmission: exposure to contaminated blood and blood products or by sexual contact; at risk for contracting hepatitis D.
            (b) Incubation period: 40 to 180 days; MOST have clinically unrecognizable symptoms; MOST recover fully.
         (3) Hepatitis C:
            (a) Transmission: exposure to contaminated blood and blood products or by sexual contact.
            (b) Incubation period: 15 to 150 days; symptoms are SAME as HB but LESS severe; however, progresses to chronic hepatitis in HALF of all infected persons.
         (4) Hepatitis D:
            (a) Transmission: exposure to contaminated blood and blood products or by sexual contact.
            (b) Incubation period: 30 to 50 days; virus depends on HB virus (HBV) for its replication; infection with BOTH viruses occurs at same time (thus considered a "piggy-back" virus).
         (5) Hepatitis E:
            (a) Transmission: fecal-oral route, contaminated food and water and sewage (not shellfish like hepatitis A).

(b) Incubation period: 14 to 60 days and slight or asymptomatic course; no long-term consequences in MOST cases (EXCEPT liver necrosis develops in many acutely infected pregnant women).

d. Treatment: palliative.

C. Pancreatic disorders:

1. Diabetes mellitus (DM, hyperglycemia): multifactorial disease leading to high blood glucose levels.

a. Types and pathogenesis: can be present for 10 to 20 years before diagnosis.

(1) Prediabetes: blood glucose levels are higher than normal but NOT yet at the high levels of type 2; includes BOTH impaired glucose toleration and impaired fasting glucose.

(2) Type 1 (insulin-dependent diabetes mellitus [IDDM], juvenile onset):

(a) MORE serious type; autoantibodies against insulin produce pancreatic beta cells so pancreas fails to secrete adequate insulin.

(b) Many serious complications over time.

(c) Requires daily insulin injections.

(3) Type 2 (non-insulin-dependent diabetes mellitus [NIDDM], mature onset):

(a) LESS serious type; target cells fail to respond to insulin.

(b) May have many serious complications over time, MORE in females; associated with obesity.

(c) May be controlled by dietary changes, but may need drug therapy, including insulin injections.

(4) Latent autoimmune diabetes of adulthood (LADA, type 1.5): slowly progressive form of type 1 DM, often diagnosed as type 2 DM, but positive for pancreatic islet antibodies, especially to glutamic acid decarboxylase (GAD); does not immediately require insulin for treatment; patients often not overweight, have little or no resistance to insulin UNLIKE type 2.

(5) Gestational (pregnancy); usually does NOT continue after birth of child.

b. Signs and symptoms: polyuria (increased urination), glycosuria (sugar in urine), polyphagia (increased hunger), polydipsia (increased thirst), increased amount of ketone bodies in the blood, acidosis (increased acidity of blood plasma), weight loss, poor wound healing, risk for infections.

c. Oral complications (ALL at increased risk with poorly controlled blood sugar): *Candida albicans* infections, xerostomia (dry mouth),

---

Box 6-1 Monitoring Levels of Blood Glucose

<70 mg/dL: Too low; tendency toward hypoglycemia. Take 15 mg of carbohydrates (glucose source) and wait 15 minutes. If this level continues, need for immediate medical consult. Risk for emergency.

70-99 mg/dL: Normal levels.

100-125 mg/dL: Prediabetes; recommend medical consult.

126-240 mg/dL: Higher levels; monitor infection level, insulin intake, stress level, food level.

>240 mg/dL: Too high; tendency toward hyperglycemia. If this level continues, need for immediate medical consult. Risk for emergency.

Levels can vary per person and situation (before and after meals and medications); only average levels noted here.

---

parotid gland enlargement, increased slight caries rate from dry mouth, as well as increased moderate to severe periodontal disease, tooth loss and mobility.

d. Systemic complications: related neural, visual, and kidney disorder because of fibrosis of blood vessels.

e. Diagnostic and monitoring tests (Box 6-1):

(1) Self-monitoring blood glucose (SMBG): recommended for ALL types; MORE frequently required for those on intensive insulin therapy or pregnant, having hard time controlling levels, with increased ketones in urine, or with intercurrent illness.

(2) Glycosylated hemoglobin (GHb): measures how much glucose attaches to hemoglobin (Hb) on red blood cells (RBCs) (HbA1c or A1c test); reflects average blood glucose levels over 3 to 4 months; >9% to 20% indicates poor control and the need to reassess the present treatment.

(3) Fasting plasma glucose (FPG): measures blood glucose levels after fast; ≥126 mg/dL is diagnostic; casual (nonfasting) of ≥200 mg/dL with classic symptoms is diagnostic but is confirmed on separate day; impaired glucose metabolism (prediabetes) has <126 mg/dL.

(4) Blood urea nitrogen (BUN) and serum creatinine: to determine any related renal damage.

(5) pH levels: to determine severity of diabetic ketoacidosis.

(6) Serum electrolytes: to determine biochemical imbalances that interfere with muscle and cardiovascular system (CVS) function.

(7) Oral glucose tolerance test (OGTT): for diagnosing gestational (pregnancy) type diabetes.

f. Treatment (See Chapter 9, Pharmacology: drug therapy for DM):

g. Risk factors:
 (1) Disturbance in balance between glucose and insulin occurs when diabetes is uncontrolled, which can lead to poor wound healing, which in turn can increase the risk of bacterial, viral, and fungal infections.
 (2) Local anesthetics with vasoconstrictors are recommended for ALL but the most complicated procedures.
h. Barriers to care: NO greater than others unless complications exist.
i. Professional care and homecare:
 (1) Thoroughly assessing oral health, as well as monitoring diabetic control; including use of diabetes risk assessment test kit (BIOSAFE), FDA-approved home use or professional use diabetic test kit (includes immediate FPG and HbA1c test from self-collected finger-prick blood sent to lab, with patient consent form; professional lab report is faxed to the dental office and paper mailed to the patient).
 (2) Antibiotic premedication may be advised in cases of uncontrolled diabetes or extensive infection before dental care (determined during medical consult).
 (3) Scheduling short dental appointments soon after morning meals (1½ hours).
 (4) Preparing for diabetic emergency (glucose source MUST be available in emergency kit).

j. Patient or caregiver education:
 (1) MUST understand that controlling oral disease means controlling blood sugar levels and overall need for drug therapy and even reduced complications.
 (2) Preventive oral health procedures and need for frequent recall; MUST control any oral infections.
 (3) Daily mineralizing fluoride and calcium product supplementation.
2. Pancreatitis: inflammation of gland.
 a. Etiology: protein- and lipid-digesting enzymes in pancreas that digest organ itself; severe cases are associated with alcoholism.
 (1) Acute: causes severe abdominal pain with sudden onset, nausea, vomiting, elevated serum levels of amylase and lipase, rapidly developing shock, pancreatic enzymes in urine.
 (2) Chronic: causes severe pain, malabsorption, DM.
 b. Treatment: acute centers on controlling systemic consequences of shock; chronic centers on treating symptoms.
3. Pancreatic cancer: early diagnosis difficult because of nonspecific and varied symptoms; MOST not diagnosed until advanced; prognosis is generally regarded as poor; MAINLY in males, smokers, persons with periodontal disease.

CLINICAL STUDY

Age	37 YRS	**SCENARIO**
Sex	☐ Male ☒ Female	A patient new to the dental practice is at the end of the 2-hour afternoon appointment. She starts complaining of a headache, reports feeling weak, and becomes more nervous and somewhat confused.
Height	5'10"	
Weight	210 LBS	
BP	112/68	
Chief Complaint	"I was so nervous about this dental appointment that I forgot to eat lunch today."	
Medical History	Diabetes mellitus (well controlled) for 2 years / Osteopenia for 1 year	
Current Medications	250 mg chlorpropamide (Diabinese) qd / OTC calcium supplement with vitamin D qd	
Social History	Interior decorator	

1. What type of diabetes does the patient have? What type of drug is she taking? When should it be taken?
2. What is the American Society of Anesthesiologists (ASA) classification of this patient at the beginning of the appointment?
3. What emergency has begun to occur during this appointment?
4. Describe the steps that should be followed to manage this situation.
5. How could this emergency have been avoided?

1. Patient has type 2 diabetes mellitus (DM), most often controlled by diet and exercise; in some more moderately involved cases by oral hypoglycemic drug(s) such as chlorpropamide (Diabinese); even by insulin in severe cases. DM occurs when body does not make enough insulin (type 1) or when insulin that is produced no longer works properly (type 2). Insulin works by helping sugar get inside the body's cells, where it is used for energy. Physician will advise the patient of the dosage schedule depending on the time of onset of the particular insulin used to achieve best control over blood sugar levels.

2. Physical status shows that mild systemic disease such as type 2 DM equates to an ASA II classification. The ASA physical status classification determines risks and necessary modifications before dental treatment.

3. Emergency that has occurred is hypoglycemia (low blood sugar); she is now at ASA IV level. Condition is most often associated with lack of food intake; in this case she missed lunch because of anxiety associated with dental appointment. Headache, weakness, nervousness, confusion are symptoms of hypoglycemia. Condition typically occurs rapidly for patients who require insulin; onset of symptoms is slower for patients taking oral hypoglycemics.

4. Dental treatment must be stopped, and patient must be positioned upright. Source of glucose (orange juice or other glucose source such as glucose tablets or gel) should be given if patient is conscious. Source of glucose should be stored in easily accessible dental office emergency kit. If situation is allowed to progress, patient may become unconscious, in which case IM or IV administration of glucagon by the supervising dentist is indicated, if available, after EMS system is activated.

5. Both lack of lunch and stress related to appointment contributed to occurrence of hypoglycemia. It is essential to explain all dental procedures to this patient to alleviate anxiety about future appointments and encourage eating before the appointment; use of morning appointments after she eats a good breakfast and takes her prescription drugs is an effective way to deal with problem. May also want her to have a prescription to ease her dental anxiety (diazepam [Valium]) and help reduce risk of hypoglycemia.

Blood Disorders

Basic categories of blood disorders include red (RBC) and white (WBC) blood cell disorders and clotting disorders. They are related to abnormal levels, function, or structure of some blood components. Note that hemophilia is discussed under inherited disorders. Will need a <u>medical consult</u> for ALL types of blood disorders before dental care.

- See Chapters 3, Anatomy, Biochemistry, and Physiology; 8, Microbiology and Immunology: vascular system and immunology.

A. Anemias: low hemoglobin and oxygen concentration in blood.
   1. Etiology: excess bleeding, hemolysis, iron or other nutrient deficiency, improper formation of new RBCs.
   2. Forms and pathogenesis:
      a. Pernicious (B_{12} deficiency, type of megaloblastic anemia): too few RBCs; factor for RBC formation is missing; treated with injections of missing intrinsic factor.
      b. Sickle-cell (sickle-cell disease): genetic hemolytic anemia; usually confined to African-Americans; RBCs are sickle (crescent) shaped and CANNOT function properly; lower level of anemia present with sickle-cell trait (person has ONLY one copy of mutation).
      c. Hypochromic (iron deficiency anemia): too little hemoglobin per RBC; treated with iron supplementation.
      d. Hemolytic: rupture of RBCs; may be genetic or environmental; NO effective treatment for genetic forms; treatment for environmentally induced forms centers on control of environmental factors.
      e. Aplastic: faulty bone marrow; treated with transfusion or stem cells from bone marrow transplantation.
      f. Secondary: from another disease; cell numbers are normal but hemoglobin level is low.
   3. Oral signs: bleeding oral tissues, angular cheilitis, pale skin and oral mucosa, erythematous burning tongue with loss of BOTH filiform and fungiform lingual papillae.
   4. Risk factors: excessive bleeding and trauma.
   5. Barriers to care: nonexistent; in severe cases fatigue may keep patient from appointments.
   6. Professional care and homecare: observation of signs and symptoms of anemia and appropriate referral; with sickle-cell anemia, needs <u>medical consult</u> for possible antibiotic premedication before dental care.
   7. Patient or caregiver education: appropriate care of anemia by following physician's orders and practicing good oral hygiene to decrease risk of infection.
B. Polycythemia: overproduction of circulating RBCs.
   1. Primary: hyperactive bone marrow and elevated hematocrit, blood viscosity, blood pressure, cardiac workload; treatment involves bloodletting and radiation therapy to reduce RBC numbers.
   2. Secondary: associated with need to compensate for inadequate blood oxygen levels caused by heart disease, emphysema, living at high altitude, or increased oxygen demand by muscles (in athletes); treated by controlling symptoms.
C. Thrombocytopenia: FEWER platelets (thrombocytes) in blood with SAME clinical signs as anemia; can be caused by decreased production in bone marrow, increased destruction, disease, or as a side effect of drugs.

D. Diseases of WBCs and bone marrow:
1. Agranulocytosis: severe reduction in number of granulocytes (basophils, eosinophils, neutrophils); results in greatly reduced immune system.
2. Leukopenia: abnormally low levels of WBCs.
3. Neutropenia: abnormally low levels of neutrophils (granulocytic WBCs):
   a. Etiology: congenital (discussed later), immunological, chemicals (drugs) or radiation therapy that suppresses bone marrow; acute disease is adverse reaction to toxic levels of drug or to bone marrow–suppressing radiation therapy.
   b. Systemic signs: lymphadenopathy; fever and chills; prostration; jaundice; bleeding **ulcers** of rectum, oral cavity, vagina; proper identification of disease is by blood test; WBC counts drop to one fifth to one tenth.
   c. Measured by absolute neutrophil count (ANC), which would be $<1800/mm^3$.
   d. Oral signs: infections, painful ulcerations, bleeding gingival lesions with rapid periodontal destruction.
   e. Infections can be fatal, so must be treated quickly; invasive oral procedures, including oral prophylaxis, should NOT be performed.
   f. Treatment: transfusions to restore WBC counts, antibiotics to control infections.
4. Leukemia: cancer of red bone marrow, lymphatic tissue, or WBCs.
   a. Etiology: largely unknown, although radiation, genetics, viruses implicated.
   b. Types and pathogenesis (Table 6-1):
      (1) Acute: rapid increase of immature WBCs that crowd out normal cells.
      (2) Chronic: excessive buildup of relatively mature, but still abnormal, WBCs that takes months and years to progress.
   c. Systemic signs: pallor (pale color) of skin and lining mucosa, bone and joint pain, abnormal bleeding that leads to bruising, enlarged lymph nodes, hepatomegaly, splenomegaly, anemia.
   d. Oral signs: red, tender gingival tissues, spontaneous sulcular bleeding, **petechiae** and **ecchymosis,** risk for infections.
   e. Treatment: chemotherapy.
5. Multiple myeloma (MM): cancer of plasma cells, which are immune system cells in bone marrow that produce antibodies and immunoglobulins (MAINLY IgG).
   a. Etiology: unknown, does not have hereditary basis, but family members may have increased risk.
   b. Systemic signs: elevated calcium level, renal failure, anemia, bone lesions (skull radiograph shows "punched-out" radiolucencies), with bone pain and increased risk of infection (Figure 6-2).
   c. Treatment: includes bisphosphonates to treat fractures and erythropoietin to treat anemia, as well as chemotherapy and transplants.
6. Burkitt's (lymphoma): cancer of B lymphocytes; one type associated with HIV and mononucleosis (Epstein-Barr virus [EBV]).
7. Langerhans cell histiocytosis X (eosinophilic granuloma, Hand-Schüller-Christian disease): rare clonal proliferation of Langerhans cells, abnormal cells from bone marrow, capable of migrating from skin to lymph nodes; affects children.

CLINICAL STUDY

Age	12 YRS	SCENARIO
Sex	☐ Male ☒ Female	During her initial intraoral examination, gingival bleeding, poor oral hygiene, three carious lesions, and two nearly exfoliated teeth are observed. Physician wants oral cavity checked for signs of infection
Chief Complaint	"My grandmother is so scared since my gums are bleeding so much!"	
Medical History	Recent diagnosis of leukemia with intensive chemotherapy scheduled in 1 week	
Current Medications	None at this time	
Social History	Grade school student studying ballet Grandmother is guardian	

1. What information must be obtained from the patient's oncologist before any dental treatment can be given?
2. What dental procedures should be completed before chemotherapy?

3. When during the several months of chemotherapy should dental treatment be scheduled?

1. Before dental treatment, oncologist should be consulted regarding blood tests (WBC count), clotting and

Table 6-1 Comparison of leukemia types

Type	Occurrence	5-Year survival rate	Overall treatment
Acute lymphocytic leukemia (ALL)*	Most in young children; also affects adults, especially those ≥65	85% in children; 50% in adults	Bone marrow and systemic disease control, prevention of spreading, e.g., to CNS
Chronic lymphocytic leukemia (CLL)*	Most in adults >55; sometimes in younger adults, but almost never children; most are men	75%	Incurable
Acute myelogenous leukemia (AML)†	More in adults than in children; most are men	40%	Bone marrow and systemic disease control, specific treatment of CNS, if involved
Chronic myelogenous leukemia (CML)†	Most in adults; small number of children	90%	

CNS, Central nervous system.
*Also known as lymphoblastic.
†Also known as myeloid or nonlymphocytic.

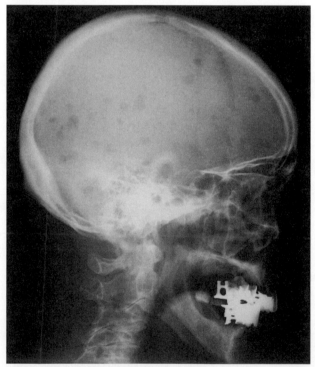

Figure 6-2 Skull radiograph of multiple myeloma showing "punched-out" radiolucencies.

bleeding factors (INR), placement of central venous catheter, when chemotherapy will begin, expected length of immunosuppression.

2. If blood counts are adequate and time is available before chemotherapy, all loose teeth and teeth close to exfoliation (shedding) should be removed, carious teeth should be restored, oral hygiene instructions and need for meticulous oral hygiene should be stressed, and oral prophylaxis should be completed. Since this is a child patient, it is important that her guardian be advised of all that is needed to maintain oral and related systemic health.

3. Dental treatment can be scheduled whenever blood counts have returned to safe levels. Safe levels are most common just before scheduled round of chemotherapy. Bleeding levels monitored by INR; INR ≤2.5 is safe for invasive dental work; older test is prothrombin time (PT). Antibiotic premedication will be needed before invasive dental procedures if catheter placement is permanent.

Bone Diseases

Diseases of the bone include osteoporosis, Paget's disease, fibrous dysplasia, cherubism, cleidocranial dysostosis (note that latter two are discussed under inherited disorders).

A. Osteoporosis: MOST common bone disease.
 1. MORE common in women and with age; other factors include low levels of sex hormones (e.g., menopause), low body weight, ethnicity (e.g., white or Asian), family history, low dietary intake of calcium and/or vitamin D, smoking, alcoholism.
 2. Drugs such as anticonvulsants or glucocorticoids can also increase risk.
 3. Reduced bone quantity and quality; loss in bone mass and decrease in bone density (i.e., increased porosity) cause the bone to weaken.
 4. EARLY loss of bone density with osteopenia; as disease progresses, bone becomes MORE fragile and even slightest trauma can cause fracture (e.g., hip fracture); resulting spinal compression fractures may result in loss of height with stooped posture (dowager's hump).
 5. May be related to oral bone loss with periodontal disease, since quality and quantity of the jaws appear to be affected.
 6. Diagnosis: dual-energy x-ray absorptiometry (DXA) measures density of spine, hip, or total body (gold standard).

7. Treatment: diet and exercise; also selective estrogen receptor modulators (SERMs) such as raloxifene (Evista). See notes on bisphosphonates and osteoradionecrosis complications.
B. Paget's disease (osteitis deformans): second MOST common bone disease after osteoporosis.
   1. Systemic signs: BOTH destruction and formation of bone in patients >50 years of age; often asymptomatic; patients may have blindness (closure of neural foramina) or deafness; MOST striking is progressive enlargement of spine, femur, and skull, MAINLY the maxilla, with tendency for bone fracture.
   2. Oral signs: teeth may loosen and migrate with jaw expansion; dentures NO longer fit (NOR do hats).
   3. Radiographs: "cotton-wool" appearance, with patchy opacities, root resorption with loss of lamina dura, enlarged maxilla.
   4. Diagnosis: elevated serum alkaline phosphatase level.
   5. Treatment: none.
C. Fibrous dysplasia: abnormal proliferation of fibrous connective tissue; COMMON in children; two types:
   1. Monostotic: ONLY one bone involved.
   2. Polyostotic (McCune-Albright syndrome): MOST severe form, affecting many bones, with "café-au-lait spots" (localized skin pigmentation).
   3. Oral signs: painless swelling of jaw; teeth may be displaced.
   4. Radiographs: unilocular or multilocular radiolucency, with "ground glass" appearance because of many irregular C-shaped trabeculae.

Neoplasia

Neoplasm is uncontrolled cellular growth resulting in a **tumor;** general term, includes either benign or malignant (cancer). Will need medical consult for ALL with neoplasm history before dental care. See later discussion of biopsy procedures and lung cancer. Treatment after radiation therapy and chemotherapy for patients in the dental office is also discussed later.
• See also Chapter 9, Pharmacology: chemotherapy.
A. Etiology: exposure to adequate concentrations of carcinogens (cancer-causing agents) that alter cellular DNA and proteins:
   1. Exogenous factors: chemicals (including drugs), radiation, viruses, other environmental factors.
   2. Endogenous factors: genetic factors (genome of cells), hormonal factors, immune system factors, nutritional factors, aging.
B. Tissues at risk for neoplastic change: tendency for cells to undergo neoplasia is roughly related to cell's involvement in physiological replacement; MUST have adequate time for initiation, transformation, growth of mass.

C. Classification:
   1. **Benign neoplasia** (suffix "-oma" added after tissue type [e.g., osteoma]):
      a. Single, discrete mass; solid organs or connective tissue, with formation of capsule around mass.
      b. Close resemblance to tissue of origin; mature cells with minimal to moderate cellular atypia.
      c. However, effects of benign tumors are NOT always so safe:
         (1) With endocrine growth, may cause uncontrolled hormone hypersecretion.
         (2) With cellular growth, may compress adjacent tissue (brain, spinal cord) or cause blockage of lumen (trachea, intestines), causing further serious or even life-threatening complications.
         (3) Examples:
            (a) Angioma: tumor composed of blood vessels (birthmark).
            (b) Lipoma: soft, fatty tumor that develops in adipose tissue.
            (c) Adenoma: tumor of glandular tissue.
         (4) Treatment: includes surgical removal and radiation therapy.
   2. **Malignant neoplasia** (cancer) ("carcinoma" added to tissue type for epithelial tissue [e.g., squamous cell carcinoma] and "sarcoma" for nonepithelial tissue [e.g., osteosarcoma]):
      a. Cells are neoplastic (new growth); capacity exists for invasion (going deeper in tissues) or metastasis (spread beyond original site).
      b. Frequency and significance:
         (1) In both sexes, MOST affected are lungs, digestive organs (including pancreas), sex organs.
         (2) In females, breast cancer is second MOST common; in males, prostate cancer.
      c. TNM classification of malignant tumors: cancer staging system that allows determination of prognosis and treatment (T = size of tumor, N = nodes involved, M = metastasis).
      d. Treatment (may be combined during therapy): includes surgical incision, chemotherapy, radiation therapy, stem cells from the blood or bone marrow transplantation, donor lymphocyte infusion (DLI); if treatment is ineffective in eliminating cancer, disease can be fatal.
      e. Paraneoplastic syndromes (such as fever, anorexia) occur with active cancer and those in remission after treatment; clinical pictures may vary greatly.
D. Vascular neoplasias:
   1. Hemangioma: benign vascular lesion that develops at birth or during early childhood.

a. Exophytic lesion that occurs on skin and rarely in oral mucosa (tongue or buccal mucosa).

b. MOST are compressible and some are emptiable.

c. Treatment: may require surgical removal; bleeding can be a problem.

2. Kaposi's sarcoma (KS): malignant vascular lesion MOST often associated with HIV/AIDS (see Figure 13-2).

a. Associated with CD4+ cell counts <200 cells/mm^3; AIDS diagnostic lesion.

b. Dark purple, flat, or exophytic, may be ulcerated and bleeding; various intraoral (palate and gingiva) and extraoral sites (see later discussion of vascular lesions).

3. Treatment: surgery, radiation, chemotherapy.

E. Osseous neoplasias:

1. Osteoma: small benign tumor that can occur anywhere, including oral cavity.

2. Osteosarcoma: MOST common malignant osseous neoplasia; poorly defined jaw radiolucency.

a. MOST in adults 30 to 40 years old; may cause pain, swelling, paresthesia (numbness).

b. Treatment: chemotherapy followed by surgical resection.

F. Muscle neoplasia:

1. Rhabdomyosarcoma: rare cancer that involves skeletal muscle, including in the head and neck area; MOST common in children.

G. Soft tissue neoplasias: MOST often benign and without serious pathogenesis; occur in variety of tissues, including adipose (lipoma), muscle (myoma), blood, lymphatic:

1. Fibroma (true): mesenchymal tumor associated with excessive growth of connective tissues.

a. Exophytic lesion with color matching surrounding tissues (unless traumatized); may occur on any oral tissue; MOST on buccal or labial mucosa.

b. When associated with gingiva and cells of the periodontal ligament, considered a peripheral odontogenic fibroma.

2. Lipoma: small benign tumor of fatty tissue.

H. Odontogenic neoplasias:

1. Ameloblastoma: aggressive benign epithelial tumor associated with cells of enamel organ.

a. MOST in posterior mandible; associated with presence of unerupted teeth, painless swelling, thinning periosteum with "egg shell" cracking when palpated.

b. Radiographs: multilocular bone destruction with "soap bubble" appearance; ameloblast-like cells in biopsy (Figure 6-3).

c. Treatment: wide surgical removal, including jaw.

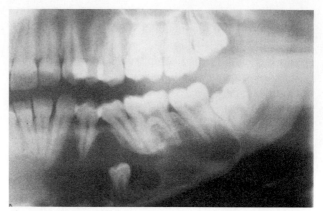

Figure 6-3 Ameloblastoma, aggressive benign jaw tumor, with "soap bubble" appearance in posterior mandible.

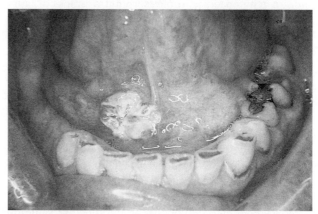

Figure 6-4 Squamous cell carcinoma of the floor of the mouth.

I. Epithelial squamous cell neoplasias:

1. Papilloma: benign, **pedunculated** or **sessile,** white warty lesion associated with squamous cells.

a. MOST on palate; may be pedunculated (have a stalk).

b. Treatment: surgical removal to rule out cancer.

2. Squamous cell carcinoma (SCC): malignancy associated with squamous cells that invades through the basement membrane; MOST common oral cancer (90%) (Figure 6-4).

a. Etiology: chronic tobacco and/or alcohol use, human papillomavirus (HPV); because of HPV, may occur in younger group as well as those ≥40 years; varies in appearance:

(1) Skin and oral signs: red and/or white papule, plaque, or ulcer that does NOT heal; pain and bleeding possible.

(2) Jaw signs: swelling, pain, numbness (paresthesia).

(3) Pharynx and larynx signs: dysphagia (difficulty swallowing), continued hoarseness, lump (mass).

(4) Salivary gland signs: small, persistent unilateral lump, little to moderate pain.

b. Location: MOST on lower lip, lateral border or base of tongue, floor of mouth, soft palate complex (including tonsillar region); MAINLY hidden areas the clinician should access thoroughly during an intraoral examination; however, if HPV involved, can be present in ANY location.

c. Diagnostic dental office tests: brush biopsy (Oral CDx), ultraviolet (UV) light kit, toluidine blue dye kit; exfoliative cytology (not recommended anymore); ALL noninvasive tests do NOT take place of surgical biopsy.

d. Pathogenesis: does NOT heal or show response to palliative treatment; may metastasize to cervical lymph nodes.

e. Verrucous carcinoma: type of SCC that is slow growing; associated with spit (smokeless) tobacco.

   (1) Associated with buccal and labial mucosa (related to placement of tobacco); NO visual difference from "chewer's" lesions, so biopsy is necessary.

   (2) Pathogenesis: does NOT invade basement membrane; unlikely to metastasize, thus with prognosis better than other SCC.

f. Treatment: surgery, radiation, chemotherapy.

3. Basal cell carcinoma (BCC): noninvasive malignancy with increase in basal epithelial cells; associated with sun exposure (actinic damage).

a. Pathogenesis: begins as small, elevated papule and then becomes more fibrous and ulcerates centrally to become small cratered lesion with indurated (hard) rolled borders on exposed areas.

b. MOST in older adults; common on exposed areas, especially lower lip.

c. Usually does NOT undergo metastasis unless less common infiltrating type.

d. Treatment: surgery, radiation, chemotherapy.

4. Melanocytic nevus (plural, nevi) (mole): blue-brown pigmented benign lesion.

a. Pathogenesis: never changes shape (symmetrical), border, color, diameter.

b. Treatment: may require a biopsy to rule out malignancy, melanoma.

5. Malignant melanoma: dark-colored skin malignancy; occasionally occurs on masticatory oral mucosa (maxillary alveolar ridge and palate).

a. Etiology: excessive exposure to sunlight; usually at site of preexisting nevus, but can be initial lesion; greater risk with family history.

b. Pathogenesis: grows aggressively, with widespread metastases; exhibits "ABCD" changes: asymmetry, border, color, diameter; may have bleeding or ulcerated surface.

c. Treatment: surgery, radiation, chemotherapy.

d. Prevention: avoidance of sun, use of sunscreen, routine examination of existing lesions.

J. Salivary gland neoplasms:

1. Pleomorphic adenoma: benign (MOST common type) with mixture of epithelial and connective tissue.

a. Asymptomatic mass associated with major or minor glands of palate; MOST with parotid gland.

b. MOST in adults ≥40 years.

c. Treatment: surgical removal.

2. Adenoid cystic carcinoma: slow-growing malignancy associated with major or minor gland.

a. "Swiss cheese–like" appearance microscopically.

b. Treatment: surgical removal.

3. Mucoepidermoid carcinoma: malignancy of epithelial and mucous cells.

a. Slow-growing mass associated with palate and parotid.

b. Treatment: surgical removal.

K. Breast cancer: second MOST common cancer in women *after* lung cancer that starts in the cells of the breast.

1. Adenocarcinoma that is classified by histological appearance; presents as metastatic disease.

2. FIRST symptom is lump that feels different from surrounding tissue; mammography or ultrasound tests for presence.

3. May secondarily involve unilateral supraclavicular lymph nodes palpated during extraoral examination, metastasis to jaws noted on radiographs as either radiolucency or opacity.

4. Treatment: surgery, radiation, chemotherapy.

L. Prostate cancer: second MOST common cancer in men *after* lung cancer, within gland of reproductive system; may cause pain, difficulty in urinating, erectile dysfunction (ED); if undergoes metastasis to jaws, may be noted on radiographs as either radiolucency or opacity.

CLINICAL STUDY ▬▬▬▬▬▬▬▬▬▬▬▬▬▬▬▬

Age	50 YRS	**SCENARIO**
Sex	☐ Male ☒ Female	The lesion noted on intraoral examination of the patient appears to be a preexisting mole that is 5 mm in diameter and has a raised, irregular, and reddened border on its anterior surface.
Height	5'10"	
Weight	140 LBS	
BP	105/70	
Chief Complaint	"My mole becomes sore and bleeds and I think it is getting larger!"	
Medical History	Past history of repeated urinary tract infections Gallbladder removed 5 years ago	
Current Medications	OTC ginseng qd	
Social History	High school teacher who spends many hours sunbathing every summer and uses tanning booths in the winter to maintain her tan, since she has very pale skin	

1. What is a likely diagnosis of the patient's condition?
2. Which of the usual signs and predisposing factors for this condition does she present?
3. How would this condition treated? What could the patient have done to prevent this condition?

1. Malignant melanoma, which is a malignancy of skin that occasionally occurs on masticatory oral mucosa (attached gingiva and hard palate); most occur on the skin at a site of existing mole (nevus) but can occur as initial lesion. Grows aggressively; dark in color; exhibits changes (ABCDs) such as asymmetry, border, color, or diameter. Caused by excessive exposure to sunlight as is shown by her lesion, which is on an exposed portion of her skin. Nevus, by contrast, is benign tumor of melanin and does not show any change in manner as this lesion does.
2. Asymmetry of lesion (flat and raised portions); irregular borders; variation in color; relatively large diameter; preexisting nevus; prolonged, frequent exposure to the sun and pale skin that burns easily.
3. Treated by surgery, radiation, chemotherapy; if surgery, patient may want to let surgeon know about her

OTC drug, since ginseng can promote bleeding and delay clot formation. Prevention includes reducing exposure to sun, using sunscreen, routine examination of existing lesions.

Biopsy Procedures

Surgical biopsy is a definitive diagnostic technique for many diseases and conditions such as neoplasia. A tissue sample surgically taken from the patient is microscopically examined and evaluated for structure and cell type. See also earlier discussion of neoplasia.

A. Indications:
   1. Any unusual or suspected lesion that CANNOT be clinically identified with certainty or has persisted for more than 2 weeks without healing.
   2. Any surgically excised tissue should be routinely evaluated.
B. Types:
   1. Excisional: *entire* suspect lesion is removed and microscopically examined.
   2. Incisional: representative *section* of suspect lesion is removed and microscopically examined; used for large lesions.

CLINICAL STUDY

Age	65 YRS	SCENARIO
Sex	☒ Male ☐ Female	The patient indicates that he noticed the sore several months ago. Intraoral examination reveals a 10-mm ulcerated red lesion located on the left lateral border of the tongue.
Height	6'2"	
Weight	195 LBS	
BP	112/72	
Chief Complaint	"This sore in my mouth really hurts!"	
Medical History	Smokes a pack of cigarettes a day Started smoking when he was 15 Consumes alcoholic beverages on the weekends	
Current Medications	None	
Social History	Farmer Volunteer firefighter	

1. What additional information is required for a proper diagnosis for the patient? What is the most likely diagnosis of the lesion?
2. Describe the histological features of this type of lesion.
3. Is this lesion likely to spread to other areas?
4. What risk factors are important in the formation of the lesion?

1. Surgical tissue biopsy is required for proper diagnosis. Surgical biopsy may confirm a squamous cell carcinoma (SCC) that is noted by its clinical signs.
2. Histologically, neoplastic squamous cells invade through epithelial basement membrane. Thus this is a carcinoma, since it involves the epithelium, unlike a sarcoma that involves nonepithelial tissues such as connective tissue like bone.
3. The SCCs of oral cavity are most likely to metastasize to lymph nodes of neck, cervical nodes, on the same side as the lesion.
4. Tobacco and alcohol use are two key risk factors associated with this case, as well as age; it is important to note that patients usually smoke or drink almost double the amount they report to their healthcare professionals.

Cancer Patient Care

Cancer will develop in just less than half of Americans. Oral cancer rates are increasing, and younger populations are being affected. Dental care is IMPORTANT part of overall treatment protocols for cancer therapy. Will need medical consult before dental care.

A. *Localized* oral and/or pharyngeal cancer concerns:
1. Surgery:
   a. Acute (short-term) complications: pain, fistula formation, speech alteration, nutritional deficiency, infection, and psychosocial impact.
   b. Long-term complications: pain, disfigurement, malocclusion, temporomandibular disorder, speech alteration, nutritional deficiency, infection, and psychosocial impact.
2. Radiation therapy to the oral cavity and salivary glands:
   a. Acute (short-term) complications: oral mucositis (discussed later), loss of taste, xerostomia (caused by salivary hypofunction), infection, nutritional deficiency.
   b. Long-term complications: continued xerostomia, caries from radiation, trismus, osteoradionecrosis (discussed later); altered growth and arrested tooth development occur in children.
3. Chemotherapy:
   a. Acute (short-term) complications: mucositis (discussed later), myelosuppression, infection.
   b. Long-term complications: NONE after chemotherapy is completed and acute complications are resolved.
B. *Systemic* cancer concerns (requiring chemotherapy and/or bone marrow transplantation, monoclonal antibody therapy):
1. Chemotherapy for systemic malignancies: higher risk for oral complications with leukemia, lymphoma, solid tumors than in chemotherapy for

other malignancies (new therapies are using short-term higher dose therapy in some cases).

2. Monoclonal antibody therapy by infusion (along with drugs, radioactive materials): made in laboratory from a single type of immune system cell to kill or stop cancer growth; complications same as with other treatments.

3. Blood cell or bone marrow transplant: stem cells (immature blood-forming cells) are transplanted by infusion to replace cells that were destroyed during cancer treatment; for complications see below.

4. Complications associated with intensive chemotherapy and/or bone marrow transplantation:
   a. Cytotoxic drug effects include temporary destruction of healthy tissues, including oral mucosa (mucositis).
   b. Myelosuppression results in low WBC count, which increases risk for oral and systemic infections; hemorrhage in response to low platelet counts and clotting factors may also occur; measured by ANC.
   c. Include temporary xerostomia, loss of appetite, nausea, pain, fatigue, graft-versus-host disease in bone marrow transplant.

C. **Oral mucositis** (OM): MOST common side effect of radiation and/or chemotherapy; painful inflammation and ulceration of mucous membranes lining digestive tract, including oral cavity.

1. Treatment is MAINLY palliative; palifermin (Kepivance), human keratinocyte growth factor (KGF) for severe OM, has been shown to enhance healing; sucking crushed ice (cryotherapy) is alternative.

2. Complications caused by ulcerations:
   a. Can become infected by virus, bacteria, or fungus; may act as site for local infection and portal of entry for oral flora that, in some instances, may cause septicemia (especially in immunosuppressed).
   b. Pain and loss of taste perception make it MORE difficult to eat, which leads to increased weight loss.
   c. In approximately half with OM, it becomes so severe that it is dose limiting; planned cancer treatment must then be modified, thus compromising prognosis.

D. **Osteoradionecrosis:** bone (can include jaws, ONJ) that has died as complication of radiation therapy; damage to the small arteries reduces circulation, depriving bone of oxygen and other necessary nutrients.

1. Increased risk in cancer patients who are receiving high doses and longer therapy with IV (possibly oral) bisphosphonates for repair of primary and metastatic bone lesions and have undergone dentoalveolar trauma (such as with extractions or periodontal disease).

2. Process is gradual and may take many months or years to appear.

3. Surgery to the affected area (including oral surgery) may not allow healing.

4. Treatment: antibiotics and passibly hyperbaric oxygen therapy that produces new blood vessels in the irradiated area and stimulates wound healing.

E. Barriers to oral care:
1. Oncologists often recommend not brushing the teeth when blood counts are low and discourage dental visits to avoid the risk of infection (controversial).

2. Psychosocial concerns, complex treatment schedules, fatigue disrupting dental recall schedules.

F. Dental hygiene care:
1. *Before* cancer treatment:
   a. Assess condition of teeth, periodontal structures, oral hygiene, previous interest in dental care, psychosocial factors.
   b. If patient is scheduled for radiation therapy to the jaw bones:
      (1) Teeth can NEVER be extracted safely from irradiated bone.
      (2) Determine, with supervising dentist, which teeth can be maintained.
   c. Oral hygiene education: dental biofilm control and gentle (nonalcoholic) mouthrinses.
   d. Nutrition and dietary counseling essential; tobacco cessation recommended.
   e. Mineralizing fluoride and calcium products:
      (1) If undergoing radiation therapy to salivary glands, needs daily prescription-strength fluoride gel in brush-on form or custom fluoride trays, as well as calcium products, for mineralization.
      (2) With temporary xerostomia during chemotherapy, may benefit from OTC mineralizing fluoride and calcium products.
   f. Instrumentation SHOULD include scaling, removal of overhangs, smoothing of rough restorations.

2. *During* cancer treatment:
   a. Design alternative dental biofilm control measures for those with OM and forbidden by oncologist to use toothbrush and floss.
   b. Counsel daily cleansing and denture removal before sleep.
   c. Suggest measures to relieve xerostomia and topical anesthetics or coating agents for OM; since xerostomia is not drug related, can recommend use of prescription cholinergic agonist drugs such as pilocarpine (Salagen) and cevimeline (Evoxac).
   d. Assist with selection of nonirritating and noncariogenic foods and tobacco cessation.
   e. Encourage continued fluoride and calcium product application.

3. *After* cancer therapy:
  a. If received radiation therapy to salivary glands and/or jaw bones:
     (1) Encourage frequent recalls, scheduled according to individual need, for prophylaxis and homecare evaluation.
     (2) Encourage palliative measures for xerostomia and stimulation of saliva or consider prescriptions (discussed earlier).
     (3) Reinforce need to continue daily fluoride and calcium product applications; encourage excellent homecare.
     (4) Recommend daily jaw exercises to prevent trismus.
     (5) Discuss nutritional care and provide tobacco cessation counseling.
     (6) Caution to avoid ALL future surgical procedures to irradiated bone.
  b. If received chemotherapy and/or bone marrow transplantation:
     (1) Monitor blood counts until recovers from immunosuppression; place on regular dental hygiene recall.
     (2) Encourage excellent oral hygiene.
     (3) Consider mineralizing fluoride and calcium products until xerostomia is resolved.
     (4) Provide tobacco cessation counseling.

CLINICAL STUDY

Age	55 YRS		Scenario
Sex	☒ Male ☐ Female		The patient has a well-fitting maxillary partial denture. Teeth #6 through #11 have localized moderate chronic periodontitis, and teeth #19 through #29 have localized severe chronic periodontitis. Dental biofilm level is moderate, with heavy calculus and stain. He brushes his teeth twice daily and rinses with Listerine once each day.
Height	5'11"		
Weight	222 LBS		
BP	120/80		
Chief Complaint	"What can I do to make sure my teeth survive this therapy?"		
Medical History	Stage III squamous cell carcinoma of the retromolar pad and left lateral tongue, with metastasis to left side of the neck Scheduled to receive a 7000-cGy dose of radiation therapy Drinks alcohol occasionally and smokes two packages of cigarettes daily		
Current Medications	None		
Social History	Mission minister who has been overseas for 20 years		

1. Identify five acute complications that this patient may experience as result of radiation therapy.
2. Name common long-term complications associated with radiation therapy to the head and neck.
3. What dental and dental hygiene treatments should be completed before the initiation of radiation therapy?
4. Two years after radiation therapy the patient complains of pain in the left mandible and an open sore beneath his denture. What may be the problem?

1. Five acute complications that the patient may experience as result of radiation therapy include thickened saliva (which causes dry mouth), alteration in taste sensation, oral mucositis (OM, inflamed tissue), *Candida* infection, muscle tightness (trismus).
2. Common long-term complications associated with radiation therapy to the head and neck include xerostomia (dry mouth resulting from salivary hypofunction), osteoradionecrosis (nonhealing tissues and bone), trismus that limits mouth opening, temporomandibular joint pain, and rampant caries in remaining teeth.
3. Before initiation of radiation therapy, all mandibular teeth should be extracted and bone and tissues should be allowed to heal; all remaining teeth should be thoroughly scaled as needed to remove deposits and promote healing. Maxillary denture must be cleaned twice daily, and patient should be instructed on the importance of meticulous homecare, including toothbrushing and flossing. Custom fluoride trays should be fabricated and tobacco cessation encouraged. Patient should be encouraged to use another mouthrinse that does not contain alcohol (Listerine does unless labeled otherwise), although gentle mechanical removal of dental biofilm is the most important factor in keeping his oral health.

4. The patient later complains of pain in the left mandible and open sore beneath denture, most likely caused by denture irritation and osteoradionecrosis, respectively. Patient should be immediately referred to oral surgeon who is aware that patient has undergone radiation therapy to the area.

Diseases of Cardiovascular System

Coronary heart disease, cerebrovascular disease, and hypertension are the three MOST common diseases of CVS. American College of Cardiology (ACC) and AHA suggest the evaluation of cardiac risk during dental care using major clinical predictors, rather than relying on time passed since cardiac event. They recommend determining functional capacity (FC), which is measured in metabolic (MET) equivalents such as ability to (1) climb flight of stairs; (2) walk up a hill; (3) run short distance (these activities that are all equal to 4 METs). Will need a medical consult for ALL with history or presence of cardiovascular disease (CVD) before dental care. See CD-ROM for a WebLink to ACC/AHA 2007 guidelines on perioperative cardiovascular evaluation and care for noncardiac surgery.

- See Chapters 8, Microbiology and Immunology: CVS infections; 9, Pharmacology: cardiac drugs; 10, Medical and Dental Emergencies: CVS emergencies, vital signs; 16, Special Needs Patient Care: stroke patient.

A. Coronary artery atherosclerosis (coronary heart disease [CHD]):
1. Etiology: primary injury to the endothelium of artery leads to deposition of platelets and serum lipoproteins and to proliferation of smooth muscle cells in artery wall.
2. May have anginal episodes; considered unstable or severe if not relieved by rest.
3. Complications: plaque formation may lead to occlusion of coronary arteries, which may result in myocardial infarction (MI, heart attack); MI considered a MAJOR clinical predictor of increased perioperative CVD risk; acute if less than 7 days previously and recent if more than 7 days but less than 1 month.
4. Risk factors: sex, heredity, diet, hypertension, smoking, obesity, DM.
5. Treatment: drugs to lower serum lipid levels and blood pressure, reduction of risk factors, bypass surgery, heart transplant.
6. Association of periodontal disease with established CHD, thus the emphasis on oral health to decrease risk of further damage to the CVS.

B. Cerebrovascular disease (CVD): atherosclerosis of blood vessels in the brain; may result in cerebrovascular accident (CVA, stroke).

C. Hypertension (high blood pressure [HBP]): multifactorial disease that involves heredity and environment;

may have significant effects on many organs, including heart, kidneys, blood vessels, brain:
1. Essential (idiopathic, primary) with unknown etiology; secondary results from such diseases as renal disease and damage and DM.
2. Treatment: drug therapy and environmental manipulation.

D. Congenital heart disease: malformation of the heart and blood vessels that occurs during fetal development:
1. Includes defects of valves, ventricular septum, atrial septum, and patent ductus arteriosus, displacement of the great vessels of the heart.
2. Etiology: heredity; infection with rubella or taking of drugs during pregnancy.
3. May have difficulty with exertion, inhibited growth.
4. May require antibiotic premedication before invasive dental procedures.

E. Cardiac dysrhythmia: irregular heartbeat caused by unreliable sinoatrial node, cardiac arrest, various dysrhythmias, heart blockage, or other disease:
1. Treatment consists of drugs and/or implantation of pacemaker.
2. Antibiotic premedication during FIRST 6 months after pacemaker implantation.
3. NO contraindication to ultrasonic because of shielding (ALL are shielded, ONLY metal detectors are a problem); AVOID electronic pulp testing.

F. Congestive heart failure (CHF): failure of diseased heart to meet needs of the body; causes fluids to build up in body tissues:
1. Etiology: related to underlying heart valve damage, ischemic heart disease.
2. Symptoms: shortness of breath with minimal exertion, fatigue, ankle and/or abdominal swelling.
3. Causes of sudden death: dysrhythmias, pulmonary embolism, acute myocarditis, acute hypertensive crisis.

G. Oral signs: no greater than for others unless patient is severely debilitated; certain drugs (calcium channel blockers) are associated with gingival hyperplasia.

H. Risk factors: infection (rheumatic or congenital heart disease), side effects of drugs, vasoconstrictors (lowered amounts), increased risk of emergency.

I. Barriers to care: transportation difficulties when the condition restricts mobility; may need to rely on others; economic issues may be present if income is restricted because of disability or fixed income.

J. Professional care risks are determined *after* medical consult:
1. Antibiotic premedication may be needed before invasive dental procedures.
2. Withhold emergency or elective surgery (or periodontal procedures by dental hygienist) for 4 to 6 weeks after MI and determine FC.

3. Dental care should be delayed unless patient <u>can meet 4 METs capacity</u> and/or further medical testing has been completed to quantify level of cardiac risk in treatment.
4. Use of stress reduction protocol that includes adequate pain control, pretreatment with anxiety premedication, use of nitrous oxide sedation (see Chapter 14, Pain Management).
5. Continued use of concurrent drug therapy, which possibly includes statins, as well as antiplatelet therapy.
6. Caution when administering local anesthetics because of possible interactions with drugs (see Chapter 14, Pain Management).
7. Adjusting chair appropriately (more upright, 45°) because some are NOT able to recline in supine position.
8. Long appointments should be avoided with CVD; blood pressure is lowest in the afternoon so appointments then or when patient is well rested are preferred.

K. Patient or caregiver education: daily meticulous homecare, frequent dental recall, need to take <u>antibiotic premedication</u> *before* appointments and cardiac drugs *as* prescribed.

Respiratory Diseases

Asthma and chronic obstructive pulmonary disease (COPD) are significant respiratory diseases. Lung cancer and cystic fibrosis are also discussed. Will need <u>medical consult</u> with respiratory disease or its history before dental care.

- See Chapters 8, Microbiology and Immunology: tuberculosis; 9, Pharmacology: respiratory disorder and disease drugs; 10, Medical and Dental Emergencies: respiratory emergencies in the dental setting.

A. Asthma: severe bronchoconstriction that results in airway obstruction.
1. Dental complications:
   a. Local anesthetics that contain vasoconstrictors (sulfite preservatives, vasoconstrictor antioxidants) or sulfite compounds, such as articaine (Septocaine, Zorcaine), should NOT be administered because of risk of allergic reactions.
   b. Can be sedated with nitrous oxide because of increased levels of oxygen present and relaxation effects.
   c. May use inhaler for acute attacks; patient should be instructed to rinse the mouth thoroughly after using and expectorate to avoid increasing systemic absorption and reduce tooth staining and taste alteration; bring to appointments in case of emergency need.
   d. Use acetaminophen (FIRST choice) as substitute for its analgesic and antipyretic effects to avoid aspirin-induced attack.

2. Treatment: adrenergic agonists (beta$_2$ agonists), corticosteroid inhalers, methylxanthines, anticholinergics, cromolyn (Intal, Nasalcrom).

B. Chronic irreversible airway obstruction (COPD): occurs with BOTH chronic bronchitis and emphysema.
1. Bronchitis:
   a. Acute: bronchitis: infection caused by viruses and bacteria; may last several days or weeks and lead to chronic condition.
   b. Chronic: cigarette smoking or breathing fumes and dusts causes chronic inflammation of airways and excess sputum, with cough (productive, yellow or greenish mucus), dyspnea (shortness of breath), chest tightness.
2. Emphysema: destruction of alveoli; airspace enlargement and airway collapse.
   a. Etiology: MOST commonly cigarette smoking.
   b. Chronic cough, trouble breathing during exercise, hard to catch breath, barrel-chest appearance (caused by using accessory muscles for respiration).
   c. Dental management focuses on prevention of respiratory depression.
      (1) More upright chair position may be necessary (45°).
      (2) Relative contraindication for nitrous oxide sedation from respiratory depressive effects of high oxygen administration (NO contraindication to local anesthetic use); need <u>medical consult</u>.
      (3) Rubber dam use may result in the feeling of compromised air exchange; provide low continuous flow of oxygen during treatment.
      (4) Concurrent CVD may require special management.
      (5) Oral signs: drug related and may include *Candida* infection and xerostomia.
   d. Treatment: palliative and to prevent complications; may include tobacco cessation, reduction of respiratory allergens and irritants, inhalation therapy with bronchodilators (inhalers), oxygen, drugs (adrenergic agonists, methylxanthines, corticosteroids, anticholinergics), possibly surgery.

C. Lung cancer: squamous cell carcinoma, adenocarcinoma, small cell carcinoma, or large cell undifferentiated carcinoma; either develops in lungs or metastasizes to lungs from lymph nodes or other sites (e.g., oral cavity).
1. Etiology: associated with tobacco (cigarette, pipe smoking, spit [smokeless] tobacco) or other pollutants (e.g., uranium, asbestos).
2. Symptoms include chronic coughing, coughing up blood, frequent pulmonary infections, Cushing's

syndrome, clubbing of fingers, dyspnea, weight loss.

3. Treatment: tobacco cessation, surgical removal of cancerous site, chemotherapy and/or radiation therapy.

D. Cystic fibrosis (CF): autosomal recessive hereditary disease that affects mainly lungs and digestive system, causing progressive disability:
   1. Thick mucus production and incompetent immune system; results in frequent lung infections.
   2. Diminished secretion of pancreatic enzymes causes poor growth, fatty diarrhea, fat-soluble vitamin deficiencies.
   3. Treatment: no cure; early death (twenties to thirties); lung transplant as worsens.

E. Oral signs of respiratory disease: xerostomia and candidiasis from inhalants or other drugs, ulcerations, lymphadenopathy.

F. Risk factors for respiratory disease:
   1. Infections, especially with long-term steroid use.
   2. Exposure to asthma provokers, such as sulfites and stress.
   3. Dyspnea breathing in supine position, may need to sit MORE upright (especially during emergency care) at 45°.
   4. Persistent coughing.
   5. Risk of lung infection with aspiration of aerosols from ultrasonics because of immunosuppression; aerosol use should be minimized; condition should be observed at all times.
   6. Relative contraindications (need <u>medical consult</u>):
      a. Use of sedatives, antihistamines, aspirin (EXCEPTION is asthma).
      b. Tranquilizers, nitrous oxide sedation, general anesthetics (EXCEPTION is asthma).

G. Barriers to care for respiratory diseases:
   1. Lack of communication because of embarrassment about condition (e.g., tuberculosis, emphysema).
   2. Transportation difficulties, if walking even short distances is difficult.
   3. Weather may exacerbate certain respiratory conditions and may require rescheduling of appointments.

H. Professional care and homecare for respiratory diseases:
   1. Recognition of communicability of tuberculosis and need to avoid aerosol production.
   2. Awareness of and ability to deal with respiratory difficulties associated with asthma and COPD.
   3. Need for relaxed dental environment to prevent asthmatic and other complications.
   4. Placement of drugs, especially bronchodilators, in close proximity.

5. Overall health and options for fatal prognosis of lung cancer and CF.

I. Patient or caregiver education: need for meticulous oral hygiene, daily mineralizing fluoride and calcium supplementation as needed, saliva substitutes, increased water intake for xerostomia.

Renal Disease

Renal disease is disease of the kidney, which alters filtering ability. It is caused by infection, autoimmune disease, or developmental disorder. Patients have unusually high levels of toxic urine components in blood. As disease worsens, may need dialysis to clean the blood and prevent death. With renal disease or its history, will need a <u>medical consult</u> before dental care; may need *antianxiety, antibiotic,* or *steroidal premedication.*

• See Chapter 3, Anatomy, Biochemistry, and Physiology, renal system.

A. Oral signs:
   1. Mucositis, candidiasis, hemorrhage, petechiae.
   2. If oral hygiene is poor, increase in dental caries, calculus development, periodontal disease.
   3. Halitosis, enamel hypocalcification.

B. Risk factors: infections, malnutrition, possible drug interactions, metabolism.

C. Barriers to care: economic; finances may be limited because of high medical costs and inability to maintain employment.

D. Professional care and homecare:
   1. Need to check vital signs and prevent drug interactions; do NOT use same arm as for shunt.
   2. May need *antianxiety, antibiotic,* or *steroidal premedication* because of shunt or organ transplant (all determined with <u>medical consult</u>).
   3. Tendency for bleeding; dental treatment after dialysis and NOT before; NO treatment on day of dialysis because of drugs given (anticoagulants).
   4. Possible interactions with local anesthetics (metabolism difficulties); may need reduced amounts.
   5. Slow healing.

E. Patient or caregiver education:
   1. Meticulous oral hygiene to reduce the incidence of infection.
   2. Frequent recall appointments for examination and prophylaxis.
   3. Daily mineralizing fluoride and calcium product supplementation.
   4. Dentifrices with antigingivitis, anticaries, anticalculus properties, unless mucosal irritation results.

Gastrointestinal Disease

Gastrointestinal (GIT) diseases include gastroesophageal reflux disease (GERD), ulcers. Both diagnosed by upper gastrointestinal (GI) radiographic series (barium) and/or endoscope. May need a <u>medical consult</u> for all patients with GIT disease if there are any questions before dental care.

- See Chapter 3, Anatomy, Biochemistry, and Physiology: GIT system.

A. GERD: mucosal damage produced by abnormal reflux in esophagus:
  1. Caused by transient or permanent changes in barrier between esophagus and stomach.
  2. Heartburn caused by acid in esophagus, burning discomfort behind breastbone (sternum), cough, hoarseness, voice changes, chronic earache, burning chest pains, nausea, or sinusitis.
  3. Complications: stricture formation, Barrett's esophagus, and esophageal ulcers; could even lead to esophageal cancer, especially in adults >60 years old.
  4. Treatment: physicians recommend lifestyle modifications (weight loss and diet change, sleeping on left side and elevating head) in addition to or instead of H2-receptor antagonists and/or proton pump inhibitors.

B. Peptic ulcer disease (PUD): sore on lining of stomach or duodenum, beginning of small intestine:
  1. Caused by bacterial infection *(Helicobacter pylori)* or use of long-term nonsteroidal antiinflammatory drugs (NSAIDs), such as aspirin (Empirin) and ibuprofen (Advil, Motrin, Pamprin).
     a. *H. pylori* weakens protective mucous coating, allowing acid to get through to sensitive lining beneath, with both acid and bacteria irritating lining and causing ulceration; diagnosed through blood, breath, stool, tissue tests.
  2. Dull, gnawing ache comes and goes for several days or weeks in empty stomach (2 to 3 hours after meal, middle of night); relieved by eating and antacids.
  3. Complications: perforation, bleeding, or obstruction of gastric portions.
  4. Treatment: combination of proton pump inhibitors with two antibiotics (e.g., clarithromycin [Biaxin], amoxicillin [Amoxil, Larotid, Polymox], metronidazole [Flagyl]), and possibly three if severe case.

Neurological Disorders

Many diseases affect the nervous system, especially the central nervous system (CNS) and its cranial nerves. May need medical consult with neurological disorder or history if there are any questions before dental care.

- See Chapters 10, Medical and Dental Emergencies: seizure; 16, Special Needs Patient Care: neurological and orthopedic disabilities.

A. Trigeminal neuralgia (tic douloureux): unilateral severe pain triggered by touch (trigger zone[s]).
  1. Unknown etiology, with damage to myelin sheath, results in erratic or excessive electrical impulses, activating pain regions or deactivating pain inhibitory regions in brain, associated with maxillary and mandibular divisions of fifth cranial (trigeminal) nerve.
  2. MOST in women ≥50 years.
  3. Treatment: surgery reserved for severe conditions; ice pack over area to numb it; drugs:
     a. Anticonvulsants are MOST effective; pain relievers usually do NOT help; may be potentiated with adjuvant such as muscle relaxer and antispastic agent baclofen (Kemstro and Lioresal) or clonazepam (Klonopin); baclofen may also help patient eat more normally if jaw movement tends to aggravate symptoms.
     b. If anticonvulsants and surgical options have both failed or are ruled out as to use, pain may be treated long term with opioid such as methadone (Dolophine); low doses of some antidepressants can be effective in treating neuropathic pain; may try Botox injections.

B. Bell's palsy (facial palsy): temporary unilateral facial paralysis, with drooping on affected half.
  1. Unknown etiology; may be an infection involving nerve tissue; usually resolves in 2 weeks.
  2. Malfunction of seventh cranial nerve (facial) that controls the muscles of facial expression.
  3. Treatment: palliative, possibly prednisone (Deltasone and/or acyclovir (Zovirax); eye care is imperative to prevent complications.

C. Epilepsy (seizure disorder): common chronic neurological group of disorders; with recurrent unprovoked seizures:
  1. Unknown etiology, with episodic abnormal electrical activity in brain.
  2. Treatment: anticonvulsant drugs (antiepileptic drugs [AEDs]) can be taken daily to prevent seizures altogether or reduce frequency.
     a. ALL have side effects that are idiosyncratic and others that are dosage dependent.
     b. NOT possible to predict who will suffer from side effects or at what dose the side effects will appear.
  3. Systemic signs:
     a. Aura (predication) for oncoming seizure (includes lights, sounds, smells).
     b. Seizures:
        (1) Petit mal: simple type with staring, trembling, or jerking motions with NO loss of consciousness.
        (2) Grand mal: complex type with a trance-like stage, impairment of consciousness, involuntary motor movements followed by confusion, irritability, extreme fatigue, NO memory of the seizure.
        (3) Status epilepticus: life-threatening condition in which the brain is in a state of persistent

seizure, with either continuous unremitting seizure lasting longer than 5 to 10 minutes or recurrent seizures without regaining consciousness between seizures for >30 minutes; associated with poor compliance (adherence to medication regimen), alcohol withdrawal, metabolic disturbances, and possibly a tumor or abscess.

4. Oral signs and concerns:
   a. Gingival hyperplasia resulting from phenytoin (Dilantin) use; dental biofilm control is vital for prevention and limitation of gingival overgrowth.
   b. Trauma from seizure activity such as cheek, tongue, or lip biting, falling, and tooth chipping (from biting instruments or clenching teeth).
   c. Risk factors:
      (1) Trauma from seizure activity during dental procedures.
      (2) Development of gingival hyperplasia because of phenytoin (Dilantin) use; surgical excision of gingival overgrowth may be required.
      (3) Drowsiness from drug usage; may inhibit memory.
      (4) Drug interactions (e.g., between phenytoin and barbiturates, doxycycline, others).
   d. Barriers to care:
      (1) Economic cost, particularly if disability affects employability.
      (2) Lack of transportation, if unable to drive.
      (3) Lack of communication, if fear of or embarrassment about having a seizure in public is strong.
   e. Professional care and homecare:
      (1) Frequent (even monthly) oral prophylaxis, depending on severity of the gingival condition.
      (2) Calm atmosphere, with careful preparation for dental appointments; medical consult may be necessary.
      (3) Demonstration and explanation of thorough homecare procedures, including sulcular brushing and flossing.
   f. Patient or caregiver education:
      (1) Discussion of oral health and need for excellent oral biofilm control.
      (2) Repetition of instruction if memory is impaired by drugs.
      (3) Positive reinforcement to bolster self-esteem.

D. Tourette syndrome (TS): inherited neuropsychiatric disorder with onset in childhood, characterized by presence of multiple physical (motor) tics (sudden, repetitive, stereotyped, nonrhythmic movements, such as eye blinking, coughing, throat clearing, sniffing, facial movements) and at least one vocal (phonic) tic. In most cases medication is unnecessary; no effective medication for every case of tics, but there are medications and therapies that can help when use is warranted, although many have severe side effects.

E. Glaucoma: group of eye diseases of second (II) cranial nerve (optic nerve), involve loss of retinal ganglion cells in characteristic pattern of optic neuropathy.
   1. Etiology: raised intraocular pressure is significant risk factor, as well as age, family history, race (African-American, Asian), diabetes mellitus, or gender (female); may be due to unstable ocular blood flow, possibly related to hypertension (high blood pressure).
   2. Visual signs: involves loss of visual field; often occurs gradually and may be recognized ONLY when advanced; once lost, damaged visual field can never be recovered; glaucoma is second leading cause of blindness.
   3. Diagnosis: dilated eye examination to check nerve; includes measurements of intraocular pressure via tonometry, changes in size and shape of eye, and examination of nerve to look for visible damage; if damage is suspected, formal visual field test should be performed.
   4. Treatment: if intraocular pressure is present, can be lowered with drugs, usually eye drops (like pilocarpine), or surgery if severe; poor compliance with drugs and follow-up visits is MAJOR reason for vision loss. Some drugs may have "hidden beta blockers"; therefore patient might experience xerostomia (dry mouth).

F. Neurofibromatosis type 1 (NF-1) (von Recklinghausen's disease): rare genetic (autosomal dominant) disorder affects nerve cell growth, with multiple cutaneous and subcutaneous tumors that appear in late childhood and medium-brown, flat discolorations of the skin, known as café-au-lait spots.

Immunological Disorders

Immunological disorders include hypersensitivity, acquired immune deficiency, erythema multiforme, lichen planus, and various autoimmune diseases. Will need medical consult for patients with immunological disorder before dental care.
• See Chapter 8, Microbiology and Immunology: immunology and HIV/AIDS.
A. Hypersensitivity (allergy):
   1. Allergic response that varies from a slight cell-mediated response to anaphylaxis.
   2. Mucositis and dermatitis (rash, hives) on oral mucosa and skin; reaction from rubber latex contact may occur in BOTH patients and healthcare providers.

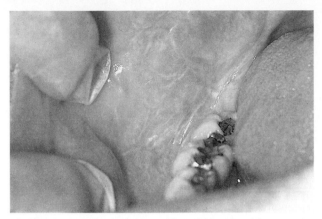

Figure 6-5   Lichen planus with Wickham's striae on the buccal mucosa.

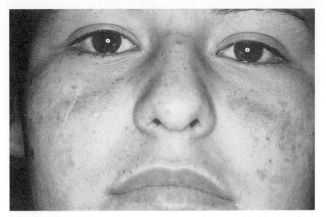

Figure 6-6   Systemic lupus erythematosus with "butterfly" rash over bridge of nose.

3. Treatment: ranges from none to drugs such as diphenhydramine (Benadryl) and epinephrine and medical assistance for emergency conditions (see Chapter 10, Medical and Dental Emergencies).

B. Erythema multiforme (EM): may affect both oral mucosa and skin (epidermoid bullosa).
 1. Lesions on skin resemble a target, consisting of concentric rings of erythema (redness), alternating with normal color.
 2. Oral: red **macules** and ulcerations with hemorrhagic crusting of lips.
 3. MOST in young adults and males; severe form is Stevens-Johnson syndrome.
 4. Treatment: topical corticosteroids.

C. Lichen planus: benign, chronic disease that affects skin and oral mucosa (Figure 6-5).
 1. Forms: atrophic, reticular, erosive, plaquelike:
  a. Reticular form: thin white lines called Wickham's striae MAINLY on buccal mucosa; consist of white papules in linear form.
  b. Erosive form: large, painful ulcerations.
 2. Associated with hepatitis C virus; develops after exposure to potential allergens such as drugs, dyes, other chemicals.
 3. Symptoms increased with emotional stress, possibly because of related changes in immune system.
 4. Biopsy reveals that epithelial layer has separated from connective tissue in erosive and bulbous forms.
 5. Treatment: ranges from palliative to help speed healing of the skin lesions to drug therapy:
  a. If symptoms are slight, NO treatment may be needed.
  b. Possible risk of cancerous change.
 6. Drug therapy:
  a. Antihistamines, topical corticosteroids (such as triamcinolone [Azmacort]) or oral corticosteroids (such as prednisone [Deltasone]) to reduce inflammation and suppress immune responses.

b. Corticosteroids may be injected directly into a lesion.
c. Topical retinoic acid cream (Retin-A, form of vitamin A) and other ointments and creams with occlusive dressings may reduce itching and inflammation and aid healing.
d. Lidocaine mouthwashes may anesthetize mouth temporarily, making eating more comfortable with erosive forms.
e. Ultraviolet (UV) light therapy.

D. Hodgkin's lymphoma: malignancy (cancer) of lymph tissue found in lymph nodes, spleen, liver, bone marrow.
 1. Etiology: unknown; MOST common at 15 to 35 and 50 to 70 years old.
 2. FIRST sign is enlarged lymph node, which appears without a known cause; can spread to nearby lymph nodes and later may spread to the lungs, liver, or bone marrow.
 3. Diagnosis: lymph node biopsy with Reed-Sternberg cells.
 4. Treatment: radiation and chemotherapy.

E. Autoimmune diseases: common in women:
 1. Scleroderma: chronic disease with excessive deposits of collagen in the skin and other organs.
  a. MOST evident symptom is hardening of the skin and oral mucosa with associated scarring; can also have Raynaud's syndrome, vasoconstricting disorder affecting fingers and toes.
  b. Can be fatal as result of heart, kidney, lung, or intestinal damage.
  c. Presence of detectable antinuclear antibody.
 2. Systemic lupus erythematosus (SLE): chronic and progressive disease that affects oral mucosa, skin, organs.
  a. Displays classic sign of "butterfly" rash over bridge of nose, also arthritis, dermatitis, glomerulonephritis, anemia, inflamed spleen and/or lymph nodes; if ONLY rash, discoid form (Figure 6-6).

b. Autoantibodies to own deoxyribonucleic acid (DNA) (antinuclear antibodies).

c. MOST common cause of death: kidney failure (degeneration of kidneys).

3. Benign mucous membrane pemphigoid (BMMP) (cicatricial pemphigoid): rare chronic, vesicular disease of oral cavity.

a. Produces **bullae** (large **vesicles**) that rupture easily; cause discomfort; MOST often on gingiva (desquamative gingivitis).

b. May produce positive Nikolsky's sign (tissue desquamation with gentle pressure, LESS common than with pemphigus), areas of ulceration; some forms leave scarring (less common in oral cavity) that can cause blindness.

c. Affects older adults, women MORE than men; biopsy reveals oral epithelium separated from lamina propria.

d. Treatment: a team of medical specialists is required for overall care; primary aim is to stop vesicle formation, promote healing, and prevent scarring (cicatricial form is difficult to treat because it can affect so many different parts of the body).

4. Pemphigus vulgaris: autoimmune disease that affects skin and oral mucosa (NOT as much as BMMP).

a. Intraepithelial formation of bullae that do NOT rupture easily, possibly positive Nikolsky's sign (MORE common than with pemphigoid,-BMMP); smear shows Tzanck cells.

b. Biopsy reveals breakdown of cellular adhesion between epithelial cells (acantholysis affecting desmosomes and hemidesmosomes), which allows symptoms to develop; MOST in middle age.

c. Treatment: corticosteroids.

5. Sjögren's syndrome: affects salivary and lacrimal glands, resulting in decrease in BOTH saliva and tears.

a. Has xerostomia *and* xerophthalmia (dry eyes).

b. May have parotid gland enlargement and Raynaud's syndrome, vasoconstricting disorder affecting fingers and toes (pain with bluish coloring).

c. Rheumatoid arthritis also present or other autoimmune disease; positive reaction to rheumatoid (RA) factor, antibody to IgG (see Chapter 16, Special Needs Patient Care).

d. Treatment: palliative; nonsteroidal antiinflammatory agents are used for arthritis; in severe cases gold injections, corticosteroids, other immunosuppressive drugs; can recommend use of prescription drugs such as pilocarpine (Salagen) and cevimeline (Evoxac), since dryness is not drug related.

CLINICAL STUDY

Age	65 YRS	Scenario
Sex	☐ Male ☒ Female	The patient states that this condition has occurred several times during the past few years. Visual examination of her oral cavity reveals several erythematous areas surrounding grayish white lesions on the gingiva. A negative Nikolsky's sign is also noted during the intraoral examination. Patient does not mention any other new health problems.
Height	5'2"	
Weight	121 LBS	
BP	110/74	
Chief Complaint	"My mouth burns and my gums are bleeding all the time now. And when I eat, the blisters in my mouth break open."	
Medical History	Past history of polio as a child	
Current Medications	ibuprofen for backaches pm	
Social History	Dry cleaning business owner, widow	

1. What is the most likely diagnosis of this patient's condition? Why?

2. Identify the common signs and symptoms associated with this condition.

3. Describe the treatment for this condition.

4. How does the presence of a negative Nikolsky's sign distinguish this condition from pemphigus vulgaris?

5. What other indicators assist in the differential diagnosis?

1. Condition most likely is benign mucous membrane pemphigoid (BMMP), autoimmune disorder that results in development of vesiculobulbous lesions on the gingiva, floor of the mouth, hard palate. Lesions

easily rupture, giving appearance of desquamative gingivitis, causing soreness. Lesions eventually heal, sometimes causing scarring. Tends to occur in older adults; chronic condition with periods of exacerbation and remission.

2. Common signs and symptoms of disorder include vesicles that easily rupture, reddened and ulcerated gingiva, burning, mouth soreness, recurrence of condition after remission, and scarring (however, less in oral cavity). Scarring can involve blindness.

3. Treatment is palliative. During active stages, tooth-brushing may be impossible; thus 0.2% chlorhexidine rinse is recommended. Topical anesthetics may be needed to encourage proper nutrition. Topical and/or systemic corticosteroids are prescribed based on se-verity of condition.

4. Both BMMP and pemphigus vulgaris may exhibit a positive Nikolsky's sign; noted histologically as sepa-ration of surface epithelium from underlying con-nective tissue; clinically shows tissue desquamation (removal) with gentle pressure. However, BMMP is associated with it less often than pemphigus vulgaris.

5. Although biopsy would confirm diagnosis of BMMP rather than pemphigus vulgaris, the fact that she has had previous oral lesions with no mention of skin lesions or other concerns indicates that BMMP is most likely diagnosis. Other autoimmune disorders such as Sjögren's syndrome and lupus erythemato-sus (systemic [SLE] and discoid) may occur in as-sociation with pemphigus vulgaris, as well as skin lesions.

TRAUMATIC ORAL LESIONS

Traumatic injury, by either chemical or physical means, can result in oral lesions. Includes attrition, abrasion, erosion, burns, tobacco-associated lesions, salivary gland obstruc-tion, connective tissue hyperplasias, ulcerations, and others.

• See Chapter 13, Periodontology: occlusal trauma.

A. Attrition: physiological wear of dentition accelerated by abnormal grinding (bruxism) and/or clenching.

1. FIRST sign is disappearance of mamelons and then MAINLY wear facets on cusp tips and incisal edges of anteriors and facets on occlusal cusps of posteri-ors; also staining of dentin-exposed worn surfaces.

2. May also result from abrasion from porcelain crowns, bridges, or denture materials on surfaces of opposing teeth (unrestored, amalgam, resins, etc.), as well as the use of spit (smokeless) tobacco (sand).

3. Bruxism may also be associated with gingival reces-sion, temporomandibular disorders (TMD), hypertro-phy (enlargement) of masseter muscle, mandibular tori, hypersensitivity because of exposed dentin and unsightly stained tooth material.

4. Prevention: occlusal splint (nightguard) and dis-cussion of habits.

5. Treatment: full coverage if restorations and/or tooth structure is compromised.

B. Abrasion: slow wear of dentition associated with abrasive substances, abnormal habit.

1. Caused by improper use of toothbrush and/or abrasive dentifrice; causes notch at exposed root surface, particularly at canine and premolar area.

2. May also be caused by repetitive habit (bobby pins, needles, musical instruments, pipe smokers), especially on incisors.

3. May lead to hypersensitivity because of exposed dentin and increased risk of caries.

4. Prevention: discussion of oral hygiene methods and habits.

5. Treatment: patient education and restorative care if indicated.

C. Erosion: loss of tooth structure because of a chemical action differing from soft tissue erosion after rupture of vesicle or bulla.

1. In bulimia or chemotherapy, result of emesis (vom-iting) of stomach acids, causes loss of enamel on maxillary lingual surfaces of teeth (perimolysis) and rising of existing restorations.

2. May be acid from industrial work (battery, plating, soft drink manufacturing).

3. Also is influenced by diet (citrus sucking, cocaine or methamphetamine use, soft drink overuse, espe-cially diet soft drink because of low pH) and can be noted in early childhood caries (ECC).

4. Prevention: discussion of diet and recommenda-tion for counseling if eating disorder is present.

5. Treatment: removing cause; fluoride and mineral (topical calcium replacement) application; rinsing the mouth with water (NOT brushing in acids) and thoroughly cleaning the teeth immediately after vomiting episodes also lessen effects of acid; may need full-coverage restorative therapy for esthetics and function.

D. Abfraction: wedge-shaped lesions at the cervical areas of teeth (especially premolars).

1. May be related to fatigue, flexure, fracture, and deformation of tooth as the result of biomechanical forces such as grinding [bruxism] and/or clenching, torquing of tooth and/or bite discrepancy.

2. Weakened tooth structure is more at risk for abra-sion, hypersensitivity because of exposed dentin and caries; mainly in older adults.

3. Prevention: occlusal splint (nightguard).

4. Treatment: restorative care with composite or glass ionomer materials, but forces may result in dislodging the restoration.

E. Temporomandibular joint disorder (TMD): con-ditions that affect musculoskelature of joint area; result in pain and dysfunction of masticatory system.

1. May affect muscles ONLY (extracapsular) or joint (intracapsular).
2. Etiology is multifactorial; stress is a frequent factor; others include arthritis, psychological problems, macrotrauma or microtrauma to joint.
3. Four primary diagnostic categories:
   a. Muscle and facial disorders of masticatory system; include trismus, myalgia, spasms, dyskinesia (abnormal movement), bruxism.
   b. Disorders of the TMJ; include conditions that cause internal derangements impeding function of joint (e.g., arthritis) (see Chapter 16, Special Needs Patient Care).
   c. Disorders of mandibular mobility, which include joint adhesions, ankylosis, and muscular fibrosis.
   d. Disorders of maxillomandibular growth, which are less common and include both neoplastic and nonneoplastic conditions.
4. Oral habits can be significant factors in production, especially in acute cases:
   a. Amount of damage produced by habit is relative to intensity and duration.
   b. Bruxism, clenching (see earlier discussion).
5. Signs and symptoms:
   a. Pain and tenderness in muscles of mastication.
   b. Pain and tenderness of the joint itself.
   c. Functional limitation of the joint.
6. Prevention and treatment: bite plane splint, antidepressants, physical therapy; surgery is last resort.
F. Oral burns: initiated by heat or chemical exposure, causing tissue necrosis of oral mucosa; MAINLY from hot foods (bagels in the East, pizza in the Midwest, coffee in the West):
   1. Can also involve "aspirin burn" from aspirin placed on oral mucosa to ease dental pain, phenol from dental procedures, live electric cords, use of hydrogen peroxide if not diluted or strong whitening products.
   2. Include white or ulcerated lesions of the oral mucosa; thermal burns on the palate are red.
   3. Treatment: analgesics, topical anesthetics; severe cases, surgery.
G. Tobacco-related oral lesions:
   1. Spit (smokeless) tobacco (chewer's) lesions: symptomatic, wrinkled, white lesions located in mucobuccal fold at tobacco placement; clinical presentation does NOT indicate level of carcinogenic changes.
   2. Nicotinic stomatitis: whitened hard palate with raised red dots (minor salivary gland inflammation); caused by heat of smoking and/or hot foods.
   3. Treatment: tobacco cessation if needed and possible biopsy to assess for SCC, spit tobacco lesions.

H. Crack cocaine smoking:
   1. Lesions from hot smoke located at midline of hard palate; vary from ulcers to keratotic lesions to exophytic reactive lesions (will also have nasal ulcerations and saddle nose appearance if snorting crack).
   2. Necrotic ulcers of the nose, tongue, and epiglottis related to smoking free-base cocaine have also been reported; epistaxis (nosebleeds) or discharge (constant wiping); saddle nose from chronic use.
   3. Treatment: substance abuse therapy.
I. Salivary gland duct obstruction: obstruction of a salivary gland duct by salivary stone (sialolith) and/or severance of the duct to prevent drainage.
   1. Translucent or bluish (because of fluid within) superficial swelling:
      a. Mucocele: smaller on labial mucosa of lower lip or tongue, involving minor gland.
      b. Ranula: larger on one side of the floor of the mouth; resembles a "frog's belly" with submental swelling related to eating, involving mainly submandibular and sublingual.
   2. Treatment: removal of the obstruction; surgery if necessary.
J. Oral connective tissue hyperplasia (reactive):
   1. Pyogenic granuloma (pregnancy tumor, if female): proliferation of connective and vascular tissue (see Figure 11-7).
      a. Located on gingiva; also on lip, tongue, buccal mucosa.
      b. Formation may be related to hormonal changes (MOST during pregnancy) combined with chronic irritants such as dental biofilm.
      c. SIMILAR in clinical appearance to peripheral giant cell granuloma; however, this lesion contains multinucleated giant cells and may lead to bone destruction.
      d. Treatment: if NOT spontaneously reduced (after birth of child), surgical excision.
   2. Denture-induced hyperplasia: proliferation of connective tissue associated with removable prosthesis.
      a. Two forms:
         (1) Epulis fissuratum: folds of tissue near denture flange (edge) from ill-fitting dentures.
         (2) Inflammatory papillary hyperplasia: nipple-like fibrous papillary projections of tissue located on palate.
      b. Treatment: surgical removal of excess tissue and a prosthesis reline or new denture, if necessary.
   3. Gingival hyperplasia: proliferation of free or attached gingival tissue, in response to local irritants (e.g., dental biofilm, calculus).
      a. Varies from soft to fibrous gingiva; color may also vary from pink to red because of increased vascularity.

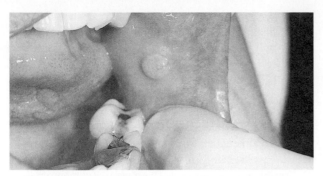

Figure 6-7 Irritation fibroma on the buccal mucosa.

b. Result of hormonal changes, including puberty and pregnancy, hypothyroidism, or heredity; exacerbated by poor oral hygiene.

c. Side effect of certain drugs: phenytoin (Dilantin) for seizures with epilepsy, calcium channel blocker such as nifedipine (Procardia, Adalat, Nifedical) for cardiac disease caused by hypertension (high blood pressure) or angina, immunosuppressant cyclosporine to prevent rejection after transplant of organs and tissue.

d. Can occur with pericoronitis when associated with partially erupted third molars ("wisdom teeth") as a flap of tissue (operculum); has more inflammation and bleeding present.

e. Treatment: gingivoplasty, gingivectomy (including removal of operculum), and oral hygiene instruction; in addition, debridement and irrigation, as well as antibiotic therapy, may be used initially to treat pericoronitis.

4. Irritation fibroma: dense connective tissue growth related to chronic irritation (Figure 6-7):
   a. Asymptomatic, exophytic growth with color similar to that of adjacent tissues.
   b. Located on the buccal or labial mucosa, gingiva, tongue.
   c. Treatment: surgical removal and possibly biopsy to rule out malignancy.

5. Frictional keratosis: chronic rubbing and friction against an oral mucosal surface may result in hyperkeratosis.
   a. Results in an opaque, white appearance and represents a protective response.
   b. Treatment: identification of trauma, eliminating cause, observing resolution; may take awhile to resolve on keratinized surfaces (e.g., attached gingiva), possible biopsy to rule out malignancy.

K. Oral ulcerations:
   1. Recurrent aphthous ulcers (RAU, "canker sores") that heal within 7 to 10 days:
      a. Painful oral lesions on lining mucosa (unattached nonkeratinized such as buccal and labial mucosa); in contrast, herpes lesions ("fever blisters") on masticatory oral mucosa (attached keratinized such as attached gingiva, hard palate).
      b. MOST often recur and may be associated with history of trauma (sharp food, toothbrush edge) or emotional stress; may be immune or bacteria related; increased incidence during tobacco cessation.
      c. Forms:
         (1) Minor: single lesion ≤1 cm in diameter; MOST common form; treated by antibacterial topical application with occlusal dressing.
         (2) Major: single lesion ≥1 cm in diameter; more destructive and can cause scarring; treated by application of topical steroids during prodromal and preulcerative period.
         (3) Herpetiform: small clusters of lesions; may coalesce into larger irregular lesions.
      d. Prevention: avoiding causative factor.
      e. Treatment: protection of lesion and topical antiseptic to reduce secondary infection.
   2. Traumatic ulcers: result of occlusal trauma (biting), irritation from orthodontic and removable appliances, trauma from food.
      a. Diagnosed using history; heal within 2 weeks (rule out carcinomatous growth).
      b. Treatment: removing cause of trauma; may need biopsy if clinically suspect.
   3. Blood-related lesions with NO treatment because they resolve by healing (may need to reassure patient):
      a. Hematoma ("blood blister"): red to purple mass produced by accumulation of blood within tissue resulting from trauma to a large blood vessel (e.g., lesion after local anesthetic injection, especially inferior alveolar nerve block, or after extraction of a difficult tooth).
      b. Ecchymosis ("bruise"): reddened to purple area with slight height; changes color during breakdown of clot.
      c. Petechiae: red spots caused by escape of small amount of blood.

L. Necrotizing sialometaplasia: benign necrotic condition of salivary glands.
   1. Moderately painful prolonged swelling and ulceration at junction of hard and soft palates.
   2. Caused by blockage of the blood supply to the area of the lesion that heals slowly; deep biopsy may be needed to confirm diagnosis.
   3. Treatment: palliative.

M. Traumatic neuroma: injury to peripheral nerve resulting from anesthetic injection, oral surgery, or other trauma.
   1. Painful lesion on palpation or constant pain possible in adults; MOST common in mental foramen region.

2. Diagnosis based on a biopsy and microscopic examination.
3. Treatment: surgical removal; recurrence is rare.
N. Amalgam tattoo:
1. Flat, bluish gray lesion of oral mucosa caused by amalgam particles embedded into tissues during restorative procedures; may have radiopaque appearance.
2. MOST on the gingiva and edentulous alveolar ridge of mandibular posterior region.
3. Treatment: none; biopsy may be necessary to rule out pigmented malignancy.

Periapical Inflammation and Pathology

Inflammation and pathological changes of the periapical tissues occur as periapical abscesses, cysts, and granulomas, condensing and alveolar osteitis, chronic hyperplastic pulpitis. **Abscess** is a localized collection of suppuration (pus) in a cavity formed by disintegration of tissues. A TRUE **cyst** is an abnormal closed epithelium-lined cavity in the body, containing liquid or semisolid material. Developmental cysts are discussed later.
- See Chapters 11, Clinical Treatment: pulpal evaluation; 13, Periodontology: periodontal and pericoronal (pericoronitis) abscesses.
A. Periapical (endodontic) abscess: acute inflammatory condition that develops in the pulp or surrounding periapical tissues.
1. Etiology: trauma, caries, spread of infective microorganisms to pulp; MOST cases result in pulpal necrosis.
2. May cause severe pain, exudate with fistula formation; may have suppuration (pus); often is difficult to distinguish from acute periodontal abscess.
3. Radiographic late finding, changes ranging from slight to distinct periapical radiolucency; located usually at apex but may follow lateral canal.
4. In MOST cases, involves a nonvital tooth; pain differs from that of periodontal abscess in that it is sharp and intermittent rather than dull and continuous; may or may NOT test positive on electric pulp tester for vitality (vitalometer with a scale of 1 to 10; the closer to 1, the healthier the tooth).
5. Treatment: endodontic therapy (root canal), extraction.
B. Periapical granuloma: involves chronic growth of granulation tissue located in periapical region.
1. Asymptomatic; late radiographic changes range from slight to distinct periapical radiolucency.
2. Treatment: endodontic therapy, extraction.
C. Periapical cyst (radicular cyst): epithelial-lined tissue cavity associated with periapical granuloma:
1. Result of proliferation of the epithelial rests of Malassez; tissue remains from Hertwig's epithelial root sheath (HERS).

2. Asymptomatic; late radiographic change indicates distinct periapical radiolucency, similar to periapical granuloma; associated with badly decayed teeth or endodontically treated teeth (in contrast, periodontal cyst usually results from trauma and is around a healthy tooth).
3. May be differentiated from periapical granuloma ONLY by biopsy.
4. Treatment: endodontic therapy, extraction; residual cyst can form.
D. Peripheral cemental dysplasia (cementoma[s]): disordered increased production of cementum and bone.
1. Radiolucent to radiopaque appearance that changes over time; can be similar to periapical disease, but tooth is vital and asymptomatic; noted FIRST on radiograph.
2. MOST in anterior teeth and in adults ≥30 years.
3. Treatment: none indicated; may need to take radiographs and perform pulp testing over time to rule out periapical disease.
E. Condensing osteitis (focal sclerosing osteomyelitis):
1. Indicated by formation of dense periapical bone, often in response to low-grade dental infection.
2. Asymptomatic; may have radiopacity in periapical region inferior to roots of teeth, with possible radiolucency either surrounding or central to it.
3. MOST with permanent mandibular first molar.
4. Treatment: none; biopsy rules out other lesions.
F. Chronic hyperplastic pulpitis (pulp polyp): asymptomatic hyperplasia of pulp:
1. Often is associated with a large carious lesion in children and young adults.
2. Treatment: pulpotomy, extraction.
G. Alveolar osteitis ("dry socket"): painful lesion in area of extraction with foul odor, bad taste, increased bleeding.
1. Usually mandibular third molar ("wisdom tooth").
2. Result of lack of proper blood clot formation after extraction; may NOT have followed postextraction recommendations (NO hot food, drink through straw).
3. Treatment: irrigation and placement of medicated dressing, possibly antibiotic coverage.
H. Ludwig's angina: serious, potentially life-threatening cellulitis involving infection of soft tissues of floor of the mouth.
1. Usually bacterial infection, *Streptococcus* or *Staphylococcus;* route of infection from mandibular third molars and/or pericoronitis (opposed to cavernous sinus thrombosis, which can also be related to spread of dental infection but involves infected thrombus transported into venous sinus of the brain, usually by way of infected maxillary teeth).

2. Usually occurring in immunocompromised adults with untreated or invasive dental infections.
3. Pain and swelling of the tongue, which raises it from the floor of the mouth, with bilateral swelling of submandibular and sublingual spaces, malaise, fever, dysphagia (difficulty swallowing), and in severe cases stridor (difficulty breathing).
4. Treatment: appropriate antibiotic drugs, monitoring and protection of airway in severe cases, and where appropriate, emergency maxillofacial surgery.

DEVELOPMENTAL DISORDERS OF ORAL CAVITY

Developmental disorder is a disturbance or lack of development of a structure; such disorders of the oral cavity include odontogenic and nonodontogenic cysts and other abnormalities within the oral cavity. See earlier discussion of periapical cysts and associated lesions.

- See Chapters 3, Anatomy, Biochemistry, and Physiology: systemic developmental disorders; 4, Head, Neck, and Dental Anatomy: orofacial development and disorders; 16, Special Needs Patient Care: developmental disabilities.

A. Odontogenic cysts, related to tooth development:
  1. Eruption cyst: bluish soft tissue swelling around newly erupting crown (NO radiographic features):
     a. MOST with a primary tooth; guardians may be concerned and need reassurance.
     b. Treatment: none (dissipates during eruption process).
  2. Dentigerous (follicular) cyst: associated with reduced enamel epithelium; leads to cyst formation around crown of unerupted tooth.
     a. Well-defined, unilocular radiolucency associated with a tooth; MOST with impacted third molar ("wisdom tooth").
     b. Treatment: surgical removal of cyst and extraction.
  3. Primordial cyst develops in place of a tooth and is caused by disturbance of enamel organ.
     a. Well-defined, unilocular or multilocular radiolucency; MOST in third molar region.
     b. Treatment: surgical removal.
  4. Odontogenic keratocyst: lined by BOTH epithelium and keratin; capable of moving and resorbing teeth.
     a. Type of primordial and dentigerous cyst.
     b. Well-defined, multilocular radiolucency; MOST in mandibular third molar region.
     c. Treatment: surgical removal; high rate of recurrence (because smaller cysts bud off).
  5. Lateral periodontal cyst: asymptomatic soft tissue or osseous cyst indicated by swelling in interdental papillae:

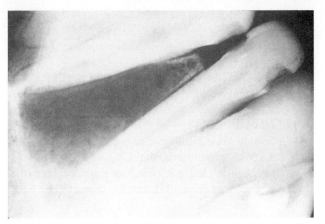

Figure 6-8 Globulomaxillary cyst, pear-shaped radiolucency between maxillary lateral and canine, with root divergence.

     a. Radiolucency; MOST in mandibular canine or premolar area.
     b. Treatment: surgical removal.
B. Nonodontogenic cysts: related to facial development (fissural), NOT to tooth development.
  1. Nasopalatine cyst: cystic transformation of epithelial remnants in nasopalatine ducts; MOST common of group.
     a. Asymptomatic, heart-shaped midline radiolucency, within incisive papilla or duct, like large incisive foramen; teeth test vital, no divergence of roots.
     b. MOST in adults between 40 and 60 years.
     c. Treatment: surgical removal.
  2. Globulomaxillary cyst: cystic transformation of epithelial remnants trapped at line of fusion between globular process of median nasal process and maxillary process (Figure 6-8):
     a. Asymptomatic; teeth test vital, indicating that periapical pathology is NOT likely.
     b. Pear-shaped radiolucency between maxillary lateral and canine; may cause root divergence.
     c. Treatment: surgical removal.
  3. Nasolabial cyst: cystic transformation of epithelial remnants trapped between fusion of globular, lateral nasal, and maxillary processes:
     a. Soft-tissue cyst located in nasolabial fold causing facial swelling; no radiographic features.
     b. MOST in 40- to 50-year-olds.
     c. Treatment: surgical removal.
  4. Median palatine cyst (rare): cystic transformation of epithelial remnants trapped between fusion of palatal process of maxilla:
     a. Midline asymptomatic, fluctuant swellings.
     b. Well-defined, unilocular, midline radiolucent lesion that is slightly posterior to incisive papilla.
     c. Treatment: surgical removal.

5. Epidermoid and dermoid cysts: consist of ONLY epithelial cells (epidermoid cyst) or a combination of epithelium, mesoderm, endoderm (dermoid cyst):
   a. BOTH occur in the mandible; noted MORE in young adults.
   b. Treatment: surgical removal.
C. Other cysts:
   1. Simple bone cyst (traumatic bone cyst): unknown etiology, possibly trauma.
      a. Well-defined, unilocular or multilocular radiolucency; located between mandibular molar roots.
      b. MOST in young adults.
      c. Treatment: surgical removal.
   2. Aneurysmal bone cyst: possibly a localized exaggerated vascular proliferative response to repair bone.
      a. Soap bubble radiographic appearance; may cause bone expansion.
      b. May follow previous lesion; MOST in young adults.
      c. Treatment: surgical removal (bleeding noted).
   3. Static bone cyst (lingual mandibular bone concavity): NOT considered a true cyst because has no epithelial lining:
      a. Depression in the medial side of the mandible, location for sublingual salivary gland.
      b. Radiolucency in the posterior mandible; MOSTLY discovered accidentally on radiographs.
      c. Treatment: none; may want to monitor by radiographs.
D. Dental developmental abnormalities: MOST do not require treatment but can cause possible problems with esthetic concerns (may need coverage by crowns or veneers, possibly whitening) and spacing in dentition or endodontic therapy complications.
   1. Hypodontia: lack of one or more teeth (tooth bud[s]).
      a. Partial lack is fairly common condition; MOST in third molar regions, maxillary laterals, mandibular premolars of permanent dentition; lateral incisors of primary dentition.
      b. Treatment: placement of fixed or removable prostheses (e.g., implants, bridges, partial dentures).
   2. Anodontia (complete lack of tooth formation or buds): rare; complete dentures are placed as the jaws grow.
   3. Supernumerary teeth: formation of extra teeth (bud[s]).
      a. Often smaller in size (microdont) and remain unerupted; extra tooth in arch; MOST in maxillary arch:

(1) Mesiodens: between maxillary central incisors.
(2) Distomolars: distal to third molar.
(3) Paramolars: buccally or lingually by molars.
   b. Treatment: extraction if it will NOT damage erupted teeth.
4. Gemination: single tooth bud forms into two joined teeth.
   a. Has one root with canal and two crowns; falsely macrodontic.
   b. MOST in primary mandibular incisors; normal number of teeth in arch.
   c. Treatment: asymptomatic and does NOT require treatment; however, may cause crowding with resultant need for orthodontics.
5. Fusion: joining of two tooth germs to form a single tooth.
   a. MORE than one root canal may be present; falsely macrodontic.
   b. MORE in primary than permanent dentition; associated with anterior teeth; one LESS tooth in arch.
   c. Treatment: asymptomatic and does NOT require treatment; however, may cause crowding with resultant need for orthodontics.
6. Dens in dente (dens invaginatus): invagination of the enamel organ into dental papilla:
   a. Occurs along lingual surface (cingulum); MOST in maxillary lateral incisor.
   b. Increased risk of pulpal exposure and endodontic therapy.
   c. Treatment: none but MUST monitor for pulpal changes.
7. Microdontia: smaller tooth (teeth).
   a. Rare to occur in entire dentition; genetic predisposition.
   b. MOST with single teeth but bilaterally, especially maxillary lateral incisors (peg lateral) or molars (peg molar).
   c. Treatment: none, but spacing may be a problem; full-coverage crown for esthetic purposes.
8. Enamel pearl (projection): exophytic area of enamel on root surface.
   a. Result of displaced ameloblasts during root formation.
   b. Located near cementoenamel junction (CEJ); MOST in mandibular molars, especially in furcation areas.
   c. May be mistaken for calculus and can be noted as radiopacity on root.
   d. Treatment: surgical removal if needed.
9. Enamel hypoplasia: incomplete enamel formation (quantity affected) that is caused by disturbances or damage to ameloblasts during enamel formation (very sensitive Barney-like cells).

a. May vary from pits to complete grooving of teeth; can be noted on radiographs as thin or absent enamel.

b. Turner's tooth: single affected tooth, usually canine or premolar, as result of trauma.

c. Also noted with congenital syphilis, tetracycline stain, amelogenesis imperfecta; can be combined with hypocalcification with fluorosis.

10. Enamel hypocalcification: incomplete enamel calcification (quality affected) that is cause by a disturbance or damage to ameloblasts during enamel formation.

a. May vary in color from white to brown (mottled enamel); NOT noted on radiographs.

b. Turner's spot ("sparkle spot"): single affected area.

c. Also noted with amelogenesis imperfecta (MOST common type); can be combined with hypoplasia with fluorosis.

11. Dental fluorosis: excessive intake of fluoride through fluoride added to the water supply or from other sources (see Chapter 17, Community Oral Health, for more information).

a. Damage in tooth development occurs between ages of 6 months to 5 years; usually permanent teeth affected; occasionally primary teeth may be involved.

b. Noted with yellowing of teeth, white spots, and pitting or mottling (multicolor disturbance) of enamel; combination of BOTH enamel hypoplasia and hypocalcification is possible.

c. In children, fluorosis appears most frequently as "snowcapping," a parchment-white-colored area on the incisal or occlusal surface.

d. In mild cases, few white flecks or small pits; more severe, may be brown stains; Dean's fluorosis index is MOST commonly used classification system.

e. By the time the physician and/or dentist recognizes fluorosis in the permanent teeth, it is too late to prevent its appearance on most of the other teeth, including those yet to erupt, because fluoride has already been incorporated into their enamel; therefore, providing the appropriate amount of fluoride during the first 6 years of life is the best method to prevent both caries and fluorosis.

f. MORE prevalent in rural areas where drinking water is derived from shallow wells and hand pumps; also MORE likely to occur in areas where the drinking water has a fluoride content of >1 ppm and calcium intake is poor.

12. Dilaceration: curvature of the root; may be caused by trauma during tooth development.

a. MOSTLY with third molars ("wisdom teeth").

b. Treatment: none; a challenge during extraction and endodontic therapy.

13. Taurodontism: formation of elongated pulp and short root (looks like bull's teeth).

a. Results from improper invagination of HERS.

b. Radiographs show teeth with elongated pulps and short roots; increased risk in molars of Native Americans and Eskimos.

c. Treatment: none.

14. Concrescence: joining of teeth by cementum.

a. Result of trauma and crowding in the area during development, MOST with molars.

b. Treatment: none indicated; can complicate extraction.

CLINICAL STUDY

Age	26 YRS	Scenario
Sex	☒ Male ☐ Female	On visual intraoral examination, acute inflammation is noted in the gingival tissues surrounding his newly erupting terminal molar, with moderate levels of dental biofilm. A panoramic radiograph is taken, and development of the third molar is assessed. In addition, a nickel-sized well-defined corticated radiolucency is noted between the roots of the maxillary right lateral incisor and canine; the roots of the teeth are also spread apart from each other.
Height	6'3"	
Weight	185	
BP	100/74	
Chief Complaint	"I really hurt in my lower right jaw. What is going on?"	
Medical History	Multiple broken bones resulting from parasailing Testicular cancer when a teenager Father recently died of pancreatic cancer	
Current Medications	Tylenol for headaches prn	
Social History	Physical therapist taking care of patient's invalid mother with early-onset Alzheimer's	

1. Name the condition the patient is experiencing in the molar regions of his oral cavity. What has caused his condition? What can this condition lead to if not treated properly?
2. What can be done to alleviate the patient's discomfort?
3. What is indicated by the radiolucency located between the roots of the maxillary lateral incisor and canine?
4. Why does the lesion have radiolucency? How is the lesion treated?

1. The patient is experiencing pericoronitis (pericoronal abscess) with gingival hyperplasia in molar regions. Condition occurs when bacteria such as with dental biofilm collect beneath flap of hyperplastic gingival tissue (operculum) that commonly covers most distal surface of newly erupting molars (especially third molars, "wisdom teeth") and cause acute infection, with pain and inflammation. If not treated promptly, can lead to Ludwig's angina, a serious, potentially life-threatening infection of soft tissues of floor of the mouth.
2. Discomfort can be relieved by gentle irrigation of sulcus with saline solution, warm water, or diluted hydrogen peroxide. Debridement of the area at initial appointment, using topical anesthetic, is recommended if patient can tolerate it. If not, debridement should occur during second visit, when inflammation has subsided somewhat. Use of systemic antibiotics may also be indicated if there are systemic signs of infection. Surgical removal of the tooth or operculum may be necessary to prevent recurrence. Prevention includes discussion of oral hygiene care in patients who are at risk for condition, such as having a partially erupted third molar.
3. Radiolucency located between roots of maxillary right lateral and canine is most likely a globulomaxillary cyst. Asymptomatic; thus teeth remain vital. Roots of adjacent teeth often diverge because of pressure from the cyst.
4. Radiolucency is from this developmental disorder, since it is noncalcified with no bony involvement. Treated by surgical excision.

Inherited Disorders

Several inherited disorders have an effect on the oral cavity. Included are disorders that affect the periodontium and teeth.

- See Chapter 16, Special Needs Patient Care: muscular dystrophy, Down syndrome.
A. Von Willebrand disease (VWD): hereditary coagulation abnormality; MOST common of all inherited bleeding disorders and can affect both women and men.
   1. Deficiency of multimeric protein factor that is required for platelet adhesion; ALL clinical signs of bleeding when organs are stressed or traumatized.
   2. Treatment: none indicated; however, ALWAYS at increased risk for bleeding; prophylactic treatment is sometimes given before surgery.
B. Hemophilia: type A (MOST common, classic) is X linked; transmitted from unaffected daughters to grandsons, thus affects ONLY men:
   1. Deficiency in blood clotting factors: type A, factor VIII deficiency; type B, factor IX deficiency; type C, factor XI deficiency.
   2. Type B (Christmas disease) and others are LESS common forms, but ALL affect only men.
   3. Oral signs: spontaneous gingival bleeding, petechiae, ecchymoses (see earlier notes on bleeding disorders such as anemia).
C. Cyclic neutropenia: autosomal dominant disorder: results in decreased neutrophil (polymorphonucleocyte [PMN]) production that tends to occur every 3 weeks (cyclic) and lasts 3 to 6 days at a time.
   1. Caused by changing rates of cell production by the bone marrow.
   2. Oral signs: severe ulcerative gingivitis, tongue and oral mucosa ulcers, increased risk of periodontal disease.
D. Papillon-Lefèvre syndrome: autosomal recessive disorder: results in aggressive periodontal disease with advanced bone destruction and tooth loss.
E. Hereditary fibromatosis: associated with several disorders (e.g., MAINLY Laband's syndrome):
   1. Causes gingival fibromatosis, nail dysplasia, joint hypermobility; disease develops soon after tooth eruption.
   2. May be present as a generalized enlargement of the gingival tissue, which eventually may cover the dentition completely; tissue is firm and slightly lighter in color than surrounding gingiva.
   3. Treatment: oral hygiene instruction, surgical removal of excess tissue.
F. Osseous disorders:
   1. Cherubism: autosomal dominant disorder that develops early in life.
      a. Bilateral facial swelling, multilocular, soap bubble bilateral radiolucency of the mandible.
      b. Associated with abnormal tooth development and eruption.
   2. Cleidocranial dysostosis (dysplasia): autosomal dominant disorder; does NOT affect intelligence.
      a. Hypoplasia of clavicles (touch shoulders together); underdeveloped premaxilla; low nasal bridge; occipital, parietal, and frontal bossing; short forearms and fingers.
      b. Supernumerary teeth, malformed teeth, abnormal eruption sequence.

3. Osteogenesis imperfecta: autosomal dominant disorder; presence of multiple bone fractures and loss of enamel because of abnormal dentin formation.

G. Dental disorders:
1. Amelogenesis imperfecta: autosomal recessive disorder: malformation of enamel, thin, pitted, mottled, snow-capped or yellowish, and poorly calcified.
   a. Causes: heredity, childhood illness, nutritional deficiency, drugs.
   b. Treatment: often requires placement of esthetic veneers.
2. Dentinogenesis imperfecta: autosomal dominant disorder: defect in the odontoblasts.
   a. Type I with osteogenesis imperfecta; type II is indicated by opalescent, blue to brown dentition.
   b. Noted in both primary and permanent dentitions; may cause enamel to fracture easily because of unsupportive dentin.
   c. Lack of pulp chamber and root canal formation, bell-shaped crowns, severe incisal or occlusal wear noted on radiographs.
3. Ectodermal dysplasia: X-linked recessive disorder:
   a. Conical or missing incisors.
   b. Lack of body hair and sweat glands; looks aged (old person appearance).
4. Dentin dysplasia: autosomal dominant condition described as type I or type II:
   a. Type I: short roots with nearly complete obliteration of pulp noted on radiographs.
   b. Type II: similar to type I on radiographs; however, also has large coronal pulps filled with abnormal dentin.
   c. Either type may cause tooth loss because of short roots and periapical lesions.

Oral Variations of Normal

Oral variants of normal are conditions that are NOT always evident but so frequently noted that they are NOT considered pathological.

A. Fordyce granules (Fordyce's spots): asymptomatic clusters of yellow **lobules** of sebaceous glands:
1. MOST on buccal mucosa and lower lip; MOST in adults ≥20 years.
2. Treatment: none.
B. Tori (single, torus): either palatal or mandibular exophytic nodular osseous growth on hard palate or bilaterally on lingual surface of mandible; asymptomatic, slow growing:
1. Palatal occur MORE often in women (with LESS risk of osteoporosis); mandibular appear on radiographs as radiopaque areas in mandibular premolar region.
2. Etiology related to genetics and possibly grinding (bruxism).

3. Treatment: none unless surgical removal for a dental prosthesis or growth interferes with speech.
C. Pigmentation (physiological, melanosis): asymptomatic, symmetrical, brown lesion located on oral mucosa, MOST on gingival tissues:
1. Greater incidence in dark-skinned individuals; nonphysiological pigmentation is also associated with Addison's disease, Peutz-Jeghers syndrome, smoking, melanomas.
2. Treatment: none, although diagnostic tests for associated diseases and syndromes or to rule out melanoma may be appropriate.
D. Linea alba: asymptomatic, bilateral line (band) of raised white tissue at level of occlusal plane on buccal mucosa; also on the labial mucosa:
1. Caused by chronic grinding (bruxism) and/or clenching habit that produces hyperkeratosis and epithelial hyperplasia.
2. Treatment: none, but does help in evaluation of habit.
E. Leukoedema: generalized, opalescent white film covering buccal mucosa bilaterally; caused by cellular edema in prickle cell layer:
1. MOST in ethnic groups (e.g., African-Americans); disappears with pressure on tissues.
2. Treatment: none.
F. Lingual thyroid nodule: small, nodular mass located slightly posterior to circumvallate lingual papillae:
1. Caused by entrapped thyroid tissue.
2. Treatment: surgical removal possible if concern; possibly biopsy.
G. Fissured tongue: deep grooves or **fissures** on dorsal tongue surface:
1. Increased with certain syndromes such as Down syndrome.
2. Treatment: oral hygiene instruction on cleaning tongue.
H. Geographic tongue (benign migratory glossitis): map-like appearance of **erythema,** surrounded by a white or yellow border on dorsal or lateral surface of the tongue as result of desquamation of filiform lingual papillae:
1. Caused by sensitivity of tissue, MOST likely because of stress, heredity, or nutritional factors.
2. Treatment: none; may want to stress gentle oral hygiene of the tongue (must remove all maps of Italy-ah!).
I. Median rhomboid glossitis (central papillary atrophy): flat or slightly raised benign lesion on tongue dorsum:
1. NO filiform present; related to chronic candiasis infection.
2. Thus no treatment with antifungals because of refractory nature.

J. Black hairy tongue: hypertrophy (elongation) of fili-form lingual papillae on ventral surface:
1. May be caused by long-term use of alcoholic mouthrinses, broad-spectrum antibiotics, steroids; color change may be attributed to bacteria, chemicals (hydrogen peroxide, antacids), tobacco use, foods, or drugs.
2. Treatment: oral hygiene instruction on cleaning tongue (without dentifrice); removal of cause; referral to physician, if needed.
K. Lingual varicosities: vascularities that appear as red or purple areas on the ventral or lateral surface of the tongue:
1. MOST in older adults.
2. Treatment: none.

Review Questions

1 Which of the following is TRUE regarding the cellular response to injury?
A. Duration of an injury has little impact on the cellular response to injury.
B. Response to injury is the same in all cell types.
C. Cell necrosis will occur if cell membrane integrity is compromised.
D. Cell necrosis will occur only if the cellular genetic apparatus is damaged.

2 Which of the following causes an irreversible injury that leads to cell death?
A. Swelling of cytoplasm
B. Fragmentation of nucleus
C. Condensation of cytoplasm
D. Brief hypoxia

3 The cardinal signs of inflammation include all of the following, EXCEPT one. Which one is the EXCEPTION?
A. Pain
B. Heat
C. Redness
D. Swelling
E. Odor

4 Which one of the following factors involved in tissue repair is CORRECTLY defined?
A. Angiogenesis is the formation of new blood vessels.
B. Fibrosis is the formation of a new epithelial layer.
C. Remodeling is the formation of a fibrous collagen patch.
D. Chemotaxis is the secretion of collagen-degrading enzymes.

5 What circulatory system changes take place during inflammation?
A. Decrease in blood vessel permeability
B. Release of chemical mediators such as histamine
C. Constriction of arterioles
D. Inhibition of diapedesis of leukocytes

6 Which of the following statements is CORRECT concerning tissue regeneration?
A. Regeneration is accomplished by the formation of a fibrous connective tissue scar.
B. In terms of tissue function, repair is more desirable than regeneration.
C. Regeneration is the replacement of damaged cells with parenchymal cells of the same type.
D. The type of cell injured has little impact on whether the tissue heals by regeneration or repair.

7 One of the following is NOT a necessary condition for neoplasia formation. Which one is the EXCEPTION?
A. Exposure to adequate concentrations of carcinogens
B. Susceptible host tissue
C. Adequate time for establishment
D. Existence of a genetic defect

8 Which of the following statements is CORRECT regarding the designation for neoplasia?
A. For benign neoplasia, the suffix "-oma" is added to the tissue name.
B. For malignant neoplasia, the suffix "-oma" is added to the tissue name.
C. Benign neoplasia of squamous epithelium is called a squamous cell carcinoma.
D. Malignant neoplasia of bone tissue is called an osteoma.

9 Which one of the following is considered an endogenous carcinogen?
A. Radiation
B. Viruses
C. Chemicals
D. Genetic anomalies

10 The process by which cells with cancer potential establish themselves and give rise to cancer is called
A. initiation.
B. transformation.
C. metastasis.
D. promotion.

11 What is the MOST common site for cancer in women?
A. Lungs
B. Uterus
C. Breast
D. Colon

12 A 14-year-old boy was hospitalized for an osteosarcoma that metastasized to the lungs. Which one of the following statements regarding this case is CORRECT?
A. Cancer in the lungs most likely originated in the liver.
B. Osteosarcoma is a benign tumor.
C. Metastasis of the osteosarcoma was most likely by blood.
D. Metastasis is the best criterion for classifying a tumor as benign.

13 Which of the following statements concerning psoriasis is CORRECT?
    A. Refers to many acute or chronic inflammations of the skin
    B. Presents as raised papules or patches with silvery scales and thickened skin
    C. Bacterial infection with multiple facial lesions from plugged sebaceous glands
    D. Most commonly located on the trunk and neck

14 A 16-year-old male presents with numerous pus-containing pimples on his face and neck. All of the following are noted regarding this condition, EXCEPT one. Which one is the EXCEPTION?
    A. Condition is acne of the skin.
    B. Condition is caused by a viral infection of the sebaceous glands.
    C. Hormonal factors are involved in this condition.
    D. Condition is caused by a bacterial infection of the sebaceous glands.

15 Which of the following statements BEST describes the relationship between acne and seborrheic dermatitis?
    A. Both acne and seborrheic dermatitis are skin diseases that affect the sebaceous glands and hair follicles.
    B. Both acne and seborrheic dermatitis are bacterial skin infections.
    C. Acne is a bacterial skin infection, and seborrheic dermatitis is a viral skin infection.
    D. Both acne and seborrheic dermatitis are autoimmune disorders.

16 Which of the following conditions would be considered with the presence of a yellow, itchy, raised lesion on the skin around the face and neck of a 3-year-old?
    A. Acne
    B. Seborrheic dermatitis
    C. Impetigo
    D. Psoriasis

17 Pituitary hyperfunction is a characteristic of which of the following diseases?
    A. Acromegaly
    B. Diabetes insipidus
    C. Graves' disease
    D. Cushing's syndrome

18 Which of the following is a manifestation of hypopituitarism?
    A. Oversecretion of growth hormone
    B. Acromegaly
    C. Hyperactive thyroid gland
    D. Copious urine production

19 Which of the following glands is associated with Graves' disease?
    A. Pituitary gland
    B. Thyroid gland
    C. Pancreas
    D. Adrenal glands

20 Which of the following could be considered a causal factor for Cushing's syndrome?
    A. Administration of glucocorticoid steroids by a physician
    B. Destruction of the thyroid gland as treatment for disease
    C. Atrophy of the adrenal glands
    D. Autoimmune hypertrophy of the parathyroid glands

21 Which of the following tumors is considered the MOST common cause of hyperparathyroidism?
    A. Pituitary adenoma
    B. Parathyroid adenoma
    C. Thyroid adenoma
    D. Medullary carcinoma of adrenal gland

22 One of following is NOT a complication of cirrhosis of the liver. Which one is the EXCEPTION?
    A. Hyperglycemia
    B. Ascites
    C. Splenomegaly
    D. Jaundice

23 Characteristics of type 1 diabetes mellitus include all of the following, EXCEPT one. Which one is the EXCEPTION?
    A. Insulin dependence
    B. Mature onset
    C. Juvenile onset
    D. More serious than type 2

24 Which of the following is a manifestation of chronic pancreatitis?
    A. Nutrient malabsorption
    B. Chronic constipation
    C. Severe jaundice
    D. Diverticula of the intestine

25 What is another term for hypochromic anemia?
    A. Secondary anemia
    B. Hemolytic anemia
    C. Iron-deficiency anemia
    D. Aplastic anemia

26 Which type of anemia is characterized by the rupturing of erythrocytes?
    A. Pernicious
    B. Hypochromic
    C. Aplastic
    D. Hemolytic

27 One of the following statements is NOT correct regarding hemophilia. Which one is the EXCEPTION?
    A. Low blood hemoglobin concentration is present.
    B. Genetic blood disease is present.
    C. Blood disease is characterized by improper blood clotting.
    D. Treatment includes transfusion and administration of clotting proteins.

28 Patients with type 1 diabetes mellitus
    A. have non-insulin-dependent diabetes.
    B. can control the disease with oral insulin.
    C. are at increased risk for infection.
    D. typically have low blood glucose levels.

29 One of the following is NOT a common oral manifestation of diabetes mellitus. Which one is the EXCEPTION?
    A. Parotid enlargement
    B. *Candida* infection
    C. Xerostomia
    D. Atrophic tongue
    E. Periodontitis

30 When treating the patient with diabetes mellitus, a dental professional should do all of the following, EXCEPT one. Which one is the EXCEPTION?
A. Schedule appointments before a meal
B. Consult with the treating physician
C. Limit the length of the appointment
D. Be prepared for an emergency

31 All of the following are correct regarding primary polycythemia, EXCEPT one. Which one is the EXCEPTION?
A. Primary polycythemia is an increase in the number of circulating erythrocytes.
B. Hyperviscosity of the blood is a manifestation of primary polycythemia.
C. Emphysema is a cause of primary polycythemia.
D. Treatment for primary polycythemia includes bloodletting.

32 Which of the following conditions is noted for bone marrow infiltration by malignant cells, an increased number of immature leukocytes in the blood, and treatment by chemotherapy?
A. Leukemia
B. Primary polycythemia
C. Secondary polycythemia
D. Hemophilia

33 Which of the following is the MOST common oral manifestation of renal disease?
A. Herpes
B. Lichen planus
C. Halitosis
D. Angular cheilitis

34 A medical consult is necessary before treating a patient with renal disease. One of the following is NOT a reason for consultation for this patient. Which one is the EXCEPTION?
A. Premedication needs
B. Bleeding tendency
C. Drug interactions
D. HIV status

35 Common causes of respiratory disease include all of the following, EXCEPT one. Which one is the EXCEPTION?
A. Cigarette smoking
B. Allergy
C. Cystic fibrosis
D. Infection
E. Diabetes mellitus

36 The dental patient with respiratory disease is at risk when exposed to all of the following, EXCEPT one. Which one is the EXCEPTION?
A. Aerosols
B. Sulfites
C. Stress
D. Inhalants

37 All of the following are risk factors associated with oral cancer, EXCEPT one. Which one is the EXCEPTION?
A. Denture irritation
B. Heavy alcohol use
C. Age
D. Tobacco

38 Patients who undergo chemotherapy for acute leukemia are NOT at an increased risk for oral infections. All patients who undergo chemotherapy for cancer will experience oral complications that are directly related to drug activity.
A. Both statements are true.
B. Both statements are false.
C. The first statement is true, the second is false.
D. The first statement is false, the second is true.

39 Angular cheilitis, pale oral mucosa, and glossitis are signs of
A. anemia.
B. leukemia.
C. hemophilia.
D. jaundice.

40 When treating the patient with hemophilia, the dental professional should do all of the following, EXCEPT one. Which one is the EXCEPTION?
A. Consult with the patient's physician
B. Treat with replacement factor
C. Prevent infectious disease transmission
D. Instrument in small segments over several appointments
E. Scale the entire mouth in one appointment

41 The patient with a cardiac condition
A. may have difficulty breathing in a supine position.
B. should not be administered local anesthetics.
C. is at high risk for oral candidiasis.
D. may have difficulty communicating.

42 For which condition would radiographic diagnosis be conclusive?
A. Alveolar osteitis
B. Periapical abscess
C. Periapical granuloma
D. Condensing osteitis

43 Which of the following lesions closely resembles or is slightly lighter in color than the tissue on which it is located?
A. Pyogenic granuloma
B. Oral fibroma
C. Papillary hyperplasia
D. Peripheral giant cell granuloma

44 Which of the following lesions is noted to be a bilateral, lobulated, exophytic bone located in the lingual mandibular premolar area?
A. Condensing osteitis
B. Genial tubercles
C. Mandibular tori
D. Ranula

45 Which of the following lesions is observed as a radiopaque area at the apex and is often associated with a restored or carious tooth?
A. Periapical granuloma
B. Focal sclerosing osteomyelitis
C. Periapical abscess
D. Compound odontoma

46 Which of the following is noted clinically as a targetlike lesion?
   A. Lichen planus
   B. Ectodermal dysplasia
   C. Erythema multiforme
   D. Lupus erythematosus

47 Which of the following is noted for a loss of lingual tooth structure associated with bulimia?
   A. Attrition
   B. Erosion
   C. Bruxism
   D. Abrasion

48 Which of the following is a cluster of sebaceous glands observed on the buccal mucosa?
   A. Lipomas
   B. Linea alba
   C. Mucoceles
   D. Fordyce granules

49 One of the following could NOT occur in response to a hypersensitivity to latex. Which one is the EXCEPTION?
   A. Contact mucositis
   B. Angioedema
   C. Contact dermatitis
   D. Lichen planus

50 Which term BEST describes a freckle?
   A. Pedunculated
   B. Sessile
   C. Macule
   D. Papule

51 Which of the following lingual papillae has desquamation and is associated with geographic tongue?
   A. Fungiform
   B. Filiform
   C. Circumvallate
   D. Foliate

52 Acantholysis and positive Nikolsky's sign are BOTH associated with which one of the following conditions listed below?
   A. Lupus erythematosus
   B. Pemphigus vulgaris
   C. Tuberculosis
   D. Pemphigoid

53 Which cyst is MOST commonly located between the maxillary canine and lateral incisor teeth?
   A. Dentigerous cyst
   B. Radicular cyst
   C. Globulomaxillary cyst
   D. Lateral periodontal cyst

54 What is the union of two teeth by cementum?
   A. Gemination
   B. Fusion
   C. Dilaceration
   D. Concrescence
   E. Dens in dente

55 What is the MOST likely etiology for basal cell carcinoma?
   A. Heredity
   B. Tobacco
   C. Alcohol
   D. Sunlight

56 Hutchinson's incisors and mulberry molars are both associated with which condition listed below?
   A. Congenital syphilis
   B. Amelogenesis imperfecta
   C. Ectodermal dysplasia
   D. Tuberculosis

57 What developmental disorder is located between tooth #8 and #9?
   A. Turner tooth
   B. Dens in dente
   C. Microdont
   D. Mesiodens

58 Improper invagination of the Hertwig's epithelial root sheath may cause which of the conditions listed below?
   A. Enamel pearl
   B. Peg lateral
   C. Talon cusp
   D. Taurodontism

59 Which tooth is MOST likely involved in microdontia?
   A. Maxillary central incisor
   B. Mandibular lateral incisor
   C. Maxillary lateral incisor
   D. Mandibular third molar

60 What is the pseudocyst that forms in the mandibular premolar or molar region and is caused by a bone depression adjacent to a salivary gland?
   A. Simple bone cyst
   B. Static bone cyst
   C. Salivary cyst
   D. Traumatic bone cyst

61 All of the following may cause gingival hyperplasia, EXCEPT one. Which one is the EXCEPTION?
   A. Cyclosporine
   B. Tetracycline
   C. Nifedipine
   D. Phenytoin

62 Which of the following X-linked recessive disorders presents with a lack of body hair and sweat glands and may be associated with missing or cone-shaped incisors?
   A. Dentin dysplasia
   B. Dentinogenesis imperfecta
   C. Amelogenesis imperfecta
   D. Hypohidrotic ectodermal dysplasia

63 Which of the following is associated with the loss of lamina dura and a cotton-wool radiographic appearance of bone?
   A. Fibrous dysplasia
   B. Type 1 diabetes mellitus
   C. Osteogenesis imperfecta
   D. Paget's disease

64 Which of the following is an autosomal dominant disorder characterized by opalescent blue or brown crowns?
   A. Amelogenesis imperfecta
   B. Ectodermal dysplasia
   C. Dentin dysplasia
   D. Dentinogenesis imperfecta

65 What is a macule?
   A. Uncovered wound of cutaneous or mucosal tissue that exhibits tissue disintegration and necrosis
   B. Soft tissue lesion in which the epithelium above the basal layer is denuded
   C. Permanent mark or cicatrix remaining after a wound heals
   D. Circumscribed area of mucosa distinguished by color from its surroundings

66 What is a papule?
   A. Superficial, elevated, solid lesion that is less than 1 cm in diameter
   B. Flat, solid raised area that is larger than 1 cm in diameter
   C. Solid mass of tissue larger than 1 cm in diameter that has the dimension of depth
   D. Solid mass of tissue smaller than 1 cm in diameter that has the dimension of depth

67 Squamous papilloma presents as what type of lesion in the oral cavity?
   A. Macule
   B. Nodule
   C. Plaque
   D. Papule

68 A circumscribed, fluid-filled elevation in the epithelium that is less than 1 cm in diameter is termed a
   A. pustule.
   B. vesicle.
   C. bulla.
   D. cyst.

69 What is a soft tissue variant of the dentigerous cyst that forms around an erupting tooth crown called?
   A. Eruption cyst
   B. Congenital epulis
   C. Dental lamina cyst
   D. Natal teeth

70 What are teeth that are considerably smaller than normal called?
   A. Macrodontia
   B. Fusion or gemination
   C. Dens invaginatus
   D. Microdontia

71 A bony exostosis that is located midline of the hard palate is called what?
   A. Maxillary abscess
   B. Palatal torus
   C. Nasopalatine duct cyst
   D. Pleomorphic adenoma

72 Which of the following is a central nervous system disorder present with a loss of consciousness?
   A. Autism
   B. Cerebral palsy
   C. Epilepsy
   D. Mental retardation

73 An aura is commonly associated with
   A. epileptic seizure.
   B. myocardial infarction.
   C. anorexia nervosa.
   D. Sjögren's syndrome.

74 A biopsy allows an examination of both surface and deep or internal cells of the lesion. Exfoliative cytology allows an examination of only the surface cells of the lesion.
   A. Both statements are true.
   B. Both statements are false.
   C. The first statement is true, the second is false.
   D. The first statement is false, the second is true.

75 Which one of the following is an advantage of exfoliative cytology?
   A. Is effective on keratinized lesions
   B. Indicates need for biopsy
   C. Gives false-negative results
   D. Does not involve cutting into the tissue

Answer Key and Rationales

1 (C) Cellular response to injury depends on multiple factors, including the type, duration, and severity of the injury; cell type; and biochemical considerations such as cell membrane, genetic apparatus, protein integrity.

2 (B) Damage to nucleus of the cell and therefore to genetic apparatus of the cell is considered irreversible cell injury. Cytoplasmic changes that occur without loss of cell membrane integrity are normal signs of reversible cell injury. Prolonged hypoxia may cause irreversible cell damage. Brief hypoxia is manifested as cytoplasmic swelling without damage to cell membrane.

3 (E) Odor is NOT one of the (cardinal) signs of inflammation, which include heat, redness, pain, swelling, loss of function.

4 (A) Angiogenesis is the proliferation of local blood vessels into site of tissue damage. Fibrosis is formation of fibrous collagen patch in and around damaged tissue. Remodeling is generation of collagen-degrading enzymes. Chemotaxis is the movement of white blood cells (WBCs) toward chemical substance that attracts them.

5 (B) Pathogenesis of inflammation has circulatory and cellular changes; includes increases in blood flow and blood vessel permeability because of release of chemical mediators. Cellular changes include emigration (diapedesis) of leukocytes (WBCs) and phagocytosis.

6 (C) Injured tissues heal by regeneration and repair. Regeneration is replacement of injured cells with parenchymal cells of the same type. Repair is healing with formation of a connective tissue scar. Type of cell injured is primary factor that determines whether tissue healing is by regeneration or repair. Some tissues, such as epithelial tissues, have high capacity for regeneration. Other tissues, such as cardiac muscle and nervous tissue, have very limited capacity for regeneration and healing by repair.

7 (D) Neoplasia formation occurs ONLY if certain conditions are met, including exposure to adequate concentrations of carcinogens; susceptible host tissue; and adequate time for neoplasia initiation, transformation, and growth. Existence of a genetic defect is NOT a necessary condition.

8 (A) For a benign neoplasia, the suffix "-oma" is added to name of the tissue (with EXCEPTION of malignant melanoma, which is ALWAYS cancerous). For malignant neoplasia in nonepithelial tissue, term "sarcoma" is added to tissue name. For malignant neoplasia in epithelial tissue, term "carcinoma" is added to tissue name. Malignant neoplasia of bone is an osteosarcoma.

9 (D) Endogenous carcinogens include genetic factors, hormonal imbalances, immunological and nutritional factors, and aging. Radiation, viruses, and chemicals are considered exogenous carcinogens.

10 (B) Transformation occurs when cells with cancer potential establish themselves and give rise to cancer. Initiation occurs when cells undergo an alteration or series of alterations to acquire autonomous growth potential. Metastasis is spread of cancerous cells to new site. Promotion is NOT part of process of cancer development.

11 (C) MOST common site for malignancy (cancer) in women is the breast. In men, MOST common site for malignancy (cancer) is the prostate gland. Second MOST common site in both is the lungs.

12 (C) Osteosarcoma is a malignant tumor of bone tissue. Metastasis is the primary criterion for classifying a tumor as malignant. Osteosarcomas metastasize by blood, and secondary tumors often develop in the lungs.

13 (B) Psoriasis is a type of dermatitis with raised papules or patches with silver scales. Cause is unknown, although tends to run in families. Lesions are MOST commonly located on extremities and lead to thickened skin.

14 (B) Condition is MOST likely acne, a bacterial infection of the sebaceous glands. MOST common during adolescence, has hormonal and hereditary components, and may be aggravated by stress and/or drugs. Viruses do NOT cause acne.

15 (A) Acne and seborrheic dermatitis are BOTH skin diseases that affect the sebaceous gland and hair follicles. Acne is caused by bacteria and is thus considered an infectious disease. Seborrheic dermatitis is a multifactorial disorder and is NOT an infectious disease.

16 (C) Impetigo is a highly contagious infectious disease that is common in children. Appears as yellow, itchy, raised pustules around the head and neck. Acne lesions are raised but are NOT yellow or itchy. Seborrheic dermatitis exhibits redness, itching, and scaling; psoriasis lesions are raised, scaly patches on the extremities.

17 (A) Gigantism and acromegaly occur when the pituitary gland oversecretes growth hormone. Diabetes insipidus is caused by pituitary hyposecretion. Graves' disease is caused by hypersecretion of the thyroid gland. Cushing's syndrome is caused by hypersecretion of the adrenal glands.

18 (D) Hypopituitarism has a hypoactive pituitary gland. Caused by agenesis, atrophy, and/or destruction of secretory cells in the pituitary gland. Lack of antidiuretic hormone (ADH) from the pituitary leads to copious (large amount of) urine production. Oversecretion of growth hormone, acromegaly, and hyperactive thyroid gland are ALL characteristics of hyperpituitarism.

19 (B) Graves' disease is associated with hyperthyroidism and is an autoimmune hypertrophy of the thyroid gland. Manifestations (signs) include hypersecretion of thyroxine, which leads to exophthalmos, tachycardia, severe weight loss.

20 (A) Cushing's syndrome is the hypersecretion of adrenal gland hormones, such as glucocorticoids. Administration of glucocorticoid steroids by a physician in inappropriate amounts could lead to elevated blood levels of glucocorticoids and Cushing's syndrome.

21 (B) Parathyroid adenoma is the primary cause of hyperparathyroidism. Adenoma is a tumor in secretory epithelium that often leads to hypersecretion by affected epithelial cells.

22 (A) Hyperglycemia is NOT a complication of cirrhosis of the liver. MOST common complications include jaundice, hepatic encephalopathy, ascites (fluid accumulation in abdominal cavity), splenomegaly, bleeding.

23 (B) Characteristics of type 1 diabetes mellitus (DM) include insulin dependency and juvenile onset, more serious than type 2. Mature onset is typical of type 2 DM.

24 (A) Pancreatitis may lead to an inadequate secretion of pancreatic juices, necessary for digestion of nutrients in the intestine. Malabsorption is KEY manifestation (sign) of chronic pancreatitis.

25 (C) Anemia is a blood disorder with low blood oxygen and hemoglobin levels; there are several types. Hypochromic has too little hemoglobin per erythrocyte (red blood cell [RBC]); often is caused by iron deficiency. Hemolytic has RBCs that rupture too easily. Pernicious has too few RBCs present. Aplastic has faulty red bone marrow. Secondary occurs as consequence of another condition.

26 (D) Hemolytic anemia has RBCs that rupture too easily and is due to hemolysis, abnormal breakdown of RBCs either in blood vessels (intravascular hemolysis) or elsewhere (extravascular). Numerous possible causes, ranging from relatively harmless to life threatening. General classification is either acquired or inherited. Treatment depends on cause and nature of breakdown.

27 (A) Hemophilia is the improper clotting of blood. Genetic disease with prolonged bleeding after even minor injuries. Treatment includes blood transfusion and administration of blood-clotting proteins. Low blood hemoglobin concentration is a characteristic of anemia.

28 (C) With type 1 DM, patients are at increased risk for infection. Require daily injections of insulin to reduce HIGH blood glucose levels.

29 (D) Atrophic tongue is NOT a common oral manifestation (sign) of DM. Tongue often is edematous, and parotid gland may be enlarged. Xerostomia, *Candida* infection, periodontitis are common.

30 (A) Schedule appointments for a patient with DM after morning meal, when blood glucose is MORE stable, to reduce possibility of emergency. Before treatment, medical consult with treating physician regarding level of blood glucose control and need for antibiotic premedication (prophylaxis). Appointments should be short. Keep orange juice or glucose tablets or gel as glucose replacement in emergency kit in case of DM emergency.

31 (C) Primary polycythemia is oversecretion of erythrocytes by hyperactive bone marrow. Factors such as emphysema, heart disease, and living at high altitude may lead to secondary polycythemia.

32 (A) Leukemia is a cancer of bone marrow. MOST common manifestations (signs) are malignant cells in the bone marrow, increased number of immature leukocytes in the blood, complications such as joint pain, unusual bleeding, hepatomegaly, splenomegaly. Polycythemias involve red blood cells, and hemophilia involves blood-clotting factors.

33 (C) Halitosis (bad breath) is a COMMON oral manifestation (sign) of renal disease. Herpes is a common viral infection that is NOT specifically associated with renal disease. Lichen planus is a chronic inflammatory disease associated with systemic diseases such as hypertension and diabetes mellitus. Angular cheilitis is associated with nutritional deficiency, candidal infection, and immunocompromised states but NOT specifically with renal disease.

34 (D) Medical consult is necessary before treating patients with renal disease. May be indication for need for antibiotic, steroidal, or antianxiety premedication, as well as tendency to bleed and any drug interactions. The HIV status is ONLY of peripheral significance.

35 (E) COMMON causes of respiratory disease include tobacco use such as cigarette smoking, allergy, cystic fibrosis, and infection. Diabetes mellitus (DM) is NOT associated with respiratory disease.

36 (D) Inhalers contain medicaments that help dilate the bronchioles and result in easier breathing. Dental patient with respiratory disease is at risk for breathing difficulty when exposed to aerosols (from ultrasonic scaler), sulfites (which provoke asthma), and stress (which can also provoke asthma).

37 (A) Denture irritation has NEVER been proved to cause squamous cell carcinoma (SCC). With oral cancer can experience denture sores or trauma from intraoral changes associated with cancer. Age, tobacco, and heavy alcohol use have been identified as MAJOR risk factors for oral SCC.

38 (B) Both sentences are false. With acute leukemia, patient undergoes myelosuppressive chemotherapy, which causes suppression of the immune system. LESS than half who receive chemotherapy experience oral complications. Certain chemotherapy drugs have little effect on the mucosal tissues and do NOT cause significant immunosuppression.

39 (A) Angular cheilitis, pale oral mucosa, glossitis are signs of anemia. Leukemia is manifested as gingival bleeding, risk for infection, and gingival hypertrophy. Hemophilia is associated with excessive gingival bleeding. Jaundice is associated with yellow skin and sclera (white of eye) tones from hemoglobin breakdown and liver disease.

40 (E) When providing dental care with hemophilia, especially when procedures may cause bleeding or when inflammation is present, the entire dentition should NOT be scaled in one appointment. To minimize bleeding, instrumentation should occur in a series of small segments over several appointments. Before treatment, medical consult is needed, replacement factor should be given (according to physician's recommendation), and infection control protocols, using standard precautions, should be in place.

41 (A) With a cardiac condition, may have difficulty breathing in a supine position, thus patient chair should be adjusted upright (45°). Caution should be taken when administering local anesthetics because of possible drug interactions; however, MOST individuals with cardiac conditions have NO difficulty with local anesthetics and vasoconstrictors if the latter is reduced in amount. Patients with cardiac conditions are NOT at high risk for oral candidiasis or communication difficulties.

42 (D) Condensing osteitis and focal sclerosing osteitis have a characteristic radiopaque appearance. Dry socket (alveolar osteitis) would NOT indicate periapical change. BOTH periapical abscess and periapical granuloma may exhibit similar radiographic appearance, ranging from slight radiolucency to very distinct periapical radiolucency.

43 (B) Fibroma is similar in color to adjacent tissues. Because of increase in vascularity, pyogenic granuloma, papillary hyperplasia, and peripheral giant cell granuloma are all MORE erythematous than the surrounding tissue.

44 (C) Mandibular torus is a lobulated overgrowth of dense bone located in mandibular premolar region. Condensing osteitis is NOT exophytic; ranula is associated with a blocked salivary gland duct and would be located in the floor of the mouth; genial tubercles are normal anatomical landmark located inferior to the mandibular central incisors on the lingual surface of the jaw.

45 (B) Focal sclerosing osteomyelitis is observed as an apical radiopacity. BOTH periapical granuloma and abscess would be observed as a radiolucency; compound odontoma would exhibit collection of tooth-like radiopacities between two teeth.

46 (C) ONLY erythema multiforme (EM) exhibits targetlike lesion on the skin but occasionally on oral mucosa. EM is a skin condition of unknown etiology but may be mediated by deposition of immune complex (mostly IgM) in the superficial microvasculature of the skin and oral mucous membrane that usually follows antecedent infection or drug exposure.

47 (B) Chronic bulimia presents with erosion of maxillary anterior lingual tooth structure, caused by emesis (vomiting) of gastric acids (chemical wearing of tooth). Tooth loss associated with attrition and bruxism is caused by physiological wear of the incisal edge or occlusal surface and is NOT associated with tooth loss because of acid exposure. Tooth loss associated with abrasion occurs at the location of the repetitive habit (e.g., cementoenamel junction of the buccal surface from toothbrush abrasion).

48 (D) Fordyce granules (Fordyce's spots) appear as a yellow cluster on the buccal mucosa; this is a normal variation. Linea alba, also a normal variation, is a white line on the buccal mucosa corresponding to the occlusal plane. Mucocele is a clear vesicle caused by trauma to minor salivary gland, and lipoma is a single neoplasia composed of mature fat cells.

49 (D) Lichen planus is an autoimmune disease. Contact mucositis, dermatitis, and angioedema are ALL examples of a hypersensitivity response; may occur after latex exposure in sensitive individual.

50 (C) Macule is a flat lesion. Pedunculated lesion has a stalk. Sessile lesion is a broad-based lesion. Papule is an elevated lesion.

51 (B) Migratory, reversible desquamation of the filiform lingual papillae is noted with geographic tongue (benign migratory glossitis). No changes in fungiform, foliate, and circumvallate lingual papilla. Name is due to condition resembling a map.

52 (B) Pemphigus vulgaris is a separation of the epithelial tissue; removal of epithelium may be noted when gauze is rubbed across the lesion (positive Nikolsky's sign). Lesions associated with systemic lupus erythematosus, tuberculosis, and pemphigoid do NOT exhibit acantholysis (separation of epithelial cells) and Nikolsky's sign is less likely positive for pemphigoid than pemphigus.

53 (C) Globulomaxillary cyst is located between maxillary canine and lateral incisors. Dentigerous and radicular cysts may be located in a variety of locations; lateral periodontal cyst is located in mandibular canine and premolar area.

54 (D) Two neighboring teeth joined ONLY by cementum is concrescence. Germination is incomplete formation of two teeth from one; fusion is combination of BOTH cementum and dentin; dilaceration is abnormal root curvature; dens in dente is invagination of enamel organ during tooth development.

55 (D) Basal cell carcinoma (BCC) is associated with sun exposure. Heredity, alcohol, and tobacco are associated with squamous cell carcinoma rather than basal cell carcinoma. BCC is the MOST common form of skin cancer; can be destructive and disfiguring. Risk for BCC is increased for individuals with a family history of the disease and with high cumulative exposure to UV light via sunlight or exposure to carcinogenic chemicals, especially arsenic. Treatment is surgery, topical chemotherapy, radiation, cryosurgery, photodynamic therapy; rarely life threatening.

56 (A) Irregularly shaped mandibular incisors (Hutchinson's) and mandibular first molars (mulberry) may develop as a result of congenital syphilis. Both ectodermal dysplasia and amelogenesis imperfecta may cause defects in enamel, but they are NOT confined to incisors and first molars. Lesions associated with tuberculosis do NOT affect dental hard tissue but instead soft tissue (Ghon and ulcer lesions).

57 (D) Supernumerary (extra tooth) located between the maxillary incisors (#8 and #9) is a mesiodens, a developmental disorder. Microdont is a small tooth that could be located in a variety of locations. Dens-in-dente would NOT be located between central incisors.

58 (D) Taurodontism is caused by a decrease in normal invagination of Hertwig's epithelial root sheath (HERS) and is located ONLY in multirooted teeth. Peg lateral is a microdontic maxillary lateral incisor; talon cusp is a tooth with accessory cusp; enamel pearl is a small formation of enamel on root surface caused by misplaced ameloblast activity.

59 (C) Maxillary lateral incisor is MOST common microdont; maxillary third molar is also a common microdont. Both mandibular third molar and lateral incisor are seldom associated with microdontia.

60 (B) Static bone cyst is identified on a radiograph as a small, well-defined radiolucency in the lower posterior region of the mandible, NOT a true cyst because it is a bone depression caused by the adjacent salivary gland and is NOT lined by epithelium. Simple and traumatic bone cysts are true cysts. Salivary gland cysts do occur in the molar and premolar areas; NOT specific to these areas. Blockage of a salivary gland duct may also be noted with salivary gland cysts.

61 (B) Tetracycline taken during tooth formation may cause intrinsic tooth discoloration but does NOT cause gingival hyperplasia. Nifedipine (Adalat, Nifedical, Procardia), cyclosporine, and phenytoin (Dilantin) have been shown to cause gingival hyperplasia.

62 (D) Missing or conical incisors are associated with the hereditary disorder ectodermal dysplasia. Lack of sweat glands and thinning body hair are also characteristic. Dysplasia of tooth structure is noted in dentin dysplasia, amelogenesis imperfecta, and dentinogenesis imperfecta; however, cone-shaped incisors and ectodermal changes are NOT characteristics of these disorders.

63 (D) Radiographic evidence reveals cotton-wool appearance and loss of lamina dura with Paget's disease. With type 1 diabetes mellitus, may show evidence of bone loss associated with periodontal disease; with fibrous dysplasia, may show a diffuse radiopacity. Osteogenesis imperfecta presents with abnormally formed bones that fracture easily and abnormal dentin formation.

64 (D) Dentinogenesis imperfecta type II, also known as hereditary opalescent dentin, exhibits crowns that appear opalescent brown to blue. Anodontia, NOT opalescent teeth, is characteristic of ectodermal dysplasia. Dentin dysplasia (radicular type) exhibits normal tooth color. Coronal dentin dysplasia exhibits amber translucent teeth in the primary dentition and normal color in the permanent dentition. Amelogenesis imperfecta has poorly calcified, mottled, or thin enamel that appears yellowish brown.

65 (D) Macule is a circumscribed area of mucosa distinguished by color from its surroundings. Ulcer is an uncovered wound of cutaneous or mucosal tissue that exhibits tissue disintegration and necrosis. Erosion is a soft tissue lesion with denuded epithelium above basal layer that leaves a depressed, moist, glistening lesion. Scar tissue is permanent mark remaining after wound heals.

66 (A) Papule is a superficial, elevated, solid lesion that is ≤1 cm in diameter. May be of any color and may be attached by a stalk or firm base. Plaque is a flat, solid raised area that is ≥1 cm in diameter. Tumor is a solid mass of tissue larger than 1 cm in diameter that has the dimension of depth. Nodule is a solid mass of tissue ≤1 cm in diameter that has the dimension of depth.

67 (D) Squamous oral papilloma presents a papule type of lesion. Papule is a superficial, elevated, solid lesion that is ≤1 cm in diameter. May be of any color and may be attached by a stalk or firm base. Macule is a circumscribed area of mucosa distinguished by color from its surroundings, such as a melanoma. Nodule is a solid mass of tissue that is ≤1 cm in diameter and has the dimension of depth. Plaque is a flat, solid raised area that is ≥1 cm in diameter like early lesion of basal cell carcinoma.

68 (B) Vesicle is a circumscribed, fluid-filled elevation in the epithelium that is <1 cm in diameter. Fluid of the vesicle consists of lymph or serum but may contain blood. Pustule is a circumscribed elevation filled with purulent exudate resulting from an infection, ≤1 cm in diameter. When diameter of a vesicle is ≥1 cm, it is a bulla. Cyst is an epithelially lined mass located in the oral mucosa, as well as dermis and even subcutaneous tissue. Cysts result from entrapment of epithelium or remnants of epithelium that grow to produce a cavity.

69 (A) Eruption cyst is soft tissue variant of the dentigerous cyst that forms around an erupting tooth crown. Children <10 years are MOST commonly affected. Appears as a small, dome-shaped, translucent swelling overlying an erupting primary tooth. Congenital epulis is a benign, soft tissue polypoid growth arising from the edentulous alveolar ridge. Remnant of the dental lamina that does NOT develop into a tooth bud may degenerate to form dental lamina cyst. Natal teeth are present at birth or erupt within 30 days of birth.

70 (D) Microdontia teeth are smaller than normal. Condition is usually noted bilaterally and is seen in families; may occur as an isolated finding, in relative condition, or in a generalized pattern. Occurs MOST with maxillary lateral incisor (peg lateral) and third molars. Macrodontic teeth are larger than normal. Fusion is the union of two tooth buds at the level of the dentin to form one tooth. Germination occurs when single tooth bud forms into two teeth (one root with canal and two crowns). BOTH fusion and gemination can leave teeth that are larger (false macrodontia). Dens invaginatus (dens in dente) is a developmental anomaly in which enamel organ invaginates into dental papilla along lingual aspect; MOST are in maxillary lateral incisors.

71 (B) Maxillary abscess can form on palate but would consist of soft tissues, UNLIKE the palatal torus, which is hard bony exostosis. Nasopalatine duct cyst is heart-shaped midline radiolucency, within incisive papilla or duct. Pleomorphic adenoma can ALSO form on palate but is a benign salivary gland tumor with mixture of epithelial and connective tissue cells.

72 (C) Loss of consciousness is associated with epilepsy, as are convulsive episodes. Individuals with cerebral palsy, mental retardation (intellectual disability), or autism alone are NOT prone to convulsions or loss of consciousness.

73 (A) Aura (predication) often precedes an epileptic seizure and is NOT typically associated with myocardial infarction, anorexia nervosa, or Sjögren's syndrome.

74 (A) Both statements are true. Biopsy examination includes BOTH surface and deep internal cells of lesion. Exfoliative cytology permits ONLY examination of surface cells, allowing potential for false negative. Statements highlight one of MAIN differences between the two types of tests and show advantage of biopsy.

75 (D) Patients respond favorably to exfoliative cytology, since it does NOT involve cutting the tissue. Unfortunately, it has a number of significant disadvantages as a diagnostic tool, such as limitations on kinds of lesions evaluated and frequent false negatives, and is NOT considered definitive.

CHAPTER 7

Nutrition

NUTRIENTS AND DEFICIENCIES

Nutrients are substances obtained from food and promote growth, maintenance, or repair. Six classes of nutrients include **macronutrients** (biomolecules) of proteins, carbohydrates, and lipids, as well as vitamins, minerals, and water. For **Acceptable Macronutrient Distribution Ranges** (AMDRs), adults should obtain 10% to 35% of calories from protein, 45% to 65% from carbohydrates, and 20% to 35% from lipids (fat). Acceptable ranges for children are SIMILAR, except that infants and younger children need higher proportion of fat (25% to 40%).

For vitamins and minerals, **Dietary Reference Intakes** (DRIs), issued by the Institute of Medicine of the National Academy, are the *average* daily dietary intake level sufficient to meet nutrient requirements of nearly ALL (~98%) healthy individuals (includes Recommended Dietary [Daily] Allowance [RDA]) (Table 7-1). RDIs (Reference Daily Intakes) and DVRs (Daily Recommended Values) are comparable standards and can be combined to create DVs (Daily Values), as published by the FDA.

Malnutrition is an imbalance between nutrients the body needs and nutrients it receives. Includes **overnutrition** (consumption of *too* many calories or *too* much of specific nutrient) and **undernutrition** (deficiency MAINLY of calories or protein). Deficiencies of vitamins and minerals are usually considered separate disorders. When calories are deficient, however, vitamins and minerals are also likely to be. **Calorie** or kilocalorie (kcal) is a unit of measurement for energy, in this case food energy. Energy is measured by heat expenditure; 1 kilocalorie is the amount of heat produced to raise temperature of 1 kilogram of water 1° C.

- See CD-ROM for Chapter Terms and WebLinks.
- See Chapters 3, Anatomy, Biochemistry, and Physiology: biomolecules; 6, General Pathology, and 16, Special Needs Patient Care: nutrition-related conditions and diseases.

Proteins

Proteins are organic compounds that are composed of amino acids, building blocks of proteins. Contain carbon, hydrogen, oxygen, nitrogen. MAIN function is to build tissue and replace cells. Presence of proteins affects ALL body activities.

A. Types:
   1. Amino acids (20) held together by peptide bonds; carboxyl (COOH) group of one amino acid is linked to an amino (NH_2) group of another.
      a. The 9 essential (indispensable) amino acids (EAAs) CANNOT be synthesized by the body and must be obtained from the diet; nitrogen balance can be achieved from proper proportions and adequate amounts of these.
      b. The 11 nonessential (dispensable) amino acids (NEAAs) can be synthesized by the body ONLY when nitrogen is present.
   2. Complete proteins (high-quality): foods that consist of ALL the essential amino acids in sufficient amounts; completely supply the needs of the body for maintenance, repair, and growth; are found in meat, fish, poultry, eggs, cheese, milk.
   3. Incomplete proteins (low-quality): foods that lack one or more essential amino acids; include plant proteins; when ONLY food eaten, can support life but NOT normal growth.
   4. Complementary proteins: two or more proteins that combine to compensate for deficiencies in amino acid content; use of whole grains IMPORTANT.

B. Physiology and metabolism of proteins: see Chapter 3, Anatomy, Biochemistry, and Physiology

C. Functions of proteins:
   1. Role in overall body needs; assist in growth, maintenance, construction, and repair of body tissue.
   2. Provide essential components of hormones and enzymes and provide precursors of antibodies.
   3. Provide energy source when carbohydrate and fat intake is inadequate: 4 kcal per gram (g).
   4. Regulate acid-base balance.

D. Role in oral health:
   1. Essential for cell growth; thus IMPORTANT in growth and development of the oral cavity.
   2. Maintain pulp.
   3. If absent, result is crowded and/or rotated teeth because of inadequate growth of bone.
   4. Deficiency can lead to disturbances in tooth development such as with kwashiorkor or marasmus (see later discussion) or damage to the periodontium (as with kwashiorkor).

Table 7-1 Acceptable macronutrient distribution ranges (AMDRs) and dietary reference Intakes (DRIs) for adults per day*

Macronutrient	Females	Males
Protein	46 g	56 g
Carbohydrates	130 g	Same
Lipids	None	Same
Vitamin A (retinol)	700 μg	900 μg
Vitamin D	5 μg (AI)†	Same
Vitamin E	15 mg‡	Same
Vitamin K	90 μg (AI)	120 μg
Thiamine (vitamin B_1)	1.1 mg	1.2 mg
Riboflavin (vitamin B_2)	1.1 mg	1.3 mg
Niacin (vitamin B_3)	14 mg	16 mg
Pantothenic acid (vitamin B_5)	5 mg (AI)	Same
Pyridoxine (vitamin B_6)	1.3 mg	Same
Cobalamin (vitamin B_{12})	2.4 μg	Same
Vitamin C (ascorbic acid)	75 mg§	90 mg§
Biotin	30 μg (AI)	Same
Folate (folacin, folic acid)	400 μg	Same
Calcium	1000 mg (AI)	Same
Phosphorus	700 mg	Same
Magnesium	310 mg	400 mg
Sodium	500 mg	Same
Chloride	750 mg	Same
Potassium	2000 mg	Same
Sulfur	None	Same

AI, Adequate intake.
*Includes adequate intake or Estimated Average Requirement (EAR), where NO DRI has been established, expected to satisfy needs of 50%.
†5 μg = 200 IU (International Units).
‡Tolerable upper intake limit (UL) is 1000 mg/day.
§Smokers should add 35 mg to these values.

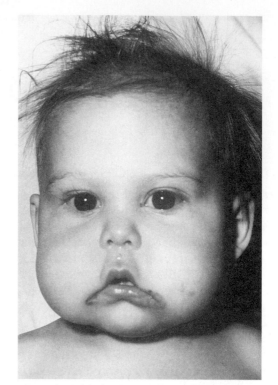

Figure 7-1 Kwashiorkor is a severe protein deficiency even with calories from carbohydrates, without severe wasting of body fat, but with apathy, failure to grow, and edema.

G. Nutrient sources of proteins:
 1. Complete proteins: meat, fish, poultry, eggs, milk.
 2. Incomplete proteins: legumes, grains, vegetables, soybeans.
H. Nutritional deficiency and diseases related to proteins:
 1. Phenylketonuria (PKU):
  a. Liver CANNOT metabolize essential amino acid phenylalanine into nonessential amino acid tyrosine.
  b. Toxic by-products build up in the body and damage developing nervous system of infant, causing intellectual disability (mental retardation).
  c. Managed by restricting phenylalanine to only enough to support normal growth; supplement tyrosine; avoid aspartame (Nutrasweet, Equal).
 2. Protein-energy (calorie) malnutrition (PEM, PCM) or undernutrition:
  a. Marasmus: inadequate food intake; MOST common in children 6 to 18 months of age in impoverished nations; impairs brain development and learning; MAINLY causes severe wasting and weakening of muscles; NO edema.
  b. Kwashiorkor: severe protein deficiency even with calories from carbohydrates; begins at approximately 2 years; WITHOUT severe wasting of body fat; symptoms include apathy, failure to grow and gain weight, listlessness, changes in hair color, edema in abdomen and legs (causes

5. Can help neutralize acids produced by dental biofilm (dental plaque).
E. Role in periodontal health or disease:
 1. IMPORTANT in maintaining health of periodontium.
 2. Essential for cellular defenses against bacteria in subgingival dental biofilm.
 3. Essential for healing and repair of tissue after periodontal trauma or surgery.
F. Dietary requirements for proteins: 0.8 g per kg of body weight for adults:
 1. DRI for adults: 46 g (female) and 56 g (male) per day.
 2. Increased during periods of growth, pregnancy, lactation.
 3. Increased during episodes of trauma, fear, anxiety, surgery, fever.

swelling); associated with necrotizing peri-odontal disease (Figure 7-1).

  c. Starvation: MOST extreme form of marasmus (and undernutrition), results from partial or total lack of essential nutrients for a long time (see self-starvation under patient with eating disorder).

  d. Cachexia: severe wasting away of muscle and fat tissue as a result of excessive production of substances called cytokines, produced by immune system in response to a disorder; MOST common with cancer and AIDS.

  e. Adult PEM (PCM): alcoholics (with nutritional liver disease), long-term bedridden or hospital patients, persons taking certain drugs that decrease appetite (diuretics) or increase metabolism (thyroxine).

    (1) Oral effects of PEM (PCM):

      (a) Tooth development decreased.

      (b) Salivary composition and flow affected.

      (c) Connective tissue and bone development affected.

      (d) Acid production increased.

3. Overconsumption of proteins (e.g., Atkins diet, with low carbohydrates):

  a. May affect calcium balance if inadequate calcium.

  b. Increase in water consumption.

  c. Additional fat stores.

  d. Stress to liver and kidneys owing to presence of excess ketones, especially if already damaged.

  e. Halitosis.

4. Possible deficiency in poorly planned strict vegan diets (consisting ONLY of plant foods); adequate as long as caloric intake is adequate and variety of foods is eaten.

  a. Easier to achieve with diets that include dairy products and eggs (lacto-ovo-vegetarian).

  b. Harder to achieve with diets consisting ONLY of fruits and vegetable oils (fruitarian diets).

Carbohydrates

Carbohydrates are organic compounds (contain carbon) that also contain the elements hydrogen and oxygen. Provide energy during metabolism (you burn 20 calories per hour chewing gum).

A. Types of carbohydrates:

  1. Simple carbohydrates:

    a. **Monosaccharides** (single sugars):

      (1) Pentoses (C5) act as coenzymes in energy production (e.g., ribose, deoxyribose).

      (2) Hexoses (C6) have MAJOR nutritional importance.

      (3) Glucose (blood sugar or dextrose) is the form used MOST efficiently by the body; obtained from ALL plant carbohydrates; serves MAINLY as fuel for the brain; found in honey, fruits, corn syrup; however, ALL sugars are converted to glucose, so do NOT need these to feed the brain.

      (4) Fructose (levulose, fruit sugar) is the sweetest of ALL sugars; closely related to glucose structurally; found in honey, fruits, corn syrup; changed to lactic acid by *Streptococcus mutans*.

      (5) Galactose, derived from hydrolysis of lactose; constituent of many plant polysaccharides; during lactation, body converts glucose to galactose in mammary tissue to synthesize lactose in breast milk.

    b. **Disaccharides** (double sugars; two monosaccharides):

      (1) Lactose (milk sugar) is composed of glucose and galactose; obtained from milk products.

      (2) Sucrose (table sugar; cane and beet sugar) composed of glucose and fructose; obtained from sugar beets, sugarcane, or maple syrup.

      (3) Maltose (plant sugar) is composed of two molecules of glucose; forms as starch in grains and breaks down during germination; ferments alcohol.

  2. Complex carbohydrates (long chains of sugars):

    a. Polysaccharides:

      (1) Starch (mixture of amylose and amylopectin) is the MOST important carbohydrate. Digestible by humans; stores energy in plants; breaks down at slower rate than monosaccharides and disaccharides; found in rice, wheat, corn, rye, potatoes, legumes.

      (2) Glycogen is the animal equivalent of starch; provides food storage system for ALL forms of animal life; stored in liver, where it regulates blood sugar, and in muscle, where it serves as an energy source for muscle contraction.

      (3) Insulin is produced by pancreas; stores energy.

      (4) Dextran forms a substrate for dental biofilm (dental plaque); serves as energy source for dental caries–producing bacteria such as *Streptococcus mutans;* makes dental biofilm sticky.

    b. Fibers:

      (1) Cellulose: provides fibrous framework for plants; good source of fiber; NOT digestible and therefore provides roughage and bulk to aid in peristalsis and elimination of water; found in fruits, legumes, ALL vegetables.

(2) Hemicellulose: group of fibers that are insoluble (do NOT easily dissolve in water); MAIN constituent of cereal fibers.

(3) Pectin: responsible for thickening of jams and fruit preserves; keeps salad dressing from separating; found in vegetables and fruits, especially citrus fruits and apples.

B. Physiology and metabolism of carbohydrates: see Chapter 3, Anatomy, Biochemistry, and Physiology.

C. Functions of carbohydrates:

1. Provide energy (4 kcal/g).
2. Spare proteins so they can supply energy when necessary, but MAIN function is to build tissue, replace cells.
3. Aid in oxidation (burning) of fats to prevent ketosis (partial fat breakdown; leads to increased ketone levels in bloodstream).
4. Furnish fiber for peristalsis; also provide bulk, reduce risk of cardiovascular disease, prevent constipation and diverticular disease.
5. Aid in formation of intercellular substance (ground substance) and collagen.
6. Aid in formation of nonessential amino acids.

D. Dietary requirements for carbohydrates:

1. DRI: 130 g/day; infants require MORE carbohydrates to prevent use of protein for energy.
2. Maximum intake level of ≤25% from added sugars.
3. Dietary fiber recommended intake: ≤50 years 25 g (female) and 38 g (male)/day; >50 years is 30 and 21 g/day, respectively, owing to decreased food consumption.

E. Nutrient sources of carbohydrates:

1. Milk, cereals, breads provide starch.
2. Leafy vegetables provide cellulose and hemicellulose.
3. Vegetables such as root tuber and seed (potatoes, beans, beets, squash) provide starch and sucrose.
4. Fruits provide MAINLY glucose and fructose.
5. Sugar, honey, corn syrups provide monosaccharides and disaccharides.
6. Sweeteners:
   a. Sucrose: disaccharide found in table sugar, beet sugar, cane sugar.
   b. High-fructose corn syrup (HFCS): 40% to 90% fructose; made by treating corn starch with acid and enzymes to break it down into glucose, which then is changed into fructose; possibly tied to obesity.
   c. Turbinado sugar: partially refined version of raw sugar; has a slight molasses flavor.
   d. Brown sugar: white sugar that contains some molasses; molasses is either added or not totally removed.
   e. Maple syrup: boiled sap from sugar maple trees.

7. Alternative sweeteners:
   a. Sugar alcohols are sugarlike compounds (nutritive sweeteners) that, like carbohydrates, yield 4 kcal/g of energy; metabolized MORE slowly than sucrose by bacteria in the mouth and therefore do NOT promote caries; CANNOT be used at same time as disulfiram (Antabuse) prescribed for treatment of alcohol abuse and alcohol dependence.
   b. Xylitol: derived from cellulose products such as wood straw or pulp cane; may produce diarrhea when taken in excess; equivalent to sucrose in sweetness; used in sugarless gums and foods, since does NOT promote caries; also reduces bacterial tooth adherence and secretion of acids and promotes tooth remineralization; must follow manufacturer's instructions when used for anticaries purposes.
   c. Sorbitol: from glucose by hydrogenation; used in foods, especially diabetic foods and sugarless gums; NOT readily absorbed by the small intestine and therefore can cause diarrhea.
   d. Mannitol: from mannose and galactose by hydrogenation; used in sugarless gums and candies; NOT readily absorbed by the small intestine; may cause diarrhea.

8. Artificial sweeteners include noncarbohydrate, noncaloric, or low caloric:
   a. Sucralose (Splenda): 600 times sweeter than sucrose, twice as sweet as saccharin and four times as sweet as aspartame; stable under heat and can be used in baking and products that require longer shelf-life; NOT recognized by body as carbohydrate, so does NOT affect blood glucose levels or insulin response (useful for diabetics); essentially inert molecule that passes through body without being broken down for calories.
   b. Aspartame (Nutrasweet, Equal): composed of two amino acids (phenylalanine and aspartic acid) and methanol; used ONLY in beverages, gelatin desserts, and sugarless gum; CANNOT be used in baking (low-calorie sweetener yields 4 kcal/g).
   c. Saccharin: derived from coal-tar compounds; 500 times sweeter than sucrose; widely used in soft drinks and table sweeteners; may cause cancer, and therefore products must contain a warning label.
   d. Acesulfame-K: 200 times sweeter than sucrose; used in sugarless gum, powdered drink mixes, gelatin puddings, nondairy creamers; can be used in baking.

F. Nutritional management of disease and deficiency related to carbohydrates. See Chapter 6, General and Oral Pathology.

1. Diabetes mellitus (DM): metabolic endocrine disorder with high blood glucose level as result of insufficient or ineffective insulin function; results in tissue damage; diet considerations will be guided by diabetic nutrition counselor.
   a. Non-insulin-dependent (MAINLY type 2):
      (1) Restrict calories and reduce weight.
      (2) Engage in regular exercise (assists muscles in taking up MORE glucose).
      (3) Space meals evenly throughout the day.
      (4) Avoid alcohol consumption.
   b. Insulin-dependent (MAINLY type 1):
      (1) Requires careful nutritional assessment; SHOULD eat regular meals with precise carbohydrate-to-protein-to-fat ratio.
      (2) Intensive insulin therapy, including regular blood glucose monitoring.
      (3) Regular exercise.
2. Reactive hypoglycemia (low blood glucose levels):
   a. Occurs in reaction to ingestion of food, 1 to 4 hours after meal:
      (1) Initial symptoms include weakness, rapid heartbeat, sweating, anxiety, hunger; caused by release of epinephrine (hormone), which is triggered by falling blood glucose level.
      (2) Fasting sets in gradually and affects the brain and central nervous system (CNS); symptoms then include headache, fatigue, blurred vision, confusion; are NOT related to epinephrine release.
   b. Prevention: eat regular meals with protein, fat, complex carbohydrates that contain soluble fiber; AVOID concentrated sweets.
   c. Management: eat balanced meals at regular intervals (this is the diet for NDHBE time!).
3. Lactose intolerance: intestinal condition with reduced lactose digestion because of deficiency of digestive enzyme lactase, which hydrolyzes lactose to glucose and galactose in the intestine.
   a. When lactase is absent in small intestine, lactose travels to large intestine, where bacteria break it down into gas and acids.
   b. Symptoms: cramps, abdominal distention, gas symptoms, diarrhea after consumption of dairy products.
   c. Management:
      (1) Eat smaller servings of milk products.
      (2) Include fat in meals; slows digestion and leaves MORE time for lactase action.
      (3) Eat cheese; lactose is lost when milk is processed into cheese.
      (4) Consume yogurt with active bacteria cultures; lactose is digested by yogurt.
4. Dental caries:
   a. Dental biofilm (dental plaque) bacteria break down sucrose and glucose into lactic acid as result of enzymatic activity of streptococci and lactobacilli.
      (1) *Streptococcus mutans* initiates process; synthesizes polysaccharides (glycogen, dextran, levan) for future fermentation.
         (a) Polysaccharides are used for energy when needed.
         (b) Dextrans form substrate and serve as energy source.
         (c) Demineralization begins at 5.5 pH.
      (2) *Lactobacillus acidophilus* extends process.
   b. Fermentable carbohydrate ingestion: concentration of sugars in food is KEY factor in caries development.
      (1) Sugar-rich foods: cariogenic activity of sucrose, glucose, fructose is similar; physical form of food also affects activity (oral clearance time of liquids is faster than that of solids and retentive sweets; thus sugared liquids are generally less cariogenic).
      (2) Concentration of 0.8 M must be present for sugar to pass through 1 mm of dental biofilm and undergo harmful fermentation (e.g., 1-M solution of sugar contains 342.3 g of sugar in water).
      (3) Starch-rich foods: if left on teeth for long periods, will degrade to organic acids and can contribute to acid levels.
   c. Salivary flow rate: inadequate salivary flow (e.g., xerostomia) interferes with oral clearance time of cariogenic foods, decreasing natural salivary buffers and initiating caries development.
   d. Daily food intake frequency: development related to between-meal snacking; eating sweets with a meal makes them less cariogenic.

CLINICAL STUDY

Scenario: The 8-year-old patient is in the dental office for a 6-month oral prophylaxis maintenance appointment. When asked more about the child's health, the mother said the girl even wet her bed a couple of nights ago. The mother also notes that she has recently had an increased appetite yet has lost weight. "My daughter had a severe chest cold about 2 months ago and now she is waking up frequently during the night to urinate."

1. What is the most likely diagnosis of the patient's condition?

2. Identify the usual causes and predisposing factors for this condition.

3. What is the best treatment plan for this condition?

4. Is this condition preventable? And if so, how?

5. What type of nutritional management would be recommended for the patient?

1. Type 1 diabetes mellitus (DM).
2. Condition that may trigger onset of type 1 DM is a viral infection. Infection may affect immune response that attacks the pancreas, leading to inability to make insulin. Symptoms include polyuria (frequent urination), increased appetite (polyphagia), thirst (polydipsia), weight loss.
3. Treatment plan would include insulin therapy, regular blood glucose monitoring, careful nutritional assessment.
4. DM cannot be prevented but can be controlled by drugs and diet. Although viral infection may play a part in the development of type 1 DM, its determination as a cause cannot always be made.
5. The patient requires careful nutritional assessment by a diabetic nutrition counselor; should eat regular meals with precise carbohydrate-to-protein-to-fat ratio; needs intensive insulin therapy, including regular blood glucose monitoring and regular exercise.

Lipids

Lipids (fats) are organic compounds composed of carbon, hydrogen, oxygen. Types include triglycerides (fats and oils), phospholipids, sterols (cholesterol). MAIN function is to provide energy.

A. Types of lipids:
1. True fats are composed of glycerol (trihydroxy alcohol) that is attached to one, two, or three fatty acids to form monoglycerides, diglycerides, or triglycerides, respectively.
   a. Saturated fatty acid carries maximum number of hydrogen atoms; remains solid at room temperature; increases serum cholesterol.
      (1) Stearic acid in beef and lard.
      (2) Palmitic acid in animal fat and palm oil.
      (3) Myristic and lauric acid in coconut oil.
   b. Monounsaturated fatty acid contains a point of unsaturated linkage (with NO hydrogen atom); viscous in form; NO effect on serum cholesterol.
      (1) Oleic acid sources include olive oil, shortening, lamb, canola oils.
   c. Polyunsaturated fatty acid contains two or more points of unsaturation; liquid in consistency (includes oils); decreases serum cholesterol.
      (1) Omega-6 fatty acids are linoleic; found in corn, cottonseed, safflower, and sunflower oils, tofu.
      (2) Omega-3 fatty acids are linolenic; found in fatty fish oils, green leafy vegetables, soybean products (tofu).
   d. Essential fatty acids (i.e., linoleic and linolenic acids) must be obtained from diet; regulate blood pressure, assist in clot formation, maintain cell membranes, make hormone-like substances, support functioning of the retina.
2. Compound lipids are compounds added to glycerol and fatty acids.
   a. Phospholipids are built on backbone of glycerol, with one fatty acid replaced by a compound that contains phosphorus.
      (1) Lecithin is found in cells and participates in fat digestion in the intestine; acts as an emulsifier by mixing oil with water (e.g., in salad dressings, mayonnaise); found in egg yolk.
   b. Lipoproteins are produced in the liver and allow cholesterol, triglycerides, phospholipids to be transported in the bloodstream.
      (1) Chylomicrons are made in the intestine after fat absorption; contain triglycerides and a small amount of protein.
         (a) Transport newly absorbed lipids from intestinal cells to the bloodstream by way of the lymphatic system.
         (b) During circulation, cells remove lipid content and therefore become smaller.
         (c) Liver picks up and breaks down chylomicrons and assembles new lipoproteins known as very low-density lipoproteins (VLDLs).
      (2) VLDLs: the liver coats cholesterol and triglycerides with a shell of protein and lipids.
         (a) VLDLs leave the liver, and triglycerides are broken down into fatty acids and glycerol by the enzyme lipase.
         (b) VLDLs become much heavier as triglycerides are released.
         (c) VLDLs gather cholesterol from other lipoproteins and become low-density lipoproteins (LDLs).
      (3) **Low-density lipoproteins** (LDLs): composed MOSTLY of cholesterol; contain a few triglycerides; larger, lighter, MORE lipid filled than VLDLs ("bad guys") (see note with nicotinic acid later).
         (a) Cells absorb LDLs from the bloodstream and break them down; MOST LDLs are taken up by liver cells when a diet is low in saturated fats and cholesterol.

(b) Scavenger cells in blood vessels engulf LDLs that are NOT taken up; over time, cholesterol builds up on inner blood vessel walls and plaque develops.

(c) Blood supply to organs is subsequently cut off (ischemia), which may result in cardiovascular disease (CVD), myocardial infarction (MI, heart attack), or cerebrovascular accident (CVA, stroke).

(4) **High-density lipoproteins** (HDLs): produced by liver and intestine; smaller, denser; contain high amount of protein ("good guys").

(a) HDLs travel in the bloodstream and pick up cholesterol.

(b) Cholesterol is transported by way of other lipoproteins back to liver for excretion.

(c) High HDL levels slow development of CVD.

3. Cholesterol (sterol):

a. Capable of forming esters with fatty acids.

b. Makes IMPORTANT hormones (estrogen, testosterone).

c. Makes bile, emulsifier needed for digestion.

d. Found ONLY in animal foods.

e. Liver can make what the body needs; high levels raise total plasma cholesterol level.

4. Fat replacements (artificial fats):

a. Olestra: made by adding fatty acids to sugar; yields NO energy to the body; may lower blood serum cholesterol levels; reduces absorption of vitamin E; has NO kilocalories; may cause diarrhea.

b. Simplesse: whey protein product; feels like fat in the mouth but contains NO fatty acids; CANNOT be used in cooking; contains 1.3 kcal/g.

c. Hydrogenation: process that reduces amount of fat per serving (e.g., diet margarine).

d. Gums: derived from plant sources and added to thicken products such as diet salad dressings.

B. Physiology and metabolism of lipids: see Chapter 3, Anatomy, Biochemistry, and Physiology, and Chapter 9, Pharmacology, for control of LDLs.

C. Functions of lipids:

1. Provide energy (9 kcal/g) (used for energy by body *after* readily available carbohydrates are used up).

2. Store energy.

3. Insulate to maintain body temperature and protect organs.

4. Transport fat-soluble vitamins to small intestine and aid in absorption.

5. Produce satiety (feeling of fullness).

6. Provide flavor and texture to foods.

D. Dietary requirements of lipids: ≤25% to 35% of total kcal (AMDR); NO DRI.

1. Saturated: <10% total kcal.

2. Monounsaturated: ~10% total kcal.

3. Polyunsaturated: ~10% total kcal.

4. Essential fatty acids: 1% to 3% total kcal.

5. Cholesterol: ≤300 mg/day.

E. Nutrient sources of lipids:

1. Saturated: animal fat and palm oil.

2. Monounsaturated: olive oil, shortening, lamb.

3. Polyunsaturated: soybean, cottonseed, and vegetable oils.

4. Cholesterol: animal foods.

5. Essential fatty acids: vegetable oils; recommendation is 1 tablespoon per day.

F. Nutritional management of deficiency and disease related to lipids:

1. Atherosclerosis: degenerative disease that produces hardening of large and medium arteries.

a. Formation of plaques:

(1) Includes formation of atheromata, deposits on inner walls of arteries.

(2) With age, plaque becomes fibrotic and narrows blood vessels.

(3) Eventually ischemia occurs, leading to decreased blood supply, development of CVD with complications.

b. Risk factors:

(1) Total blood cholesterol >240 mg/100 mL.

(2) LDL cholesterol >160 mg/100 mL.

(3) HDL cholesterol <35 mg/100 mL.

(4) Men >45 years; women >55 years.

(5) Smoking and family history.

(6) Hypertension.

c. Management:

(1) Reduce saturated fat in diet (intake <10% of total kilocalories lowers LDL cholesterol level); maintain polyunsaturated and monounsaturated fat intake at ~10% of total kilocalories.

(2) Increase consumption of dietary fiber (20 to 35 g per day).

(3) Lose weight; then maintain desirable body weight.

(4) Stop smoking.

(5) Eat LESS cholesterol (<300 mg per day).

(6) Replace foods rich in animal fat, butter, coconut oil, hydrogenated (solid) fat with LESS hydrogenated forms; low-fat (or fat-free, nonfat in some cases) food recommendations:

(a) Meat, fish, poultry: lean cuts; trim fat; grill, roast, or bake; tuna packed in water.

(b) Dairy: low-fat or nonfat milk, cheese, yogurt, nonfat frozen yogurt.

(c) Fruits and vegetables: nonfat salad dressing; steamed vegetables; fruit for dessert.

(d) Breads and cereals: jelly on bread instead of butter or margarine; avoid croissants, coffee cake, sweet rolls.

2. Obesity (see weight control section):
    a. Decrease fat and calorie intake.
    b. Excess weight of 30% increases risk of CVD, high blood pressure (HBP), DM, cancer.

Vitamins

Vitamins are organic nutrients needed by the body in small quantities. They do NOT contribute energy to the body but are facilitators of body processes. **Fat-soluble vitamins** include A, D, E, and K; **water-soluble vitamins** include the Bs and C. Note that DRI is for adults.

A. *Fat-soluble vitamins:* soluble in fats and fat solvents; mineral oils interfere with absorption; NOT readily excreted and so can build up to toxic levels; stored in liver and fatty tissues:
    1. Vitamin A (retinol):
        a. Function:
            (1) IMPORTANT for night vision; retinol forms rhodopsin (visual pigment).
            (2) Facilitates transcription of DNA to RNA.
            (3) Antioxidant properties help prevent damage to cells by free radicals.
            (4) Necessary for immune defenses.
            (5) Promotes normal growth and development.
            (6) Facilitates absorption of calcium at intestine.
            (7) Assists in maintenance of epithelial cells such as those of oral mucosa.
            (8) Assists in formation of ameloblasts and odontoblasts.
        b. DRI: 700 micrograms (µg or mcg) (female) and 900 µg (males).
        c. Nutrient sources:
            (1) Preformed vitamin A (retinoids; animal form) is found in liver, body fat of fish, egg yolk, butter, cheese, cereal, crackers, vitamin A–fortified milk.
            (2) Provitamin A (carotenoids; from plant-derived precursor carotene) is converted in body to vitamin A; MOST potent form is beta-carotene (antioxidant); found in orange-yellow and dark green fruits and vegetables (e.g., carrots, spinach, apricots, broccoli).
        d. Nutritional deficiency and disease: night blindness (nyctalopia); dry, rough skin or dry oral mucosa; glossitis; pulp calcification; enamel hypoplasia; defective dentin; acne and skin problems treated with isotretinoin (Accutane), which can dry oral cavity.
        e. Toxicity: irritability; enlarged liver and spleen; dry skin; bone and joint pain; xerostomia; damage to red blood cells (RBCs) and lysosomes; increased risk of hip fractures because of stimulation of osteoclasts and inhibition of osteoblasts.

    2. Vitamin D (calciferol):
        a. Functions as a hormone:
            (1) Absorbing calcium and phosphorus.
            (2) Promoting mineralization of teeth and bones.
            (3) Regulating proper serum levels of calcium and phosphorus.
        b. DRI: 5 µg (adequate intake [AI]).
        c. Nutrient sources:
            (1) Sunlight: liver makes a vitamin D precursor (7-dehydrocholesterol) that surfaces on the skin, is activated by sunlight, and is converted into vitamin D_3 (cholecalciferol).
            (2) Ultraviolet light.
            (3) Fortified milk, butter, cod-liver oil, fatty fish.
            (4) Vitamin D_2 (ergocalciferol): derived from plants, especially yeasts and fungi.
        d. Nutritional deficiency and disease:
            (1) Rickets in children: softening of the bones (failure to calcify normally); bowed legs; enlarged head, joints, rib cage; deformed pelvis.
            (2) Osteomalacia in adults: calcium is taken from bones to make up for insufficient absorption by the intestine; bowed legs, bent posture, and pain in ribs, pelvis, legs.
        e. Toxicity: occurs with high blood calcium levels; nausea, weight loss, constipation, weakness, vomiting, loss of appetite, mental confusion.
    3. Vitamin E (tocopherol):
        a. Functions:
            (1) Antioxidant: prevents oxidation of vitamin A, beta-carotene, vitamin C, unsaturated fatty acids.
            (2) Protects RBCs from damage.
            (3) Necessary for neural and muscular structure.
            (4) Necessary for cellular respiration.
        b. DRI: 15 mg/day, 1000 mg/day upper limit (UL); NO proven need for supplementation.
        c. Nutrient sources:
            (1) Plant (vegetable) oils: safflower, cottonseed, peanut.
            (2) Green leafy vegetables.
            (3) Legumes, nuts, whole grains.
            (4) Apricots, apples, peaches.
        d. Nutritional deficiency and disease: erythrocyte hemolysis (breakdown of RBCs), anemia.
        e. Toxicity: relatively safe; increased levels may lead to increased bleeding, especially in those prone (drugs, medical history, etc.).
    4. Vitamin K:
        a. Function: synthesizes blood-clotting factor prothrombin (PT).
        b. DRI: 90 µg (AI) (female) and 120 µg (male)/day.

c. Nutrient sources: green leafy vegetables; meat and dairy; also synthesized by intestine.

d. Nutritional deficiency: hemorrhage; for females, reduced bone mass.

e. Toxicity: eating large amounts in foods can counteract benefits of blood-thinning agents such as warfarin (Coumadin), heparin, or aspirin for CVD.

B. *Water-soluble vitamins:* easily excreted; LESS likely to reach toxic levels; NOT stored in body; need daily amounts.

1. Thiamin (B_1):

   a. Functions:

      (1) Essential in metabolism of carbohydrates and aids in metabolism of fats and proteins.

      (2) Assists in proper functioning of nervous and cardiovascular systems.

   b. Properties: sensitive to heat; avoid overcooking.

   c. DRI: 1.1 mg (female) and 1.2 mg (male)/day.

   d. Nutrient sources: whole grains (wheat germ), pork, sunflower seeds, nuts, legumes (peanuts, soybeans), organ meats.

   e. Nutritional deficiency and disease: causes beriberi, which used to be present only in those whose diet was polished white rice in Asia but is now rare and associated ONLY with alcoholics, because drinking heavily can lead to poor nutrition, making it harder to absorb and store vitamin; two types: wet, affecting cardiovascular system, and dry, affecting nervous system.

   f. Presents with limb swelling, elevated pulse, heart failure; Wernicke-Korsakoff syndrome (jerky gait, disorientation, impaired short-term memory) occurs among alcoholics.

2. Riboflavin (B_2):

   a. Functions: aids in metabolism of carbohydrates, fats, and proteins; assists in adenosine triphosphate (ATP) formation.

   b. Properties: sensitive to light; milk SHOULD be stored in cardboard or opaque containers.

   c. DRI: 1.1 mg (female) and 1.3 mg (male)/day.

   d. Nutrient sources: milk products, grains, organ meats, green vegetables (e.g., broccoli, turnip greens, asparagus), meat, poultry, fish, enriched food.

   e. Nutritional deficiency and disease: glossitis, angular cheilosis, dermatitis, anemia.

3. Niacin (B_3):

   a. Functions:

      (1) Coenzyme that assists in energy metabolism.

      (2) Aids normal functioning of CNS.

      (3) Maintains healthy skin and oral mucosa; however, essential for growth of cariogenic bacteria.

      (4) Supplemental nicotinic acid (2 to 3 g/day; >1000 mg may cause facial flush if NOT sustained release) assists in reducing LDL cholesterol and tryglycerides, increasing HDL cholesterol levels.

   b. Properties: amino acid tryptophan from B_6 can be converted to niacin, one of the MOST stable vitamins.

   c. DRI: 14 mg (female) and 16 mg (male)/day.

   d. Nutrient sources:

      (1) Meat, poultry, fish.

      (2) Enriched breads and cereals.

      (3) Legumes (peanuts, soybeans), seeds, nuts.

      (4) Milk, eggs.

   e. Nutritional deficiency and disease:

      (1) Pellagra: dementia, diarrhea, dermatitis (rough, painful skin), death (considered the "4 Ds").

      (2) Gastrointestinal disturbances, loss of appetite.

      (3) Stomatitis, glossitis, inflamed gingiva, fissured tongue.

   f. Toxicity: blood vessel dilation (flushing) caused by increased blood flow (reduced by use of analgesics), headache, nausea, vomiting, blurred vision, fainting.

4. Pantothenic acid (B_5):

   a. Functions:

      (1) Aids in metabolism of carbohydrates, fats, proteins for energy.

      (2) As coenzyme A, assists in fatty acid metabolism and initiates fatty acid synthesis.

      (3) Aids in formation of hormones and nerve-regulating substances.

   b. Properties: easily destroyed by heat.

   c. DRI: 5 mg/day (AI).

   d. Nutrient sources: liver, eggs, whole grains, legumes, broccoli.

5. Pyridoxine (B_6):

   a. Functions:

      (1) Involved in carbohydrate, protein, fat metabolism.

      (2) Converts tryptophan to niacin.

      (3) Aids in synthesis of hemoglobin and neurotransmitters.

      (4) Regulates blood glucose.

   b. Properties: stable to heat.

   c. DRI: 1.3 mg/day.

   d. Nutrient sources:

      (1) Animal sources: meat, fish, poultry.

      (2) Fruits and vegetables: bananas, cantaloupe, broccoli.

      (3) Whole grain products.

   e. Nutritional deficiency and disease: weakened immune system, weakness, irritability, insomnia, dermatitis, anemia, angular cheilitis, glossitis.

   f. Toxicity: uncommon; long-term megadoses result in sensory nerve damage, numbness in extremities, walking difficulties.

6. Cobalamin (B$_{12}$):
   a. Functions:
      (1) Assists folate metabolism.
      (2) Maintains myelin sheaths that insulate nerve endings.
      (3) Essential for the proper functioning of ALL cells.
   b. Properties:
      (1) Intrinsic factor (protein): made in stomach; needed for absorption; prevents pernicious anemia.
      (2) Extrinsic factor: must be obtained through foods; prevents pernicious anemia.
   c. DRI: 2.4 μg/day.
   d. Nutrient sources: found exclusively in foods of animal origin (meat, liver, eggs, cheese).
   e. Nutritional deficiency and disease:
      (1) Can occur in strict vegetarians, those with diets consisting ONLY of plant foods (see earlier discussion under protein deficiency), persons who chronically abuse nitrous oxide and alcohol.
      (2) Loss of absorption with stomach surgery (such as weight loss surgery) (see later discussion).
      (3) Deficiency: pernicious anemia (type of megaloblastic anemia) with weakness, glossitis, hemorrhagic gingiva, stomatitis, xerostomia, bone loss, apathy.

7. Vitamin C (ascorbic acid):
   a. Functions:
      (1) Promotes synthesis of protein collagen in connective tissue, bone, teeth, blood vessels; assists in wound healing.
      (2) Acts as antioxidant, reducing formation of cancer-causing nitrosamines in stomach; keeps folate coenzymes intact.
      (3) Promotes iron absorption.
      (4) Protects the body from infections.
      (5) Maintains integrity of the capillaries (reduces capillary fragility).
   b. Properties: CANNOT be stored in the body for long periods.
   c. DRI: 75 mg (female) and 90 mg (male)/day.
   d. Nutrient sources: citrus fruit (oranges), tomatoes, cantaloupe, strawberries, mangoes, broccoli, peppers.
   e. Nutritional deficiency and disease:
      (1) Scurvy: deficiency with ruptured blood vessels, swollen and bleeding gingiva with "scorbutic" glossitis, delayed wound healing, rough skin (Figure 7-2).
      (2) DRI for smokers is 35 mg/day higher, since they are under increased oxidative stress

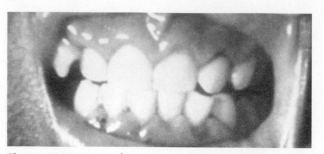

Figure 7-2 Scurvy from water-soluble vitamin C deficiency, with swollen and bleeding gingiva.

from toxins and generally have lower blood levels of vitamin C.
   f. Toxicity:
      (1) Nausea, abdominal cramps, diarrhea.
      (2) May interfere with cobalamin (B$_{12}$) absorption.
      (3) *Rebound* scurvy can occur after megadoses are reduced.

8. Biotin:
   a. Functions: coenzyme form assists in energy metabolism and serves as carrier of carbon dioxide, thus promoting synthesis of glucose and fatty acids.
   b. Properties: avidin, protein that is present in raw egg whites, can bind to biotin and interfere with its absorption.
   c. DRI: 30 μg/day (AI).
   d. Nutrient sources: egg yolk, yeast, liver, cereals; also synthesized by intestinal bacteria.
   e. Nutritional deficiency and disease:
      (1) Glossitis, papillary atrophy, oral mucosal pallor.
      (2) Severe deficiency may lead to nausea, muscle pain, loss of appetite and sleep.

9. Folate (folacin, folic acid):
   a. Functions:
      (1) Assists in forming DNA and protein.
      (2) Manufactures RBCs.
   b. Properties: easily destroyed by processing and heating.
   c. DRI: 400 μg/day.
   d. Nutrient sources: liver, dark green leafy vegetables, fruits (oranges, orange juice, cantaloupe).
   e. Nutritional deficiency and disease:
      (1) Birth defects: neural tube disorders (NTDs) such as spina bifida.
      (2) Megaloblastic anemia.
      (3) Impaired cell division and immune response.
      (4) Gastrointestinal tract (GIT) deterioration and diarrhea.
      (5) Glossitis and periodontal disease.
      (6) Lowered resistance to *Candida albicans*.
   f. Toxicity: kidney damage.

CLINICAL STUDY ▬▬▬▬▬▬▬▬▬▬▬▬▬▬▬▬▬▬▬▬▬

Age	27 YRS	**SCENARIO**
Sex	☐ Male ☒ Female	The patient is in the dental office for an oral prophylaxis appointment. Her oral cavity shows signs of slight gingivitis.
Height	5'4"	
Weight	135 LBS	
BP	114/58	
Chief Complaint	"I am concerned for the health of my baby."	
Medical History	Two weeks pregnant but has not seen her physician History of spina bifida in family	
Current Medications	None	
Social History	Lawyer	

1. Identify the typical causes of and predisposing factors for spina bifida.
2. How can this condition be prevented?
3. What food sources are essential in preventing spina bifida?

1. Folic acid (folate, folacin) deficiency during pregnancy is associated with increased risk of spina bifida. Because folate is necessary for nucleic acid synthesis, deficiency may impair cell growth, causing anomalies of fetus. Defects usually occur within first 6 weeks after conception.
2. The patient must see a physician as soon as possible. Most women are encouraged to increase folate consumption even before conceiving. Adequate intake of foods containing folate is important; however, prenatal vitamins containing folate may be prescribed.
3. Food sources high in folate include fruits and vegetables, especially green leafy vegetables. Raw vegetables are usually better than cooked vegetables because cooking easily destroys folate. Orange juice is also a good source of folate.

Minerals

Minerals are inorganic nutrients used to build the body and regulate functions. They yield NO energy to the body but assist in regulating the release of energy.

A. **Macrominerals** (major minerals): needed in amounts >100 mg/day.
  1. Calcium (MOST abundant mineral in the body):
    a. Functions:
      (1) Forms and maintains bones and teeth.
      (2) Aids in blood coagulation.
      (3) Assists in muscle contraction or relaxation.
      (4) Maintains normal functioning of the nervous system.
      (5) Regulates cellular metabolism.
    b. Properties:
      (1) Proper absorption requires vitamin D (most supplementations include it).
      (2) Parathyroid hormone (PTH) maintains normal level of serum calcium.
      (3) DRI: 1000 mg/day (AI).
      (4) Nutrient sources:
        (a) Dietary: dairy products, milk, yogurt, cheese.
        (b) Calcium-fortified orange and fruit drinks; calcium supplements.
      (5) Nutritional deficiency and disease: women are MOST likely to be at risk.
        (a) Osteoporosis: bone disease that develops MORE commonly in women with decreased bone density (osteopenia is early indication of loss of bone density).
        (b) Calcium tetany: failure of the muscles to relax after contraction.
        (c) Rickets in children: deficiency leads to stunted growth.
        (d) Affects HBP.
        (e) Weight loss surgery may adversely affect absorption.
        (f) Prevention: vitamin D hormone or hormone calcitonin, meeting DRI requirements, exercising regularly, AVOIDING alcohol and/or smoking.
      (6) Toxicity: nausea, vomiting, severe constipation, kidney stone formation, irregular heartbeat, tingling, xerostomia, fatigue,

increased blood pressure; may inhibit iron and zinc uptake.

2. Phosphorus: second MOST abundant mineral in body.
  a. Functions:
    (1) Assists in formation of bones and teeth.
    (2) Involved in the transfer and release of high-energy phosphates.
    (3) Regulates acid-base balance.
    (4) Releases energy from carbohydrates, protein, fat metabolism.
    (5) Plays active role in cell protein synthesis.
  b. Properties: absorption is affected by vitamin D and PTH.
  c. DRI: 700 mg/day.
  d. Nutrient sources: milk, cheese, bakery products, meats.
  e. Nutritional deficiency and disease: uncommon; risk is greater among elderly, strict vegetarians, alcoholics; presents with hypocalcification and muscle weakness.

3. Magnesium:
  a. Functions:
    (1) Calcium homeostasis.
    (2) IMPORTANT to structural integrity of heart muscle.
    (3) Assists in mineralization of bones and teeth.
    (4) Facilitates operation of enzymes.
    (5) Assists in production of energy.
  b. Properties: vitamin D enhances its absorption.
  c. DRI: 310 mg (female) and 400 mg (male)/day.
  d. Nutrient sources: nuts, legumes, whole grains, dark green leafy vegetables.
  e. Nutritional deficiency and disease: risk is greater among women:
    (1) Vomiting, diarrhea, tetany, weakness, convulsions.
    (2) Alveolar bone reduction, hypoplasia of enamel and dentin.

4. Sodium:
  a. Functions:
    (1) Retains body water.
    (2) With chloride and potassium, aids in maintenance of acid-base and fluid balance.
    (3) Facilitates transmission of nerve impulses and muscle contraction.
  b. Properties: possibly contributes to HBP, which can lead to CVD and complications (MI and CVA); HBP may be controlled by lifestyle management in its early stages and managed in its later stages by:
    (1) Limiting intake of processed foods.
    (2) Restricting intake of sodium to 3 g/day (sea salt has LESS sodium).
    (3) Exercising.

c. DRI: 500 mg/day.
d. Nutrient sources: table salt, animal meat, salt-water fish, eggs, dairy, processed foods.
e. Nutritional deficiency and disease are rare in United States, but with restriction of intake: muscle cramps, mental apathy, dizziness, decreased appetite, nausea.

5. Chloride:
  a. Functions:
    (1) Aids in maintaining normal acid-base and fluid balance.
    (2) Component of hydrochloric acid in the stomach and necessary for digestion.
    (3) Assists in maintenance of nerve functions.
  b. Properties: negative ion of extracellular fluid.
  c. DRI: 750 mg/day.
  d. Nutrient sources: table salt, processed foods, water.
  e. Nutritional deficiency and diseases:
    (1) Caused by starvation, fever, diarrhea, vomiting.
    (2) Muscle cramps, mental apathy, decreased appetite.

6. Potassium:
  a. Functions:
    (1) Maintains fluid-electrolyte balance and cell integrity.
    (2) Assists in the transmission of nerve impulses.
    (3) Aids in muscle contraction (including heart muscle) and electrical conductivity of heart.
    (4) Assists in carbohydrate and protein metabolism.
    (5) Reduces adverse effects of sodium on blood pressure.
    (6) Reduces risk of kidney stones and possibly reduces bone loss.
  b. DRI: 2000 mg/day.
  c. Nutrient sources:
    (1) Inside ALL living cells, both plant and animal.
    (2) Fresh fruits (banana, oranges) and vegetables (yams).
    (3) Milk, meat, whole grains, dried beans, legumes (peanuts, soybeans).
  d. Nutritional deficiency and disease:
    (1) Hypokalemia: caused by dehydration, diabetic acidosis, vomiting, diarrhea, diuretics, steroids.
    (2) Leads to muscle weakness, cramps, loss of appetite, constipation, mental confusion, apathy.
  e. Toxicity: muscle weakness, cardiac arrest.

7. Sulfur:
   a. Functions:
      (1) Aids in maintaining normal acid-base balance.
      (2) Stabilizes shape of proteins by forming bridges between sulfur molecules (creates rigid proteins in hair, nails, skin).
   b. Properties: component of amino acids and vitamins biotin and thiamin (B_1).
   c. DRI: none.
   d. Nutrient sources: ALL protein-containing sources; found in preserved foods and naturally on certain fruit (grapes).
   e. Nutritional deficiency and disease: protein deficiency occurs *before* sulfur deficiency.

B. **Trace elements:** remaining elements necessary for health, and have safe adequate intakes (SAEs) of <100 mg/day.
   1. Iron: IMPORTANT in hemoglobin in RBCs, bonds to oxygen in lungs and carries it throughout body; deficiency causes hypochromic anemia, with risk of bleeding, feeling of tiredness at the end of the day.
   2. Fluorine: helps make teeth resistant to caries by hardening outer enamel.
   3. Zinc: involved in growth, healing of wounds, male sexual development.
   4. Iodine: IMPORTANT in function of thyroid gland; iodine deficiency causes endemic goiter and enlarged gland and can result in learning deficiencies; iodine deficiency uncommon because of addition to table salt (not usually included in sea salt, unless noted).
   5. Cobalt: contained in cobalamin (B_{12}).
   6. Copper: deficiency can cause anemia and bone disease, changes in hair color, problems with immune system.
   7. Manganese: vital for bones, reproductive system, nervous system.
   8. Chromium: involved in metabolism of sugar.
   9. Also small amounts of boron, molybdenum, selenium, tin, nickel, etc.

C. Lead poisoning can result from ingestion of old paint chips by children; will cause anemia and blue lines in gingiva.

CLINICAL STUDY

Age	62 YRS	SCENARIO
Sex	☐ Male ☒ Female	After an initial examination of the patient, a panoramic radiograph is taken and thinning of the posterior border of the mandible is noted. The patient is then questioned regarding her diet. She states that she has never been a milk drinker.
Height	5'2"	
Weight	112 LBS	
BP	112/74	
Chief Complaint	"My lower partial denture does not fit as well anymore."	
Medical History	Fractured radius from fall 6 months ago Menopausal for 1 year Smokes pack and half a day of cigarettes	
Current Medications	None	
Social History	Photographer for travel magazine	

1. What is the most likely diagnosis of the patient's condition?
2. Identify the most common causes of and predisposing factors for this condition.
3. What is the best treatment plan for this condition?
4. Is this condition preventable? If so, how?

1. Osteoporosis, a bone disease that develops more commonly in women with decreased bone density (osteopenia is early indication of loss of bone density).
2. Genetics is a factor in the development of osteoporosis and in the attainment of bone mass. Early menopause is a predictor for the development of osteoporosis (note that menopause is earlier for smokers by at least 5 years). Other contributing factors include deficiencies in calcium and/or vitamin D, lack of physical activity, cigarette smoking, excessive intake of protein and/or caffeine.
3. Traditional treatment plan includes estrogen replacement (controversial), calcium and/or vitamin D supplements, regular exercise; exercise (weight bearing) may increase bone mass.
4. Adequate calcium intake is necessary throughout individual's life; DRI 1000 mg/day for adults.

Water

Water, main constituent of the body, makes up 50% to 60% of total body weight. MOST of water is located in the cells. Required on a daily basis to maintain necessary levels; have enough if urine is clear enough to read through.

A. Functions:
  1. Removes waste products, including urea (by-product of protein metabolism, contains nitrogen) and stabilizes ALL body fluids.
  2. Maintains body temperature.
  3. Serves as solvent for minerals, vitamins, glucose, amino acids and acts as lubricant around joints.
  4. Participates in chemical reactions and transports inorganic nutrients.
  5. Maintains normal kidney function and electrolyte balance, reducing risk of kidney stones.
B. Dietary requirements: ~3.7 L/day for adults.
C. Nutrient sources: MORE water and beverages.
D. Nutritional deficiency and disease: survival without water is limited to 2 to 3 days. Dehydration is caused by:
  1. Lack of water intake.
  2. Vomiting and/or diarrhea.
  3. Blood loss.
  4. Malfunctioning kidneys.
E. Toxicity (by dehydration) is characterized by:
  1. Dizziness and nausea.
  2. Sodium retention.
  3. Hypertension.

EFFECTS OF NUTRIENTS ON CELLS OF ORAL TISSUES

Nutrients significantly affect the function and health of oral tissues by providing components for synthesis, repair, immunity.

Periodontal and Dental Health

Several nutrients are needed for the formation and maintenance of the health of the periodontium and other dental tissues. MANY deficiencies are noted in the tongue as glossitis (smooth inflamed tongue), since it affects the sensitive lingual papillae on dorsum as well as other dental tissues.

A. Iron, vitamin C, zinc are needed for collagen synthesis and wound healing:
  1. Collagen is MAIN component of periodontium and hard dental tissues.
  2. Sources:
     a. Iron: beef, liver, beans.
     b. Vitamin C: citrus, broccoli, peppers.
     c. Zinc: red meats, shellfish.
B. Folate and protein are needed for cell formation:
  1. Junctional epithelial cells, which have a rapid turnover.
  2. Sources:
     a. Folate: asparagus, broccoli, liver.
     b. Protein: meat, fish, poultry.

C. Vitamin A maintains the integrity of the tissues:
  1. Synthesizes protein matrix for tissues, also for enamel and dentin.
  2. Sources: carrots and squash.

Repair Process

Speed and effectiveness of the repair process are greatly influenced by nutrients such as proteins, vitamins, minerals (see later discussion on postsurgical diet). Repair is an important part of posttreatment of the periodontium and other dental tissues.

A. Zinc speeds wound healing and the repair process; sources include oysters, shrimp, crab, bran cereal, lean pork, lamb, ham, hamburger.
B. Calcium, phosphorus, vitamin D all promote bone density and calcify the protein matrix of cementoblasts, ameloblasts, and odontoblasts; sources include milk and hard cheeses.
C. Protein and vitamin C are involved in connective tissue formation; sources for protein include animal sources and water-packed tuna; sources for vitamin C include citrus fruits and green vegetables.

Immune Mechanisms

Proteins are needed for the immune system and aid in controlling infection, important factors in periodontal health and protection against periodontal disease.

WEIGHT CONTROL AND ENERGY

Weight control is achieved when the calories gained from food equal the energy needs of body. One kilocalorie is amount of heat produced to raise the temperature of 1 kg of water 1° C. Weight control MUST be done with healthy intent.

A. Basal metabolism rate (BMR):
  1. Rate of energy utilization in the resting state is MOST closely related to lean body mass; measured from O_2 consumption (CO_2 production) of a person awake, at rest, after an overnight fast.
  2. Includes energy needed for breathing, beating of the heart, circulation, muscle tone, body temperature; influenced by such factors as age, gender, body size, infection, injury, surgery, hormone levels. (~70% of total energy expenditure is due to basal life processes; ~20% comes from physical activity, ~10% from thermogenesis, or digestion of food).
  3. Thyroid gland is the MAJOR gland that regulates metabolism; higher thyroid hormone levels increase the metabolic rate.
B. Degree of physical activity is the voluntary component of energy.
  1. Varies from sedentary to strenuous activity (we weigh less on top of mountain than at sea level, so let's all move!).

2. Influenced by such factors as intensity and length of activity and size of individual.

C. **Specific dynamic activity** (SDA):
   1. Energy required to digest and absorb food.
   2. Contributes ~10% of total kilocalories consumed.

Eating Disorders

Include serious eating disorders such as anorexia, bulimia, bulimorexia, compulsive overeating, obesity. Requires multidisciplinary care (dental, medical, psychosocial, nutritional consults).

A. **Anorexia nervosa:** syndrome that involves extreme loss of weight (20% to 40% below average) as result of self-starvation (protein-energy malnutrition [PEM], protein-calorie malnutrition [PCM]), excessive exercise, aversion to food, altered eating habits, and/or chronic use of laxatives or suppositories in response to a distorted body image.
   1. Etiology: unknown, but disorder is associated with psychosocial pressures; occurs MAINLY in young women with low self-esteem; can prove fatal.
   2. Outpatient treatment, in conjunction with antidepressant and antianxiety drugs, is common.
   3. Decreased heart rate, malnutrition, dehydration, constipation, diarrhea; often occurs in individuals with family history of depression or bipolar disorder.
   4. May cause dry skin and nails, with excessive growth of facial and appendage hair (hirsutism), called lanugo ("downy"), which helps to insulate the body against heat loss.
   5. Amenorrhea: absence of a menstrual cycle in response to hormonal changes.
   6. Oral signs: dental caries, xerostomia, and oral lesions from malnutrition.
   7. Risk factors for oral health: medical crises and emotional stress.
   8. Barriers to care: lack of communication because of denial, guilt, fear of gaining weight, lack of compliance; may include economic barriers because of cost of repairing damage.
   9. Professional care and homecare: fluoride in custom tray and use of mineralizing calcium products are recommended if xerostomia or vomiting is problem.
   10. Patient education: prevention of further damage to the teeth; discussion of influence of diet on caries; recommendation for daily mineralizing fluoride and calcium products.

B. **Bulimia nervosa:** compulsive disorder that involves periods of starvation, bingeing, purging; person has a perceived lack of control over eating behavior; affected individuals engage in an average of two episodes a week.
   1. Etiology: unknown but is likely to be stress related, affecting young women.
   2. **Bingeing** may be followed by purging activity (vomiting with laxative and diuretic abuse) in those who are fearful of gaining weight.

3. Purging is responsible for MORE of the oral and medical complications associated with this disorder, including erosion, anemia, cardiac problems, GIT disturbances, renal failure, failure to ovulate.
4. Diuretic use can cause reduction in salivary flow and development of angular cheilitis; laxative use can lead to metabolic acidosis and dependence on laxatives for adequate bowel function.
5. Body weight is normal or slightly overweight, with malnutrition, dehydration, cardiac dysrhythmias, calluses noted on knuckles.
6. Family history of alcoholism and drug abuse is common; may have depression.
7. Oral signs:
   a. Dental erosion (perimolysis) and thermal sensitivity on maxillary anteriors from vomiting, dishing of lingual surfaces, raised appearance of restoration margins, appearance of anterior open bite (See Chapter 6, General and Oral Pathology).
   b. Dental caries from gastric acids.
   c. Xerostomia from prescribed antidepressants, laxative and/or diuretic abuse.
   d. Palatal trauma lesion from forced vomiting.
   e. Angular cheilosis; enlarged interdental papillae as result of constant irritation from acidic vomitus.
   f. Parotid salivary gland enlargement, with change in shape of face (round) and jaw (square).
8. Risk factors for oral health: denial of the problem, emotional stresses, xerostomia, vomit acid.
9. Barriers to care:
   a. Lack of communication because of denial, guilt, fear of gaining weight, and lack of compliance; also results from clinician's inability to gain patient's trust and confidence and failure to refer patient to physician and/or psychiatrist.
   b. Economic barriers may be involved because of cost of repairing damage (Figure 7-3).

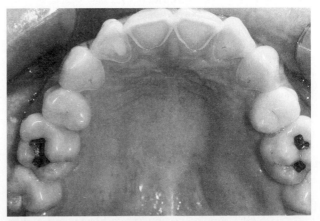

Figure 7-3 Loss of enamel on lingual surfaces as result of bulimia. Repaired using veneer crowns. (From Bath-Balogh M, Fehrenbach MJ: Illustrated dental embryology and anatomy, ed 2, St. Louis, 2007, Saunders/Elsevier).

10. Professional care and homecare: restoration of carious teeth with glass ionomer restorative (to leach fluoride ions) where possible, sealing of eroded areas with composite resins, assessment of progression of erosion (whether by study models and/or intraoral photos), use of mineralizing neutral sodium fluoride and calcium products.

11. Patient education:
    a. Discussion of oral and medical problems associated with purging, diuretics, and laxative use.
    b. Need to neutralize vomit acid by rinsing with tap water, or possibly a mix of water with sodium bicarbonate or magnesium hydroxide may be used.
    c. Discouragement of toothbrushing or flossing immediately after vomiting to reduce abrasion.
    d. Use of saliva substitutes and sugarless gums (possibly with xylitol) to increase salivary flow.
    e. Daily use of mineralizing fluoride and calcium products.

12. Daily vitamin and mineral supplementation may be recommended when gingival tissue appears unhealthy or when angular cheilitis is present.

C. Bulimorexia: combination of anorexia and bulimia (binge eating followed by starvation).
   1. Involves signs and symptoms of both anorexia and bulimia.
   2. Medical complications, oral signs, risk factors, barriers to care, professional care, and patient education are the same as for anorexia nervosa and bulimia.

D. Diabulimia: bulimia in insulin-dependent diabetics who purge to keep sugar levels under control.

E. **Compulsive overeating:** chronic uncontrolled episodes of overeating without other signs of eating disorder.
   1. Overeating in response to stress, feelings of anxiety, or depression.
   2. Bingeing on foods that are easy to eat in large portions (e.g., noodles, rice).
   3. Eating foods categorized as "junk" foods, such as ice cream and chips.
   4. Characteristics:
      a. Eating large quantities in isolation to induce a sense of well-being.
      b. Grazing in some individuals with lack of preoccupation with weight.
      c. Difficulty expressing and dealing with feelings.
   5. Management:
      a. Dietary:
         (1) Eat until full (a must) but not beyond.
         (2) Avoid diets that may encourage more bingeing.
      b. Psychological:
         (1) Focus on responding to hunger rather than emotions.
         (2) Identify personal needs and express them.

F. **Obesity:** excessive body weight caused by excessive nutrient intake (overnutrition) and sedentary lifestyle.
   1. Evaluated in absolute terms by measuring body mass index (BMI).
   2. Etiology:
      a. Positive energy balance (kilocalorie intake exceeds expenditure).
      b. Genetics: child with one obese parent has HIGH risk of becoming obese, child with two obese parents has HIGHER risk.
      c. Development of excess fat cells during childhood; theory includes that:
         (1) During childhood, increased number of fat cells develops in response to excess kilocalorie intake (hyperplasty).
         (2) After puberty, fat cells enlarge (hypertrophy).
      d. Set-point theory: body chooses a weight and defends its set-point by internal factors.
      e. Psychological factors (e.g., finding comfort in eating).
      f. Physical activity (i.e., lack of energy expenditure).
   3. Prevention and weight control:
      a. Losing weight involves:
         (1) Controlling energy intake and eating low-fat carbohydrate foods such as fresh fruits, vegetables, whole grains, and some nonfat (fat free).
         (2) Drinking adequate water to satisfy thirst and fill the stomach.
         (3) Still meeting DRI nutritional needs; avoiding diet drinks that contain high amounts of acid and may falsely increase need for "sweet" items.
      b. Behavior modification (changing eating behavior):
         (1) Become aware of current behaviors.
         (2) Stimulus control; change environment to minimize stimuli for eating (e.g., shopping after eating to avoid poor choices).
         (3) Cognitive restructuring; altering one's state of mind regarding eating (e.g., avoiding excuses for overeating such as having difficult day).
         (4) Self-monitoring (i.e., keeping diary of foods and eating patterns); complies BEST when involved in decision making.
         (5) Contingency management; developing plan for responding in environment where overeating is MOST likely to occur (e.g., party where snacks are served).
      c. Physical activity:
         (1) Increases energy output and controls appetite.
         (2) Aids in stress reduction and increases basal metabolism.
         (3) Increases self-esteem.

4. Risk for CVD (especially HBP, high blood cholesterol, triglyceride levels [combined hyperlipidemia]), DM type 2, sleep apnea, osteoarthritis; possibly periodontal disease.
5. May have media-driven diet with all its restrictions and implications (discussed earlier under each nutrient, especially noted is overconsumption of proteins).
6. May undergo or have had bariatric procedure (weight loss surgery [WLS]; gastric bypass or Lap-Band) performed to modify GIT to reduce nutrient intake or absorption; need to have nutritional blood tests done regularly.
   a. Diet is soft and limited by smaller size stomach.
   b. Loss of stomach lining may adversely affect absorption of calcium, zinc, cobalamin (B$_{12}$), and other nutrients; may increase risk for osteopenia, osteoporosis, and ultimately osteomalacia.
   c. May have acidic oral cavity with certain surgeries and poor diet that increases caries risk.
   d. Poor fit of dentures because of rapid weight loss after surgery.
   e. AVOID drugs that can cause ulceration or trauma to GIT such as nonsteroidal antiinflammatory agents or drugs (e.g., NSAIAs, NSAIDs, ibuprofen).

NUTRITIONAL COUNSELING

Counseling for weight control and proper health and nutrition involves diet counseling, diet management, nutritional counseling. Nutritional counseling by dental hygienists MAINLY involves maintenance of a healthy oral cavity; patients with serious systemic nutritional problems, such as DM or eating disorder, need to be referred initially to a nutritional counselor.

A. Diet counseling:
1. Patient selection:
   a. Patient MUST be willing to change and/or improve eating habits.
   b. Patient has a need for dietary improvement.
2. Communication techniques are necessary to create motivation in patient.
   a. Maintain good eye contact.
   b. Use effective verbal and nonverbal methods of communication; tone of voice, gestures, and facial expressions can communicate sincerity and concern to patient.
   c. Adapt education to patient's needs and understanding.
3. Patient interview:
   a. Purpose:
      (1) Understand the problem.
      (2) Determine factors that contribute to the problem.
      (3) Understand the personality and motivation of the patient.

4. Counseling approaches:
   a. Directive: decisions are made by counselor; patient is passive.
   b. Nondirective: counselor assists in understanding needs and recommends changes; patient is involved in planning, implementing, evaluating diet.
B. Principles of diet management:
1. Food diary:
   a. Patient keeps a 3-, 5-, or 7-day food diary (including weekend); records ALL meals and between-meal snacking (MOST common; BEST representation of normal diet).
   b. Patient keeps a 24-hour food diary (NOT representative of normal diet).
   c. Food frequency checklist represents consumption of certain foods per week; MORE representative than 24-hour but not as representative as food diary, since limited in scope.
2. Interview:
   a. Assess MAIN problem or complaint.
   b. Ascertain routine and habits.
   c. Review medical history for any changes or problems; may reveal systemic conditions or drug intake that can influence medical health, including ability to digest and/or metabolize food.
   d. Evaluate diet.
      (1) Review adequacy of food intake.
      (2) Determine amount of foods that contain sugar and frequency of intake.
      (3) Look for food items or herbal supplements that can interfere with prescription drugs (e.g., grapefruit juice).
   e. Assess clinical signs of deficiencies or diseases:
      (1) Dental caries.
      (2) Gingivitis and periodontal diseases, especially necrotizing forms.
      (3) Other signs such as dry skin, hair loss, stomatitis, angular cheilosis, glossitis may need to be referred to a nutritional counselor.
   f. Dental hygiene diagnosis: try to determine possible causes for clinical signs.
3. Follow-up:
   a. Review a second 3-, 5-, or 7-day diet plan.
   b. Compare second plan with first.
   c. Emphasize good changes patient has made.
C. Nutritional management:
1. Dental caries:
   a. Cariogenic factors associated with diet:
      (1) Frequency of between-meal snacking; MORE frequent the exposure to sugar, MORE cariogenic the diet (BEST to eat sugar-rich foods at mealtime).
      (2) Physical form of food; solid and retentive forms have SLOWER oral clearance time

and therefore are MORE cariogenic than liquid forms; sticky food forms (raisins etc.) have slower oral clearance as well.

 (3) Amount of sugar added to foods and beverages (e.g., to cereals, coffee).

 (4) Acidic foods also promote demineralization (e.g., soft drinks and sports drinks, especially citrus and/or diet).

b. Dietary recommendation:

 (1) Eat nutritionally balanced diet and eliminate sugary snacks.

 (2) Restrict sugar to mealtimes and avoid prolonged exposure to dietary acids.

 (3) Eat hard cheeses to help neutralize pH.

 (4) Use fluoride rinses and calcium products to promote remineralization process.

 (5) Use xylitol in form of gum and candy (according to manufacturer's instructions).

c. Dietary modifications: use USDA's MyPyramid and the Dietary Guidelines for Americans 2005 (see CD-ROM):

 (1) Helps to determine recommended servings and establish needs to meet body's requirements for essential nutrients.

 (2) Allows modification of the American diet with four themes: variety, proportionality, moderation, activity.

2. Chronic periodontitis:

a. Dietary recommendation:

 (1) Considerations:

  (a) Evaluate information obtained for any factors that may interfere with nutritional status.

  (b) Determine eating patterns and food habits.

  (c) Patient should assist in determining revised diet.

b. Procedure:

 (1) Patient determines deficiencies and makes appropriate choices to improve diet.

 (2) Direct patient to choices that can benefit periodontium.

 (3) Stress importance of decreasing sugar-rich foods in diet.

 (4) Instruct patient to add variety to meal planning and to focus on nutritionally sound foods that the patient likes.

c. Dietary recommendations:

 (1) Goals:

  (a) Assist patient in meeting stress of surgery.

  (b) Aid wound healing and recovery time.

  (c) Increase resistance to infections.

 (2) Preoperative diet before nonsurgical and surgical periodontal therapy:

  (a) Recommend increased intake of vitamin C 1 week before to condition tissues to heal; sources include supplementation, orange juice, pepper, broccoli.

  (b) Recommend adequate amounts of carbohydrates to spare protein.

  (c) Avoid OTC herbal supplements that can promote bleeding such as gingko, garlic.

 (3) Postoperative diet before nonsurgical and surgical periodontal therapy:

  (a) First postoperative day: fluids such as water, juices, broths; recommend MORE frequent feedings.

  (b) Second postoperative day: blended fruits and vegetables, oatmeal, ice cream, milk, milk shakes, eggs, and/or meat broths.

3. Necrotizing periodontal disease, bacterial infection of the periodontium, associated with poor oral hygiene.

a. Diet consists of empty-calorie and sugar-rich foods because of decreased ability to chew.

b. Dietary recommendation:

 (1) Recommend food sources or supplementations that contain protein, calcium, folate, iron, zinc, vitamins A and C.

 (2) Patient should eat six to eight small meals per day (one or two foods at each meal).

c. Dietary modification:

 (1) Use USDA's MyPyramid and the Dietary Guidelines for Americans 2005 for serving recommendations (see CD-ROM).

 (2) Choose good food sources high in nutrients.

 (3) Initially, menus should consist of liquids and soft foods.

d. Avoid spicy foods.

4. Diet after dental whitening (bleaching): avoidance of foods that may cause dentinal hypersensitivity (hot and spicy) or staining (red wine, fast food colorings) until teeth have had time to rehydrate by saliva; 24 to 48 hours recommended.

Review Questions

1 Which of the following characterizes a complete protein?
A. Adequate in all the essential amino acids
B. Synthesized by the body
C. Provided through plant foods
D. A dispensable amino acid

2 All of the following conditions are examples of negative nitrogen balance, EXCEPT one. Which one is the EXCEPTION?
A. Infection
B. Anorexia nervosa
C. Blood loss
D. Pregnancy

3 Phenylketonuria is a condition that
  A. involves protein-energy malnutrition.
  B. restricts the consumption of aspartame.
  C. ineffectively metabolizes phenylalanine to threonine.
  D. involves a disorder in carbohydrate metabolism.

4 Kwashiorkor is a disease that
  A. occurs most commonly in children in underdeveloped countries.
  B. presents without severe wasting of body fat.
  C. occurs in children 6 to 12 months of age in underdeveloped countries.
  D. is not characterized by edema.

5 What is the MAIN function of carbohydrates?
  A. Repair body tissues
  B. Neutralize acid-base
  C. Provide energy
  D. Regulate metabolism

6 One gram of carbohydrate yields
  A. 9 kcal.
  B. 7 kcal.
  C. 5 kcal.
  D. 4 kcal.

7 Sorbitol, which is a sugar alcohol used in diabetic foods and sugarless gum, is made from
  A. fructose.
  B. glucose.
  C. galactose.
  D. mannitol.

8 Which of the following foods would be MOST cariogenic?
  A. Dried apricots
  B. Soda pop
  C. Cake
  D. Milk

9 Which of the following allows lipids to be transported in the blood?
  A. Bile
  B. Phospholipids
  C. Lipoproteins
  D. Water

10 A high level of which lipoprotein actually slows down the development of cardiovascular disease?
  A. Chylomicron
  B. Very low-density lipoprotein
  C. Low-density lipoprotein
  D. High-density lipoprotein

11 All of the following are characteristics of cholesterol, EXCEPT one. Which one is the EXCEPTION?
  A. Is a phospholipid
  B. Can be made by the body
  C. Acts as an emulsifier
  D. Increases the risk of heart disease

12 Important functions of dietary lipids include
  A. providing essential fatty acids and aiding in absorption of B vitamins.
  B. aiding in absorption of B vitamins and providing satiety.
  C. providing essential fatty acids, aiding in absorption of B vitamins, and providing satiety.
  D. providing essential fatty acids, providing satiety, and aiding in absorption of vitamins A, D, E, and K.
  E. providing essential fatty acids, preventing night blindness, and aiding in absorption of B vitamins.

13 Overconsumption of the following foods can increase the risk of atherosclerosis, EXCEPT one. Which one is the EXCEPTION?
  A. Butter
  B. Coconut oil
  C. Beef
  D. Skim milk

14 Risk factors associated with atherosclerosis include all of the following, EXCEPT one. Which one is the EXCEPTION?
  A. Hypertension
  B. LDL cholesterol of 120 mg/100 mL
  C. Total blood cholesterol greater than 240 mg/100 mL
  D. Smoking

15 Fat-soluble vitamins include all of the following, EXCEPT one. Which one is the EXCEPTION?
  A. A
  B. E
  C. C
  D. K
  E. D

16 Preformed vitamin A is found in which of the following food sources?
  A. Carrots
  B. Body fat of fish
  C. Broccoli
  D. Cauliflower

17 Rickets is a disease associated with which vitamin deficiency?
  A. A
  B. D
  C. E
  D. C

18 Which of the following is a function of vitamin E?
  A. Aids in the prevention of night blindness
  B. Promotes the mineralization of teeth
  C. Acts as an antioxidant
  D. Synthesizes prothrombin

19 Which of the following is a function of water-soluble vitamins?
  A. Aid in the metabolism of energy-producing nutrients
  B. Assist with immune defenses
  C. Regulate serum levels of calcium and phosphorus
  D. Absorb calcium and phosphorus

20 The amino acid tryptophan can be converted into which water-soluble vitamin?
  A. Riboflavin
  B. Pantothenic acid
  C. Thiamin
  D. Niacin

21 Interference with the intrinsic-extrinsic factor leads to a deficiency in which vitamin?
  A. Cobalamin
  B. Folate
  C. Biotin
  D. Pantothenic acid

22 A strict vegetarian diet MOST likely will be deficient in which vitamin?
  A. Cobalamin
  B. Folate
  C. Biotin
  D. Thiamin

23 A disease caused by vitamin C deficiency is
  A. beriberi.
  B. pernicious anemia.
  C. scurvy.
  D. pellagra.

24 One of the following characteristics is NOT true concerning calcium. Which one is the EXCEPTION?
  A. Aids coagulation
  B. Assists in muscle contraction and relaxation
  C. An intake of 400 mg/day is recommended
  D. Vitamin D assists in its absorption

25 Which of the following is the MOST abundant mineral in the body?
  A. Calcium
  B. Phosphorus
  C. Copper
  D. Fluorine
  E. Magnesium

26 Which of the following is the BEST food source of magnesium?
  A. Citrus fruits
  B. Dairy products
  C. Dark yellow vegetables
  D. Whole grains and nuts

27 The functions of sodium include all of the following, EXCEPT one. Which one is the EXCEPTION?
  A. Nerve impulse conduction
  B. Maintenance of acid-base balance
  C. Retention of body water
  D. Used to invoke an immune response

28 Which of the following minerals is used to preserve foods?
  A. Sodium
  B. Chloride
  C. Sulfur
  D. Phosphorus

29 Body water possesses all of the following characteristics, EXCEPT one. Which one is the EXCEPTION?
  A. Is found extracellularly as well as intracellularly
  B. Makes up 85% of total body weight
  C. Assists in maintaining body temperature
  D. Acts as a lubricant around joints

30 Several nutrients have an effect on the cells of the oral tissues. Which of the following nutrients assists in speeding up wound healing?
  A. Zinc
  B. Folate
  C. Calcium
  D. Phosphorus

31 With regard to energy measurement, 1 kcal is the amount of heat produced to raise the temperature of
  A. 1 g of water 1° C.
  B. 1 kg of water 1° F.
  C. 1 kg of water 1° C.
  D. 1 g of water 1° F.

32 One of following activities is NOT included in the measurement of the basal metabolism rate (BMR). Which one is the EXCEPTION?
  A. Breathing
  B. Maintaining body temperature
  C. Beating of the heart
  D. Digesting food

33 Which of the following is the major gland that affects the BMR?
  A. Thyroid
  B. Endocrine
  C. Hypothalamus
  D. Sebaceous

34 For an individual to lose weight, a reduction in energy intake must take place. The individual should also decrease physical activity.
  A. Both statements are true.
  B. Both statements are false.
  C. The first statement is true; the second is false.
  D. The first statement is false; the second is true.

35 The individual with anorexia nervosa is usually
  A. male.
  B. female and exercises excessively.
  C. female and aware that her behavior is abnormal.
  D. female, and condition is often difficult to diagnose because of a lack of physical signs.

36 Bulimia is an eating disorder that involves
  A. weight loss 40% to 60% below desirable body weight.
  B. mostly male political candidates.
  C. episodes of binge eating followed by purging.
  D. decreased heart rate in response to a decreased metabolism.

37 Compulsive overeating is associated with
  A. eating large quantities of food and purging.
  B. eating large quantities of food in response to stress or an emotional outlet.
  C. an aversion to all forms of food.
  D. a fear of becoming overweight.

38 The BEST counseling technique for increasing patients' involvement and responsibility in making their own decisions
  A. is directive.
  B. is nondirective.
  C. involves motivation.
  D. involves listening.

39 Which of the following is the BEST example of a nondirective approach?
  A. Counselor makes all recommendations for a diet modification program and the patient accepts.
  B. Patient is involved in the diet analysis and evaluation and the counselor makes recommendations for diet modification.
  C. Patient is involved in the diet analysis, evaluation, and diet modification program and the counselor explains each process to the patient.
  D. Counselor provides information regarding the diet analysis, evaluation, and diet modification and the patient accepts all recommendations.

40 The recommended number of days for recording a diet diary is
  A. 2 to 3 days.
  B. 4 to 7 days.
  C. 7 to 10 days.
  D. 14 days.

41 The basic diet for patients recovering from periodontal surgery is a
  A. diet that is nutritionally adequate and modified for the patient's chewing ability.
  B. clear liquid diet with supplements of vitamins A and E.
  C. diet high in fiber with six to eight glasses of water.
  D. diet that consists of foods recommended in the Food Guide Pyramid and high in vitamin C and cobalamin.

42 The MOST common barrier to care for the patient with an eating disorder is
   A. communication.
   B. transportation.
   C. economic.
   D. physical.

43 The MOST devastating oral effects of eating disorders are related to
   A. excessive exercising.
   B. binge eating.
   C. frequent purging.
   D. malnutrition.
   E. laxative use.

44 Which of the following should immediately follow a purging incident?
   A. Rinsing with tap water
   B. Brushing with baking soda
   C. Brushing with fluoride gel
   D. Flossing

45 Which of the following is correct concerning the condition hypokalemia?
   A. Restriction of the consumption of aspartame
   B. Ineffective metabolism of phenylalanine to threonine
   C. Lack of potassium
   D. Lack of calcium

46 An adult patient who is deficient in vitamin D could suffer from osteomalacia. A patient deficient in calcium could suffer from osteosclerosis.
   A. Both statements are true.
   B. Both statements are false.
   C. The first statement is true, the second is false.
   D. The first statement is false, the second is true.

47 Mineral oils interfere with the absorption of which of the following vitamins?
   A. Vitamin A
   B. Vitamin C
   C. Vitamin B_6
   D. Vitamin B_{12}

48 Two types of food diaries are commonly used today. The 24-hour food diary and the 7- to 10-day food diary are the diaries MOST commonly used today.
   A. Both statements are true.
   B. Both statements are false.
   C. The first statement is true, the second is false.
   D. The first statement is false, the second is true.

49 Water makes up 50% to 60% of total body weight but is NOT the main constituent of the body. Water is required on a daily basis.
   A. Both statements are true.
   B. Both statements are false.
   C. The first statement is true, the second is false.
   D. The first statement is false, the second is true.

50 Which of the following is a major mineral?
   A. Vitamin A
   B. Boron
   C. Selenium
   D. Calcium

Answer Key and Rationales

1 **(A)** Animal proteins are considered complete (high-quality) proteins. Composition of human tissue MORE closely resembles that of animal tissue than that of plant tissue. Tissue similarities enable the human body to use animal proteins MORE effectively for its MAIN functions: body maintenance, repair, growth. Animal proteins contain ALL the essential amino acids in amounts that are sufficient for the body.

2 **(D)** Nitrogen balance refers to balance between input and output of nitrogen. If the body is NOT growing or in need of extra protein to recover from illness or infection, ONLY enough protein is needed to equal input to output. Negative protein balance exists when output is greater than input (as occurs with semistarvation, infection, fever, blood loss). However, if the body is growing, as during childhood, pregnancy, or recovery from illness, MORE protein will be necessary to supply the body's needs for tissue repair. Increased need for protein intake is defined as positive protein balance.

3 **(B)** Phenylketonuria (PKU) is a disease in which the liver is NOT able to metabolize the essential amino acid phenylalanine into the nonessential amino acid tyrosine. By-products of phenylalanine build up in the body, damaging the nervous system and therefore causing intellectual disability (mental retardation). Recommended that individuals with PKU NOT consume aspartame because it contains high levels of phenylalanine.

4 **(B)** Kwashiorkor is a disease caused by protein-energy malnutrition and characterized by a severe protein deficiency. Affected children who are approximately 2 years old and raised in underdeveloped countries show evidence of edema in the abdomen and legs but NO severe wasting of body fat. Other signs include listlessness, failure to grow and gain weight, changes in hair color.

5 **(C)** Main function of carbohydrates is to provide energy. Although proteins can provide energy, use of carbohydrate energy spares proteins for MAIN function, to repair body tissues. Carbohydrates also aid in oxidation of lipids to prevent ketosis. Polysaccharides and fibers provide for normal peristalsis. One of main functions of water-soluble B vitamins is to regulate metabolism of carbohydrates. Minerals such as phosphorus help regulate acid-base balance.

6 **(D)** Energy yield for carbohydrates is 4 kcal/g (same as for proteins). However, fats can be broken down and used as energy source, yielding 9 kcal/g.

7 **(B)** Sorbitol is a sugar alcohol made from glucose through hydrogenation. Sugar alcohols are carbohydrates and yield approximately same energy as sucrose (4 kcal/g); both are nutritive sweeteners. Advantage that sugar alcohols have over sucrose is that they do NOT promote caries because they are NOT easily metabolized by bacteria in the mouth. Fructose is a monosaccharide and sweetest of ALL sugars; found in honey, fruits, and corn syrup. Mannitol is another sugar alcohol made from mannose and galactose.

8 (A) Consistency of food plays a role in caries development. Food with sticky consistency will remain on the teeth longer and have slower clearance time. Dried apricots, like raisins, are a dried fruit and remain on the teeth longer than other foods. Retention is a factor contributing to the initiation and progression of dental decay. Although soda pop, cake, and milk contain moderate to large amounts of sugar, they are cleared from the oral cavity MORE quickly.

9 (C) Lipoproteins are a means of transportation through the bloodstream for cholesterol, triglycerides, and phospholipids. Lipoproteins include chylomicrons, very low-density lipoproteins, low-density lipoproteins, and high-density lipoproteins.

10 (D) High-density lipoproteins (HDLs) are capable of transporting cholesterol back to the liver, where it can be disposed of. Contain higher level of protein, making them smaller and denser than very low-density and low-density lipoproteins. HDLs are often referred to as "good" cholesterol because elevated levels of HDLs are associated with low risk of heart and vessel disease.

11 (A) Cholesterol is a sterol, one of three main types of lipids. It is synthesized in the liver and makes bile to aid in the digestion (emulsification) of fats. Because dietary cholesterol elevates blood cholesterol, it may increase risk of coronary disease.

12 (D) Dietary lipids have essential functions in the body. They provide a concentrated source of energy: 9 kcal/g. In addition, they assist with the absorption of fat-soluble vitamins and provide insulation, essential fatty acids, flavor and texture to foods, and a sense of satiety. Deficiency in fat-soluble vitamin A may cause night blindness.

13 (D) Skim milk is considered nonfat food source. Butter, coconut oil, beef contain high levels of saturated fat. High intake of saturated fats (>30% of daily intake) is associated with development of atherosclerosis, disease characterized by plaque buildup on arterial walls, which increases risk of cardiovascular disease. To reduce amount of fat from diet, reduce amount of saturated fats. Can be accomplished by eating such foods as fish, skinless poultry, low-fat or nonfat dairy products.

14 (B) Atherosclerosis obstructs blood flow along arterial walls. High blood pressure (HBP) is evidence that heart is applying MORE pressure to circulate the blood because of narrowing of walls of arteries from plaque buildup. Smoking is also risk factor for cardiovascular disease (CVD), as is low-density lipoprotein cholesterol (LDL) reading ≥160 mg/100 mL and total blood cholesterol >240 mg/100 mL. Men who are >45 years and women who are >55 are also at greater risk for this disease.

15 (C) Fat-soluble vitamins include A, D, E, and K. These vitamins are soluble in fat and NOT readily excreted, so they can build up in toxic amounts. ALL B vitamins and vitamin C are water soluble.

16 (B) Preformed vitamin A (retinoid) is found in animal sources. Provitamin A (carotenoid) is found in plant foods, especially deep green and yellow fruits and vegetables.

17 (B) Rickets is a bone disease that affects children as a result of vitamin D deficiency. Bones soften because of failure to calcify normally; include bowed legs.

18 (C) Vitamin E is a fat-soluble antioxidant; protects other substances from oxidation. Also protects RBC membranes.

19 (A) Water-soluble vitamins must be consumed regularly because they are easily excreted or lost in cooking and therefore readily dissolved. Although vitamins do NOT provide energy, they play an active role in energy metabolism. Carbohydrates, lipids, proteins require vitamin input for energy metabolism.

20 (D) Niacin is found in protein foods such as fish, beef, turkey, and chicken. However, 1 mg of niacin can be converted from 60 mg of the amino acid tryptophan.

21 (A) Intrinsic factor is made in the stomach and is needed for absorption of cobalamin (B_{12}). If intrinsic factor becomes inadequate or halts because of surgical removal of the stomach (weight loss surgery), absorption will be affected. Results in deficiency, causing pernicious anemia. Deficiency in extrinsic factor, which must be obtained from food, also causes pernicious anemia but can be prevented by altering diet to include animal foods.

22 (A) Strict vegetarian will be deficient in cobalamin (B_{12}) because major source is almost exclusively animal-derived foods.

23 (C) Scurvy is a disease caused by vitamin C deficiency. Deficiency in vitamin C is NOT uncommon because this water-soluble vitamin is NOT stored for long periods. FIRST sign of a deficiency is bleeding gingiva. Subsequently the muscles begin to degenerate and the skin takes on a dry and scaly appearance. Takes approximately 10 mg of vitamin C per day to prevent overt scurvy; however, DRI for adults is 90 mg/day (males) and 75 mg/day (females).

24 (C) Although MAJOR function of calcium is to form and maintain bones, it has other IMPORTANT functions. Aids in the contraction of muscles and in the blood coagulation process. Also may reduce the risk of colon cancer. MOST of its absorption is in the upper intestine, with assistance of active vitamin D hormone. Recommended daily allowance for both calcium and phosphorus is 1000 mg/day.

25 **(A)** Calcium is MOST abundant mineral found in the body (followed by phosphorus). The bones and teeth store 99% of the body's calcium. Plays a vital role in keeping bones healthy and in preventing bone disease, such as osteoporosis, in later life.

26 **(D)** Magnesium facilitates the operation of enzymes and assists with the relaxation of muscles after contraction. Foods rich in magnesium include dark green leafy vegetables, whole grain breads and cereals, nuts, legumes, and seafood.

27 **(D)** Sodium, MAJOR mineral, is active in maintaining the acid-base balance in the body. Along with calcium, potassium, and magnesium, plays a vital role in nerve conduction. Sodium also helps retain water by triggering a thirst reaction when it is consumed. Thirsty individual will drink MORE water to help balance the sodium-water ratio.

28 **(C)** Sulfur is present in ALL proteins and in the vitamins biotin and thiamin. Aids in maintaining a normal acid-base balance in the body. Sulfur compounds preserve foods.

29 **(B)** Water is the MAIN constituent of the body and comprises 50% to 60% of total body weight. Required on a daily basis and flows in and out of cells through cell membranes. Roles include removal of waste products, maintenance of body temperature, transport of inorganic nutrients, lubrication around joints, maintenance of normal kidney function.

30 **(A)** Adequate zinc intake is essential for the proper development of sexual organs and bone. Also is needed for DNA and protein metabolism and assists with wound healing.

31 **(C)** Energy is measured by heat expenditure. One kilocalorie is the amount of heat produced to raise the temperature of 1 kilogram of water 1° C.

32 **(D)** Basal metabolism requirement (BMR) is ~60% to 70% of the total energy used by the body. Minimal amount of energy is necessary to maintain life at rest. The BMR involves circulation, beating of the heart, breathing, maintaining body temperature. Does NOT include specific dynamic activity, which is the energy required for the digestion of food.

33 **(A)** MAJOR gland that affects the BMR is the thyroid gland. Higher thyroid hormone levels increase the metabolic rate.

34 **(C)** First statement is true; the second is false. Reduction in weight can be accomplished by a reduction in energy input together with an increase in physical activity (energy output). Increase in physical activity controls the appetite, aids in stress reduction, increases the BMR, raises self-esteem.

35 **(B)** Anorexia nervosa is an eating disorder that is characterized by self-starvation (PEM, PCM). Individual, usually female, has a distorted body image (believes self to be overweight). Tendency to exercise excessively, and weight is usually 20% to 40% below desirable body weight. Individual has low self-esteem, is competitive in nature, and is NOT aware of problem.

36 **(C)** Bulimia is an eating disorder that involves episodes of binge eating followed by purging by means of vomiting and/or use of diuretics. Individual is usually female, maintains normal body weight, is aware that behavior is abnormal.

37 **(B)** Compulsive overeating is uncontrolled episodes of overeating without other signs of eating disorder. Individual eats foods that are easy to consume in large portions, such as noodles, rice, and foods that are categorized as "junk" foods. MOST who compulsively overeat do so in response to stress and feelings of depression.

38 **(B)** MOST effective counseling approach when decisions are needed is nondirective. Counselor assists the patient in understanding the needs and changes recommended, and subsequently patient is active participant in planning, implementing, evaluating the changes.

39 **(C)** Directive approach in diet counseling involves a passive participant and decisions made by the counselor. In a nondirective counseling approach, counselor assists with the process but patient is active participant in analysis, evaluation, modifications of diet.

40 **(B)** Diet diary should be recorded for 5 days and should include a weekend. This gives sufficient data for a review of adequacy of food intake and determination of foods that contain sugar and frequency of their consumption.

41 **(A)** Diet after recovering from periodontal surgery should include MORE frequent feedings and MOSTLY fluids on first day. On FIRST day after surgery, should consume plenty of water, juices, and broths. Diet on second day can include blended fruits and vegetables, oatmeal, dairy products such as milk shakes, ice cream. For protein, may have meat broth and eggs. Comfort in chewing will determine what can be consumed.

42 **(A)** Communication is MOST common barrier to care with eating disorder. Denial, shame, guilt, lack of compliance, fear of weight gain are typical reasons for NOT wishing to discuss eating disorder. Transportation and physical barriers are insignificant, but economic considerations may be problematic when dentition has been damaged from behaviors associated with eating disorders, particularly vomiting.

43 **(C)** Frequent purging (vomiting) is responsible for the MOST devastating oral effects of eating disorders. Purging is associated with severe erosion of enamel surfaces, high incidence of caries, sensitivity to sweets and temperatures. Excessive exercising, bingeing, malnutrition, laxative use ALL have fewer direct effects on the oral cavity.

44 (A) Immediately after purging incident, should rinse with tap water (water mixed with sodium bicarbonate or magnesium hydroxide may be used) to neutralize vomit acid. Brushing and flossing are contraindicated immediately after vomiting because the tooth enamel is weakened and brushing and flossing may abrade surface.

45 (D) Lack of potassium causes hypokalemia. Lack of calcium would cause osteopenia and osteoporosis. Liver CANNOT metabolize essential amino acid phenylalanine into nonessential amino acid tyrosine with phenylketonuria (PKU).

46 (C) First statement is true, and second statement is false. Osteosclerosis results from living in an overfluoridated area for a very long period; lacking calcium puts a person at risk of osteoporosis.

47 (A) Vitamin A is a fat-soluble vitamin, and others are water soluble. Mineral oils interfere with absorption of fat-soluble vitamins.

48 (C) First statement is true, and second statement is false; 3-, 5-, or 7-day food diary is the MOST common today.

49 (D) First statement is false, second is true. Water makes up 50% to 60% of total body weight but is main constituent of the body; however, water is required on a daily basis. The body loses water ALL the time, and it must be replaced daily.

50 (D) Calcium is a major mineral (macromineral) essential for strong bones and teeth. Boron is MAINLY an essential plant nutrient, ONLY trace mineral in animals; physiological role in animals is poorly understood. Selenium is also a trace mineral. Vitamin A is a vitamin essential for vision.

CHAPTER 8

Microbiology and Immunology

MICROBIOLOGY

Microorganisms are life forms that normally CANNOT be seen with the unaided human eye. Possess characteristics common to ALL cellular life in terms of physiology, morphology, reproduction. Inhabit MOST niches of environment. Normal inhabitants of human body (normal flora). A medically IMPORTANT microorganism is one that inhabits human host and is considered a **pathogen** (causes disease).

• See CD-ROM for Chapter Terms and WebLinks.

Microbiology Classification

Microbiology spectrum includes prokaryotes, eukaryotes, viruses. Classification of prokaryotes and eukaryotes employs Latin binomial system of genus and species. Ultrastructures have important MAIN differences.

A. **Prokaryotes** (bacteria) possess a relatively simple cellular structure and are MORE primitive cells.
   1. Propagate by binary fission (split into two).
   2. Operationally classified into divisions and classes based primarily on morphological and physiological characteristics; divided into two major taxa: eubacteria and archaeobacteria.
      a. Eubacteria (true bacteria): comprise bacteria of MOST importance to medicine; smallest bacteria.
         (1) Mycoplasmas: smallest free-living bacteria.
         (2) Rickettsias and chlamydials, obligate intracellular parasites: smallest members of bacteria.
      b. Archaeobacteria: primitive nonpathogenic bacteria normally associated with extreme or unusual environments (e.g., thermophilic, halophilic, methanogenic bacteria).
B. **Eukaryotes:** possess relatively complex cellular structure, MORE highly evolved than prokaryotes.
   1. **Fungi:** NOT photosynthetic; include number of pathogenic **molds** and **yeasts.**
   2. **Protozoa** and **helminths:** NOT photosynthetic; include some pathogens.
   3. Algae: photosynthetic; do NOT include pathogens.
C. **Viruses:** acellular life forms that are principally composed of proteins and nucleic acid; NOT a cell, so cannot be classified as either prokaryote or eukaryote.

   1. ALL are **parasites** and require viable (living) host cell for replication; replicate once inside the cell and NOT by binary fission.
   2. Classification by shape (symmetry), type of nucleic acid, type of host cell, type of vector (agent of transmission), and/or associated disease produced.

Microbial Metabolism

Microbial metabolism includes sum total of all biochemical reactions that occur in the cell.
• See Chapter 3, Anatomy, Biochemistry, and Physiology: body metabolism.
A. Exoenzymes:
   1. Enzymes that are excreted into external cellular environment.
   2. Break down polymers and other molecules into subunits that are small enough to be transported into the cell.
   3. May be potent exotoxins (e.g., *Clostridium botulinum* and *C. tetani* produce lipases that affect central nervous system [CNS]).
   4. Examples:
      a. Carbohydrases degrade polysaccharides to individual sugar residues.
      b. Proteases degrade proteins to amino acids.
      c. Lipases degrade lipid molecules.
      d. Hemolysins lyse red blood cells.
B. Transport of molecules for metabolism:
   1. Includes transport of individual molecules to the cell and concentration of these molecules within the cell.
   2. Includes four MAIN transport mechanisms:
      a. Passive diffusion: random movement of molecules into and out of the cell, progressing from higher to lower concentration gradient (e.g., diffusion of water); cellular energy and carrier proteins are NOT involved.
      b. Facilitated diffusion: transport of molecules, such as sugars, mediated by carrier protein that follows a concentration gradient; cellular energy is NOT expended.
      c. Active transport: mediated by a carrier protein, requires expenditure of cellular energy to move molecules into the cell against a concentration gradient.

d. Group translocation (phosphotransferase system): moves molecules into the cell against concentration gradient:
   (1) Carrier protein and energy (form of phosphoenol pyruvate) are involved, and substrate (e.g., glucose molecule) becomes phosphorylated in the process.
   (2) Molecule becomes negatively charged (e.g., glucose-phosphate), then retained inside the cell.
   (3) MOST efficient and MOST common form of transport in bacteria.

C. Metabolism:
   1. Involves metabolic pathways; once inside the cell, a molecule (e.g., glucose) enters metabolic pathways.
   2. Includes two major classes of metabolic reactions:
      a. Catabolic reactions: degradative reactions that:
         (1) Produce energy (adenosine triphosphate [ATP]).
         (2) Produce carbon skeletons.
         (3) Produce reducing power.
      b. Anabolic reactions: biosynthetic reactions that:
         (1) Use up energy (ATP).
         (2) Use up carbon skeletons.
         (3) Use up reducing power.

D. Oxidation-reduction reactions: employed in cellular metabolism:
   1. Compound is oxidized when gives up or loses electrons; reduced when receives or gains electrons.
   2. Reactions are simultaneous; when molecule is oxidized, another is simultaneously reduced.

E. Energy production (catabolism):
   1. Bacteria produce cellular energy, MAINLY in form of ATP, by passing pair of electrons through the cell.
   2. Molecule that gives up the pair of electrons and becomes oxidized is called the electron donor.
   3. Molecule that ultimately receives these electrons after they pass through the cell is called the final electron acceptor.
   4. Molecules that accept and transfer these electrons (within the cell) from the donor to the final electron acceptor are called electron carriers; typical electron carrier involved in energy metabolism is nicotine adenine dinucleotide (NAD).
   5. When the electron donor (e.g., glucose) becomes oxidized, NAD receives the pair of electrons (and protons) and becomes reduced to $NADH_2$; however, the cell is limited in number of oxidized NAD molecules; soon all would become reduced to $NADH_2$ and energy metabolism would cease.
   6. The reduced $NADH_2$ molecule MUST be able to donate its electrons to an acceptor to regenerate oxidized NAD; thus defines fermentation and respiration:
      a. Fermentation: organic molecule serves as final electron acceptor.
      b. Respiration: inorganic molecule serves as final electron acceptor.

F. Fermentation: energy-inefficient process that results in the production of two ATPs from the partial oxidation of one glucose molecule.
   1. Strictly anaerobic process:
      a. Glucose (electron donor) enters glycolytic pathway.
      b. Glycolysis occurs, resulting in oxidation of 1 glucose molecule (C6) into 2 pyruvate molecules (C3) and net production of 2 reduced $NADH_2$ molecules and 2 molecules of ATP, which is referred to as substrate level phosphorylation.
      c. Pyruvate, organic compound, is central "hub" of fermentation reactions and serves as final electron acceptor in simplest fermentation; reduced $NADH_2$ donates its electrons directly to pyruvate, reducing it to lactic acid (C3), which is released into external environment.
   2. Accomplished by microorganisms capable of carrying out fermentations that result in a wide variety of metabolic end products, including CO_2, H_2, organic acids, and alcohols.
   3. Ability or inability of organism to ferment different substrates is one of KEY features that enable distinction among bacterial species.

G. Respiration: energy-efficient process that results in production of 38 ATPs from complete oxidation of 1 glucose molecule.
   1. Can be either aerobic or anaerobic process:
      a. Glucose (C6) enters the glycolytic pathway, with same result as in fermentation: 2 ATP, 2 $NADH_2$, and 2 pyruvate (C3) molecules are formed.
      b. Pyruvate becomes decarboxylated and bound to coenzyme A, resulting in acetyl-CoA, CO_2, and production of 1 reduced $NADH_2$ molecule.
      c. Acetyl-CoA feeds into tricarboxylic acid (TCA) cycle; one turn of the TCA cycle results in production of 2 CO_2 molecules and 4 reduced $NADH_2$ molecules.
      d. Second pyruvate molecule generated by glycolysis undergoes same series of reactions; at this point glucose is completely oxidized to 6 molecules of CO_2; 2 ATPs have been produced and a total of 12 reduced $NADH_2$s have been formed; cells then regenerate oxidized NAD and generate MORE energy by means of the electron transport system.

e. Electron transport chain is made up of a series of electron transfer molecules (cytochromes) that are located in cytoplasmic membrane:

(1) Reduced $NADH_2$ donates its electrons and protons to electron transport chain, becoming reoxidized to NAD.

(2) Passage of the electrons through electron transport chain results in production of 3 ATP molecules, producing oxidative phosphorylation.

(3) At the end of electron transport chain the electrons and protons combine with O_2, reducing it to H_2O.

(4) Overall, there are a total of 12 reduced $NADH_2$ molecules, which results in the production of 36 ATPs (3×12) in addition to the 2 ATPs produced from glycolysis, for a total production of 38 ATPs from 1 glucose molecule.

H. Differences *between* aerobes and anaerobes:

1. *Aerobic* respiration:

a. Carried out by bacterium that can use O_2 as the final electron acceptor in respiration.

b. Involves a combination of O_2, electrons, and protons at the terminus of the electron transport chain, resulting in the formation of toxic intermediates, superoxide anions (O_2^-), and hydrogen peroxide (H_2O_2).

c. Requires bacterium that can grow aerobically to possess two enzymes for removal (conversion) of these toxic products.

(1) Superoxide dismutase: converts O_2^- into H_2O_2

(2) Catalase (peroxidase): subsequently converts H_2O_2 into H_2O and O_2.

2. *Anaerobic* respiration:

a. Carried out by bacteria that possess electron transport chain but lack either or both superoxide dismutase and catalase and are unable to remove toxic by-products of aerobic respiration.

b. Uses oxidized inorganic compounds other than O_2 as final electron acceptor; some common inorganic compounds used in anaerobic respiration include sulfate (SO_4), sulfur (S), nitrate (NO_3), and carbon dioxide (CO_2).

I. Anaerobic fermentation enables bacteria that lack components of, or do NOT have, electron transport chain to grow anaerobically by means of fermentation.

J. Biosynthesis (anabolism): fermentation and respiration produce energy for driving biosynthetic (anabolic) reactions of the cell for necessary synthesis of nucleic acids, proteins, carbohydrates, and lipids.

Microbial Observation

Observation of microorganisms may be either macroscopic or microscopic, depending on total number of organisms.

A. *Macroscopic* observation is necessary when organisms are in large numbers:

1. Turbidity (cloudiness) in liquid cultures.

2. Colonial morphology occurs when grown on solid surface such as agar agar Petri dish:

a. Defined as mass of cells that arise from single cell.

b. May provide distinguishing characteristics of organism in terms of color (pigmentation), texture, size, shape.

B. *Microscopic* observation of individual cells is required because of small size:

1. Bacteria may range in size from ~10 μm (size of a red blood cell) to 0.1 μm (micrometer = 10^{-6} of a meter); viruses are even smaller; range in size from ~0.25 μm to as small as 15 nm (nanometer = 10^{-9} of a meter).

2. Compound microscopes (two or more lenses) provide enlargement (magnification) and allow distinguishing of fine details (resolving power).

3. Resolving power is dependent on wavelength of light and employed with decreasing wavelength, resulting in higher resolving power.

C. Bright field microscopy (via compound microscope): uses visible light and oil immersion:

1. MOST commonly used microscopy type (magnification = ~1000× and resolution = ~0.25 μm).

2. Specimens MUST be stained to be observed.

D. Dark field microscopy: observes living, unstained specimens; oblique light increases contrast so specimens appear bright against dark background.

E. Phase-contrast microscopy: observes unstained specimens; contrast is amplified by detection of small differences in refractive indices between specimen and surrounding medium; some dental offices offer this to show dental biofilm during oral hygiene discussion.

F. Fluorescence microscopy: visualizes objects that fluoresce, i.e., emit light, when exposed to light of different wavelength:

1. Detects fluorescent objects illuminated by ultraviolet or near-ultraviolet light; specimens absorb light and emit visible light.

2. Fluorescent dyes conjugated with specific antibodies are basis of immunofluorescence; employed in identification of microorganisms and BEST for tracking of antigen-antibody complexes.

G. Electron microscopy (EM): takes advantage of short wavelength of electrons:

1. Greatly increases magnification and resolving power.

2. BEST for observation of cellular ultrastructure and viruses.
   a. Transmission EM: BEST for thin sections of specimens.
   b. Scanning EM (SEM): BEST for whole cells and cells attached to surfaces.

Specimen Preparation and Staining

Specimens MUST be prepared and then stained to be seen under light microscope because refractive index of MOST organisms is clear. Basic dyes (e.g., crystal violet, methylene blue, safranin) are positively charged and combine with negatively charged cell constituents. Acidic dyes (e.g., eosin, nigrosin, basic fuchsin) possess negative charge and combine with positively charged cell components.

A. Specimens MUST be heat fixed to slide for bright field microscopy so that cells adhere and are NOT washed off during staining procedures.
B. Simple staining: employs single stain, such as methylene blue or crystal violet; useful ONLY to distinguish cellular morphology.
C. Differential stains: employ two different-colored stains to indicate cellular morphology and distinguish between groups of organisms and/or cellular structures.
   1. **Gram stain:** separates ALL bacteria into two groups: **gram-positive** (purple-blue) cells or **gram-negative** (red-pink) cells; stain reflects differences in cell wall structure.
      a. MOST important staining procedure in microbiology, first step in bacterial identification.
      b. Procedure has four steps:
         (1) Crystal violet (purple) is primary stain.
         (2) Iodine is mordant that helps to "fix" primary stain to cells.
         (3) Alcohol is wash that decolorizes ONLY gram-negative cells.
         (4) Safranin (red) is counterstain that enables observation of colorless gram-negative cells.
   2. **Acid-fast stain:** BEST used to differentiate mycobacteria, causative agents of tuberculosis, which appear red, from other bacteria, which appear blue.
      a. Primary stain MUST be heated into cell and is NOT washed out, even with acid alcohol, because of hydrophobic waxy nature of cell wall; thus the stain is acid "fast."
      b. Procedure has three steps:
         (1) Carbolfuchsin (red) is primary stain heated into cell.
         (2) Wash with 3% HCl in alcohol that decolorizes non-acid-fast cells.
         (3) Methylene blue is counterstain that enables observation of the non-acid-fast cells.

Bacterial (Prokaryotic) Structure and Function

Small bacteria possess variety of shapes and sizes and internal or external structures that aid in survival and are useful in identification of different bacteria. Survival is KEY to involvement with infectious processes.
A. Cellular shape:
   1. Coccus (plural, cocci), spherical:
      a. Diplococci (pairs): *Streptococcus pneumoniae.*
      b. Chains of cocci: *Streptococcus mutans, Streptococcus pyogenes.*
      c. Random clusters: *Staphylococcus aureus.*
   2. Bacillus (plural, bacilli), cylindrical rods:
      a. Large rods: *Bacillus subtilis, Clostridium botulinum.*
      b. Small rods: *Escherichia coli, Salmonella, Shigella.*
      c. Chains aligned end to end: *Streptobacillus moniliformis.*
      d. Fusiform types (threadlike): rods with pointed ends.
      e. Filamentous types (threadlike): branching bacillus rods.
   3. Spirillum (plural, spirilla) (spirochetes), cylindrical with an amplitude (spiral with axial fibrils):
      a. *Leptospira, Treponema, Borrelia.*
      b. Vibrios have a comma shape: *Vibrio cholerae.*
   4. Palisade arrangement ("snapping division"): *Corynebacterium diphtheriae.*
   5. **Pleomorphic** (lack a defined cell shape): *Mycoplasma pneumoniae.*
B. Cellular ultrastructure:
   1. Internal cellular structures:
      a. Chromosomal DNA: circular and haploid; possesses MOST cellular genes and genetic information.
      b. **Plasmids:** autonomously self-replicating, small, circular DNA molecules, may be transferred from cell to cell and may contain genes for resistance to multiple antibiotics; NOT present in all bacteria.
      c. Ribosomes: composed of 30S and 50S subunits, which make up 70S ribosomal RNA required for protein synthesis, distributed throughout the cytoplasm.
      d. Inclusion bodies: noted in some bacteria; consist of energy storage molecules, such as poly-beta-hydroxybutyrate, that form granules or refractive bodies.
   2. Cytoplasmic membrane encompasses cytoplasm:
      a. Composed of lipids, proteins, ions; provides hydrophobic matrix; exists as bilayer.
      b. Provides permeability barrier and support for transporting proteins, as well as electron transport system.

3. Cell wall surrounds the cytoplasmic membrane, which provides cellular shape and rigidity.
   a. Cell wall: prevents cell from lysing because of increased internal osmotic pressure.
   b. Periplasmic space: region between cytoplasmic membrane and cell wall; contains various enzymes and proteins associated with transport.
4. Cell surface structures external to the cell wall:
   a. **Capsule:** generally composed of polysaccharides; thick, tightly bound structure found in some; when present, may be antigenic and may protect against phagocytosis and desiccation.
   b. **Slime layer:** composed of polypeptides; exists as relatively thin layer over the cell surface of some; loosely bound and in some instances MUST be present to provide virulence in bacteria.
   c. **Glycocalyx:** surrounds the surface of some; composed of a macromolecular network of primarily polysaccharide molecules; provides cellular adhesion to surfaces such as tooth enamel (e.g., *Streptococcus mutans*).
   d. **Flagella:** long (as long as 70 μm), thin protein (flagellin) filaments extending from the cell surface; provide bacterial motility by turning in a circular motion.
      (1) Allow movement toward or away from chemical substances (chemotaxis).
      (2) Bacteria without flagella MUST depend on brownian motion (random activity by van der Waals forces) for movement.
   e. **Pili** (singular, pilus) and **fimbriae** (singular, fimbria): short, proteinaceous, hairlike structures that extend from the cell surface; associated with gram-negative bacteria.
      (1) Pili: involved with the cell-to-cell transfer of genetic material between bacteria.
      (2) Fimbriae: provide cell-to-cell adhesion (e.g., pellicle formation, clumping together of cells).
   f. **Endospore:** large, generally spherical structure that forms within the cytoplasmic interior of the cell; one spore is formed per cell and one bacterium is produced per spore upon germination.
      (1) Spore coat: contains large amounts of dipicolinic acid and divalent cations (Ca^{++}).
      (2) Spores: means of survival and NOT reproduction; formation is induced by deteriorating growth conditions.
         (a) Spores resist high temperatures, desiccation, ultraviolet light, and disinfectants and are major reason for elaborate and harsh sterilization procedures; prevalent throughout environment and

may remain viable for thousands of years (the Dick Clark of the microbial world).
         (b) *Bacillus* (aerobic) and *Clostridium* (anaerobic) are the two MAJOR genera of spore-forming bacteria.
C. Chemical differences in cell wall structure *between* gram-positive and gram-negative bacteria:
   1. Peptidoglycan (murine) is present in BOTH gram-positive and gram-negative cells:
      a. Three-dimensional macromolecular net that surrounds the cytoplasmic membrane.
      b. Composed of a polysaccharide backbone (repeating *N*-acetyl glucosamine/*N*-acetyl muramic acid subunits) to which amino acid chains are attached (to muramic acid residues).
      c. Amino acid chains are further cross-linked to amino acid chains on adjacent peptidoglycan molecules by additional amino acid residues, thus providing three-dimensional structure.
         (1) Gram-positive bacteria possess thick, highly cross-linked peptidoglycan layers because of high internal osmotic pressures; stains purple (e.g., *Streptococcus* and *Actinomyces* species; susceptible to antibiotic cillins and sporins).
         (2) Gram-negative bacteria possess thin, sparsely cross-linked peptidoglycan layers because of relatively low internal osmotic pressures with lipopolysaccharides and lipoproteins; stay red-pink (e.g., *Escherichia coli, Salmonella, Neisseria gonorrhoeae*).
   2. Gram-positive wall macromolecules:
      a. Teichoic acid: polymers of repeating glycerol phosphate and ribitol phosphate residues attached to peptidoglycan; may serve as antigenic determinants or receptor sites for bacterial viruses.
      b. Lipoteichoic acids: structures similar to teichoic acid, but with diglyceride residue(s) on one end that provide an anchor into the cytoplasmic membrane.
      c. Various polysaccharides may bind to peptidoglycan.
   3. Gram-negative wall macromolecules: lipid-enriched outer membrane is formed externally to the peptidoglycan layer by the presence of lipopolysaccharides and lipoproteins.
      a. **Lipopolysaccharides** (LPS) (endotoxins): complex lipid molecule linked to a polysaccharide chain oriented on the outer surface of the peptidoglycan, with polysaccharide chains extending into the environment.
         (1) Antigenic and may serve as receptor sites for bacterial viruses.

(2) Important NOT only in systemic infections but also in initiation and progression of periodontal disease.

b. Lipoproteins: lipid and extended amino acid chains oriented in a manner similar to that of LPS.

c. Porins: globular hollow proteins that form pores in the lipid-rich outer membrane.

D. Mycobacterial (acid-fast) cell walls *differ* from those of typical gram-positive and gram-negative cells:

1. Waxes (wax D) and mycolic acids cover peptidoglycan layer; creates hydrophobic surface layer correlated with staining reaction of the bacteria (e.g., causative agent of tuberculosis).

2. Basis for the formulations of many disinfectants is whether they can break down this strong cell wall (see later discussion in chapter).

Bacterial Growth and Nutrition

Bacterial growth is the increase in the numbers of bacterial cells by binary fission. Growth is influenced by the physical environment and the availability of essential nutrients. This is important NOT only in pathogenesis of systemic infections but also with development of infectious oral disease (periodontal disease and caries) and its MAIN etiological factor, dental biofilm (dental plaque).

A. Bacterial growth:

1. **Generation time:** amount of time it takes a single cell to divide into two cells (~30 minutes for a typical bacterium growing under ideal conditions).

   a. Cell numbers expressed as log to the base 10 (e.g., $1 \times 10^7 = 10$ million cells) for convenience because of the large number of bacterial cells that may be attained under ideal growth conditions.

   b. Measured by visually observing turbidity of a culture, increase in optical density, and increase in protein concentration, or by direct cell counts in a Coulter counter.

2. Bacterial growth curve has four phases:

   a. Lag phase: on inoculation into a new medium, cells do NOT immediately divide; cells swell, begin metabolic preparation for growth in the new medium, and use ATP.

   b. Exponential (logarithmic, log) phase: cells divide and generation time is at a minimum; ALL cells are viable (alive) and use nutrients; Gram stain is MOST reliable during this phase; antibiotics and infection control agents such as disinfectants are MOST effective.

   c. Stationary phase: number of dying cells equals number of dividing cells (constant population numbers); endospore formation may begin; nutrients are being depleted (used up) and toxic metabolic products are increasing.

d. Death (decline) phase: cells begin dying exponentially; now the nonviable cells outnumber the viable ones and nutrients are depleted.

B. Nutritional requirements for bacterial growth:

1. Include liquid water, inorganic elements, carbon, energy source for growth and reproduction.

2. Bacteria may be physiologically classified based on how they derive their carbon and/or energy (sorry, they do not drink coffee to keep them going like some of you are doing right now!).

   a. **Heterotrophs:** obtain carbon from an organic compound (e.g., glucose).

   b. Autotrophs: obtain carbon from inorganic source (e.g., CO2).

   c. Phototrophs: derive energy from light.

   d. **Chemotrophs:** derive energy from the oxidation of chemical compounds.

3. Bacteria may be further subdivided based on the carbon plus the energy source:

   a. Photolithotrophs: obtain energy from light and carbon from CO_2.

   b. Photoorganotrophs: obtain energy from light and carbon from organic compounds.

   c. Chemolithotrophs: obtain energy from inorganic compounds (e.g., sulfur, iron) and carbon from inorganic CO_2.

   d. Chemoorganotrophs: obtain BOTH energy and carbon from organic compounds, often from the same molecule (e.g., glucose).

   e. **Saprophytes:** grow on dead organic matter.

   f. Parasites: grow on living organic matter.

C. Media for bacterial growth:

1. May be liquid or solidified by addition of 1.5% agar agar (obtained from kelp); inert to bacterial metabolism.

2. May be identified as one of several media based on its composition:

   a. Defined medium: exact concentration and exact composition of all compounds added are known.

   b. Complex medium: exact concentration of components added is known; exact composition of all constituents is NOT known.

   c. Selective medium: agents are added that inhibit growth of one group of bacteria but NOT another.

   d. Differential medium: distinguishes between different organisms.

   e. Differential and selective medium: contains components of BOTH selective and differential mediums.

   f. Enriched media: for fastidious (difficult to culture) organisms; contain such complex components as serum and red blood cells.

   g. Reducing media and special techniques are necessary for the cultivation of anaerobic organisms that CANNOT be grown in the presence of oxygen.

(1) Reducing agents such as thioglycollate, hydrogen sulfide, cysteine are added to remove oxygen from the medium.

(2) Air may be replaced with nitrogen, hydrogen, and/or carbon dioxide in special jars; hydrogen generator and palladium catalyst used to remove oxygen; employed for cultivating organisms on agar agar plates.

D. Factors that influence microbial growth:
1. Oxygen requirements for growth and reproduction:
    a. **Aerobes** (*need* O₂): require and use oxygen.
    b. **Anaerobes** (*NO* O₂): grow in absence of oxygen; exposure to oxygen may be toxic.
    c. **Facultative anaerobes** (*okay* O₂ or *NO* O₂): use oxygen or grow in absence oxygen.
    d. **Microaerophiles** (*low* O₂): require and use oxygen but in low concentrations.
2. Hydrogen ion concentration (pH): MOST bacteria grow optimally near neutrality, pH 7.0 (see Chapter 3, Anatomy, Biochemistry, and Physiology).
    a. Acidophiles: grow ONLY at acidic values, ~0 to 4.0 pH.
    b. Alkalophiles: grow ONLY in alkaline values, > 9.0 pH.
    c. Aciduric: tolerate an acid environment (e.g., *Streptococcus mutans*).
    d. Acidogenic: produce weak acids by fermentation (e.g., *Streptococcus mutans*).
3. Osmotic pressure: MOST bacteria grow optimally at salt concentrations near salinity (0.9%).
E. Microbial growth relationships:
1. May be beneficial, harmful, or benign metabolic interactions between microorganism and host; interactions (Table 8-1) (just like the cast of "Friends").
2. Involve growing on or within other organisms (hosts), including humans.
F. Bacterial genetics: microorganisms vary in the composition of their DNA and RNA and in the way their genetic codes are expressed, similar to the cells of the human body.
1. Genetic transfer between bacteria:
    a. Involves the passage of DNA from a donor bacterial cell to a recipient cell.

Table 8-1 Microbial interactions

Term	Microorganism	Host
Symbiosis	Benefits	Benefits
Commensalism	Benefits	Benign
Parasitism	Benefits	Benign or harmed
Pathogenesis	Benefits	Harmed

b. Spontaneous mutations occur infrequently in a population, but recipient bacteria may instantly acquire new genes, which allows changes to the genetic constitution and capabilities of the organism.
c. Incoming DNA may be degraded by nucleases of the recipient or may be exchanged and integrated with existing sequences in the recipient DNA by recombination.
2. Types of transfer between bacteria:
    a. Transformation: gene transfer mediated by free "naked" DNA.
    b. Transduction: gene transfer mediated by bacteriophages (bacterial viruses).
    c. Conjugation: plasmid-mediated gene transfer, which requires cell-to-cell contact.
3. Significance of conjugation and gene transfer: NOT only can these plasmids become donated and spread like an infection throughout a bacterial population, but they may be transferred between different genera of bacteria and between species of the same genus.

INFECTIOUS DISEASES

Microorganisms generally MUST breach host defense barriers to initiate disease-causing reactions and transfer to new hosts, whether it involves bacteria or viruses. EXCEPTION is transmission by ingestion of preformed microbial (bacterial) toxin that can cause **toxemia** (poison in the bloodstream) (see later discussion). There are many overlaps between the routes of transmission of infectious materials, since the overwhelming goal of the microorganism is to survive at ANY means; there are also nonspecfic and specific host defenses.

Each route of transmission is discussed here with the MOST common examples of infectious disease that have practical association with MAJOR risks for exposure in the dental setting. Risk factors for NOT achieving oral health are also listed when involved. Infection control protocol and standard precautions to prevent transmission are discussed later.

A. Nonspecific host defenses: constitute first-line barriers and reactions against invading microorganisms:
1. Physical defenses of skin cells and hair.
2. Chemical defenses:
    a. Acidic pH present in stomach (acid secretion), vagina (microbial flora), and skin (lipids).
    b. Microbe-digesting enzymes at mucosal sites (e.g., lysozyme), including oral mucosa.
    c. Blood proteins termed "acute phase" proteins, which harm microbes by being deposited on their surface and facilitating clearance by phagocytosis.

3. Biological defenses:
   a. Phagocytic cells, which internalize and degrade potential pathogens.
   b. **Complement:** series of proteins that damage microbial membranes and facilitate clearance by phagocytosis.
B. Specific host defenses: immune system recognizes and responds to microbes and microbial toxins (discussed later).
C. Common ways for infection transmission:
   1. **Contact:**
      a. Direct contact with other infected host(s), which occurs during patient care; especially involves hands, such as NOT washing after restroom use and between patients.
      b. Nondirect contact: occurs with a contaminated intermediate object, usually inanimate, e.g., contaminated instruments or gloves that are NOT changed between patients.
   2. Droplet (airborne): travel on dust particles or respiratory droplets that may become aerosolized (sneeze, cough, laugh, or exhale); increased with aerosol production generated in dental practice, e.g., ultrasonic use.
   3. **Vehicle:** transmitted to host by contaminated items, e.g., food, water, drugs, devices, equipment; includes fecal contamination of food, water, or hands.
   4. Many infections are transmitted from insects or other living carriers (vector borne).
D. MORE common infection transmission routes:
   1. MOST common route is via respiratory system, oral mucosa, eyes (do NOT ever touch your eyes at workplace).
      a. Facilitated by the absence of protective skin cells.
      b. Potential access to various body cells (e.g., epithelial cells, lymphocytes, macrophages).
   2. Second MOST common route is fecal-oral (see handwashing discussion).
   3. Skin protection can be breached by cuts or abrasions of unprotected skin, e.g., reschedule patients with open infected lesions until healed.
   4. Other infections are transmitted by sexual mode; protection afforded by intact skin is bypassed.
   5. Perinatal route from the mother to the fetus and/or newborn (congenital infections).

Bacterial Infections

Many infections are bacterial in origin, but many have vaccinations developed against them or are sensitive to antibiotics and other infection control procedures. However, resistant strains are now a developing problem in healthcare. See later discussion on antibiotics.
• See Chapters 6, General and Oral Pathology: oral infections, infectious peptic ulcers; 9, Pharmacology:

antibiotic premedication patient; 17, Community Oral Health: epidemiology.
A. Group A *Streptococcus* (e.g., "strep throat") infection: caused by *S. pyogenes* transmitted by ANY route, but MOST commonly from infected person (or carrier) via respiratory droplets or skin contact; nasal discharge is IMPORTANT source.
   1. Pathogenesis: site dependent, with rapid spreading; attachment to pharyngeal epithelium in the case of sore throat, with disease ranging from local skin infections to fatal bacteremia and toxic shock syndrome.
   2. Diagnosis: strep throat, pharyngitis, tonsillitis, redness and edema of mucous membranes, purulent exudate, fever, enlarged cervical lymph nodes; isolation of streptococci in smears or cultures; rapid detection of group A streptococcal antigen from throat swabs is available; may have symptoms of rheumatic fever (see below), including carditis, polyarthritis, subcutaneous nodules.
   3. Prevention: unavailable.
   4. Treatment: penicillin (Pen-Vee K) for 10 days.
   5. Epidemiology of rheumatic fever: in a few cases, untreated strep throat may progress to rheumatic fever; mechanism responsible is antigenic cross-reaction with heart tissue (see later discussion of infective endocarditis), then immune response becomes directed against heart antigens (rheumatic heart disease).
B. Tuberculosis (TB): caused by *Mycobacterium tuberculosis* transmitted by respiratory route (droplets produced by coughing).
   1. Pathogenesis: chronic infection spreads throughout the body via lymphatics and blood, with growth of bacteria in monocytes and intracellular growth, which stimulates T-cell lymphocytic response and results in cell-mediated hypersensitivity and associated tissue damage, causing fibrosis and the calcification of granulomas in the lungs and possibly liver and kidneys.
   2. Symptoms: fever, night sweats, chills, malaise, cough, lymphadenopathy of cervical and submandibular lymph nodes; weight loss is common.
      a. With lung, coughing and spitting blood.
      b. With CNS: may include meningitis.
      c. Oral: ulcer on tongue (common and highly infectious lesion).
   3. Diagnosis: by fever, fatigue, and specific organ involvement; examination of smears and culture; tuberculin ("TB") skin testing using PPD (purified protein derivative) reveals positive cell-mediated response to antigens.
   4. Prevention: bacille Calmette-Guérin (BCG) vaccination, NOT recommended because of questionable efficacy, also now renders tuberculin skin test false positive; avoidance of close contact

with infectious persons is first defense; long-term therapy with antibiotics is second defense.

   a. Can be transmitted from patient to patient if infection control procedures such as <u>standard precautions</u> are NOT followed.

   b. Avoid elective dental care for patients with active TB; includes first 2 weeks of therapy or until tests are negative.

5. Treatment: antibiotics (isoniazid [INH, Nydrazid], rifampin [Rifadin, Rimactane], pyrazinamide [PZA], or ethambutol [Myambutol]); requires long course (6 to 9 months) to eliminate disease; additional drugs if antibiotic resistance.

6. Epidemiology: close contact and massive exposure enhance transmission rate; immunosuppression, such as with acquired immunodeficiency syndrome (AIDS), leads to enhanced susceptibility.

   a. Increased risk for healthcare personnel, including dental healthcare personnel.

   b. Patients with human immunodeficiency virus (HIV)-positive history and undiagnosed pulmonary infection SHOULD be suspected of having TB.

   c. Poor compliance has resulted in emergence of multidrug-resistant strains (MDR-TB), especially with HIV infection.

C. *Actinomyces* infection: caused by *Actinomyces israelii* (MOST common) and *A. naeslundii,* gram-positive, rod-shaped, anaerobic or facultatively anaerobic; part of normal oral flora.

1. Pathogenesis: **opportunistic infection** (see later discussion in this chapter) that follows injury, introducing contaminated debris into tissues in immunocompromised, with facial swelling ("lumpy jaw") and abscess formation in soft tissues becomes fibrotic ("wooden") and can then discharge tangled masses of bacteria ("sulfur granules") (Figure 8-1).

2. Treatment: antibiotics such as penicillin (Pen-Vee K) or amoxicillin (Amoxil, Larotid, Polymox) for 6 months to year; surgery if extensive.

D. Meningitis: inflammation of the membranes (meninges) of brain and spinal cord; MAINLY caused by group B streptococci, *Escherichia coli, Neisseria meningitidis, Haemophilus influenzae,* and *Streptococcus pneumoniae* (but also caused by enteroviruses, mumps virus, fungi, parasites), with transmission by contact with another individual or other outside source or as result of invasion by microorganisms normally present (normal flora).

1. Pathogenesis: occurs after microbial invasion of CNS.

2. Diagnosis:

   a. Clinical, including fever, irritation, headache, neurological signs.

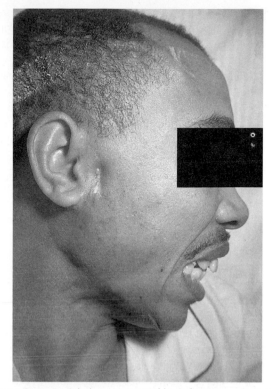

Figure 8-1 Facial abscess caused by infection with *Actinomyces israelii.*

   b. Lab analysis of cerebrospinal fluid (CSF) for cells, elevated protein level, and depressed glucose level.

   c. Lab identification of bacteria present in CSF is critical for rapid institution of antibiotic therapy.

3. Prevention:

   a. Vaccines for several causative microbes (e.g., *H. influenzae, S. pneumoniae, N. meningitidis*).

   b. Prophylactic use of antibiotics for close contacts.

4. Treatment:

   a. Prompt use of appropriate antibiotics, antifungals, or antiparasitics.

   b. Antiviral therapy when involving herpes simplex virus.

5. Epidemiology:

   a. Occurs in all age groups; neonatal meningitis (group B streptococci or *E. coli*) has HIGH fatality rate.

   b. Use of *H. influenzae* vaccine has greatly reduced incidence of childhood form caused by *H. influenzae.*

   c. AIDS patients are at risk for meningitis caused by *Cryptococcus neoformans.*

E. Legionnaire's disease: caused by gram-negative bacillus; *Legionella pneumophila* is MAIN species transmitted to humans by way of infected water supply, primarily by aerosol.

1. Pathogenesis: infection of lower respiratory tract; results in toxic effects on lung cells and stimulation of inflammatory responses; exacerbates tissue damage.
2. Diagnosis: lab culture, detection of bacterial antigen and seroconversion.
3. Prevention: decontamination of contaminated water supplies by heating or chlorination.
4. Treatment: antibiotic erythromycin (Robimycin, E-Mycin, E.E.S.) for symptomatic infections.
5. Epidemiology: bacterium common in aquatic systems; dissemination by aerosols (e.g., from evaporative condensers, cooling towers, nebulizers) plays important role in outbreaks; immunosuppression appears to play a role in susceptibility; risk factors are greater for healthcare facilities.

F. Infective (bacterial) endocarditis (IE): inflammation of lining of heart, MAINLY from infected valves (especially mitral) that may lead to massive sepsis (blood infection), with all signs of infection (mainly fever); ends in fatality.
   1. Pathogenesis: presence of artificial (prosthetic) valves is MAJOR risk factor, with or without heart transplant; valves need replacement because of congenital disease, IE, rheumatic heart disease, or drugs (phen-fen).
      a. Bacteremia (bacteria in the blood) from invasive procedures, e.g., surgery, dentistry, intravascular medical or drug abuse devices, that allow entry of infectious agents.
      b. Caused by *Staphylococcus aureus* (MOST common) or *Streptococcus viridans;* however, other microorganisms can be involved; thus name is now "infective" instead of bacterial.
      c. Risk factors besides valvular complication: past history of IE, cancer, diabetes mellitus (DM), corticosteroid use, IV drug use, alcoholism, renal failure, systemic lupus erythematosus (SLE).
   2. Diagnosis: repeated blood cultures.
   3. Treatment: early intervention is KEY; prolonged bactericidal antimicrobial therapy, parenterally in high dosages (see discussion below on MRSA).
   4. Prevention: antibiotic premedication (prophylaxis) before invasive procedures in high-risk patients, excellent oral hygiene, monitoring past history of disease (high risk for recurrence).

G. Prosthetic (artificial) joint infection: caused by *Staphylococcus aureus* or *S. epidermidis* (NOT viridans group streptococci), the MAJOR oral bacterial species involed.
   1. Pathogenesis: bacteremias from invasive procedures cause hematogenous seeding of total joint implants (ALL joint surfaces are replaced), BOTH in early postoperative period and for 2 years (critical period) following implantation or continually for persons at risk such those with comorbidities and immunocompromised health (e.g., diabetes mellitus, systemic lupus erythematosus).
   2. Diagnosis: redness, warmth, and inflammation around affected area, which may be stiff, drain pus, lose range of motion; radiographs and magnetic resonance imaging (MRI) scans, as well as blood samples and aspirated fluid for culturing.
   3. Prevention: antibiotic premedication before invasive procedures in high-risk patients, excellent oral hygiene, monitoring past history of disease (high risk for recurrence).
   4. Treatment: early intervention is KEY; prolonged bactericidal antimicrobial therapy, administered parenterally in high dosages (see discussion below on MRSA).

H. Methicillin-resistant *Staphylococcus aureus* (MRSA) infections: caused by gram-positive *S. aureus* ("staph") bacteria transmitted by contact.
   1. Pathogenesis: deep wound infection in older adults, chronically ill, persons with weakened immune systems; leads to serious skin and soft tissue infections, pneumonia.
   2. Diagnosis: small red bumps that resemble pimples, boils, or spider bites, quickly turning into deep, painful abscesses that require surgical draining; tissue sample, nasal secretions, detection of organism's DNA.
   3. Prevention: isolation of infections in healthcare settings, standard precautions for healthcare personnel with emphasis on washing hands, basic hygiene practices after sports, special precautions with immunocompromised, testing if suspected, CORRECT use of basic antibiotics.
   4. Treatment: antibiotic vancomycin and others already proved effective against particular strains, such as gentamicin (Garamycin); resistant to all β-lactam antibiotics (penicillins [Pen-Vee K], amoxicillin [Amoxil], cephalosporins [Keflex]).
   5. Epidemiology: now community acquired (CA-MRSA), NOT only in healthcare setting (i.e., hospital).

I. Osteomyelitis: infection of bone and bone marrow, usually caused by pyogenic bacteria or mycobacteria.
   1. Subclassified on basis of causative organism, route, duration, anatomical location; *Staphylococcus aureus* MOST common.
   2. Pathogenesis: microorganisms may be disseminated to bone hematogenously (i.e., via the bloodstream).
      a. Spread contiguously to bone from local areas of infection, such as cellulitis, or are introduced by penetrating trauma, including such

iatrogenic causes as joint replacement, internal fixation of fractures, or endodontically treated teeth.

b. Leukocytes release enzymes that lyse bone while trying to heal area; pus spreads into the bone's blood vessels, impairing the flow, and areas of devitalized infected bone, known as sequestra, form the basis of a chronic infection.

c. The body commonly tries to create new bone around area of necrosis; new bone is an involucrum.

3. Treatment: prolonged antibiotic therapy via IV.

CLINICAL STUDY

Age	42 YRS	**SCENARIO**
Sex	☒ Male ☐ Female	The patient presents at a walk-in medical and dental clinic with weight loss, fever, oral sore. A sputum smear shows the presence of acid-fast bacilli. A chest radiograph shows evidence of pulmonary lesions. Two days later, a test the patient took on his skin is determined to be positive; however, he says he has never received any vaccinations since he was a baby.
Height	5'10"	
Weight	140 LBS	
BP	98/67	
Chief Complaint	"I am coughing all the time now."	
Medical History	Serious car accident 5 years ago Smokes cigars when he can get them Used to abuse alcohol	
Current Medications	None	
Social History	Homeless for the last 5 years Past work as a taxi driver	

1. Does the patient pose a risk to healthcare personnel, and if so, what precautions could be taken?
2. What oral lesion may be present in his mouth?
3. What is the significance of the patient's positive skin test?
4. How would therapy for condition be handled?

1. Close contact and heavy exposure enhance tuberculosis (TB) transmission by respiratory droplets, so healthcare personnel are at greater risk. Limiting droplet exposure by wearing facemasks helps reduce the risk of acquiring TB. Also, using a high- to intermediate-level disinfectant against the microorganism (tuberculocidal) on surfaces that are not covered with disposables will help prevent transmission, as will other standard precautions. However, the patient should not be treated differently from other patients; standard precautions should be strictly followed for all patients. Unless it is necessary, such as with emergency care, elective dental care should wait until he is on drug therapy and no longer contagious. This includes the first 2 weeks of drug therapy or until tests are negative.
2. Common oral sign of secondary TB is a tongue ulcer with irregular border, which is a highly infectious lesion. Confirmed by biopsy and culturing, it resolves after treatment.

3. Positive TB test indicates active immunity (with T-cell lymphocytes and cell-mediated immunity [CMI]) to tubercle bacillus, *Mycobacterium tuberculosis*. Based on the symptoms and results of the other lab tests and no other past medical history of vaccination, active infection with TB is likely.
4. Therapy would consist of immediate antibiotic therapy and monitoring of compliance with drug therapy, which consists of pyrazinamide (PZA) combined with INH (Nydrazid) and rifampin (Rifadin, Rimactane). Ethambutol (Myambutol) is being added to the usual three-drug therapy regimen. Therapy requires long course (6 to 9 months) to eliminate disease; additional drugs may be added if antibiotic resistance develops. Compliance is very important for eradication of the infection but will be difficult for this patient to maintain in his present homeless situation.

Bacterial Toxins

Some bacteria may cause disease in humans because of toxic (poisonous) properties present in protein molecules (toxins), which they carry and release, producing a toxemia. Disease from toxin exposure may NOT require bacterial replication in the body, because in some cases exposure to the toxin alone is sufficient.

A. Enterohemorrhagic *Escherichia coli* infection: from toxin-producing enteric gram-negative rod, transmitted via contaminated food by fecal-oral route (food poisoning).
  1. Pathogenesis: production of toxins, which cause hemorrhagic colitis and hemolytic-uremic syndrome (HUS, with kidney failure, hemolytic anemia, thrombocytopenia); NOT usually the harmless strains that are part of normal gut flora, producing vitamin K or preventing establishment of pathogenic bacteria within intestine.
  2. Diagnosis: strain-specific immunological detection and growth in culture.
  3. Prevention: thoroughly cooking ground beef, which is MOST common source.
  4. Treatment: rapid administration of antibiotics, reconstitution of fluid and electrolyte imbalances, treatment of disseminated intravascular coagulation.
  5. Epidemiology: fatal cases may occur; children and debilitated are MOST susceptible.
B. Staphylococcal food poisoning: toxin (enterotoxin): from half of *Staphylococcus aureus* strains.
  1. Pathogenesis: toxin action on gut nerves, stimulates vomiting and diarrhea.
  2. Diagnosis: by symptoms and epidemiology, may be assayed.
  3. Prevention: complicated by normal presence of *S. aureus* on skin and mucous membranes; use of antiseptics and good personal hygiene may help control spread to food; antibiotic therapy for carriers has limited use because of emergence of drug resistance and need for long-term therapy; heating of contaminated food may be sufficient to destroy the bacteria, although toxin remains active.
  4. Treatment: symptomatic because of short incubation period (1 to 8 hours) after exposure to toxin.
C. Whooping cough (pertussis): toxin from *Bordetella pertussis,* gram-negative bacterium transmitted in respiratory droplets.
  1. Pathogenesis: colonization of ciliated cells in the respiratory mucosa, followed by production of bacterial toxins; MOST likely play a role in cell damage.
  2. Diagnosis: lab culture, demonstration of specific IgA antibodies, molecular detection of DNA.
  3. Prevention: vaccination with whole-cell vaccines, effective but occasionally toxic; LESS toxicity with acellular vaccines.
  4. Treatment: antibiotic erythromycin (Robimycin, E-Mycin, E.E.S.) reduces infectious period to 5 to 10 days but has LITTLE effect on the disease.
  5. Epidemiology:
    a. Period of highest infectivity occurs soon after infection, when levels of bacteria are highest, but remains infectious for as much as 5 weeks.
    b. In addition to paroxysmal cough, encephalopathy and bronchopneumonia occasionally develop; disease has been stemmed by vaccination in developed countries ONLY; recovery is associated with immune protection; increased numbers are due to LACK of vaccination by choice.
D. Toxic shock syndrome (TSS): toxin (TSST) from some strains of *Staphylococcus aureus;* tampon-associated disease; toxin absorbed into blood after growth of bacteria in tampon; however, any staphylococcal infection that produces enterotoxin or TSST may cause TSS.
  1. Pathogenesis: by activation of large numbers of T lymphocytes by TSST; superantigen causes release of inflammatory cytokines.
  2. Diagnosis: based on fever, shock, rash; lab detection of bacteria and/or enterotoxin; also indicated by organ system failure.
  3. Prevention: use less absorbent tampons, change more often.
  4. Treatment: antibiotics and supportive measures.
  5. Epidemiology: recognition of relationship between TSS and highly absorbent tampons has led to reduced incidence; sporadic cases continue to occur and require rapid recognition.

ORAL MICROORGANISMS

Many microorganisms are found in a healthy oral cavity. Vary according to age and location as noted in the Human Oral Micro-biome Database (HOMD).
A. Appearing soon after birth: coliform bacteria (disappear soon after), *Streptococcus, Staphylococcus, Lactobacillus, Neisseria*.
B. Appearing with tooth eruption: *Actinomyces* species (teeth-occlusal) and streptococci: *S. sanguis* (MAINLY tongue dorsum, teeth-occlusal), *S. salivarius* (MAINLY saliva, tongue dorsum), *S. mutans* (teeth—MAINLY smooth surfaces), *S. mitior* (ALL nonkeratinized tissue).
C. Dental biofilm (dental plaque): see Chapter 13, Periodontology, for complete description and discussion.

Viruses

Viruses are the smallest and simplest infectious agents. Genome consists of RNA or DNA (NOT both). Structurally, composed of protein molecules; some proteins are glycosylated or associated with lipids. Obligate intracellular parasites, requiring host cell's metabolic apparatus for reproduction. Two major groups: (1) infect prokaryotic (bacterial) cells, bacteriophages; (2) infect ONLY eukaryotic cells.
A. Composition and morphology of virions (complete infectious virus particles):

1. Nucleic acid may be single-stranded (ss) or double-stranded (ds) forms of either DNA or RNA.
2. Viral capsid: protein that surrounds nucleic acid; capsomers: capsid subunits.
3. Some viruses have an envelope that surrounds the capsid and contains lipid acquired from membrane of host cell; BOTH viral proteins and glycoproteins are embedded in the lipid envelope, serving as antigens and virulence factors.

B. Classification of viruses: increasingly based on nucleic acid sequence homology; periodically updated as molecular data become available.
   1. Traditional classification has been based on size, symmetry, type of nucleic acid, and virus-host interactions such as cellular location of replication (nucleus or cytoplasm), type of disease associated with the virus (e.g., hepatitis), tissue site from which the virus was isolated.
   2. Includes different families of viruses, classified according to criteria above; clinically IMPORTANT examples:
      a. Bacteriophages: plant viruses, animal viruses.
      b. Picornaviruses (small "RNA" viruses): polio and a common cold virus (rhinovirus).
      c. Reoviruses (dsRNA): rotavirus, which causes diarrheal illness.
      d. Orthomyxoviruses (ssRNA): influenza virus.
      e. Rhabdoviruses (ssRNA): rabies virus.
      f. Retroviruses (ssRNA): human immunodeficiency virus (HIV).
      g. Herpesviruses (dsDNA): herpes simplex virus (HSV).
      h. Hepadnaviruses (dsDNA): hepatitis B virus (HBV).

C. Replication within host cell requires several basic steps (similar to creature in the movie "Alien"):
   1. Attachment (or adsorption): virus attachment to host cell surface, mediated by interaction between viral proteins and host cell surface receptor molecules.
   2. Penetration: virus enters the cell through endocytosis or direct passage through cell membrane.
   3. Uncoating: virus disassembles and releases its nucleic acid inside cell.
   4. Multiplication: viral nucleic acid replication and production of viral proteins, as virus takes over some of the host cell biochemical machinery.
   5. Maturation of virus particles: viral nucleic acid and proteins are packaged into mature virions and released from the cell through rupture or budding of cell membranes.

D. Pathogenesis can be divided into the following categories:
   1. Harmful effects of virus replication on host cells (structural and biochemical damage).
   2. Genetic effects on the host (e.g., carcinogenesis).
   3. Induction of harmful host immune responses (immunopathology) as infected host attempts to fight the virus.

E. Detection by culture of viruses in appropriate host cells (bacterial, plant, or animal) grown in lab:
   1. Important tool for detection of viruses and determination of their concentration by virus titration.
   2. May cause microscopically visible damage and cytopathic effects.
   3. By structural analysis: electron microscopy BEST used for definitive identification of viruses.
   4. By genetic technology: allows specific identification of viral nucleic acid sequences in cells or tissues (e.g., by polymerase chain reaction [PCR], using viral-specific probes to amplify and detect viral nucleic acid).
   5. By presumptive identification of specific virus infection: determining specific host immune response that occurs during infection (e.g., determination of HIV infection by identifying HIV-specific antibodies in the blood of infected individual).

F. Antiviral therapy: see later discussion with each infectious disease discussed; generally designed to interfere with viral replication (e.g., viral-coded enzyme) and not actually destroy viral particle.

Viral Infections

The closer that an infectious agent's physiology is to ours, the MORE difficult it is to treat. Viruses, although simple, tend to be difficult to treat because they become part of our cells and take over the cells' machinery. Attacking the virus ultimately means attacking our cells, since they replicate once inside the cell. See later discussion of antivirals. **Persistent virus infection** is an infection that may involve latency or some other mechanism that promotes continuous internal infection.

• See Chapter 9, Pharmacology: specific antivirals.

A. Influenza (flu): caused by RNA virus (orthomyxovirus) transmitted by aerosols of respiratory secretions.
   1. Pathogenesis: virus replication in airway cells; inflammatory immune response contributes to tissue damage.
   2. Diagnosis: fever, malaise, headache, cough; detecting virus antigens in cells from nasopharynx.
   3. Prevention: vaccination; protects some but NOT all individuals; vaccine preparation is complicated by mutations and antigenic strains that arise.
   4. Treatment: amantadine (Symmetrel) and rimantadine (Flumadine), antivirals that hasten recovery from some cases if started early.
   5. Epidemiology: yearly epidemics (higher rate than expected) and occasional worldwide pandemics (epidemic that spreads over a specific region).

B. Polio: caused by RNA virus (picornavirus) transmitted by oral route, from virus present in water or from close contact with carriers who shed the virus in pharyngeal secretions and feces.
   1. Pathogenesis: infection of tonsils and small intestine cells, invasion of CNS, damage of nerve cells, which leads to muscle paralysis; MAINLY self-limiting infections; immunity to the same strain of virus occurs after recovery; reactivation in adult as postpolio syndrome (PPS).
   2. Diagnosis: symptoms ranging from minor to major, including paralysis; isolation of the virus or demonstration of seroconversion.
   3. Prevention: vaccination with BOTH live-attenuated and killed vaccines.
   4. Treatment: none, supportive.
   5. Epidemiology: worldwide pandemic; susceptibility of children.
C. Rubeola ("measles"): caused by RNA virus (paramyxovirus) transmitted by respiratory route; involves local infection followed by viremia and systemic spread.
   1. Pathogenesis: replication of virus in various body cells, including skin (rash), respiratory tract, conjunctiva; virus may persist for years; rarely, causes fatal brain infection.
   2. Diagnosis: Koplik spots (early-appearing red spots with blue-white centers on buccal mucosa), fever, sneezing, cough, skin rash (head and neck moving downward); virus isolation or seroconversion.
   3. Prevention: immune protection after natural infection is lifelong; vaccination with measles immunoglobulin is highly effective and passive prophylaxis.
   4. Treatment: none, supportive.
   5. Epidemiology: by age 12, MOST unvaccinated children have had measles and thus become immune; vaccination has greatly reduced the incidence in developed countries.
D. Rubella ("German measles"): caused by RNA virus (togavirus) transmitted by contact with respiratory secretions or directly to fetus.
   1. Pathogenesis: virus replication in respiratory and other body cells.
   2. Complication: congenital rubella with growth retardation; mental retardation; malformations of the heart and eyes; deafness; and liver, spleen, and bone marrow problems.
   3. Diagnosis: typical rash (starts on face, then proceeds downward) and lymphadenopathy; specifically by virus isolation and seroconversion.
   4. Prevention: protective immunity occurs after infection or vaccination; live-attenuated rubella virus vaccine NOT for use during pregnancy, must be given *before*.
   5. Treatment: none, supportive.

   6. Epidemiology: occurs sporadically in United States; vaccine has greatly reduced incidence.
E. Mumps: caused by RNA virus (paramyxovirus) transmitted by respiratory route (droplets), local virus replication, viremia, systemic dissemination.
   1. Pathogenesis: virus replication in parotid gland, testes (after puberty), ovaries, brain, kidneys, other organs.
   2. Diagnosis: malaise, MAINLY parotid (parotitis) or other salivary gland enlargement; specifically, by isolation of virus or seroconversion.
   3. Complication: orchitis, painful inflammation of testicles, possibly with sterility.
   4. Prevention: **immunization** is effective; combination vaccine for measles-mumps-rubella (MMR).
   5. Treatment: none, supportive.
   6. Epidemiology: worldwide epidemics (primarily children); vaccine use has greatly reduced incidence and complications.
F. Varicella (chickenpox) and herpes zoster (shingles): caused by varicella zoster virus (VZV).
   1. Pathogenesis:
      a. Chickenpox caused by acute infection with VZV.
      b. Shingles caused by reactivation of dormant virus in tissue of cranial nerve V (trigeminal) (SIMILAR to reactivation of herpetic gingivostomatitis and/or recurrent herpes labialis from dormant virus in nerve tissue).
      c. Chickenpox: skin lesions; oral lesions may occur; shingles: unilateral painful vesicles or ulcers on oral/genital mucosa; facial area served by ophthalmic division of trigeminal is MOST commonly affected; may be associated with immunodeficiency.
      d. Complications: in eyes can cause blindness or on skin may result in neuralgia (painful area).
   2. Prevention: vaccines for BOTH chickenpox and shingles.
   3. Treatment: supportive, possibly antivirals such as acyclovir (Zovirax).
G. (Infectious) mononucleosis ("mono", "kissing disease"): caused by Epstein-Barr virus (EBV), DNA herpes virus (HHV-4) transmitted by saliva to pharynx and/or salivary glands.
   1. Pathogenesis: 30- to 50-day incubation period, virus replicates in epithelial and B-lymphoid cells, development of enlarged lymph nodes and spleen, persistence of virus in B lymphocytes, suppression of EBV by immunity.
   2. Diagnosis: headache, malaise, fatigue, sore throat, palatal petechiae (red spots), enlarged spleen and lymph nodes; virus isolation and seroconversion.
   3. Prevention: vaccine NOT available.
   4. Treatment: none, supportive.
   5. Epidemiology: COMMON infection, establishes lifelong persistence; associated with two types of

cancers, Burkitt's lymphoma and nasopharyngeal carcinoma.

Molds and Yeasts (Fungi)

Molds and yeasts are eukaryotic cells that may reproduce either asexually or sexually. MOST are saprophytes (grow on dead organic matter), but many are parasites (grow on living material), which are pathogenic for plants and animals. Some produce potent mycotoxins or aflatoxins that may cause liver tumors. Others are responsible for such afflictions as ringworm, athlete's foot, trench mouth, and thrush. Mold and yeast isolation and culture generally employ techniques similar to those used for bacteria.

A. Molds (mycelium): grow by production of hyphae; mycelia: forming cottonlike tangled mass.
   1. Two types:
      a. Nonseptate: long, stringlike cells that do NOT contain cross-walls.
      b. Septate: similar but contain perforated cross-walls.
   2. Identification: based primarily on morphology and modes of reproduction (e.g., types of asexual and sexual spores produced).
B. Yeasts: special class of egg-shaped, elliptical, single-celled molds, larger than bacteria; do NOT produce mycelia.
   1. Reproduce asexually by cell division called budding; asexual spores are NOT produced; sexual spores (ascospores) may be produced by some upon two-cell mating.
   2. Can grow anaerobically by fermentation, with production of alcohol (ethanol) and $CO2$.
   3. Examples:
      a. *Saccharomyces:* important in bread, wine, and beer production.
      b. *Candida albicans:* agent of thrush and oral candida (see discussion below).

Fungal Infections

Metabolically versatile and grow on typical media as well as on cork, hair, paint, even polyvinyl plastics. Fungal spores are everywhere and are MAINLY responsible for contamination of bacterial cultures and media, as well as infections (there is a fungus among us).

A. Histoplasmosis: caused by *Histoplasma capsulatum* transmitted by inhalation.
   1. Pathogenesis: pulmonary infection; with intracellular growth of fungus, may disseminate to lymph nodes, liver, bone marrow, or brain, causing life-threatening infection in immunocompromised persons and infants.
   2. Diagnosis: culture from blood, sputum, bone marrow, CSF, or by biopsy and histological examination.

3. Treatment of progressive disease: antifungal amphotericin B (Fungilin, Fungizone, Fungisome, Amphocil, Amphotec); ONLY half is achieved in immunocompromised.
   4. Epidemiology: fungus resides in soil and is endemic in central United States as well as tropical world areas, transported to air and inhaled so that fungal spores may spread from alveoli to lymph nodes, resulting in disseminated disease, which may appear years after initial infection in immunocompromised hosts.
B. Candidiasis: caused by overgrowth of *Candida albicans;* however, normal flora present in oral cavity.
   1. Pathogenesis: long-term antibiotics, corticosteroid use, DM (sugar in blood), immunodeficiency (see later discussion); serious infection that can be life threatening and may occur in immunocompromised such as patients with cancer, transplant, AIDS.
   2. Types:
      a. Acute pseudomembranous candidiasis (thrush): curdlike superficial plaque easily removed, leaving raw, bleeding area of oropharyngeal region.
      b. Angular cheilitis: cracking and/or redness with labial commissures (corners of mouth); may be mixed infection with staphylococcal bacteria.
      c. Chronic hyperplastic candidiasis: MORE penetrating and enlarged tissue form.
      d. Acute atrophic candidiasis: reduced tissue form associated with antibiotic use.
      e. Chronic atrophic candidiasis: associated with full or partial dentures; flat red outline mimics denture shape.
      f. Systemic: MAINLY genital but can be involved any body tissues.
   3. Diagnosis: by symptoms, microscopic examination, culturing.
   4. Treatment: antifungal topical (e.g., nystatin [Mycostatin]), with caries risk from sugar content, and/or use of systemic drugs such as amphotericin B (Fungilin) and clotrimazole (Diflucan); correct denture care to reduce incidence of fungal infections (see Chapter 15, Dental Biomaterials).
   5. Epidemiology:
      a. Using long-term antibiotics can lead to eliminating natural competitors for resources and increase severity.
      b. Solely treating with drugs may NOT give desired results, and other underlying causes require consideration; may need to control health factors (e.g., DM, HIV), change environmental pH, hygiene, diet, other factors.

CLINICAL STUDY

Age	68 YRS
Sex	☒ Male ☐ Female
Height	5'6"
Weight	225 LBS
BP	115/95
Chief Complaint	"My upper denture still feels sore even after last week's adjustment."
Medical History	Tired and seeming to gain weight in last year but his whole family is overweight
Current Medications	None
Social History	Plumber

SCENARIO

The patient visits his dental office for an oral prophylaxis of his mandibular teeth. Intraoral examination reveals several new white patchy lesions that adhere to his buccal mucosal surfaces and erythematous mucosa underlying his upper denture. Microscopic examination of a small specimen mixed with saline and placed on a slide under low-power resolution reveals ovoid cells, some of which appear singly and some of which are budding. When the specimen is cultured in the lab where it was sent by the dentist, irregular cream-colored colonies rapidly appear. Further investigations by the patient's family physician after referral reveal a fasting blood sugar concentration of 200 mg/dL.

1. The patient is diagnosed with a fungal infection. Which of the data mentioned are important to the diagnosis? What organism is the likely cause of the infection?
2. What is the likely source of the fungal infection?
3. What is the most important factor in the patient's susceptibility to this oral infection?
4. What strategies for treating the patient would be appropriate?

1. Gross and microscopic appearance of lesion and growth in culture are consistent with oral *Candida albicans* infection. Patient's type is chronic atrophic candidiasis, which is associated with full or partial dentures and has a flat red outline mimicking denture shape. May be misdiagnosed as a denture sore from physical irritation by denture; however, it does not heal after the denture has been adjusted.
2. *C. albicans* is ubiquitous (environmental exposure is common), and likely source was endogenous (from *Candida* harbored in or on his body). *C. albicans* thus represents opportunistic pathogen and causes clinical disease during breakdown in host defenses.
3. Fasting blood glucose level of 200 mg/dL suggests diagnosis of diabetes mellitus (DM) type 2 (normal = 70 to 110 mg/dL). DM is known to increase susceptibility to some infections, including opportunistic *C. albicans*.
4. Several antifungals, both topical and systemic, including amphotericin B (Fungilin), nystatin (Mycostatin), clotrimazole (Diflucan), may be useful in helping to clear oral infection. DM must be evaluated by physician and treated by nutritional therapy through diabetic nutritional counselor and possibly appropriate drug therapy for both fungal infection and uncontrolled DM. Medical examination may want to look signs of

any systemic infections. Risk of caries from sugar in drugs (if physician is comfortable prescribing a drug with sugar for this patient), as well as correct denture care, should be discussed and then monitored by the dental staff. Annual intraoral examination would reveal recurrent or resistant oral fungal lesions in the future.

PARASITES

Parasites are eukaryotic animals that are found in two subkingdoms, protozoa and metazoa. Protozoa are unicellular organisms. Metazoa comprise all the parasites other than protozoa. Important group of the metazoa are the helminths, which are worms. Classification of parasites is based on morphology, cytoplasmic structure, locomotion, organelles, life cycles, reproduction.

A. Protozoa: unicellular but may be found in groups as colonies; range from ~10 to 200 μm in length.
 1. Nutritionally holozoic; ingest solid food particles through mouth or opening, reproduce asexually or sexually.
 2. Classified based primarily on mode of locomotion, transmitted by ingestion but sometimes by penetration of skin; cyst formation may occur (helps with transmission of parasitic forms).
 3. Protozoa classes:
  a. Mastigophora (flagellates) move by means of flagella; MAJOR pathogens include:
   (1) *Giardia lamblia:* giardiasis, intestinal infection with cramps and diarrhea; fecal-oral transmission.
   (2) *Trichomonas vaginalis:* trichomoniasis, genitourinary infection; sexually transmitted disease (STD).
   (3) *Trypanosoma gambiense:* African sleeping sickness; tsetse fly transmission.

b. Sarcodina: flexible amoebas; major pathogen is *Entamoeba histolytica,* which causes amebic dysentery and has fecal-oral or sexual transmission.

c. Sporozoa: nonmotile; major pathogens include:
   (a) *Plasmodium malariae:* malaria; transmission from mosquito to the bloodstream.
   (b) *Toxoplasma gondii:* toxoplasmosis, fatigue syndrome; transmission by cat feces or undercooked meat.

d. Ciliata (ciliates): move by means of cilia; major pathogen is *Balantidium coli,* which causes severe dysentery and has fecal-oral transmission.

B. Helminths: multicellular complex organisms; elongated and bilaterally symmetrical worms; macroscopic in size.
   1. Classes: include tapeworms, flukes, roundworms.
   2. Pathogens: *Trichinella spiralis* causes trichinosis in intestine and muscles; transmitted by ingestion of larvae in meat, especially pork.

Parasitic Infections

Medical parasitology involves study of parasitic protozoa, helminths, anthropoids.

A. *Giardia lamblia* infection: caused by protozoan found in small intestine of humans; transmission occurs by ingestion of fecally contaminated food or water that contains *Giardia* cysts; may survive for weeks or months.
   1. Pathogenesis: attachment of the parasite to wall of small bowel; occurrence of persistent infections, with weakness, abdominal pain, weight loss; however, may be asymptomatic.
   2. Diagnosis: microscopic examination of stool specimens.
   3. Prevention: personal hygiene and disinfection of water through filtration, boiling, and chlorination.
   4. Treatment: antibiotic quinacrine hydrochloride (Atabrine) and/or metronidazole (Flagyl).
   5. Epidemiology: epidemics in institutional settings and outbreaks in wilderness areas (which suggest transmission from animal sources [zoonosis]).

B. *Toxoplasma gondii* infection: caused by protozoan that infects wide range of animals, including the cat family; transmitted to humans by exposure to cat feces (which carry oocyst), by eating undercooked meat that contains tissue oocysts, or from mother to fetus (in utero).
   1. Pathogenesis: asymptomatic infection in humans; development of congenital toxoplasmosis when nonimmune mothers are infected during pregnancy.
      a. Immunosuppression, associated with toxoplasmosis.

   b. Damage to macrophages and other body cells in which *T. gondii* replicates.
   2. Diagnosis: prenatal toxoplasmosis in pregnant woman, which is associated with blindness and other defects, including neurological damage, in newborn; microscopic examination, animal inoculation, and seroconversion.
   3. Prevention: avoidance of cat feces; proper cooking of meats.
   4. Treatment: antibiotics, including sulfonamides (sulfa drugs, sulfisoxazole [Gantrisin] and trimethoprim-sulfamethoxazole [TMP-SMX, Bactrim, Septra]) and pyrimethamine (Daraprim).
   5. Epidemiology: MOST natural infections occur from eating undercooked meat containing tissue cysts or from eating food contaminated with cat feces.

Vector-Borne Infections

Many infections are transmitted from a **vector** (insect such as tick, mosquito, or flea that spreads infection). Carriers acquire an infectious agent from an infected individual or waste and pass it to a susceptible individual, either directly (e.g., bite) or indirectly (e.g., food or environment). Others than those discussed here include Lyme disease (deer tick) and West Nile (mosquitoes).

A. Malaria: tropical disease caused by mosquito-borne transmission of parasite (genus *Plasmodium*), with transmission occurring in cycle, from mosquito to human.
   1. Pathogenesis: internal growth of parasite through life cycle, resulting in chronic infection and damage to red blood cells and other body sites; those with sickle-cell disease NOT affected (reason for maintenance of disease in populations).
   2. Diagnosis: examination of stained blood specimens; hematological and liver function tests may be BEST.
   3. Prevention: avoidance of mosquito bites, eradication of mosquitoes, prophylactic use of antimalarial drugs, treatment of infected individuals; vaccines under development.
   4. Treatment: antimalarial chloroquine, drug of choice for acute attacks; resistance may occur, necessitating other drugs (suffix "-ine") for therapy or prophylaxis.
   5. Epidemiology: has been resistant to eradication in tropical areas; may be transmitted via contaminated needles, by blood transfusions, from mother to fetus (in utero).

B. Hepatitis A infection: caused by RNA virus (hepatovirus, HAV) transmitted via fecal-oral route; commonly caused by contamination of water or food, including shellfish (unlike hepatitis E).
   1. Pathogenesis: target organ is liver; causes necrosis of liver cells and inflammatory changes.

2. Diagnosis: elevated levels of liver enzymes (aminotransferase); anti-HAV antibodies.
3. Prevention: prophylaxis by administration of immunoglobulins, type of passive immunity; NO vaccine is available.
4. Treatment: none, supportive.
5. Epidemiology: common occurrence in families, institutions, camps, and armed forces; short incubation period of 15 to 45 days; onset is abrupt, with recovery by means of immune response.

CLINICAL STUDY

Scenario: The 5-year-old patient's mother, contacted by phone by the receptionist, wants to wait to schedule the child's routine dental examination. Three weeks after starting at her new daycare center because her mother just started back to work, she abruptly developed fever and general malaise of several days' duration. After obtaining some lab data, the patient's physician diagnoses hepatitis A virus infection. Her mother says, "My daughter is just not feeling well."

1. What was the likely source of the hepatitis A virus infection for the patient?
2. What lab tests would help in the diagnosis of this infection?
3. What is the likely outcome of this case for the patient? When will the patient be feeling better enough for her dental appointment?
4. Are other family members or other children at risk for this infection? If so, what might help prevent infection?

1. Transmission of hepatitis A virus (HAV) is primarily by fecal-oral route. Case history suggests likely exposure in institutional daycare setting, most likely from contaminated food or water.
2. Lab determination of elevated blood levels of aminotransferase; increases in antibodies to HAV would confirm the diagnosis.
3. Complications of HAV infection are uncommon; within a few weeks, her healthy immune system will clear infection.
4. Her family and other children are at risk for HAV infection. Because contamination occurs through fecal-oral route, handwashing and aseptic handling of foods and drink are essential. Family members may receive antibodies or immunoglobulins (Igs) as preventive or prophylactic measure, a type of passive immunity.

Infections Transmitted Sexually or by Blood and Body Fluids

A variety of microorganisms have adapted to sexual transmission, whereby protection afforded by intact skin is bypassed and exchange of body fluids that contain infectious agents or infected cells may occur. In these sexually transmitted diseases (STDs) or sexually transmitted infections (STIs), microbial exposure of fragile mucous membranes in body cavities allows direct infection of target cells near the site of exposure and also facilitates access to blood, particularly in cases of concurrent infection or trauma. Blood transfusions and sharing of contaminated needles during recreational drug injection also facilitate cross-infection between individuals.

- See Chapter 13: Periodontology: acute herpetic gingivostomatitis; 6, General and Oral Pathology: hepatitis discussion.
A. Gonorrhea: caused by *Neisseria gonorrhoeae;* sexually transmitted; infects MOSTLY mucous membranes of urethra in males or cervix in females.
   1. Pathogenesis: invasion of epithelial cells and cell damage associated with inflammatory response; dissemination to various body sites (e.g., brain, heart, joints, peritoneal cavity).
   2. Diagnosis: gram-negative diplococci, culture of oxidase-positive colonies, immunological studies (fluorescent antibody staining; agglutination), or reaction with DNA probes.
   3. Prevention: NO vaccine available; condoms are effective in preventing transmission.
   4. Treatment: cephalosporin (ceftriaxone [Rocephin] and quinolone (ciprofloxacin [Cipro]) antibiotics (quinolone resistance is becoming widespread).
   5. Epidemiology: STD or STI often acquired from asymptomatic sex partner.
B. Syphilis: caused by *Treponema pallidum;* sexually transmitted, and ALL oral lesions are highly contagious at each stage.
   1. Pathogenesis: complex; may involve almost ANY tissue in the body; three stages possible unless treated:
      a. Primary: occurs at site of entry (usually mucous membrane); characterized by oral and/or genital chancre (ulcer) that eventually heals.
      b. Secondary: follows weeks to months later by dissemination of bacteria to various tissues; results in development of new contagious lesions, which heal within several weeks after appearance because of immunological defenses; presence of oral mucous patch, painless ulcers (Figure 8-2).
      c. Tertiary: occurs years later; infection reemerges in cardiovascular system (CVS) or CNS in body tissues as gumma (soft tissue lesion) with resultant dementia and may be fatal.
   2. Diagnosis: physical symptoms, microscopic identification of spirochetes, positive serological finding (detection of antisyphilis antibodies).
   3. Oral signs in infected offspring (congenital form): Hutchinson's triad, which consists of Hutchinson's teeth (mulberry molars, with constricted or poorly developed crowns and incisors, with

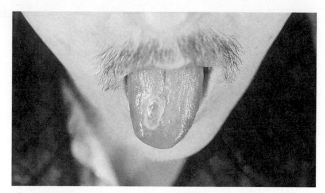

Figure 8-2 Oral mucous patch on dorsum of tongue from infection with *Treponema pallidum* with syphilis.

screwdriver or bell-shaped shaped crowns and notched incisal edge), eighth cranial nerve deafness (labyrinthine disease), interstitial keratitis.

4. Prevention: vaccines are NOT yet effective; tracing of contacts and prophylactic treatment with penicillin (Pen-Vee K); condoms are effective in preventing transmission.

5. Treatment: antibiotic penicillin (Pen-Vee K).

C. Herpes simplex infection: caused by two subtypes of DNA virus family, which are HSV type 1 (HSV-1) and HSV type 2 (HSV-2); transmitted BOTH nonsexually (primarily HSV-1) and sexually (primarily HSV-2) through breaks in the skin or direct mucosal contact with infected lesions; weeping of lesions may easily spread infection to other sites (intraoral and/or extraoral) or other persons.

1. Pathogenesis: virus-induced cell death and inflammation; two forms possible:

   a. Primary infection (acute herpetic gingivostomatitis): skin and/or oral mucous membranes; dormant virus in nerve tissues; reactivation presents as edematous, red, painful gingival tissues, with vesicles (blisters), MOST in children 6 months to 6 years.

   b. Secondary infection: reactivation from dormant nerve presents as recurrent vesicles that break to ulcer(s) ("cold sores," "fever blisters"); MOST often on lip (labialis; Figure 8-3) or perioral tissues or on fingers (whitlow); however, lesions may also be noted on keratinized oral mucosa (e.g., palate and gingiva).

   c. Reactivation from dormant virus in nerve tissue is SIMILAR to that of the pathogenesis of herpes zoster (chickenpox in childhood to herpes zoster in adulthood); reactivation triggered by tissue trauma (physical, chemical, or by excessive sunlight), as well as an immunocompromised or stressed state.

2. Diagnosis: by symptoms as noted; however, initially may be asymptomatic or may present with fever, malaise, gingival inflammation; specific virus isolation and seroconversion.

3. Treatment: antivirals acyclovir (Zovirax), valacyclovir (Valtrex), and famciclovir (Famvir).

4. Epidemiology: widespread (HSV-1 greatest incidence); LESS common: encephalitis, meningitis, neonatal herpes.

D. Human papillomavirus (HPV) infection: caused by DNA viruses that initially infect epithelial cells of skin and/or mucous membranes, transmitted by intimate contact.

1. Pathogenesis: range of clinical lesions, include oral and skin wart, plantar wart, flat wart, genital condyloma, oral and laryngeal papilloma; tumor resulting from virus infection of epithelial cells; linked with premalignant or malignant (cancer) oral and/or genital lesion(s) MAINLY in young persons and transmitted sexually.

2. Diagnosis: clinical appearance and/or viral type detection.

3. Prevention: avoidance of sexual contact effective for genital infection; vaccination (Gardasil, Cervarix) of certain populations.

4. Treatment: removal or destruction of wart lesion by cryotherapy, surgery, cone biopsy, electrosurgery (LEEP).

5. Epidemiology: majority of genital cancers are associated with types 16 and 18.

E. Hepatitis B infection: caused by DNA virus (HBV) transmitted by blood transfusion, IV drug use, sexual and/or oral, mother to fetus (in utero), occupational exposure (healthcare personnel), present in blood, saliva, semen, vaginal fluids.

1. Pathogenesis: long onset, chronic liver infection, leads to liver dysfunction and cancer.

2. Diagnosis:

   a. By symptoms; vary and include jaundice, rash, and arthritis.

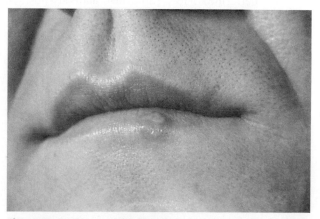

Figure 8-3 Herpes labialis lesion on lower lip from infection with herpes simplex virus (HSV-1).

b. By specific immunological tests for viral antigens and antivirus antibodies or detection of elevated blood levels of some liver enzymes.

3. Transmission in dental setting, from patient to dental professional, through:
   a. Injuries from contaminated sharps.
   b. Splatter of contaminated blood and saliva onto open oral mucosa or skin.
   c. Spread of contaminated blood to open lesions by ungloved hands or torn gloves.

4. Prevention: postexposure prophylaxis with passive injection of hepatitis B immune globulin (HBIG) without seroconversion after vaccination; Recombivax is currently used HBsAg, derived from yeast cells; avoidance of exposure to body fluids; HBV vaccination.

5. Treatment: none, supportive; specific therapy NOT available.

6. Epidemiology: MOST recover completely; 5% to 10% become chronic carriers with higher risk for liver cancer.

F. Hepatitis C infection: caused by RNA virus (HCV) transmitted like HBV, by blood transfusion, IV drug abuse, mother to fetus (in utero), sexual or oral, occupational exposure (healthcare personnel); present in blood, saliva, semen, vaginal fluids.

1. Pathogenesis: little is known; replicates over time, causing mild disease in ~10% of recipients.

2. Diagnosis: viral nucleic acid, using virus-specific cDNA probe and seroconversion.

3. Transmission in dental setting: SAME as HBV.

4. Prevention: NO vaccine.

5. Treatment: antiviral interferon (INF)-alpha and ribavirin; type of natural protein (cytokine) produced by immune system can be used to inhibit viral replication in infected cells.

6. Epidemiology:
   a. MOST common cause of transfusion-associated hepatitis; blood donor screening currently performed to eliminate antibody-positive donors.
   b. Over 75% of infected persons become chronically infected carriers.
   c. Chronic active hepatitis develops in ~50%; can progress to cirrhosis and liver cancer.

G. AIDS: caused by HIV retrovirus (contains reverse transcriptase, which mediates transcription of viral RNA into DNA); various strains exist; MOST AIDS patients in North America are HIV-1 infected, with transmission occurring via sexual contact from contaminated body fluids, by IV from contaminated needles or surgical implements that penetrate skin, or from mother to fetus (in utero).

1. Pathogenesis: HIV replication in CD4+ T cells, macrophages, and other body cells.

   a. Prolonged asymptomatic incubation period (~10 years average) for MOST HIV-infected people, during which the immune system becomes progressively impaired from reduction in CD4+ cells, leading to neurological and physical symptoms.
   b. Development of AIDS-defining infections and/or cancer follows, resulting in death if untreated, generally within few years.
   c. Early-stage symptoms: weight loss (wasting), fever, diarrhea, generalized lymphadenopathy (enlarged lymph nodes), night sweats, nausea; later stages: encephalopathy, dementia, neoplasia, opportunistic infections, gastrointestinal (GIT) disorders.

2. Oral signs:
   a. Persistent generalized lymphadenopathy (PGL), angular cheilitis, dental erosion from frequent vomiting (side effect of AZT use), xerostomia (drug induced), caries, bleeding.
   b. Hairy leukoplakia: opportunistic infection with Epstein-Barr virus (EBV), DNA herpes virus, presenting as bilateral white patch on lateral tongue with corrugated or "hairy" appearance (Figure 8-4); NO treatment needed unless for esthetic purposes (acyclovir).
   c. Other opportunistic infections (especially with LOW CD4+ lymphocyte counts): candidal, severe and recurrent aphthous and/or herpetic infections, severe and chronic gingival and aggressive periodontal infections (with linear gingival erythema [LGE] of the marginal tissues), oral warts.
   d. Kaposi's sarcoma (see Chapter 6, General and Oral Pathology, and Figure 13-2).

3. Risk factors: vomiting and xerostomia from infection and/or drug use and risk of infection.

4. Diagnosis:
   a. Case-defining infections (e.g., cytomegalovirus [CMV], *Pneumocystis carinii,* candidiasis,

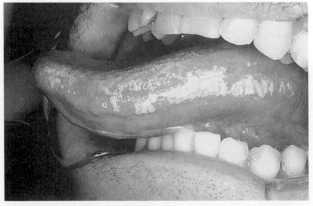

Figure 8-4 Hairy leukoplakia on the lateral tongue from opportunistic infection from Epstein-Barr (EBR) virus in person with HIV infection and AIDS diagnosis.

histoplasmosis, TB, toxoplasmosis, cryptococcosis); one or more opportunistic infections.
  b. Presence of HIV RNA in blood and reduced blood CD4+ cells; positive **enzyme-linked immunosorbent assay** (ELISA) screen for anti-HIV antibodies in blood (i.e., seroconversion).
  c. Confirmation of anti-HIV antibodies in blood by **immunoblot** (MORE specific antibody test), history of exposure; acute disease occurs 2 to 4 weeks after infection and is characterized by fever, adenopathy, pharyngitis, rash.
5. Prevention:
  a. Avoidance of contact with blood and other body fluids (tears, saliva, semen, vaginal secretions, amniotic fluid, urine, cerebrospinal fluid) of HIV-infected individuals; screening of blood used for transfusion.
  b. Virus is easily killed outside the body (MORE easily than HBV or *Mycobacterium tuberculosis*).
6. Treatment of HIV infection:
  a. Frequent assays of HIV RNA level in blood and determination of blood CD4+ cell counts.
  b. Highly active antiretroviral therapy (HAART), type of combination therapy, includes reverse transcriptase inhibitors, such as AZT, D4T, ddI, or ddC, and one or more viral protease inhibitors; extends length of disease-free period of infection by suppressing viral replication and encouraging blood CD4+ count increases.
7. Barriers to care:
  a. Lack of communication: patient may be afraid to provide accurate or thorough medical information; attitudes and fears of dental professionals may interfere with communication.
  b. Transportation problems, if debilitated.
  c. Economic difficulties because of the high costs of drugs, medical visits, and hospitalizations; also may be caused by loss of employment.
8. Professional care and homecare:
  a. <u>Medical consult</u> regarding blood counts and risk of bleeding; know blood CD4+ cell counts and current INR, if needed.
  b. Careful orofacial examination for signs of infection and focus on maintenance of oral health.
  c. Frequent professional oral prophylaxis and dental examination to reduce opportunity for secondary (opportunistic) infections.
  d. Avoiding creation of aerosols during instrumentation (especially with sonics and ultrasonics).
  e. Diet counseling, if xerostomia and vomiting occur, should emphasize adequate nutrition with noncariogenic foods to reduce caries risk.
  f. Tobacco cessation counseling, as needed, to reduce periodontal disease risk.
  g. Treating patient and caregivers with respect, kindness, compassion.
9. Patient or caregiver education:
  a. Meticulous, frequent daily homecare, including flossing and brushing; self-care may be impossible during later stages of disease.
  b. Prevention of dental disease to promote oral and systemic health.
  c. Use of daily chlorhexidine mouthrinse and systemic antibiotics if severe gingivitis or periodontitis is present.
10. Epidemiology:
  a. Worldwide epidemic; highest transmission groups in North America include homosexual males and IV drug users who share needles; in Africa greatest risk is via heterosexual transmission.
  b. Fatality rate is high; more than half are due to immunodepressed state.
H. Cytomegalovirus (CMV) infection: caused by DNA herpes virus transmitted by sexual contact and close oral and respiratory contact (saliva and urine shedding).
  1. Pathogenesis: subclinical, 4- to 8-week incubation period, followed by infectious mononucleosis–like syndrome.
    a. Involves congenital and perinatal infections, may result in severe fetal and newborn infections.
    b. Causes severe infection in immunosuppressed hosts, such as transplant recipients, patients with AIDS or cancer.
  2. Diagnosis: malaise, myalgia, fever, lymphocytosis, atypical lymphocytes; virus isolation and seroconversion.
  3. Prevention: unavailable.
  4. Treatment of CMV retinitis: ganciclovir (Cytovene) and foscarnet (Foscavir), Cidofovir (Vistide), Valganciclovir (Valcyte).
  5. Epidemiology: prevalence, determined by antibody (demonstration of immune response to infection), is ~50% to 100%; latent infection is lifelong, with intermittent shedding.

CLINICAL STUDY

Age	69 YRS	SCENARIO
Sex	☒ Male ☐ Female	During an extraoral examination of a patient of record in the dental office, a cluster of blisters in noted on lower lip; lymphadenopathy is also noted.
Height	6'4"	
Weight	225 LBS	
BP	115/95	
Chief Complaint	"I had a slight fever a few days ago and my lower lip felt odd."	
Medical History	Prostate cancer in remission after 10 years Cataract surgery 5 years ago	
Current Medications	None	
Social History	Semiretired with landscaping business	

1. What are the most likely diagnosis and cause of the patient's condition?
2. What common signs of inflammation are associated with the condition? Is this an acute or chronic inflammation?
3. Identify the major functions of inflammation. During the healing process of the patient's condition, are tissues restored by regeneration or by repair?
4. What other locations might exhibit the condition? How long does this condition last?
5. Are prodromal conditions present? Are they signs or symptoms of the condition? Was the patient's job a factor in this condition?

1. In recurrent herpes simplex (herpes labialis, "cold sore," "fever blister"), etiological agent (cause) is herpes simplex virus (HSV). Virus exists in a latent or quiescent state in trigeminal ganglion, and infection follows stimulus.
2. Common signs of inflammation include fever, pain, swelling. Functioning of lip is often limited because of discomfort. These are signs (not symptoms) because they are objective evidence of disease that can be discerned by clinician or patient. Acute inflammation that is immediate response to viral attack and results in redness, vesicle formation (increased vessel permeability), movement of leukocytes to the area (mainly neutrophils).
3. Major functions of inflammation are neutralization or destruction of injurious agent, cleansing of necrotic debris, initiation of repair and regeneration. During healing process, most epithelial tissues are restored by regeneration.
4. Herpes labialis occurs on vermilion border of lips; however, recurrent herpes may occur on keratinized masticatory mucosa, such as hard palate and gingival tissues. In contrast, aphthous ulcers (canker sores)

appear on nonkeratinized lining mucosa. Herpetic condition lasts for 1 to 2 weeks.
5. Prodromal conditions, such as pain, burning, or tingling, occur before vesicle development; these are symptoms of the condition, since they are subjective information about disease by patient. Landscaping job is a factor for condition because excessive exposure to sunlight is one of several stimuli known to trigger viral activity.

IMMUNOLOGY

Immunology is controlled by the immune system, which protects the body from both harmful infections and the development of some tumors. Bone marrow stem cells generate the immune cells on a continuous basis throughout life. Body produces BOTH specific and nonspecific immune factors. Thus either immunosuppression or immunodeficiency predisposes the individual to infections and some types of cancers.

• See CD-ROM for Chapter Terms and WebLinks.

Antigens

Antigens (immunogens) are molecules that are recognized as foreign and potentially harmful by the immune system. Present on all invading microorganisms; are constituents of bacterial toxins; are targets for specific protective immune reactions.

Lymphocytes

Lymphocytes are the KEY antigen-specific cells of the immune system. Antigen receptors on their surface recognize the presence of foreign microbial invaders, which triggers their responses. Produce antigen-specific molecules that focus immune responses on foreign microorganisms that have entered the body. Help activate antigen-nonspecific inflammatory responses produced by macrophages, neutrophils (polymorphonuclear leukocytes [PMNs]), and other cells. Combined immune responses neutralize or destroy agents of pathogenic infections, as well as some tumors. All cells of immune system originate from bone marrow stem cells.

- See Chapter 3, Anatomy, Biochemistry, and Physiology: white blood cells.

A. Lymphoid tissue and cell interactions:

1. **B lymphocytes** are highly dependent on bone marrow because much of their maturation occurs there (Figure 8-5).
2. **T lymphocytes** mature in the thymus.
3. B and T lymphocytes migrate to secondary lymphoid tissue (e.g., lymph node, spleen).
   a. Secondary lymphoid tissues are sites of interaction with trapped antigen, also considered sites of initiation of immune responses (Figure 8-6).
   b. Accessory cells (e.g., macrophages, dendritic cells) present antigen to lymphocytes, thereby facilitating immune responsiveness.
4. Three functional types of lymphocytes:
   a. B cells produce antibodies (**immunoglobulins, class of blood proteins that contains antibodies**) from subpopulation of plasma cells.
      (1) An immunoglobulin (Ig) or **antibody** chemically binds to specific antigenic determinants known as epitopes.
      (2) Humoral immunity is mediated by antibodies:
         (a) IgG: major blood antibody; crosses placenta to protect newborn.
         (b) IgA: protects mucosal sites (e.g., gastrointestinal and genitourinary tracts); present in tears, saliva, breast milk (secretory type), or blood (serum type).
         (c) IgM: first antibody produced during immune response.

(d) IgE: attacks parasites and harms MOSTLY by causing allergies.
(e) IgD: participates in immune regulation.
(3) Antibodies may bind to surface of microbes and thereby trigger:
   (a) Neutralization.
   (b) Destruction by way of complement activation or phagocytosis by macrophages and PMNs.
   b. T cells specifically recognize microbial antigens and carry out cell-mediated immunity (CMI).
      (1) T cells are also involved in:
         (a) Helping B cells respond by secreting cytokines (regulatory protein molecules), which stimulate B cells.
         (b) Killing virus-infected cells by recognizing the presence of viral antigen on the surface of the infected target cells; kill tumor cells by a similar mechanism.
         (c) Stimulating phagocytosis of microbes by macrophages and PMNs through release of activating cytokines.
   c. NK cells (natural killer cells) mature also in the bone marrow; large cells that are involved in first line of nonspecific host defense; kill tumor or virally infected cells and thus are NOT considered part of the immune response.

Development of Immunity

Immune responses occur when antigens are recognized by lymphocytes. Primary immunity describes the first contact with an antigen; may occur by natural infection or by vaccination; takes time (varies, several days to weeks) for immunity to develop after primary immunization. Secondary immunity is the subsequent rapid, highly vigorous immune response to a second contact with the same antigen, by way of reexposure or booster vaccination.

Vaccination

Vaccination (active immunization) is exposure to antigens in a manner designed to stimulate protective immunity. See later discussion of required or suggested vaccinations for dental personnel.

A. Killed vaccines: heat- or chemical-treated microorganisms or toxins; safe but in some cases may be LESS effective than live-attenuated vaccines.
B. Live-attenuated vaccines: genetically altered microorganisms that have lost virulence but still undergo limited replication.
C. Molecular vaccines: composed of critical antigenic determinants, derived as recombinant (from cloned bacteria or yeast) or synthetic peptides; **adjuvants** may be used to stimulate immune responses (types I and III—see later discussion).

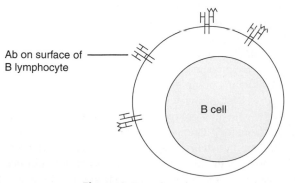

Antigenic determinant (epitope)

Ab on surface of B lymphocyte

B cell

Figure 8-5 B lymphocyte.

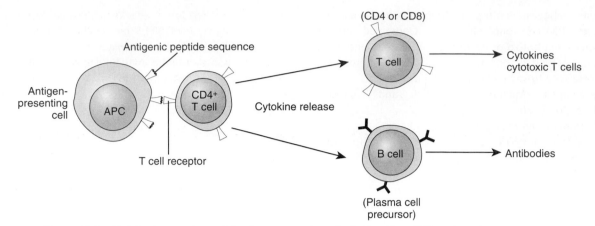

Figure 8-6 Cellular interactions of the immune system, including B and T lymphocytes.

Passive Immunization

Passive immunization is the transfer of protective antibodies (immunoglobulins) into individual. Protection is immediately established but MAINLY short lived because of antibody catabolism. A common form of postexposure prophylaxis after possible exposure to infection (e.g., hepatitis viruses A/B, HBIG) or toxin (e.g., snakebite). Also occurs naturally during pregnancy, when maternal antibodies are transported into fetus, and during nursing, when breast milk antibodies are ingested.

Allergies

Allergies (hypersensitivities) are immune reactions with pathological inflammatory side effects.
• See Chapter 10, Medical and Dental Emergencies: allergic emergencies in a dental setting.
A. Types of hypersensitivity reaction based on cells involved:
1. Type 1: IgE-mediated humoral reaction induces basophils and mast cells to release chemical mediators of inflammation (includes histamine).
   a. Asthma and hay fever are common.
   b. Anaphylaxis is an emergency that requires immediate treatment with epinephrine; drugs (e.g., penicillin, Pen-Vee K) and stings and bites may cause anaphylaxis.
   c. Rubber latex allergy:
      (1) Increasing incidence; may occur in anyone, but at-risk groups include healthcare personnel (including dental healthcare personnel [DHCP]) and other people who work with rubber latex; MORE women than men.
      (2) Contact with hospital gloves, catheters, tourniquets, dental dams, balloons, baby bottle nipples, condoms, or other rubber latex items may sensitize individual to rubber latex molecules.

(3) Powdered rubber latex gloves may facilitate inhalation of rubber latex molecules bound to cornstarch powder, which become airborne, setting stage for an allergic (hypersensitivity) response to inhaled rubber latex molecules; occasionally, severe or life-threatening hypersensitivity reactions occur and require emergency medical treatment (use of epinephrine or other drugs).
(4) DHCP should be familiar with the signs and symptoms of rubber latex sensitivity; DHCP exhibiting symptoms of this type of rubber latex allergy need medical consult because further exposure could result in a serious allergic reaction.
(5) Procedures should be in place for minimizing rubber latex–related health problems among DHCP and patients while protecting them from infectious materials; should include reducing exposures to rubber latex–containing materials by using appropriate work practices, training and educating DHCP, monitoring symptoms, and substituting other products without rubber latex where appropriate.
2. Type II and III: IgG antibodies involved in humoral reactions:
   a. By attaching to cell surface antigens and activating complement to injure or kill cells.
   b. By forming circulating immune complexes, which lodge in capillaries to then incite inflammatory damage.
3. Type IV **(delayed-type hypersensitivity):** T cells release inflammatory cytokines, which stimulate tissue damage as seen in cell-mediated reactions in tuberculosis (also BOTH TB skin test and TB

vaccine) and transplant rejection; includes allergy to nickel in restorations.

B. Treatment of allergies:
1. Drugs that suppress inflammation.
   a. Antihistamines.
   b. Corticosteroids.

2. Avoidance of allergen (e.g., food allergy such as peanuts, use other products that do not contain rubber latex in dental setting).
3. Desensitization: exposure to allergen by a different route, which alters immune response (e.g., modulating from IgE to IgG) such as by use of allergy injections.

CLINICAL STUDY

Age	27 YRS		**SCENARIO**
Sex	☒ Male ☐ Female		The patient has returned from his travels late for his 6-month recall appointment. Because he has not had dental radiographs taken during the past 18 months, four bitewing radiographs are taken. Upon returning from discussing the radiographs with the supervising dentist, the dental hygienist observes that the patient's lips appear swollen and he complains that he is having difficulty breathing. His breathing appears labored and is noisy (wheezing).
Height	6'2"		
Weight	205 LBS		
BP	116/67		
Chief Complaint	"I don't want to wear dentures like my dad."		
Medical History	Allergy to milk, eggs, bee stings, pollen Carries EpiPen (self-administered epinephrine)		
Current Medications	cetirizine (Zyrtec) 10 mg qd		
Social History	Semipro golfer		

1. What is the most likely cause of the patient's symptoms?
2. What should be done immediately?
3. What office preparations are necessary to ensure that the patient does not have the same experience during his next dental appointment?
4. DHCP can also have this response. What precautions can minimize the risk its development?

1. The patient appears to be having anaphylactic reaction. Swelling of lips indicates that he has had contact with an allergen, since he has a strong allergenic history. Because rubber latex is a common allergen, exposure to powders on rubber latex gloves is a likely cause of this response.
2. Activate dental office emergency plan. Inform the supervising dentist, activate emergency medical service (EMS) system, and provide oxygen if necessary. Supervising dentist must determine whether appropriate drugs from the emergency kit should be administered. Patient may self-administer epinephrine with use of the EpiPen; recommended to also have in kit.
3. DHCP must identify all rubber latex–containing instruments, equipment, and protective devices (anything that contacts patient) before seeing this patient again. DHCP should order replacement devices that do not contain rubber latex to ensure safe care for all their patients. Many dental settings are becoming rubber latex free.

4. Use of powder-free, hypoallergenic gloves helps to prevent rubber latex allergies. Residual rubber latex proteins are the allergens responsible for the rubber latex allergic response. These proteins bind to powder used to facilitate glove application and are then transmitted to the wearer. Hypoallergenic gloves are specially treated to remove most of residual rubber latex proteins responsible for allergic response. DHCP must wash hands after wearing any rubber latex gloves. Oil-based lotions (e.g., petroleum, mineral oil, lanolin, coconut oil) should not be worn because these oils break down glove barrier and cause release of more allergens, as do same lubricants on lips.

Autoimmunity

Autoimmunity occurs when an individual's immune system develops a breakdown in the normal control mechanisms that prevent immune reactions against "self"-antigens. Spectrum of autoimmunity ranges from mild, transient responses to potentially fatal responses. May be organ specific (e.g., directed against a particular endocrine gland, such as the thyroid) or more generalized (e.g., directed against DNA). May be successfully treated with immunosuppressive and/or antiinflammatory drugs such as corticosteroids or aspirin.
- See Chapter 6, General and Oral Pathology: autoimmune disorders.

A. Body is self-tolerant:
1. When lymphocytes that are reactive for self-antigens develop in the body, they are automatically eliminated, which provides protection from internal immune attack.
2. If mechanisms that normally eliminate self-reactive lymphocytes break down, surviving self-reactive lymphocytes may lead to autoimmune disease (i.e., clinically apparent immune reaction to self-antigen).
3. Reasons for breakdown in self-tolerance are NOT clear; some autoimmune disease may have a genetic basis because the major histocompatibility complex (MHC, gene locus present in all mammals that codes for immunologically important cell surface proteins; this protein class is human leukocyte antigen [HLA] in humans) governs immune recognition and regulation; viral or bacterial infection may trigger some autoimmune diseases.

B. Examples:
1. Hashimoto thyroiditis: hypothyroidism with antithyroid autoantibodies.
2. Type 1 diabetes mellitus (DM): autoantibodies against pancreatic insulin-producing beta cells.
3. Multiple sclerosis (MS): etiology unknown, but autoimmune responses are caused by demyelination of CNS.
4. Myasthenia gravis (MG): muscle weakness with autoantibodies that disrupt nerve connections to muscle.
5. Rheumatoid arthritis (RA): etiology unknown, but has autoantibodies against antibodies ("rheumatoid factors").
6. Systemic lupus erythematosus (SLE): anti-DNA antibodies are present.
7. Sjögren's syndrome: affects salivary and lacrimal glands, resulting in a combination of dry mouth and dry eyes.

Immunodeficiencies

Immunodeficiency is a breaksown of one or more immune system components; leads to NOT being able to fend off infection or cancer. Severity varies: may NOT be clinically apparent (detected ONLY by lab test), may be mild and treatable with drugs, or may be severe enough to cause death as noted with some more uncommon types (Table 8-2).
A. Severity is often related to the location of the cellular defect:
1. Failure of lymphocyte stem cells to develop properly leads to a wide-ranging immunodeficiency.
2. Defect late in the developmental pathway of lymphocytes may lead to a selective immunodeficiency (e.g., the inability to produce ONLY a single immunoglobulin isotype, such as IgA).

Table 8-2 Immunodeficiency types and clinical associations

Name or type	Clinical associations
Selective IgA deficiency	Mild to severe infections at mucosal sites (respiratory, gastrointestinal, genitourinary) because of low levels of IgA
X-linked hypogammaglobulinemia	Reduced levels of circulating antibodies (immunoglobulins) leading to chronic bacterial infections
DiGeorge syndrome	Absence of the thymus leading to T-lymphocyte deficiency, viral infections, and increased susceptibility to some cancers
Severe combined immunodeficiency (SCID)	Absence of functional T and B lymphocytes is potentially fatal

3. May involve any of the molecules, cells, tissues, or organs that constitute the complex immune defenses, including B and T lymphocytes, phagocytic cells, complement molecules.
   a. Primary: intrinsic (genetic) defects in immunity; caused by inheritance or mutation:
      (1) Severe combined immunodeficiencies (NO functional B or T lymphocytes).
      (2) Variety of disorders linked to the X chromosome (generally B-cell disorders).
   b. Secondary: result of an insult to the immune system:
      (1) Malnutrition.
      (2) Trauma from burns or toxin exposure.
      (3) Virus infection (e.g., HIV with AIDS).
      (4) Long-term antibiotic or immunosuppressant therapy.
      (5) Radiation and chemotherapy.
B. Complications:
1. Opportunistic infection: infection with microbes of normally low virulence that usually do NOT cause pathological changes, such as actinomycosis, MRSA, candidiasis (see earlier discussions).
2. Reactivated infection: previous exposure does NOT stimulate lifelong protective immunity, such as HBV.
3. Incidence of some cancers is higher.
C. Treatment: immunotherapy:
1. Passive administration of pooled Igs (also used for prophylaxis for some viruses after contamination, such as hepatitis A or B [HBIG after needlestick injury]).

2. Transplantation of human stem cells (e.g., from bone marrow or other sources), used with severe combined immunodeficiency (SCID).
3. Immune stimulators (e.g., cytokines) (also treat some cancers).
4. **Immunosuppression,** drugs or antibodies directed against immune cells (may also treat autoimmunity or graft rejection).

MICROORGANISM CONTROL BY ANTIBIOTICS AND OTHER CHEMOTHERAPEUTIC AGENTS

Antibiotic is a natural chemotherapeutic compound that is produced by a bacterium or mold (may also be synthetically produced), inhibits growth of or even kills bacteria or molds, and may be taken internally or used topically. Similarly, antimetabolites are involved against bacteria's normal functions and antifungals inhibit or destroy fungal growth. In contrast, antivirals do not kill the virus but interfere with viral replication so that the virus cannot continue to reproduce to the level at which normal cellular functions are disabled.

- See Chapter 19, Pharmacology: specific chemotherapeutic agents.

A. Antibiotics:
1. Ideal antibiotic:
   a. Broad spectrum; has ability to inhibit wide range of microorganisms.
   b. Prevents development and spread of organisms resistant to antibiotic.
   c. Selective for pathogenic organism and NOT detrimental to human host (e.g., does NOT cause allergy or toxicity).
   d. Does NOT eliminate the normal flora of the human host.
   e. Has NOT been found.
2. Antibiotics that act by inhibiting cell wall biosynthesis:
   a. Includes IMPORTANT group of agents because bacteria possess peptidoglycan but eukaryotic (human) cells do NOT; without a complete peptidoglycan, bacterial growth will stop or cells will lyse.
   b. Inhibitors of earlier stages of peptidoglycan biosynthesis: cycloserine, vancomycin, ristocetin, bacitracin.
   c. Beta-lactam antibiotics inhibit peptidoglycan cross-linking, last stage of peptidoglycan biosynthesis: active site of all of these antibiotics is the lactam ring, internal amide bond; effective primarily on gram-positive bacteria:
      (1) Penicillin (Pen-Vee K):
         (a) FIRST antibiotic discovered; can be rendered ineffective by penicillinase, enzyme produced by resistant bacteria that opens lactam ring on penicillin molecule.
         (b) Can cause serious allergy (including anaphylaxis); original molecule was chemically modified in attempt to overcome resistance and allergy problems, resulting in derivatives such as ampicillin (Polycillin), methicillin (Staphcillin), cloxacillin (Tegopen, Cloxapen), dicloxacillin (Dynapen, Pathocil).
         (c) Ampicillin (Polycillin) is used for <u>antibiotic premedication</u> for infective endocarditis (IE) if NO history of allergy.
      (2) Cephalosporins, monobactams, carbapenems:
         (a) Other classes of lactam antibiotics; some have broader spectrum.
         (b) Cephalosporins: cephalexin (Keflex), ceftriaxone (Rocephin), cefazolin (Ancef), cefadroxil (Duricef), cefaclor (Ceclor), cefuroxime (Ceftin).
         (c) Cephalexin (Keflex), ceftriaxone (Rocephin), or cefazolin (Ancef) is used as <u>antibiotic premedication</u> for infective endocarditis (IE) in individuals who are allergic to penicillin (Pen-Vee K).
3. Antibiotics that act on cell membranes:
   a. Agents are few in numbers because bacterial and eukaryotic membranes are very similar, which makes targeting cell membrane difficult.
   b. Include topically applied agents:
      (1) Polyene antibiotics:
         (a) Molecules that contain many double bonds; complex with sterols in the membrane, causing disruption.
         (b) BEST for fungal infections because bacteria do NOT contain sterols in the membrane.
         (c) Include amphotericin B (Fungilin) and nystatin (Mycostatin).
      (2) Polymyxins (polymyxin B):
         (a) Small polypeptides that disrupt membranes by a detergent-like action.
         (b) MOST often combined with other agents to provide broad-spectrum antibiotics.
         (c) BEST for stopping infection with severe burns; highly neurotoxic and nephrotoxic, very poorly absorbed from GIT.
4. Antibiotics that act on DNA synthesis; inhibitors of DNA gyrase:
   a. Toxic to BOTH bacteria and the human host because of the universal structure of DNA and its biosynthesis; bacteria do differ from eukaryotes in that the DNA is circular and the enzyme DNA gyrase is required for supercoiling and DNA stability.

b. Include nalidixic acid, basis for class called quinolones and novobiocin.

5. Antibiotics that act on protein synthesis:
   a. Inhibits bacteria at the level of protein synthesis.
   b. Antibiotic action involving transcription:
      (1) Bacteria and eukaryotic cells differ in structure of their ribosomal RNA; bacteria possess 70S ribosomes made up of 30S and 50S subunits and eukaryotes possess 80S ribosomes made up of 40S and 60S subunits.
      (2) Prolonged use of these antibiotics may have detrimental side effects because mitochondria of eukaryotic cells possess 70S ribosomes.
      (3) Inhibitor, so few clinically useful antibiotics are produced because of universal nature of the transcription process.
         (a) Rifampin (Rifadin, Rimactane) inhibits initiation of mRNA synthesis by inhibiting RNA polymerase; primary agent when combined with others in therapy for mycobacterial (TB) infections.
   c. Antibiotic action involving translation:
      (1) Binding to 30S ribosome:
         (a) Aminoglycosides (e.g., streptomycin, neomycin [Mycifradin], kanamycin [Kantrex], gentamicin [Garamycin], tobramycin) contain unusual amino sugars in their structures and are bactericidal because they bind irreversibly to the 30S ribosomal subunit.
         (b) Tetracyclines (e.g., tetracycline [Achromycin, Sumycin], doxycycline [Vibramycin], minocycline [Minocin]) are broad-spectrum antibiotics that contain a series of cyclohexyl rings in their structure and are bacteriostatic because of binding reversibly to 30S ribosomal subunit.
      (2) Binding to 50S ribosome: inhibits by blocking transpeptidation or translocation; generally are bacteriostatic.
         (a) Chloramphenicol, quite toxic; reserved for typhoid fever and infectious agents that are resistant to LESS toxic antibiotics.
         (b) Macrolides (e.g., erythromycin [Robimycin, E-mycin, E.E.S.], clarithromycin [Biaxin], azithromycin [Zithromax]) are effective on gram-positive bacteria and antibiotic of choice for mycoplasmal infections and Legionnaire's disease; azithromycin (Zithromax) and

clarithromycin (Biaxin) are used for antibiotic premedication for infective endocarditis (IE).
         (c) Clindamycin (Cleocin), spectrum similar to the macrolides; used in dental medicine as substitute for penicillin (Pen-Vee K) and for *Bacteroides* infections; used for antibiotic premedication for infective endocarditis (IE); however, may cause pseudomembranous colitis.

6. Reasons for *judicious* (careful) use of antibiotics:
   a. Have potentially harmful side effects (e.g., allergy, liver damage, bone deposition, nerve damage).
   b. Viruses are NOT affected by antibiotics.
   c. Indiscriminate use of antibiotics and unnecessary placement into the environment ultimately select for organisms that become increasingly resistant to the antibiotic, thereby reducing usefulness (see later dicussion).

B. Antimetabolites: are NOT strictly considered antibiotics but are chemically derived chemotherapeutics that stereochemically resemble metabolic intermediates that block important biosynthetic pathways in bacteria.
   1. Sulfonamides (sulfa drugs, sulfisoxazole [Gantrisin] and trimethoprim [combined SMX-TMP: Bactrim, Septra]), which resemble paraaminobenzoic acid (PABA); intermediate; reversibly block (bacteriostatic) folic acid biosynthesis in bacteria; highly allergenic.
   2. Isoniazid (INH): stereochemically resembles niacin and nicotinamide; appears to block synthesis of these two coenzymes; used in treatment of TB with other drugs.

C. Antifungals and antivirals: see Chapter 19, Pharmacology, for more discussion.

D. Chemotherapeutic drug resistance:
   1. Mechanisms for antibiotic resistance:
      a. Enzymatic inactivation (e.g., penicillinase).
      b. Modification of the agent's binding site.
      c. Decreased cell permeability or loss of ability to transport the agent into the cell.
      d. Overproduction of biosynthetic intermediates that are inhibited by the agent.
   2. Origins of antibiotic resistance:
      a. Random natural genetic mutations followed by selection.
      b. Gene transfer: multiple antibiotic resistance genes are carried on plasmids, which may be transferred from an antibiotic resistant donor bacterium to antibiotic sensitive bacterium, rendering recipient immediately resistant to antibiotics.
   3. Increasing antiviral and antifungal agent resistance is also occurring (CDC monitors changing influenza viruses).

CONTROL OF MICROORGANISMS BY CHEMICAL AND PHYSICAL AGENTS

Microbial growth is controlled by the use of both chemical and physical agents. Agents range from those that inhibit or slow growth to those that kill microorganisms.

Infection Control Agents

Effectiveness of these agents depends on a number of factors.

- See Chapter 12, Instrumentation: instrument processing and sterilization, biological monitoring.
A. Effectiveness of controlling agents is modified by:
   1. Number of microorganisms present.
   2. Concentration of the agent.
   3. Temperature during treatment.
   4. Duration of exposure to the agent.
   5. Environment (e.g., microorganisms trapped in pus or dried blood).
B. Cell death by chemical or physical agents:
   1. Does NOT occur instantly or simultaneously for members of a microbial population; usually exponential; may take an extended time to eliminate the last remaining cell or endospore.
   2. Resisted MOST by endospores.
C. Physical agents and effects:
   1. Moist heat:
      a. **Pasteurization:** process of disinfection applied to dairy products, wines, beers.
         (1) Items are heated to temperature high enough to kill only known pathogenic organisms that might be present.
         (2) Milk, for example, is pasteurized when heated at 65° C for 30 minutes, eliminates possible presence of *Mycobacterium tuberculosis* (agent of TB), *Brucella abortus* (agent of abortion), and *Coxiella burnetii* (agent of Q-fever); all can be transmitted through milk.
         (3) Many bacteria survive pasteurization, which is why milk eventually sours.
      b. Autoclaving: process of sterilization that uses steam under pressure.
      c. Dry heat: process of sterilization that uses electric dry air oven.
   2. Cold temperatures:
      a. Refrigeration ONLY slows microbial growth and metabolism.
      b. Freezing stops microbial growth and kills some but NOT all cells of a microbial population; deep freezing at -70° C is also the BEST means of preserving many microbial cultures.
   3. Ionizing radiation (gamma rays):
      a. Penetrates cells, can react with macromolecules, but reacts primarily with water molecules in the cell; when hit by a gamma ray, water molecule is converted into hydroxyl radical ($\cdot$OH) and hydride radical ($\cdot$H), which are potent oxidizing and reducing agents, respectively.
      b. BEST for sterilizing many items that would be destroyed by high temperatures, such as plastic Petri dishes, sutures, prosthetic devices, brachioscopes.
   4. Ultraviolet (UV) light:
      a. Absorbed by thymine molecules present in the DNA of the cell; subsequently forms thymine dimers that inhibit DNA replication.
      b. NO effect on bacterial endospores, which are resistant; does NOT penetrate glass, plastic, or other materials.
      c. BEST for disinfecting surfaces and sometimes air.
   5. **Filtration:**
      a. Employs membrane filters with pore sizes in the approximate range to retain bacteria and viruses.
      b. BEST for sterilization of sensitive material that would be destroyed by other means, such as antibiotic solutions, vitamins, serum, biological fluids.
      c. High-efficiency particulate air (HEPA) filters are used to filter the air flowing into aseptic environments and out of potentially contaminated ones (e.g., containment facilities).
D. Chemical agents and effects:
   1. MOST chemical agents are disinfectants because endospores may NOT be killed by these agents.
   2. Many are mild enough to be used as topical skin antiseptics.
   3. **Detergents:** disrupt cellular membrane.
      a. When cationic, possess a net positive charge; examples: cetylpyridinium chloride and benzalkonium chloride, representatives of quaternary amine compounds.
      b. When anionic, possess net negative charge; examples: soap and sodium lauryl sulfate.
      c. When nonionic, lack a charge; examples: Triton-X and Tween compounds, which are fairly ineffective disinfectants.
   4. Phenolic compounds: work by disrupting membranes and ultimately precipitating proteins.
      a. Based on the phenol nucleus, which by itself is caustic.
      b. Types:
         (1) Cresols: methylated phenol derivatives in mixture form; example: Lysol.
         (2) Halogenated diphenyls: two phenol molecules linked together with additional chlorine molecules; examples: hexachlorophene (pHisoHex) and hexylresorcinol (ST-37 in mouthwash).

5. Alcohols, which disrupt cellular membranes and precipitate cellular proteins.
   a. A 100% alcohol is NOT effective because ONLY serves to dehydrate the cell.
   b. A 70% isopropyl alcohol is MOST commonly used, made by dilution with water.
6. Heavy metal compounds:
   a. Contain mercury or silver molecule; react reversibly with sulfhydryl groups of proteins to form mercaptide bonds; are bacteriostatic.
   b. Examples: mercury-containing merbromin (Mercurochrome) and merthiolate (Metaphen), silver nitrate.
7. Oxidizing agents:
   a. React irreversibly with active hydrogen molecules of proteins, such as sulfhydryl groups, to form covalently linked disulfide bonds; are bactericidal.
   b. Include iodine, chlorine, hypochloric acid (bleach), hydrogen peroxide.
8. Alkylating agents:
   a. React with reactive hydrogen molecules in the cell, such as sulfhydryl groups, by adding (alkylating) hydroxy methyl or hydroxy ethyl groups to these residues; are bactericidal.
   b. Include formaldehyde (solution), glutaraldehyde (solution), ethylene oxide (gas).
      (1) Chemical vapor: uses combination of chemicals (alcohol, formaldehyde, ketone, acetone, and water) instead of water alone to create a vapor for sterilizing.
      (2) Ethylene oxide: MAJOR gaseous sterilant for sterilizing nonbiological materials at room temperature.

INFECTION CONTROL PROTOCOL

Planned system of preventing disease transmission is an important element of dental setting protocol. MOST diseases that are transmissible in the dental setting are difficult or impossible to cure; consequently, preventing transmission from patient to patient, from patient to clinician or **dental healthcare personnel** (DHCP), and from DHCP to patient is of MOST importance. DHCP refers to ALL paid or unpaid personnel in dental healthcare setting who might be occupationally exposed to infectious materials, including body substances and contaminated supplies, equipment, environmental surfaces, water, or air; includes dentists, dental hygienists, dental assistants, dental laboratory technicians (in-office, commercial), students and trainees, contractual personnel, and other persons NOT directly involved in care but potentially exposed to infectious agents (e.g., administrative, clerical, housekeeping, maintenance, or volunteer personnel).

DHCP SHOULD become familiar with the hierarchy of controls that categorizes and prioritizes prevention strategies. Personnel subject to occupational exposure SHOULD receive infection control training on initial assignment, whenever new tasks or procedures affect their occupational exposure, and at a minimum annually. Education and training should be appropriate to the assigned duties of specific DHCP. Dental practices SHOULD develop written infection control program to prevent or reduce the risk of disease transmission. This should include establishment and implementation of policies, procedures, practices (in conjunction with selection and use of technologies and products) to prevent work-related injuries and illnesses among DHCP, as well as healthcare-associated infections among patients.

Program SHOULD include principles of infection control and occupational health, reflect current science, and adhere to relevant federal, state, and local regulations and statutes. Infection control coordinator (e.g., dentist or other DHCP) knowledgeable or willing to be trained should be assigned responsibility for coordinating the program. Health status of DHCP can be monitored by maintaining records of work-related medical evaluations, screening tests, immunizations, exposures, postexposure management; records MUST be kept in accordance with all applicable state and federal laws.

• See CD-ROM for related guidelines and terminology.

A. Dental patients and DHCP can be exposed to pathogenic microorganisms:
   1. High to moderate risk: cytomegalovirus (CMV), hepatitis B (HBV), hepatitis C (HCV), herpes simplex virus types 1 and 2 (HSV-1, -2), *Mycobacterium tuberculosis* (TB), staphylococci, streptococci, other viruses and bacteria that colonize or infect oral cavity and respiratory tract.
   2. Low risk: HIV transmission in dental settings in United States compared with HBV/HCV and others.
      a. Risk increases with exposure to large volume of blood, as indicated by deep injury with a device that was visibly contaminated with patient's blood, or procedure that involved needle placed in a vein or artery.
      b. Risk increases if exposure was to blood from patient with terminal illness, possibly reflecting higher titer of HIV in late-stage AIDS.
B. Pathogenic microorganisms transmitted in dental settings through:
   1. Direct contact with blood, oral fluids, or other patient secretions.
      a. Splatter involved in delivery (rinsing mouth, using prophy angle to polish, debridement with sonic and ultrasonic scalers).
      b. Contaminants through capillary action for next patient:
         (1) Ultrasonic and sonic scalers and high-speed handpieces and air-polishing devices.

(2) Air-water syringes and dental unit water-lines (may serve as contaminated biofilm reservoir).

(3) Self-contained water units, antiretraction valves, and backflow preventive devices help eliminate risk that patient will draw back contaminated water.

c. Needlestick and sharps injuries; open skin wound or mucous membrane.

2. Inhalation of airborne microorganisms that can remain suspended in the air for long periods.

a. Aerosols created by:

(1) Coughing, sneezing, or breathing.

(2) Prophy angles, brushes, or cups.

(3) Using BOTH controls on air-water syringes.

(4) Ultrasonic and sonic scalers; high-speed handpieces and air-polishing devices.

(5) Failure to use high-volume evacuation (HVE, high-speed suction).

b. Containing and reducing the production of aerosols MUST be considered (see later discussion).

3. Indirect contact with contaminated objects (e.g., instruments, equipment, or environmental surfaces).

4. Contact of conjunctival, nasal, or oral mucosa with droplets (e.g., spatter) containing microorganisms generated from an infected person and propelled short distance (e.g., by coughing, sneezing, or talking).

C. Infection through any of these routes requires that all of the following conditions be present:

1. Pathogenic organism of sufficient virulence and in adequate numbers to cause disease.

2. Reservoir or source that allows the pathogen to survive and multiply (e.g., blood).

3. Mode of transmission from the source to the host.

4. Portal of entry through which the pathogen can enter the host.

5. Susceptible host (i.e., one who is NOT immune).

D. Occurrence of these events provides the chain of infection; effective infection control strategies such as standard precautions prevent disease transmission by interrupting one or more links in the chain.

E. Avoiding occupational exposures to blood is the MAIN way to prevent transmission of HBV, HCV, and HIV to DHCP in healthcare settings.

Standard Precautions

Standard precautions as discussed by the Centers for Disease Control (CDC) in "Guidelines for Infection Control in Dental Health-Care Settings—2003" integrate and expand the elements of past "universal" precautions into a standard of care designed to protect DHCP and patients from pathogenic microorganisms that can be spread by blood or any other body fluid, excretion, or secretion. Standard precautions apply to contact with (1) blood; (2) all body fluids, secretions, and excretions (except sweat), regardless of whether contaminated by blood; (3) nonintact skin; and (4) mucous membranes. Saliva has ALWAYS been considered a potentially infectious material in dental infection control; thus NO operational difference exists in clinical dental practice between "universal" precautions and standard precautions.

• See CD-ROM for related information about standard precautions.

• See Chapters 5, Radiology: radiology practice protocol; 11, Clinical Treatment: clinical practice protocols; 15, Dental Biomaterials: lab control protocols.

A. Taking and reviewing detailed patient medical histories:

1. Complete, updated histories are important for the protection of all parties involved in providing and receiving dental care.

2. Medical histories identify prescription and over-the-counter (OTC) drugs.

3. Drugs the patient is taking can give clues to present medical status and enable dental care professionals to explain possible impact on oral health that the condition or the drugs may have.

4. Combination of written and oral questions gives patient an opportunity to explain condition.

5. Noting specialties of listed physicians gives clues as to medical conditions the patient is monitoring.

a. Increased trust between patient and provider promotes patient honesty in divulging medical history.

b. Dental office MUST maintain the confidentiality of patients' medical records (see Chapter 18, Ethics and Jurisprudence).

B. Appropriate immunization of DHCP (see earlier discussion of immunology and the CD-ROM):

1. HBV vaccination:

a. Full-time, part-time, temporary, and probationary employees MUST begin series during first 10 working days of employment.

b. New employees can continue to provide patient care during 6 months needed to complete series; new employees may refuse, but MUST read and sign "Refusal for Hepatitis B Vaccination" form.

(1) Vaccinations MUST be made available to employee free of charge and at reasonable time and location; licensed physician or other healthcare professional MUST supervise administration.

(2) Employees who receive vaccination MUST have appropriate documentation in medical

records; primary immunization with hepatitis B vaccine usually consists of three IM doses; second and third doses should be given 1 and 6 months after first, respectively.

(3) Vaccine is administered unless employee has proof of HBV antigens or antibodies to HBV antigens; vaccinated individuals should be tested after last injection to verify positive immune response.

2. Vaccination recommended for influenza, measles, mumps, rubella, varicella (chickenpox) (see CD-ROM).

3. Note that CDC does NOT recommend routine immunization against TB (i.e., inoculation with bacille Calmette-Guérin [BCG] vaccine) or hepatitis A (HAV); NO vaccine exists for HCV.

C. DHCP handwashing hygiene:
1. MUST be washed between patients, *before* donning and *after* removing gloves; using antimicrobial liquid soap provides additional protection by leaving protective layer.
   a. Short handwashing method: wash hands twice (rinsing in between) for 15 seconds at beginning of each day; between patients, wash for 15 seconds.
   b. Surgical hand scrub: before surgical procedures, scrub hands and forearms for 5 minutes, repeatedly washing with antimicrobial soap and soft brush and rinsing off debris; dry with a sterile towel.
   c. Whenever gloves are punctured or torn, hands MUST be washed and covered with new gloves.
   d. If the hands are NOT visibly soiled, alcohol-based hand rub is adequate; rubs are rapidly germicidal when applied to the skin but should include such antiseptics to achieve persistent activity as chlorhexidine, quaternary ammonium compounds, octenidine, or triclosan.
2. Keeping nails short; majority of microflora on the hands are found under and around fingernails.
   a. Nails should be short enough to allow DHCP to thoroughly clean underneath them and prevent glove tears; sharp nail edges or broken nails are also MORE likely to increase glove failure.
   b. Long artificial or natural nails can make donning gloves MORE difficult and can cause gloves to tear MORE readily.
3. Jewelry worn on hands should NOT interfere with glove use (e.g., impair ability to wear correct-sized glove or alter glove integrity).
D. Respiratory hygiene or cough etiquette (additions added): see CD-ROM for more information.

E. **Personal protective equipment** (PPE) of DHCP: DHCP MUST remove PPE before leaving patient-care areas.
1. Gloves:
   a. Single-use examination (nonsterile): rubber latex, vinyl, or nonvinyl materials; should extend over the cuffs of long-sleeved treatment gowns. Rubber latex allergy discussed earlier.
      (1) Single-use sterile: BEST used in conjunction with surgical procedures.
      (2) Single-use plastic overgloves: worn over treatment gloves to prevent cross-contamination (e.g., of charts, drawers, writing instruments).
   b. Multiple-use utility: *heavy* rubber latex or neoprene; BEST used during handling of contaminated instruments, cleaning of operatories, or handling of chemicals.
   c. Glove use protocols:
      (1) MUST be used whenever contact with blood, saliva, mucous membranes, or blood-contaminated objects is a possibility.
      (2) Hands MUST be washed before and after wearing gloves; defective gloves MUST be changed immediately (accompanied by appropriate handwashing) and between patients or during long appointments.
      (3) MUST not be reused between patients; MUST not be washed or disinfected and then reused.
      (4) Prevent herpetic whitlow (digital herpes simplex infection) (Figure 8-7).
2. Masks: glass fiber mat and synthetic fiber mat are MOST effective types.
   a. Dome masks with elastic bands provide space between the mask and mouth and reduce moistening of the mask (increasing effectiveness); surgical masks (ear-loop or tie-on type) filter smaller particles BETTER but become moist quicker, thus compromising clinician protection.

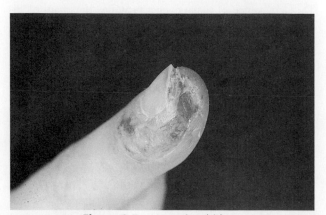

Figure 8-7 Herpetic whitlow.

b. American Society for Testing and Materials (ASTM) identifies masks according to three levels of protection (low, medium, or high); high-performance masks provide MOST protection for use in procedures where heavy to moderate amounts of fluid, spray, and/or aerosols are produced, especially with high- and low-speed handpieces and ultrasonic scalers.

c. Mask use protocols:

(1) Place and adjust before handwashing and change between patients.

(2) Avoid touching during appointment and continuing to wear after completion of procedures for protection against particulate matter or microorganisms in ambient air.

(3) Avoid contamination with disinfectants or other chemicals; avoid touching of mask proper, dangling mask around neck, or removing over the head by elastic or ties.

3. Protective eyewear and/or face shield:

a. Prescription eyewear offers LESS protection because of open top, sides, and bottom.

b. Safety glasses and goggles cover all areas around the eye, offer MOST protection from splatter, and are shatter resistant.

c. Face shields ensure maximum coverage, but mask MUST also be worn for protection from inhalation of contaminants.

d. Reasons for wearing protective eyewear:

(1) Prevention of disease transmission (e.g., conjunctivitis, ocular herpes, HBV).

(2) Protection against penetrating eye injury.

(3) Protection against chemical splatter (e.g., disinfectants, chemicals with a low pH).

(4) Patient protection (e.g., against chemical splatter, oral debris, dropped instruments).

e. Eyewear use protocols:

(1) Wear eyewear for ALL clinical appointments; clean and disinfect between patients.

(2) AVOID touching protective eyewear during care delivery to reduce possibility of contamination.

4. Protective clothing:

a. Types of protective clothing: reusable or disposable gowns or uniforms, surgical gowns (BEST choice), laboratory coats.

b. Selection of protective clothing:

(1) Any protective clothing MUST cover street clothing, fit closely around BOTH neck and wrists, cover the arms.

(2) Protective clothing made from synthetic material is MORE protective, since it is MORE fluid resistant.

c. Protective clothing protocols:

(1) Wear whenever contamination with blood or bodily secretions is likely (e.g., from aerosolization of blood, saliva, respiratory secretions, and microorganisms during ultrasonic scaling or polishing of teeth).

(2) Change daily or more often if visibly soiled; MUST avoid wearing outside of healthcare facility.

(a) Limit handling as much as possible after wearing; place in bags for transportation to laundering facility.

(b) MUST be thoroughly laundered between wearings separately from other clothing and using commercial laundry detergent, highest water temperature (60° to 70° C), machine dried at highest temperature (>110° C).

Procedures Related to Standard Precautions

Certain procedures or protocols MUST be performed on a daily basis to maintain standard precautions in the dental setting.

• See Chapter 12, Instrumentation: instrument processing.

A. Infection control protocol methods: involve sterilization and/or disinfection.

1. **Sterilization** (destruction of ALL forms of life) of reusable dental instruments; recommended for ALL dental instruments in critical category (e.g., scalers, burs, bone chisels, scalpels) and in semicritical category (if heat stable) (discussed later).

2. **Disinfection** (destruction of pathogens but NOT of spores) of instruments unable to withstand heat of sterilization; MUST be high-level disinfection for heat-unstable instruments in semicritical category; can be used for noncritical surfaces (discussed later).

a. Disinfection of environmental surfaces in the operatory:

(1) Disinfect according to categories of critical surfaces (Table 8-3).

(a) Critical surfaces: items that are used to penetrate soft tissue or bone (e.g., scalpels); MUST be sterilized.

(b) Semicritical surfaces: touch intact mucous membranes or oral fluids but do NOT penetrate tissues (e.g., scalers); require sterilization or high-level disinfection.

(c) Noncritical surfaces: contact ONLY the skin (do NOT contact mucous membranes) (e.g., lead [or lead equivalent] apron); require intermediate disinfection.

(2) Involves identifying surfaces that MUST be disinfected after treatment (e.g., patient chair,

Table 8-3 Levels of disinfection

Level of disinfection	Action	Use
High	Kills some but not all bacterial spores and is tuberculocidal; disinfectant and sterilizant agents registered by the Environmental Protection Agency are high-level disinfectants	Critical instruments that have touched mucous membranes, have penetrated soft tissue but not touched bone, or will not withstand sterilization
Intermediate	Kills HBV, HIV, *Mycobacterium tuberculosis* (var. *bovis*); does not kill spores	Noncritical instruments that have contact with intact skin.
Low	Kills most bacteria, some fungi, some viruses; does not kill spores or *M. tuberculosis* (var. *bovis*)	General cleaning

clinician chair, dental light, countertops, tray tables, handpiece and air-water syringe supports, ALL tubing, knobs, drawers used); some can be isolated using plastic wrap or bags to reduce time and effort needed to prepare treatment area for next patient.

  b. Disinfection technique (Table 8-3):

   (1) MUST wear multiple-use utility gloves (heavy rubber, nitrile, or neoprene) and PPE when disinfecting treatment areas.

   (2) Uncovered or contaminated surfaces SHOULD be precleaned using cleaner (detergent) or cleaner-disinfectant; BEST to use high- to intermediate-level tuberculocidal disinfectant registered by the Environmental Protection Agency (EPA) for BOTH cleaning step and disinfecting step.

   (3) Surfaces should be wiped to dislodge accumulations; then SHOULD wiped again with the disinfectant and remain wet for recommended amount of time (≤10 minutes depending on manufacturer).

   (4) Criteria for agent(s) used for disinfection (see later discussion):

    (a) MUST be water-based disinfectant and EPA-registered hospital disinfectant labeled viricidal and fungicidal (high to intermediate level); MUST kill *Mycobacterium tuberculosis* (TB organism very resistant to disinfection because of tough cell wall).

    (b) MUST be compatible with treatment area surfaces and remain active in presence of organic matter.

    (c) MUST be accepted by ADA Council on Scientific Affairs as effective disinfectant for dental environment.

   (5) Environmental surfaces that CANNOT be disinfected should be covered to prevent contamination during patient care, recovered between patients to break chain of infection; plastic coverings should be removed and disposed of properly, while DHCP are still gloved.

 B. Reducing the oral microflora population with preprocedural antimicrobial mouthrinse before treatment:

  1. Includes mouthrinses with alcohol, chlorhexidine gluconate, essential oils, or povidone-iodine.

  2. Can reduce level of oral microorganisms in aerosols and spatter generated during routine dental procedures with rotary instruments (e.g., dental handpieces, ultrasonic scalers).

 C. Minimizing aerosolization of microorganisms with use of high-volume evacuation (HVE, high-speed suction) with evacuation of debris, as well as ultrasonic and polishing use; AVOID use of both controls on air-water syringe and use of dental dams, if possible.

 D. Care and disinfection of dental unit waterlines:

  1. All retraction valves SHOULD be replaced with anti-retraction valves; should be checked to ensure proper function; may become stuck (open) over time.

  2. Waterlines SHOULD be flushed at beginning of each day for 3 to 5 minutes to reduce bacterial counts (e.g., for handpieces, ultrasonic scalers, air-water syringes).

  3. Waterlines SHOULD be flushed for 20 to 30 seconds between patients to eliminate bacterial accumulation (if unit has been NOT been used for some time, should be flushed for 3 to 5 minutes).

 E. Appropriate disposal of dental sharps and biohazardous waste generated during care delivery to prevent the transmission of disease (discussed later).

CLINICAL STUDY

Scenario: A new dental assistant is employed in the dental office, after graduating from high school last week at age 18. She has had no education or experience in dental assisting but has held a dental office receptionist position for 3 months. Between patients, she carefully washes her gloves. She wears the same facemask throughout the day, even though it appears moist and has a small bloodstain on it. At the end of the day, the dental assistant walks out of the dental office without changing her clothes.

1. What training should the dental assistant have had before participating in patient treatment?
2. What immunization issues must be addressed if the dental assistant is to continue employment at the dental office?
3. Identify mistakes that the dental assistant made on her first day of work.
4. What implications do these mistakes have regarding the dental assistant's health and the health of the patients?

1. The assistant should have had comprehensive training in the dental office's infection control policy and procedures, including discussion of standard precautions, before she began seeing patients. She does not understand the concepts of cross-contamination, chain of infection, or use of personal protective equipment (PPE).
2. The assistant must review her personal immunization record to verify her present status. She must be up to date with immunizations against measles, mumps, rubella, tetanus. She must also begin the hepatitis B vaccination series (or sign a waiver of refusal) within 10 days of employment to maintain employment in the dental office. She can continue employment while she receives the three-dose regimen. She would also be well advised to receive influenza vaccine to help prevent future sickness and missed workdays.
3. The assistant was washing and reusing her rubber latex gloves. She was not changing her mask between patients or when it became soiled or damp. She wore her office uniform home after work. Because she was violating these infection control protocols, she may have been violating others and contaminating the dental office with infectious agents.
4. Her health was in danger because of her lack of knowledge of both infection control protocols and standard precautions. She has been endangering the health and well-being of both patients and fellow staff members since her employment began. Her family and friends are also at risk for infection from contaminated items and surfaces (including her uniform and her skin) that she brought outside of the dental office.

Care and Disposal of Waste

Infectious waste, according to the EPA, consists of blood, blood-soaked items, tissue, extracted teeth, and sharps. The ADA and the Occupational Safety and Health Administration (OSHA) have further categorized waste generated in the dental setting into two types, biohazardous waste and biomedical waste. These guidelines are categorized under Occupational Exposure to Bloodborne Pathogens and Hazard Control (2001-2003).
A. Biohazardous waste:
  1. Blood, blood-soaked items, blood-caked items, and items soaked or caked with other potentially infectious material, including teeth and other body tissues NOT required for microscopic examination.
  2. Sharps: include used and unused syringe needles, glass and plastic local anesthetic cartridges, broken instruments, scalpel blades, burs, disposable syringes, broken glass, and suture needles (see later discussion).
  3. Disposal of biohazardous waste:
    a. Involves separating this waste from biomedical waste.
    b. Involves determining which disposal options (incineration, burial, sterilization) are available and which is the MOST cost effective.
    c. Involves labeling infectious waste with biohazard label to alert those who will handle the waste container and inform them of its contents.
    d. Involves discarding sharps in a puncture-resistant container for disposal.
B. Biomedical waste:
  1. Waste generated during course of care delivery that does NOT qualify as biohazardous.
  2. Includes gloves, masks, patient napkins (bibs), surface barriers, paper towels that do not fit criteria noted above.
  3. Disposal of biomedical waste involves same procedures as disposal of regular trash, unless state and local regulations stipulate different handling procedures.

Handling Sharps and Occupational Exposure Incident (Needlestick Protocol)

Every sharp dental instrument should be considered potentially infectious and should be handled with safety and injury prevention in mind. If occupational exposure occurs, protocol MUST be followed as referenced in 2004 CDC document "Exposure to Blood: What Health Care Workers Need to Know."
• See Chapter 12, Instrumentation: instrument processing.
A. Sharps:
  1. Include used and unused syringe needles, scalpels, burs, broken instruments, suture needles, local anesthetic cartridges, broken glass, sharp wires.
  2. Considered biohazardous (infectious) waste and therefore MUST be disposed of in a puncture-proof,

leak-resistant container kept *within* operatory according to local, state, or federal regulations (whichever take precedence).

3. MUST be handled carefully to avoid occupational exposure (puncture of skin with contaminated sharps).

B. Needle recapping: MUST use safe method/device.

1. Occupational exposures often happen during handling of syringe after local anesthesia administration.

2. AVOID recapping needles using ONLY two-handed technique; do NOT bend or break needles after use on trays or in tops of sharps containers because of risk of needlestick.

C. Occupational exposure incident (including needlestick protocol):

1. Consists of eye, mouth, mucous membrane, nonintact skin, or parenteral contact with blood or other potentially infectious materials during the performance of an employee's duties.

2. Wounds and skin sites that have been in contact with blood or body fluids should be washed with soap and water; mucous membranes should be flushed with water.

3. Exposure incidents might place DHCP at risk for hepatitis B virus (HBV), hepatitis C virus (HCV), or human immunodeficiency virus (HIV) infections, therefore should be evaluated immediately following treatment of the exposure site by qualified healthcare professional.

4. Employers should follow all federal (including OSHA) and state requirements for recording and reporting occupational injuries and exposures. Should include the following details:

   a. Details about the exposure source: whether the patient was infected with hepatitis B virus (HBV) and hepatitis B e antigen (HBeAg) status, hepatitis C virus (HCV), or human immunodeficiency virus (HIV); if source was infected with HIV, stage of disease, history of antiretroviral therapy, viral load, if known.

   b. Details about exposed person (e.g., hepatitis B vaccination and vaccine response status).

   c. Details about counseling, postexposure management, follow-up.

   d. If this information is NOT known from medical record, source patient should be asked to obtain serological testing for HBV, HCV, HIV.

5. After conducting this initial evaluation of the occupational exposure, qualified healthcare professional MUST decide whether to conduct further follow-up on individual basis using ALL of information obtained.

CLINICAL STUDY

Scenario: A new dental hygienist has been employed for 9 months after taking a year off to have a child. She is nearly an hour behind schedule because of unforeseen scheduling problems. Her final appointment of the day is with the dentist's sister, who is scheduled to receive two quadrants of nonsurgical periodontal therapy. The dental hygienist helps the supervising dentist administer local anesthesia. While she is recapping the needle, the cap, which she is holding in her left hand to put over the needle, slips and she accidentally sticks herself in her left index finger. A pool of blood the size of a dime forms under her glove. She proceeds with completion of the appointment and subsequently dismisses the patient.

1. What is the primary cause of this needlestick injury?
2. How should the dental hygienist have handled the situation immediately after the injury occurred?
3. What is the protocol that must be followed after a needlestick injury?
4. Is any follow-up required after a needlestick injury?
5. When do most needlestick injuries occur?

1. This needlestick injury was a direct result of using a two-handed recapping technique.

2. After the injury occurred, the hygienist should have stopped treating the patient, carefully removed and disposed of her gloves in biomedical waste, washed the needlestick area thoroughly with soap and water, and applied a bandage to the injury. She subsequently should have asked the patient to immediately accompany her to a medical setting where both could have blood drawn to test for infectious agents.

3. Immediately after an occupational exposure incident such as a needlestick, the hygienist as an employee must complete an exposure incident form, be evaluated by a healthcare professional, and possibly have herself and the patient tested for HBV, HCV, and HIV. Her dentist employer must send her job description, a report of incident, relevant medical information for both the hygienist and patient, and a copy of OSHA's bloodborne pathogens standard to the healthcare provider. She should be counseled on test results, infectious status, and associated risks. She should be given recommendations for postexposure management.

4. The hygienist must be provided with a report containing her healthcare provider's written opinion regarding the incident. Depending on the circumstances surrounding the incident, she may need to given prophylactic drug therapy and be medically reexamined in 6 months.

5. Most needlestick injuries occur during the recapping of used needles. Must recap using a safe method or device, unlike what the hygienist did this time.

Review Questions

1 *Candida albicans* has all the following characteristics EXCEPT one. Which one is the EXCEPTION?
  A. Reproduced by budding
  B. Yeast organism
  C. Causative agent of thrush
  D. Inhibited by penicillin

2 The rigidity and shape of the bacterial cell are caused by the
  A. capsule.
  B. peptidoglycan layer.
  C. lipopolysaccharide layer.
  D. teichoic acid layer.

3 Which of the following sequences is correct for staining a bacterial smear with the Gram stain?
  A. Crystal violet, alcohol, iodine, safranin
  B. Crystal violet, iodine, alcohol, safranin
  C. Safranin, iodine, alcohol, crystal violet
  D. Safranin, alcohol, iodine, crystal violet

4 One of following is NOT a characteristic of mycobacteria. Which one is the EXCEPTION?
  A. Acid fast
  B. Lacks cell wall
  C. Possesses mycolic acids and waxes in the wall structure
  D. Causes tuberculosis

5 The term "sterilization" means the killing of
  A. spores.
  B. microbes that cause disease.
  C. all life.
  D. fungus.

6 Multiple antibiotic resistance may be rapidly spread through bacterial populations by
  A. transformation.
  B. transduction.
  C. high-frequency recombination.
  D. plasmids.

7 What does penicillin effectively inhibit?
  A. Cell wall synthesis
  B. Cytoplasmic membrane
  C. Nucleic acid
  D. Transcription

8 How is a bactericidal agent recognized?
  A. Action is irreversible
  B. Does not kill bacteria and only stops bacterial growth
  C. Effective only on dead cells
  D. Action is reversible

9 The central intermediate that leads to the production of different fermentation products by bacteria is
  A. pyruvate.
  B. ATP.
  C. lactate.
  D. NADH.

10 One of the following statements is INCORRECT regarding bacterial respiration. Which one is INCORRECT?
  A. May occur anaerobically
  B. Organic compound serves as the final electron acceptor
  C. May occur aerobically
  D. Produces more energy in the form of ATP than does fermentation

11 A facultative anaerobe grows in the presence of
  A. oxygen.
  B. no oxygen.
  C. oxygen or no oxygen.
  D. low concentrations of oxygen.

12 What is the antibiotic of choice in the treatment of a topical yeast or fungal infection?
  A. Nystatin
  B. Hexachlorophene
  C. Tetracycline
  D. Penicillin

13 What is the principal agent currently used for gaseous sterilization?
  A. Formaldehyde
  B. Isopropyl alcohol
  C. Gamma rays
  D. Ethylene oxide

14 Identification of bacterial species depends on all of the following, EXCEPT one. Which one is the EXCEPTION?
  A. Presence of plasmids
  B. Nutritional requirements
  C. Biochemical characteristics
  D. Staining and morphology

15 Transduction as a means of gene transfer between bacteria is mediated by
  A. bacteriophages.
  B. cell-to-cell contact.
  C. free DNA.
  D. yeasts.

16 What are the enzymes needed for the breakdown of hydrogen peroxide to H_2O and O_2?
  A. Autotrophs
  B. Heterotrophs
  C. Aerobes
  D. Anaerobes

17 A virus can be distinguished from all other microorganisms by virtue of its
  A. ability to be isolated from the blood.
  B. need to replicate intracellularly.
  C. resistance to antibodies.
  D. possession of only one type of nucleic acid.

18 Prokaryotic cells differ in structure from eukaryotic cells in that prokaryotes each possess
  A. a nuclear membrane.
  B. mitochondria.
  C. 70S ribosomes.
  D. 80S ribosomes.

19 One of following statements regarding the control of microorganisms is INCORRECT. Which one is INCORRECT?
  A. Widespread and indiscriminate use of antibiotics may select for bacteria that are resistant to antibiotics.
  B. An antibiotic that inhibits a large variety of different organisms is said to possess a broad spectrum.
  C. Tetracyclines are inhibitors of bacterial cell wall biosynthesis.
  D. Viruses are not affected by antibiotics.

20 By what means do bacteria usually reproduce?
  A. Endospores
  B. Mitosis
  C. Binary fission
  D. Budding

21 What is the source of carbon for a heterotrophic bacterium?
   A. Glucose
   B. Hydrogen gas
   C. Carbon dioxide
   D. Hydrogen sulfide

22 In which phase of bacterial growth is the number of newly formed cells equal to the number of dying cells?
   A. Lag
   B. Exponential
   C. Stationary
   D. Death

23 What do aminoglycoside antibiotics (e.g., streptomycin) inhibit?
   A. Transcription
   B. Cell wall biosynthesis
   C. Translation
   D. DNA replication

24 Elaborate and harsh procedures are required for sterilization because of the possible presence of
   A. viruses.
   B. endospores.
   C. capsules.
   D. flagella.

25 Which one of the following antibiotics is different from ALL of the others in its mode of action?
   A. Erythromycin
   B. Tetracycline
   C. Cephalosporin
   D. Streptomycin

26 Yeasts possess all of the following characteristics, EXCEPT one. Which one is the EXCEPTION?
   A. Reproduce asexually
   B. Reproduce sexually
   C. Unicellular organisms
   D. Produce mycelia

27 Which type of microorganism may be found growing deep inside a wound and on its surface?
   A. Aerobe
   B. Anaerobe
   C. Facultative anaerobe
   D. Microaerophile

28 Biologically active solutions such as antibiotics and vitamins are BEST sterilized by
   A. autoclaving.
   B. ethylene oxide.
   C. filtration.
   D. gamma radiation.

29 All of the following infective agents would have penicillin as antibiotic of choice for treatment, EXCEPT one. Which one is the EXCEPTION?
   A. *Streptococcus pneumoniae*
   B. *Mycoplasma pneumoniae*
   C. *Staphylococcus aureus*
   D. *Bacillus subtilis*

30 Tuberculosis is characterized by all of the following, EXCEPT one. Which one is the EXCEPTION?
   A. Rapidly cured by antibiotic therapy
   B. Emergence of drug-resistant *M. tuberculosis*
   C. Susceptibility is enhanced by HIV infection
   D. Efficient airborne transmission

31 Antibodies are BEST characterized by which of the following?
   A. Lack of antigen specificity
   B. Production of T lymphocytes
   C. Specific interaction with antigenic determinants
   D. Absence from blood

32 B lymphocytes have which important characteristic?
   A. Absence of cell wall cytokine receptors
   B. Inability to produce antibodies
   C. Maturation centered in the thymus
   D. Clonal expansion after immunization or infection

33 All of the following are TRUE about immunoglobulin G, EXCEPT one. Which one is the EXCEPTION?
   A. Predominant antibody class found in blood plasma
   B. Mediator of specific antibacterial and antiviral immunity
   C. Produced by plasma cells
   D. Failure to bind to Fc receptors

34 Which of the following statements can be applied to phagocytic cells?
   A. Have no role in the generation of specific immunity
   B. Capable of ingesting foreign molecules in the absence of antibodies
   C. Capable of synthesizing antibodies
   D. Do not bear surface Fc receptors

35 All of these are TRUE about the complement system, EXCEPT one. Which one is the EXCEPTION?
   A. Consists of many blood proteins
   B. Helps defend the body against infection
   C. Facilitates attachment and clearance of foreign molecules by the body
   D. Genetic deficiencies do not occur

36 Allergic reactions are BEST characterized by which of the following?
   A. Subclinical symptoms
   B. Susceptibility that excludes genetic inheritance
   C. Lack of T-lymphocyte participation
   D. Mediation by IgE

37 The spectrum of antigens recognized by the immune system is
   A. restricted to immune recognition of membrane lipid molecules.
   B. highly diverse; caused by genetic mechanisms that regulate antigen receptor molecules.
   C. very narrow because most B and T cells carry the same antigen receptor molecules.
   D. unaffected by B and T cell antigen receptor molecules.

38 Immune mechanisms of host defense against infections include all of the following, EXCEPT one. Which one is the EXCEPTION?
   A. IgG-mediated neutralization of viruses
   B. Stimulation of bacterial phagocytosis by antibodies and/or complement (opsonization)
   C. IgD-mediated neutralization of bacteria
   D. Complement-mediated degradation of bacteria

39 Graft rejection is characterized by
   A. immunological tolerance to the grafted tissue.
   B. immune recognition of powerful transplantation antigens on the graft.
   C. failure of B and T cells to become activated.
   D. failure of the complement system to become activated.

40 Which of the following is CORRECT concerning the human major histocompatibility complex?
A. Known as the human leukocyte antigen complex
B. Encodes antibody molecules
C. Identical among all humans
D. Encodes T-cell receptor molecules

41 Genetic typing of a person's HLA genes
A. has no role in controlling the likelihood of graft rejection.
B. has no role in the diagnosis of certain autoimmune diseases.
C. can be performed using cellular, serological, or genetic technology.
D. cannot yet be performed because HLA alleles are uncharacterized.

42 Which of the following are known characteristics of CD4+ T cells?
A. Greater in number in individuals with AIDS
B. Known as "helper" T cells
C. Nonresponsive to vaccine injections
D. Unable to produce interleukin-2

43 Cytokines are cells that are
A. protein molecules produced by lymphocytes, macrophages, and other cells.
B. normally not involved in regulating immune responses.
C. not involved in the inflammatory process.
D. produced only during humoral immune responses.

44 Cytotoxic T cells are cells that
A. recognize and kill virus-infected and tumor cells.
B. release killer antibody molecules.
C. are not antigen specific.
D. bear the CD4 cell surface marker.

45 Immunological protection of a newborn is
A. unnecessary because of vigorous nonspecific and innate protection.
B. transferred to the baby only after birth by contact with foreign antigens.
C. passively transferred to the baby in utero by maternal IgG antibodies.
D. unaffected by nursing.

46 Systemic lupus erythematosus is characterized by all of the following, EXCEPT one. Which one is the EXCEPTION?
A. Autoimmunity
B. Circulating anti-DNA antibodies of unknown origin
C. Lack of effect by sex hormones
D. Immune complex–mediated damage to the kidneys

47 All of the following describe immune complexes, EXCEPT one. Which one is the EXCEPTION?
A. Are found during infections
B. Are formed in response to virus infections
C. Are associated with complement activation
D. Result in tissue repair when deposited in blood vessels

48 Hemolytic disease occurs in newborns of Rh-negative mothers and is characterized by all of the following, EXCEPT one. Which one is the EXCEPTION?
A. Father whose erythrocytes bear the Rh+ phenotype
B. Mother whose erythrocytes bear the Rh+ phenotype
C. Maternal antibodies stimulated by paternal erythrocyte antigens, which are recognized as foreign by the mother
D. Antibody-mediated attack against red cells made by the newborn

49 Determination of which of the following characterizes specific serological diagnosis of an infection?
A. Seroconversion after vaccination
B. Blood B-cell counts
C. Specific blood antibody response to antigens
D. Elevated total blood IgG levels

50 For which of the following is the ELISA test used as a screening tool?
A. HIV RNA
B. CD4+ T cells
C. Cytotoxic T cells
D. Anti-HIV antibodies

51 Which of the following is a CORRECT statement concerning bone marrow transplantation?
A. Replaces body stem cells, leading to regeneration of the immune system
B. Effective only for B-cell regeneration; T cells and phagocytes are not affected
C. Treatment of choice for anaphylactic reactions
D. Cannot introduce infections into the recipient

52 Important oral signs of HIV infection include all of the following, EXCEPT one. Which is the EXCEPTION?
A. Aphthous ulcers
B. Dental caries
C. Necrotizing ulcerative gingivitis
D. Oral hairy leukoplakia

53 Current therapy for HIV infection is based on all of the following, EXCEPT one. Which one is the EXCEPTION?
A. Treatment with viral reverse-transcriptase inhibitors
B. Management with viral protease inhibitors
C. Reduction of viral load
D. Human bone marrow transplant

54 Which of the following characterizes the secondary immune response?
A. Predominance of IgM
B. High-affinity IgG
C. Absence of IgA
D. Unrelated to booster vaccination

55 Which of the following is a CORRECT statement concerning the process of antigen presentation to CD4+ T cells?
A. Not necessary for helper T-cell activation, because CD4+ T cells recognize soluble antigen
B. Occurs only in the thymus
C. Necessary for the immune response to T-dependent antigens
D. Does not depend on recognition of MHC molecules

56 All of the following are B cell–dependent mechanisms of cytotoxicity, EXCEPT one. Which one is the EXCEPTION?
A. IgM complement activation
B. ADCC
C. CTL activity
D. K cells

57 Monoclonal antibodies may have all of the following properties, EXCEPT one. Which one is the EXCEPTION?
A. Products of single clone of B cell
B. React with a single antigenic determinant
C. Have little antitumor activity
D. Specific for one epitope

58 The hemagglutination test of blood erythrocytes from the following individuals would be positive in all cases, EXCEPT one. Which one is the EXCEPTION?
  A. Blood group A–positive person tested with anti-A antibody
  B. Blood group A–negative person tested with anti-A antibody
  C. Newborn with hemolytic disease
  D. Person with autoimmune hemolytic anemia

59 Which of the following is the BEST treatment for a patient with severe combined immunodeficiency?
  A. Transplantation with purified donor T cells
  B. Transplantation with purified donor stem cells
  C. Passive immunization with pooled human gamma globulins
  D. Periodic injections of interleukin-2

60 Secretory component is a substance that is
  A. produced by T cells; stabilizes the T-cell receptor.
  B. required for IgE binding to mast cells.
  C. required for cross-linking of IgM monomers.
  D. produced by epithelial cells; protects IgA.

61 The serum protein electrophoresis pattern of a patient with a history of recent infections shows abnormally elevated gamma globulins. Subsequent serum immunoelectrophoresis shows an elevation of the IgM band. The MOST likely diagnosis of this patient is
  A. hypogammaglobulinemia.
  B. DiGeorge syndrome.
  C. Waldenström's macroglobulinemia.
  D. T-cell lymphoma.

62 What condition is associated with multi-drug-resistant tuberculosis?
  A. Systemic lupus erythematosus
  B. Acquired immunodeficiency disease syndrome
  C. Trisomy 21
  D. Bullous pemphigoid

63 All of the following routes are involved in HIV transmission, EXCEPT one. Which one is the EXCEPTION?
  A. Exposure to contaminated blood, blood products, or blood-contaminated body fluids
  B. Infected mother to unborn child
  C. Intimate sexual contact involving the exchange of semen or vaginal secretions
  D. Casual contact with a recently seroconverted HIV-positive individual

64 An important deterrent against the transmission of disease in the dental office is
  A. requiring that patients undergo HIV testing.
  B. refusing to treat patients from high-risk groups.
  C. vaccinating office staff who are exposed to bloodborne pathogens for HBV.
  D. asking whether patients have AIDS during the medical history.

65 All of the following are methods of reducing airborne transmission of infectious agents, EXCEPT one. Which one is the EXCEPTION?
  A. Having the patient use an antimicrobial mouthrinse
  B. Using high-volume suction during ultrasonic scaling procedures
  C. Wearing protective clothing, gloves, and mask
  D. Mouth rinsing using both controls on an air-water syringe

66 Laundering of contaminated protective clothing requires
  A. cool water temperatures, a commercial laundry detergent, and a cool dryer.
  B. tepid water temperatures, a commercial laundry detergent, and a warm dryer.
  C. warm water temperatures, a commercial laundry detergent, and a warm dryer.
  D. hot water temperatures, a commercial laundry detergent, and a hot dryer.

67 Waterlines in the dental office are BEST disinfected by flushing for
  A. 1 to 3 minutes at the beginning of the day and for 10 to 15 seconds between patients.
  B. 3 to 5 minutes at the beginning of the day and for 20 to 30 seconds between patients.
  C. 5 to 10 minutes at the beginning of the day and for 35 to 45 seconds between patients.
  D. 10 to 15 minutes at the beginning of the day and for 50 to 60 seconds between patients.

68 Biomedical waste includes all of the following, EXCEPT one. Which one is the EXCEPTION?
  A. Extracted teeth
  B. Gloves
  C. Patient napkins
  D. Facial masks

69 Biohazardous waste is
  A. disposed of with regular trash.
  B. incinerated, buried, or sterilized.
  C. placed in plain packaging.
  D. disposed of with biomedical waste.

70 All of the following are common oral manifestations of AIDS, EXCEPT one. Which one is the EXCEPTION?
  A. Hairy leukoplakia
  B. Candidiasis
  C. Kaposi's sarcoma
  D. Angular cheilitis
  E. Lichen planus

71 The major barrier to care for the patient with HIV/AIDS is
  A. communication.
  B. transportation.
  C. economic.
  D. physical.

72 One of the following does NOT meet the criteria for a diagnosis of acquired immune deficiency syndrome. Which one is the EXCEPTION?
  A. Kaposi's sarcoma
  B. Histoplasmosis
  C. Herpes simplex
  D. Mouth rinsing using both controls on an air-water syringe
  E. Lymphoma of the brain

73 Which of the following lesions is produced by herpes zoster and eventually ulcerates and causes intense pain?
  A. Vesicle
  B. Pustule
  C. Bulla
  D. Cyst

74 All of the following are statements regarding acquired immune deficiency syndrome, EXCEPT one. Which one is the EXCEPTION?

A. Fatal syndrome that develops after infection by virus.

B. Best classified as an autoimmune disease.

C. Contracted by contact with contaminated blood.

D. Late-stage symptoms include increased opportunistic infections.

75 In treatment of a patient with AIDS who has pseudomembranous candidiasis, which of the following drugs would be MOST likely be prescribed?

A. Acyclovir

B. Corticosteroid

C. Ketoconazole

D. Chlorhexidine

Answer Key and Rationales

1 (D) Penicillin (Pen-Vee K) is NOT effective in treatment of *Candida* infections because organism is a yeast, eukaryotic cell. Thrush is a *Candida* infection common in infants. Penicillin inhibits peptidoglycan biosynthesis in bacterial cell walls, and peptidoglycan is found ONLY in prokaryotic cells.

2 (B) Peptidoglycan is three-dimensional macromolecular structure of the cell wall that surrounds cytoplasmic membrane and provides shape and rigidity to bacterial cells. Because of high osmotic pressure within the cell, bacteria normally would lyse without this structure.

3 (B) Correct order of reagents used in Gram stain is crystal violet (primary stain), iodine (mordant), alcohol (which decolorizes gram-negative cells), and safranin (counterstain). Gram-positive bacteria retain primary stain and appear purple-blue. Gram-negative bacteria are decolorized and take up counterstain; appear red-pink.

4 (B) Mycobacteria possess a peptidoglycan cell wall covered with mycolic acids and waxes. Hydrophobic surface is responsible for positive acid-fast staining reaction characteristic of causative agent of tuberculosis, *Mycobacterium tuberculosis*. Mycoplasmas are organisms that LACK cell wall and are smallest free-living bacteria.

5 (C) Sterilization is killing of all life, including bacterial endospores. Major sterilization agents include high temperatures (use of an autoclave or dry air oven), gamma radiation, ethylene oxide. Disinfectants are usually harsh agents, including chemical agents and ultraviolet (UV) light, that kill MOST but NOT all organisms.

6 (D) Plasmids are small, circular, self-replicating DNA molecules that may contain multiple genes that code for resistance to different antibiotics. Plasmids may be transmitted from a donor bacterium to a recipient by conjugation. Thus a bacterium sensitive to antibiotics may receive plasmid from donor cell and become immediately resistant to antibiotics. Transformation, transduction, high-frequency recombination are mechanisms for transfer of chromosomal genes.

7 (A) Penicillin (Pen-Vee K) specifically inhibits biosynthesis of bacterial cell wall peptidoglycan. Inhibits cross-linking of peptidoglycan chains, disrupting integrity of three-dimensional structure; effective ONLY on actively growing cells.

8 (A) Bactericidal agent is one that binds irreversibly with microorganism, resulting in death of bacterium. Bacteriostatic agent binds reversibly to bacterium, stopping growth, but does NOT kill organism.

9 (A) Pyruvate is end product of glycolytic pathway in which sugar such as glucose (C6) is broken down into two molecules of pyruvate (C3), resulting in net production of two ATP molecules and two reduced $NADH_2$ molecules. During simplest fermentation, pyruvate is the organic compound that serves as final electron acceptor and is thus reduced to fermentation product, lactate, central "hub" in fermentation reactions.

10 (B) By definition, inorganic compound serves as final electron acceptor in respiration, whereas organic compound serves this function in fermentation. Bacterial respiration may occur aerobically, employing oxygen, or may occur anaerobically, using other inorganic compounds (e.g., sulfate, nitrate); produces MORE energy from one glucose molecule in the form of ATP (38 net) than does fermentation (2 net).

11 (C) Facultative anaerobe is bacterium that may grow either aerobically, in presence of oxygen, or anaerobically, in absence of oxygen. Aerobe grows ONLY in presence of oxygen, and anaerobe grows ONLY in absence of oxygen; microaerophile requires limited amounts of oxygen for growth.

12 (A) Nystatin (Mycostatin) and amphotericin B (Fungilin) are polyene antibiotics (antifungals) that complex with sterol, thereby disrupting membranes of eukaryotic cells such as yeast. Bacterial cells are NOT affected by these antibiotics because sterol is absent. Tetracyclines such as tetracycline (Achromycin, Sumycin), doxycycline (Vibramycin), and minocycline (Minocin) and penicillin (Pen-Vee K) act ONLY on prokaryotic cells. Hexachlorophene (Nabac, Phisohex, Septisol) is NOT an antibiotic but a disinfectant.

13 (D) Ethylene oxide is BEST used for room-temperature gaseous sterilant for materials that may be destroyed by other means. Used as a sterilant for foods and medical supplies. Colorless flammable gas or refrigerated liquid with a faintly sweet odor.

14 (A) Plasmids are NOT present in all microorganisms and NOT routinely useful for purposes of identification. Identification depends on Gram stain and morphology (e.g., rods, cocci), biochemical characteristics (such as ability to grow on different substrates), metabolic end products, requirement for oxygen, specific nutritional requirements.

15 (A) Transduction occurs upon replication within host bacterium when piece of host cell chromosomal DNA is mistakenly incorporated into phage capsid instead of phage DNA. Upon infection of new host cell, this piece of DNA is injected and thus transferred to the new bacterial cell. Conjugation is process of gene transfer mediated by cell-to-cell contact, and transformation is incorporation of free "naked" DNA into recipient cell.

16 (C) For bacteria to grow aerobically, using oxygen as final electron acceptor (respiration), enzymes catalase and superoxide dismutase are required to break down toxic intermediates that form at end of electron transport chain. Superoxide dismutase converts superoxide anions (toxic) to hydrogen peroxide (toxic), and the peroxide is converted to water and oxygen. Without these enzymes, bacteria grow anaerobically. Autotrophs are bacteria that use carbon dioxide as carbon source; heterotrophs derive carbon from organic compounds.

17 (D) Distinguishing feature of viruses is that they contain either DNA or RNA but NOT both as do cellular lifeforms. Able to replicate themselves from information contained in DNA or information in RNA.

18 (C) Prokaryotes (bacteria) possess 70S ribosomes. Others are characteristic of MORE complex eukaryotic cells. MANY useful antibiotics specifically inhibit bacterial protein synthesis because they specifically bind to 70S ribosomes, but NOT to 80S ribosomes of eukaryotic cells.

19 (C) Tetracyclines such as tetracycline (Achromycin, Sumycin), doxycycline (Vibramycin), minocycline (subgingival: Arestin, oral: Minocin) inhibit bacterial protein synthesis. Penicillins (Pen-Vee K) and other beta-lactam antibiotics inhibit cell wall biosynthesis. Others are all CORRECT and should be remembered when administering antibiotics.

20 (C) Bacteria reproduce by binary fission. Eukaryotic cells reproduce by mitosis, and yeasts do so by budding. Endospores are NOT a mode of reproduction in bacteria but are a means of survival.

21 (A) Organic compounds serve as the carbon source for heterotrophic bacteria. Carbon dioxide is the carbon source for autotrophic bacteria. Although hydrogen and hydrogen sulfide may serve as energy source for chemolithotrophic bacteria, they do NOT contain carbon.

22 (C) Dividing and dying bacteria are in balance during stationary phase of growth. NO growth during the lag phase. Rapid growth and division of the cell occur during exponential phase, and cells die exponentially during death phase.

23 (C) Aminoglycoside antibiotics specifically inhibit protein synthesis at level of translation by binding to the 30S ribosomal subunit. Antibiotics such as rifampicin inhibit protein synthesis at level of transcription. Nalidixic acid is inhibitor of DNA synthesis, and beta-lactam antibiotics (e.g., penicillin, Pen-Vee K) inhibit cell wall biosynthesis.

24 (B) Bacterial endospores are MOST resistant form of life known. They resist heat, ultraviolet light, desiccation. Viruses are killed by much milder conditions; capsules and flagella are bacterial structures that are easily destroyed by physical and chemical procedures.

25 (C) Cephalosporins such as cephalexin (Keflex), cefadroxil (Duricef), cefaclor (Ceclor), cefuroxime (Ceftin), cefazolin (Ancef), ceftriaxone (Rocephin) are beta-lactam antibiotics that inhibit cross-linking in peptidoglycan biosynthesis. Erythromycins such as Robimycin, E-Mycin, E.E.S.; tetracyclines such as tetracycline (Achromycin, Sumycin), doxycycline (Vibramycin), and minocycline (subgingival: Arestin, oral: Minocin); and streptomycin are ALL inhibitors of bacterial protein synthesis.

26 (D) Yeasts do NOT produce mycelia; they are unicellular fungi. Yeasts may reproduce asexually, by budding, or sexually, by the production of ascospores.

27 (C) Facultative anaerobes may grow on surface of wound, in presence of air, or deep in a wound, where anaerobic conditions exist. Anaerobes grow only deep in wound, and aerobes grow only on surface. Microaerophiles might be expected to grow just below surface.

28 (C) Sterilization by filtration is necessary for biologically active solutions. Alternative methods such as autoclaving, ethylene oxide, or gamma radiation would be TOO severe and would destroy biological activity.

29 (B) Penicillin (Pen-Vee K) inhibits cell wall biosynthesis. Mycoplasmas are bacteria that LACK a cell wall and are therefore NOT affected by any of the cell wall antibiotics. Others possess typical cell walls and are inhibited by penicillin.

30 (A) Drug resistance is significant problem in treating tuberculosis (TB), as is drug compliance, because patient may feel better soon after initiating therapy; however, eradication of *M. tuberculosis* may take MANY months of treatment. TB is a growing problem in immunocompromised, including those with human immunodeficiency virus (HIV) infection. Infected may cough up large numbers of organisms, and these may survive for long periods of time because of outer waxy coat of this bacterium, which makes airborne transmission relatively efficient.

31 (C) KEY property of antibodies (produced ONLY by plasma cells after these cells are produced by B cells) is specific reactivity with antigens, which allows targeting of specific pathogens while avoiding autoimmune responses. Antibodies are soluble proteins that circulate in blood, facilitating contact with pathogens that invade the body.

32 (D) Production of antibodies by B lymphocytes is greatly influenced by cytokines (e.g., IL-2, produced by T cells). B lymphocytes are generated by bone marrow and mature there and in secondary sites such as lymph nodes. Contact with antigens, either naturally or by immunization, selects specific clones of B lymphocytes for expansion.

33 (D) Plasma cells represent terminal stage of B-cell differentiation; secrete antibodies that find way into blood (IgG has highest concentration in blood) and other body sites (e.g., mucosal sites where antibody is MAINLY IgA, secretory); may mediate immune reactions against bacteria, viruses, and other pathogens. Fc receptor binding is MAJOR mechanism that helps phagocytic cells clear pathogens.

34 (B) Phagocytic cells (e.g., macrophages, neutrophils) help in generation of specific (B and/or T cell) immunity by processing antigen molecules, presenting antigen fragments to B and T cells, and releasing cytokines. However, phagocytic cells do NOT synthesize antibodies, although they are rich in surface Fc receptors, which helps interaction with antibodies and immune complexes.

35 (D) Complement system is complex biochemical system that comprises MORE than 30 protein molecules. When activated by contact with antigens and/or antibodies, complement helps stimulate inflammation and magnify immune reactions; also attaches to and helps clear foreign molecules and pathogens from the body. Various complement proteins may be adversely affected by genetic mutations.

36 (D) Clinical spectrum of allergy is broad and includes potentially fatal allergic reactions (e.g., anaphylaxis caused by food or drug allergy). Genetic factors that affect susceptibility to allergy include HLA genes. Although T cells may participate in some types of allergies (e.g., delayed-type hypersensitivity), some of the MOST severe allergies are caused by antibodies (immunoglobulin [Ig]).

37 (B) Diversity is hallmark of immunity, being generated by recombination at V(D)J genes that encode for antibodies and T cell receptors. Results in the generation of antibodies that specifically recognize antigens of virtually ANY molecular structure.

38 (C) Immune mechanisms of host defense are multifactorial. Include antibody reactions (e.g., direct neutralization and complement activation) and opsonization (facilitation of clearance of bacteria and other foreign invaders by phagocytic cells). IgG is major mediator of virus neutralization. Although bacteria may be inhibited by IgG, IgA, or IgA antibodies, binding to critical receptors, IgD has NO known direct antimicrobial function. IgD is involved in developmental regulation of immune responses.

39 (B) Tolerance is LACK of immune reactivity to specific antigens (e.g., self-antigens). Graft rejection is characterized by active immunity against antigens carried by the graft; MOST potent appear to be transplantation (MHC) antigens, which activate T and B cells to react against the graft. Complement may play IMPORTANT role in graft rejection, either through direct activation by graft cells or through antibodies that react against graft.

40 (A) MHC is generic term for gene complex, also known as human leukocyte antigen complex (HLA). Carries alleles (specific DNA coding sequences), which are highly diverse. Antibodies and T-cell receptors are encoded on separate and distinct gene regions outside HLA complex.

41 (C) HLA typing is IMPORTANT method used to match graft donors and recipients and to help diagnose autoimmune diseases (and some cancers) that have been linked to certain MHC alleles. Classical cellular and serological typing techniques are being replaced with the molecular detection of HLA gene sequences.

42 (B) CD4 denotes the "helper" T-cell phenotype. CD4+ T cells are destroyed in AIDS (MOST likely because HIV replicates within these cells). Because CD4+ T cells are IMPORTANT for immune responses and in the production of cytokines such as IL-2, their destruction leads to susceptibility to infections.

43 (A) Many cell types, including B and T lymphocytes and macrophages, produce cytokines. Cytokines are IMPORTANT regulators of immunity and participate in ALL phases of immune responses.

44 (A) Cytotoxic (CD8+) T cells are capable of killing other cells by a specific protein-killing mechanism unrelated to antibodies, which are NOT produced by T cells. Antigen-specific T-cell killing allows these cells to be directed against virus-infected or tumor cells.

45 (C) Immune system of a newborn is NOT fully mature. Without passive maternal protection, acquired in utero (maternal IgG crosses placenta) and during nursing (from breast milk antibodies and cells), newborn would NOT be able to cope effectively with exposures to infection. By ~6 months of age, immune system has reached stage in which it is likely to respond well to contact with MOST foreign antigens.

46 (C) Anti-DNA antibodies are found in the blood of persons with systemic lupus erythematosus (SLE), MOSTLY female; thus sex hormones exert influence on development of SLE, although it is NOT known why anti-DNA antibodies develop. Clinical spectrum of this autoimmune disease is broad. In MORE severe cases, kidney failure may occur from BOTH the deposition of immune complexes in kidney and the stimulation of inflammatory responses.

47 (D) As in the example of systemic lupus erythematosus (SLE), immune complexes may precipitate tissue damage, and the activation of complement is a major pathway for this occurrence. Nonpathogenic immune complexes circulate at low levels (e.g., as result of immune responses to microorganisms and their antigens) and are cleared in healthy individuals without causing dangerous immune reactions.

48 (B) When an Rh-negative mother is exposed to paternal Rh+ antigen during pregnancy (usually because of expression of RhD antigen by erythrocytes of the developing fetus, which leak into the maternal circulation before or during birth), the mother may become sensitized to the RhD antigen. During subsequent pregnancies, maternal IgG anti-RhD antibodies may enter the fetus and damage fetal red blood cells, resulting in hemolytic disease of the newborn. Prophylactic treatment consists of injecting mother with anti-RhD antibodies at approximately time of birth; passively administered antibodies bind to paternal antigen and inhibit development of maternal anti-RhD antibodies. Reactions to blood group antigens other than RhD may also occur.

49 (C) Determination of specific antibody responses to pathogens (e.g., anti-HIV detection by enzyme-linked immunosorbent assay [ELISA]) is powerful tool for detecting human exposure and infection. However, specific antibody response that occurs as result of vaccination would NOT necessarily indicate infection because immunization itself could be responsible for seroconversion. Blood B-cell counts and IgG levels are nonspecific measures of immunity and do NOT reveal specific exposures.

50 (D) Enzyme-linked immunosorbent assay (ELISA) screening for HIV infection detects specific immunity that occurs during HIV infection, as represented by circulating IgG or IgM anti-HIV antibodies. False-positive ELISA reactions may occur because of blood antibodies that cross-react with HIV antigens, even in the absence of HIV infection. Blood HIV RNA detection by molecular techniques and measurement of CD4+ T cells in the blood by cytochemistry BOTH provide important correlates of disease progression but are NOT carried out by ELISA.

51 (A) By providing a new source of functional stem cells, bone marrow transplantation may effectively treat a variety of immune system disorders, including those that affect B and T cells and phagocytes. Transmission of infection—particularly but NOT exclusively virus infection—from the donor to the recipient is one of the risks of this procedure.

52 (B) Dental caries is NOT indicative of human deficiency virus (HIV) infection, although it may occur when oral hygiene is inadequate or may be caused by xerostomia (dry mouth) from drug use. Aphthous ulcers (canker sores) are common in HIV infection. LESS common but still prevalent in HIV infection are necrotizing ulcerative gingivitis (NUG), necrotizing periodontal disease with anaerobic infection, treatable with systemic metronidazole (Flagyl), and oral hairy leukoplakia (white lesions on the lateral surfaces of the tongue involving filiform lingual papillae) caused by Epstein-Barr virus (EBV), treatable (if desired, not needed) by acyclovir.

53 (D) Bone marrow transplant from a human donor has NOT been developed as a human deficiency virus (HIV) treatment because the donor cells might be infected with HIV. Central goal of current HIV therapy is to reduce the viral load present in the body (measured by the HIV RNA copy number in the blood) by using highly active antiretroviral therapy (HAART); this includes reverse transcriptase inhibitors, such as AZT, D4T, ddI, or ddC, and one or more viral protease inhibitors and extends length of disease-free period of infection by suppressing viral replication and encouraging blood CD4+ count increases.

54 (B) IgG is present MAINLY during the secondary immune response. IgM is present MAINLY during primary immune response (first Ig produced), but the affinity of ALL antibody isotypes, including IgA, increases during secondary immune response, which for some vaccinations requires a "booster shot."

55 (C) Antigen presentation to CD4+ T cells occurs at many lymphoid sites. Necessary for the generation of immunity to T-dependent antigens and the activation of T-helper activity because CD4+ T cells CANNOT recognize soluble antigen. CD4+ T cells recognize antigen in combination with MHC molecules that are present on the antigen-presenting cell surface.

56 (C) Cytotoxic T-lymphocyte (CTL) activity is independent of antibody, but IgM activation of complement, antibody-dependent cell-mediated cytotoxicity (ADCC), and K cells all require antibody for role in cytotoxicity.

57 (A) Monoclonal antibodies are obtained from cultures of cloned cells; products of a single clone of B cells that react with a single antigenic determinant or epitope. Epitope, also known as antigenic determinant, is the part of a macromolecule that is recognized by the immune system, specifically by antibodies and B cells. Epitopes are useful as an antitumor treatment in some cases of leukemia.

58 (B) For the cases listed in A, C, and D, erythrocytes will carry either antigen (the A antigen for A) or antibodies (maternal anti-RhD for C; autoantibody for D), which results in positive hemagglutination test.

59 (B) Transplantation with stem cells (or stem cell–containing tissue) provides the ONLY mechanism for reconstituting the immune system with severe combined immunodeficiency (SCID). Administration of T cells ONLY puts patient at risk for graft-versus-host disease. Passive immunizations or cytokine injections have too limited an effect to provide significant benefit with SCID because all functional B and T cells are absent.

60 (D) Secretory component is produced by epithelial cells located near mucosal sites, becomes attached to IgA, and provides protection from degradation at mucous membranes (such as oral mucosa in oral cavity).

61 (C) Waldenström's macroglobulinemia is B-cell tumor characterized by overproduction of IgM, which in this case was observed on protein electrophoresis and isoelectric focusing. Hypogammaglobulinemia is B-cell deficiency, and DiGeorge syndrome is absence of the thymus, neither of which would result in elevated serum IgM.

62 (B) Multi-drug-resistant tuberculosis is ALWAYS associated with AIDS and is resistant to rifampin (Rifadin, Rimactane) and isoniazid (INH, Nydrazid). Trisomy 21 (Down syndrome) is a genetic disorder with extra chromosome 21. Affected persons have NO epicanthic eye fold, shorter stature, heart abnormalities, intellectual disability (mental retardation), and greater tendency to develop periodontal disease. Systemic lupus erythematosus (SLE) is chronic autoimmune disease of unknown cause. Skin lesions are MOST common sign of SLE (butterfly rash over nose, erythematous lesions on fingertips), and oral lesions include bleeding gingiva and reddened lesions with white striae radiating from center.

63 (D) HIV is commonly transmitted through contact with blood, from infected mother to unborn child or fetus (in utero), and through secretions of intimate sexual contact. HIV is transmitted ONLY through the exchange of body fluids (e.g., saliva, semen, vaginal secretions, blood). Casual contact with HIV-infected individual (carrying on conversation, standing nearby, riding in elevator) is NOT a risk factor for transmission of HIV virus.

64 (C) Staff immunizations against hepatitis B (HBV) are effective way to deter the transmission of communicable disease in the dental office. Human immunodeficiency (HIV) testing provides professional with ONLY momentary view of HIV status because detection of seroconversion takes several weeks to months and because test does NOT detect any other disease. Testing has NO impact on spread of communicable disease in the dental office. Discriminating against patients from perceived "high-risk" groups is illegal and unethical. One CANNOT tell whether a person is infected with HIV by appearance. Although knowing whether patient has acquired immunodeficiency syndrome (AIDS) may be important when considering treatment choices and regimens, knowing HIV status has NO effect on transmission of communicable disease in the dental office. Standard precautions protect BOTH patients and healthcare providers from infectious diseases transmissible in the dental office.

65 (D) Mouth rinsing using BOTH controls on an air-water syringe *increases* aerosolization of infectious agents in the treatment area. Others help to *reduce* airborne transmission of infectious agents.

66 (D) Contaminated protective clothing should be washed with hottest water temperatures available and dried at highest temperature the garment can withstand.

67 (B) Recommended flushing times are 3 to 5 minutes at beginning of the day (or if the unit has NOT been used for a few hours) and 20 to 30 seconds between patients. Longer rinse times are NOT harmful but are NOT an efficient use of time.

68 (A) Extracted teeth, blood-soaked sponges and gauze, sharps, and tissue removed from patients are considered biohazardous wastes. ALL others fall into category of biomedical waste.

69 (B) Biohazardous waste is treated differently from biomedical waste and MUST be incinerated, buried, or sterilized. Biomedical waste can be disposed of with regular trash.

70 (E) Hairy leukoplakia, candidiasis, Kaposi's sarcoma, and angular cheilitis are common oral manifestations of AIDS. Lichen planus is chronic inflammatory disease of unknown cause that is often associated with systemic diseases such as diabetes mellitus and hypertension but NOT commonly associated with AIDS.

71 (A) Communication is MAJOR barrier to care for patient with HIV/AIDS. Fear of healthcare providers' attitudes may prevent patient from fully disclosing health status. Transportation, economic, physical barriers may arise as patient becomes MORE debilitated with disease.

72 (C) Herpes simplex infection would NOT be considered an indicator of acquired immune deficiency syndrome (AIDS) unless herpes simplex infection persisted longer than 1 month. Others are IMPORTANT in AIDS diagnosis.

73 (A) Herpes zoster produces vesicle (blister) as a virus-infected, circumscribed, fluid-filled elevation in epithelium ≤1 cm in diameter. Acne can produce pustule, circumscribed elevation filled with purulent exudate resulting from infection. Pemphigus vulgaris produces bulla (plural, bullae); diameter of large vesicle is ≥1 cm. TRUE cysts result from entrapment of epithelium or remnants of epithelium that grow to produce a cavity, such as that of nasopalatine cyst; MUST be lined by epithelium.

74 (B) Acquired immune deficiency syndrome (AIDS) is NOT considered autoimmune disease because immune system is NOT attacking own tissues. Rather, AIDS is syndrome that develops as result of infection by human immunodeficiency virus (HIV).

75 (C) Recommended treatment for pseudomembranous candidiasis consists of either topical or systemic ingestion of an antifungal agent, such as nystatin (Mycostatin), ketoconazole (Nizoral), or fluconazole (Diflucan). Acyclovir (Zovirax) is an antiviral reserved for viral infections, and Lidex (fluocinonide), a corticosteroid, is often used to soothe the pain of oral ulcerations. Chlorhexidine (Periogard) is frequently prescribed in HIV/AIDS to assist in controlling the intraoral bacterial load.

CHAPTER 9

Pharmacology

PHARMACOLOGICAL PRINCIPLES AND CONCEPTS

Understanding a pharmacological effect on a patient and possible interaction with other drugs is essential to safe dental care. Thorough medical history helps identify adverse effects and potential drug interactions with current **prescription** (Rx) drugs, dental drugs, **over-the-counter** (OTC) drugs. Dental settings are advised to have the current *Physician's Desk Reference* (PDR) Index for reference information concerning drug information by brand and generic names, product categories, manufacturers.

- See CD-ROM for Chapter Terms and WebLinks.
- See Chapters 6, General and Oral Pathology: disease states; 14, Pain Management: physical classification system; 8, Microbiology and Immunology: antibiotics; 10, Medical and Dental Emergencies: allergy-related emergencies in a dental setting; 11, Clinical Treatment: contraindications, xerostomia.

A. Dosage:
1. Effective dose: produces 50% of maximum response or specific response in 50% of subjects (ED_{50}).
2. Lethal dose: kills 50% of subjects (LD_{50}); certainly lethal dose (CLD): amount of drug likely to cause death.
3. **Therapeutic index** (TI): measurement of safety (= LD_{50}/ED_{50}); larger the number, safer the drug.
4. **Maximum recommended dose** (MRD): established by manufacturer (in milligrams per pound).

B. Administration: latest is **time-released drug** with ingredients released at predictable rate:
1. Topical: local effect applied directly where action is desired; includes eye drops and ear drops, epicutaneous, enema, vaginal.
2. Enteral: desired effect is systemic (nonlocal), given by way of the digestive tract; includes oral, by tube, sublingual, rectal administration.
3. Parenteral: desired effect is systemic, given by routes other than digestive tract; includes transdermal, intradermal, intravenous (IV), subcutaneous (SC), intramuscular (IM), intrathecal, intraperitoneal, inhalation.

C. **Pharmacokinetics** ("ADME" scheme):
1. Absorption: process of a substance entering the body.
2. Distribution: dispersion or dissemination of substances throughout fluids and tissues of the body.
3. Metabolism: irreversible transformation of substance and its daughter metabolites.
4. Excretion: elimination of substances from the body.

D. **Indications** (therapeutic uses):
1. Valid reasons to use drug (test, drug, procedure, or surgery).
2. Strictly regulated by Food and Drug Administration (FDA).

E. Reactions to drugs:
1. **Potency:** strength of a drug in terms of ability to achieve particular result.
2. Produces BOTH desired (therapeutic effect) and adverse effects (reaction, side effect) on the body.
   a. Desired effect(s):
      (1) **Pharmacological effect**(s): act on target organs to achieve therapeutic response.
      (2) **Therapeutic effect**(s): dose related, predictable.
   b. Adverse effect(s) (reaction[s]):
      (1) **Side effect**(s) or unintended consequence(s) specifically arising from drug therapy; unpredictable and dose related (e.g., xerostomia [dry mouth], gingival hyperplasia).
      (2) Act on nontarget organs (e.g., vomiting with antibiotic erythromycin [Robimycin, E-Mycin, E.E.S.] and topical fluoride products).
   c. Interactions:
      (1) **Synergism:** combination action of two drugs gives a greater total effect than sum of individual drug's effects (e.g., codeine with acetaminophen for pain relief, alcohol and diazepam to cause respiratory depression).
      (2) **Agonist:** drug that causes an effect by interacting with a receptor.
      (3) **Antagonist:** drug that counteracts another drug's effect on a receptor (e.g., at neuromuscular junctions).
   d. **Tolerance:** Decreased susceptibility to effects of a drug because of repeated use (e.g., painkillers, intoxicants, or antibiotics); when occurs, MORE drug is needed to produce same pharmacological effects.

3. Toxicology:
   a. Unpredictable and dose related; acts on target organs and involves extended pharmacological effect(s) (e.g., hepatotoxicity with antineoplastic methotrexate [Rheumatrex Dose Pack, Trexall]).
   b. **Drug allergy** reaction(s): immunological response; NOT predictable or dose related; four types:
      (1) Type I (immediate hypersensitivity): occurs immediately (within minutes) after exposure to previously encountered antigen (e.g., allergy to penicillins [Pen-Vee K], preservative [sodium metabisulfite] for epinephrine in local anesthetics); can be life threatening if produces anaphylaxis, must activate emergency medical services (EMS) system.
      (2) Type II (cytolytic or cytotoxic): inhibits or prevents cell function; results in cell destruction; may be result of blood transfusion or drug-induced anemia.
      (3) Type III (Arthus): occurs within 6 to 8 hours after exposure (SIMILAR to serum sickness); symptoms include urticaria (hives, wheals), lymphadenopathy, fever (e.g., allergy to topical benzocaine, penicillins, sulfonamides).
      (4) Type IV (cell-mediated delayed hypersensitivity): occurs within 48 hours, results in an inflammatory reaction such as contact dermatitis (e.g., allergy to penicillins, poison ivy).
      (5) Idiosyncratic (individual) reactions: abnormal and have genetic causes.

F. **Contraindications:**
   1. Conditions and factors that increase risks involved in using particular drug (carrying out medical procedure or engaging in particular activity); may be absolute or relative; opposite of indication.
      a. Absolute contraindication: situation that makes particular treatment or procedure inadvisable. Example: aspirin [Bayer, Ecotrin, Empirin, Bufferin] is an absolute contraindication for an infant or child because of danger that it can cause Reye's syndrome; can substitute acetaminophen.
      b. Relative contraindication: situation that makes particular treatment or procedure somewhat inadvisable but does NOT rule it out. Example: nitrous oxide sedation during pregnancy is a relative contraindication because of concerns for developing child; should not be used unless deemed absolutely necessary because it is preferable to other general anesthetics; NOT classified in Pregnancy Risk Category (PRC); need medical consult (discussed later).

G. Excretion:
   1. MOST drugs are excreted by means of renal route.
   2. Extrarenal excretion routes include lungs, gastrointestinal (alimentary) tract (GIT), saliva, breast milk, sweat.
   3. Lactating: many drugs are excreted into breast milk, such as tetracyclines, and can affect newborn, medical consult needed; safest drugs SHOULD be considered.

Prescription Writing

Effective prescription writing requires accurate diagnosis; proper selection of drug, dosage form and route of administration; proper size and timing of dose; precise dispensing; accurate labeling; and correct packaging. Prescription is provided by a physician, osteopath, dentist, or other approved practitioner. Note that OTC drugs do not require a prescription but must be included with drug history.

A. Prescription form and written contents:
   1. Prescriber's full name, address, telephone number, DEA number (can be preprinted); group practices may contain multiple prescribers' names to be circled or checked.
   2. Superscription: dated order includes name, address, and age of patient; with symbol ℞ (means prescription, capital R with a cross on diagonal) that separates superscription from inscription.
   3. Inscription: body of prescription; contains name and amount and/or strength of each ingredient for prescribed drug.
   4. Subscription: directions to pharmacist in short sentence.
   5. Signatura (sig or signa, "write"): contains directions to patient; can be written out or abbreviations can be used (Table 9-1), with prescriber's signature.

Table 9-1 Pharmacological abbreviations for prescription writing

Abbreviation	Meaning
a.c.	Before meals
b.i.d.	Twice daily
h.s.	At bedtime
q.d.	Once per day
q.i.d.	4 times per day
q.o.d.	Every other day
q6h	Every 6 hours
p.c.	After meals
p.o.	By mouth
p.r.n.	As needed
sl.	Sublingual
stat	Immediately
supp	Suppository
t.i.d.	3 times per day
u.d.	As directed

Table 9-2 Controlled substances*

Schedule	Abuse potential	Medical use	Examples
I	High	None except research	Heroin, hallucinogens, opium derivatives
II: Requires prescription; nonrefillable	High (severe dependence possible)	Legal medical uses	Oxycodone, amphetamines, morphine
III: Requires prescription; five refills in 6 months	Lower than Schedule I and II drugs (moderate dependence possible)	Legal medical uses	Codeine, anabolic steroids
IV: Requires prescription; five refills in 6 months	Low (limited dependence possible)	Legal medical uses	Benzodiazepines, barbiturates
V: Requires prescription; five refills in 6 months	Lower than Schedule IV drugs	Legal medical uses	Codeine cough syrups

*Drug schedules (classifications) issued as part of the Controlled Substances Act in 1970. The Drug Enforcement Administration determines which drugs are added to and removed from the schedules.

6. Labeling: when drug name is to be included, "label" box is checked.
7. Refills: designated by number.
8. Proprietary (**brand name,** trade) vs. nonproprietary **(generic name):** indication of desire or willingness to dispense type of drug known by **chemical name** (brand, generic).
B. Laws affecting prescription writing by types of drugs:
   1. **Restricted drugs:** available without prescription but kept at pharmacy service counter because of labeling or abuse risk (e.g., drugs containing pseudoephedrine, such as Claritin-D).
   2. **Legend drugs:** may NOT be dispensed by a pharmacist without prescription from physician, osteopath, dentist, or other approved practitioner; FDA and state drugs are legend; label carries the legend, "Caution! Federal law prohibits dispensing without a prescription."
   3. **Controlled drugs:** require further safeguards for storage, in addition to requiring a prescription; refills are also limited; BOTH state and federal government agencies promulgate (make public) the regulations (see Table 9-2 for Controlled Substances Act).
      a. Federal agency is Drug Enforcement Administration (DEA).
      b. State agency is Division of Narcotics and Dangerous Drugs (DHHR).

DRUG EFFECTS ON AUTONOMIC NERVOUS SYSTEM

MANY drugs exert their effects on the autonomic nervous system (ANS). There are two ANS systems: sympathetic division (SANS) and parasymphathetic division (PANS).
• See Chapter 3, Anatomy, Biochemistry, and Physiology: ANS.

A. The SANS enables the body to function during emergencies or respond to stressful situations (engage in "fight-or-flight"):
   1. By means of the release of its neurotransmitters, which include norepinephrine and epinephrine.
   2. These neurotransmitters subsequently stimulate the SANS receptors, which include alpha (α)- and beta (β)-receptors:
      a. Stimulation of α-receptors causes vasoconstriction of the skin and skeletal muscles.
      b. Excitation of β_1-receptors causes stimulation of the heart muscle and glycogenolysis.
      c. Stimulation of β_2-receptors causes smooth muscle relaxation, which results in bronchodilation of the lungs.
B. The PANS enables the body to maintain bodily functions during normal daily activities (engage in "stay-and-play"):
   1. By means of the release of the neurotransmitter acetylcholine (ACh).
   2. The ACh subsequently stimulates its receptor sites (muscarinic and nicotinic) to enhance body function.
C. Prolonged stressful situations can cause chronic SANS stimulation and depression of PANS with diarrhea, constipation, difficulty maintaining sexual arousal, depressed immune system (see Chapter 16, Special Needs Patients: mental illness).

ADRENERGICS

Adrenergics stimulate α- and β-receptors and include epinephrine, levonordefrin, isoproterenol, ephedrine, dopamine III.
• See Chapters 11, Medical and Dental Emergencies: emergency kit for the dental setting; 14, Pain Management: vasoconstrictor use.
A. Pharmacological effects:
   1. Excitation of CNS.

2. Effects on cardiovascular system (CVS):
   a. Hypertension (high blood pressure [HBP]), dysrhythmias, tachycardia (increased pulse rate).
   b. Blood vessel vasodilation with β_2-receptors, vasoconstriction with α_1-receptors.
3. Hyperglycemia from β_1 stimulation increases glycogenolysis, decreases release of insulin.
4. Bronchodilation, mydriasis (pupil dilation), xerostomia (dry mouth).

B. Therapeutic uses:
1. Vasoconstriction:
   a. Increases duration of local anesthetic actions and decreases systemic location and toxicity.
   b. Controls bleeding through hemostasis, nasal decongestants (due to α-receptors).
2. Treatment of cardiac arrest by epinephrine (because of β_1-stimulation).
3. Bronchodilation (because of β_2-receptors) for treatment of asthma and emphysema.
4. Stimulation of central nervous system (CNS) by methylphenidate (Ritalin) or pemoline (Cylert) for treating attention deficit–hyperactivity disorder (ADHD).

C. Adverse reactions:
1. CNS stimulation, resulting in anxiety and tremors.
2. Heart palpitations and dysrhythmias.
3. HBP (if drug affects α-receptors).

D. Drug interactions:
1. Decreased pressor effect with haloperidol, phenothiazines, thioxanthenes, diuretics.
2. Cardiac dysrhythmias with halogenated general anesthetics, cardiac glycosides, tricyclic antidepressants (TCAs).
3. HBP with β-blockers from blocking β-adrenergic effects of epinephrine.

E. Contraindications:
1. Narrow-angle glaucoma from an increase in intraocular pressure.
2. Cardiac dysrhythmias.

ADRENERGIC BLOCKERS

Adrenergic blockers inhibit α- and β-receptors, including (1) α-adrenergic blockers such as tolazoline (Priscoline) and phentolamine (Regitine); (2) β-adrenergic blockers, including nonspecific blockers such as propranolol (Inderal) and nadolol (Corgard) and specific blockers such as metoprolol (Lopressor) and atenolol (Tenormin); (3) α- and β-adrenergic blockers such as labetalol (Normodyne, Trandate). See later discussion of patient with CVD.

A. Pharmacological effects:
1. α-Blockers inhibit vasoconstriction in blood vessels (α-receptor effects).
2. β-Blockers competitively block the effects of adrenergics on β-receptors and may inhibit specific β-receptors or be nonspecific receptor site inhibitor.

B. Therapeutic uses:
1. α-Blockers:
   a. Peripheral vascular disease (PAD) or Raynaud's syndrome.
   b. Pheochromocytoma, catecholamine-secreting tumor of adrenal medulla.
2. β-Blockers and α_1-selective blockers:
   a. HBP, angina pectoris, dysrhythmias, migraine headaches, alcohol withdrawal, myocardial infarction (MI, heart attack) prophylaxis, anxiety syndromes.

C. Adverse reactions:
1. Few occur because receptor effects are MORE site specific.
2. Xerostomia, nausea, vomiting.
3. Hypotension (low blood pressure).

D. Drug interactions (see also antiadrenergics under antihypertensives):
1. Effects of β-blockers:
   a. Decreased by sympathomimetics, nonsteroidal antiinflammatory drugs (NSAIAs/NSAIDS), rifampin (Rifadin, Rimactane).
   b. Increased by calcium channel blockers.

E. Contraindications:
1. Hypersensitivity, asthma.
2. Congestive heart failure (CHF).

CHOLINERGICS

Cholinergics stimulate body functions by direct action (choline esters) or indirect action (inhibition of acetylcholinesterase). Include pilocarpine (Salagen) and bethanechol (Urecholine).

A. Pharmacological effects:
1. Effects on the CVS:
   a. Bradycardia (slow pulse rate), hypotension (direct effect on heart), tachycardia (rapid pulse rate).
   b. HBP (indirect effect on blood vessels).
2. Nausea, diarrhea, dyspepsia (indigestion).
3. Miosis (pupil constriction), decreased intraocular pressure.

B. Therapeutic uses:
1. Xerostomia.
2. Glaucoma by decreasing intraocular pressure.
3. Urinary retention after surgery by increasing secretions and activity of GIT.
4. Myasthenia gravis (MG) by decreasing muscle weakness.

C. Adverse reactions: increased salivation, lacrimation, urination, defecation.

D. Drug interactions:
1. Reduced effects with anticholinergics.
2. Enhanced effects with cholinergics.

E. Contraindications:
1. Severe cardiovascular disease (CVD) from its CVS effects.

2. Peptic ulcer, asthma, obstruction of GIT or urinary tract by increasing secretions.
3. Uncontrolled hyperthyroidism, with impaired drug metabolism.
4. Patients with MG taking cholinesterase inhibitors (neostigmine [Prostigmin]).

ANTICHOLINERGICS

Anticholinergics (parasympathomimetics) inhibit body functions by blocking muscarinic cholinergic receptors. Include atropine (oral, Sal-Tropine; ophthalmic, Atropair) and propantheline bromide (Pro-Banthine).
A. Pharmacological effects:
　1. The CNS effects are dose dependent:
　　a. High doses result in stimulation.
　　b. Therapeutic doses result in depression.
　2. The CVS effects are dose dependent:
　　a. High doses result in tachycardia (vagal blockade).
　　b. Small doses result in bradycardia.
　3. Smooth muscle relaxation results in bronchodilation and constipation.
　4. Exocrine gland by reducing secretions in the respiratory tract, genitourinary tract, GIT.
　5. Include mydriasis and cycloplegia (blurred vision).
B. Therapeutic uses:
　1. Preoperative drug to inhibit salivary and bronchial secretions, producing dry field.
　2. Eye examinations with relaxation of the lens and mydriasis.
　3. Blocking of vagal slowing of the heart in response to general anesthetics.
　4. Parkinson-like tremors caused by smooth muscle relaxation from antipsychotics.
　5. Motion sickness; also sleep aid with depression of CNS.
　6. GIT disorders with decreasing secretions and hypermotility (e.g., gastric ulcers).
C. Adverse reactions:
　1. Xerostomia, photophobia (light sensitivity), cycloplegia (paralysis of the lens).
　2. Signs of CNS stimulation, tachycardia, hyperpyrexia (high fever).
　3. Urinary and GIT stasis.
D. Drug interactions:
　1. Increased anticholinergic effects with TCAs, antihistamines, antidepressants, opioids, antipsychotics.
　2. Decreased absorption of ketoconazole (Nizoral).
E. Contraindications:
　1. Prostatic hypertrophy or intestinal or urinary obstruction or retention because drug increases urinary retention.
　2. For CVD because of tachycardia, vagal blockade.
　3. Glaucoma (narrow-angle) from an increase in intraocular pressure.

ANXIETY AND PAIN MANAGEMENT

Management of pain and anxiety during dental treatment uses antianxiety drugs, analgesics, anesthetics, sedatives.

Antianxiety Drugs

Main purpose of antianxiety (tranquilizer) drugs is to decrease anxiety through depression of the CNS. Drugs are also noted with therapeutic uses.
A. Benzodiazepines (BZDs) (suffixes "-lam," "-pam"):
　1. Pharmacological effects:
　　a. Antianxiety and anticonvulsant effects and muscle relaxation.
　　b. Anterograde amnesia (temporary memory impairment).
　　c. Wide therapeutic index makes overdose poisoning rare (compared with barbiturates).
　2. Therapeutic uses:
　　a. Anxiety associated with depression and panic attacks with diazepam (Valium), alprazolam (Xanax), temazepam (Restoril), triazolam (Halcion).
　　b. Insomnia by means of CNS depression with flurazepam (Dalmane).
　　c. Alcohol withdrawal (agitation, tremors [delirium tremens, DTs]) with chlordiazepoxide (Librium), lorazepam (Ativan), oxazepam (Serax).
　　d. Epileptic seizures with clonazepam (Klonopin), diazepam (Valium).
　　e. <u>Antianxiety premedication</u> in dentistry with diazepam (Valium) or alprazolam (Xanax); also memory loss of stressful dental procedures.
　3. Adverse reactions:
　　a. Xerostomia.
　　b. Depression of CNS, which results in sedation and fatigue.
　　c. Thrombophlebitis, if given IV.
　　d. Possible physical and psychological addiction; occurs less often than with barbiturates.
　　e. Possible teratogenicity, especially during first trimester.
　4. Drug interactions:
　　a. Increased effects with alcohol and CNS depressants.
　　b. Decreased effects with smoking.
　　c. Avoid with antifungals.
　　d. Increases effects of digoxin (Lanoxin) and phenytoin (Dilantin) (particularly with clonazepam [Klonopin]).
　5. Contraindications:
　　a. Drug addiction, narrow-angle glaucoma, hypersensitivity, pregnancy.
　　b. Psychosis (experience CNS stimulation), chronic pain (because of possible abuse and addiction).

B. Barbiturates (among first antianxiety drugs):
  1. Classified (by length of action):
     a. Ultrashort acting: methohexital (Brevital) and thiopental sodium (Pentothal).
     b. Short acting: pentobarbital (Nembutal) and secobarbital (Seconal).
     c. Intermediate acting: amobarbital (Amytal) and butabarbital (Butisol).
     d. Long acting: phenobarbital (Luminal).
  2. Pharmacological effects:
     a. Depression of CNS, which results in sedation.
        (1) Higher doses result in greater CNS depression, including respiratory and CVS depression.
     b. Anticonvulsant effect.
     c. Stimulate microsomal liver enzymes to stimulate metabolism of other drugs metabolized by liver.
  3. Therapeutic uses (by duration of action):
     a. Ultrashort-acting barbiturates: short-term general anesthesia.
     b. Short-acting and intermediate acting barbiturates: replaced by benzodiazepines for antianxiety and insomnia.
     c. Long-acting barbiturates: treatment of seizures with epilepsy.
  4. Adverse reactions:
     a. Like alcohol, barbiturates are intoxicating:
        (1) Mild: slurred speech, loss of coordination, stumbling, staggering, shallow breathing, fatigue, frequent yawning, irritability.
        (2) High: unpredictable emotional reactions and mental confusion, severely impaired judgment, mood swings.
     b. Mental effects depend on amount and strength; person falls asleep but drug remains in system for long time.
  5. Drug interactions:
     a. Decreased effects of acetaminophen (Tylenol), β-blockers, oral contraceptives, doxycycline (Vibramycin), phenytoin (Dilantin), steroids, TCAs, warfarin (Coumadin).
     b. Increased effects with disulfiram, monoamine oxidase inhibitors (MAOIs), propoxyphene (Darvon).
     c. Increased CNS depression with alcohol and other CNS depressants.
  6. Contraindications:
     a. Hypersensitivity.
     b. Porphyria (excess amount of porphyrins); can stimulate and increase the production of porphyrins.
     c. Chronic pain and drug addiction (because of risk of further abuse and addiction).
C. Chloral hydrate (orally): sedation of children.
D. Meprobamate: dental anxiety disorders and as muscle relaxant for acute temporomandibular disorders (TMD) with muscle spasms.
E. Zolpidem (Ambien): nonbenzodiazepine sedative hypnotic that is used as short-term sleep aid for insomnia: SAME adverse effects and drug interactions as other sedatives.

CLINICAL STUDY

Age	45 YRS		SCENARIO
Sex	☒ Male ☐ Female		The patient is scheduled for an oral prophylaxis today. He has generalized dental biofilm and slight calculus deposits throughout, with only slight to moderate gingivitis.
BP	105/57		
Chief Complaint	"I hate being here but I know that I have to keep up my mouth."		
Medical History	Myasthenia gravis (MG) Rheumatoid arthritis (RA)		
Current Medications	prednisone (Deltasone) 20 mg qod neostigmine (Prostigmin) 5 mg qd diazepam (Valium) 10 mg before dental appointments		
Social History	Science fiction writer		

1. What types of drugs are prednisone (Deltasone) and neostigmine (Prostigmin), and why is he taking them?
2. What type of drug is diazepam (Valium)? Identify its common uses.
3. What are the oral signs of MG that are possible for him?

4. Why does the patient especially need to avoid stress that a dental appointment might bring on, as well as avoid any dental infections?

1. Prednisone (Deltasone) is a corticosteroid, antiinflammatory drug. It treats various diseases of allergic,

inflammatory, autoimmune origin. Patient takes prednisone to treat RA, an inflammatory joint disease. Neostigmine (Prostigmin) is an anticholinesterase muscle stimulant that markedly improves muscle strength by improving muscle contraction; he takes it to treat MG, disease of muscular weakness.

2. Diazepam (Valium) is a benzodiazepine (BZD), antianxiety, anticonvulsive drug. He takes it as an antianxiety premedication to help cope with dental anxiety.

3. MG affects facial and cervical musculature, leading to loss of control of facial muscles and resulting in difficulty with smiling, eating, swallowing, speaking, vision; when severe, can cause respiratory distress.

4. Crisis can occur as result of infection (oral included), emotional stress (such as dental care), and surgery. It could involve a myasthenic crisis, which includes loss of swallowing and speaking ability and difficulty breathing and seeing; caused by undermedication, underlying illness, risk factors, or worsening of disease. Or it could involve a cholinergic crisis: related to overmedication with anticholinesterase, occurs within hour of drug use, causes increased muscle weakness, gastrointestinal upset, respiratory difficulties. Both crises require the dental office to provide basic life support and activate EMS system.

Analgesics

Analgesics inhibit perception of pain. Nonopioids reduce pain perception by inhibiting prostaglandin synthesis; MORE effective if they are taken before onset of pain. Opioids depress pain perception in CNS by binding with opioid receptors (Tables 9-3, 9-4, and 9-5).

- See Chapter 11, Medical and Dental Emergencies: emergency kit (aspirin).
A. Nonopioids:
  1. Salicylates: aspirin (Bayer, Ecotrin, Empirin, Bufferin) and long-acting diflunisal (Dolobid).
     a. Pharmacological effects:
        (1) Analgesia for mild-to-moderate pain relief; antipyretic effect (reduces fever).
        (2) Antiinflammatory effect (from inhibition of prostaglandin synthesis), decreases vasodilation and swelling.
        (3) Antiplatelet effect (from reduction of platelet aggregation), results in reduced clotting.
        (4) Uricosuric effect; high doses (MORE than 5 g/24 hours) cause increase in uric acid secretion in urine.
     b. Therapeutic uses:
        (1) Analgesia for mild-to-moderate pain.
        (2) Reduction of fever (antipyretic effect).

Table 9-3 Drug interactions with commonly used analgesics

Drug	Interactions
NSAIA	Decrease antihypertensive effects of ACE inhibitors (captopril), beta blockers, loop diuretics, and thiazide diuretics Increase effects of anticoagulants Increase effects of digoxin Increase effects of phenytoin Increase effects of lithium Increase methotrexate toxicity Increase effects of sympathomimetics Nephrotoxicity with cyclosporine Probenecid increases NSAIA concentrations Salicylates decrease NSAIA concentrations
Salicylates (aspirin [Bayer, Ecotrin, Empirin, Bufferin])	Alcohol increases gastrointestinal ulceration and bleeding time Corticosteroids decrease salicylate concentrations Decrease antihypertensive effects of ACE inhibitors (captopril), beta blockers, loop diuretics, and thiazide diuretics Decrease NSAIA concentrations Decrease uricosuric effect of probenecid and sulfinpyrazone Increase effects of anticoagulants Increase effect of sulfonylureas and exogenous insulin, thereby increasing hypoglycemic effect Dose >2 g per day displaces VA from binding site, thereby increasing VA effect Nizatidine increases salicylate concentrations
Acetaminophen (Tylenol)	Alcohol increases hepatotoxicity Beta blocker (propranolol) increases effects of acetaminophen Oral contraceptives decrease half-life

ACE, Angiotensin converting enzyme; *NSAIA,* nonsteroidal antiinflammatory agent; *VA,* valproic acid.

Table 9-4   Nonopioids: comparison of analgesic efficacy

Drug	Dose (mg)	Dosing interval (hr)	Peak (hr)
Acetaminophen (Tylenol)	325-650	4-6	0.5-2
Aspirin (Bayer, Ecotrin, Empirin, Bufferin)	650	4-6	1-2
Ibuprofen (Advil, Motrin, Pamprin)	400	4-6	1-2
Diflunisal (Dolobid)	Loading dose: 1000; subsequent doses: 500	8-12	1-2
Naproxen sodium (Aleve, Anaprox)	250-500	6-8	2-3

Table 9-5   Analgesic drug combinations and uses

Drug name	Opioid component	Nonopioid component	Dental use
Hydrocodone a/APAP (Bancap HC, Dolacet, Vicodin)	Hydrocodone	Acetaminophen	Mild to moderate pain; posttreatment pain control
Acetaminophen w/codeine (Capital w/codeine, Phenaphen w/codeine, Tylenol w/codeine)	Codeine	Acetaminophen	Mild to moderate pain; posttreatment pain control
Propoxyphene N/APAP (Darvocet-N 100, Wygesic, Roxicet)	Propoxyphene napsylate	Acetaminophen	Mild to moderate pain; posttreatment pain control
Percocet (Tylox)	Oxycodone	Acetaminophen	Moderate to severe pain; posttreatment of postoperative pain
Hydrocodone w/aspirin (Lortab ASA, Alora 5/500, Azdone)	Hydrocodone	Aspirin	Mild to moderate pain; posttreatment pain control
Oxycodone w/aspirin (Percodan, Codoxy, Percodan-Demi, Roxiprin)	Oxycodone	Aspirin	Moderate to severe pain; posttreatment of postoperative pain

(3) Reduction of pain and swelling (antiinflammatory effect); also treats inflammatory conditions such as arthritis.

(4) Prevention of post–myocardial infarction (MI, heart attack) (because of antiplatelet effect) at low-dose (LD) levels.

c. Adverse reactions:

   (1) GIT irritation, MOST common (caused by *direct* irritation of stomach mucosa).

   (2) Bleeding levels monitored by international normalized ratio (INR); INRs ≤2.5 are safe for invasive dental work; older test is prothrombin time (PT).

   (3) Asthmatics; use acetaminophen (FIRST choice) as substitute for its analgesic and antipyretic effects to avoid aspirin-induced attack.

d. Drug interactions:

   (1) Increased risk of bleeding with anticoagulants.

(2) Increased risk of GIT complaints with NSAIAs, corticosteroids, alcohol.

(3) Increased risk of hypoglycemia with oral antidiabetics.

(4) Decreased effects of gout drugs such as probenecid (Benemid, Probalan) and sulfinpyrazone (Anturan).

(5) Increased risk of toxicity with methotrexate (Rheumatrex Dose Pack, Trexall), lithium (Lithobid, Eskalith), zidovudine (AZT; Retrovir).

e. Contraindications:

   (1) Hypersensitivity.

   (2) GIT bleeding and bleeding disorders (because of GIT irritation and antiplatelet effect); peptic ulcers (because of GIT irritation).

   (3) Children with flulike symptoms (Reye's syndrome [abnormal accumulations of fat begin to develop in the liver and other

organs of the body, along with a severe increase of pressure in the brain] can occur during some viral infections).

   (4) Can be toxic if larger doses taken, especially if expired (will smell like vinegar).

2. NSAIAs (NSAIDs): naproxen (Naprosyn; OTC: Aleve, Anaprox), ibuprofen (OTC: Advil, Motrin, Pamprin), etodolac (Lodine), ketorolac (Toradol), indomethacin (Indocin), celecoxib (Celebrex).

   a. Pharmacological effects:

      (1) Analgesic, antipyretic, antiinflammatory effects SIMILAR to aspirin (Bayer, Ecotrin, Empirin, Bufferin).

   b. Therapeutic uses: control of mild to moderate pain, fever, inflammatory conditions such as RA.

   c. Adverse reactions:

      (1) Stomach mucosa irritation SIMILAR to aspirin's effect on GIT; xerostomia.

      (2) Inhibition of platelets; occur ONLY for drug's duration.

      (3) Depression of the CNS, including sedation, dizziness, depression.

      (4) Teratogenicity (can interfere with closure of ductus of fetal heart [ductus arteriosus]).

   d. Drug interactions:

      (1) Decreased effects of antihypertensives.

      (2) Increased effects of oral anticoagulants, lithium (Lithobid, Eskalith), digoxin (Lanoxin), phenytoin (Dilantin), sympathomimetics.

      (3) Increased risk of toxicity with methotrexate (Rheumatrex Dose Pack, Trexall) and cyclosporine.

      (4) Raises serum concentration of hypoglycemic agents.

      (5) May cause GIT ulcers with corticosteroids.

   e. Contraindications:

      (1) Hypersensitivity to ANY antiinflammatory drugs.

      (2) Blood clotting problems (because of antiplatelet effect).

      (3) Renal disease (caused by higher risk of adverse renal reactions); GIT disorders, such as peptic ulcer; asthma.

      (4) Celecoxib (Celebrex) is a COX II inhibitor: increased risk of MI/CVA (cardiovascular accident, stroke) but can be taken with low-dose aspirin (Bayer, Ecotrin, Empirin, Bufferin).

3. Acetaminophen (*N*-acetyl-para-amino-phenol [NAPP]; OTC: Tylenol).

   a. Pharmacological effects:

      (1) Analgesic and antipyretic effects SIMILAR to aspirin (Bayer, Ecotrin, Empirin, Bufferin) and NSAIAs.

      (2) Little or NO antiinflammatory effect occurs (UNLIKE other NSAIAs).

   b. Therapeutic uses: reduction of mild to moderate pain and fever; as substitute for its analgesic and antipyretic effects to avoid aspirin-induced attack in asthmatics.

   c. Adverse reactions:

      (1) Hepatotoxicity and nephrotoxicity (associated with long-term use, excessively high doses).

         (a) Minimum toxic dose is 10 g (140 mg/kg), but liver damage occurs with one 5.85-g dose.

         (b) Chronic excessive use (MORE than 4 g/day) can cause transient hepatotoxicity.

         (c) Safe dose for chronic alcoholics should NOT exceed 4 g/day; should be 2 g/day or less if hepatotoxicity has occurred (occurs in some chronic alcoholics who take the therapeutic dose).

   d. Drug interactions: rare at therapeutic doses.

   e. Contraindications:

      (1) Hypersensitivity.

      (2) Hepatic and renal disease.

B. Opioids: morphine (MS Contin), hydromorphone (Dilaudid), meperidine (Demerol), propoxyphene (Darvon), codeine (various cough preparations), oxycodone (OxyContin; with acetaminophen [Percocet], with aspirin [Percodan]) (Table 9-4).

1. Pharmacological effects:

   a. Analgesic effect for relief of moderate to severe pain; sedative effect for relief of mild anxiety.

   b. Antitussive effect (cough suppression); antidiarrheal effect (caused by increase in smooth muscle tone in GIT); constipating.

   c. Depress CNS by interacting with opioid receptors.

2. Therapeutic uses: analgesia for moderate to severe pain, cough suppression, sedation, anxiety relief.

3. Adverse reactions are related to the drug's potency (greater potency, greater risk of adverse reactions):

   a. Addicting; can be abused.

   b. Drowsiness, sedation, and (occasionally) stimulation; decreased rate and depth of respiration (causing death with overdose).

   c. Increased intracranial pressure (because of cranial vasodilation); bradycardia and orthostatic hypotension.

   d. Nausea, emesis (vomiting), constipation; urinary retention.

   e. Miosis (pupil constriction); may be used to determine abuse or overdose.

4. Drug interactions: increased sedation and respiratory depression with other CNS depressants such as MAOIs, TCAs, alcohol.
5. Contraindications:
   a. Hypersensitivity.
   b. Respiratory problems, including asthma and emphysema (because of respiratory center depression).
   c. Chronic pain (abuse and addiction may occur).
   d. Head injury (caused by increase in intracranial pressure).
C. Semisynthetic opioids: hydrocodone (Vicodin, Lorcet):
   1. Derived from two of the naturally occurring opiates, codeine or thebaine.
   2. Combined with paracetamol (acetaminophen, Tylenol), aspirin (Bayer, Ecotrin, Empirin, Bufferin), ibuprofen (Advil, Motrin, Pamprin), homatropine methylbromide (hydrocodone compounds).
   3. Purpose of the noncontrolled drugs in combination:
      a. Provide increased analgesia because of synergy.
      b. Limit intake by causing unpleasant and often unsafe side effects at higher than prescribed doses.
   4. Pharmacological effects and therapeutic uses: narcotic analgesic and antitussive.
   5. Adverse so reactions, drug interactions, contraindications: SAME as opioids.
      a. Addicting, so can be abused.
      b. Liver problems caused by larger amounts of acetaminophen (Tylenol).
D. Opioid antagonists:
   1. Short-acting naloxone (Narcan): used to reverse respiratory depression caused by opioids.
   2. Long-acting naltrexone (ReVia, Trexan): used for opioid addiction after detoxification.

Anesthetics and Sedatives

Anesthetic, local (with or without vasoconstrictors) and systemic, as well as sedatives to control pain.
• See Chapter 14, Pain Management: local anesthetics, vasoconstrictors, drug for reversal of local anesthesia, nitrous oxide sedation.
A. Local anesthetics:
   1. Pharmacological effects:
      a. Reversibly blocked peripheral nerve conduction.
      b. Depressed cardiac conduction and excitability that results in hypotension.
   2. Therapeutic uses:
      a. Topical: 20% benzocaine (preinjection or surgical gel, liquid, or spray, Americaine, Lanacaine, Hurricane; oral gel, Anbesol, Orajel) and 5% lidocaine (preinjection or surgical gel, Topicaine; patch, Lidoderm; preinjection or anesthetic cream 2.5% with prilocaine 2.5%, EMLA):

(1) Esters can result in topical allergies (from PABA) (see earlier discussion).
(2) Overall, can increase plasma levels with overuse and lead to toxicity.
   b. Periodontal gel: 2.5% lidocaine, 2.5% prilocaine (Oraqix) for site-specific soft tissue anesthesia; *see state regulation if can be used by dental hygienist:*
      (1) LOW levels in plasma, NO allergenic potential; MRD 5 cartridges or 8.5 mg, with 1 cartridge usually used per quadrant.
      (2) Used with caution in patients with severe impairment of renal or hepatic function; NOT used with pregnant woman or under age 18.
      (3) Indications: nonsurgical periodontal therapy, substitution for injection when injection is contraindicated.
      (4) Technique:
         (a) Apply on gingival margin around selected teeth using blunt-tipped applicator; wait 30 seconds and fill periodontal pockets until becomes visible.
         (b) Wait another 30 seconds before starting treatment.
   c. Lidocaine transoral delivery system (Denti-Patch): 46.1 mg of lidocaine for site-specific soft tissue anesthesia.
      (1) Onset of action is 5 to 10 minutes; duration of action is ~45 minutes.
      (2) Indications: preinjection anesthesia (especially in palatal areas), nonsurgical periodontal therapy, substitution for injection when injection is contraindicated.
      (3) Technique:
         (a) Remove plastic backing.
         (b) Isolate and dry targeted area for 30 seconds.
         (c) Apply with pressure for 30 seconds.
   d. Injected for soft and hard tissue anesthesia:
      (1) Esters:
         (a) Procaine (Novocaine) and propoxycaine.
         (b) Withdrawn from market (because of increased allergenic potential).
      (2) Amides:
         (a) Shorter-acting injectables: 2% lidocaine (Xylocaine, Anestacaine), 2% and 3% mepivacaine (Carbocaine), 4% prilocaine (Citanest), 4% articaine (Septocaine, Zorcaine).
         (b) Longer-acting injectables: 2% bupivacaine (Marcaine), 1.5% etidocaine (Duranest).

3. Adverse reactions:
   a. Talkativeness, apprehension, tremors, seizures (sometimes followed by CNS depression, respiratory and CVS depression, coma).
   b. Hematoma at site of injection (especially if piercing pterygoid plexus of veins, maxillary artery).
   c. Allergy, ranging from a rash to anaphylaxis; allergic reactions to esters occur MORE often than those to amides; if there is an allergy to BOTH esters and amides, first-generation antihistamine diphenhydramine (Benadryl) can be used for a local anesthetic effect.
   d. Metabolism of amides occurs primarily in liver; esters hydrolyzed by pseudocholinesterase, a plasma enzyme.
   e. BOTH amides and esters are excreted by kidneys.
4. Drug interactions: additive effect with CNS depressants.
5. Contraindications:
   a. Hypersensitivity; sulfite compounds in articaine (Septocaine, Zorcaine).
   b. May cause allergic reactions in asthmatics and/or sensitivity to sulfites.
B. Vasoconstrictors (inclusion in some local anesthetics): epinephrine, levonordefrin (Neo-Cobefrin).
1. Pharmacological effects:
   a. Cardiac stimulation and lipolysis in response to β_1-receptor stimulation.
   b. Bronchodilation in response to β_2-receptor stimulation.
   c. Epinephrine causes vasoconstriction of blood vessels in response to α_1 receptor stimulation.
2. Adverse reactions: tremors, anxiety, palpitations, HBP.
3. Therapeutic effects:
   a. Epinephrine is available with ALL amides EXCEPT mepivacaine, which is available ONLY with levonordefrin (Carbocaine with Neo-Cobefrin).
      (1) Available at 1:20,000 (with levonordefrin), 1:50,000, 1:100,000, 1:200,000 (with epinephrine).
      (2) An MRD of 0.2 mg per appointment for healthy patients.
      (3) Used MAINLY at 1:100,000 for nerve blocks and 1:50,000 for infiltrations; higher levels do NOT increase effectiveness, only hemorrhage control.
   b. Increased duration of local anesthetics because of decreased absorption into CVS.
   c. Decreased absorption of local anesthetics into CVS because of blood vessel constriction.
   d. Epinephrine has hemostatic properties (stoppage of bleeding) by blood vessel constriction.

4. Drug interactions:
   a. HBP, when used in conjunction with nonselective β-blockers.
   b. Vasoconstriction is enhanced with TCAs when epinephrine is given IV.
   c. Increase in blood glucose with oral antidiabetics.
5. Contraindications:
   a. Absolute: hypersensitivity to sulfite compounds that serve as preservative antioxidants may cause allergic reactions in asthmatics and/or sensitivity to sulfites (red wine, aged cheese).
   b. Relative: CVD patient who undergoes elective dental treatment should:
      (1) Receive a local anesthetic with a vasoconstrictor to increase pain control and its duration, which lowers patient stress level (decreasing endogenous epinephrine).
      (2) Receive an MRD of 0.04 mg of vasoconstrictor per appointment (equal to one cartridge of 1:50,000, two cartridges of 1:100,000, or 4 cartridges of 1:200,000).
C. General anesthetics:
1. Pharmacological effects: depress CNS.
   a. Guedel's stages:
      (1) Stage I: analgesia (reduced pain sensation).
      (2) Stage II: delirium and excitement (unconsciousness and involuntary movement).
      (3) Stage III: surgical anesthesia.
      (4) Stage IV: respiratory and medullary paralysis (death occurs if NOT reversed).
   b. Flagg's phases (BETTER description of anesthesia levels):
      (1) Induction phase: occurs before surgery.
      (2) Maintenance phase: begins when depth of anesthesia necessary for operation is achieved; continues until procedure is completed.
      (3) Recovery phase: occurs at end of operation, continues through postoperative period until patient is fully responsive.
2. Adverse reactions:
   a. Dysrhythmias, cardiac arrest, HBP, hypotension.
   b. Respiratory depression and arrest.
   c. Teratogenicity, with chronic exposure.
   d. Hepatotoxicity, with chronic exposure.
D. General anesthetics:
1. Nitrous oxide, inhalation gas (relatively odorless, colorless).
   a. Pharmacological effects:
      (1) Analgesia and amnesia, affecting the CNS, with NO significant effect on the respiratory system.
      (2) Used instead in MOST cases for mild to moderate (conscious) sedation and NOT

at usual general anesthetic levels (less than 50%, standard of care) during nonsurgical dental treatment.

b. Adverse reactions:
   (1) Peripheral vasodilation.
   (2) Nausea and vomiting, especially if patient consumes large meal before.
   (3) Diffusion hypoxia may result in headache or other adverse reactions if patient does NOT receive 5 minutes of 100% oxygen when sedation is terminated.
   (4) Neuropathy and paresthesia result with abuse; symptoms include numbness of hands and legs, as well as liver and kidney problems.
   (5) Inhalation volatile liquids.

c. Absolute contraindications:
   (1) Recent ophthalmic surgery during which gas was administered (C3F8, perfluoropropane or SF6, sulfur hexafluoride).
       (a) Gas bubble in the eye is associated with perfluoropropane use within the past 8 weeks or with sulfur hexafluoride use within the past 14 days.
       (b) Can disrupt the bubble and cause blindness.
   (2) Cystic fibrosis.
   (3) Lack of patient cooperation or existence of communication barrier (such as differing language).
   (4) Patients with head trauma or shock.
   (5) Patients who fear nitrous oxide or those who must ALWAYS be in control (NEVER talk anyone into use).

d. Relative contraindications:
   (1) Respiratory obstruction and congested airway (NO exchange of gas possible through nasal passages).
   (2) Chronic obstructive pulmonary disease (COPD) (CANNOT tolerate receiving additional oxygen).
   (3) Emotional instability, mental illness (altered sense or euphoria may occur); poor patient communication.
   (4) Pregnancy because of concerns for developing fetus unless it is absolutely necessary because other general anesthetics cannot be used; NOT classified in Pregnancy Risk Category (PRC); chronic exposure reduces fertility in women; spontaneous abortion or miscarriage may occur.
   (5) Contagious disease (e.g., tuberculosis, hepatitis) if nonautoclavable tubes are used.

2. Benzodiazepines (BZDs): diazepam (Valium), midazolam (Versed):

a. Pharmacological effects: used IV for conscious sedation, short-duration sedation; often used for oral surgery; also used as adjunctive drug in balanced anesthesia technique or for antianxiety premedication before appointment.
b. Adverse reactions: thrombophlebitis with diazepam (Valium); using water-soluble midazolam (Versed) reduces risk.

3. Halogenated ether, enflurane (Ethrane).
a. Pharmacological effects: produces greater skeletal muscle relaxation than halothane.
b. Adverse reactions:
   (1) Respiratory depression, hypotension, myocardial contractility depression.
   (2) Dysrhythmias (occur less often than with halothane).
   (3) Depressed renal function.
   (4) Possible seizure activity.

4. Halogenated hydrocarbon, halothane (Fluothane).
a. Pharmacological effects:
   (1) Fruity odor; is nonflammable, nonexplosive.
   (2) Safe for asthmatics because does NOT irritate bronchioles.
b. Adverse reactions:
   (1) Incomplete muscle relaxation; depression of renal function.
   (2) Uterine muscle relaxation; possible bradycardia, hypotension, dysrhythmias.

5. Halogenated ether, isoflurane (Forane).
a. Pharmacological effects:
   (1) Does NOT cause liver toxicity.
b. Adverse reactions:
   (1) Respiratory depression, hypotension, muscle relaxation.
   (2) Deeper levels of anesthesia result in respiratory acidosis.

6. Ultrashort-acting IV barbiturates: thiopental (Pentothal), methohexital (Brevital), thiamylal (Surital):
a. Pharmacological effects: IV results in rapid onset of action; barbiturates are NOT analgesics; local anesthetics are required for pain control.
b. Adverse reactions: bronchospasm, laryngospasm, hiccups, increased muscle activity, delirium on recovery.
c. Contraindications: porphyria and status asthmaticus.

7. Ketamine (Ketalar): chemically related to phencyclidine (PCP):
a. Pharmacological effects: produces dissociative anesthesia (patient fails to respond to environment but is NOT asleep).

   b. Adverse reactions:
      (1) HBP and tachycardia, nausea, excessive salivation; atropine (Sal-Tropine) may be required for dry field.
      (2) Can cause hallucinations and delirium during recovery.
   c. Contraindications: HBP and CVD.
8. Opioids: sufentanil (Sufenta), fentanyl (Sublimaze), alfentanil (Alfenta), morphine (MS Contin).
   a. Pharmacological effects: does NOT cause significant peripheral vascular resistance or CVD changes.
   b. Adverse reactions: respiratory depression, which is reversible with naloxone, opioid antagonist.
9. Innovar: neuroleptics, combination of antipsychotic (droperidol) with opioid analgesic (fentanyl).
   a. Pharmacological effects: droperidol causes sedation and catatonia; drug combination produces wakeful anesthetic state.
   b. Adverse reactions:
      (1) Boardlike chest, which requires ventilatory assistance for respiratory depression.
      (2) Tremors.
   c. Contraindications:
      (1) Parkinson's disease.
      (2) Pulmonary insufficiency.

INFECTION MANAGEMENT

Infection management drugs include oral antimicrobials, antibiotics, antifungals, antivirals, antituberculins. Discussion of antibiotic premedication follows this discussion.
• See Chapter 11, Clinical Treatment: oral antimicrobials.

Antivirals

Antivirals (suffix "-vir") inhibit replication of viral DNA, which is necessary for viruses to reproduce themselves. These drugs reduce rate of viral growth but will NOT destroy inactive virus already present. NOT curative, and must be used either prophylactically or early in development of infection. However, drug therapy must normally be initiated within 48 hours of onset of infection to provide any benefit. Tend to be narrow in spectrum and have limited efficacy.
• See also Chapter 8, Microbiology and Immunology: for more information on viruses and related infections.
A. Antiherpetic virals:
   1. Pharmacological effects and therapeutic uses:
      a. Infections with herpesvirus types 1 and 2 and varicella-zoster virus (chickenpox, shingles).
      b. Should be used at the first signs of an outbreak:

         (1) Acyclovir (Zovirax): topically, orally, parenterally.
         (2) Valacyclovir (Valtrex): orally; longer duration of time than acyclovir; converted to acyclovir in body.
         (3) Penciclovir: topically (Denavir) and by IV.
         (4) Famciclovir (Famvir): longer duration of time than acyclovir (Zovirax); converted to penciclovir in body.
   2. Adverse reactions: suprainfections, resistant strains.
B. AIDS antivirals:
   1. Include combination drug therapy, highly active antiretroviral therapy (HAART) with reverse transcriptase inhibitors, such as AZT, D4T, ddI, or ddC, and one or more viral protease inhibitors; HAART extends length of disease-free period of infection by suppressing viral replication and encouraging blood CD4+ count increases.
   2. Adverse reactions; these toxicities LIMIT use:
      a. Headache, nausea, diarrhea, anemia.
      b. Peripheral neuropathy and oral ulcers.
C. Foscarnet (Foscavir), ganciclovir (Cytovene), cidofovir (Vistide), valganciclovir (Valcyte) in treatment of cytomegalovirus (CMV) retinitis in immunosuppressed patients, primarily HIV-positive patients and transplant recipients.
D. Interferons (IFN): type of natural proteins (cytokines) produced by immune system; can be used to inhibit viral replication in infected cells; treat hepatitis C and multiple sclerosis.
E. Amantadine (Symmetrel) and rimantadine (Flumadine): antivirals that hasten recovery from some influenza cases if started early.

Antifungals

Antifungals inhibit or destroy fungal growth.
• See Chapters 6, General and Oral Pathology; 8, Microbiology and Immunology: fungal infections.
A. Nystatin (Mycostatin), amphotericin B (Fungilin), clotrimazole (Mycelex), ketoconazole (Nizoral), fluconazole (Diflucan) (suffix "-zole"):
   1. Therapeutic uses: candidiasis:
      a. Cream, lotion, solution to apply to the skin; oral suspensions.
      b. Lozenges (troches) to dissolve in the mouth.
      c. Vaginal tablets and vaginal cream.
   2. Adverse reactions: troches may contain sugar for taste compliance, which increases the risk for caries.
B. Ketoconazole (Nizoral):
   1. Adverse reactions (occur MORE often):
      a. GIT irritation, MOST common (nausea and vomiting).

b. Hepatotoxicity, MOST serious reaction.

c. Headache, photophobia, allergic reactions.

2. Drug interactions:

a. Decreased effects with anticholinergics, H_2 blockers, antacids, rifampin (Rifadin, Rimactane).

b. Cardiac toxicity occurs with terfenadine and astemizole (Hismanal).

3. Contraindications: hypersensitivity.

C. Fluconazole (Diflucan):

1. Therapeutic uses:

a. Prophylactic for immunocompromised patients to prevent candidiasis.

b. Nonresponsive candidal infections; treatment of vaginal infections.

D. Echinocandins (caspofungin [Cancidas]): inhibit synthesis of cell wall glucan (similar to penicillin when given for bacteria, but for fungi), which can be used in case of azole-resistant *Candida,* with long half-life and low side effects.

Antibiotics

Antibiotics prevent or control bacterial growth; they are seldom dual prescribed. Oral antibiotics decrease effectiveness of oral contraceptives (birth control pills [BCP]); female dental patients of childbearing age when prescribed should be asked to use alternative birth control method until the start of the next menstrual cycle. Also, care must be used when prescribing oral antibiotics to patients with history of lower GIT disorders (colitis, diverticulitis, inflammatory bowel disorder [IBS]), since they are MORE likely to develop serious diarrhea. **Superinfections** (such as community-associated methicillin-resistant *Staphylococcus aureus* [CA-MRSA]) and resistant strains are other recent considerations with use, since they lower the **spectrum** of the drug. (See later discussion of antibiotic premedication.)

• See Chapter 8, Microbiology and Immunology: drugs and related microorganisms.

A. Penicillins: three subgroups: narrow-spectrum, penicillinase-resistant, extended-spectrum (broad- or wide-spectrum).

1. Pharmacological effects:

a. Interfere with bacterial wall synthesis.

b. Bactericidal.

2. Narrow-spectrum penicillins: penicillin G and penicillin VK (Pen-Vee K, V-Cillin K).

a. Therapeutic uses (Penicillin VK, MOST frequently used antibiotic in dentistry; BETTER oral absorption):

(1) Ear, skin, respiratory, and urinary tract infections.

(2) Aggressive periodontal disease, periodontal abscesses, soft tissue infections, osteomyelitis.

3. Penicillinase-resistant penicillins: cloxacillin (Tegopen, Cloxapen), methicillin (Staphcillin), dicloxacillin (Dynapen, Pathocil), still narrow spectrum.

a. Therapeutic uses: infections caused by penicillinase-producing bacteria.

4. Extended-spectrum (broad- or wide-spectrum) penicillins: as ampicillin (Polycillin, Omnipen, Totacillin) and amoxicillin (Amoxil, Larotid, Polymox) (suffix "-cillin").

a. Therapeutic uses:

(1) Infections caused by gram-positive and some gram-negative bacteria (*Escherichia coli* and *Haemophilus influenzae*), but NOT penicillinase-resistant.

(a) Ampicillin (Polycillin, Omnipen, Totacillin): drug used in the 2007 American Heart Association (AHA) antibiotic premedication regimen for patients unable to take oral drug (adults 2 g, children 50 mg/kg IM or IV, 30 to 60 minutes before procedure) to prevent infective endocarditis (IE) in certain at-risk patients.

(b) Amoxicillin (Amoxil, Larotid, Polymox) is used MORE often in dentistry; uses SIMILAR to those of Penicillin VK; first drug of choice for the 2007 AHA antibiotic premedication regimen for patients able to take oral drug (adults 2 g, children 50 mg/kg PO, 30 to 60 minutes before procedure) to prevent IE in certain at-risk patients; multidrug therapy for peptic ulcers caused by *Helicobacter pylori* bacteria.

(c) Amoxicillin with clavulanic acid (CA) (Augmentin): CA combines with penicillinase so drug is NOT inactivated.

b. Adverse reactions:

(1) SIMILAR to other antiinfectives: allergic reaction, GIT irritation, superinfection (because of resistance from penicillinase-producing bacteria).

(2) Candidiasis, glossitis, stomatitis, taste alteration, xerostomia, black hairy tongue.

c. Drug interactions:

(1) Increased anticoagulant effect (especially with warfarin [Coumadin]).

(2) Decreased antimicrobial effectiveness with tetracyclines and erythromycin (Robimycin, E-Mycin, E.E.S.).

(3) Increased plasma levels with disulfiram (Antabuse) for alcoholism and probenecid (Benemid) for gout.

d. Contraindications: hypersensitivity (range from rash to anaphylaxis; see Chapter 8).

B. Tetracyclines: tetracycline (Achromycin, Sumycin), doxycycline (Vibramycin), minocycline (subgingival: Arestin, oral: Minocin) (suffix "-cycline").

1. Pharmacological effects:
   a. Inhibits protein synthesis.
   b. Bacteriostatic.
2. Therapeutic uses:
   a. Sexually transmitted diseases and infections (STDs/STIs) such as syphilis, gonorrhea.
   b. Doxycycline at low-dose (LD) levels:
      (1) Reduced level for antiinflammatory effects (reduced activity of collagenase) and NOT for antibiotic activity.
      (2) Used for dermatological lesions such as acne and rosacea (Oracea) and periodontal disease (Periostat), since it concentrates in gingival crevicular fluid.
3. Adverse reactions:
   a. Tetracycline causes permanent intrinsic yellow or brown staining of teeth if taken during developmental period involving enamel calcification; minocycline produces bluish gray stain in adults (see below).
   b. Systemic minocycline can cause black pigmentation of jaws (including palate); pigment appears bluish through mucosal tissues.
   c. GIT irritation, including nausea, vomiting, diarrhea, xerostomia.
   d. Superinfection.
   e. Increased risk of liver damage when tetracycline is given IV.
   f. Nephrotoxicity (with older tetracyclines).
   g. Photosensitivity (because of exaggerated response of skin and eyes to sun exposure).
4. Drug interactions:
   a. Older tetracyclines show chelation and thus less effectiveness when concomitantly administered with dairy products (Ca), mineral supplements (Fe, Ca, fortified foods), antacids (Ca, Mg, Al).
   b. LESS pronounced effect with dairy products with the newer synthetic forms doxycycline (Vibramycin) and minocycline (Minocin), but AVOID concomitant use of mineral supplements and antacids.
   c. Enhanced effect of oral sulfonylureas, which results in hypoglycemia.
   d. Increased effect of anticoagulants.
5. Contraindications:
   a. Hypersensitivity.
   b. Should NOT be prescribed for children younger than 8 years or pregnant or nursing women (because of intrinsic stain of developing teeth).

C. Cephalosporins: cephalexin (Keflex), cefadroxil (Duricef), cefaclor (Ceclor), cefuroxime (Ceftin), cefazolin (Ancef), ceftriaxone (Rocephin).

Box 9-1 Patients at Potential Increased Risk of Hematogenous Total Joint Infection

All patients during first 2 years after prosthetic joint replacement
Immunocompromised and immunosuppressed patients:
- Inflammatory arthropathies (e.g., rheumatoid arthritis, systemic lupus erythematosus)
- Drug-induced immunosuppression
- Radiation-induced immunosuppression
Patients with comorbidities:
- Previous prosthetic joint infections
- Malnourishment
- Hemophilia
- HIV infection
- Insulin-dependent (type 1) diabetes

---

1. Pharmacological effects:
   a. SAME as for penicillins: interfering with bacterial cell wall synthesis.
   b. Bactericidal.
2. Therapeutic uses:
   a. Infections caused by gram-positive, penicillinase-producing, and some gram-negative bacteria such as *Salmonella* and *E. coli*; respiratory and urinary tract infection; otitis media.
   b. BOTH cefazolin (Ancef) and ceftriaxone (Rocephin) can be used for the 2007 AHA antibiotic premedication regimen if patient is unable to take oral drug and allergic to penicillin (Pen-Vee K) or ampicillin (Polycillin) (adults 1 g, children 50 mg/kg IM or IV, 30 to 60 minutes before procedure) to prevent IE in certain at-risk patients.
   c. Cephalexin (Keflex) or other cephalosporin can be used for the 2007 antibiotic premedication regimen if patient is allergic to penicillin (Pen-Vee K) or ampicillin (Polycillin) (adults 2 g, children 50 mg/kg PO, 30 to 60 minutes before procedure) to prevent IE in certain at-risk patients.
   d. Antibiotic premedication (prophylaxis) for prevention of hematogenous total joint infection if patient has had surgery within past 2 years, is immunocompromised or immunosuppressed, or has a medical history of comorbidities (Box 9-1).
3. Adverse reactions:
   a. SAME oral effects as penicillins.
   b. Allergic reactions (ranging from rash to anaphylaxis; see Chapter 8).
   c. Local reactions: localized pain and swelling in response to IM.
   d. GIT irritation; includes diarrhea (can be pseudomembranous colitis), nausea, vomiting.
   e. Nephrotoxicity; hemostasis impairment; superinfections.

4. Drug interactions: decreased effectiveness with tetracycline and erythromycin (Robimycin, E-Mycin, E.E.S.).

5. Contraindications: hypersensitivity (including cross-sensitivity reaction in patients allergic to penicillin [Pen-Vee K]).

D. Clindamycin (Cleocin):

1. Pharmacological effects: inhibit protein synthesis; bacteriostatic.

2. Therapeutic uses:

a. Infection by *Bacteroides fragilis* and gram-positive organisms.

b. Drug of choice for the 2007 AHA <u>antibiotic premedication</u> regimen for patients allergic to penicillin (Pen-Vee K) or ampicillin (Polycillin), either able to take oral drugs or NOT (adults 600 mg, children 20 mg/kg PO, IM, or IV, 30 to 60 minutes before procedure), to prevent IE in certain at-risk patients.

3. Adverse reactions:

a. Allergic reactions, GIT irritation.

b. Superinfections.

4. Drug interactions:

a. Decreased effectiveness with erythromycin (Robimycin, E-Mycin, E.E.S.).

b. Increased effects of nondepolarizing muscle relaxants.

5. Contraindications:

a. Hypersensitivity.

b. Ulcerative colitis, enteritis (because of GIT irritation).

E. Macrolides: erythromycin (Robimycin, E-Mycin, E.E.S.), clarithromycin (Biaxin), azithromycin (Zithromax, Z pack, descending doses) (suffix "-mycin"; do NOT confuse with aminoglycosides).

1. Pharmacological effects:

a. Interfere with protein synthesis; wide distribution, long-lasting effects.

b. Bacteriostatic.

2. Therapeutic uses:

a. Mild to moderate respiratory tract infections, otitis media, Legionnaire's disease, STDs.

b. Alternate choice for orofacial infections caused by aerobic gram-positive bacteria.

c. BOTH clarithromycin (Biaxin) and azithromycin (Zithromax) can be used for the 2007 AHA <u>antibiotic premedication</u> regimen for patients allergic to penicillin (Pen-Vee K) or ampicillin (Polycillin) (adults 500 mg, children 15 mg/kg PO, 30 to 60 minutes before procedure) to prevent IE for certain at-risk patients.

3. Adverse reactions:

a. GIT irritation with standard therapeutic doses.

b. Allergic reactions are uncommon.

4. Drug interactions:

a. Increased serum concentrations with digoxin (Lanoxin, leading to toxicity), warfarin (Coumadin, increased bleeding), carbamazepine (Tegretol), cyclosporine (Neoral, Sandimmune, Gengraf).

5. Contraindications: hypersensitivity.

F. Aminoglycosides (suffix "-mycin"; do NOT confuse with macrolides):

1. Pharmacological effects:

a. Inhibit protein synthesis.

b. Bactericidal.

2. Therapeutic uses (MOST given IM/IV):

a. Gentamicin (Garamycin) for gram-negative infections that require hospitalization (e.g., bone, respiratory tract, urinary tract infections), including methicillin-resistant *Staphylococcus aureus* (MRSA).

b. Neomycin (Mycifradin) as topical for skin infections.

c. Also includes streptomycin, kanamycin (Kantrex), tobramycin (eye drops).

3. Adverse reactions (excessive blood levels): ototoxicity for cranial nerve VIII (auditory); BOTH balance and auditory functions affected.

G. Metronidazole (Flagyl):

1. Pharmacological effects:

a. Inhibits protein synthesis.

b. Bactericidal.

2. Therapeutic uses:

a. Dentistry: infections caused by anaerobes such as *Bacteroides* organisms and aggressive periodontal disease treatment.

b. Medical: intestinal amebiasis, trichomoniasis, giardiasis.

3. Adverse reactions:

a. Metallic taste, black hairy tongue, xerostomia.

b. Effects on the CNS, including dizziness, headache, vertigo.

c. Nausea, vomiting, diarrhea.

d. Renal toxicity; carcinogenicity in animals but has been discounted.

4. Drug interactions:

a. Disulfiram (Antabuse) reactions occur with alcohol and alcohol-containing products; antimicrobial rinses (e.g., chlorhexidine, Listerine) that contain alcohol are contraindicated.

b. Decreased effects with phenobarbital (Luminal).

5. Contraindications:

a. Hypersensitivity.

b. CNS disorders (because of CNS effects).

c. Renal disease (because of renal toxicity).

H. Sulfonamides (sulfa drugs): sulfisoxazole (Gantrisin) and trimethoprim-sulfamethoxazole (TMP-SMX, Bactrim, Septra).

1. Pharmacological effects: prevent use of PABA to make folic acid.
2. Therapeutic uses:
   a. Drug of choice for treating *Pneumocystis jiroveci (carinii)* pneumonia with acquired immunodeficiency syndrome (AIDS).
   b. Urinary tract infection, otitis media.
3. Adverse reactions:
   a. Skin rash, photosensitivity.
   b. Hematological reactions (e.g., leukopenia, thrombocytopenia).
4. Contraindications: hypersensitivity.
I. Quinolone such as ciprofloxacin (Cipro):
   1. Pharmacological effects: inhibits bacterial portion.
   2. Therapeutic uses: effective against gram-negative bacteria.
   3. Adverse reactions: AVOID dental light in eyes.

Antituberculins

Antituberculins inhibit spread of tuberculosis (TB) in patients; usually three or more are given concurrently. May be involved in directly observed therapy short-course (DOTS), in which healthcare professional administers medication for compliance.
• See Chapters 6, General and Oral Pathology, and 8, Microbiology and Immunology: tuberculosis.
A. Rifampin (Rifadin, Rimactane):
   1. Therapeutic uses: when administered with other antituberculosis drugs, reduces development of antituberculosis drug resistance.
   2. Adverse reactions:
      a. Stomatitis, discolored (red-orange) saliva and urine, nausea, vomiting, diarrhea.
      b. Thrombocytopenia (low platelet count).
   3. Drug interactions:
      a. Increased hepatotoxicity with alcohol and acetaminophen (Tylenol).
      b. Decreased effect of ketoconazole (Nizoral).
   4. Contraindications: hypersensitivity to drug(s).
B. Isoniazid (INH) (Nydrazid):
   1. Therapeutic uses:
      a. Treatment and prevention.
      b. Can be used alone for prevention or with rifampin (Rifadin, Rimactane) and pyrazinamide (PZD) for treatment (see below).
   2. Adverse reactions:
      a. Xerostomia.
      b. Effects on the CNS: peripheral neuropathy, toxic encephalopathy, convulsions.
      c. Hepatotoxicity, vitamin B_6 deficiency.
      d. Hematological effects: hemolytic anemia, thrombocytopenia, agranulocytosis.
   3. Drug interactions:
      a. Increased hepatotoxicity with alcohol or acetaminophen (Tylenol).
      b. Decreased effects of ketoconazole (Nizoral).
   4. Contraindications: hypersensitivity to drug(s).
C. Pyrazinamide (PZA): combined with INH (Nydrazid) and rifampin (Rifadin, Rimactane).
D. Ethambutol (Myambutol): with other drugs noted above; contraindicated for patients with optic neuritis because of optic neuropathy.
E. Rifapentine (Priftin): taken once a week during last 4 months of drug therapy.

MANAGEMENT OF SPECIAL PATIENTS
Patients Receiving Antibiotic Premedication

The American Heart Association (AHA) has 2007 guidelines on antibiotic premedication or prophylaxis for patients at risk, Recommendations for the Prevention of Infectious Endocarditis (Box 9-2 and Table 9-6; also see CD-ROM). Patients with cardiac conditions associated with highest risk of adverse outcome from infective endocarditis (IE), such as patients with artificial heart valves, history of endocarditis, certain serious congenital heart conditions, or hypertrophic cardiomyopathy, as well as heart transplant patients in whom problem with heart valve develops, should receive antibiotic premedication (prophylaxis) before invasive dental procedures (may have wallet card). For patients with history of pathological (organic) heart murmur or documented case of such heart murmur, premedication with antibiotics is NOT necessary before invasive dental procedures. Specific antibiotic coverage has already been discussed.

The American Academy of Orthopaedic Surgeons (AAOS) and the American Dental Association (ADA) published an advisory statement regarding use of antibiotic premedication (prophylaxis) to prevent infection in persons with total joint replacements who are undergoing dental procedures, Antibiotic Prophylaxis for Dental Patients with Total Joint Replacements (see CD-ROM and Box 9-1). Antibiotic prophylaxis is NOT indicated for dental patients with pins, plates, and screws. Antibiotic prophylaxis is NOT routinely indicated for MOST dental patients with prosthetic joints.

Patients who have received total prosthetic (artificial) joints (hips, shoulders, knees) need antibiotic premedication before invasive dental procedures ONLY for the 2 years after the joint has been placed or if they continue to have immunocompromised or immunosuppressed tendencies or problem, rejection, or infection in joint after placement. Recommendation for prophylaxis includes those with inflammatory arthropathies such as rheumatoid arthritis (RA) and systemic lupus erythematosus (SLE), drug- or radiation-induced immunosuppression, or comorbidities such as previous prosthetic joint infections, malnourishment, hemophilia, HIV infection, type 1 insulin-dependent diabetes mellitus (DM), malignancy (cancer).
• See Chapter 8, Microbiology and Immunology: infective endocarditis, prosthetic joint infection.

Box 9-2 Antibiotic Premedication (Prophylaxis) for Cardiac Conditions and Dental Procedures to Reduce Risk of Infective Endocarditis

CARDIAC CONDITIONS NEEDING ANTIBIOTIC PREMEDICATON

Prosthetic cardiac valve

Previous infective endocarditis

Congenital heart disease only in the following categories:

- Unrepaired cyanotic congenital heart disease, including those with palliative shunts and conduits
- Completely repaired congenital heart disease with prosthetic material or device, whether placed by surgery or catheter intervention, during first 6 months after procedure
- Repaired congenital heart disease with residual defects at site or adjacent to site of prosthetic patch or device (which inhibits endothelialization)

Cardiac transplantation recipients with cardiac valvular diseases, since endothelialization of prosthetic material occurs within 6 months after procedure

CARDIAC CONDITIONS *NOT* NEEDING ANTIBIOTIC PREMEDICATION

Heart murmur (functional and pathological)

Bypass graft surgery history

Pacemaker

Mitral valve prolapse with or without insufficiency

Rheumatic heart disease

Bicuspid valve disease

Calcified aortic stenosis

Congenital heart conditions such as ventricular septal defect, atrial septal defect, and hypertrophic cardiomyopathy

DENTAL PROCEDURES FOR WHICH ANTIBIOTIC PROPHYLAXIS IS RECOMMENDED IN PATIENTS WITH CARDIAC CONDITIONS LISTED ABOVE

All dental procedures that involve manipulation of gingival tissue or the periapical region of teeth, or perforation of the oral mucosa

DENTAL PROCEDURES OR EVENTS FOR WHICH ANTIBIOTIC PROPHYLAXIS IS *NOT* RECOMMENDED

Routine anesthetic injections through noninfected tissue; taking dental radiographs; placement of removable prosthodontic or orthodontic appliances; adjustment of orthodontic appliances; placement of orthodontic brackets; shedding of primary teeth and bleeding from trauma to the lips or oral mucosa

Modified from Wilson W, Taubert KA, Gewitz M, et al: Prevention of infective endocarditis: guidelines from the American Heart Association Rheumatic Fever, Endocarditis, and Kawasaki Disease Committee, Council on Cardiovascular Disease in the Young, and the Council on Clinical Cardiology, Council on Cardiovascular Surgery and Anesthesia, and the Quality of Care and Outcomes Research Interdisciplinary Working Group, Circulation 116:1736, 2007.

CLINICAL STUDY

Age	60 YRS	**SCENARIO**
Sex	☒ Male ☐ Female	The patient is due to return for a recall examination and oral prophylaxis appointment. To facilitate the appointment, his chart is reviewed before scheduling and he is called to update his medical history. He is taking two drugs now, and he also has additions to his list of cardiac complications.
Medical History	History of infective endocarditis (IE) Allergy to penicillin (Pen-Vee K)	
Current Medications	digoxin (Lanoxin) 0.5 mg qd OTC loratadine (Claritin) 10 mg prn	
Social History	Chef	

1. The patient takes digoxin (Lanoxin) for the treatment of which type of condition? What type of drug is this?
2. Does the patient require prophylactic antibiotic treatment before his appointment? If so, what antiinfective agent should be prescribed and why?
3. Why is the patient taking loratadine (Claritin)? What type of drug is this?

1. Digoxin (Lanoxin) is used to treat congestive heart failure (CHF) and is a cardiac glycoside. This must

be an addition that he needs to discuss and add to his medical history.

2. Yes, he will be undergoing an invasive dental procedure(s); the 2007 AHA Recommendations for the Prevention of Infectious Endocarditis should be followed because of his history of IE, since he is at increased risk for IE. Amoxicillin (Amoxil, Larotid, Polymox) should NOT be used because of his history of penicillin (Pen-Vee K) allergy. However, azithromycin (Zithromax) or clarithromycin (Biaxin),

Table 9-6 American Heart Association recommendations for the prevention of infectious endocarditis: antibiotic premedication (prophylactic) regimens recommended for dental procedures

Situation	Agent	Regimen: single dose 30 to 60 minutes before procedure	
		Adults	**Children**
Oral	Amoxicillin	2 g	50 mg/kg
Unable to take oral medication	Ampicillin	2 g IM or IV	50 mg/kg IM or IV
	Cefazolin or ceftriaxone	1 g IM or IV	50 mg/kg IM or IV
Allergic to penicillins or ampicillin: oral regimen	Cephalexin*,†	2 g	50 mg/kg
	Clindamycin	600 mg	20 mg/kg
	Azithromycin or clarithromycin	500 mg	15 mg/kg
Allergic to penicillins or ampicillin and unable to take oral medication	Cefazolin or ceftriaxone†	1 g IM or IV	50 mg/kg IM or IV
	Clindamycin	600 mg IM or IV	20 mg/kg IM or IV

Modified from Wilson W, Taubert KA, Gewitz M, et al: Prevention of infective endocarditis: guidelines from the American Heart Association Rheumatic Fever, Endocarditis, and Kawasaki Disease Committee, Council on Cardiovascular Disease in the Young, and the Council on Clinical Cardiology, Council on Cardiovascular Surgery and Anesthesia, and the Quality of Care and Outcomes Research Interdisciplinary Working Group, Circulation 116:1736, 2007.
IM, Intramuscular; *IV,* intravenous.
*Or other first- or second-generation oral cephalosporin in equivalent adult or pediatric dosage.
†Cephalosporins should NOT be used in individual with history of anaphylaxis, angioedema, or urticaria with penicillins or ampicillin.

which can usually be used in these patients, should be avoided for this particular patient because of potential drug interactions. Azithromycin (Zithromax) and clarithromycin (Biaxin) belong to the macrolide family of antibiotics. Digoxin (Lanoxin) in combination with these antibiotics tends to increase drug availability, thereby increasing the risk of digoxin (Lanoxin) toxicity. Therefore the drug of choice in the AHA regimen, clindamycin (Cleocin) (for adults 600 mg PO, 30 to 60 minutes before procedure) could be prescribed by the supervising dentist, since the patient can take oral drugs. However, a medical consult would be warranted in this case.

3. Loratadine (Claritin), an H_1 receptor antagonist, is used to treat rhinitis and seasonal allergies. This must be the other medical condition that he wants to add to his medical history.

Patients with Cardiovascular Disease

Patient with cardiovascular disease (CVD) has damage or disease of the heart and blood vessels. Includes hypertension (high blood pressure [HBP]; MOST common CVD), congestive heart failure (CHF), dysrhythmias, angina pectoris.

• See Chapter 6, General and Oral Pathology: CVD; 11, Medical and Dental Emergencies: emergency kit drugs in dental settings.

A. Antihypertensives:
  1. General pharmacological effect:
    a. Lower blood pressure by relaxing the blood vessels so heart does NOT have to pump as hard.
    b. Control chest pain by increasing supply of blood to heart.
  2. General therapeutic uses:
    a. Control of HBP.
  3. General adverse reactions:
    a. Xerostomia.
    b. CNS depression.
    c. Orthostatic hypotension.
  4. Diuretics: first-line intervention for HBP (suffixes "-mide," "-nide").
    a. Thiazide-type diuretics: hydrochlorothiazide (HCTZ) (Lopressor):
      (1) Specific pharmacological effect:
        (a) Increase secretion of sodium and water.
        (b) Thus lower blood volume and blood pressure.
      (2) Specific therapeutic uses:
        (a) Used in combination with other antihypertensives (see below).
      (3) Specific adverse reactions:
        (a) Hypokalemia (low blood potassium); thus must have potassium supplement.
        (b) Hyperglycemia (high blood glucose).
        (c) Hyperuricemia (excessive uric acid in the body), increased urination.
      (4) Drug interactions:
        (a) Decrease in hypotensive effect with NSAIAs.
    b. Loop diuretics: furosemide (Lasix).
      (1) Specific pharmacological effects:
        (a) Inhibit absorption of sodium and chloride in loop of Henle and distal renal tube.
        (b) Thus increase excretion of water and sodium.

(2) Specific therapeutic uses:
  (a) Also CHF and edema present with heart, liver, or kidney disease.
  (b) Impaired kidney function.
  (c) Used if patient does NOT respond to thiazides.
(3) Specific adverse reactions and drug interactions:
  (a) SAME as thiazides.
c. Potassium-sparing diuretics: spironolactone (Aldactone).
  (1) Adverse reactions:
    (a) Hyperkalemia (high blood potassium).
    (b) Increased urination.
    (c) Tumors in lab animals.
  (2) Drug interactions: SAME as thiazides.
d. Thiazides combined with potassium sparing diuretics: Maxzide, Dyazide.
  (1) Specific therapeutic uses: reduce incidence of hypokalemia.
5. Adrenergic blockers (see also under earlier discussion of adrenergic blocker):
  a. β-blockers (suffix "-olol"):
    (1) Specific pharmacological effects:
      (a) Reduce the workload of the heart by decreasing arterial pressure.
      (b) Thus decrease venous return, decrease preload and myocardial oxygen demand.
    (2) Specific therapeutic uses:
      (a) Also angina pectoris, migraine headache prophylaxis, MI prophylaxis.
    (3) Specific adverse reactions:
      (a) Fatigue, sleep disturbances, sexual dysfunction (impotence).
      (b) If discontinued suddenly, spontaneous rebound HBP.
    (4) Drug reactions:
      (a) Decrease effects of sulfonylureas (oral hypoglycemics).
      (b) Decrease antihypertensive effects with NSAIAs, barbiturates, penicillins, rifampin (Rifadin, Rimactane), salicylates.
      (c) Mask tachycardia from hypoglycemia caused by insulin and hypoglycemics
      (d) Slow metabolism of lidocaine (Xylocaine); may lead to toxicity (need to limit dose).
  b. Nonselective β-blockers: propranolol (Inderal):
    (1) Specific pharmacological effects: block BOTH β-receptors.
    (2) Specific adverse reactions and contraindications:
      (a) Bronchospasm; NOT used with patients who have HBP with impaired pulmonary function such as COPD and asthma.

(b) Decrease glycogenolysis and glucagon secretion; NOT preferred for insulin-dependent DM.
(3) Drug interactions: HBP and bradycardia occur when used with epinephrine (need to reduce amounts with local anesthesia use).
c. Selective (cardioselective) β-blockers: atenolol (Tenormin), metoprolol (Lopressor, Toprol XL):
  (1) Specific pharmacological effects: block MORE β_1 receptors at lower doses.
  (2) Therapeutic uses:
    (a) NO effect on insulin; preferred for insulin-dependent DM.
    (b) NO bronchoconstrictor effects; used for patients with HBP along with impaired pulmonary function such as COPD and asthma.
    (c) Less likely to interact with vasoconstrictors in local anesthetics than nonselective β-blockers.
  (3) Drug interactions: reduced antihypertensive effects with COX inhibitors like ibuprofen (Advil) and naproxen (Aleve).
d. Centrally acting antiadrenergics stimulate central α-adrenergic receptors: clonidine (Catapres) and methyldopa (Aldomet).
  (1) Specific adverse reactions: sedation.
  (2) Drug interactions:
    (a) Increase CNS depression when used with CNS depressants.
    (b) Decrease hypotensive effect when used with NSAIAs and sympathomimetics.
e. α_1-Selective blockers: prazosin (Minipress, Hypovase).
6. Angiotensin-converting enzyme (ACE) inhibitors: captopril (Capoten), enalapril (Vasotec), lisinopril (Zestril, Prinivil) (suffix "-pril"):
  a. Specific pharmacological effects:
    (1) Prevent formation of angiotensin II, powerful body vasoconstrictor.
    (2) Inhibit breakdown of bradykinin; result is vasodilation, lowering of blood pressure.
    (3) Decrease secretion of aldosterone, which decreases retention of sodium and water; thus act like diuretic to lower blood pressure.
  b. Specific therapeutic uses: used when first-line interventions (diuretics, β-blockers) are NOT effective or are contraindicated.
  c. Specific adverse reactions:
    (1) Neutropenia (abnormal decrease in neutrophils in blood).

Table 9-7 Drugs that cause gingival hyperplasia

Generic name	Brand name	Drug classification
Diltiazem	Cardizem, Dilacor, Tiazac	Calcium channel blocker
Nifedipine	Procardia, Adalat, Nifedical	Calcium channel blocker
Verapamil	Isoptin, Calan, Bosoptin	Calcium channel blocker
Phenytoin	Dilantin	Hydantoin

    (2) Cough, dysgeusia (altered taste that may lead to caries), xerostomia.

    (3) Hypotension, teratogenicity.

  d. Drug interactions: decreased effect with indomethacin (Indocin) and possibly other NSAIAs.

7. Calcium channel blockers: diltiazem (Cardizem, Dilacor, Tiazac), nifedipine (Procardia, Adalat, Nifedical), verapamil (Isoptin, Calan, Bosoptin), amlodipine (Norvasc; with atorvastatin [Lipitor], Caduet; with valsartan [Diovan], Exforge; with benazepril, Lotrel) (suffix "-dipine").

  a. Specific pharmacological effects:

    (1) Inhibit calcium ions from entering voltage-sensitive channels with vascular smooth muscle and myocardium during depolarization, relaxing the muscles.

    (2) Vasodilate coronary and peripheral arterioles, lowering blood pressure.

    (3) Reduce spasm in coronary arteries, promote vasodilation.

  b. Specific therapeutic uses:

    (1) BEST in patients with asthma, DM, Pelizaeus-Merzbacher disease.

    (2) Also used for angina pectoris and dysrhythmias.

  c. Adverse reactions:

    (1) Hypotension, dizziness, lightheadedness, nausea.

    (2) Gingival hyperplasia (Table 9-7); LESS common with amlodipine (Norvasc).

    (3) Inhibition of platelet function; increased bleeding should be monitored during invasive or surgical dental procedures.

  d. Drug interactions:

    (1) Increased effects with antifungals, clarithromycin (Biaxin), doxycycline (Vibramycin), erythromycin (Robimycin, E-Mycin, E.E.S.).

    (2) Decreased effects with indomethacin (Indocin), ibuprofen (Advil, Motrin, Pamprin), possibly other NSAIAs.

8. Angiotensin II receptor blockers: irbesartan (Avapro), losartan (Cozaar), valsartan (Diovan) (suffix "-sartan").

  a. Specific pharmacological effects (SIMILAR to ACE inhibitors):

    (1) Block binding of angiotensin 1 to II.

    (2) Block vasoconstriction and aldosterone-secreting effects of angiotensin II, lowering blood pressure.

  b. Specific therapeutic uses:

    (1) Alternatives to ACE inhibitors because of fewer side effects.

    (2) Reduce kidney damage that can occur with DM; thus BETTER for patients with DM.

  c. Adverse reactions:

    (1) Oral lesions.

    (2) Nausea, vomiting, dyspepsia.

    (3) Orthostatic hypotension in early stages of use.

  d. Drug reactions: decrease effects when given with antifungal ketoconazole (Nizoral).

9. Vasodilators: minoxidil (Loniten) and hydralazine (Apresoline).

  a. Specific pharmacological effects: relax smooth muscles of arterioles.

  b. Adverse reactions: hirsutism (hair growth, reversing baldness).

  c. Drug interactions: toxicity with sympathetic blockers, β-blockers, diuretics.

B. Digitalis glycoside: digoxin (Lanoxin):

1. Pharmacological effects: increases cardiac contractility and output.

2. Therapeutic uses:

  a. Commonly prescribed.

  b. Used in treatment of CHF (inability of the heart to pump efficiently).

3. Adverse reactions:

  a. Sensitive gag reflex, nausea, vomiting.

  b. CNS effects: headache, drowsiness, fatigue, muscular weakness.

  c. Blurred vision and photophobia; dysrhythmias; hypotension.

  d. Narrow therapeutic index.

4. Drug interactions:

  a. Possible dysrhythmias when used in conjunction with epinephrine or levonordefrin.

  b. Digoxin (Lanoxin) toxicity when used in conjunction with macrolides or tetracyclines.

5. Contraindications:

  a. Hypersensitivity.

  b. Ventricular fibrillation and tachycardia.

C. Antiarrhythmics: disopyramide (Norpace, Rythmodan), lidocaine (Xylocaine; used parenterally), propranolol (Inderal):

1. Pharmacological effects: suppression of dysrhythmias by various mechanisms, depending on drug classification.
2. Therapeutic uses: treat cardiac dysrhythmias (altered rhythmic contractions of cardiac muscle).

D. Antianginals: nitroglycerin (NTG, Nitrostat), isosorbide dinitrate (Isordil), β-blockers (see antihypertensives), calcium channel blockers (see antihypertensives).
   1. Pharmacological effects: reduction of oxygen consumption, which decreases work of heart and thus relieves anginal pain.
   2. Therapeutic uses:
      a. Treat angina pectoris, caused by insufficient oxygen supply to myocardium, resulting in chest pain.
      b. Patient's own supply should be brought to each dental appointment but may NOT be current.
      c. Thus NTG (metered spray or tablet form) should be part of dental office emergency kit (do NOT refrigerate).
   3. Adverse reactions to NTG:
      a. Xerostomia, headache.
      b. Orthostatic hypotension.
   4. Drug interactions: increased hypotensive effects with alcohol, opioids, benzodiazepines, phenothiazines, erectile dysfunction (ED) drugs (discussed later).
   5. Contraindications: hypersensitivity to NTG (Nitrostat) or nitrites.

E. Antihyperlipidemics (hypolipidemics, lipid-lowering drugs [LLD]): MOST common type of drug prescribed in recent years:
   1. General pharmacological effects:
      a. Result in lowered plasma cholesterol during treatment of hyperlipidemias.
      b. Reduce arteriosclerosis (plaque stabilization), improve coronary endothelial function, inhibit platelet thrombus formation.
   2. Statins (HMG-CoA reductase inhibitors): lovastatin (Mevacor, Altocor), atorvastatin (Lipitor), simvastatin (Zocor) (suffix "-statin").
      a. Specific pharmacological effects:
         (1) Inhibit enzyme HMG Co-A reductase in liver, rate-limiting step in cholesterol synthesis.
         (2) Decrease synthesis of cholesterol.
         (3) Clearance of harmful low-density lipoproteins (LDL) and triglycerides.
         (4) Increase plasma levels of desired high-density lipoproteins (HDL) in some patients.
      b. Specific therapeutic uses (drug of choice):
         (1) Lipitor: primary CVD: risk of MI and CVA, multiple risk factors (HBP and/or smoking, low HDL), type 2 DM.
         (2) Zocor: secondary CVD.
      c. Adverse reactions:

(1) Headaches, flatulence (excess gas in GIT), abdominal pain, constipation, diarrhea.
(2) May have myalgia (muscle soreness) that would affect oral care; adjustments in patient positioning in dental chair and/or shorter appointments.
(3) Elevated liver enzyme levels (monitored).
   d. Drug interactions:
      (1) Myalgia (diffuse muscle pain) and myositis (muscle tissue inflammation), leading to rhabdomyolysis (muscle weakness and deterioration) with acute renal failure (dose-related) with macrolide antibiotics (erythromycin [Robimycin, E-Mycin, E.E.S.], clarithromycin [Biaxin]), azole antifungals (itraconazole, ketoconazole), or combined with other antihyperlipidemics or large quantities of grapefruit juice (guess it does not pay to want to watch your waistline!).
      (2) Increased effects of levothyroxine (Synthroid), digoxin (Lanoxin), ethinyl estradiol; AVOID taking with alcohol.
   3. Ezetimibe (Zetia); in combination with simvastatin: Vytorin:
      a. Pharmacological effects:
         (1) Inhibits absorption of cholesterol within small intestines.
         (2) Reduces dietary cholesterol, resulting in decrease in hepatic cholesterol stores.
         (3) Increases cholesterol clearance from blood, causing reductions in LDL, total levels and triglycerides, increases in HDL.
      b. Therapeutic uses: high cholesterol levels.
      c. Adverse reactions: SAME as simvastatin.
   4. Fibrates: bezafibrate (Bezalip), ciprofibrate (Modalim), gemfibrozil (Lopid), fenofibrate (TriCor).
      a. Specific pharmacological effects:
         (1) Class of amphipathic carboxylic acids.
         (2) Increase desired high-density lipoproteins (HDL); combined therapy with statins.
      b. Adverse reactions and drug interactions: SAME as statins.
   5. Niacin (vitamin B_3):
      a. Specific pharmacological effects: blocks breakdown of fats (decreasing free fatty acids in the blood).
      b. Adverse reactions: facial flushing (decreased with NSAIAs).

F. Antithrombotics include anticoagulants and antiplatelets. American Dental Association has stated that these rarely need to be discontinued before MOST dental procedures to prevent adverse reactions of bleeding (see below); there is a greater risk of thromboembolic events than uncontrollable bleeding if drugs are temporarily stopped. If risks of drug are too great, <u>medical consult</u> is needed.

1. Anticoagulants: warfarin (Coumadin):
    a. Pharmacological effects:
        (1) Interfere with blood clotting factors (those dependent on vitamin K).
        (2) Thus reduce risk of thrombus and embolism formation.
    b. Therapeutic uses:
        (1) Post-MI treatment.
        (2) Treatment of pulmonary emboli (blood clots in the lung).
        (3) Treatment of thrombophlebitis (vein inflammation).
        (4) Treatment of atrial dysrhythmias.
    c. Adverse reactions:
        (1) Gingival bleeding and hemorrhage; can be serious problem during dental work, especially with surgical procedures (extractions); however, see note above.
        (2) Monitored by international normalized ratio (INR); INRs ≤2.5 are safe for invasive dental work; older test is prothrombin time (PT).
    d. Drug interactions:
        (1) Increased effects with salicylates, metronidazole (Flagyl), erythromycin (Robimycin, E-Mycin, E.E.S.), NSAIAs.
        (2) Decreased effects with barbiturates and vitamin K.
    e. Contraindications: blood disorders.
2. Antiplatelets: clopidogrel (Plavix), ticlopidine (Ticlid), aspirin (Bayer, Ecotrin, Empirin, Bufferin) (also low-dose compounds, see earlier discussion):
    a. Pharmacological effects:
        (1) Inhibits platelet aggregation.
        (2) Thus reduce risk of thrombosis and embolism formation.
    b. Therapeutic uses:
        (1) Clopidogrel (Plavix) and ticlopidine (Ticlid) are MORE effective than low-dose aspirin compounds at preventing MI and CVA in patients at risk.
        (2) Clopidogrel (Plavix) used for those unable to tolerate GIT effects of aspirin; has replaced ticlopidine (Ticlid) for those who are allergic to or intolerant of aspirin.
        (3) Adverse reactions: SAME as for warfarin (Coumadin) and aspirin, but lower GIT effects; see earlier notes.
    c. Drug interactions:
        (1) Toxicity with some herbal supplements and NSAIAs.
        (2) Increased effects also with aspirin (Bayer, Ecotrin, Empirin, Bufferin), with other herbal supplementals, and with other NSAIAs, antiplatelets, anticoagulants.
        (3) Decreased effects of atorvastatin (Lipitor) and macrolides (erythromycin [(Robimycin, E-Mycin, E.E.S.], clarithromycin [Biaxin]).

G. Erectile dysfunction (ED) drugs: sildenafil citrate (Viagra, Revatio), tadalafil (Cialis), vardenafil (Levitra), ALL resulting in increased inflow of blood; concurrent use of NTG (Nitrostat) or amyl nitrate would lead to serious hypotension, so monitor BP during dental appointment; may have hearing loss or vision impairment with chronic use.

CLINICAL STUDY

Age	29 YRS	**SCENARIO**
Sex	☐ Male ☒ Female	A recall patient apologizes for missing her last 6-month recall appointment. Today at this appointment, her mandibular anterior gingiva is visibly hemorrhagic.
Height	5'9"	
Weight	205 LBS (previous 180 LBS)	
BP	148/98 (previous 120/76)	
Chief Complaint	"My gums bleed when I brush them."	
Medical History	Took dexfenfluramine (Redux) in past Artificial mitral valve placed 4 months ago	
Current Medications	None	
Social History	Party planner	

1. What type of drug is dexfenfluramine (Redux), and why was it prescribed?
2. What might explain the change in the patient's blood pressure readings? Why did the drug cause her heart valve to be replaced?
3. Should the patient receive dental treatment at this recall appointment?

1. Dexfenfluramine (Redux) is an anorexiant. It suppresses appetite and was prescribed as an aid to weight loss.
2. Although one adverse effect of dexfenfluramine (Redux) is hypertension (high blood pressure [HBP]), this effect usually disappears after the drug is discontinued. Moderate weight gain after discontinuing drug might be her cause of HBP. A more serious cause might be primary pulmonary HBP, which is a side effect of the drug and is associated with dyspnea, angina, syncope, edema of the lower extremities, and possible congestive heart failure (CHF). Her diastolic reading is considered stage 1 (mild) HBP. Fenfluramine (Pondimin) and dexfenfluramine (Redux) in combination with phentermine (commonly referred to as phen-fen) were both removed from the market because of their adverse effects on the heart valves when taken long term, causing disease. In the case of valve disease associated with fenfluramine and dexfenfluramine, leakiness is problem; valvular damage may ultimately produce severe heart and lung disease. Drug caused so much permanent damage to her mitral valve that it needed to be replaced with artificial valve.
3. She should not receive invasive dental treatment (including oral prophylaxis) at this time because of possibility of significant oral bleeding. This is because of her artificial heart valve, as well as having had cardiac surgery within the last 6 months. Patient must be premedicated with antibiotics before any invasive dental procedure according to 2007 American Heart Association (AHA) Recommendations for the Prevention of Infective Endocarditis (IE) (see recommendations below). Patient should be also immediately referred by the dentist to her cardiologist because of her HBP reading, especially in consideration of her complex medical history and signs of oral inflammation.

Patients with Mental Illness

Patients with mental illness or disability include those who are treated for mental disorders that affect ability to recognize reality. MOST medications for these disabilities cause xerostomia and taste alterations, which must be taken into account to reduce risk of caries; bruxism (grinding) may also be present. In some cases, antidepressants may be associated with worsening symptoms of depression or suicidal thoughts or behavior, particularly early in treatment or when there is a change in dosage; be sure to refer patient to healthcare providers if there are any of these signs.

- See Chapters 6, General and Oral Pathology; 16, Special Needs Patient Care: discussion on specific mental illnesses.
A. Antipsychotics:
   1. Phenothiazines: chlorpromazine (Thorazine), mesoridazine (Serentil), prochlorperazine (Compazine), thioridazine (Mellaril).
   2. Phenylbutylpiperadines: haloperidol (Haldol) and pimozide (Orap).
   3. Dibenzapine derivatives: clozapine (Clozaril), loxapine (Loxitane), olanzapine (Zyprexa), and quetiapine (Seroquel).
   4. Benzisoxidil group: risperidone (Risperdal) and ziprasidone (Geodon).
   5. Pharmacological effects:
       a. Calm emotions and slow down psychomotor responses.
       b. Act as antiemetics (antivomiting drugs) by depressing chemoreceptor zone; mainly prochlorperazine.
   6. Therapeutic uses:
       a. Treatment of psychoses (e.g., schizophrenia, obsessive-compulsive disorder [OCD], bipolar disorder [manic-depressive illness]).
       b. Preoperative relaxation; nausea and vomiting.
   7. Adverse reactions:
       a. Orthostatic hypotension and tachycardia.
       b. Sedation (tolerance develops).
       c. Extrapyramidal effects (body movements) such as Parkinson-like symptoms, e.g., tremors, rigidity, akathisia (increased motor restlessness); acute dystonia: muscle spasms of the face, tongue, back, and neck; tardive dyskinesia: involuntary, abnormal movement of tongue, lips, face, and neck; seizures (because of lowered seizure threshold).
   8. Drug interactions:
       a. Additive effect with CNS depressants, including barbiturates, alcohol, general anesthetics, opioid analgesics.
       b. Hypotension and tachycardia with epinephrine IV; epinephrine can be safely administered as a vasoconstrictor in local anesthetic.
       c. Increased anticholinergic effects (xerostomia) with anticholinergics.
       d. Increased photosensitivity with tetracycline.
   9. Contraindications: hypersensitivity.
B. First-generation antidepressants, TCAs: amitriptyline (Elavil), nortriptyline (Pamelor, Aventyl), imipramine (Tofranil) (suffix "-triptyline")
   1. Pharmacological effects (onset of action may take several weeks):
       a. Mild sedation and fatigue in normal patients.
       b. Elevation of mood and decreased depression in depressed patients.

2. Therapeutic uses:
   a. Treatment of depression.
   b. Combination with phenothiazines.
   c. Nortriptyline is prescribed if less sedation is desired.
3. Adverse reactions:
   a. Drowsiness (tolerance may develop), confusion, sometimes tremors.
   b. Blurred vision and constipation (tolerance does develop).
   c. Avoid with narrow-angle glaucoma, enlarged prostate (benign prostatic hyperplasia), or certain types of heart disease (HBP, dysrhythmias, MI, since higher risk of heart attack).
   d. May affect blood sugar levels; with DM, check blood sugar levels more often.
4. Drug interactions:
   a. Increased anticholinergic effects with antihistamines and phenothiazines.
   b. Increased effects of epinephrine and CNS depressants; used with caution if history of seizures or thyroid problems.
C. Second-generation antidepressants, selective serotonin reuptake inhibitors (SSRIs) (suffix "-ine"):
1. General pharmacological effects:
   a. Increase extracellular neurotransmitter serotonin by inhibiting its reuptake into presynaptic cell.
   b. Increase serotonin available to bind to the postsynaptic receptor.
   c. Result in elevated mood, improved sleep, satiety after eating.
2. General therapeutic uses:
   a. Used in the treatment of depression, anxiety disorders (social anxiety, panic attacks, OCD, eating disorders), chronic pain (acute temporomandibular disorder [TMD]).
   b. Personality disorders; also premature ejaculation problems.
3. Adverse reactions:
   a. Fewer CVD and CNS problems than with TCAs.
   b. Must be tapered off when discontinued.
4. Drug interactions:
   a. Contraindicated with concomitant use of MAOIs (serotonin disorder) or other CNS antidepressants such as alcohol.
   b. Increased bleeding complications with NSAIAs.
5. Contraindications:
   a. Liver impairment, pregnancy.
   b. Box warning for suicide risk in children and adolescents is required.
6. Specific drugs' pharmacological effects and therapeutic uses:

   a. Fluoxetine (Prozac): does NOT have adverse interactions with vasoconstrictors.
   b. Trazodone (Desyrel, Molipaxin, Trittico, Thombran, Trialodine): CNS stimulation, NOT depression; nausea, diarrhea, aphthous stomatitis.
   c. Bupropion (Wellbutrin, Zyban: tobacco cessation): increases seizures; xerostomia, vivid dreams (does develop tolerance).
   d. Sertraline (Zoloft, Lustral): dizziness and nausea; may increase effects of certain drugs.
   e. Paroxetine (Paxil): libido difficulties, anticholinergic effects.
   f. Escitalopram (Lexapro): used for MAJOR depressive disorders and generalized anxiety disorders.
D. Other antidepressants:
1. Monoamine oxidase inhibitors (MAIOs): moclobemide (Aurorix, Manerix), phenelzine (Nardil), isocarboxazid (Marplan).
   a. Pharmacological effects:
      (1) Brain's three neurotransmitters, known as monoamines (serotonin, norepinephrine, dopamine), are broken down by monoamine oxidase, a liver and brain enzyme.
      (2) The MAIOs inhibit the activity of monoamine oxidase, thus preventing breakdown of monoamine neurotransmitters and increasing availability to ease depression.
   b. Therapeutic uses: powerful older antidepressant.
      (1) Reserved as *last* line of defense (because of potentially lethal dietary and drug interactions) when antidepressant drugs (e.g., SSRIs and TCAs) have been tried unsuccessfully.
      (2) Patch: selegiline (Emsam) applied transdermally; drug does NOT enter GIT, decreasing dangers of dietary interactions.
   c. Adverse reactions:
      (1) React with many foods containing tyramine (e.g., aged cheeses, fish, wines, smoked meats).
      (2) Nausea and vomiting, HBP, fever.
      (3) NOT for patients with CVD, epilepsy, bronchitis, asthma, or HBP or those who resist following stringent diet.
   d. Drug reactions:
      (1) The SSRIs (serotonin disorder), TCAs, disulfiram, β-blockers (life-threatening reactions).
      (2) AVOID use of levonordefrin (vasoconstrictor with mepivacaine local anesthetic agent, Carbocaine with Neo-Cobefrin).
2. Lithium (Lithobid, Eskalith): treats bipolar disorder (manic-depressive illness); works by decreasing abnormal activity in brain; toxicity can be

avoided if blood levels are monitored; NSAIAs increase drug's toxicity.

3. Venlafaxine (Effexor): bicyclic antidepressant; NO adverse interactions with vasoconstrictors; <u>box warning for suicide risk</u>.

4. Nefazodone (Serzone): NO adverse interactions with vasoconstrictors; serious and possibly fatal reactions with use of MAOIs.

Patients with Seizure Disorders

Patients who suffer from seizure disorders such as epilepsy are treated with anticonvulsants (antiepileptics [AEDs]) to depress the CNS, preventing seizures. Adverse reactions include CNS depression and stimulation (in young and elderly individuals), xerostomia, gingival hyperplasia, nausea and vomiting, teratogenicity, gingival hyperplasia (Table 9-7).

- See Chapters 6, General and Oral Pathology: seizures, epilepsy, gingival hyperplasia; 13, Periodontology: surgery for gingival hyperplasia; 16, Special Needs Patient Care: related discussion on specific seizure disorders.

A. Phenytoin (Dilantin):
  1. Adverse reactions:
    a. Gingival hyperplasia (Table 9-7).
    b. Vitamin D and folate deficiencies.
    c. Rashes; can cause Stevens-Johnson syndrome.
  2. Drug interactions:
    a. Decreased effects with barbiturates and carbamazepine (Tegretol).
    b. Decreases effects of steroids and doxycycline (Vibramycin).

B. Carbamazepine (Tegretol):
  1. Other pharmacological effects:
    a. Anticholinergic, antiarrhythmic, antineuralgic, antidiuretic, muscle relaxant.
  2. Therapeutic uses: also treats trigeminal neuralgia (tic douloureux).
  3. Adverse reactions:
    a. Glossitis, constipation.
    b. Aplastic anemia, thrombocytopenia, leukocytosis; lab monitoring of blood is necessary.
    c. Rashes, photosensitivity, erythema multiforme, abnormal liver function.
  4. Drug interactions:
    a. Decreased effect of phenobarbital (Luminal), benzodiazepines, doxycycline (Vibramycin), warfarin (Coumadin), oral contraceptives.
    b. Increased effect with erythromycin (Robimycin, E-Mycin, E.E.S.), isoniazid (Nydrazid), propoxyphene (Darvon), calcium channel blockers, cimetidine (Tagamet).

C. Valproic acid (VPA, Depakene, Depakote).
  1. Adverse reactions:

a. Hepatotoxicity, increased bleeding time; bleeding levels monitored by international normalized ratio (INR); INRs ≤2.5 are safe for invasive dental work; older test is prothrombin time (PT).
    b. Constipation.
  2. Drug interactions:
    a. Additive effect with CNS depressants.
    b. Increased bleeding when taken with salicylates and NSAIAs.

D. Phenobarbital (Luminal): used as anticonvulsant agent by itself or in combination with other anticonvulsants (e.g., phenytoin [Dilantin]).

E. Benzodiazepines (BZDs): clonazepam (Klonopin) and diazepam (Valium); diazepam (Valium) used to treat recurrent tonic-clonic seizures and untreated statis epilepticus (see earlier discussion on BZDs).

Patients with Endocrine Disorders

Endocrine disorders include adrenal gland disorders, diabetes mellitus (DM), thyroid disorders, female hormonal disorders.

- See Chapters 2, Anatomy, Biochemistry, and Physiology; 6, General and Oral Pathology: related discussion on specific endocrine disorders.

A. Adrenocorticosteroids (corticosteroids):
  1. Types:
    a. Glucocorticoids: hydrocortisone, prednisone (Deltasone), triamcinolone (Kenalog, Kenacort, Aristocort, Atolone), dexamethasone (Decadron); used MORE often.
    b. Mineralocorticoids, which affect water and electrolyte balance (hydrocortisone has SAME effect) (suffixes "-sone," "-one," "-ide").
  2. Pharmacological effects:
    a. Affect carbohydrate metabolism, which decreases inflammatory response.
    b. Allergic reactions, immunosuppression.
    c. Osteoporosis (thinning bone).
  3. Therapeutic uses:
    a. Replacement drug therapy for Addison's disease (adrenal gland insufficiency).
    b. Cushing's syndrome (hyperadrenocorticism) with resulting "moon face," "buffalo hump," truncal obesity.
    c. Antiinflammatory effects treat dermatitis, acute asthma, systemic lupus erythematosus (SLE), scleroderma, rheumatoid arthritis (RA), severe and acute allergic reactions, TMD.
    d. Used to treat emergencies such as shock and adrenal crisis; dental patient may need MORE steroids; <u>medical consult</u> needed.
    e. Used to treat aphthous stomatitis and noninfectious inflammatory oral lesions (e.g., erythema multiforme, lichen planus, pemphigus).
  4. Adverse reactions:
    a. Decreased resistance to infections.

b. Delayed wound healing.

c. Development of osteoporosis.

d. Adrenal crisis (including hypertension, circulatory collapse, and death) as a result of abrupt drug withdrawal and stress; may be avoided by premedication with additional steroids.

e. Weight gain and hyperglycemia; increased stomach acid.

f. Behavioral changes, including agitation, euphoria, depression.

5. Drug interactions:

a. Decreased effects with barbiturates and rifampin (Rifadin, Rimactane).

b. Increased adverse reactions with alcohol, salicylates, NSAIAs.

6. Contraindications:

a. Psychosis because of effects on behavior during presence or withdrawal of the drug.

b. Infection because of antiinflammatory effects may mask symptoms of infection; also may decrease resistance to infection.

c. Peptic ulcers because of stimulation of gastric acid secretions.

d. CVD because of HBP associated with mineralocorticoids.

e. Do NOT use topical preparations on open wounds, burns, or large areas; dermal absorption from use in these areas may approach SAME effects as oral dose.

B. Drugs for the treatment of DM:

1. For type 1 DM: insulin (MOST given SC/SQ: thigh, abdomen, upper arm; rotating sites):

a. Rapid acting: Humulin R.

b. Intermediate acting: Humulin L and Humulin N (NPH).

c. Long acting: Humulin U.

d. Mixed: Humulin 70/30; MOST common combination is Humulin R and NPH.

(1) Insulin pumps: external for certain patients who need intensive insulin therapy, syringe filled with a predetermined amount of short-acting insulin, plastic cannula, needle and pump that periodically deliver the desired amount.

2. For type 2 DM: oral hypoglycemics (suffixes "-ide," "-gliatazone"):

a. First-generation: sulfonylureas class: tolbutamide (Orinase), chlorpropamide (Diabinese).

b. Second-generation: sulfonylureas class: glyburide (DiaBeta, Micronase), glipizide (Glucotrol).

c. Third-generation: biguanides class: metformin (Glucophage, Fortamer, Riomet); α-gluocosidase inhibitors class: acarbose (Precose), miglitol (Glyset); thiazolididinediones (TZD) class: pioglitazone (Actos), rosiglitazone (Avandia) and metformin with glipizide (Metaglip), with glyburide (Glucovance), with rosiglitazone (Avandamet), with pioglitazone (Actoplus Met); meglitinide class (repaglinide (Prandin), nateglinide (Starlix).

d. Exenatide (Byetta): mimics GLP-1 incretin, insulin secretagogue with glucoregulatory effects; used in monotherapy or in combination, injected with prefilled pen (from ugly Gila monster spit—who would believe it!); unlike sulfonylureas and meglitinides, increases insulin synthesis and secretion in presence of glucose only, lessening hypoglycemia risk and causing significant weight loss; being used to treat insulin resistance.

e. Sitagliptin (Januvia): class of dipeptidyl peptidase–IV (DPP-4) enzyme inhibitors that degrade GLP-1 and GIP incretin hormones, which stimulate insulin release in response to increased blood glucose levels following meals to enhance glycemic control; indicated for type 2 DM as monotherapy or in combination; lower side effects (e.g., less hypoglycemia, less weight gain) in control of blood glucose values.

3. Pharmacological effects:

a. Reduce hepatic glucose production, decrease intestinal absorption of glucose.

b. Improve insulin receptor sensitivity, improving glucose utilization in the periphery.

c. Metformin also reduces LDL and raises HDL; useful for patients with CVD.

4. Adverse reactions:

a. Hypoglycemia (when insulin overdose results in insulin shock); especially noted with combination therapy; meglitinide less than for sulfonylureas.

b. Hyperglycemia (insufficient insulin); less common, treated in the hospital.

c. GIT complications.

5. Drug interactions:

a. Increased hypoglycemia with salicylates, NSAIAs, alcohol.

b. Hyperglycemia with corticosteroids and epinephrine.

6. Contraindications:

a. Hepatic and/or renal disease.

b. Cardiac and/or respiratory insufficiencies.

c. Alcohol abuse, severe infections, pregnancy.

C. Thyroid gland replacements: levothyroxine (Synthroid, Levoxyl, Levothroid, Unithroid) and liotrix (Euthroid, Thyrolar).

1. Pharmacological effects:

a. Maintain the function of organ systems.

b. Regulate metabolism and control energy use.

2. Therapeutic uses:

a. Hypothyroidism: hypofunction that requires thyroid replacement therapy for treatment; suppresses thyroid-stimulating hormone (TSH).

3. Drug interactions:
   a. Increased sensitivity to opioids and sedatives.
   b. Increased effects of anticoagulants (warfarin [Coumadin]).
   c. Toxicity with TCAs.
   d. Decreased absorption with antacids, sucralfate (Carafate).
   e. Decreased serum levels with antiseizure drugs and rifampin (Rifadin, Rimactane).
   f. Decreased effects of sulfonylureas.
D. Antithyroid drugs: methimazole (Tapazole), iodide, radioactive iodine; used to treat hyperthyroidism (such as Graves' disease); hyperfunction results from excess hormones circulating in the blood (thyrotoxicosis, thyroid storm, emergency condition).
E. Female sex hormones:
   1. Progesterones: synthetic, medroxyprogesterone (Provera, Depo-Provera) oral and parenteral, levonorgestrel (Norplant) implants.
      a. Pharmacological effects: prepares uterus for implantation after fertilization.
      b. Therapeutic uses:
         (1) Contraception (birth control pill [BCP]); occurs by inhibition of ovulation and thus pregnancy.
             (a) Inhibits release of follicle-stimulating hormone (FSH) and luteinizing hormone (LH).
             (b) Combination with estrogen or alone.
         (2) Treatment of endometriosis, dysmenorrhea, dysfunctional uterine bleeding, premenstrual tension.
         (3) Treatment of postmenopausal symptoms (in combination with estrogen).

   c. Adverse reactions:
      (1) Nausea and vomiting (tolerance does develop).
      (2) Edema and weight gain.
      (3) HBP; increased with tobacco use.
      (4) Increased incidence of dry socket with extraction, increased crevicular gingival fluid and gingivitis levels.
      (5) Uterine bleeding and thrombophlebitis (inflammation of vein); increased with tobacco use.
   d. Drug interactions: decreased effectiveness of BCP when taking antibiotics.
   2. Estrogens (synthetic: Premarin, Estraderm), oral tablets, creams, transdermal patches; includes estradiol.
      a. Pharmacological effects:
         (1) Female sex characteristics, puberty changes, reproductive development, preparation for conception.
         (2) Increased fat deposition, salt and water retention, bone cell activity (osteoblasts).
      b. Therapeutic uses:
         (1) Contraception (see progesterone discussion above) with BCP.
         (2) Treatment of menstrual disturbances (e.g., dysmenorrhea, dysfunctional uterine bleeding).
         (3) *Short-term* treatment of acute symptoms of menopause (hot flashes, sleep disturbances) from a depletion of estrogen.
      c. Adverse reactions: SIMILAR to progesterone.
      d. Drug interactions: increase effects of corticosteroids.

CLINICAL STUDY

Age	34 YRS	**SCENARIO**
Sex	☐ Male ☒ Female	The patient is scheduled for four appointments for quadrant scaling of nonsurgical periodontal therapy after diagnosis of generalized moderate chronic periodontitis based on the AAP classification of periodontal disease. These procedures will require the administration of local anesthesia. Patient calls to make the appointments and provide an update of her medical history.
Height	5'8"	
Weight	110 LBS (previous 135 LBS)	
BP	130/95 (taken at physician's office)	
Chief Complaint	"So that is my medical history! When are we going to start with the therapy?"	
Medical History	Recent diagnosis of Graves' disease, poorly controlled Seasonal allergies GIT distress	
Current Medications	methimazole (Tapazole) 40 mg tid famotidine (Pepcid) 20 mg qd	
Social History	Ballroom dancer	

1. What gland in the body does Graves' disease involve, and what are some common symptoms of the disease?
2. Why does the patient take methimazole (Tapazole) and famotidine (Pepcid)?
3. Are there any changes in dental treatment for this patient in regard to local anesthetic?

1. Graves' disease is a thyroid disorder that causes hyperthyroidism; more common in females and diagnosed between 30 and 40 years of age. Symptoms include enlarged thyroid gland (goiter), exophthalmos (forwardly displaced eyes), hyperactivity, weight loss, tachycardia.
2. Methimazole (Tapazole) is an antithyroid agent that is used to suppress hyperactivity of the thyroid gland that is present with Graves' disease. Famotidine (Pepcid) is an H_2-receptor antagonist that treats GIT disorders such as heartburn and acid indigestion; acts by decreasing gastric secretions.
3. Changes in dental treatment include avoidance of epinephrine in local anesthetic until hyperthyroidism of Graves' disease is controlled, since drug may cause thyrotoxicosis, thyroid storm. Thyroid storm can be fatal and associated with fever, tachycardia, arrhythmia, hypermetabolism, and other serious complications. Treatment may have to wait until the patient has moved from ASA IV status to ASA III and able to have elective dental treatment. Medical consult would confirm this need to wait.

Osteoporotic Patients

Postmenopausal osteoporosis is prevented and treated with bisphosphonates (suffix "-dronate"). Also used to treat bone loss that results from glucocorticoids (prednisone, cortisone) therapy and Paget's disease. Those given orally include alendronate (Fosamax), risedronate (Actonel); those given by IV (injectables): ibandronate (Boniva), pamidronate (Aredia), and zoledronic acid (Zometa). Orals are taken on empty stomach with water ONLY; injectables are for those who CANNOT sit upright. May be combined with vitamin D and/or calcium supplementation. Teriparatide (Forteo) and raloxifene (Evista) offer alternatives to bisphosphonate therapy.
• See Chapter 12, Clinical Treatment: menopausal and geriatric patient.
A. Pharmacological effects:
   1. Alendronate and risedronate increase bone mass, reducing spine, hip, and other fractures.
   2. Ibandronate reduces spine fractures.
   3. Teriparatide increases bone density and strength (synthetic parathyroid hormone).
   4. Raloxifene alters cycle of bone formation and bone tissue loss.

B. Adverse reactions:
   1. GIT complications: difficulty swallowing, erosion and inflammation of esophagus, gastric ulcer.
   2. Hypocalcemia.
   3. Rare: jaw osteonecrosis (damage to blood supply causes bone to die), especially noted with injectables in cancer patients; risk is considerably lower in people who take them orally for osteoporosis.
   4. Forteo may cause impaired thinking and reactions; avoid smoking.
   5. Evista listed in pregnancy category "X" for teratogenicity.
C. Drug interactions: calcium, antacids, and iron can reduce absorption.

Allergic Patients

Patients who suffer from allergies use drugs to control symptoms. See later discussion of respiratory drugs.
• See Chapter 6, General and Oral Pathology, and Chapter 8, Microbiology and Immunology: allergic reactions; 11, Medical and Dental Emergencies: allergic emergencies in dental setting.
A. First-generation H_1-receptor antagonists: diphenhydramine (Benadryl), clemastine (Tavist), dimenhydrinate (Dramamine), doxylamine (Unisom), chlorpheniramine (Chlor-Trimeton, Piriton), hydroxyzine hydrochloride (Atarax). Diphenhydramine is part of dental office emergency kit.
   1. Pharmacological effects:
      a. Decreased vasodilation, bronchodilation, pain, itching (antihistamine effects).
      b. Antiemesis, xerostomia, sedation (stimulation can occur).
      c. Diphenhydramine provides local anesthetic effect.
   2. Therapeutic uses:
      a. Control of symptoms of allergic reactions; however, if anaphylaxis occurs, epinephrine rather than antihistamine should be used for bronchodilation.
      b. OTC sleep aids (e.g., diphenhydramine in Nytol, Phendry, Compoz, Sleep-Eze, Sominex, Unisom).
      c. Preoperative sedation; may also be used as antiemetics.
   3. Adverse reactions:
      a. Drowsiness.
      b. Xerostomia, nausea, constipation.
   4. Drug interactions:
      a. Increased effects of CNS depressants, including alcohol.
      b. Increased anticholinergic effect occurs with anticholinergics, phenothiazines, TCAs.
   5. Contraindications:
      a. Hypersensitivity.

b. Acute asthma attack; epinephrine is MORE effective for latter.

B. Second-generation (selective) H_1-receptor antagonists: loratadine (Claritin), cetirizine (Zyrtec); third-generation (selective) H_1-receptor antagonists: desloratadine (Clarinex), fexofenadine (Allegra).
   1. Pharmacological effects:
      a. Antihistaminic and anticholinergic actions SIMILAR to first-generation drugs but without sedation.
      b. NO CVS effects.
      c. Little evidence for advantage of second- over third-generation that have been developed from second-generation.
   2. Therapeutic uses:
      a. Treatment of rhinitis.
      b. Seasonal allergy symptoms.
   3. Adverse reactions:
      a. Xerostomia.
      b. Constipation.
   4. Drug interactions: SAME as for first-generation.

C. Leukotriene-receptor antagonist: montelukast (Singulair).
   1. Pharmacological effects:
      a. Blocks leukotriene receptor sites.
      b. Prevents leukotrienes from producing airway edema and inflammation, causing bronchoconstriction.
   2. Therapeutic uses:
      a. Treats mild or early forms of asthma as alternative to steroids (carrying rescue bronchodilators still recommended).
      b. Treats season allergy symptoms.
   3. Adverse reactions: dream abnormalities, drowsiness, irritability, restlessness.
   4. Drug interactions:
      a. Chewable form contains phenylalanine (contraindicated for phenylketonuria).
      b. Seizure drugs may decrease effects.

Patients with Gastrointestinal Tract Disorders

Patients with GIT disorders present with vomiting, nausea, constipation, diarrhea, gas, gastric acid complications.
- See Chapter 6, General and Oral Pathology; related discussion on GIT disorders.

A. Emetics: induce vomiting (emesis) to treat poisoning (e.g., OTC syrup of ipecac); abused with eating disorders.

B. Antiemetics: reduce nausea and vomiting (e.g., prochlorperazine [Compazine]); are used with nitrous oxide and other general anesthetics if there is risk of these adverse reactions; can cause CNS sedation and xerostomia.

C. Laxatives: increase GIT motility to treat constipation (e.g., milk of magnesia); abused with eating disorders.

D. Antidiarrheals: reduce GIT motility to treat diarrhea (e.g., Lomotil, Imodium, any opioid); may have xerostomia.

E. The H_2-receptor antagonists (antihistamines, OTC): cimetidine (Tagamet), ranitidine (Zantac), famotidine (Pepcid), nizatidine (Axid) (suffix "-tidine").
   1. Pharmacological effects:
      a. Decreased gastric acid secretions; pain is relieved.
      b. NO further damage to esophageal lining from gastric secretions.
   2. Therapeutic uses:
      a. Treat gastric ulcers resulting from NSAIAs and gastroesophageal reflux (GERD).
   3. Adverse reactions:
      a. Nausea, diarrhea, constipation.
      b. Cimetidine (Tagamet) and ranitidine (Zantac) may cause tachycardia and bradycardia.
   4. Drug interactions:
      a. Decreased absorption with ketoconazole (Nizoral).
      b. Cimetidine (Tagamet) results in increased blood levels of metronidazole (Flagyl), alcohol, lidocaine (Xylocaine), opioids.
      c. Cimetidine (Tagamet) inhibits diazepam (Valium), warfarin (Coumadin).
      d. AVOID ulcerogenics such as NSAIAs and glucocorticoids.

F. Proton pump inhibitors (PPIs): first-generation (OTC): omeprazole (Prilosec); second-generation: lansoprazole (Prevacid), esomeprazole (Nexium), pantoprazole (Protonix) (suffix "-prazole").
   1. Pharmacological effects:
      a. Bind to proton pump in parietal cells of stomach to reduce gastric acid secretions; pain is relieved.
      b. Neutralize gastric acid after it has been released; protect gastric mucosa from damage.
   2. Therapeutic uses:
      a. Treat erosive esophagitis and GERD.
      b. Treat gastric ulcers associated with use of NSAIAs, maintenance therapy for healed ulcers, used with antibiotics for ulcers caused by *Helicobacter pylori*.
      c. Lansoprazole (Prevacid) for limited nighttime and pantoprazole (Protonix) for daytime and nighttime heartburn relief and with long-term use of NSAIAs to prevent GIT ulceration.
   3. Adverse reactions:
      a. Xerostomia, esophageal candidiasis, mucosal atrophy of tongue.
      b. Nausea, diarrhea, constipation.
   4. Drug interactions:
      a. Decrease absorption of weak bases that require acid for absorption such as antiretrovirals, iron salts, systemic azole antifungals.

b. Esomeprazole (Nexium) increases levels of some benzodiazepines (e.g., diazepam [Valium]).

c. Pantoprazole (Protonix) increases effects of SSRIs, some oral hypoglycemics, phenytoin (Dilantin), warfarin (Coumadin).

Patients with Respiratory Disease

Asthma and chronic obstructive pulmonary disease (COPD) are serious respiratory diseases. COPD includes chronic bronchitis and emphysema. For these patients it is difficult to make analgesic choice: aspirin (Bayer, Ecotrin, Empirin, Bufferin) compounds may precipitate attack, so NSAIAs may be contraindicated and opioids cause bronchoconstriction; acetaminophen may be the drug of choice, possibly mixed with a weak opioid. Patients using inhaler should be instructed to rinse thoroughly after using and expectorate, which avoids increasing systemic absorption, reduces tooth staining, reduces risk for candidal infection (with inhalers containing steroid), and reduces taste alteration. Patient MUST bring own inhalers to appointments; however, many personal inhalers may NOT be current, so should be provided for in the dental office emergency kit.

- See Chapters 6, General and Oral Pathology, and 8, Microbiology and Immunology: respiratory disorders and diseases; 11, Medical and Dental Emergencies: respiratory emergencies in a dental setting.

A. The β_2-adrenergic (sympathomimetic) agonists by way of tablets, liquids, inhalers: albuterol (Proventil, Ventolin), metaproterenol (Alupent), salmeterol (Serevent inhaler with fluticasone, Advair Diskus).
1. Pharmacological effects:
   a. Bronchodilation by means of β_2-receptor stimulation in the lungs.
   b. NO antiinflammatory effects.
2. Therapeutic uses:
   a. NOT used alone for treatment of asthma and COPD.
   b. For rescue use ONLY with immediate relief during an attack.
3. Adverse reactions:
   a. Xerostomia, nervousness, insomnia, tachycardia with selective adrenergic β_2-agonists.
   b. However, fewer adverse reactions occur with these selective drugs than with nonselective adrenergic agonists (epinephrine and isoproterenol) that can be administered during an acute attack.
   c. Overuse can lead to hyperreflexive airway, resulting in drug failure during respiratory crisis.
4. Drug interactions:
   a. Increased CVS effects with MAOIs, antidepressants, sympathomimetics (amphetamines, dopamine).

b. Increased risk of malignant arrhythmias with inhaled anesthetics.
   c. Decreased effects with nonselective β-blockers (propranolol, Inderal).

B. Methylxanthine: aminophylline (Phyllocontin, Truphylline), theophylline (Theo-dur, Slo-bid), caffeine.
1. Pharmacological effects: bronchodilation, CNS stimulation, diuresis.
2. Adverse reactions:
   a. Nausea, vomiting.
   b. Anxiety, cardiac palpitations, increased respirations.
3. Drug interactions:
   a. Increased effects with erythromycin (Robimycin, E-Mycin, E.E.S.).
   b. Increased dysrhythmias with CNS stimulants.
   c. Decreased effects with barbiturates, carbamazepine (Tegretol), ketoconazole (Nizoral).

C. Corticosteroid inhalers (metered dose inhalers [MDIs]): triamcinolone (Azmacort, Aerobid), beclomethasone (Qvar, Beclovent, Vanceril); used for acute and maintenance therapy; MDI provides drug directly to pulmonary tissues, lowering dose necessary for effect.

D. Cromolyn (Intal, Nasalcrom): effective ONLY for prevention of acute bronchospasm; NOT a treatment.

E. Anticholinergics: atropine (past asthma drug) and ipratropium bromide (Atrovent): newer drug causes fewer adverse reactions than atropine, used MAINLY for emphysema.

Pregnant Patients

Many drugs can pass through the placental barrier, such as tetracyclines that affect the newborn. However, some medical conditions such as gestational diabetes, hyperthyroidism, or hypertension may require drug therapy to ensure optimal health of mother and fetus. Important to AVOID any unnecessary drugs with pregnant patient and obtain a medical consult if use of any drugs is needed in a dental setting. See FDA Pregnancy Risk Category (PRC) and dental drug examples of each category in Table 9-8. See Chapter 11, Clinical Treatment, for a related discussion.

Patients with Cancer

Cancer patients may undergo chemotherapy (antineoplastics) and/or radiation therapy to eradicate cancerous (malignant) growth (see Chapter 6, General and Oral Pathology: cancer treatment).

Immunocompromised Patients

Patients undergoing immunosuppressive therapy or with autoimmune disease may be taking certain potent drugs.
- See also Chapters 6, General and Oral Pathology, and 8, Microbiology and Immunology: immunocompromised

Table 9-8 FDA use-in-pregnancy ratings with dental drug examples*

PRC	Rating notation	Category interpretation	Dental drug example*	Possible negative outcome[†]
A	Controlled studies show no risk	Adequate, well-controlled studies in pregnant women have failed to demonstrate a risk to the fetus in any trimester of pregnancy.	None	
B	No evidence of risk in humans	Adequate, well-controlled studies in pregnant women have not shown increased risk of fetal abnormalities despite adverse findings in animals, or, in the absence of adequate human studies, animal studies show no fetal risk. The chance of fetal harm is remote but remains a possibility.	Local anesthetics: etidocaine (Duranest), lidocaine (Xylocaine), prilocaine (Citanest) Pain relievers: acetaminophen (Tylenol), ibuprofen (Advil, Motrin, Pamprin), naproxen (Aleve, Anaprox)[‡] Antibiotics: amoxicillin (Amoxil, Polymox), cephalexin (Keflex), clindamycin (Cleocin), erythromycin: base (E-Mycin), estolate (Ilosone), ethylsuccinate (E.E.S.), metronidazole (Flagyl), penicillin V-potassium (Pen-Vee K)	Delayed labor and prolonged pregnancy in mother
C	Risk cannot be ruled out	Adequate, well-controlled human studies are lacking, and animal studies have shown a risk to the fetus or are lacking as well. There is a chance of fetal harm if the drug is administered during pregnancy, but the potential benefits may outweigh the potential risks.	Local anesthetics: bupivacaine (Marcaine), mepivacaine (Carbocaine) Pain relievers: aspirin (Bayer, Ecotrin, Empirin, Bufferin) Centrally acting opioid analgesics: codeine with acetaminophen (Tylenol with codeine), hydrocodone and acetaminophen (Vicodin), oxycodone with acetaminophen (Percocet) Antibiotics: gentamicin (Garamycin)[‡]	Fetal bradycardia Postpartum hemorrhage and delivery complications Neonatal respiratory depression and opioid withdrawal (codeine also has multiple birth defects) Potential ototoxicity in fetus
D	Positive evidence of risk	Studies in humans, or investigational or postmarketing data, have demonstrated fetal risk. Nevertheless, potential benefits from the use of the drug may outweigh the potential risk. For example, the drug may be acceptable if needed in a life-threatening situation or serious disease for which safer drugs cannot be used or are ineffective.	Sedatives: diazepam (Valium), alprazolam (Xanax) Antibiotics: doxycycline (Vibramycin, Periostat)	Possible oral clefts in fetus with prolonged exposure Instrinsic tooth stain
X	Contraindicated in pregnancy	Studies in animals or humans, or investigational or postmarketing reports, have demonstrated positive evidence of fetal abnormalities or risks, which clearly outweighs any possible benefit to the patient.	Antibiotics: chloramphenicol (Chloromycetin)	Maternal toxicity and fetal death

FDA, Food and Drug Administration; *PRC,* pregnancy risk category.
*Nitrous oxide is not rated.
[†]Data from Moore PA: Selecting drugs for the pregnant dental patient, J Am Dent Assoc 129(9):1281, 1998.
[‡]Risk for use during third trimester.

disorders or autoimmune diseases and immune system.

A. Immunosuppressants: cyclosporines, tacrolimus, sirolimus, etanercept (Enbrel).
   1. Pharmacological effects: prevent activity of immune system.
   2. Therapeutic uses:
      a. Prevent rejection of transplanted organs and tissues (e.g., bone marrow, heart, kidney, liver).
      b. Used to treat autoimmune diseases (e.g., RA, MG, SLE, Crohn's disease, ulcerative colitis) and other nonautoimmune inflammatory diseases (e.g., long-term allergic asthma control).
   3. Adverse reactions:
      a. Risk of infections and cancer (MAJORITY of them act nonselectively).
      b. HBP, hyperglycemia, peptic ulcers, liver and kidney injury (especially with cyclosporines).
      c. Gingival hypertrophy with cyclosporines, may be even MORE severe if patient is also taking a calcium channel blocker.
   4. Drug interactions: many interactions noted; needs medical consult.

Patients with Substance Abuse

Substance (drug) **abuse** can be described as use of drugs despite adverse consequences to user or others. Dental patients with **substance** (drug) **addiction** or **drug dependence** may be problematic: (1) they may seek dental care to obtain legal but addictive drugs; (2) patients with drugs in bloodstream may be at risk for adverse drug interaction with dentally prescribed drug. Drugs that can be abused are discussed next, and alcoholic patient is discussed later.

This category does NOT include drugs that cause a discontinuation syndrome when treatment stops abruptly or several doses are missed; can cause similiar withdrawal-like symptoms ("brain zaps," "brain shocks," "brain shivers," or "head shocks") unless medication is gradually tapered off (e.g., occurs with antidepressants such as SSRIs).

• See CD-ROM for related terms.

A. Oral signs: trauma, mucositis, xerostomia, extrinsic stain, high rates of dental caries, gingival lesions, periodontal disease, often from poor oral hygiene.
B. Risk factors:
   1. May be be undergoing **withdrawal,** with **psychological dependence** and **tolerance,** which could affect overall health and attitude.
   2. Drug interaction with local anesthetics (AVOID vasoconstrictor use in cocaine and marijuana users) and ineffectiveness of local anesthetics in drug abusers.
   3. Increased risk for contracting disease such as HIV, hepatitis, STD, infective endocarditis (IE) through IV drug use (IVDA).

   4. Risk of bacteremia is higher in IV drug users, thus antibiotic premedication may be indicated.
C. Barriers to care:
   1. Communication problems related to denial of drug abuse and disordered behavior (careful attention to behavior and physical appearance may help identify condition).
   2. Transportation problems, if patient is unable to drive.
   3. Economic problems related to drug habit costs and possible unemployment.
D. Professional care and homecare:
   1. Careful assessment of patient behavior and appearance (needle marks, sniffing, agitation, dull expression, careless dress and hygiene, dilated or constricted pupils, bloodshot eyes); this needs to be done even if patient claims to be in **abstinence,** a drug-free state.
   2. Thorough intraoral examination with possible increase in risk of oral cancer owing to cohabit of tobacco and alcohol use.
   3. Awareness that patient may request pain or nitrous oxide sedation because of drug habit.
      a. Seek drugs through dental offices by requesting drugs for pain relief.
      b. Suspicions of drug abuse should be aroused when specific drugs are requested.
      c. Eliminating source of pain and prescribing NSAIAs if pain control is necessary, preferable to prescribing addicting drugs.
      d. Short-term prescribing when necessary with medical consult; NOT prescribing with history of drug addiction.
   4. Caution with use of local anesthetics to prevent reactions with illegal drugs (e.g., vasoconstrictor with cocaine use can lead to fatality).
E. Patient or caregiver education should emphasize:
   1. Responsibility for maintaining good oral hygiene and for keeping scheduled recall appointments.
   2. Prevention of oral infection is particularly important in IV drug users because of risk of bacteremia.
F. Abused drugs: many drugs can be abused, and dental professional must be aware of this possibility; alcohol abuse is considered in next section.
   1. Abuse of CNS stimulants: nicotine, caffeine, amphetamines, cocaine.
      a. Caffeine (coffee, tea, sports and soft drinks):
         (1) Physical dependence can occur with consumption of two to three cups of caffeinated drink daily.
         (2) Tolerance can develop.
         (3) Withdrawal can occur 24 hours after last intake, with headache, lethargy, irritability, anxiety, constipation.

b. Nicotine (tobacco products):

(1) Serious diseases can result from use (e.g., CVD, oral and lung cancer); use is linked with increased risk of infant clefts and caries, as well as endodontic complications.

(2) Withdrawal symptoms:

(a) Different for each person.

(b) Aphthous ulcers (canker sores) as keratinization is reduced.

(3) Drugs can be used to reduce symptoms during cessation (behavioral modification can help process):

(a) Nicotine replacement therapy (NRT): chewing gum (Nicorette), lozenges (Commit), patches (Nicoderm, Nicotrol, Prostep, Habitrol), inhaler and spray (Nicotrol) may be used to reduce physical dependence.

(b) Reduce psychological dependence by continuing to release low levels of dopamine (antidepressant bupropion, Zyban); can be used with NRT.

(c) Blocking receptors so smoking is less pleasurable (nicotinic receptor partial agonist varenicline [Chantix] box labeling involving mental states); NOT used with NRT.

(4) Quitlines have been shown to be effective in introducing cessation efforts (healthcare professionals MAINLY use 5 As; ADHA uses three steps: "Ask, Advise, Refer").

c. Amphetamines: dextroamphetamine (Dexedrine), methylphenidate (Ritalin), methamphetamine (crystal meth) (Desoxyn).

(1) Provide sense of euphoria and increased energy; tolerance to euphoria develops.

(2) Toxic symptoms: anxiety, hallucinations, paranoia, aggressiveness.

(3) Withdrawal symptoms: psychological depression and suicidal tendencies.

(4) Acute overdose: mydriasis, HBP, tachycardia, cardiac dysrhythmias.

(5) Abuse of meth may be seen in ALL age groups, including children; high lasts long time (12 hours compared with 1 hour from cocaine).

(6) Methamphetamine produces "meth mouth," erosion based on xerostomia, extended periods of poor oral hygiene, frequent consumption of high-calorie carbonated beverages, bruxism and clenching; smoking MOST damaging form of drug for causing dental destruction.

d. Cocaine (crack, rock):

(1) Creates sense of euphoria, short duration of action (1 hour).

(2) Tolerance to the drug does NOT occur; withdrawal symptoms also do NOT occur.

(3) HBP, MI, CVA, seizure, or dysrhythmias may occur.

(4) Use of vasoconstrictors (such as epinephrine in local anesthetic) is absolutely contraindicated; could be fatal.

(5) Pregnancy category "X" drug.

2. Abuse of CNS depressants: opioids, barbiturates, benzodiazepines, volatile solvents (huffing glue, gasoline), nitrous oxide, alcohol.

a. Opioids: heroin, hydromorphone (Dilaudid), morphine (MS Contin), methadone (Dolophine), oxycodone (OxyContin; with acetaminophen [Percocet], with aspirin [Percodan]).

(1) Pharmacological effects: elevated mood, euphoria, suppressed hunger, reduced sexual drive, slowed respirations, constipation, urinary retention, peripheral vasodilation.

(2) Physical dependence and tolerance develop; MORE drug is needed to achieve "high" feeling.

(3) Opioid overdose: respiratory depression, miosis, coma; overdose treated by administration of short-acting naloxone (Narcan).

(4) Withdrawal effects: lacrimation, rhinorrhea (runny nose), chills, diaphoresis, tremors, tachycardia, HBP.

(5) Treatments:

(a) Methadone maintenance programs.

(b) Counseling such as Narcotics Anonymous (NA).

b. Sedative-hypnotics: benzodiazepines (Valium), barbiturates, meprobamate (Miltown), Quaalude, Librium.

(1) Symptoms: resemble those of alcohol intoxication, with MORE respiratory depression, decreased GIT, urinary, cardiac output.

(2) Prolonged abuse: paranoia and suicidal tendencies.

(3) Withdrawal symptoms are SIMILAR to opioids but can be life threatening (withdrawal replacement drugs may include benzodiazepines).

c. Nitrous oxide: hallucinations, paresthesias of the extremities, mood swings; chronic abuse can cause death.

3. Psychedelics (hallucinogens): marijuana, lysergic acid diethylamide (LSD), phencyclidine (PCP).

a. Effects of psychedelics are psychological; disturb reality perception; tolerance develops quickly.

b. Abuse can cause lasting psychological disturbances, range from panic attacks to schizophrenic episodes to life-threatening depression.

c. Marijuana (cannabis, "weed"):
   (1) Increases pulse rate; reddening of eyes, euphoria.
   (2) Active ingredient has antiemetic effect; can be used by prescription in some states to treat nausea that occurs during cancer chemotherapy.
d. LSD overdose symptoms: mydriasis, HBP, visual distortions, hallucinations, paranoia; flashbacks can occur years after using.
e. PCP (peep, angel dust) users exhibit bizarre behavior, HBP, tachycardia; used alone or with other street drugs; associated with a high incidence of "bad trips."
4. Oral signs of drug abuse:
   a. Rampant caries and tooth loss, halitosis (bad breath), xerostomia.
   b. Trauma to the mouth, teeth, tissues; bruxism (grinding).
   c. Tissue ulceration, gingival recession, periodontal disease.
   d. Increased risk of oral cancer.

CLINICAL STUDY

Age	18 YRS	SCENARIO
Sex	☐ Male ☒ Female	The patient presents for her oral prophylaxis appointment in an agitated state. Her behavior is in direct contrast to her behavior at previous oral prophylaxis appointments. She asks the dental hygienist if he ever partied after work with all the drugs available in the dental office.
BP	112/65 (previous 100/60)	
Chief Complaint	"I want some of that laughing gas!"	
Medical History	None	
Current Medications	None	
Social History	High school student	

1. What might be the cause of the patient's unusual behavior?
2. What is "laughing gas"? Identify its drug classification and common uses. Should it be used at this appointment?
3. What is the significance of the slightly higher blood pressure at this appointment?

1. Patient's unusual behavior could have several possible causes, including anxiety, emotional disturbance, illness, fatigue, substance abuse.
2. "Laughing gas" is slang term for nitrous oxide and oxygen analgesia (sedation). Classified as CNS depressant, along with opioids, barbiturates, benzodiazepines, and alcohol. In dentistry, used to relax anxious patients during dental treatment. Before gas is administered, careful medical and dental history interview and physical assessment must be conducted to determine whether patient is using any drugs; necessary to avoid potential problems such as drug interactions (e.g., with phenothiazines, lithium [Lithobid, Eskalith], TCA) and CNS suppression.
3. Significance of slightly higher blood pressure at appointment may be one indicator of substance abuse, emotional distress, or a similar problem. Alone, vital signs offer little information; however, when combined with other information, may lead to explanation of patient's behavior. Suspicions of drug abuse should be aroused when specific drugs are requested, as well as awareness that patient may request pain or nitrous oxide sedation when not needed (procedure does not entail much pain in a teenager's oral cavity) because of drug habit.

Alcoholic Patients

Alcoholism is a chronic but treatable disease that involves compulsive abuse of ethanol-containing substances. Causes may include genetic, psychological, environmental factors.
A. Systemic complications:
   1. Impaired judgment, mydriasis, slurred speech, ataxia, seizures, coma, even death may occur.
   2. Nutritional deficiencies and cirrhosis of the liver.
   3. May have DTs during withdrawal.
   4. Chronic consumption during pregnancy causes fetal alcohol syndrome (FAS) with mild to severe developmental disturbances; thus pregnancy category "X" drug.
B. Orofacial signs:
   1. Jaundiced (yellow) skin and sclera, puffiness of the eyes.
   2. Reddened nose (rhinophyma), forehead, and cheeks.
   3. Xerostomia, reduced ability to taste, glossitis, odor of alcohol on breath.

4. Enlargement of the parotid gland and the tongue.
5. Facial and dental trauma from falls and injuries.
6. Increased risk of BOTH caries and periodontal disease from poor oral hygiene.
7. Increased risk of oropharyngeal cancer.

C. Treatment:
1. Counseling such as Alcoholics Anonymous (AA).
2. Disulfiram (Antabuse) may be used during treatment; ingestion of alcohol while taking causes the patient to become nauseated (i.e., to vomit); must AVOID alcohol-containing mouthrinses.
3. Use of β-blockers.

D. Risk factors for oral health: nutritional deficiencies, interactions with drugs, infections, trauma, oral cancer (especially if tobacco is also used); caution should be used when administering amide local anesthetics and nitrous oxide sedation.

E. Barriers to care:
1. Communication difficulties; patient may NOT appear for appointments when actively drinking.
2. Transportation problems, if patient does NOT drive or has lost driving privileges and must rely on others.
3. Economic problems if the patient is unable to hold a job or is on fixed income.

F. Professional care and homecare:
1. Use of nonalcoholic mouthrinses.
2. Possible bleeding problems from liver damage.
3. Need for increased level of oral cancer evaluation.
4. Daily supplementation with fluoride and calcium product as needed.
5. Dealing with patient's intoxication and difficulties in keeping appointments.

G. Patient or caregiver education should emphasize need for frequent recall, fluoride and calcium product supplementation, saliva substitutes, need for practicing good homecare because of the risk of infection.

Review Questions

1 The strength of a drug with regard to its ability to achieve a desired effect is termed
A. efficacy.
B. potency.
C. therapeutic effect.
D. tolerance.

2 All of the following are sites of drug elimination, EXCEPT one. Which one is the EXCEPTION?
A. Liver
B. Kidney
C. Colon
D. Lungs
E. Pancreas

3 What is an adverse reaction to a drug that is both predictable and dose related and that acts on target organs?
A. Side effect
B. Toxic reaction
C. Type I allergic reaction
D. Type III allergic reaction
E. Type IV allergic reaction

4 A patient reveals a history of asthma and uses the following drugs: propranolol, acetaminophen, cephalexin, and isoproterenol. Which of these drugs is used to treat asthma?
A. Propranolol (Inderal)
B. Acetaminophen (Tylenol)
C. Cephalexin (Keflex)
D. Isoproterenol (Isuprel)

5 At his recall appointment, John complains that his oral tissues and teeth are sensitive. He states that he chews gum more often because his mouth is dryer. Upon examination, a caries problem is detected. John reports a drug change since his last appointment. Which one of the following drugs could account for the change in his oral condition?
A. Nadolol (Corgard)
B. Digoxin (Lanoxin)
C. Temazepam (Restoril)
D. Sulfinpyrazone (Antazone)

6 A recall patient returns after receiving radiotherapy for cancer of the head and neck. The dental hygienist recognizes that the patient has salivary gland hypofunction in the form of xerostomia. The drug that may be prescribed for this condition is
A. atropine (Atropair).
B. diflunisal (Dolobid).
C. pilocarpine (Salagen).
D. prilocaine (Citanest).

7 An analgesic, antipyretic, and antiinflammatory effect occurs with all of the following drugs, EXCEPT one. What is the EXCEPTION?
A. Diflunisal (Dolobid)
B. Acetaminophen (Tylenol)
C. Naproxen (Aleve)
D. Ibuprofen (Advil)

8 Which of the following is a nonopioid drug that patients take in low doses after a myocardial infarction?
A. Aspirin (Empirin)
B. Acetaminophen (Tylenol)
C. Ibuprofen (Advil)
D. Naproxen (Aleve)

9 A recall patient who is in pain because of a dental abscess is prescribed Tylenol #3. The patient requires diazepam (Valium), an antianxiety drug, before her appointments. A possible drug interaction to be aware of is
A. decreased sedation.
B. increased sedation.
C. increased antitussive effect.
D. decreased analgesia.

10 When respiratory depression occurs because of an overdose of an opioid analgesic agent, a drug that will reverse the respiratory depression is
A. morphine (MS Contin).
B. epinephrine.
C. naloxone (Narcan).
D. ammonia inhalants.
E. lidocaine (Xylocaine).

11 All of the following are TRUE about tetracyclines, EXCEPT one. Which one is the EXCEPTION?
  A. Are used to treat aggressive periodontal disease.
  B. Photosensitivity is a side effect of their use.
  C. Chelation occurs when they are combined with calcium, magnesium, or aluminum.
  D. Tooth discoloration is not an adverse effect of their use.
  E. Use decreases the effectiveness of oral contraceptives.

12 A patient being treated for aggressive periodontal disease complains of a metallic taste, black hairy tongue, and xerostomia. The drug that is causing these conditions is
  A. amoxicillin (Amoxil).
  B. metronidazole (Flagyl).
  C. tetracycline (Tetracyn).
  D. cephalexin (Keflex).
  E. clindamycin (Cleocin).

13 A patient reports no medical conditions on her medical history but indicates that she takes isoniazid (Nydrazid) and rifampin (Rifadin). These medications indicate that she might have
  A. tuberculosis.
  B. human immunodeficiency virus infection.
  C. osteomyelitis.
  D. candidiasis.

14 A patient has aggressive periodontal disease and takes chlorpropamide (Diabinese) for type 2 diabetes. The drug of choice for treating the periodontal disease and avoiding adverse interaction with Diabinese is
  A. doxycycline (Vibramycin).
  B. metronidazole (Flagyl).
  C. penicillin V (Pen-Vee K).
  D. cephalosporin (Keflor).

15 Harry requires prophylactic antibiotic coverage for an artificial heart valve before dental treatment. He also takes digoxin (Lanoxin) to treat congestive heart failure. He is NOT allergic to penicillins. The safest antiinfective agent for Harry that follows AHA recommendations is
  A. tetracycline (Achromycin).
  B. clindamycin (Cleocin).
  C. azithromycin (Zithromax).
  D. amoxicillin (Amoxil).

16 Propranolol (Inderal) is used to treat all of the following conditions, EXCEPT one. Which one is the EXCEPTION?
  A. Angina pectoris
  B. Congestive heart failure
  C. Moderate to severe hypertension
  D. Migraine headaches
  E. Myocardial infarction prophylaxis

17 A patient reports that he is being treated for high cholesterol. He is MOST likely taking which one of the following drugs?
  A. Propranolol (Inderal)
  B. Metoprolol (Toprol XL)
  C. Simvastatin (Zocor)
  D. Atenolol (Tenormin)
  E. Nifedipine (Procardia)

18 Diazepam (Valium) is used in dentistry for all of the following therapeutic uses, EXCEPT one. Which one is the EXCEPTION?
  A. Analgesic
  B. Antianxiety
  C. Anticonvulsant
  D. Muscle relaxant

19 Phenobarbital (Luminal) is used for its anticonvulsant effect and belongs to which one of the following drug groups?
  A. Benzodiazepines
  B. Barbiturates
  C. Nonbarbiturates
  D. Phenothiazines
  E. Monoamine oxidase inhibitors

20 A patient reports that he is taking prochlorperazine (Compazine). All of the following are adverse reactions of Compazine, EXCEPT one. Which one is the EXCEPTION?
  A. Orthostatic hypotension
  B. Seizures
  C. Xerostomia
  D. Tardive dyskinesia
  E. CNS stimulation

21 A patient reports having manic-depression. Which one of the following drugs is used to treat this illness?
  A. Phenelzine (Nardil)
  B. Amitriptyline (Elavil)
  C. Lithium (Lithobid, Eskalith)
  D. Chlordiazepoxide (Librium)

22 All of the following are second-generation antidepressants, EXCEPT one. Which one is the EXCEPTION?
  A. Fluoxetine (Prozac)
  B. Amitriptyline (Elavil)
  C. Trazodone (Desyrel)
  D. Bupropion (Wellbutrin)

23 Sarah reports that she has epilepsy but cannot remember the drug she takes to treat it. She notices that her gingiva is enlarged. The drug she is MOST likely taking is
  A. cimetidine (Tagamet).
  B. fluconazole (Diflucan).
  C. phenytoin (Dilantin).
  D. diazepam (Valium).

24 Carbamazepine (Tegretol) is used as an anticonvulsant agent. Its other pharmacological effects include all of the following, EXCEPT one. Which one is the EXCEPTION?
  A. Antihypertension
  B. Anticholinergic
  C. Antidepressant
  D. Sedative
  E. Muscle relaxant

25 Prednisone (Deltasone) is prescribed to treat all of the following conditions, EXCEPT one. Which one is the EXCEPTION?
  A. Crohn's disease
  B. Rheumatoid arthritis
  C. Addison's disease
  D. Cushing's syndrome
  E. Systemic lupus erythematosus

26 A patient with type 1 diabetes mellitus complains of pain after professional prophylaxis. The dental hygienist recommends a nonopioid analgesic. Which of the following medications would have the LEAST interaction with the patient's medication?
   A. Aspirin (Empirin)
   B. Acetaminophen (Tylenol)
   C. Ibuprofen (Advil)
   D. Diflunisal (Dolobid)

27 A recall patient reveals a recent history of taking Premarin. She states that she has gained weight, and the dental hygienist discovers that the patient's blood pressure is much higher than during previous visits. These symptoms may be the result of
   A. drug interactions.
   B. allergic reactions.
   C. adverse reactions.
   D. toxic reactions.

28 A patient who reports taking levothyroxine (Synthroid) has which of the following conditions?
   A. Hypothyroidism
   B. Hyperthyroidism
   C. Cushing's syndrome
   D. Addison's disease
   E. Cancer

29 When Tom arrives for his dental appointment, he complains of itching and a rash on his arm. He reports that he took his prophylactic antibiotic an hour before his appointment. Which of the following drugs will treat this mild type IV allergic reaction?
   A. Loratadine (Claritin)
   B. Clemastine fumarate (Tavist)
   C. Prednisone (Deltasone)
   D. Ibuprofen (Advil)
   E. Diphenhydramine (Benadryl)

30 A patient with cardiovascular problems has seasonal allergies. Which antihistamine agent has little or no effect on the cardiovascular system and can be safely used for this patient?
   A. Nizatidine (Axid)
   B. Loratadine (Claritin)
   C. Hydroxyzine (Atarax)
   D. Famotidine (Pepcid)

31 When oral surgery is performed, a long-acting local anesthetic is usually needed. Which of the following would be the drug of choice?
   A. Procaine (Novacaine)
   B. Bupivacaine (Marcaine)
   C. Lidocaine (Xylocaine)
   D. Prilocaine (Citanest)
   E. Mepivacaine (Marcaine)

32 Adding a vasoconstrictor to a local anesthetic does all of the following, EXCEPT one. Which one is the EXCEPTION?
   A. Creates hemostasis
   B. Constricts blood vessels
   C. Increases duration of anesthetic
   D. Increases absorption into cardiovascular system

33 When nitrous oxide is used during nonsurgical dental treatment, which of the following is the desired effect?
   A. Loss of consciousness
   B. Conscious sedation
   C. General anesthesia
   D. Respiratory depression
   E. Local anesthesia

34 After terminating the use of nitrous oxide, a patient complains of a headache. Which of the following has occurred?
   A. Diffusion hypoxia
   B. Neuropathy
   C. Allergic reaction
   D. Toxic reaction

35 All of the following are inhalation volatile liquids that are used as general anesthetics, EXCEPT one. Which one is the EXCEPTION?
   A. Halothane (Fluothane)
   B. Enflurane (Ethrane)
   C. Methohexital (Brevital)
   D. Isoflurane (Forane)

36 The MAIN adverse reaction that occurs with the use of an opioid agent as a general anesthetic is
   A. significant cardiovascular change.
   B. excessive salivation.
   C. hypertension.
   D. respiratory depression.
   E. bronchospasm.

37 Abuse occurs with all of the following central nervous system depressant drugs, EXCEPT one. Which one is the EXCEPTION?
   A. Alcohol
   B. Morphine (MS Contin)
   C. Diazepam (Valium)
   D. Nicotine (Camels)
   E. Oxycodone (Percodan)

38 Antineoplastics usually produce all of the following oral conditions, EXCEPT one. Which one is the EXCEPTION?
   A. Mucosal pain
   B. Gingival recession
   C. Gingival hemorrhage
   D. Xerostomia
   E. Mucosal ulceration

39 An asthmatic patient returns for a recall appointment. The patient forgets to bring her inhaler but remembers that it is a corticosteroid inhaler. The active agent in the inhaler is
   A. triamcinolone (Azmacort).
   B. albuterol (Proventil).
   C. metaproterenol (Alupent).
   D. isoproterenol (Isuprel).

40 Asthmatic patients may have allergic reactions when they are given local anesthetics that contain vasoconstrictors. Such reactions may be caused by which of the following in dental cartridges?
   A. Epinephrine
   B. Lidocaine (Xylocaine)
   C. Sodium bisulfite
   D. Sodium sulfate

41 Common oral manifestations of substance abuse include all of the following, EXCEPT one. Which one is the EXCEPTION?
A. Xerostomia
B. Trauma
C. Lichen planus
D. Extrinsic stain
E. Mucositis

42 In the treatment of a patient who is a suspected substance abuser, the safest pain control modality is
A. local anesthetic.
B. local anesthetic with vasoconstrictor.
C. nitrous oxide analgesia.
D. general anesthesia.

43 All of the following are conditions associated with alcoholism, EXCEPT one. Which one is the EXCEPTION?
A. Reddened nose
B. Puffy eyes
C. Yellow skin
D. Dry mouth
E. Fruity breath

44 Prophylactic antibiotics are required for the prevention of infective endocarditis in all of the following conditions, EXCEPT one. Which one is the EXCEPTION?
A. Mitral valve prolapse with valvular regurgitation
B. Past history of infection
C. Prosthetic cardiac valves
D. Valve disorders after heart transplant

45 Diffusion hypoxia may result with headache or other adverse reactions because patient did not receive 5 minutes of 100% oxygen when nitrous oxide sedation terminated.
A. Both the statement and reason are correct and related.
B. Both the statement and reason are correct but NOT related.
C. The statement is correct, but the reason is NOT.
D. The statement is NOT correct, but the reason is correct.
E. NEITHER the statement NOR the reason is correct.

46 Ketamine produces dissociative anesthesia because the patient continues to respond to environment but is not asleep.
A. Both the statement and reason are correct and related.
B. Both the statement and reason are correct but NOT related.
C. The statement is correct, but the reason is NOT.
D. The statement is NOT correct, but the reason is correct.
E. NEITHER the statement NOR the reason is correct.

47 Antimicrobial rinses (e.g., chlorhexidine, Listerine) are contraindicated in a recovering alcoholic taking disulfiram (Antabuse) because reactions occur with antifungal-containing products.
A. Both the statement and reason are correct and related.
B. Both the statement and reason are correct but NOT related.
C. The statement is correct, but the reason is NOT.
D. The statement is NOT correct, but the reason is correct.
E. NEITHER the statement NOR the reason is correct.

48 Digitalis glycoside (Lanoxin) is used in treatment of glaucoma because it decreases kidney output.
A. Both the statement and reason are correct and related.
B. Both the statement and reason are correct but NOT related.
C. The statement is correct, but the reason is NOT.
D. The statement is NOT correct, but the reason is correct.
E. NEITHER the statement NOR the reason is correct.

49 Diazepam (Valium) is a benzodiazepine given as premedication before dental treatment. A history of infective endocarditis requires premedication before dental treatment.
A. Both statements are true.
B. Both statements are false.
C. The first statement is true, the second is false.
D. The first statement is false, the second is true.

50 Contraception using birth control pills occurs because of inhibition of ovulation and thus pregnancy.
A. Both the statement and reason are correct and related.
B. Both the statement and reason are correct but NOT related.
C. The statement is correct, but the reason is NOT.
D. The statement is NOT correct, but the reason is correct.
E. NEITHER the statement NOR the reason is correct.

Answer Key and Rationales

1 **(B)** Potency of a drug refers to strength, which enables it to achieve desired effect. Efficacy is ability, NOT strength, to produce desired effect. Therapeutic effect is clinically desirable action of a drug. Tolerance occurs when no effect takes place because of decreased susceptibility to drug after continuous use.

2 **(E)** Pancreas aids in digestion of foods and regulation of carbohydrate metabolism; however, unlike liver, kidney, colon, and lungs, does NOT function to eliminate drugs from body.

3 **(B)** Toxic reactions and side effects (adverse reactions), unlike allergic reactions, are predictable and dose related. However, toxic reactions, unlike side effects, act on target organs because they are extension of drug's pharmacological effect.

4 **(D)** Isoproterenol (Isuprel), adrenergic (sympathomimetic) agent, affects β_2-receptors in lungs to enhance bronchodilation. Propranolol (Inderal) is a nonselective β-adrenergic blocker that treats cardiovascular diseases. Acetaminophen (Tylenol) is a nonopioid analgesic, and cephalexin (Keflex) is a cephalosporin antiinfective agent.

5 **(A)** Nadolol (Corgard) is a nonspecific β-adrenergic blocker. Common adverse reaction is xerostomia, which can cause an increase in caries and sensitivity. Digoxin (Lanoxin), a cardiac glycoside, temazepam (Restoril), a benzodiazepine, and sulfinpyrazone (Antazone), a uricosuric agent, are NOT associated with xerostomia as an adverse reaction.

6 **(C)** Pilocarpine (Salagen) is a cholinergic (parasympathomimetic) agent that mimics action of ACh (a neurotransmitter) on parasympathetic receptors, thereby increasing salivary excretion. Atropine (Atropair) is an ophthalmic anticholinergic agent that decreases tears. Diflunisal (Dolobid) is a nonsteroidal antiinflammatory agent (NSAIA) that is used

for analgesia. Prilocaine (Citanest) is an amide local anesthetic.

7 (B) Acetaminophen (Tylenol) is a nonopioid analgesic with antipyretic but no antiinflammatory effects. Others are NSAIAs, nonopioid analgesics that possess ALL three stated effects.

8 (A) Aspirin (Bayer, Ecotrin, Empirin, Bufferin) is a nonopioid agent that irreversibly reduces platelet adhesiveness. When used at low dose (other compounds), it prevents unwanted clotting and helps to prevent occurrence of myocardial infarction (MI, heart attack). Others are also nonopioids but do NOT have irreversible platelet effects.

9 (B) Tylenol #3 contains codeine, an opioid analgesic that depresses CNS. Diazepam (Valium) is a benzodiazepine that depresses CNS. When combined, produce additive effect of CNS depression.

10 (C) Naloxone (Narcan) is an opioid antagonist that competes with opioids at receptor sites and thus reverses opioid respiratory depression. Morphine (MS Contin) is an opioid analgesic, NOT antagonist. Epinephrine, lidocaine (Xylocaine), and ammonia inhalants also are NOT opioid antagonists.

11 (D) Permanent tetracycline staining does occur if the drug is given in the period of enamel calcification during tooth development.

12 (B) Metronidazole (Flagyl) is an antiinfective agent. Drug of choice for aggressive periodontitis that may produce ALL three oral effects. Amoxicillin (Amoxil) and tetracycline (Tetracyn) are antiinfectives that treat aggressive periodontitis but that do NOT have ALL three oral effects. Cephalexin (Keflex) and clindamycin (Cleocin) are antiinfectives but are NOT used to treat aggressive periodontitis.

13 (A) Tuberculosis treatments often combine isoniazid (Nydrazid) and rifampin (Rifadin, Rimactane) for their antituberculosis synergistic effects. Drug combination also is used prophylactically in patients who test positive in response to tuberculosis skin test (Mantoux test).

14 (B) Drugs of choice for aggressive periodontitis are metronidazole (Flagyl) and tetracyclines such as doxycycline (Vibramycin). Tetracyclines combined with oral sulfonylureas such as chlorpropamide (Diabinese) result in hypoglycemia. ONLY remaining drug of choice for this patient is metronidazole (Flagyl) because penicillins (Pen-Vee K) and cephalosporin are NOT appropriate for treating aggressive periodontal disease.

15 (D) Amoxicillin (Amoxil, Larotid, Polymox), NOT clindamycin (Cleocin), is first drug of choice in the 2007 American Heart Association (AHA) regimen for prevention of infective endocarditis (IE). Patient is at risk for IE from artificial heart valve. NO adverse drug interactions between amoxicillin

(Amoxil, Larotid, Polymox) and digoxin (Lanoxin), and patient is NOT known to be allergic to penicillin. Combining digoxin (Lanoxin) with azithromycin (Zithromax) may cause increased blood levels of digoxin (Lanoxin), which leads to toxicity, since digoxin belongs to family of macrolide antibiotics. Tetracyclines are NOT drug choice in AHA regimen.

16 (B) Propranolol (Inderal) is an antiadrenergic nonselective β-blocker that treats angina pectoris, hypertension, and migraines and can be used for myocardial infarction (MI, heart attack) prophylaxis. NOT a digitalis glycoside; CANNOT treat congestive heart failure (CHF).

17 (C) Simvastatin (Zocor) is an antihyperlipidemic used to treat hyperlipidemia (high cholesterol). Propranolol (Inderal), an antiadrenergic nonselective β-blocker, metoprolol (Lopressor) and atenolol (Tenormin), antiadrenergic β₁-blockers, and nifedipine (Procardia), calcium channel blocker, ALL treat cardiovascular diseases, NOT hyperlipidemia.

18 (A) Diazepam (Valium) is a benzodiazepine (sedative-hypnotic) agent that is used for anxiety control, for <u>antianxiety premedication</u>, for treatment of seizures, as muscle relaxant; it has NO analgesic effects.

19 (B) Phenobarbital (Luminal) is a long-acting barbiturate that treats epilepsy.

20 (E) Prochlorperazine (Compazine), a phenothiazine, is an antipsychotic agent that depresses, rather than suppresses, central nervous system.

21 (C) Lithium (Lithobid, Eskalith) is an antipsychotic agent that treats manic-depressive illness, now considered bipolar disorder, which cycles between moods of depression or mania. Phenelzine (Nardil), antidepressant monoamine oxidase inhibitor (MAOI), and amitriptyline (Elavil), tricyclic antidepressant (TCA), treat depression other than that with bipolar disorder. Chlordiazepoxide (Librium) is a benzodiazepine that treats anxiety.

22 (B) Amitriptyline (Elavil) is a tricyclic antidepressant (TCA), NOT a second-generation antidepressant. Others are second-generation antidepressants.

23 (C) Phenytoin (Dilantin) is an anticonvulsant agent. Gingival hyperplasia is one of its common adverse reactions. Cimetidine (Tagamet) is an H₂ antagonist that treats ulcers. Fluconazole (Diflucan) is an antifungal that treats candidiasis. Diazepam (Valium), benzodiazepine, is used as adjunct in seizure control, NOT associated with gingival hyperplasia as adverse reaction.

24 (A) Carbamazepine (Tegretol) can create hypertension; NOT classified as cardiovascular disease (CVD) drug.

25 (D) Prednisone (Deltasone), glucocorticoid with antiinflammatory and immune-suppressing effects, treats diseases listed, EXCEPT for Cushing's syndrome. Cushing's syndrome results from hypersecretion of glucocorticoids by adrenal cortex; therefore prednisone is contraindicated for this disease.

26 **(B)** NO adverse drug interaction occurs when acetaminophen (Tylenol) is combined with insulin. Insulin combined with salicylates (aspirin [Bayer, Ecotrin, Empirin, Bufferin] and diflunisal [(Dolobid] or NSAIAs (ibuprofen [Advil, Motrin, Pamprin]) may increase hypoglycemia.

27 **(C)** Premarin, estrogen, is associated with several adverse reactions, including nausea, vomiting, uterine bleeding, weight gain, thrombophlebitis, hypertension (high blood pressure).

28 **(A)** Levothyroxine (Synthroid) is a thyroid gland agent. Administered to patients who have hypothyroidism (insufficient production of thyroid hormone) and require thyroid replacement therapy. Cushing's syndrome and Addison's disease are associated with adrenal cortex abnormalities. Cancers are treated with antineoplastics.

29 **(E)** Diphenhydramine (Benadryl) is an H_1-receptor antagonist (antihistamine). When a type IV allergic reaction creates a rash by releasing histamine, administration of an antihistamine blocks histamine and decreases allergic reaction. Loratadine (Claritin) and clemastine fumarates (Tavist) are antihistamines that treat seasonal allergies. Prednisone (Deltasone) is a steroid, and ibuprofen (Advil, Motrin, Pamprin) is a nonopioid analgesic.

30 **(B)** Loratadine (Claritin) is second-generation H_1-receptor antagonist (antihistamine). Claritin has NO effect on CVS and therefore can be administered to patients with cardiovascular problems. Nizatidine (Axid) and famotidine (Pepcid) are H_2 antihistamines that treat ulcers. Hydroxyzine (Atarax) is an antianxiety antihistamine.

31 **(B)** Bupivacaine (Marcaine) and etidocaine (Duranest) are longer-acting amide local anesthetic drugs. Others are considered shorter-acting drugs.

32 **(D)** Vasoconstrictor constricts blood vessels, thereby decreasing absorption of local anesthetic agent into CVS and increasing duration of agent. Vasoconstrictor also creates hemostasis because of blood vessel constriction.

33 **(B)** Nitrous oxide is not used at the level of a general anesthetic for most nonsurgical dental treatment (standard of care recommends use at less than 50%). When it is used properly, conscious (moderate) sedation should occur with NO significant effect on respiratory system.

34 **(A)** Diffusion hypoxia results in a headache if patient does NOT receive at least 5 minutes of 100% oxygen at the termination of the nitrous oxide sedation.

35 **(C)** Methohexital (Brevital) is ultra-short-acting barbiturate used as an IV agent, NOT an inhalation volatile liquid.

36 **(D)** Primary adverse reaction associated with opioids is respiratory depression, which can be reversed with opioid antagonist such as naloxone (Narcan).

37 **(D)** Nicotine is abused, is a CNS stimulant, NOT a depressant.

38 **(B)** Gingival recession does NOT occur because of antineoplastic agent use but because of other factors in patient's oral cavity.

39 **(A)** Triamcinolone (Azmacort) is a corticosteroid inhaler that achieves significant improvement in pulmonary function. Others are adrenergic agonists that create bronchodilation by means of β_2-receptor stimulation in lungs.

40 **(C)** Sodium bisulfite is antioxidant (preservative) for vasoconstrictor (epinephrine) in dental local anesthetic (such as lidocaine) cartridges. Preservative may be catalyst for allergic reactions in asthmatic patients who receive local anesthetics with vasoconstrictors. Sodium sulfate is natural sulfate found in body.

41 **(C)** Common oral manifestations (signs) of substance abuse include xerostomia, oral and facial trauma, extrinsic stain, mucositis. Lichen planus is an inflammatory disease of unknown origin associated with systemic diseases such as hypertension (high blood pressure) and diabetes mellitus.

42 **(A)** With suspected substance abuser, AVOID use of epinephrine because may interact with cocaine and other drugs. Safest pain control modality is local anesthetic without vasoconstrictor. Nitrous oxide analgesia (sedation) is safe to use but does have potential for abuse and for transmission of infectious diseases (such as hepatitis B or C) if tubing is NOT sterilized. General anesthesia is NOT recommended because of concern for patient safety and dental practice risk management. For general pain control, over-the-counter (OTC) pain relievers are recommended.

43 **(E)** Fruity breath is NOT one of conditions associated with alcoholism. Reddened nose (rhinophyma), puffy eyes, yellow skin (jaundice), and dry mouth (xerostomia) are associated with alcoholism.

44 **(A)** Functional heart murmurs involve NO tissue damage and therefore NO risk of infective endocarditis. American Heart Association (AHA) recommends that antibiotic premedication be given before any invasive dental procedure for patients with prosthetic heart valves, past history of infection, valve disorders after heart transplant, and NOT mitral valve prolapse with regurgitation.

45 **(A)** Both statement and reason are correct and related. Diffusion hypoxia may result with headache and other adverse reactions because patient did NOT

receive 5 minutes of 100% oxygen when nitrous oxide sedation terminated.

46 (C) Statement is correct, but reason is NOT. Ketamine produces dissociative anesthesia because patient continues to fail to respond to environment but is NOT asleep.

47 (C) Statement is correct, but reason is NOT. Antimicrobial rinses (e.g., chlorhexidine, Listerine) that may contain alcohol are contraindicated in a recovering alcoholic taking disulfiram (Antabuse) because reactions occur with alcohol and alcohol-containing products.

48 (E) Neither statement nor reason is correct. Digitalis glycoside (Lanoxin) is used in treatment of congestive heart failure (CHF) with its inability of the heart to pump efficiently because digitalis increases cardiac contractility and output.

49 (A) Both statements are true. Diazepam (Valium) is a benzodiazepine and antianxiety drug that is given as an <u>antianxiety premedication</u> to help cope with dental anxiety. Infective endocarditis (IE) is a serious infection; patients with past history of it need <u>antibiotic premedication</u> before invasive dental treatment.

50 (A) Both statement and reason are correct and related. Contraception using birth control pills occurs by inhibition of ovulation and thus pregnancy.

CHAPTER 10

Medical and Dental Emergencies

EMERGENCY PREVENTION

The combination of pain, stress, infection, and anesthesia use in the dental setting may contribute to medical emergencies. Evaluation includes completion of a comprehensive health history, in-depth history of present illness, assessment of vital signs, physical assessment, and thorough emergency preparation in the dental setting. Instances of when to request a <u>medical consult</u> regarding a patient and/or when to consider a situation an emergency and <u>activate the **Emergency Medical Service** (EMS) system</u> are discussed in this chapter.

- See CD-ROM for Chapter Terms and WebLinks.
- See Chapters 6, General and Oral Pathology: pathological disorders risk for emergencies; 8, Microbiology and Immunology: allergic reactions in a dental setting; 9, Pharmacology, drugs in emergency kit in a dental setting; 14, Pain Management: local anesthesia and nitrous oxide administration emergencies in a dental setting.

HEALTH HISTORY

Patient's health history includes BOTH medical and dental history, as well as in-depth history of present illness. Crucial to BOTH the diagnosis and treatment of and prognosis for conditions experienced by dental patients. Modifying dental treatment as indicated by the health history creates less risk of emergencies in the dental setting.

- See Chapters 9, Pharmacology: antibiotic premedication and *Physician's Desk Reference;* 11, Clinical Treatment: health history; 18, Ethics and Jurisprudence: related ethical concerns.
- A. Identifies changes in drugs and/or conditions that may require <u>antibiotic premedication</u> (e.g., valvular replacement and/or congenital heart disease or transplant).
- B. Identifies precautions, allergies, or conditions that may contraindicate or modify treatment.
- C. Includes record of vital signs.
- D. May assist in identification of oral manifestations associated with some drugs or systemic diseases.
- E. Assists in planning treatment according to physiological and psychological status.
- F. Serves as medicolegal document.

Vital Signs

Vital signs include blood pressure reading, pulse rate, respiration rate, temperature reading (if needed), pupil size. Obtained as a baseline for patient. Specific vital signs are

retaken as needed. Information in the following is taken from the "7th Report of the Joint National Committee on Prevention, Detection, Evaluation, and Treatment of High Blood Pressure" (2003).

- See Chapter 3, Anatomy, Biochemistry, and Physiology: physiology of blood pressure; Chapter 6, General and Oral Pathology: high blood pressure.
- A. Blood pressure: force exerted by circulating blood on the walls of blood vessels.
  1. Measured in terms of air pressure required to compress large artery to point of shutting off blood flow, reading recorded in fractions of millimeters of mercury (mm Hg), although mercury is NO longer used in most modern vascular devices because of possible toxicity. Measurements for healthy adult patient are usually <120/80; cannot feel blood pressure level.
     a. **Systolic pressure:** heart contracts (works):
        (1) Is <120 mm Hg.
        (2) FIRST pulse sound heard when pressure is released from the cuff.
     b. **Diastolic pressure:** heart dilates (rests):
        (1) Is <80 mm Hg.
        (2) Last pulse sound heard when pressure is released from the cuff.
  2. **Prehypertension** ("high normal"):
     a. 120 to 139/80 to 89 mm Hg.
     b. Treat as usual, but recommend that patient schedule a consult with physician.
     c. Usually involves changes in lifestyle to reduce risk of further complications.
  3. **Hypertension** (high blood pressure [HBP]):
     a. Indicated by sustained readings that are ≥140/90 mm Hg.
     b. Can occur for either systolic or diastolic or both.
     c. HBP can have two stages:
        (1) Stage 1: Mild HBP (140 to 159/90 to 99 mm Hg):
           (a) Repeat, patient may have "white-coat" syndrome (elevated arterial pressure specifically during medical exams, probably because of anxiety) or may have raced to appointment.
           (b) NO change in dental care treatment plan.
           (c) MUST refer to physician unless other signs of HBP are present or patient is in denial.

(2) Stage 2: Moderate to severe HBP (>160/>100 mm Hg):
  (a) Ask patient if taking prescribed antihypertensive drug(s); patient may NOT be compliant, since "feels better."
  (b) May NOT be able to perform elective dental care; may need <u>immediate medical consult</u>.
(3) If ≥180/≥110 mm Hg: <u>activate EMS system</u> and treat as emergency.
4. Blood pressure affected by:
  a. Heart rate (HR), stroke volume, total peripheral resistance.
  b. Exercise, eating, stimulants, pain, stress, anxiety, patient positioning.
  c. Drugs being taken, such as antihypertensives or others (e.g., monoamine oxidase inhibitors [MAOIs]).
  d. Recordings taken from right and left arm may differ.
5. Technique for taking blood pressure reading: instruments used to measure blood pressure include stethoscope and sphygmomanometer (cuff size is determined by arm size, cuff too small or large will give false HBP reading); SIMILAR for digital devices; need to wait 2 to 3 minutes between readings for all types.
  a. Cuff placed snugly 1 inch above antecubital fossa, NO clothing between cuff and arm.
  b. Cuff pumped until radial pulse is NO longer felt; note this point (estimated systolic number) and release the pressure.
  c. Cuff then repumped to 10 to 30 mm Hg above previously recorded point (maximum inflation level).
  d. Pressure released slowly until systole (FIRST pulse sound) is heard.
  e. Continues to release pressure slowly until diastole (last pulse sound) is heard (must listen ALL the way down because at times there is a gap in the sounds).
  f. Patient is informed of reading, which is recorded in patient record.
B. Pulse rate frequency of the heart beat or rate, measured in beats per minute (BPM):
1. Taken from radial artery if patient is *conscious* (easy access) and from common carotid artery in *unconscious* patient (more accurate) for adults and brachial artery on infants but ONLY by EMS system personnel; fingers used for palpation, since thumb has own pulse.
2. Taken for 30 seconds if within range (number is multiplied by 2 if the rate is regular); if increased or irregular, taken again for 1 minute.
3. Measurements for healthy patients: adults 60 to 90 BPM; children 80 to 110 BPM.
4. Affected by age, exercise, stress, drugs, stimulants, fasting, long-term illness, emotional state.
5. Unusual pulse rates:
  a. **Tachycardia:** faster than normal; >100 BPM for adult.
  b. **Bradycardia:** slower than normal; <60 BPM for adult.
  c. **Pulsus alternans:** beats are alternately weak and strong.
  d. **Premature ventricular contractions (PVCs):** longer than normal pause or a skip noted between beats; if MORE than 5 per minute, cause for concern as this may represent a heart block.
6. AVOID palpating carotid pulse unless EMS personnel (lack indicates death), since stimulating its baroreceptors with vigorous palpation can provoke severe bradycardia or even stop the heart in some sensitive persons; BOTH should not be palpated at the same time to AVOID risk of fainting or brain ischemia.
C. Respiration rate: obtained by counting number of breaths for 30 seconds (number is multiplied by 2 if rate is regular), one exhalation and one inhalation together count as one breath; if increased or irregular, taken again for 1 minute.
1. Measurement for healthy patient: adults 14 to 20 breaths/min; children 18 to 30 breaths/min.
2. Normal rates can be altered if patient knows that breathing is being observed; overall rates can be affected by anxiety, pain, excitement, infection, presence of fever.
3. Rate, rhythm, quality (if strong, labored, shallow, deep) should be noted MAINLY for those who present with medical history of respiratory symptoms, e.g., asthma, emphysema, congestive heart failure, or allergic reactions.
4. Unusual respiration rates:
  a. **Dyspnea:** difficult or labored breathing.
  b. **Hyperventilation:** increased rate and depth of respirations that result in decreased level of carbon dioxide.
  c. **Kussmaul breathing:** heavy, labored breathing, either rapid or slow; occurs during hyperglycemic incident.
D. Temperature reading: taken with covered thermometer when needed because of signs of clinical infection or inflammation:
1. Measurement in healthy patient: 97.0° to 99.6° F (36.1° to 37.6° C).
2. Fever: elevated temperature by at least a full degree; occurs with infection, acute inflammation, shock, or changes in temperature exposure.

a. Hyperthermia: >105.8° F; with infection or overexposure to heat.

b. Hypothermia: <96.0° F; with shock or overexposure to cold.

E. Pupil size: evaluate for signs of constriction, dilation, evenness during extraoral examination.

1. Dilated pupils (mydriasis): indication of shock, heart failure, hallucinogens, or amphetamine use.

2. Constricted or pinpoint pupils (miosis): with morphine, heroin, or barbiturate use.

3. Loss of evenness (two pupils with different sizes): with concussion.

ASA Physical Classification

Emergencies may be minimized or prevented by the pretreatment evaluation of physical classification status. The **ASA** (American Society of Anesthesiologists) **physical status classification** is used to determine risks and necessary modifications before treatment.

A. ASA I: healthy.

1. Able to walk up one flight of stairs or two level city blocks without distress.

2. Little or no anxiety; little or no risk.

B. ASA II: mild systemic disease or healthy ASA I who demonstrates a MORE extreme anxiety and fear toward dentistry.

1. Able to walk up one flight of stairs or two level city blocks but will have to stop after completion because of distress.

2. History of well-controlled disease, which includes non-insulin-dependent diabetes mellitus (DM), HBP, epilepsy, asthma, or thyroid conditions; ASA I with a respiratory condition, pregnancy, active allergies.

3. Minimal risk during treatment.

C. ASA III: severe systemic disease that limits activity but is NOT incapacitating.

1. Able to walk up one flight of stairs or two level city blocks, but MUST stop enroute because of distress.

2. History of controlled chronic disease, which includes angina pectoris, myocardial infarction (MI), cerebrovascular accident (CVA), congestive heart failure (CHF) or cardiac surgery more than 4 to 6 weeks in the past, slight chronic obstructive pulmonary disease (COPD), controlled insulin-dependent DM/HBP (with drugs).

3. May need medical consult before elective treatment.

4. If dental care is indicated or allowed, stress reduction protocol and other treatment modifications are indicated.

D. ASA IV: severe systemic disease that limits activity and is a constant threat to life.

1. NOT able to walk up one flight of stairs or two level city blocks; distress is present even at rest.

2. History of uncontrolled acute or chronic disease, which includes unstable angina pectoris, MI/CVA within the last 4 to 6 weeks, severe CHF, moderate to severe COPD, and uncontrolled HBP, epilepsy, DM, or thyroid condition.

3. Pose significant risk, since patients in this category have a severe medical problem of GREATER importance to the patient than the planned dental treatment.

4. Whenever possible, NO elective dental care should be performed; should be postponed until medical condition has improved to at least ASA III; will need medical consult before emergency treatment.

E. ASA V: moribund; NOT expected to live longer than 24 hours, hospitalized, terminally ill; elective dental treatment is definitely contraindicated; however, emergency care or palliative treatment may be necessary.

F. ASA VI: died, and organs are to be harvested.

G. Emergency operation of any variety modifies classifications (e.g., ASA III-E).

H. Those who demonstrate a MORE extreme anxiety and fear toward dentistry have a baseline of ASA II even before their medical history is considered; situation raises ASA one level each time.

PREPARATION FOR MEDICAL EMERGENCIES IN DENTAL SETTING

When emergency situations occur, mandatory that ALL personnel in the dental setting know procedures to be followed, location and use of the emergency kit and oxygen, possibly a portable defibrillator and pulse oximeter, and are able to provide basic life support (BLS). MAIN management of emergency involves BLS; drugs delivered are of secondary importance. Kit can be assembled by personnel or purchased as a unit and MUST not contain expired drugs. Personnel are MORE likely to be familiar with one they have organized, which is MORE likely to contain articles that meet needs of particular dental setting. Kit MUST be readily available during treatment time.

ALL staff must be trained to use emergency kit's contents. Periodic emergency drills and posting the telephone numbers of EMS or other appropriately trained healthcare providers is also recommended at the dental setting. *Many states require all dental settings to have portable automated external defibrillator (AED).*

A. Basic emergency kit: MUST include:

1. Noninjectable drugs:

a. Nitroglycerin (sublingual tablets or nitrolingual aerosol spray) for angina attacks.

b. Bronchodilator (asthma inhaler).

c. Glucose source (e.g., orange juice, oral glucose gel or tablets).

d. Aspirin, prevents additional platelet activation and interferes with platelet adhesion and cohesion with cardiac events.

e. Secondary (additional): aromatic ammonia (amyl nitrate), can be used to stimulate breathing.

2. Injectable (IV) drugs:
   a. Epinephrine (1:1000; EpiPens are also recommended) for allergic responses.
   b. Diphenhydramine (Benadryl), histamine blocker.
   c. Secondary (additional): glucagon, hormone that converts stored glycogen into glucose and releases it into the bloodstream.

3. Oxygen with positive pressure administration capability:
   a. Oxygen cylinder (size E) SHOULD be available to deliver 100% oxygen for 30 minutes (5 liters/min with a nasal cannula).
   b. For patient who is NOT breathing, delivery requires pocket mask and demand-valve resuscitator (alternative is Ambu bag); full masks of clear material that provide tight seal are necessary.

B. AED: portable electronic device that automatically diagnoses potentially life-threatening cardiac arrhythmias of ventricular fibrillation and ventricular tachycardia.

1. Arrhythmia can be treated by application of electrical therapy, which stops arrhythmia, allowing heart to reestablish effective rhythm.

2. When turned on or opened, unit will instruct user to connect the electrodes (pads) to patient:
   a. Once pads are properly attached, everyone should AVOID touching victim to prevent false readings by unit.
   b. Pads allow unit to examine electrical output from heart and determine if patient is in viable, shockable rhythm (either ventricular fibrillation or ventricular tachycardia); if device determines that a shock is viable, will use battery to charge internal capacitor in preparation to deliver shock.

C. Pulse oximeter: indirectly measures oxygen saturation and changes in blood volume in skin, producing a photoplethysmograph; useful for monitoring patients during surgical procedures.

1. BEST for simplicity and speed for patients with respiratory and cardiac problems.

2. Monitor displays percentage of arterial hemoglobin in the oxyhemoglobin configuration (possibly heart rate); acceptable normal ranges are from 95% to 100%; for a patient breathing room air at not far above sea level, estimate of arterial pO_2 can be made from blood-oxygen monitor SpO_2 reading.

3. NOT a complete measure of respiratory sufficiency; example: patient with hypoventilation (poor gas exchange in the lungs) given 100% oxygen can have excellent blood oxygen levels while still suffering from respiratory acidosis caused by excessive carbon dioxide.

4. NOT a complete measure of circulatory sufficiency; example: if insufficient blood flow or insufficient hemoglobin in the blood (anemia), tissues can suffer hypoxia despite high oxygen saturation in the blood that does arrive.

MEDICAL EMERGENCIES IN DENTAL SETTING ■

COMMON medical emergencies that may occur in the dental setting include syncope, hyperventilation, airway obstruction. *After* emergency, patient should be called at home or at hospital later in the day to ensure well-being. Cardiovascular and other less common emergencies in the dental setting are discussed later.

Syncope and Orthostatic Hypotension

A. **Syncope** (fainting): MOST common dental setting emergency; MOST common cause of loss of consciousness.

1. MOST often associated with a form of stress.

2. Caused by decreased oxygen flow to the brain, which in turn is caused by:
   a. Psychogenic factors: stress, unwelcome news, noxious smell or sight of a needle or blood (MOST common cause in dental setting).
   b. Nonpsychogenic factors: poor health or exhaustion.

3. Presyncope stage:
   a. Pallor, dizziness, and nausea.
   b. Lowered blood pressure (hypotension) and increased pulse rate (tachycardia).

4. Syncope symptoms:
   a. Loss of consciousness, shallow breathing, dilated pupils.
   b. Lowered blood pressure (hypotension) and thready pulse.

5. As with ALL emergencies that involve unconscious patient, may lead to airway obstruction and death if improperly recognized and treated.

6. Treatment:
   a. Place in **Trendelenburg position** (subsupine with feet elevated higher than head), EXCEPT for pregnant patient (on side before feet are elevated); usually ensures recovery (Figure 10-1).
   b. Maintain open airway to prevent airway obstruction by tongue; imperative for unconscious patient.
   c. Use of aromatic ammonia inhalant (amyl nitrate), as needed, to provide stimulus for breathing; caution is necessary during use to prevent burning of tissue.
   d. Administration of oxygen.
   e. Carefully monitor until vital signs return to baseline; mandatory because syncope is LIKELY to recur soon after recovery; vomiting MOST commonly occurs after unconsciousness.

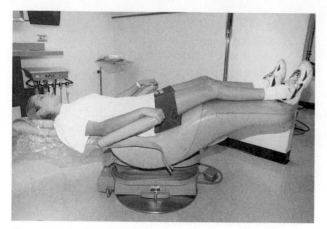

Figure 10-1 Trendelenburg position with patient in a sub-supine position and feet elevated higher than head.

 f. NO further dental treatment should take place for 24 hours.

 7. Prevention: place supine during treatment; use of relaxation techniques and pharmacological means such as use of <u>antianxiety premedication</u> such as diazepam (Valium) and/or nitrous oxide sedation to relieve stress (see Chapter 14, Pain Management).

B. **Orthostatic** (postural) **hypotension:**
 1. May occur when patient sits up quickly from being in a supine position and may result in loss of consciousness (second MOST common cause of unconsciousness).
  a. Sitting upright or standing can lead to a drop in blood pressure; with standing, systolic drops at <25 mm Hg, diastolic drops at <10 mm Hg.
  b. Highest risk: antihypertensives predispose patient (see discussion on angina and nitroglycerin).
  c. Also at risk: patients who are elderly, pregnant, have Addison's disease, or are under nitrous oxide or diazepam (Valium) IV sedation.
 2. Patient usually asymptomatic just before incident and returns to consciousness *after* lying down.
 3. Treatment:
  a. Check vital signs and administer oxygen at 5 liters/min through nasal cannula, if needed.
  b. Reposition slowly from supine position when patient feels recovered.
 4. Prevention: bring ALL patients slowly up after being supine; especially if at risk.

C. Hyperventilation: in dental setting usually related to anxiety.
 1. Increased rate and depth of respirations, which results in decreased level of carbon dioxide.
  a. Other symptoms: tightness of chest, sensation of suffocating, dizziness, tingling in fingers.

  b. Does NOT usually occur in children, since anxiety is released by other means (e.g., crying, refusing to cooperate).
  c. May lead to syncope and then vomiting; vicious cycle.
 2. Treatment:
  a. Calm and place in upright position; respiratory emergencies SHOULD be managed with patient upright, if conscious.
  b. Restore carbon dioxide:
   (1) Have patient try to regulate breathing: inhale, hold breath, then exhale.
   (2) Have patient breathe (called rebreathing) into a paper bag or headrest cover (NOT plastic); patient should hold bag and breathe 6 to 10 times/min.
   (3) ONLY emergency situation in which oxygen does NOT benefit patient; further decreases carbon dioxide levels, which then slows return to normal.
  c. Administration of tranquilizer drug such as diazepam (Valium) by supervising dentist in severe cases, if available.
 3. Prevention: same as syncope.

D. Airway obstruction or foreign body airway obstruction (FBAO):
 1. Occurs MORE easily in dental setting because of supine position; includes cotton rolls, extracted teeth or fragments, restorative materials, vomit.
 2. Types of FBAO:
  a. Partial FBAO with adequate air exchange:
   (1) Occurs when airway is NOT completely blocked, allows patient to cough forcibly and talk.
   (2) Requires NO treatment but must be monitored closely.
  b. Partial FBAO with poor air exchange:
   (1) Patient is NOT able to cough forcibly, and wheezing occurs during inhalation.
   (2) May lead to complete FBAO and SHOULD be treated the same (see next).
  c. Complete FBAO:
   (1) Patient is NOT able to talk; may exhibit universal distress signal of hands clasped at throat.
   (2) Symptoms include cyanosis (blue face from lack of oxygen) and loss of consciousness when the object is NOT removed.
  d. Treatment for conscious adult or child with complete or partial FBAO with poor air exchange is the SAME:
   (1) Ask "Are you choking?" and "Can you speak?"
   (2) Perform Heimlich maneuver: stand behind patient, wrap both arms around the patient

and deliver abdominal thrusts (position flat portion of one fist between navel and bottom of rib cage; wrap other hand around fist), push inward and upward until object is expelled or patient becomes unconscious.

(3) For pregnant or obese patient: chest thrusts in SAME manner on lower portion of the sternum.

(4) <u>Activate EMS system</u> if patient becomes unconscious:

   (a) Help patient to the floor or perform abdominal thrusts in the chair, straddling patient's hips or standing close to hips at one side (if in dental unit).

   (b) Place heel of one hand between navel and bottom of rib cage; position other hand above first, interlacing fingers; push inward and upward five times; then move to head and open airway.

   (c) After abdominal thrusts, repeat process of lifting chin, moving tongue, feeling for and possibly removing the object.

   (d) If airway is still NOT clear, repeat abdominal thrusts as often as necessary; if object has been removed but patient is still NOT breathing, <u>provide BLS</u> and start CPR as needed (see Table 10-1).

(5) In ALL cases, <u>referral to hospital emergency unit</u> because of risk of laryngeal edema.

  e. Prevention: use rubber dam and suction; exercise care when working with small objects in the mouth; do NOT use instruments that can break off easily.

CLINICAL STUDY

Age	33 YRS	**SCENARIO**
Sex	☐ Male ☒ Female	The patient dreads dental appointments but currently experiences less anxiety because she has been following 6-month oral prophylaxis schedule and her appointments take less time. Her dental health is good. After her medical history is updated and her vital signs are obtained, bitewing radiographs are taken. While the dental hygienist leaves the operatory to discuss the case with the office manager, the patient remains seated in an upright position. Upon returning to the patient, the dental hygienist notes that she is breathing rapidly, and she complains of tightness in her chest and tingling in her fingers.
BP	122/82	
Chief Complaint	"I just hate being here and I hate all that happens here!"	
Medical History	Varicose veins removed 6 months ago Knee surgery 5 years ago Achilles' tendon rupture and repair 2 years ago	
Current Medications	None	
Social History	Physician at free clinic Husband recently died in a freak accident	

1. What is the patient most likely experiencing?
2. How should this emergency be handled?
3. Is oxygen indicated? Why or why not?
4. What can further emergency complications can result from this type of breathing?

1. Probably experiencing hyperventilation, indicated by increased rate of respiration, dizziness, chest tightness, tingling in fingers. Most often occurs in the dental setting because of anxiety. Anxiety about dental appointments was a problem, although the patient believed it had lessened. Her recent personal loss and stressful career must also be taken into consideration.
2. Treatment includes calming her and keeping her positioned upright. Rapid rate of breathing results in decreased level of carbon dioxide. To restore carbon dioxide, patient should inhale, hold her breath, and then exhale. If this is ineffective, should breathe into paper bag 6 to 10 times/min (known as rebreathing); important to allow her to hold bag in position.
3. Hyperventilation is one emergency in which administration of oxygen is not indicated; although oxygen would not harm her, it would not benefit her.
4. May lead to syncope and then vomiting, which can become a vicious cycle.

Allergic Reactions

Allergic reactions, including asthmatic attacks, are common in a dental setting. MOST are due to increased sensitivity to allergen (antigen, foreign) that has entered the body (type I [immediate] hypersensitivity).

A. Allergic reactions:
1. Immune system then releases chemicals, such as histamine from mast cells, resulting in varying degrees of reaction.
2. Skin reactions generally are NOT considered true emergencies; however, MUST be monitored for

potential advancement; reactions may be localized or generalized, severity and type of reaction are related to type and amount of allergen to which patient is exposed.

3. If reaction occurs immediately after exposure, is MORE severe; when reaction occurs MORE than 60 minutes after exposure, LESS severe.

4. Types of hypersensitivity and allergic reactions:

   a. Contact dermatitis: occurs when skin is exposed to an allergen.

      (1) Results in erythema, edema, vesicle formation; usually acute and localized but can spread.

      (2) Treatment includes removing cause; referral to dermatologist or allergist; supervising dentist may administer an antihistamine (histamine blocker) such as diphenhydramine (Benadryl) or chlorpheniramine (Chlor-Trimeton) to reduce reaction in an emergency situation.

   b. Urticaria (hives): appears as raised areas of edema, accompanied by pruritus (itching).

      (1) Caused by ingestion of food or drug or by direct skin contact with allergen.

      (2) Treated by removing cause; referral to dermatologist or allergist; supervising dentist may administer antihistamine (histamine blocker), such as diphenhydramine (Benadryl) or chlorpheniramine (Chlor-Trimeton), to reduce reaction.

   c. **Angioedema:** initially may be mistaken for hives.

      (1) Localized, unilateral, colorless and painless swellings of face or neck without well-defined borders of hives; allergic reaction to food or drug; affects tissues of the hands, face, genitals; rarely results in pain or itching.

      (2) Treated by removing cause; referral to dermatologist or allergist, supervising dentist may administer antihistamine, such as diphenhydramine (Benadryl) or chlorpheniramine (Chlor-Trimeton), to reduce reaction; localized, mild allergic reactions should be treated with oral histamine blocker for minimum of 3 days because of risk of recurrence.

   d. **Anaphylaxis** (anaphylactic reaction): MOST severe allergic reaction.

      (1) Level depends on amount of allergen to which patient is exposed, acquired sensitivity, route of entry; occurs almost immediately after exposure; may be fatal despite treatment.

      (2) Can be caused by foods, drugs (MOSTLY penicillin and related antibiotics), rubber latex, or other environmental factors.

   (3) With allergy to local anesthetic agent (rare), MUST be determined if true allergic reaction or some other adverse reaction occurred.

      (a) Allergic reaction occurs MORE often in response to ester injectable local anesthetic agents (e.g., procaine was removed from American market for this reason); allergic reactions to amide agents are rare; NO longer using injected ester agents, so has become rare with injectables.

      (b) Allergy to preservative sodium metabisulfite (antioxidant for the vasoconstrictor) must also be considered; using plain local anesthetic, such as 2% lidocaine (Xylocaine), 3% carbocaine (Mepivacaine), or 4% prilocaine (Citanest), without any vasoconstrictor will prevent almost ALL local anesthetic-related allergic reactions.

      (c) Increased sensitivity to articaine (Septocaine) from sulfites in agent for some patients with history must be considered, MORE in asthmatic population; may want to AVOID use in sensitive or asthmatic patients.

      (d) Localized reaction to topical benzocaine is also possible, since this is an ester; will need to use amide (lidocaine or prilocaine) for topical use instead (see earlier discussion).

   (4) Symptoms affect different body systems and may occur separately or simultaneously:

      (a) Begins rapidly as a skin response (pruritus, urticaria, angioedema); angioedema in mouth may result in airway obstruction.

      (b) Gastrointestinal system may respond with spasms, cramps, nausea, diarrhea; respiratory system exhibits varying degrees of laryngeal edema, which is MOST common cause of death from anaphylaxis.

      (c) Circulatory system involvement includes hypotension, shock, cardiac arrest.

   (5) Treatment for anaphylaxis:

      (a) Place in supine position, administer oxygen at 5 liters/min through nasal cannula; provide BLS as needed.

      (b) Activate EMS system; epinephrine administration (0.3 mg every 5 minutes for adults, 0.15 mg for children; in some cases of systemic allergic reactions, clinical signs of bronchospasm and hypotension persist after FIRST dose of epinephrine) by supervising dentist when diagnosis is definite.

   (c) Because of urgent nature of epinephrine administration in anaphylactic shock, prefilled syringes provide quicker, MORE foolproof method for administering; autoinjectors (EpiPen) are available to inject single adult or pediatric dose when pressed against the thigh (even through clothing) by patient or supervising dentist.

   (d) Since MORE than one dose may be needed, must have MORE than one dose of epinephrine available in the kit (see earlier discussion); <u>referral to emergency unit via ambulance</u> is essential.

B. Asthma attack: respiratory emergency that affects individuals of ALL age groups, often is triggered by anxiety; may occur suddenly or slowly and may be allergic or nonallergic in nature.

1. Identification requires distinguishing asthma (wheezing upon *expiration*) from airway obstruction (wheezing upon *inspiration*).
2. If medical records indicate history of asthma, patient is MORE likely experiencing an asthmatic attack.
3. Involves narrowing of bronchioles (airway) in response to overproduction of mucus and smooth muscle contraction.
4. Results in difficulty breathing because IgE causes histamine release from mast cells, then affects respiratory system.
5. Symptoms of asthma attack: sweating, coughing, nervousness, tightness of the chest, struggling for air (wheezing on expiration).
6. Treatment for asthma attack:
   a. Position upright.
   b. Use bronchodilator (patient's if possible and is current; from emergency kit, if needed); dilates bronchi and bronchioles, increasing airflow; for quick relief, use of short-acting β_2-agonists (SABAs) such as albuterol (Proventil).
   c. Administration of oxygen at 5 liters/min through nasal cannula, allowing patient to position mask.
   d. Administration of epinephrine by supervising dentist if bronchodilator is NOT effective (see above discussion).
   e. <u>Provide BLS and/or referral to hospital emergency unit</u>, if necessary.
7. Prevention: AVOID trigger for attack if possible; prepare for emergency; reduce patient stress.

CLINICAL STUDY

Scenario: A healthy 12-year-old boy recently experienced trouble breathing after eating a peanut butter sandwich. His mother relates this experience at his next dental appointment when asked if there has been any change in his medical history. She says that his symptoms included wheezing and a swollen face. His parents took him to the local hospital emergency unit, where his blood pressure was 60/40 mm Hg and his breathing was labored. He received an injection of epinephrine (adrenaline), and minutes later his blood pressure normalized and his breathing difficulty abated.

1. Describe the pathogenesis and etiology of the young boy's clinical presentation.
2. What lab tests would help confirm the diagnosis?
3. What role did epinephrine play in facilitating his recovery?
4. What preventive measures should he and his mother take in the future?

1. Patient had an allergic response to peanuts, based on his symptoms and the case history. Therefore the presumptive diagnosis is anaphylactic response. Pathogenesis is that of a type I (immediate) hypersensitivity response: after having become sensitized to peanut antigens, upon subsequent exposure he produced an IgE response that triggered anaphylaxis.
2. Tests to confirm and further explore this diagnosis would include skin test with peanut antigens (to see whether responds with wheal and erythema) and radioallergosorbent test (RAST), which specifically seeks out blood IgE antibodies that are reactive with particular antigens.
3. Epinephrine was the solution to his emergency because this drug causes decrease in mast cell degranulation, vasoconstriction, and maintenance of blood pressure and respiratory rate, resulting in rapid inhibition of type I allergic or hypersensitivity response. Other drugs that could be administered as second line of treatment include corticosteroid, such as prednisone, and bronchodilators in inhalers such as albuterol (Preventil).
4. Future medical precautions would include avoiding peanuts and carrying self-injectable emergency epinephrine pen (EpiPen), because peanuts may be hidden component of some foods (especially ethnic foods) and thus difficult to avoid entirely.

Cardiovascular Emergencies

Although NOT as common as the medical emergencies discussed previously, emergencies related to the cardiovascular system (CVS) can occur; they are the MOST serious. CVS emergencies include angina pectoris, heart attack, cardiac arrest, and stroke and can occur in the dental setting. BLS is also discussed (Table 10-1).

Table 10-1 Basic life support (by lay rescuer), ABCDs (see notes below)

ABCDs	Adult CPR (8 years and older)	Child CPR (1 to 8 years old)	Infant CPR (less than 1 year old)*
Airway	Establish unresponsiveness; activate EMS system, and locate AED if possible. Open airway using head-tilt, chin-lift.	Establish unresponsiveness; call for help. Open airway using head-tilt, chin-lift.	Establish unresponsiveness; call for help. Open airway using head-tilt, chin-lift.
Breathing†	Determine breathlessness within 5 to 10 seconds. No breathing: give two ventilations (1 second per breath) with enough volume to produce visible chest rise.	Determine breathlessness within 5 to 10 seconds. No breathing: give two ventilations (1 second per breath) with enough volume to produce visible chest rise.	Determine breathlessness within 5 to 10 seconds. No breathing: give two ventilations (1 second per breath) with enough volume to produce visible chest rise.
Circulation‡	Begin compressions, pressing 1½ to 2 inches in center of chest, between nipples, using two hands, with heel of one hand, second hand on top. Give 100 compressions per minute, allowing chest to recoil; 30 compressions followed by two breaths. Continue until AED arrives, there is movement, or EMS arrive.	Begin compressions, pressing ⅓ to ½ of chest depth in center of chest, between nipples, using two hands, with heel of one hand, second hand on top. Give 100 compressions per minute, allowing chest to recoil; 30 compressions followed by two breaths. After five cycles, activate EMS. Continue until AED arrives, there is movement, or EMS arrive.	Begin compressions, pressing ½ to 1 inch of chest depth, just below nipple line, using two fingers. Give 100 compressions per minute, allowing chest to recoil, 30 compressions followed by two breaths. After five cycles, activate EMS system, continue with compressions and breathing until EMS arrive.
Definitive care/defibrillation	Use adult pads. When attempting defibrillation with AED, deliver one shock followed by immediate CPR, beginning with chest compressions. Check rhythm after giving five cycles (about 2 minutes).	Use child pads if available, adult pads when not. When attempting defibrillation with AED, deliver one shock followed by immediate CPR, beginning with chest compressions. Check rhythm after giving five cycles (about 2 minutes).	Not recommended to use AED because of age.

AED, Automated external defibrillator; *CPR,* cardiopulmonary resuscitation; *EMS,* emergency medical services.
*Different values for newborn infant.
†Breathing is performed only on adults who experience lack of oxygen because of drowning, drug overdose, or carbon monoxide poisoning; breathing is still used on children, since they are more likely to have trouble breathing if they unexpectedly collapse.
‡To maximize effectiveness of compressions, victim should lie supine on hard surface (e.g., backboard or floor), with rescuer kneeling beside victim's thorax.

A. Angina pectoris: chest pain caused by decreased oxygen flow to the heart (anoxia).
  1. Prevention: remind patients with history of angina to bring own nitroglycerin (NTG) to dental appointment (watch expiration of patient's supply).
  2. Symptoms:
    a. Includes chest pain, which may spread to jaws and teeth, even edentulous arches.
    b. Lasts 3 to 5 minutes after cause of the pain is removed; person will remain still in attempt to relieve pain.
  3. Types:
    a. Stable angina: often caused by emotional upset or physical exertion.
      (1) With constant duration and intensity of pain, quickly relieved by administration of NTG.
      (2) Ointment, patch, or pill forms of NTG may be prescribed by physician to prevent or reduce number of angina episodes; NOT recommended for rapid treatment of angina because work slowly; MUST use sublingual NTG for quick relief.
    b. Unstable angina: can occur when victim is at rest.
      (1) Episodes have greater intensity, longer duration, MORE frequent occurrence.
      (2) NOT relieved by administration of NTG.
    c. Treatment for either type of angina in dental setting:
      (1) Calm patient and position as comfortably as possible.
      (2) Administer oxygen at 5 liters/min through nasal cannula, as needed.

(3) Administer NTG sublingually (beneath tongue), as needed; works as a vasodilator; emergency kit should contain it:
    (a) Sublingual tablet has shorter shelf-life; may be used for 6 months after container opened; metered spray form has longer shelf-life; one metered spray is equal to 1 tablet.
    (b) Ammonia inhalant (amyl nitrite) can be used; provides significant vasodilation in 10 seconds (however, side effects are greater).
(4) Usually 1 to 3 sublingual tablets (or SAME number of sprays) relieve pain in 1 to 2 minutes; BEST to follow patient's instructions for NTG use; pain should NOT return.
(5) Side effects include orthostatic (postural) hypotension and headache resulting from antihypertensive effects.
(6) If NO relief occurs after tablets or sprays or if angina returns after relief, MI may be occurring.

B. Myocardial infarction (MI, heart attack): also known as coronary thrombosis or coronary occlusion (acute coronary syndrome) (depending on etiology).
  1. Death of portion of heart muscle (irreversible necrosis), caused by decrease or lack of oxygen flow to that part of heart muscle (prolonged ischemia).
  2. May be caused by atherosclerosis with occlusion (blocking) of coronary arteries or by thrombosis (blood clot) in artery that supplies heart muscle.
  3. INCREASED risk with stressful situation; however, MOST often occurs while victim is at rest; may follow preexisting anginal condition.
  4. Symptoms of MI:
    a. Diffuse crushing pain in chest, arm, neck, shoulder, lower jaw, especially left side, since pain can spread from chest to other areas.
    b. Pain is of greater intensity and duration than angina pectoris; LESS intense symptoms for women.
    c. Patient typically moves around in attempt to alleviate discomfort; other symptoms include dizziness, shortness of breath, cold and clammy skin, weakness, fatigue, anxiety, denial of possible MI.
  5. Treatment for MI:
    a. Position however patient is MOST comfortable.
    b. Administer NTG if have not done already; angina pectoris that is NOT relieved by NTG may lead to cardiac arrest; if conscious, patient can be asked to chew aspirin (at least 160 mg and up to 325 mg), which prevents additional platelet activation and interferes with platelet adhesion and cohesion.
    c. Activate EMS system.

    d. Administer oxygen at 5 liters/min through nasal cannula.
    e. Provide BLS as indicated (Table 10-1).
    f. May need administration of morphine sulfate IV by supervising dentist to alleviate pain and attendant anxiety, if available.
  6. Considerations after MI:
    a. Withholding emergency or elective surgery (or periodontal procedures by dental hygienist) for 4 to 6 weeks and then determining functional capacity (FC).
    b. Dental care should be delayed unless patient can meet 4 METs (metabolic equivalents) and/or further medical testing has been completed to quantify level of cardiac risk in treatment; medical consult before ALL dental treatment.
    c. May start taking drugs, including anticoagulants (heparin [Calciparine, Liquaemin] and warfarin [Coumadin]); antiplatelets (aspirin and clopidogrel [Plavix], dipyridamole [Aggrenox, Persantine]); digitalis (Crystodigin, Lanoxin); and NTG; these have associated side effects (e.g., increased bleeding) (see Chapter 9, Pharmacology).

C. Sudden cardiac arrest (SCA, sudden death): abrupt, unexpected cessation of breathing and circulation.
  1. Causes of SCA:
    a. Cardiovascular disease (CVD), drug overdose, electrocution, drowning.
    b. Anaphylactic shock, hypoxia.
  2. Symptoms of SCA: NO pulse or respiration, cyanotic tissues, dilated pupils, unconsciousness.
  3. Treatment of SCA for adult, child, or infant: provide BLS through CPR (Table 10-1).

Cerebrovascular Accident

A. Cerebrovascular accident (CVA, stroke): classified according to cause, such as cerebral embolism, hemorrhage, infarction, or thrombosis.
  1. Symptoms: headache together with confusion, impaired speech, paralysis, unconsciousness; vary in relation to area affected and type of CVA and do NOT regress.
  2. CVA is NOT a common dental office emergency; predisposing factors include HBP, DM, CVD, and history of transient ischemic attacks (TIAs).
  3. Treatment for CVA:
    a. If patient is conscious, allow to remain upright; if unconscious, position supine, with head slightly elevated.
    b. Activate EMS system.
    c. Monitor vital signs (blood pressure will be elevated).
    d. Administer oxygen at 5 liters/min through nasal cannula to unconscious patient; for

conscious, administer oxygen ONLY when respiratory difficulty exists; <u>provide BLS</u> as needed.

4. Other considerations after CVA:
   a. High incidence of recurrence; thus patients with history pose greater risk in the dental office; management involves recording vital signs at each appointment; high blood pressure readings are of concern.
   b. Withholding emergency or elective surgery (or periodontal procedures by dental hygienist) for 4 to 6 weeks and/or further medical testing has been completed to quantify level of risk in treatment; <u>medical consult</u> before ALL dental treatment.

c. Physical limitations during appointment (understanding, speech, and movement) and with oral hygiene care treatment by drugs such as anticoagulants (heparin [Calciparine, Liquaemin], warfarin [Coumadin]), antiplatelets (aspirin and clopidogrel [Plavix], dipyridamole [Aggrenox, Persantine]) with possible side effects (increased bleeding).

B. Transient ischemic attack (TIA, temporary or incipient stroke):
   1. Similar to a CVA yet lasts for ONLY few minutes; symptoms regress, NO permanent neurological damage results.
   2. NOT mini-strokes but precursors to CVA; patient remains conscious but experiences confusion.
   3. MUST make medical referral.

CLINICAL STUDY

Age	54 YRS		SCENARIO
Sex	☒ Male ☐ Female		The patient is in the dental office for his recall oral prophylaxis appointment. Shortly after the patient is placed in a reclining position and treatment is begun, the patient asks to sit up. He appears pale, is short of breath, and says that his chest hurts. He takes 3 tablets of nitroglycerin sublingually, but his chest still hurts.
Height	5'10"		
Weight	195 LBS		
BP	158/94		
Chief Complaint	"I feel fine and can't wait anymore to have my teeth cleaned, since it has been a whole year."		
Medical History	Myocardial infarction 5 years ago Past cigar smoker Bypass heart surgery 4 years ago Angina pectoris (occasional)		
Current Medications	nifedipine (Procardia) 10 mg tid nitroglycerin sl prn		
Social History	Tax accountant		

1. What term describes the pain in the patient's chest?
2. How should this condition be treated?
3. What is indicated by the continued presence of chest pain after the patient's use of nitroglycerin tablets?
4. What type of drug is nitroglycerin?
5. What other drug should be administered?
6. Describe how this situation is managed if the patient loses consciousness.

1. Chest pain is angina pectoris and is caused by decreased oxygen supply to the heart. Pain may spread to jaws and teeth, even edentulous arches.
2. Treatment of angina includes administration of nitroglycerin (NTG) tablets beneath tongue (sublingual). It is best to follow patient's instruction for administering drug, if possible. Relief often results within 90 seconds.

While patient is experiencing angina, should be placed in whatever way patient is most comfortable. Oxygen should be administered to any patient who is experiencing chest pain. Can also use metered NTG spray form (1 spray equals 1 tablet). Many patients carry expired drugs, so it is important to have these emergency drugs ready in the emergency kit in a dental office.

3. When angina pectoris is not relieved after three NTG tablets or spray cycles, myocardial infarction (MI, heart attack) must be considered. Although this patient does exhibit predisposing factors for a cerebrovascular accident (stroke, CVA), such as hypertension (high blood pressure [HBP]) and cardiovascular disease (CVD), presence of nonresponding angina pectoris is strongly suggestive of MI and not of CVA.

4. A vasodilator and the most effective drug in the treatment of angina, NTG increases blood flow to coronary arteries by decreasing coronary artery resistance. It may result in orthostatic (postural) hypotension and/or headache.
5. If conscious, patient can be asked to chew aspirin (at least 160 mg and up to 352 mg), which prevents additional platelet activation and interferes with platelet adhesion and cohesion.
6. If patient loses consciousness, management includes BLS of cardiopulmonary resuscitation (CPR). First, the dental setting must activate EMS system; position patient supine, open airway, assess breathing, and begin chest compressions as needed. Chest compressions are given on center of chest, between nipples, pressing 1½ to 2 inches and watching chest recoil between compressions; must give 100 compressions per minute. Breathing is performed only on adults who experience lack of oxygen because of drowning, drug overdose, or carbon monoxide poisoning; breathing is still used on children, since they are more likely to have trouble breathing if they unexpectedly collapse. To maximize effectiveness of compression, victim should lie supine on hard surface (e.g., backboard or floor), with rescuer kneeling beside victim's thorax.

Seizures, Hypoglycemia, and Hyperglycemia

Other common medical emergencies that may be encountered in the dental setting include seizures, hypoglycemia, hyperglycemia.
A. Seizures:
1. MOST caused by epilepsy; other causes include prolonged high fever, alcohol or drug withdrawal, trauma to head, congenital abnormalities, imbalance of body fluids; in dental setting, seizures caused by epilepsy may be triggered by stress.
2. Seizures are categorized according to the area of brain affected and associated symptoms:
   a. Grand mal seizure: MOST severe type, MOST common type; has three phases:
      (1) Prodromal phase (early symptom of disease): occurs before seizure activity, may result in a personality change, may include aura (scent, flicker of light, or noise) that is unique for that person (few seconds to several hours).
      (2) Convulsive (ictal) phase: loss of consciousness, associated with an epileptic cry caused by air rushing from the lungs, with tonic movements that occur as the body becomes rigid (10 to 20 seconds) and clonic movements that result from the contraction and relaxation of muscles and cause patient to jerk violently (2 to 5 minutes).
      (3) Postictal stage: patient sleeps soundly after seizure activity (10 to 30 minutes); provide BLS if needed, and may be critical at this time; snoring during sleep indicates that airway is partly blocked; gurgling sound indicates that airway MUST be suctioned for vomitus or blood, with confusion and disorientation; full recovery takes several hours.
   b. Petit mal (absence) seizure: less severe type, less common type.
      (1) Occurs MORE often in children than in adults.
      (2) Involves LOSS of awareness of surroundings for a few seconds; victim stares blankly and experiences twitching or rapid blinking.
   c. Partial seizure: jerking of one side of body because ONLY one hemisphere of brain is involved, trancelike appearance and engagement in purposeless activity.
   d. Hysterical seizure:
      (1) Occurs when there is an audience and used to manipulate others, indicates that this seizure can be triggered by emotions and anxiety.
      (2) Involves movements that are MORE controlled (e.g., repeated up-and-down movement of one arm).
   e. Status epilepticus:
      (1) With SAME symptoms present during convulsive stage of grand mal, but symptoms last longer than 5 minutes; uninterrupted, with NO recovery between episodes; may last for hours or days.
      (2) MAJOR cause of death is related directly to seizures, MUST have immediate medical referral.
3. Treatment for seizure(s): MAIN objective is to prevent patient from becoming hurt and provide support afterward.
   a. Other considerations:
      (1) Remove dental objects from mouth if possible (removable appliances are NOT recommended; may cause trauma or may be aspirated during seizure activity); do NOT place fingers in the mouth of a patient having a seizure.
      (2) If anticipating a seizure (noting aura) during prodromal phase ONLY, can place bite block or mouth prop.
      (3) Clear area surrounding patient; NO attempt should be made to restrain patient.
      (4) Place conscious patient on side afterward; for unconscious patient, place patient in supine position and maintain open airway.

(5) Patient should NOT be given anything to eat or drink; also should NOT be permitted to drive afterward.

(6) <u>Activate EMS system</u> if injury occurs during seizure or if breathing is NOT present.

b. Drugs patient might be taking include anticonvulsants, such as phenytoin (Dilantin), which may result in gingival overgrowth.

B. Hypoglycemia (low blood sugar): increased risk with history of DM; MORE common emergency with DM than hyperglycemia.

1. Caused by skipped meal, excess insulin, increased exercise, or change in routine; onset rapid for patient who requires insulin; symptoms occur MORE slowly for individuals who take oral hypoglycemic drugs.

2. With cold sweat, headache, trembling, weakness, possible personality change, nervousness, and confusion; confusion may be mistaken for inebriation.

3. Can cause potential fatal insulin shock; although can be experienced by anyone, MOST occurs with type 1 DM.

4. Treatment for hypoglycemia:

a. If patient is conscious: give glucose replacement (see earlier discussion about kit).

b. If patient unconscious:

(1) Position supine, with feet elevated; normally, breathing and circulation are maintained; pulse rate is MORE rapid but blood pressure is NOT affected.

(2) Because glucose CANNOT be administered to unconscious patient, administration of glucagon (hormone that converts stored glycogen into glucose and releases it into the bloodstream) IV or IM by supervising dentist, if available.

(a) Response occurs in 10 to 15 minutes.

(b) If parenteral administration is NOT possible, small amounts of glucose gel can be placed in the mouth in mucobuccal fold.

(c) When patient is unconscious for >30 seconds, seizure activity is MORE likely to occur; if seizure occurs, must be managed *before* hypoglycemia is treated.

c. Then <u>activate EMS system</u>, as needed.

C. Hyperglycemia (high blood sugar): LESS common emergency with DM than hypoglycemia.

1. FIRST indication of disease; reason DM is diagnosed in patients.

2. Occurs in response to little or NO insulin or when glucose level is too high; may occur with DM or with undiagnosed DM; urine samples indicate high glucose level and presence of ketones.

3. Infection, stress, illness, failure to comply with therapy, and other factors that increase need for insulin may lead to this condition.

4. At an emergency level, patient has increased thirst and urination, loss of appetite, nausea, vomiting, Kussmaul breathing, dry warm skin, and fruity, sweet odor of the breath; heart rate is rapid and weak, and blood pressure is lower than normal; when these symptoms are present, NO further dental treatment is performed and <u>medical consult</u> is needed; emergency situation; if untreated, may lead to unconsciousness (diabetic coma or ketoacidosis):

a. <u>Activate EMS system</u>; patient typically is seen immediately by physician and hospitalized; condition may advance to diabetic coma.

b. If patient's skin is dry and has ketoacidic smell, <u>administration of glucose IV or IM may be lethal</u>.

5. When it is NOT known whether nature of emergency is hyperglycemia or hypoglycemia, condition is treated as *hypoglycemia* by EMS personnel, since if NOT treated quickly, may lead immediately to serious damage or death; alternatively, permanent disability or death takes much longer to occur with hyperglycemia.

CLINICAL STUDY

Age	65 YRS	SCENARIO
Sex	☒ Male ☐ Female	The patient is following a 6-month recall schedule for oral prophylaxis and examination. His intraoral examination notes slight to moderate levels of dental biofilm and calculus deposits, with slight gingivitis.
Height	6'2"	
Weight	245 LBS	
BP	144/80	
Chief Complaint	"I am a little tired from all my travel this week, and the girls are keeping me up."	
Medical History	Type 1 diabetes mellitus for 45 years, well controlled Secondary hypertension for 2 years	
Current Medications	U-100 insulin (Humulin 70/30) bid hydrochlorothiazide (Lopressor) 100 mg bid	
Social History	Sales executive who recently adopted twin baby girls from overseas with his second wife	

1. Which of patient's medical conditions are associated with potential emergency?
2. Describe potential emergencies the dental hygienist should be aware of for this patient.
3. Is the blood pressure recorded for this appointment within normal range?

1. Hypertension (high blood pressure [HBP]), diabetes mellitus (DM), and antihypertensive drugs pose risks and may lead to an emergency.
2. Several emergencies are possible with this patient. A common emergency in the dental setting involves patient positioning. Antihypertensive drugs may increase chance of loss of consciousness caused by orthostatic hypotension (lowering of blood pressure from remaining in one position for significant period). Patients may experience dizziness, lightheadedness, loss of balance, or loss of consciousness when raised from supine position or when they stand up on their own. Important to raise patients slowly and allow them to sit upright before being dismissed. Potential for hypoglycemia or hyperglycemia (low or high blood sugar, respectively) is also of concern for patients who have DM. Individuals with insulin-dependent DM are more likely to have hypoglycemia. Conscious patients who have episode of hypoglycemia demonstrate quickly occurring symptoms of cold sweat, headache, trembling, weakness, personality change, confusion. Source of glucose, such as orange juice or other glucose source replacement, should be given to reverse symptoms. Hypoglycemia may result in insulin shock if not resolved.

3. If unconsciousness occurs because of hypoglycemia, patient will be unable to take glucose source and injection of glucagon IV or IM will be necessary by supervising dentist, if available. When chronic hyperglycemia occurs in uncontrolled or noncompliant diabetics, patient presents dry warm skin, Kussmaul breathing, fruity breath odor, increased thirst and urination. Factors that increase need for insulin, such as stress, illness, or infection, will cause hyperglycemia. If these symptoms occur, dental treatment should be stopped and medical consult should be sought. Will result in diabetic coma if not resolved. If the patient's skin is dry and patient has ketoacidic smell, administration of glucose IV or IM may be lethal. Presence of both HBP and DM also is a concern. Cerebrovascular accident (CVA, stroke) does not commonly occur in the dental setting, but having two predisposing factors (HBP and DM) does increase a patient's risk for this occurrence.

4. Blood pressure reading of 144/80 indicates higher than normal systolic reading (range is <120 mm Hg) but diastolic is within normal range (<80 mm Hg). Because systolic reading is above 140, second blood pressure reading should be taken to check accuracy; patient may have "white-coat" syndrome or raced to appointment. Reading is below level that necessitates a medical consult (160 to 179/100 to 109 mm Hg or greater). Patient may have stage 1 (mild) high blood pressure (HBP) (140 to 159/90 to 99 mm Hg). However, must refer to physician for follow-up medical consult on HBP, especially with patient's medical history.

COMMON DENTAL EMERGENCIES

Dental emergencies occur as result of dental treatment or because treatment is needed. Include avulsed tooth, displaced tooth, postsurgical hemorrhage, broken instrument tip, foreign body injuries, needlestick, burns.

- See Chapters 6, General and Oral Pathology: dry (necrotic) socket and Ludwig's angina; 8, Microbiology and Immunology: standard precautions, needlestick protocol, sharps and waste handling; 13, Periodontology: periodontal and pericoronal (pericoronitis) abscesses; 14, Pain Management: needle breakage.

A. Avulsed tooth: completely removed from socket because of trauma, may involve moderate pain or NO pain.
   1. Immediate examination in dental setting or emergency hospital unit by a dental professional.
   2. Ask patient to bring tooth along in a wet handkerchief, milk, or water or in buccal vestibule (preferred mode of transport because of maintenance of hydration in saliva); purchased transport medium for sport teams is now available.
   3. Radiograph of area to identify any remaining fragments; reimplantation of tooth and placement of splint.
   4. BETTER prognosis results when there is short time between avulsion and reimplantation.
   5. Root canal therapy, as indicated; observation of other trauma and tetanus booster may be indicated.

B. Displaced tooth: loosened in socket and visibly moves, usually associated with pain.
   1. Immediate examination in dental setting or emergency hospital unit by a dental professional.
   2. Radiograph of area to check for root fracture; applying splint depending on severity of displacement; instructing NOT to chew or bite with tooth.
   3. Observation of other trauma; identification of need for tetanus booster; application of cold packs to minimize external swelling.

C. Postsurgical hemorrhage:
   1. Primary bleeding: within 24 hours after extraction.
   2. Secondary bleeding: 24 or more hours after extraction.
   3. Prevention:
      a. Awareness of medical conditions that could cause problems (updating medical history), may be taking anticoagulant drugs ("blood thinners") such as aspirin, warfarin (Coumadin, Dicumarol).
      b. American Dental Association has stated that these rarely need to be discontinued before MOST dental procedures because adverse reactions could occur: there is greater risk of thromboembolic events than uncontrollable bleeding if medication is temporarily stopped; if risks of drug are considered too great, need medical consult.

      c. Bleeding levels monitored by international normalized ratio (INR); INRs ≤2.5 are safe for invasive dental work.
         (1) Older test is prothrombin time (PT), broad measurement of time it takes blood to clot; normal PT levels were 11 to 13.5 seconds.
         (2) Result of a PT test is now converted into standard INR units that can be compared regardless of the reagent used; MOST common INR target range for patient taking anticoagulants is 2 to 4; INR of 5 or more is typically avoided because risk of bleeding increases significantly.
      d. Instruct patient (both written and oral instruction) to refrain from tobacco and alcohol use and AVOID rinsing area, drinking from straw, or strenuous exercise for 24 hours.
   4. Treatment: control by biting on folded gauze, folded tissue, or tea bag (theophylline is a vasoconstrictor).

D. Broken instrument tip: requires removal from mouth.
   1. Clinician stops procedures, keeps patient calm, and asks patient NOT to swallow.
   2. Recovery of instrument tip:
      a. Visually examine area FIRST, then dry with cotton roll (NOT with air syringe).
      b. Examine sulcus with gentle strokes of a curet in a spoonlike manner; tip should NOT be pushed into base of sulcus.
      c. If tip is NOT located, expose periapical radiograph of suspected location of broken tip.
      d. If tip is still not located, must have immediate medical referral and radiographs of chest and gastrointestinal area; policy is essential for the management of this emergency; SHOULD include an outline of the steps to be followed; ALL personnel should be familiar with this policy.

E. Foreign body injuries to patient:
   1. Injuries caused by objects that are foreign to a particular part of the body; in dentistry, MOST often affect the eyes and respiratory tract (see earlier discussion).
   2. Typically involve polishing agents, calculus, restorative materials, chemicals, or extracted teeth.
   3. Prevention:
      a. Protective eyewear SHOULD be worn by patient during treatment.
      b. Children must be attended to at ALL times.
      c. Clinician MUST have knowledge of equipment being used and rotation direction of rubber cup when polishing.
      d. Patient should be informed of ALL procedures and role in prevention.

e. Throat pack of 4 × 4 gauze should be used to protect pharynx.

f. Clinician must use care when handling instruments and polishing pastes; pastes and other solutions should NOT be held directly over patient's face.

g. Thin instruments SHOULD be replaced to prevent breakage; rubber dam SHOULD be used as needed during treatment.

4. Treatment:

a. For cases involving aspiration, radiographs of the chest and gastrointestinal area may be necessary to locate the object. See earlier discussion of respiratory obstruction (FBAO).

b. If object has entered the eye (reacts by tearing and blinking): ask patient to look down and position upper lid over lower lid for 1 second; then pull lid upward.

   (1) If object or particle can be seen in lower lid, use moistened cotton applicator to retrieve object and flush eye using eye cup or eye washing station.

   (2) Must have immediate medical referral, especially if object CANNOT be removed; to prevent rubbing the eye, stabilize gauze over eye with adhesive tape.

F. Wounds that break the skin of clinician:

1. Slippage of instruments during treatment or cleanup; dull instruments; sudden patient movement; needlestick; bite.

2. Treatment:

a. Clean wound with soap and water; may be necessary to force puncture wound to bleed.

b. Place ice pack on area to reduce swelling.

c. Apply firm pressure to control bleeding of a laceration.

G. Foreign bodies in eye of clinician: see earlier discussion.

1. Prevention:

a. Wear protective eyewear.

b. Maintain stable fulcrum on dried surface during instrumentation and use sharp instruments.

c. Use approved method or device to recap needles.

d. Take care when passing instruments; NEVER pass instruments over the patient's face or eyes.

H. When cross-infection or contamination is a concern, use needlestick protocol for postexposure management (see Chapter 8, Microbiology and Immunology).

I. Burns that occur in laboratories and sterilization areas are MOST often caused by Bunsen burners, denture torches, autoclaves, or dry heat sterilizers.

1. Classified according to their source (e.g., heat or chemicals) or depth:

a. Superficial (first-degree) burns involve ONLY epidermis, top layer of skin, with redness, dryness, pain.

b. Deep (second- and third-degree burns) involve BOTH layers of skin, epidermis and dermis.

   (1) With redness and blisters that may open and weep, causing a wet appearance, swelling results and is painful, since exposed nerve endings are sensitive to air; scarring may occur during healing.

   (2) These wounds often become secondarily infected.

2. Basic steps of treatment:

a. Small superficial (first-degree) burns SHOULD be immersed in cool water or ice to stop burn (ice can be used ONLY for this type of burn); clean area and cover with antibiotic ointment; most often does NOT require medical attention.

b. Deep (second- and third-degree) burns must have immediate medical referral:

   (1) Cool area with large amounts of cool water.

   (2) Remove clothing from area carefully; however, cloth that sticks to the burn should NOT be removed.

   (3) Ointments, butter, oil, and other remedies should NOT be placed on deep burn that requires medical attention.

   (4) Blisters should be left intact to help prevent infection; dry, sterile bandage should be used to cover the burn loosely to prevent infection.

   (5) Must NOT allow patient to become chilled or overheated; if possible, burned area SHOULD be elevated above the heart.

   (6) Large deep burn can cause shock from pain and body fluid loss.

   (7) Must have immediate medical referral to ensure hydration, asepsis, wound management.

c. Chemical burns:

   (1) Will continue to burn as long as agent is in contact with the skin; affected area should be flushed with water (but NOT forcefully; vigorous flushing may further damage the area), and soaked clothing removed.

   (2) If an eye is affected, required eye washing station should be used to flush the eyes for 15 to 20 minutes; head should be tipped so that the affected eye is lower than the other eye.

   (3) If chemicals have been inhaled, must have immediate medical referral.

CLINICAL STUDY

Age	42 YRS	SCENARIO
Sex	☒ Male ☐ Female	The patient visits the dental office on Wednesday morning for an extraction of tooth #15. The extraction is simple and no complications are expected. After the extraction, sterile gauze is placed over the wound and patient is instructed to bite the gauze for 30 minutes. Verbal instructions for care of the extraction site are given before he is released. On Thursday afternoon, he calls the office from the road where he had to dig himself out of the snow. He is calling because the extraction site has begun to bleed.
Chief Complaint	"I am sorry I smoked, but I needed to relax after such a try-ing week."	
Medical History	Smokes one pack of cigarettes a day	
Current Medications	None	
Social History	Traveling computer specialist Tends to use sugared mints for fresh breath	

1. What verbal instructions should have been given to the patient after the extraction?
2. Is the bleeding that occurred on Thursday considered primary or secondary bleeding?
3. Describe the appropriate treatment for this situation.
4. What could the patient have done to prevent the recurrence of bleeding?
5. What could dental personnel have done to prevent the situation?

1. Patient should have been given verbal instructions to avoid all of the following for at least 24 hours: strenuous activity, rinsing the mouth, drinking from a straw, smoking, drinking alcohol.
2. Bleeding that occurs 24 hours after extraction is considered secondary bleeding; bleeding that occurs within first 24 hours is primary bleeding.
3. Treatment of postsurgical hemorrhage includes returning to the dental office if occlusion on gauze does not halt bleeding. Because bleeding has recurred, patient should not drink from straw or rinse area with warm saline rinses for 24 hours.
4. Smoking after the extraction most likely was the cause of secondary bleeding, although strenuous activity when he traveled may have been involved.
5. In cases of surgical tooth extraction, written instructions in addition to verbal instructions should be given to the patient. Although patient may indicate that he understands procedures to be followed, he may not hear or remember all instructions. In this case, he did not adhere to instruction regarding smoking.

Review Questions

1 What is the pressure in the blood vessels termed when the heart contracts?
   A. Diastolic
   B. Systolic
   C. Pulse
   D. Ventricular

2 During an emergency, which artery is used by emergency personnel to check the pulse for an unconscious adult?
   A. Femoral
   B. Brachial
   C. Carotid
   D. Radial

3 The term "premature ventricular contractions (PVCs)" refers to
   A. longer than normal pause or skip between beats.
   B. slower than normal pulse rate.
   C. alternately strong and weak beats.
   D. faster than normal pulse rate.

4 Which of the following is administered immediately by the supervising dentist when treating an anaphylactic reaction?
   A. Oxygen
   B. Epinephrine
   C. Corticosteroids
   D. Antihistamines

5 What is the possible side effect of Dilantin that can affect dental health?
   A. Gingival hyperplasia
   B. Dry mouth
   C. Increased chance of syncope
   D. Decreased prothrombin time

6 Erythema and small vesicle formation on the hands in response to wearing latex gloves are an example of
A. pruritus.
B. urticaria.
C. contact dermatitis.
D. angioedema.

7 Those who are LEAST likely to hyperventilate include
A. males.
B. children.
C. elderly.
D. females.

8 The emergency oxygen tank or cylinder in the dental office should include which size?
A. H
B. B
C. C
D. E

9 If the mask becomes fogged when oxygen is delivered to a patient, it indicates which of the following?
A. Flowmeter is set too high.
B. Mask does not fit the patient correctly.
C. Tank is empty, and no further oxygen is available.
D. Patient has started breathing.

10 What is the primary advantage of using an emergency kit assembled by office personnel?
A. Office personnel are more familiar with the contents.
B. It is less expensive than manufactured kits.
C. There is no advantage; manufactured kits are always superior and more effective.
D. Office personnel know where it is stored.

11 When blood pressure is taken, the cuff is initially inflated to 110 mm Hg, the point at which the pulse can no longer be palpated. To which level should the cuff be inflated next?
A. 90 to 110 mm Hg
B. 100 to 110 mm Hg
C. 130 to 140 mm Hg
D. 150 to 160 mm Hg

12 Which of the following is indicated for the patient who is experiencing an asthma attack?
A. Aspirin or ibuprofen
B. Bronchodilator
C. Glucagon
D. Diazepam

13 Which emergency is NOT triggered by stress?
A. Insulin shock
B. Hyperventilation
C. Epileptic seizure
D. Asthma attack
E. Anaphylaxis

14 In the prodromal phase of which type of seizure does a person experience an aura?
A. Petit mal
B. Partial
C. Grand mal
D. Hysterical

15 What is the initial treatment for syncope?
A. Positioning the patient upright
B. Administering oxygen
C. Using ammonia inhalants
D. Positioning the patient in the Trendelenburg position

16 What emergency situation occurs when a diabetic patient who requires daily insulin has increased thirst and urination, Kussmaul breathing, and a fruity, acetone breath?
A. Hyperglycemia
B. Insulin shock
C. Hypoglycemia
D. Low blood sugar

17 Which of the following procedures applies to the treatment of any emergency in the dental office?
A. Patient should always be moved from the dental chair.
B. Use of a manufactured drug kit ensures greater success.
C. Basic life support is considered primary management.
D. Oxygen administration is always necessary for ALL emergencies.
E. Administration of drugs is considered primary management.

18 What should be done in the dental office for a patient with partial airway obstruction and poor air exchange?
A. Manage the situation as for a complete airway obstruction.
B. Do not intervene; allow the patient to cough and expel the obstruction.
C. Administer back blows as needed until the object is expelled.
D. Do nothing until the patient becomes completely unconscious.

19 When performing cardiopulmonary resuscitation on an adult, how far down should the chest compressions be on the center of the chest, between the nipples?
A. ⅓ to ½ inch
B. 1 to 1½ inches
C. 1½ to 2 inches
D. 2 to 2½ inches

20 The ratio of compressions to breaths for a child victim during basic life support is
A. 15:2.
B. 15:5.
C. 30:2.
D. 30:5.

21 For a child who requires basic life support, breaths should be given within the last ____ second(s).
A. 1
B. 2
C. 5
D. 10
E. 15

22 After determining that an adult victim is unconscious, the NEXT step in this emergency situation is to
A. activate EMS system.
B. perform CPR for 1 minute and then activate EMS system.
C. determine whether the victim is breathing.
D. open the airway.

23 What is used for a child of 7 years who requires chest compressions?
A. One finger
B. Two fingers
C. One hand
D. Heel of one hand
E. Heel of one hand, second hand on top

24 A patient is being transported to the dental office after an accident during volleyball practice that resulted in an avulsed tooth. The BEST method of transporting the tooth is in
   A. a dry cloth.
   B. a glass of water.
   C. patient's vestibule.
   D. patient's cleaned hand.

25 During scaling an instrument tip breaks. What should the clinician do immediately?
   A. Examine the area closely, after drying it thoroughly with air.
   B. Ask the patient to help locate the tip with his or her tongue.
   C. Examine the sulcus, using a curet and gentle strokes.
   D. Expose a radiograph of the area.

26 You have been performing the Heimlich maneuver for a victim for some time without being able to dislodge the obstruction. As the individual becomes unconscious, you help him to the floor and activate the EMS system. It is now necessary to
   A. straddle the victim's hips, administer five abdominal thrusts, and attempt to ventilate.
   B. continue administering the Heimlich maneuver, with the victim positioned on his side.
   C. kneel beside the victim's hips and administer six to ten chest compressions.
   D. do nothing further until emergency assistance arrives.

27 For the patient who has experienced a heart attack within the last 4 weeks
   A. patient positioning is important; the patient should be more upright.
   B. the clinician should be ready to perform basic life support as needed.
   C. dental treatment should be performed only after medical consult.
   D. the clinician must determine whether angina is present.

28 At which of the following blood pressure readings is a medical consult indicated?
   A. 110/68
   B. 119/76
   C. 150/92
   D. 164/102

29 Conditions that predispose a patient to cerebrovascular accident include all of the following EXCEPT one. Which is the EXCEPTION?
   A. Diabetes mellitus
   B. Hypertension
   C. Transient ischemic attack
   D. Cardiovascular disease
   E. Epilepsy

30 An epileptic cry caused by air rushing from the lungs may occur during which stage of a grand mal seizure?
   A. Prodromal
   B. Convulsive
   C. Postictal
   D. Characteristic of hysterical seizure instead

31 A seizure may be caused by all of the following EXCEPT one. Which is the EXCEPTION?
   A. Prolonged high fever
   B. Trauma to the head
   C. Congenital abnormalities
   D. Drug withdrawal
   E. Myocardial infarction

32 Alleviating a patient's fears of dental treatment will aid in preventing each of the following EXCEPT one. Which is the EXCEPTION?
   A. Angina pectoris
   B. Myocardial infarction
   C. Anaphylaxis
   D. Hyperventilation
   E. Epileptic seizure

33 Which of the following is an example of an ASA II medical history of a patient?
   A. Uncomplicated pregnancy
   B. Uncontrolled epilepsy
   C. Controlled angina pectoris
   D. Controlled insulin-dependent diabetic

34 Which of the following is an example of an ASA III medical history of a patient?
   A. Slight COPD with exercise
   B. Myocardial infarction 7 months ago
   C. Controlled epilepsy
   D. Active allergies

35 Bleeding levels in patients at risk of hemorrhage are MORE effectively monitored by
   A. blood glucose testing.
   B. international normalized ratio.
   C. prothrombin time.
   D. reducing drugs and performing surgery.

36 A sublingual tablet of nitroglycerin has a long shelf-life; it may be used for 12 months after the container is opened. The metered spray form of nitroglycerin has a much shorter shelf-life, and one metered spray is equal to two tablets.
   A. Both statements are true.
   B. Both statements are false.
   C. The first statement is true, the second is false.
   D. The first statement is false, the second is true.

37 ASA IV classification of physical status indicates significant risk because the person has moderate systemic disease that limits activity and is a constant threat to life.
   A. Both the statement and reason are correct and related.
   B. Both the statement and reason are correct but NOT related.
   C. The statement is correct, but the reason is NOT.
   D. The statement is NOT correct, but the reason is correct.
   E. NEITHER the statement NOR the reason is correct.

38 One of the following does NOT predispose a patient to orthostatic hypotension. Which one is the EXCEPTION?
   A. Elderly
   B. Pregnancy
   C. Addison's disease
   D. Nitrous oxide or diazepam (Valium) IV sedation
   E. Getting up slowly from dental chair

39 Presyncope stage is characterized by
A. thready pulse.
B. loss of pulse.
C. tachycardia.
D. bradycardia.

40 Which type of burn involves only epidermis, the top layer of skin, along with redness, dryness, and pain?
A. Superficial
B. Deep
C. Second degree
D. Third degree

Answer Key and Rationales

1 **(B)** Systolic pressure is pressure in blood vessels when the heart contracts (work). Diastolic pressure is pressure in blood vessels when the heart dilates (rest). Pulse pressure is found by subtracting diastolic reading from systolic reading. Ventricular pressure applies to pressure within ventricular chambers of the heart, NOT within blood vessels.

2 **(C)** Common carotid artery is ONLY used to check carotid pulse for an unconscious adult in an emergency situation by trained EMS system personnel (if <60 mm Hg, artery is NOT palpable). Radial artery is used during routine appointments to check for radial pulse (if <90 mm Hg, artery is NOT palpable) on conscious patient. Note that checking for pulse such as carotid pulse is NOT a part of basic life support (BLS) or cardiopulmonary resuscitation (CPR) by nontrained personnel. Brachial artery is used during an emergency for an unconscious infant ONLY by EMS personnel. Femoral artery is NOT commonly used to check pulse in an adult. Since systolic blood pressure rarely drops low enough that carotid pulse cannot be felt, lack of a carotid pulse usually indicates death.

3 **(A)** Premature ventricular contractions (PVCs) are longer than normal pauses or skips in beat. Bradycardia is a slower than normal pulse rate (<60 BPM). Pulsus alternans is alternate strong and weak beats. Tachycardia is faster than normal pulse rate (>100 BPM).

4 **(B)** Epinephrine is drug of choice when treating severe allergic reactions such as anaphylaxis. Rapid effect after administration makes it extremely useful when time is crucial. Epinephrine is a vasopressor and bronchodilator and has antihistamine actions (prevents mast cell degranulation). Can be given by supervising dentist as an IV or can be given by supervising dentist or patient by injectable pen (EpiPen). As with MOST emergencies, oxygen can be administered (5 liters/min with a nasal cannula) but will NOT stop the reaction. Corticosteroids and antihistamines can be used in non-life-threatening allergic reactions.

5 **(A)** Phenytoin (Dilantin) can result in slight to severe gingival hyperplasia and may affect patient's oral hygiene. Other possible side effects include skin rash, drowsiness, gastric distress, restlessness. Dry mouth (xerostomia) may result from antihistamines and other drugs. There is an increased chance of loss of consciousness from orthostatic (postural) hypotension, which MOST commonly occurs with antihypertensive drugs. Bleeding may occur with increased use of aspirin. Prothrombin time (PT) is a more generalized test. Bleeding levels are monitored more effectively by international normalized ratio (INR); INRs ≤2.5 are safe for invasive dental work.

6 **(C)** Contact dermatitis is characterized by erythema and small vesicle formation on the hands, a localized allergic reaction. Pruritus, urticaria, and angioedema are other types of allergic reactions.

7 **(B)** In the dental setting, hyperventilation in response to anxiety is LEAST likely to occur in children because they release their anxiety in other ways (e.g., crying, refusing to cooperate). State of breathing faster and/or deeper than necessary, thereby reducing the carbon dioxide concentration of the blood to below normal. Hyperventilation can cause symptoms, such as numbness or tingling in the hands, feet, and lips, lightheadedness, dizziness, headache, chest pain, slurred speech, and sometimes syncope (fainting).

8 **(D)** Oxygen tanks that are part of the emergency equipment in dental settings SHOULD be at least size E, which supplies 100% oxygen for 30 minutes, administered at 5 liters/min with a nasal cannula.

9 **(D)** When oxygen mask becomes fogged during use, this indicates that patient has started breathing. Full mask made of clear material SHOULD be used; should fit the patient to provide tight seal. Setting flowmeter too high, empty tank, or improper fit of mask does NOT cause mask to fog.

10 **(A)** Office personnel will be MORE familiar with the contents of an emergency kit that they have assembled to meet the needs of their particular dental setting. Although this kit is likely to be less expensive, the cost is NOT an issue. Effective use of an emergency kit is the MOST important factor. Personnel should ALL know where the kit is stored, NO matter if purchased or NOT.

11 **(C)** When blood pressure is taken, the cuff is initially inflated until the radial pulse is NO longer felt. This is the estimated systolic number (palpatory systolic pressure) and is mentally noted as aid in hearing first systolic sound; cuff is then reinflated 10 to 30 mm Hg above this point. If pulse is NO longer palpated at 110 mm Hg, cuff is then inflated to 130 to 140 mm Hg. Inflating to only 90 to 110 mm Hg would result in loss of FIRST systolic reading; inflating to 150 to 160 is unnecessary and is uncomfortable for patient.

12 (B) Asthma attack is a respiratory emergency that often is triggered by anxiety. Overproduction of mucus and contraction of smooth muscles narrow bronchioles, making breathing difficult. Treatment includes use of a bronchodilator, which acts directly on the bronchial smooth muscle. Patient SHOULD be allowed to use own bronchodilator if possible (it is current and patient knows how to use it). Aspirin or ibuprofen may cause an asthma attack in those who are allergic to it. Glucagon is administered IV or IM by the supervising dentist to an unconscious patient who is experiencing hypoglycemia. Diazepam (Valium) can be administered IV by the supervising dentist for the treatment of severe hyperventilation, if available.

13 (E) Anaphylaxis is caused by exposure to an allergen and is NOT associated with stress. Insulin shock, hyperventilation, epileptic seizure, and asthma attack may be triggered by stress; thus it is necessary to lower anxiety as much as possible by explaining ALL procedures thoroughly, attending to patients promptly, closely monitoring patients.

14 (C) Aura, such as flicker of light, certain smell, or noise, may occur during prodromal phase of a grand mal seizure. Characteristic symptom of grand mal seizure; is NOT characteristic of petit mal, partial, or hysterical seizure. Can also occur before migraine headache; allows epileptics time to prevent injury to themselves. Time between appearance and onset of a migraine or seizure can be anything from a few seconds up to an hour; MOST who have auras have the same type of aura every time.

15 (D) Syncope (fainting) is caused by a decreased oxygen supply to the brain. Placing the patient in the Trendelenburg position (subsupine with feet elevated higher than head) typically ensures recovery by increasing blood flow to the brain and thereby replenishing oxygen. If such positioning does NOT result in recovery, ammonia inhalants (amyl nitrate) can be used to stimulate breathing, and oxygen can be administered (5 liters/min with a nasal cannula).

16 (A) Hyperglycemia (high blood sugar) is an emergency that affects patients with diabetes mellitus (DM) who require daily insulin. Results when there is little or NO insulin available and may be caused by failure to adhere to therapy, increased exercise, or infection. With increased thirst and urination, Kussmaul breathing, and the presence of a fruity odor on the breath. Loss of appetite, nausea, and vomiting may be present. Urine samples indicate high glucose levels and presence of ketones. May result in diabetic coma. Hypoglycemia (low blood sugar) and its potentially fatal end result, insulin shock, occur when level of blood glucose is low and have different characteristics.

17 (C) During treatment of any emergency, BLS is the MAIN management. Drug usage is secondary. For an unconscious patient, MUST maintain an open airway and administer breathing and chest compressions as indicated to supply the necessary oxygen to the brain. NOT always necessary to move patient from chair; positioning of the patient depends on the type of emergency. Using a manufactured drug kit does NOT guarantee successful recovery. Oxygen may be beneficial but is NOT necessary for ALL emergencies (e.g., hyperventilation).

18 (A) When an individual exhibits partial airway obstruction and poor air exchange, it indicates that he or she is unable to cough forcibly in an attempt to remove the object. This situation must be managed in the same manner as complete airway obstruction: Heimlich maneuver should be performed until the obstruction is expelled or the victim becomes unconscious. Back blows are NOT part of the Heimlich maneuver; they are part of the protocol for obstructed airway of an infant. ONLY when the victim can cough forcibly is it correct NOT to intervene. Doing nothing until a patient becomes unconscious is NOT an appropriate choice for any emergency.

19 (C) For an adult who requires BLS, chest compressions in cardiopulmonary resuscitation (CPR) are performed with two hands: heel of one hand, with the second hand on top, pressing 1½ to 2 inches in the center of the chest, between the nipples. For an infant, compressions are ½ to 1 inch of chest depth; for a child, compressions are ⅓ to ½ inch of chest depth. It is recommended that the clinician note if the chest has recoiled from compression to allow the heart to fill with blood. Do NOT allow interruptions in compressions; give ALL 100 compressions per minute.

20 (C) During BLS for children and infants, ratio of compressions to breaths is 30 to 2.

21 (A) For child who requires BLS, breaths should be given within the last 1 second. Must use enough volume to see chest rise when giving each breath; use regular breathing before breaths; do NOT use a deep breath.

22 (A) As soon as unconsciousness is established in an adult victim, the next step is to <u>activate EMS system</u>. Afterward, airway is opened and rescuer determines whether victim is breathing. If the victim is NOT breathing, chest compressions are begun to start cardiopulmonary resuscitation (CPR). Necessary to activate EMS as quickly as possible, since during (sudden) cardiac arrest (SCA), heart may undergo fibrillation and require use of special equipment transported by EMS personnel. Such equipment defibrillates the heart and allows effective compressions. Some dental settings may have portable automated defibrillator equipment (AED) and be able to start the process.

23 (E) For the child who requires chest compressions, using two hands, with heel of one hand, second hand on top, pressing ⅓ to ½ of chest depth. For an adult, it is the same two hands but pressure of 1½ to 2 inches. For infant, ONLY two fingers are necessary to perform chest compressions, pressing ½ to 1 inch of chest depth.

24 (C) BEST mode of transportation for an avulsed tooth is in patient's own buccal vestibule, since the saliva will keep the tooth moist. Other choices include a wet handkerchief, milk, or water; commercial preparations are available. For reimplantation with the BEST prognosis, do NOT to dry the tooth.

25 (C) When an instrument tip breaks during scaling, primary objective is to remove the tip from the patient's mouth. It is important for the clinician to remain calm and examine the area using gentle strokes with a curet in the sulcus. To dry the area, a cotton roll should be used. Patient should NOT swallow or attempt to locate broken tip with tongue. If the tip is NOT retrieved, radiograph should be used to aid in the location of the tip.

26 (A) When airway obstruction results in unconsciousness, the victim should be helped to the floor. Operator then should straddle the victim's hips and administer five hand thrusts to abdomen with upward and inward motion in attempt to dislodge obstruction. Thrusts are followed by attempt to ventilate. Routine is continued until object is expelled and clinician is successful in ventilating. Two additional ventilations are then given to stimulate breathing and pulse is checked.

27 (C) Withholding emergency or elective surgery (or periodontal procedures by dental hygienist) for 4 to 6 weeks after MI and then determining functional capacity (FC); dental care should be delayed unless patient can meet 4 METs (metabolic equivalents) and/or further medical testing has been completed to quantify level of cardiac risk in treatment. Patient positioning is NOT the primary consideration. Patient who experiences angina pectoris and carries his or her own nitroglycerin (NTG) should have easy access to NTG. Office personnel should be prepared to provide BLS for any patient, NOT just those with recent history of MI.

28 (D) Medical consult is indicated when systolic reading is >160 and diastolic is >100 mm Hg; this is stage 2, moderate to severe high blood pressure (HBP). Blood pressure reading of 150/92, stage 1, mild HBP, should be rechecked for accuracy by taking again; patient may have raced to appointment or have "white-coat syndrome"; must refer to physician if second reading is within same range. Readings of 110/68 and 119/76 are considered within normal range.

29 (E) Epilepsy does NOT predispose a person to cerebrovascular accident (CVA, stroke). History of diabetes mellitus (DM), hypertension (high blood pressure), transient ischemic attack (TIA), and cardiovascular disease (CVD) increase risk for CVA.

30 (B) Epileptic cry, which is caused by air rushing from the lungs, occurs during convulsive stage of grand mal seizure. Aura is characteristic of prodromal stage; patient regains consciousness during post-ictal stage. Petit mal seizures do NOT have stages.

31 (E) Myocardial infarction (MI, heart attack) typically does NOT cause seizures. Seizure may be caused by a prolonged high fever, trauma to the head, congenital abnormalities, alcohol or drug withdrawal. Other causes include epilepsy and imbalance of body fluids. Temporary abnormal electrophysiological phenomenon of the brain, resulting in abnormal synchronization of electrical neuronal activity. Can manifest as an alteration in mental state, tonic or clonic movements, convulsions, various other psychic symptoms.

32 (C) Alleviating fears of dental treatment will aid in preventing angina pectoris, myocardial infarction (MI, heart attack), hyperventilation, epileptic seizure, since ALL are risks when the patient is undergoing stress. Anaphylaxis, instead, is based on a severe allergy. Angina pectoris is chest pain caused by decreased oxygen flow to heart. MI involves death of a portion of heart muscle; caused by decrease in or lack of oxygen flow to that part of heart muscle.

33 (A) Uncomplicated pregnancy is example of ASA II; others are examples of ASA III.

34 (A) Slight COPD with exercise is example of ASA III; others are examples of ASA II.

35 (B) Bleeding levels are monitored by international normalized ratio (INR); INRs ≤2.5 are safe for invasive dental work. Older test is prothrombin time (PT). Blood glucose testing is done to monitor status of diabetics. NO need to reduce drugs if patient is at risk of hemorrhage, however, medical consult is indicated.

36 (B) Both statements are false. Sublingual tablet of nitroglycerin (NTG) has short shelf-life, may be used for 6 months after container opened. Metered spray form has longer shelf-life; one metered spray is equal to 1 tablet.

37 (C) Statement is correct, but reason is not. ASA IV classification of physical status indicates significant risk because the person has moderate systemic disease that limits activity and is a constant threat to life. Poses significant risk because patients in this category have a severe medical problem of greater importance than the planned dental treatment.

38 (E) Orthostatic (postural) hypotension occurs in elderly, pregnant women, persons with Addison's disease, and with nitrous oxide or diazepam (Valium) IV sedation. Certain antihypertensives and use of NTG predispose patient to postural hypotension, as does getting up quickly from dental chair.

39 (C) Presyncope stage has tachycardia (increased pulse rate) and NOT slower pulse rate (bradycardia); syncope by thready pulse.

40 (A) Superficial or first-degree burns involve ONLY epidermis, top layer of skin, with redness, dryness, and pain.

CHAPTER 11

Clinical Treatment

DEFINITION OF DENTAL HYGIENE PRACTICE

Dental hygiene is the science and practice of recognition, treatment, prevention of oral diseases. Hygienist is a preventive oral health professional who has graduated from an accredited program in an institution of higher education; a licensed professional who provides educational, clinical, research, administrative, therapeutic services supporting total health through promotion of optimal oral health. In practice, hygienists integrate roles of clinician, educator, advocate, manager, researcher to prevent oral diseases and promote health; hygienists work in partnership with dentists.

The distinct roles of the hygienist and dentist complement and augment the effectiveness of each professional and contribute to a cotherapist environment (see later discussion under "Motivation"). Hygienists are viewed as experts in their field, are consulted about appropriate dental hygiene interventions, are expected to make clinical dental hygiene decisions, and are expected to plan, implement, and evaluate the dental hygiene component of the overall care plan. Hygienist establishes the dental hygiene diagnosis, which is an integral component of the comprehensive dental diagnosis established by the dentist. *Each state has defined its own specific regulations for dental hygiene licensure.*

- See CD-ROM for Chapter Terms and WebLinks.
- See CD-ROM for ADHA Guidelines for the Standards For Clinical Dental Hygiene Practice (SCDHP) (2008).
- A. Process of care consists of six components (ADPIED):
  1. Assessment: systematic collection, analysis, documentation of the oral and general health status and patient needs.
  2. Dental hygiene diagnosis: component of the overall dental diagnosis; identification of existing or potential oral health problem that a dental hygienist is educationally qualified and licensed to treat.
  3. Planning: establishment of goals and outcomes based on patient needs, expectations, values, current scientific evidence.
  4. Implementation: delivery of dental hygiene services based on dental hygiene care plan in a manner minimizing risk and optimizing oral health.
  5. Evaluation: process of reviewing and documenting the outcomes of dental hygiene care, which occurs throughout the process of care.
  6. Documentation: complete and accurate recording of all collected data, treatment planned and provided, recommendations, and other information relevant to patient care, treatment.
- B. Dental hygiene process of care is a cycle in which the hygienist might pass through each of the recommended steps (ADPIED) several times during a course of treatment; over a period of months or years, a hygienist may have evaluated the process several times, altering the diagnosis and plan numerous times as the patient's condition changes.

DENTAL RECORD

The dental record is a <u>medicolegal document</u> that should be complete, accurate, and legible. From the record, it should be possible to recreate the patient's medical and dental history and oral status at initial presentation, along with periodic updates, treatment needs, treatment rendered, and any recommendations made.

- See Chapters 16, Special Needs Patients: medical disabilities; 18, Ethics and Jurisprudence: HIPAA, informed consent.
- A. Financial record demographic and insurance information.
- B. Assessment data:
  1. Medical history.
  2. Dental history:
     a. Significant past experiences.
     b. Chief complaint (CC).
     c. Attitudes about dentistry and possible anxiety.
     d. Dental biofilm control and self-care practices.
  3. Test results.
  4. Abnormal findings from extraoral and intraoral examination.
  5. Dental and periodontal chart.
  6. Radiographs and photographs.
- C. Diagnosis (treatment needs).
- D. Treatment plan and record of informed consent.
- E. Documentation of treatment (progress record):
  1. Implementation of specific treatment provided by date and signed by clinician.
  2. Evaluation of treatment outcomes.
  3. Referrals and recommendations.
  4. Future plans.
- F. Correspondence.

Health History

Health history is BEST for gathering information regarding the medical and dental history, behavior, demographics, vital signs. Listed below is only overview of what may be noted in chart. Dental history is included under assessment of the dentition.

- See Chapters 6, General and Oral Pathology: common conditions and diseases in dental setting; 8, Microbiology and Immunology: vaccinations, infectious diseases; 9, Pharmacology: antibiotic premedication; 10, Medical and Dental Emergencies: medical history, physical status classification (ASA), high blood pressure.

A. **Medical history:** review of physical health status.
1. Includes statement of chief complaint (CC), history of present and past illness, drug history.
2. Need for <u>medical consult</u> and <u>antibiotic and/or antianxiety premedication</u> MUST be assessed.
3. Information obtained by:
   a. Questionnaire vs. interview:
      (1) Questionnaire: saves time, consistent, potentially MORE thorough; however, inflexible and LACKS opportunity for development of rapport with patient; impersonal.
      (2) Interview: flexible and personable; requires good communication skills; enhances the relationship-building process between patient and clinician; time consuming and may cause embarrassment.
      (3) Combining BOTH interview and questionnaire achieves practical results and thoroughness by allowing clinician to get additional clarification and information on positive responses.
   b. Subjective vs. objective information:
      (1) **Subjective information:** impressions, feelings, attitudes from patient and clinician; patient reports (symptoms), e.g., nausea, and clinician's observations of patient, e.g., flushed skin.
      (2) **Objective information:** concrete notes, facts, data (signs), test results.

B. **Health status:** notation of existing and previous conditions.
1. Includes chief complaint (CC) and formation of physical classification status (American Society of Anesthesiologists [ASA]):
   a. CC: statement in patient's own words of why he or she is seeking dental care.
   b. Formation of ASA status: reduces risk of emergency occurring during treatment.
   c. History of present illness; may influence future treatment options and setting.
      (1) Includes description of current complaint and its signs, symptoms, onset, duration,

intensity, location, as well as related drug therapies.
      (2) May influence or contraindicate certain dental procedures.
   d. History of past illness includes:
      (1) Diseases that complicate dental treatment or might require special precautions or <u>antibiotic premedication</u> *before* treatment.
      (2) Allergy or untoward reactions to drugs.
      (3) Diseases and drugs with oral signs.
      (4) Communicable diseases.
      (5) Physiological and psychological state.
   e. Includes common medical conditions noted on medical history forms; as a result may need <u>medical consult</u>.
      (1) Confirming fax is recommended from involved healthcare professionals
      (2) Legally similar to sending certified mail, since cannot be refused by recipient; if there is no response, it is viewed as admission of silence; no need to be HIPAA qualified because it is viewed as a telephone call.

C. Medically compromised patients who can be seen in a dental setting but need MAJOR modification of dental treatment and/or need <u>medical consult</u> (drug history discussed next):
1. Patient with cardiovascular disease (CVD):
   a. Has inadequate blood circulation to heart muscle, resulting from arteriosclerosis, blocking or narrowing of blood vessels; MUST be ready for an emergency.
   b. Possibly reports angina pectoris caused by muscle pain that radiates to left arm and jaw; experiences pain with exertion and anxiety; discomfort is relieved by rest and vasodilator nitroglycerin (NTG, Nitrostat); request that patient bring NTG to dental appointment; have readily available during treatment.
   c. May use antihypertensives (includes diuretics, adrenergic blockers) that may result in xerostomia.
   d. Patient *after* myocardial infarction (MI, heart attack): attack resulted from insufficient blood supply to heart muscle caused by atherosclerosis of blood vessel walls; after cardiac episode and/or surgery, requires 4- to 6-week delay before emergency or elective dental procedures.
   e. MUST meet 4 metabolic (MET) equivalents to determine functional capacity (FC) to decrease cardiac risk during dental care; continue on CVD drug therapy during treatment.
   f. May need to lower amount of vasoconstrictor with local anesthesia.
   g. Increased risk of periodontal disease, and if present, may affect CVD.

2. Patient with hypertension (high blood pressure [HBP]): has or had elevated blood pressure; may also report symptoms of headache, dizziness, or nosebleeds:
   a. Taking antihypertensive and/or diuretic drug(s); may result in xerostomia.
   b. Can progress to arteriosclerosis, impaired renal function, cardiac enlargement, MI, cerebrovascular accident (CVA, stroke); MUST be ready for an emergency.
   c. Monitor blood pressure at each visit; refer to physician when blood pressure is stage 1: mild HBP (140 to 159/90 to 99 mm Hg); with stage 2, moderate to severe HBP (>160/ >100 mm Hg), may NOT be able to perform elective dental care; may need <u>immediate medical consult</u>.
   d. Do NOT provide dental treatment when blood pressure is ≥180/≥110 mm Hg, <u>activate EMS system</u> and treat as emergency.

3. Patient with congestive heart failure (CHF): occurs when heart muscle is weak and is unable to pump blood at an adequate rate; blood circulation is poor, resulting in congestion and pooling of blood in the organs and lower extremities.
   a. Swollen ankles from edema; shortness of breath; fatigue.
   b. May be taking digitalis glycoside (digoxin, Lanoxin) and diuretics that usually result in xerostomia.

4. Patient with cardiac dysrhythmia: had or has irregular heartbeat (too slow or fast).
   a. May have pacemaker (with or without defibrillator) and report taking digitalis glycoside (digoxin, Lanoxin) or calcium channel blocker such as diltiazem (Cardizem, Dilacor, Tiazac) or nifedipine (Procardia); may have xerostomia and gingival hyperplasia.
   b. With pacemaker, do NOT need to avoid use of ultrasonic scalers, since ALL are shielded, AVOID electric pulp testing (EPT) (discussed later).
   c. Antibiotic premedication for first 6 months after placement of pacemaker.

5. Patient with valvular heart disorder:
   a. Has or had deformity of heart valves because of past infection, drug use (such as phen-fen for weight control), congenital disorder, or heart transplant; artificial replacement of valves may have been performed.
   b. Patient with artificial (prosthetic) valve is at high risk for infective endocarditis (IE), infection of lining of heart caused by bacteremia (bacteria in blood) from invasive procedures; requires <u>antibiotic premedication</u> before invasive dental procedures.

6. Patient with diabetes mellitus (DM): has disorder of glucose metabolism resulting from relative or absolute lack of insulin; has vascular component (may have related CVD and/or renal diseases; see later discussion).
   a. Two types: type 1, can be severe and unstable; stems from lack of insulin produced from pancreas, and type 2, often NOT as severe but usually stable; develops slowly with age; frequently associated with obesity; pancreas produces adequate insulin but there is insulin insensitivity of the tissue.
   b. Dental appointment should be scheduled *after* meal and insulin therapy if taken; MUST be ready for emergency.
   c. Need to know current blood glucose levels: <70 mg/dL, too *low;* tendency toward hypoglycemia; >240 mg/dL: too *high;* tendency toward hyperglycemia; <u>medical consult</u> since is a risk for emergency.
   d. Risk factor for periodontal disease; MORE frequent maintenance appointments are required, as well as excellent oral hygiene self-care; if periodontal disease is present, may affect DM control.

7. Patient with renal disease: renal function is impaired at various levels, possibly maintained by hemodialysis or kidney transplant.
   a. Experiences MORE frequent infections, poor healing, bleeding difficulties.
   b. Surgical systemic shunts require <u>antibiotic premedication</u>.
   c. Certain drugs remain in circulation longer because of poor renal function (metabolism); care MUST be taken with drugs delivered (such as anesthetics and preventives) and prescriptions given by the dental office.

8. Patient with blood disorder or with history of difficulty with bleeding:
   a. Patients include those with anemia, deficiency of red blood cells (RBCs) resulting from vitamin or iron deficiency, bone marrow malfunction, excessive loss of blood, or RBC destruction.
   b. Also include patients with leukemia, cancer of white blood cells that do NOT function normally (cells are immature and excessive in number); thrombocytopenia may develop from chemotherapeutic treatment.
   c. Prone to infection, weakness, postappointment bleeding, hematomas, or other traumatic vascular lesions; can present with traumatic oral lesions, periodontal disease, xerostomia resulting from chemotherapy.
   d. Bleeding levels can be monitored by international normalized ratio (INR); INRs ≤2.5 are safe for invasive dental work.

9. Patient with respiratory infection or disease:
   a. May have a cold, flu, or tuberculosis (TB); may have TB oral lesion (highly contagious); if contagious, postpone dental treatment until antibiotic therapy reduces infection that may be transmitted.
   b. With emphysema or other forms of chronic obstructive pulmonary disease (COPD), may need oxygen during treatment and to be kept upright.
10. Patient with sexually transmitted disease or infection (STD, STI):
    a. Includes patients with syphilis, gonorrhea, and chlamydia acquired through sexual intercourse; note any oral or pharyngeal lesions (highly contagious).
    b. If contagious, postpone dental treatment until antibiotic therapy reduces infection that may be transmitted.
11. Patient with hepatitis A, B, C, D, E: patients ALL have inflammation of the liver resulting from viral infection; causes fatigue, nausea, tender joints, jaundice.
    a. Follow recommendations for hepatitis B vaccination for ALL dental providers *before* treating patients in any clinical setting, since carrier status is frequently unknown.
    b. HIGH risk of disease transmission to clinician and then through chain to other patients; however, dental providers MUST follow standard precautions at ALL times when treating ALL patients.
    c. May have difficulty with bleeding and metabolism of drugs because of liver damage.
12. Patient with allergy: can have reactions to substance that may be as slight as a skin rash or as severe as fall in blood pressure and anaphylactic shock (airway obstruction from tissue swelling and/or cardiac arrest).
    a. Reports reaction to known substance (allergen) such as antibiotics, rubber latex, restorative metals (especially nickel), other allergens; need to AVOID allergen.
    b. May have asthma; need to recommend acetaminophen as substitute for its analgesic and antipyretic effects to avoid aspirin induced attack, may need to alter local anesthetics (AVOID vasoconstrictor or articaine).
    c. May use inhaler for acute asthmatic attacks, so should be asked to bring to ALL appointments; instruct to rinse mouth thoroughly after using and expectorate, to reduce systemic absorption, tooth staining, and taste alteration.
    d. MUST determine cause and severity of allergic response; MUST be ready for an emergency, which includes having inhalers in emergency kit.
13. Patient with epilepsy: patient can have disturbance of electrical brain activity resulting in seizure (convulsions).
    a. Usually reports taking anticonvulsants such as phenytoin (Dilantin); may have related gingival hyperplasia.
    b. Appointments should be made when rested; confirm drug compliance and keep appointments short; MUST be ready for an emergency.
14. Patient with total joint replacement:
    a. Patient has replacement for ALL surfaces of joint (knee, hip, elbow, fingers) because of past infection or traumatic disorder, osteoporosis, or osteoarthritis.
    b. HIGH risk for prosthetic joint infection 2 years after implantation and ALWAYS for immunocompromised (such as diabetics) from bacteremia caused by invasive dental procedures and thus requires antibiotic premedication before invasive dental procedures.
15. Patient with xerostomia: if NOT drug related (such as with patients who have cancer or Sjögren's syndrome), can recommend use of prescription cholinergic agonist drugs such as pilocarpine (Salagen) and cevimeline (Evoxac); drug-related xerostomia is discussed in next section.

Drug History

Drug history provides information on drugs that may affect oral health, dental treatment, and oral hygiene self-care. Often requires use of reference text and/or online resource, such as *Physician's Desk Reference* (PDR), or a medical consult and/or pharmacist consult for further information. PDR lists all drugs by manufacturer's name, brand name, generic name.
- See Chapters 6, General and Oral Pathology: specific conditions and diseases noted in dental setting; 9, Pharmacology: drugs that affect dental care.
A. Pharmacological record: information regarding drug action, usage, contraindications, adverse reactions, warnings, precautions is reviewed.
   1. Includes record of drugs taken (including over the counter [OTC]), noting dosage and condition being treated; note if drug has impact on oral health and any contraindications for dental treatment.
   2. Common drug-induced *oral* side effects:
      a. Xerostomia (dry mouth): associated with cracked lips, sore labial commissures, inflamed smooth tongue (glossitis).
         (1) MOST common reaction to drugs; MOST commonly to drugs used to treat depression and anxiety, urinary incontinence, Parkinson's disease, as well as antihistamines, antihypertensives, antidiarrheals, muscle relaxants; BOTH prescription and OTC, such as for colds, flu, allergies.

(2) Results in thick and ropy saliva, altered taste, loss of buffering action; may be associated with burning tongue.

(3) Increases incidence of caries, especially of the root; causes difficulty with chewing, swallowing, speaking, bad breath, denture wearing.

(4) Treatment: relieving symptoms through increased water consumption (sip water), saliva substitutes, tissue lubricants, chewing sugar-free gum (especially with xylitol), air humidification; AVOID alcohol mouthrinses that can dehydrate tissues; to prevent caries, use of home fluoride applications and calcium products for additional remineralization; see earlier discussion if non–drug related.

b. Candidiasis: overgrowth of yeast organism, *Candida albicans* (see Chapter 8, Microbiology and Immunology):

(1) Increased risk with history of prolonged antibiotics, immunosuppressants, or corticosteroid therapy with immunocompromised health, denture or dental appliance wear.

(2) Frequently results in painful irritations, creating difficulty in chewing, speaking, wearing dental appliances.

(3) Treatment: antifungals such as nystatin (Mycostatin), clotrimazole (Mycelex), ketoconazole (Nizoral), fluconazole (Diflucan) that may contain sugar, increasing risk of caries; education given on proper denture care (see Chapter 15, Dental Biomaterials).

c. Drug-induced gingival hyperplasia: associated with enlarged, bulbous, and fibrotic gingival tissues:

(1) Results from anticonvulsant phenytoin (Dilantin), calcium channel blocker such as nifedipine (Procardia), or transplant rejection drugs such as cyclosporine.

(2) Can be controlled or prevented through adequate oral hygiene self-care, especially if begun before the drug regimen.

(3) May need surgery to remove excess tissues (see Chapter 13, Periodontology).

d. Additional oral signs of drugs: glossitis, erythema signs, hairy tongue, lichenoid eruptions, trigeminal neuralgia.

3. Common drugs that affect dental treatment:

a. Antihypertensives: used to reduce high blood pressure (HBP) with cardiovascular disease (CVD).

(1) Can cause orthostatic (postural) hypotension (reduced blood pressure): sit patient up slowly and keep seated for several minutes to reduce dizziness of hypotension:

(2) Monitor blood pressure at each visit (see earlier discussion).

(3) Can cause xerostomia (discussed earlier).

(4) Nifedipine (Procardia), calcium channel blocker, can cause gingival hyperplasia (discussed earlier).

(5) May need to alter local anesthetic agent.

(6) Common HBP drugs:

(a) Diuretics: hydrochlorothiazide (Lopressor), furosemide (Lasix) (see next discussion).

(b) Calcium channel blockers: diltiazem (Cardizem, Dilacor, Tiazac), nifedipine (Procardia, Adalat, Nifedical).

(c) Beta blockers: propranolol (Inderal), nadolol (Corgard), metoprolol (Lopressor), atenolol (Tenormin).

(d) Angiotensin converting enzyme (ACE) inhibitors: captopril (Capoten), enalapril (Vasotec), lisinopril (Zestril, Prinivil).

b. Diuretics: used to promote renal excretion in the treatment of CHF and HBP:

(1) Result in frequent urination and xerostomia (see earlier discussion); affects planning of appointment time and length of appointment.

(2) Common drugs: see antihypertensives and diuretics.

c. Anticoagulants and antiplatelets: used for treatment of CVD to increase blood flow by suppressing or delaying coagulation of blood:

(1) Discontinuation of drug may be hazardous because of embolus, thrombus formation.

(2) Side effects can be prolonged; spontaneous internal bleeding can occur; hematoma more likely with some local anesthesia injections (especially inferior alveolar nerve block).

(3) Requires monitoring of bleeding by INR levels (see earlier discussion) and medical consult.

(4) Common drugs: warfarin (Coumadin), clopidogrel (Plavix), aspirin (low dose).

d. Antianginals: used for treatment of angina pectoris to increase oxygen supply to heart muscle through vasodilation:

(1) Usage pattern should be established before each appointment; keep patient's NTG tablets handy during dental appointment; make dental appointment short and in morning.

(2) When combined with alcohol, can cause severe hypotension.

(3) Common drug: NTG (Nitrostat).

e. Cardiac drugs:

(1) Used with CHF; strengthen myocardial contractility.

(2) May present with swollen extremities and report shortness of breath; seat in upright (45°) position to increase ease of breathing.

(3) Common drugs: digitalis (Lanoxin), enalapril (Vasotec), captopril (Capoten).

f. Anticonvulsant drugs: used to reduce incidence of seizures with epilepsy or Down syndrome.

(1) Stimulate gingival growth, resulting in gingival hyperplasia (see earlier discussion).

(2) Common drugs: phenytoin (Dilantin).

g. Vasoconstrictors: used to alleviate symptoms of asthma and emphysema; taken as inhalants.

(1) Can cause xerostomia (see earlier discussion); frequently associated with inflamed gingival tissues because of mouth breathing (associated with asthma).

(2) Need to follow inhaler use instructions (discussed earlier).

(3) May need to alter local anesthetic agent; may need to avoid use with sulfites (vasoconstrictors, articaine).

(4) Common drugs: albuterol (Proventil, Ventolin).

h. Thyroid drugs: treat hypothyroidism (MOST common type) by increasing metabolic rate.

(1) Have NO oral side effects; patient may have goiter or surgical removal of gland.

(2) Common drugs: levothyroxine (Synthroid).

i. Antiinflammatory drugs: depress inflammatory response and treat adrenocortical insufficiency, rheumatoid arthritis (RA), and respiratory disease (emphysema):

(1) High risk for candidal infections (see earlier discussion) and oral ulcerations.

(2) Common drugs: corticosteroids such as prednisone (Deltasone).

j. Antidepressants: taken for mental disorders, weight loss, tobacco cessation, sleep disorders, temporomandibular disease (TMD).

(1) May cause xerostomia (see earlier discussion) and taste alterations; may cause bruxism with resultant attrition.

(2) May need to alter local anesthetic agent and AVOID levonordefrin (such as with TCAs; see next).

(3) Common drugs:

(a) Tricyclic antidepressants (TCAs): amitriptyline (Elavil).

(b) Selective serotonin reuptake inhibitors (SSRIs): bupropion (Wellbutrin), sertraline (Zoloft), paroxetine (Paxil), escitalopram (Lexapro).

(c) Monoamine oxidase inhibitors (MAOIs): phenelzine (Nardil).

(d) Lithium (Lithobid): treats manic-depressive illness (bipolar disorder).

k. Tranquilizers: may be taken daily or ONLY for antianxiety premedication because of anxiety and fear of dental care.

(1) Result in CVS depression; may be drowsy, fatigued, or sedated.

(2) May cause xerostomia (see earlier discussion).

(3) Long-term use can cause tardive dyskinesia, involuntary facial movements of facial muscles and/or tongue; may have bruxism with attrition.

(4) Be aware of signs of suicidal or depressive tendencies; refer immediately to physician.

(5) Common drugs: diazepam (Valium), alprazolam (Xanax).

PATIENT ASSESSMENT

Patient assessment is necessary to establish baseline information on general health; includes taking vital signs as well as performing extraoral and intraoral examination and dental and periodontal evaluations. Obtaining baseline information allows determination of treatment needs and subsequent development of treatment plan.

• See Chapter 10, Medical and Dental Emergencies: vital signs.

Patient Examination

Patient examination includes both extraoral and intraoral examination of the soft and hard tissues of the head and neck as part of the assessment of the patient. Recognition of abnormal findings may be critical in preserving the overall health. MUST be recorded in chart (see documentation discussion).

• See Chapters 4, Head, Neck, and Dental Anatomy: head and neck anatomy; 6, General and Oral Pathology: diagnosis.

A. Examination technique: includes visual observation, palpation, auscultation, olfaction.

1. Visual observation, BOTH direct and indirect (mouth mirror), to examine intraoral and extraoral structures:

a. Adopt organized, sequential pattern to AVOID omitting areas.

b. Look for abnormal color (change to red, black, blue, white, dark brown; spread of color), size (change is sudden or ongoing), or change in appearance (irregular margins, elevation, texture becomes scaly, crusty, or ulcerated).

c. Inform patient of the results of examination.

2. Palpation used to examine tissues and underlying structures:

a. Digital: one finger used to examine tissue (hard palate).

b. Bidigital: tissue grasped between finger(s) and thumb (cheeks, alveolar ridges, lips, vestibule, tongue, ducts, floor of mouth, larynx).

c. Manual: all fingers of one hand used to grasp tissue (anterior deep and superficial cervical nodes).

d. Bimanual: finger(s) and thumb from each hand applied simultaneously to examine tissues (floor of the mouth).

e. Bilateral: bilateral structures examined simultaneously to detect differences *between* sides (temporomandibular joint [TMJ], inferior border of mandible); place fingers on anterior border of jaw, palpate distally on BOTH right and left sides at same time.

f. Circular compression: fingers move in circular motion while applying pressure (occipital nodes); AVOID on palate.

3. Auscultation used to listen to body sounds to determine a change from normal:

a. TMJ sounds, such as clicking, grinding, or popping; make note if pain is associated with sounds.

b. Hoarseness or cough; make note of how long it has persisted.

c. Speech disorders, such as slurred speech, stuttering, or extra loud speech.

4. Olfaction to detect unusual smells:

a. Bad breath (halitosis): poor oral hygiene, necrotizing periodontal disease, GIT difficulties, overconsumption of proteins; MOST comes from coated tongue; encourage tongue cleaning.

b. Acetone breath: indicative of DM, from increased processing of ketones.

c. Alcohol breath: recent alcohol consumption, alcoholism.

B. Documentation (see Chapter 18, Ethics and Jurisprudence):

1. To record findings that may be significant in the overall diagnosis and recommended treatment.

2. As legal record in case of a claim or patient identification (accident or disaster).

3. As baseline data for subsequent examination and future treatment planning.

4. Standard of recording:

a. Requires adequate space to record in a brief, accurate manner.

b. Includes diagnosis and treatment alternatives and/or recommendations.

c. Summarizes patient's response, listing wants, needs, expectations.

d. Indicates treatment to be rendered:

(1) NO treatment: refuses to follow through with treatment and/or recommendations.

(2) Treatment: agrees to continue treatment.

(3) Consent: documentation of consent, including risks, benefits, alternative treatment options.

(4) Referral: patient referred to specialist by supervising dentist.

Extraoral Examination

Patient SHOULD be seated in an upright position for extraoral examination of the head, face, and neck areas, unless NOT able. Good lighting and exposure of the area being assessed are essential (e.g., patient's collar and tie loosened, glasses removed).

A. Overall physical appearance by visual examination:

1. Unsteadiness of gait: CANNOT walk at a normal pace and maintain balance because of orthopedic disabilities or influence of drugs.

2. Restricted mobility: limps while walking, which may indicate injury to hip, leg, knee, or foot or systemic disease; investigate possible surgery that required pins, joint repair, or prosthesis.

3. Imbalance: CANNOT walk without losing balance; may be due to equilibrium problem, inner ear infection, loss of muscular strength, or damage from CVA.

4. Stature: appears stiff while standing, sitting, or walking; may indicate back problem or arthritis; if assumes a slumped position, may be due to lack of muscle tone resulting from a CVA.

5. Difficulty breathing: appears out of breath while walking or right after walking; may indicate CHF, lung disease, or other systemic disorder.

B. Hair by visual examination and palpation:

1. Unusual amount: loss or thinning may be result of chemotherapy; excessive growth (hypertrichosis) caused by hormone disorder.

2. Unusual distribution: as in alopecia, with loss of hair in patches.

3. Lack of luster: poor nutrition; coarse texture with hypothyroidism.

4. Scalp lesions: psoriasis, previous injury, basal cell carcinoma (BCC); lice: small insects, nits appear as tiny white globules at hair root; spreads easily.

C. Face by visual examination and palpation:

1. General expression can indicate general mood (e.g., happy, sad, angry, indifferent).

2. Asymmetry: facial paralysis (along with lack of blinking) with CVA or Bell's palsy.

3. Drooling, lack of expression, diminished blinking: Parkinson's disease.

4. Unusual muscle twitching and loud vocal sounds: Tourette's syndrome.

5. Bruising, bleeding, or burned areas: physical abuse, anticoagulation therapy, or blood disorder.

6. Pigmentation: Addison's disease or melanoma.

D. Skin by visual examination and palpation:
1. Color: indicates general health status (e.g., illness, disease, or trauma); note paleness, redness, acne, rosacea, sunburn, patches of pigmentation.
2. Textures: unusual ones should be noted, such as scarring, clamminess, firmness, swelling, acne.
3. Lesions: should be documented, noting color, size, shape, surface texture (note any changes in pigmented nevus).

E. Eyes by visual examination and reaction to light source:
1. Pupil size: normal; dilated or pinpoint may be related to drug abuse.
2. Sclera color: if yellow, may indicate jaundice; if red and crusty, conjunctivitis.
3. Bulging (exophthalmos) or puffy and swollen eyes with edematous eyelids: possible thyroid disorder.
4. Eyes without palpebral fissures and with broad, flat nose and low-set ears: Down syndrome.

F. Nose by visual examination and palpation:
1. Obstructed airway: congestion and/or a structural defect or ulceration related to drug abuse.
2. Secretions: sinus drainage; yellow or green secretion: infection or drug use (constant wiping).
3. Red butterfly-shaped lesion over the nose: systemic lupus erythematosus (SLE).
4. Rhinophyma: overgrowth of sweat and sebaceous glands; appears red and bulbous with increased alcohol consumption.

G. Ears by visual examination and palpation:
1. Hearing loss and use of hearing aids: will require clinician to look at patient while speaking; during use of ultrasonic scaler, patient may need to turn off hearing aid.
2. Infections: may affect ability to hear; may also affect balance.
3. Tinnitus (ringing): may cause humming or buzzing in ear; may result from long-term use of aspirin, infection, or environmental noise trauma.

H. Bones, muscles, lymph nodes, glands using visual and palpation:
1. Parotid glands: bilateral circular compression for pain, swelling, enlargement, hardness; salivary flow observed at opening of duct across from maxillary first molar on buccal mucosa when gland is milked.
2. TMJ: bilateral palpation with BOTH index fingers slightly anterior to outer meatus, have patient open and close several times, slowly; note pain, clicking, popping, grinding, and restriction in opening or closing; note any deviations, including during patient interview; may have TMD.
3. Masseter and temporalis muscles: bilateral circular compression for pain, swelling, enlargements, unusual hardness; masseter may be enlarged because of bruxism and/or clenching habits.
4. Border of mandible: bimanual palpation from midline to posterior angle for changes in contour and pain.
5. Mentalis muscle: digital palpation, rolling tissue over mandible, for smoothness or restriction in swallowing movement.
6. Lymph nodes: assessed for tenderness or pain, swelling, enlargement, unusual hardness, fixed position:
   a. Occipital: bilateral palpation, with head tilted forward.
   b. Auricular (anterior and posterior), parotid (superficial), facial: bilateral palpation.
   c. Superficial cervical (submental, submandibular, anterior and external jugular): digital palpation with fingers anteriorly from midline of mandible with head down to posteriorly to angle of mandible, rolling tissue over jaw, and then down to and along sternocleidomastoid muscle (SCM), with patient's head to side.
   d. Deep cervical (superior and inferior): palpating deep tissues along SCM with thumb and fingers, with head to side.
   e. Accessory and supraclavicular: palpating continuing down into clavicular area, with shoulders up and forward.
7. Submental and submandibular salivary glands: bilateral digital palpation for asymmetry, noncontiguous borders, pain, swelling, enlargement, unusual hardness, difficulty in swallowing.
8. Larynx: bimanual palpation for unrestricted movement.
9. Thyroid gland: displacing gland to one side of neck, then combination of bimanual and manual palpation inferolaterally to cartilage ("Adam's apple") while patient sits upright; ask patient to swallow (may need glass of water) to check for mobility; note asymmetry, nodules, enlargement (goiter), or surgical removal.

Intraoral Examination

Patient should be seated in a supine position (see earlier position discussion). Use preprocedural antimicrobial mouthrinse and have client remove any pigmented lipsticks. Apply nonpetroleum lubricant to cracked and dry areas to make examination more comfortable, and remove any removable appliances. Overall, note level of saliva and whether dry mouth (xerostomia) is present.

A. Lips by visual examination and bidigital palpation:
1. Changes in size: swelling or allergic reaction (rubber latex).
2. Chapping: mouth breathing, nutritional deficiency or environmental conditions; cracking, with angular cheilitis, candidiasis, or vitamin B deficiency.

3. Blistering: ulcers; herpetic lesions; irritations, from lip biting or trauma.

4. Limited motion: scarring, trauma, or paralysis.

5. Unusual color given overall pigmentation; loss of vermilion border.

6. Abnormal texture, lack of firmness or moistness; with dehydration and sun damage.

7. Lower lip: high-risk area for oral cancer, with loss of vermilion border, fibrosis, ulceration.

B. Labial and alveolar mucosa using visual examination and bidigital palpation:

1. Ulcerated lesions: such as herpetic lesions, aphthous ulcers.

2. Tight frenum attachments: can cause gingival defects such as loss of attached gingiva (mucogingival defect).

3. Amalgam tattoo: blue or black macules of varying size on soft tissues.

4. Enlarged mucous retention cyst (mucocele): trauma to duct.

5. Hyperkeratosis: use of lozenges, drugs, or spit (smokeless) tobacco products held in mandibular vestibule; careful evaluation of changes is essential.

6. Smokeless (spit) tobacco lesion: hyperkeratinized tissue; white, sometimes corrugated, in appearance.

7. Torn or lacerated frenum (lingual frenum too): often caused by forced feedings, binding, gagging (abuse).

8. Tissue trauma: biting, abrasion, burns; horizontal bruises at commissures may indicate binding or gagging with abuse.

C. Buccal mucosa using visual examination and palpation:

1. Check parotid (Stensen's) duct using bilateral palpation: pain, enlargements, tumors, calcified areas; milk the ducts to confirm function.

2. Linea alba: white line paralleling occlusal plane with trauma; also note trauma from toothbrushing, cheek biting (irritation fibroma).

3. Wickham's striae: thin white lines with lichen planus.

D. Gingiva using visual examination and palpation:

1. Tissue trauma: caused by abrasion, burns, or cuts.

2. Infection, with redness and swelling (inflammation), such as McCall's festoons (lifesaver marginal gingiva): inadequate dental biofilm removal and presence of periodontal disease, mainly gingivitis, possibly periodontitis.

3. Fibrosis: chronic periodontal disease, drug use, or traumatic toothbrushing.

4. Exostosis (plural, exostoses): small benign bone growths projecting from alveolar process, MAINLY on maxillary facial surface.

5. Recession: loss of periodontal attachment, caused by vigorous toothbrushing, abfraction, or gingival disease or surgery.

6. Mucogingival defects:
   a. Lack of attached gingiva: tooth positioning, hereditary factors, oral habits, poor oral hygiene.
   b. Stillman's clefts (comma shaped): poor oral hygiene and occlusal trauma.
   c. High frenum attachments: muscle pull on attached gingiva.

E. Hard and soft palate using visual inspection and digital palpation:

1. Torus (plural, tori): hard protruding bony structure (benign exostosis), NOT of significance unless partial or full denture is being constructed, then may need to be reduced or removed.

2. Ulcerations: fluid-filled lesions surrounded with red halo with aphthous ulcers, burns, viral infection, or autoimmunity (broken blisters).

3. Trauma: mechanical or chemical irritation; should heal within 10 days, if not, further investigation needed to rule out pathological condition or child abuse.

4. Stomatitis: ranges from small, red, petechia-like lesions (nicotine and denture stomatitis) to generalized and granular (denture stomatitis) to ulcerative (aphthous stomatitis) to intense redness with focal bone loss (necrotizing stomatitis).

5. Petechiae: small red dots on mucous membranes, caused by trauma or systemic disease (mononucleosis on palate).

6. Fistulas: pimplelike lesions with periodontal or periapical abscess.

7. Soft palate: high-risk area for oral cancer, with red and/or white lesions, bleeding, ulceration; also area for trauma from abuse.

F. Floor of mouth using visual inspection and palpation:

1. Check submandibular (Wharton's) duct: can become blocked with mucous plugs or sialoliths (present on occlusal radiograph).

2. Varicosities: often found sublingually on elderly.

3. Large mucous retention cyst (ranula): blocked or traumatized ducts of submandibular and sublingual glands; soft, sessile, slowly enlarging mass on one side of floor of mouth; painless; once removed, may recur.

4. Limited tongue movement: ankylosis of tongue; may lead to swallowing and speech disorders.

5. High-risk area for oral cancer, with red and/or white lesions, bleeding, ulceration.

G. Tongue using visual examination and palpation:

1. Coating: varying degree of keratinization of filiform lingual papillae; food, drugs, bacteria (halitosis); staining caused by tobacco use; tongue cleaning needed.

2. Fissuring: presence of numerous grooves and crevices on dorsal surface and lateral borders of tongue; entrap food and bacteria; tongue cleaning needed; MORE common with Down syndrome.
3. Varicosities: often found on ventral surface on elderly.
4. Lateral border and ventral surface: high-risk area for oral cancer, with red and/or white lesions, bleeding, ulceration.
5. Other common lesions of the tongue:
   a. Ulcers: aphthous is MOST common, with systemic disease such as viral infections or autoimmunities or with smoking cessation.
   b. Irritation fibroma: trauma.
   c. Geographic: common benign condition involving filiform lingual papillae found on dorsum and borders; lesions are red areas with white borders; outline of lesions changes, heals, reappears in different area.
   d. Median rhomboid glossitis (central papillary atrophy): flat or lump benign lesion on dorsum, NO filiform present; related to chronic candidiasis
   e. Tongue thrust (during swallowing): anterior portion pushes between teeth; ideally SHOULD be positioned on palate behind maxillary central incisors while swallowing; retraining may be necessary if thrusting causes speech disorders or tooth positioning problems (malposed teeth).
   f. White plaques: lichen planus, candidiasis, or other systemic disease; definitive diagnosis is needed.
   g. Black hairy tongue: elongation of filiform with dark staining: long-term use of certain drugs or tobacco; long-term rinsing with undiluted hydrogen peroxide.
   h. Hairy leukoplakia: hyperkeratosis of filiform caused by Epstein-Barr virus (EBV); results in white corrugated appearance on lateral borders; associated with HIV/AIDS.
   i. Hemangiomas and lymphangiomas: developmental benign tumors creating enlargements.
   j. Macroglossia: symmetrical enlargement; developmental abnormality, cretinism, acromegaly; may be scalloped from pushing against the teeth.

CLINICAL STUDY

		SCENARIO
Age	27 YRS	The patient has minimal calculus and dental biofilm with slight gingival inflammation.
Sex	☒ Male ☐ Female	
Height	5'2"	
Weight	135 LBS	
BP	110/65	
Chief Complaint	"I know I have to keep my mouth healthy, since it impacts all of my health."	
Medical History	Hemophilia Contracted AIDS 15 years ago from blood transfusion	
Current Medications	Coagulation therapy prn Undergoing highly active antiretroviral therapy (HAART)	
Social History	Rock band member	

1. What is hemophilia, and what are its risks and treatment?
2. What additional information should be known before the patient is treated?
3. Is the patient's sister likely to have hemophilia?
4. Are there any special treatment considerations because of the patient's hemophilia or HIV status?
5. Why were hemophiliacs at risk for AIDS before 1985?
6. What HIV symptoms may be discovered during the oral examination?

1. Hemophilias are a group of disorders involving blood-clotting mechanisms. Diseases are genetic, do not produce factor VIII (hemophilia A), factor IX (hemophilia B, or Christmas disease), factor IX (hemophilia C), or von Willebrand's factor (vWF). Treatment includes coagulation therapy.
2. Additional information needed before treatment would include type and severity of hemophilia, treatment regimen for control of hemophilia, drugs being taken for hemophilia, HIV status including CD4 cell

counts (lymphocyte subset cell count), presence of any AIDS-associated conditions (includes oral signs), and any drugs (both prescription and OTC) being taken to manage HIV condition. In addition, INR numbers would be needed to ascertain bleeding levels; medical consult needed. Antifibrinolytic agents (Cyklokapron) effectively prevent oral bleeding when they are combined with a preventive dose of clotting factor and can be used with oral surgery.

3. Hemophilia A, B, and C are rare in women; however, von Willebrand's disease does occur in both men and women.

4. Standard precautions are followed for every patient. Light debridement (scaling) is only instrumentation needed in the patient's case because of minimal deposits and inflammation; may want to avoid ultrasonic scalers and use manual instrumentation, since aerosols created may be a health risk for immunocompromised patient. However, he should be seen for preventive maintenance every 3 months because of high-risk status. Excellent oral hygiene self-care and preventive therapy reduce chances for oral infection and bleeding.

5. Before 1985, blood stores used for transfusions were not required to be tested for HIV virus, and many hemophiliacs contracted virus.

6. Thorough intraoral and extraoral examination is critical for noting progression of patient's HIV status, since many early indicators of disease progression are exhibited in the mouth. Palpate for any persistent generalized lymphadenopathy (PGL) and visually observe for any skin lesions such as Kaposi's sarcoma, purpura, or herpes. Check for common oral signs of progressing AIDS virus, such as candidiasis, Kaposi's sarcoma, hairy leukoplakia, gingival inflammation (linear gingival erythema [LGE]), or necrotizing periodontal disease.

DENTITION ASSESSMENT

Along with the medical history, the **dental history** is taken to complete the patient's health history. Questions concerning the patient's experiences with dentistry, as well as needs, should be discussed and reported in the records. Then the dentition can be assessed for caries, attrition, abrasion, erosion, fracture, inflammation, necrosis, restoration, and other conditions. These assessments can involve visual, radiographic, and clinical evaluation and a variety of diagnostic tests. Dental evaluation includes a written record of the assessment of all teeth using commonly acceptable dental notation (listed below in order of notation), done manually or using software to save time and improve efficiency.

• See Chapters 4, Head, Neck, and Dental Anatomy: dental anatomy, charting, orthodontic evaluation; 6, General and Oral Pathology: oral diseases and conditions; 15, Dental Biomaterials: restorative materials.

A. Teeth are identified by numbers or symbols:
1. Universal Tooth Designation System: MOST widely accepted (and used on NDHBE).
   a. Permanent teeth: numbered #1 to #32; primary (deciduous) teeth: letters A to T.
   b. Chart clockwise for BOTH as if you are looking at patient smiling.
2. Overview of dentition:
   a. Missing teeth: determined by clinical absence (developmentally or extraction), radiographic findings, reported dental history; charted with single vertical line or with X through tooth.
   b. Unerupted permanent tooth: if completely unerupted, circled entirely; if partially erupted, ONLY that portion that is not exposed is circled (common with third molars).
   c. Supernumerary tooth is an extra tooth: charted by drawing in general location, noting as "Su."
   d. Root canal has pulp tissue removed (endodontic therapy): charted by placing vertical line through root and noting as "RC."
   e. Full or partial removable denture or removable prosthetic appliance: missing teeth are charted with vertical lines and area the appliance replaces is bracketed; labeled "PUD" (partial upper denture), "PLD" (partial lower denture), "CUD" (complete upper denture), or "CLD" (complete lower denture) (Figure 11-1).
   f. Implant: surgically placed into the bone of jaw, after healing, prosthesis (crown, bridge, denture) is constructed over implant; charted by "X" marked on root(s), with prosthesis drawn in and implant is noted as "I."
B. Restorations (uses G.V. Black's Classification) (Figures 11-2 and 11-3):
1. Temporary: placed on or in tooth for short period; includes cement, preformed crowns, or chairside-made acrylic crown; charted by outlining, shading, noting as "T."
2. Tooth-colored (esthetic) restorations: may be acrylic, composite resin, glass ionomer cements, porcelain.
   a. Composite resins can be placed on anteriors or posteriors; material cured by visible (blue) light; charted by outlining, shading, noting as "C," "CR," "GIC," or "R."
   b. Acrylic jackets: crowns; charted by outlining, shading, noting as "AJC."
   c. Porcelain: used for a crown, inlay, or veneer; charted by outlining, shading, noting as "PJC," "PI," or "Ven," respectively; if metal is used as substructure on crown, noted as "PFM" for porcelain-fused-to-metal.

Dental and Periodontal Charting

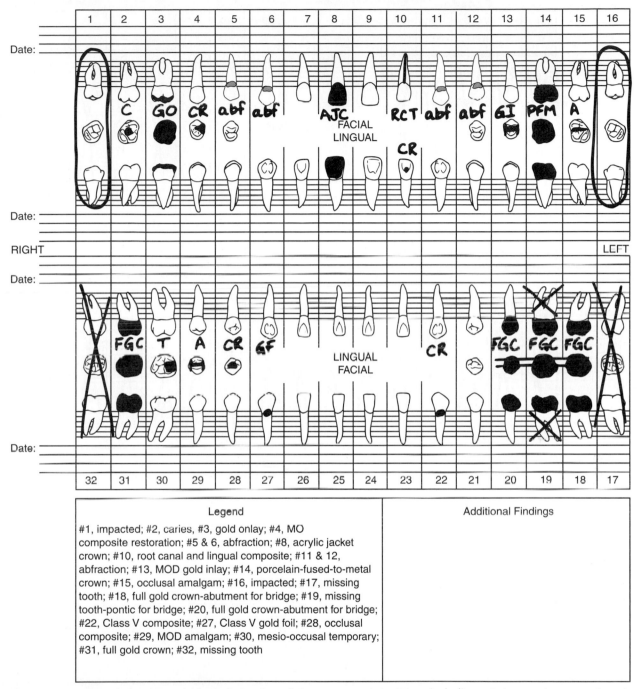

Figure 11-1 Dental charting. Anatomical charting of the permanent dentition, including missing teeth, restored teeth, carious lesions, and additional notations.

3. Enamel (pit and fissure) sealant: resin (clear or tinted) mechanically or chemically bonded (see above); charted by outlining, shading, noting as "S" or "SL."

4. Amalgam: alloy used for Class I, II, V; charted by outlining, shading, noting as "A."

5. Metal casting: made from a wax pattern of tooth preparation; classified depending on metal content:

a. Full high noble, noble, and base metal crowns; charted by outlining, shading, noting as "FGC" or "GC."

b. Three-quarter crowns; charted by outlining, shading, noting as "¾ GC."

c. Onlay (covers at least one cusp tip); charted by outlining, shading, noting as "GO."

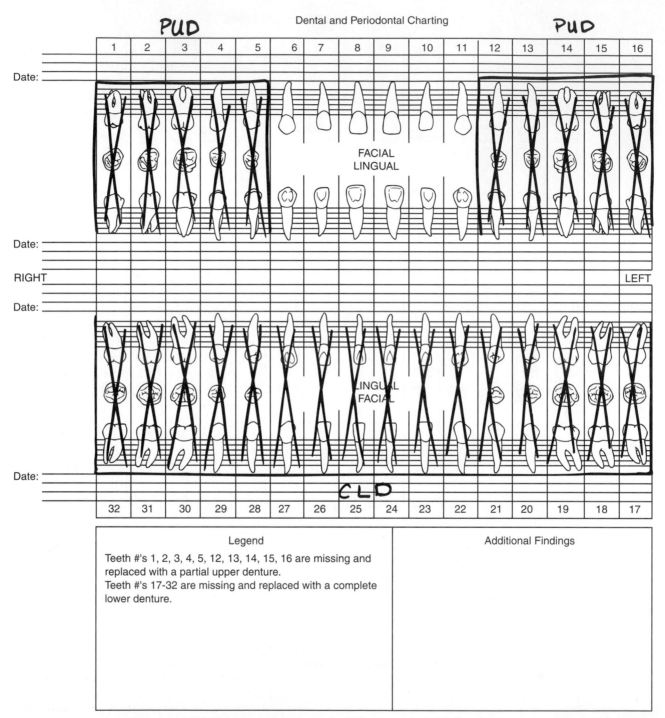

Figure 11-2 Dental charting of partially edentulous permanent dentition. Anatomical charting that demonstrates bracketing of teeth included in the partial, as well as missing teeth.

d. Inlay (lies between cusps of the teeth); charted by outlining, shading, noting as "GI."

6. Bridge (fixed denture): pontic replaces missing tooth; charted by outlining, shading crown portion, and drawing vertical line or an "X" on root; double horizontal lines are drawn to abutments (crowns adjacent to pontic for support), and abutment crowns are outlined and shaded as per material.

7. Gold foil: soft metal condensed used in any carious area, cannot withstand heavy occlusal wear, hard on pulp, seldom used because of technically demanding and time-intensive placement; charted by outlining, shading, noting as "GF."

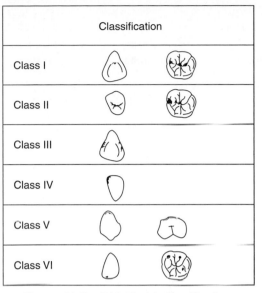

Classification		
Class I		
Class II		
Class III		
Class IV		
Class V		
Class VI		

Figure 11-3 G.V. Black's Classification.

8. Overhang: extension of restorative material beyond confines of preparation, extra bulk makes oral hygiene difficult in the area, may lead to periodontal irritation; noted as "O" or "OH" and drawn by location.

C. Dental caries are determined by visual, explorer, laser light, radiographic examination:

1. New caries: charted by outlining and shading in red and/or use of two-digit number.

a. G.V. Black's Classification (Figure 11-3):

(1) Classification by location:

(a) Class I: pits and fissures on occlusal, buccal, lingual surfaces of posteriors and lingual of anteriors.

(b) Class II: proximal surface of posteriors.

(c) Class III: proximal surface of anteriors.

(d) Class IV: proximal surface, including incisal edge of anteriors.

(e) Class V: gingival one third of facial and lingual surfaces of anteriors and posteriors.

(f) Class VI: cusp tips on molars, premolars, canines.

(2) Classification by surfaces:

(a) Simple: one tooth surface (e.g., occlusal).

(b) Compound: two tooth surfaces (e.g., mesio-occlusal [MO]).

(c) Complex: more than two surfaces (e.g., mesio-occlusal-distal [MOD]).

b. Carious lesion classification (with minimal intervention dentistry) (Figure 11-4) using two-digit numbers:

(1) Classification by site:

(a) Pits and fissures on the occlusal surface.

(b) Contact area.

(c) Cervical areas including exposed root surfaces.

(2) Classification by lesion size:

(a) Size 0: initial lesion that can be identified but has not yet resulted in surface cavitation; may be possible to undergo remineralization.

(b) Size 1: smallest minimal lesion requiring operative intervention; just beyond remineralization.

(c) Size 2: moderate-sized cavity; still sufficient sound tooth structure to maintain integrity of the remaining crown and accept occlusal load.

(d) Size 3: cavity needs to be modified and enlarged to provide some protection for remaining crown from occlusal load; already split at cusp base or, if not protected, a split is likely to develop.

(e) Size 4: cavity is now extensive following loss of cusp from posterior tooth or incisal edge from anterior.

2. Recurrent caries: new caries around previously placed restoration, charted by outlining restoration in red.

3. Decalcification: area that has started to demineralize, chalky and soft; charted by outlining, noted as "decal" or can be cross-hatched.

D. Other traumatic lesions:

1. Open contact: lack of proximal contact between two teeth, can be due to periodontal disease, unrestored carious lesion, iatrogenic dentistry, or discrepancies in alignment of permanent dentition; can cause food impaction resulting in increased caries and periodontal irritation; noted with two parallel lines between teeth.

2. Malposed teeth: located out of normal position in dental arch; caused by lack of space or unusual eruption:

a. Rotated teeth marked with arrow pointing toward surface rotated, usually marked across facial view.

b. Lingual version noted with arrow pointing from incisal edge away from facial view.

c. Labial version noted by arrow pointing toward occlusal view.

3. Attrition: loss of structure caused by tooth-to-tooth contact on occlusal and incisal surfaces, from excessive horizontal forces such as bruxism; charted by outlining, shading, noting with horizontal line across affected portion.

4. Fractured tooth: result of trauma, confirmed by using radiograph, illumination, and/or reported history; noted with red line that resembles fracture configuration.

5. Abrasion: mechanical wearing other than by mastication, such as aggressive brushing or oral habits like opening pins or biting on pen; charted by outlining, shading, noting as "abr."

Site	Size				
	No cavity 0	Minimal 1	Moderate 2	Enlarged 3	Extensive 4
Pit or fissure 1	1.0	1.1	1.2	1.3	1.4
Contact area 2	2.0	2.1	2.2	2.3	2.4
Cervical 3	3.0	3.1	3.2	3.3	3.4

Figure 11-4 Classification with caries lesions grid (with minimal invasive dentistry).

6. Abfraction: area at cervical one third that appears as a V-shaped notch, associated with occlusal forces; charted by outlining, shading, noting as "abf."
7. Erosion: chemical wear, caused by acid substance, involves several teeth and damage over a broad surface; area is bracketed and noted as "Ero."
8. Ankylosed teeth: roots that are fused to underlying bone, common on first and second primary molars, generally appear lower than occlusal plane, sound hollow when tapped; noting as "ankl."
9. Hypocalcification (enamel hypoplasia, Turner's tooth or "white spot"): area on tooth that has not completely calcified, is white or yellow (exposed dentin); pitting may also be present; caused by trauma or high fever during tooth formation or due to localized fluorosis if permanent tooth (from fluoride ingestion); noting as "hycal."
10. Dilaceration: distortion of a root and crown linear relationship usually caused by trauma; noting as drawing in shape of root.

E. Other developmental conditions are charted by making special note or drawing on chart:
1. Fusion: union of two tooth buds involving dentin along entire tooth, root, or crown; each has separate pulp canals.
2. Gemination: splitting of a single tooth germ; single root and pulp canal.
3. Dens-in-dente: enamel organ is invaginated internally ("tooth-within-a-tooth" on radiograph).

CLINICAL STUDY

Age	75 YRS	**SCENARIO**
Sex	☒ Male ☐ Female	Clinical and radiographic examinations of the patient noted the following: (1) tooth #30 has a swelling on the buccal mucosa, about 6 to 8 mm in diameter; large existing MOD amalgam; the radiograph demonstrates distal root caries, as well as a radiolucency located at the apex of the distal root, and (2) teeth #30 and #31 are in crossbite with #2 and #3.
Height	5'11"	
Weight	168 LBS	
BP	130/60	
Chief Complaint	"Not sure what is going on in my mouth with this gumboil!"	
Medical History	Bypass surgery 4 months ago	
Current Medications	captopril (Capoten) 25 mg tid hydrochlorothiazide (Lopressor) 25 mg qd	
Social History	Lived alone since wife died 6 months ago Retired chess player	

1. Does the patient need antibiotic premedication before oral prophylaxis? Are there any contraindications with his treatment because of his medical history? What is his ASA physical classification status at this time?
2. How should the lesion around tooth #30 be palpated?
3. What are common oral side effects of the patient's drugs? What recommendations can be made to help relieve these symptoms?
4. Regarding his crossbite, how are the mandibular teeth positioned relative to the maxillary teeth?

1. With history of heart bypass surgery, does not require any antibiotic premedication to protect from infective endocarditis (IE). Bypass surgery does not involve heart valve tissues, which when damaged and replaced with artificial valves are at risk for IE. However, there is 4- to 6-week delay after cardiac surgery (or any cardiac event or episode) for emergency and elective dental treatment until heart has healed. Thus any emergency treatment by supervising dentist, possibly for the lesion on #30, will need medical consult with physician before proceeding. However, presence of oral infection is serious with his medical history. Thus he is ASA IV because of recent bypass surgery. He poses significant risk, since patients in this category have severe medical problem of greater importance to patient than planned dental treatment. Whenever possible, elective dental care should be postponed until his medical condition has improved to at least ASA III. His blood pressure reading of 130/86 indicates a prehypertension level and thus may not be fully regulated with his antihypertensive drug therapy or lifestyle changes; need to mention this to patient so he can consult on it also with physician.
2. Before palpating tooth #30 and adjacent tissues, observe and note any suppuration (pus) or presence of a papule ("gumboil") that indicates a draining fistula. Use digital palpation with light pressure to examine lesion for tenderness, draining fluid (pus), or any irregular tissue (i.e., hard, firm immovable mass). Bidigital compression and circular movements can also be used to palpate submandibular area for indications of lymph node drainage and swelling.
3. Xerostomia from salivary hypofunction is likely problem for this patient because of two antihypertensive drugs he takes; captopril (Capoten) is an angiotensin-converting enzyme (ACE) inhibitor, and hydrochlorothiazide (HCTZ, Lopressor) is a thiazide-type diuretic. Changes in saliva consistency, amount, and buffering capacity are often mistakenly associated with aging adults but are most often associated with drug use rather than physiological changes. Other problems created by xerostomia include increased risk of caries (especially root caries) and irritation or dryness of the mucous membrane that causes difficulties with speaking, taste, and nutrition. Increase in water consumption by sipping it, use of artificial saliva, air humidification, water-based lubrication, sucking on sugarless candies or chewing gum (especially those with xylitol) would all help to increase saliva production or relieve mouth dryness. Brush-on or tray prescription–strength fluoride (probably sodium fluoride) should be recommended for application just before bed with directions to expectorate the excess and not rinse the mouth. Many OTC fluoride mouthrinses contain alcohol and may be contraindicated if the mucous membranes are sensitive from the xerostomia. Replacement therapy with calcium products can also be used to remineralize teeth.
4. Mandibular teeth #30 and #31 are buccal to buccal cusps of maxillary teeth #2 and #3. Thus crossbite occurs when mandibular teeth are placed facially to maxillary teeth. Normal occlusion would have #2 and #3 buccal to the mandibular buccal cusps of #30 and #31. Thus permanent maxillary first molar to mandibular arch is established when ML cusp interdigitates with central fossa of mandibular first molar.

Evaluation of Tooth Stains

Teeth normally vary in color. However, stains are TRUE discolorations of teeth. **Intrinsic stain** is within the tooth and CANNOT be removed by scaling and/or polishing, although it may be reduced by whitening (bleaching), both internally and externally. **Endogenous intrinsic stain** occurs from internal influences. **Exogenous intrinsic stain** is caused by environmental influences that result in intrinsic stain. **Extrinsic stain** occurs on the external surface of the tooth and can be removed by scaling and polishing; occurs in variety of colors. Over time, however, extrinsic stain can become intrinsic because of the uptake by exposed dentin that occurs with recession and attrition.

• See Chapters 12, Instrumentation: scaling and polishing; 15, Dental Biomaterials: tooth whitening.

A. Endogenous intrinsic stain:
  1. Fluorosis: white and/or brown spots, milky opalescence, and in extreme cases, pitting and mottling caused by excess oral fluoride intake during tooth development.
  2. Tetracycline (Tetracyn): yellow and/or brown, caused by ingestion of antibiotic during tooth development.
  3. Tetracycline derivative, minocycline (Minocin): bluish gray stain in adults.
  4. Amoxicillin (Amoxil): possibly white opacities caused by ingestion of antibiotic during tooth development.
  5. Traumatized or infected pulp: gray or black as result of blood leaching into dentin.
  6. Age: yellow caused by thinning of enamel, allowing color of underlying dentin to show through.

7. Genetic and systemic anomalies:
   a. Hypocalcification: white opacities.
   b. Amelogenesis imperfecta: white opacities, pitting.
   c. Dentinogenesis imperfecta: bluish, translucent.
   d. Dentin dysplasia: bluish, translucent.
   e. Porphyria: dark yellow or brown.
B. Exogenous intrinsic stain:
   1. Caries: white, brown, black; caused by acid-producing dental biofilm, diet, vomiting.
   2. Pulp necrosis: yellow, black, gray; caused by trauma.
   3. Restorative materials: gray, black: result of materials (amalgam, pins, posts) showing through enamel or by amalgam staining surrounding tooth.
   4. Pulpitis: pink caused by inflammation and internal bleeding within pulp chamber; internal resorption can also appear pink.
C. Exogenous extrinsic stain:
   1. Noted mainly at cervical area and facial surfaces unless otherwise noted.
   2. Can become intrinsic over time and affect the incisal and occlusal surfaces with tooth wear (attrition).
   3. Need to AVOID MOST of these factors post whitening procedures until tooth has rehydrated for effectiveness and for long-term maintenance (chromogenic agents).
      a. Yellow: caused by heavy dental biofilm buildup.
      b. Green: caused by poor oral hygiene; can become intrinsic through underlying decalcification; difficult to remove, but AVOID abrasive scaling or polishing because of possible decalcification; may also be due to staining of Nasmyth's membrane on newly erupted teeth (MOST brushes off).
      c. Black or black line: caused by iron compounds from oral fluids that embed in dental biofilm; found in clean mouths on lingual surfaces and near amalgam restorations.
      d. Brownish to black: caused by tobacco use.
      e. Orange: rare, associated with chromogenic bacteria.
      f. Tan to dark brown: from diet (food) such as red wine, tea, coffee, colas, vegetables, fruits, nuts, candies.
      g. Brown or orange-tan: caused by antimicrobials chlorhexidine (increased with staining diet) and stannous fluoride.
      h. Gray-green: associated with marijuana use.
      i. Metallic hues: vary in color and are due to ingestion of industrial dust and various foods and water.

Occlusal Evaluation

Occlusion is the contact relationship of the maxillary and mandibular teeth when the teeth are fully closed. Angle's classification of malocclusion is the MOST widely used system to initially describe the relationship of the permanent and primary teeth when in centric relation (MOST posterior position of mandible). In addition, movements of the mandible in relationship to maxilla are evaluated.
- See Chapters 4, Head, Neck, and Dental Anatomy: normal occlusion, occlusal evaluation, malocclusion; 13, Periodontology: occlusal trauma.

Dental Caries Pathogenesis and Diagnosis

Dental caries is due to irreversible solubilization of tooth mineral by acid. (See earlier discussion on classification and charting; later discussion on prevention by dental biofilm removal, fluorides, oral microbials, enamel sealants, as well as clinical care throughout a lifetime for patients.)
- See Chapters 7, Nutrition: cariogenic diet; 15, Dental Biomaterials: caries treatment; 17, Community Oral Health: caries epidemiology, community prevention programs.
A. Etiology:
   1. MAIN cause: for coronal lesions, *Streptococcus mutans* with initiation, lactobacilli with progression of the lesion (root caries discussed later).
   2. Lesser cause: dietary acids and/or other means of acidic contact, such as gastric acids.
B. Pathogenesis:
   1. Tooth surface loses some mineral (calcium, phosphate) from action of the acid at ≤5.0 pH (demineralization).
      a. From dental biofilm bacteria after ingestion of foods containing fermentable carbohydrates.
         (1) Low pH selects for aciduric organisms, such as *S. mutans* and lactobacilli, which store polysaccharide (MAINLY *S. mutans*) and continue to secrete acid (acidogenic) long after food has been removed by swallowing.
         (2) In addition, when fermentable foods are eaten frequently, low pH in dental biofilm is sustained.
      b. From dietary acids, includes citrus products, soft drinks, and sports drinks (especially diet).
      c. From gastric acids because of vomiting (bulimia, pregnancy, chemotherapy) or reflux (gastroesophageal reflux disease [GERD]) or after bariatric surgery.
   2. Normally, tooth minerals are replenished by saliva between meals (remineralization); however, when low pH is sustained, net loss of mineral from the tooth occurs, producing caries.
   3. Addition of dry mouth from drugs or systemic disorders increases acid damage caused by lessening of salivary buffering and clearance effects.

> **Box 11-1** Caries Risk Factors
>
> Dental biofilm: quantity and composition
> Previous caries experience
> Frequent exposure to fermentable carbohydrates or oral acids
> Active periodontal therapy
> Saliva: quantity and quality
> Number of periodontal pockets >3 mm
> Systemic illness or disability, cancer therapy, or stomach regurgitation
> Number of exposed roots, furcations, and crowded teeth
> Tobacco use
> Fewer than nine remaining teeth
> Low income
> Orthodontic appliances or removable partial dentures

C. Caries risk factors (Box 11-1).
1. IMPORTANT to determine a patient's risk factors for caries development so as to create a treatment plan that involves NOT just present concerns but also preventive needs (see CD-ROM for caries risk levels and treatment concerns).
2. There is overlap between caries risk and periodontal disease risk as the patient may have MORE dental biofilm, poor oral hygiene, xerostomia, gingival recession.
3. Caries risk assessment methods:
   a. Chairside culture procedures:
      (1) Tests that allow estimate of number of *S. mutans* or *Lactobacillus* organisms in saliva.
      (2) Salivary assessment tests: measure hydration, conditions, resting and stimulated pH, salivary buffering capacity, stimulated salivary flow.
   b. Software programs: assess individual patient's caries risk based on a database.
D. Diagnostic methods: explorer, mirror, air, dental light; improved with loupes and intraoral camera; other diagnostic methods:
1. Radiographs: radiolucencies in enamel and/or dentin; used MAINLY for interproximal smooth surface caries; NOT considered "gold standard" in caries diagnosis; do NOT provide definitive diagnosis and have ONLY around 50% to 70% sensitivity using visual means.
   a. Software associated with digital radiographs can analyze changes in radiographic density to identify demineralized areas by way of database and determine probability that caries is present.
2. Laser (DIAGNOdent): uses fiber optic transillumination and digital imaging fiber optic transillumination (DIFOTI), which interacts with detector,

reads out number and audible signal if there is a lesion.
   a. Numbers of 11 to 20 need preventive or restorative treatment, depending on caries risk; >21 indicates probability of subsurface lesion and need for restorative treatment.
   b. NOT able to use on coronal smooth surfaces, ONLY noncavitated suspected pit and fissure occlusal lesions.
3. Quantitative light-induced fluorescence (QLF; Inspektor Pro): uses fluorescence to determine demineralization; used on ALL coronal surfaces except interproximally.
E. Clinical signs:
1. Noncavitation (incipient stage): atraumatic white spot is present because of subsurface demineralization.
2. Early cavitation (early clinical stage): microorganisms penetrate enamel rods.
3. Late cavitation (advanced clinical stage, frank lesion): microorganisms enter dentin and approach tooth pulp using dentinal tubules; can become painful.

Types of Caries and Treatment

Caries can be classified by rate of progression or etiology (see earlier discussion with charting). Includes rampant or early childhood caries, as well as recurrent or arrested caries. Can also be classified by location, either pit and fissure or smooth surface (Figure 11-5). With pit and fissure progression, two triangles are noted histologically (one triangle in enamel, other in dentin) with bases conjoined to each other at dentinoenamel junction (DEJ), includes occlusal, facial, and lingual surfaces. With smooth surface progression, the base and apex of the two triangles join; includes interproximal or root caries.

A. **Rampant caries:** advanced or severe decay on multiple surfaces of many teeth.
1. Professional considerations:
   a. Discussion of medical implications: vomiting; xerostomia induced by drugs, including methamphetamine and sugar-laced drugs (nystatin); use of spit (smokeless) tobacco that contains sugar.
   b. Close monitoring:
      (1) Evaluate ability to remove dental biofilm at 1-week, 1-month, 3-month intervals.
      (2) Confirm home fluoride and/or calcium use at each appointment.
      (3) Have patient keep a diet diary for review at next appointment (see Chapter 7, Nutrition).
   c. Expose bitewing radiographs at MORE frequent intervals.
2. Recommendations to patient or caretaker:
   a. Dental biofilm removal with brush, floss, or other aids.

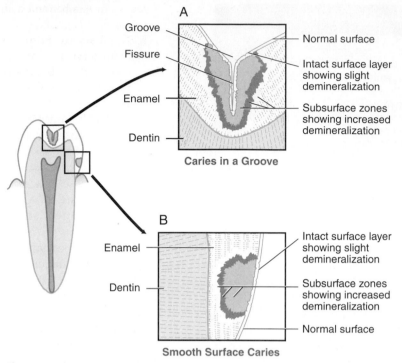

Figure 11-5 Caries process. (From Bath-Balogh M, Fehrenbach MJ: Illustrated dental embryology and anatomy, ed 2, Philadelphia, 2006, Saunders/Elsevier.)

b. Nutritional counseling: reduce frequency of ingesting simple-sugar foods; for example, decrease from three cans of sweetened, carbonated beverages daily to one can and drink beverage in 30 minutes using straw instead of sipping over 3 hours; use non-citrus-based beverages.

c. Home fluoride use with OTC or prescription mouthrinses or brush-on or tray application of foam or gels (see earlier discussion of fluoride and trays).

d. Use of mineralizing calcium products both professionally and at home, as well as xylitol products.

B. **Early childhood caries** (ECC; also, baby bottle caries tooth decay [BBTD]): shallow acute cervical lesions of primary dentition caused by dental biofilm (MAINLY *S. mutans*) and/or dietary acids from beverages in bottles for infants and young children (Figure 11-6):

1. Professional considerations:

   a. MAINLY involves primary maxillary anteriors (C, D, E, F, G, H) because of contact with nipple; tongue and saliva help cleanse other teeth.

   b. Fluoridated water has positive effect, which may be missed if bottled water used; NOT able to use fluoridated dentifrice until child will NOT swallow it.

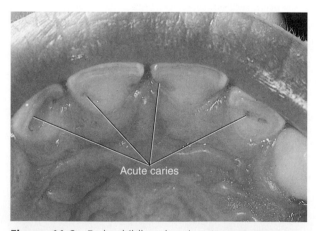

Figure 11-6 Early childhood caries. (From Bath-Balogh M, Fehrenbach MJ: Illustrated dental embryology and anatomy, ed 2, Philadelphia, 2006, Saunders/Elsevier.)

c. Breastfeeding has been proved NOT to be associated; however, because cariogenic bacteria (especially *S. mutans*) are transmitted soon after FIRST teeth erupt, decreasing guardian's levels may decrease child's risk; encourage dental visit to ensure guardian's own oral health.

d. May be at severe levels (S-ECC), which can progress and cause pulpal exposure, resulting in large restorations and early tooth loss owing to thinness of overlying enamel and dentin of primary teeth; treatment ranges from composites to stainless steel crowns to extraction.

    e. Fluoride varnish is BEST method for topical fluoride application for primary teeth (see later discussion).

    f. Prevalence is epidemic, MOST in minority and rural populations (>70%); community programs address issue with education and fluoride varnish.

  2. Recommendations to guardians:

    a. Do NOT put infant to bed with baby bottle filled with formula, milk, juice, soft drinks for long periods of time; may continue with no-spill training cup (sippy cup) in toddlers.

    b. Plain water is BEST choice for prolonged bottle use; educate guardian that infants' and toddlers' teeth SHOULD be brushed starting from first emergence after every feeding or meal.

C. **Root caries:** soft, leathery progressive, small and shallow lesions of root surfaces caused by dental biofilm (MAINLY *Actinomyces viscosus,* same microorganism as involved with occlusal; possibly *Veillonella parvulus*) and/or dietary acids.

  1. Professional considerations:

    a. Root MORE vulnerable to process than enamel because cementum begins to demineralize at 6.7 pH, which is higher than enamel's critical pH; can lead to a rapid loss of teeth despite valiant recare efforts.

    b. Formation: precipitated by conditions that cause root surface exposure:

      (1) Periodontal disease.

      (2) Malocclusion.

      (3) Mechanical trauma (toothbrush abrasion).

      (4) Orthodontic tooth movement.

      (5) Periodontal surgery.

      (6) Abfraction caused by bruxism and/or clenching.

  2. Recommendations to patients or caregivers:

    a. Significant risk factors: attachment loss, age, number of teeth, presence of coronal caries, level of oral hygiene, water fluoridation, years of education, xerostomia.

      (1) Common outcome when xerostomia is present; IMPORTANT risk factor because preventive action of saliva is diminished by such factors as buffering, washing, antibacterial, immunological (see earlier discussion).

      (2) Risk factors for xerostomia:

        (a) MOST systemic medications.

        (b) Radiation therapy.

        (c) Pathological conditions.

    b. Root caries may be prevented by:

      (1) Effective dental biofilm control.

      (2) Combination fluoride therapy, along with calcium and xylitol products.

      (3) Noncariogenic diet; reduced intake of cariogenic foods to decrease accumulation of substrate (see earlier discussion).

      (4) Frequent examinations of exposed root surfaces.

    c. Thus BOTH the geriatric patient and periodontal maintenance (PM) patient are at high risk for root caries based on number of significant risk factors listed above (discussed later).

D. **Recurrent caries** (secondary caries): appears at location with previous history of caries; frequently found on margins of dental restorations; marginal discoloration by itself is NOT a valid sign for dental caries.

E. **Arrested caries:** brown, smooth, shiny lesion that was previously demineralized but was remineralized before causing cavitation; associated with sclerotic dentin.

F. Treatment for all carious lesions:

  1. For noncavitated initial lesions:

    a. Minimally invasive dentistry (MID) using preventive mode (or nonsurgical management) by use of remineralizing therapy (discussed later) instead of repair mode (traditional restorative treatment); this therapy can arrest or repair the initial lesion so that it does not progress to cavitation and need restorative treatment.

    b. Use of enamel (pit and fissure) sealants (discussed later).

  2. For early cavitated lesions: alternative (atraumatic) restorative treatment (ART) where NOT all infected dentin is removed, as long as a secure seal can be achieved between tooth and material, then MAINLY using glass ionomer restoration with its fluoride release.

  3. For late cavitated lesions: traditional restorations.

CLINICAL STUDY

Age	19 YRS	SCENARIO
Sex	☐ Male ☒ Female	At the patient's previous dental examination and oral prophylaxis, 15 months ago, she had only one occlusal restoration placed. At this appointment the clinical and radiographic examinations reveal: (1) moderately inflamed gingival tissues, light calculus on the mandibular anteriors and posterior molars interproximally; (2) no dental biofilm deposits or stain; (3) new carious lesions on 13 of her posterior teeth (#2-M, #3-D, #4-M, #5-DO, #12-O, #13-D, #14-MOD, #15-M, #18-M, #19-D, #20-MOD, #30-M, #31-MO). Patient shows the dental hygienist a good brushing technique, brushes once a day, and flosses infrequently. However, when asked about any dietary changes, she states she ate well at school at first until the fall when she began drinking coffee with sugar and three or four sweetened, carbonated soft drinks sipped all day long to keep her awake for her studies.
Height	5'4"	
Weight	150 LBS	
BP	112/67	
Chief Complaint	"My jaw joint hurts when I open my mouth."	
Medical History	None	
Current Medications	None	
Social History	College student, comes home at breaks	

1. What is the most probable reason for the patient's dramatic increase in caries?
2. What techniques should be used to examine the TMJ area? If positive findings, what recommendation should be made?
3. How does the patient's gingival health vary from normal, healthy gingiva with respect to color, consistency, texture, and marginal contour? Why is there tissue inflammation in the absence of any dental biofilm?
4. What oral hygiene self-care regimen(s) is (are) recommended? What can be planned in the dental office to reduce her caries risk? Explain any nutritional recommendations that should be made.
5. What type of instrumentation is needed to complete the oral prophylaxis?

1. Increase in sugar consumption with coffee and soft drink is the most likely reason for increase in interproximal and occlusal caries. Sugar frequency affects acid production, thereby increasing risk for proximal and occlusal caries.
2. Use bilateral palpation to assess the TMJ. Bilateral palpation involves placing the index fingers of each hand just anterior to the outer auditory meatus of the ear and feeling the joint area as the patient opens and closes. Observation is also required to assess the TMJ for deviations in the functional movements of opening, closing, and lateral movements. Use auscultation (listening for sound) to detect clicking, crepitus, popping, and grating. Question patient regarding painful symptoms associated with jaw movements. For positive findings, refer to supervising dentist for further evaluation.
3. Healthy gingiva should appear pale pink, firm, and stippled; marginal contour should hug neck of the tooth and be 1 mm coronal to CEJ, and papilla should appear pointed or "knife-edge" in interproximal areas. Gingival tissue is likely to be red, edematous, and spongy, with some loss of stippling, and marginal contour will be swollen and possibly bulbous, indicating diagnosis of gingivitis (gingival inflammation). The patient is dental biofilm free at this appointment, most likely because she brushed her teeth more thoroughly just before this dental checkup than she typically does; previous dental biofilm buildup caused the inflammation.
4. At this dental appointment, primary need for treatment of dental caries should be addressed. Because of increased number of carious lesions, caries process should be discussed with patient. She should be encouraged to brush two or three times a day for 2 minutes each time, using fluoride dentifrice (toothpaste). She also needs to add flossing to her daily self-care. Regimen of prescription topical home fluoride applications before bedtime (brush-on or tray fluoride) is recommended. Specific directions must include not rinsing after fluoride application to allow fluoride to continue to work in higher concentrations. Because of excessive interproximal caries, it is appropriate to request that patient swish with home fluoride mouthrinse daily and use mineralizing calcium products. For her restorative treatment in the dental office, may want to include enamel sealants in any high-risk pit and fissure areas. After her restorative treatment is finished, she should schedule another appointment for examination in 3 months because of her high risk, possibly including bitewing (BW) radiographs and evaluation of caries management. Discuss the form and frequency of sugar exposures from coffee and soft drinks, explaining

that drinking soft drinks for 1 hour continually bathes the teeth with substrate bacteria used to produce an acid environment. The carbonation of the soft drink provides additional acid attack on the teeth; substrate bacteria can actually exist in such an acidic environment. Recommend reducing sugar and acid exposures by limiting amount and duration (length of time) of soft drink (whether sugared or sugar free, since latter is more acidic, and use of straw) and coffee with sugar consumption and by rinsing mouth with water after eating or drinking to reduce acid environment. Citrus-containing soft drinks cause the greatest demineralization of the enamel.

5. Manual instrumentation with anterior and posterior sickles, as well as universal or Gracey curets, is sufficient to debride for the oral prophylaxis. Ultrasonic instrumentation using thin periodontal inserts could also be used. Polishing, even by selective methods, would not be appropriate considering her caries risk and related possibility of increased levels of decalcification of the enamel surface. Thus all instrumentation should avoid the occlusal or other pit and fissured areas, as well as the cervical surfaces of the teeth. Professional fluoride application, such as with fluoride varnish, should follow instrumentation to replace any loss of surface mineralization.

Dentinal Hypersensitivity

Dentinal (dentin) **hypersensitivity** is pain caused by differing stimuli such as thermal (cold/heat), evaporative (blowing air), osmotic (sweet or sour/acid), tactile (toothbrushes, flossing, toothpick, dental instruments) on dentin of root that is exposed by gingival recession and/or on masticatory surfaces as result of attrition. Abrasion, erosion, and abfraction can further complicate the situation. Common occurrence also with periodontal patients before and/or after nonsurgical and surgical therapy, as well as post whitening. Associated pain may be sharp, short, or transient in nature with rapid onset. Hypersensitivity is a chronic condition with acute episodes. Spontaneous remission without further intervention has been shown to occur in ~20% to 45% in 4 to 8 weeks; also becomes LESS noticeable 2 to 3 weeks after nonsurgical periodontal therapy.

A. Etiology is BEST explained by hydrodynamic theory (Figure 11-7):
   1. Stimulation of open dentinal tubules at root surface causes movement of the fluid within the tubules.
   2. This movement transmits signals to the nerves in the adjacent pulp chamber, resulting in pain.
B. Pathogenesis:
   1. Root after periodontal surgery is frequently sensitive because of exposure of the root surface and eventual dissolution of smear layer approximately 7 days after exposure.

   2. Root after scaling (and root planing) is frequently sensitive because removal of cementum exposes the dentinal tubules.
   3. Post whitening, teeth may be sensitive because of evaporation of dentinal fluid in the tubules and subsequent rehydration (can be reduced by pretreatment with desensitizing agents and fluoride treatments).
   4. Protective smear layer can also be removed by dietary and gastric acids, as well as detergents found in toothpastes and rinses.
C. Management: performed professionally or at home:
   1. Professional application of the following desensitizing agents has proved effective:
      a. Protein-precipitating agents (e.g., silver nitrate, zinc chloride, strontium chloride, formaldehyde).
      b. Tubule-occluding metallic salt agents (e.g., calcium hydroxide or phosphate, potassium nitrate, fluorides, sodium citrate, iontophoresis with 2% sodium fluoride, potassium oxalate); fluoride varnish is particularly effective because its globules fill in the tubules and stay for a long period of time.
      c. Neutral noncolored fluoride treatment pre and post whitening procedure: gel or foam with trays.

STIMULATION

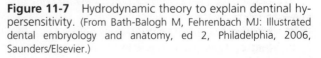

Exposed dentin
Dentinal tubule
Change in dentinal fluid
Odontoblastic process

Possible nerve location
Odontoblast cell body in pulp tissue

Pain message sent to brain

Figure 11-7 Hydrodynamic theory to explain dentinal hypersensitivity. (From Bath-Balogh M, Fehrenbach MJ: Illustrated dental embryology and anatomy, ed 2, Philadelphia, 2006, Saunders/Elsevier.)

2. Physical sealing of the tubules with composites, resins, glass ionomers, varnishes, sealants; may be used if chemical applications do NOT provide relief.

3. Desensitizing dentifrices (toothpastes) are available for home use and contain one of the following active ingredients (see later discussion under dentifrices): strontium chloride, potassium nitrate, sodium citrate, amorphous calcium phosphate. Note that fluoride-containing toothpastes do NOT have high enough fluoride concentration to have impact.

Pulpal Vitality Testing

Pulp responds to any form of stimulus, whether electrical, touch, or temperature, ONLY with pain. Normal pulp will typically respond to these pain-producing stimuli in manner consistent with similar teeth in the dentition. Pulp tissue can undergo inflammation or pulpitis as result of trauma or infection from either dental or periodontal pathological changes, either reversible or irreversible. Continuing pulpitis can lead to death of the pulp or necrosis. Tooth varies in its response to pain-producing stimuli when undergoing pulpitis and necrosis, as noted during pulp vitality testing. *Practice acts concerning pulp vitality testing vary by state.*

• See Chapters 6, General and Oral Pathology: pulpal pathology; 15, Dental Biomaterials: endodontic therapy.

A. Diagnostic categories for pulpal diseases:
   1. Reversible pulpitis: exhibits quick, sharp hypersensitive response to thermal stimulus that subsides with removal of stimulus.
   2. Irreversible pulpitis: usually indicated by lingering response to cold temperatures; may give spontaneous pain without stimulation or may be asymptomatic; pulpal damage is NOT repairable.
   3. Necrotic pulp: indicated by asymptomatic, nonvital tooth that does NOT respond to any stimuli; NOT repairable; requires endodontic therapy (root canal) or extraction.

B. General testing technique: decisions are based on a combination of all available data.
   1. Recognize that individual pulp test can give either false-positive or false-negative response.
   2. Goal is to make distinction between vital and nonvital pulps or determine existence of abnormal pulp.
   3. Recognize that pulpal pathological changes can be of dental (caries) or periodontal origin; combination of factors can occur.
   4. Test both suspected teeth and control teeth (usually adjacent teeth and contralateral tooth) for comparison data.
   5. Compare readings of all teeth tested to determine results, since same types of teeth (e.g., molars)

give similar readings in same individual but may vary widely among individuals.
   6. Record results of all tests and other pulpal assessments in record.

C. Sources of data for pulpal diagnosis: patient's subjective report of symptoms MUST always be confirmed with objective, clinical information and testing.
   1. Dental history related to tooth or teeth in question, as well as trauma, pain, mobility.
   2. Intraoral and extraoral examination: tooth fracture, large carious lesion, large restoration, lymphadenopathy, swelling, pustule (or draining fistula), tenderness.
   3. Radiographic examination by periapical film: pathological radiolucency, periodontal ligament (PDL) space widening, fracture, caries, or deep restorations (see Chapter 4, Radiology).
   4. Palpation: inflammation in periapical tissues extending into periodontium.
      a. Bidigital palpation of bone in the area of tooth apex.
      b. Use palpation of surrounding (control) teeth for comparison.
   5. **Percussion:** test for inflammatory changes in the PDL (horizontal and vertical):
      a. Use end of mirror handle or similar instrument to gently tap the teeth in both a vertical and horizontal direction; use ONLY finger pressure rather than tapping with an instrument if patient reports that the teeth are very sensitive.
      b. Ask the patient if any of the percussed teeth feel different or tender in comparison with surrounding (control) teeth.
      c. Interpretation: positive test indicates inflammation in PDL; confirmation of diagnosis by other clinical tests is needed because inflammatory changes in PDL are NOT always of pulpal origin.
      d. Can also have patient bite tongue depressor (locates fractures, too).
   6. Thermal tests for pulp vitality: see earlier diagnostic discussion.
      a. May involve use of either cold or hot thermal stimulus to test for pulpal response.
         (1) Cold test is MORE frequently used.
         (2) Heat test is helpful when the ONLY symptom is heat sensitivity and the offending tooth is NOT clearly identified.
      b. Cold test technique:
         (1) Use ice, carbon dioxide (dry ice), or a cotton-tipped applicator coated with refrigerant such as ethyl chloride.
         (2) Place cold agent on the tooth and observe any response.

(3) Remove stimulus immediately on patient response; leave on tooth a maximum of 10 seconds (20 seconds for full crown coverage).

c. Hot test technique:

(1) Lubricate selected teeth to prevent material from sticking.

(2) Heat a small amount of gutta-percha or stopping material and place on the tooth.

(3) Remove stimulus immediately on patient response; leave on the tooth a maximum of 10 seconds (20 seconds for teeth with full crown coverage).

7. Interpretation of test results:

a. Abnormal pulp status is indicated when there is different response between suspected and surrounding (control) teeth or similar teeth.

b. Diseased pulp is suspected when:

(1) NO response.

(2) Response is excessively rapid (comparative).

(3) Response is lingering or prolonged (comparative).

(4) Response is of increasing intensity (comparative).

(5) Preexisting pain is alleviated when cold is applied.

8. Electric pulp test (EPT; vitalometer) (forget what you have seen in horror movies!):

a. Absolute contraindication for patient with cardiac pacemaker because of possibility of electrical interference.

b. Technique:

(1) Place small amount of conducting material (usually dentifrice or toothpaste) on tip.

(2) Starting with control dial at lowest number (lowest electric impulse), place electrode on the tooth and have patient touch metal handle with fingers to complete circuit.

(3) Depending on equipment, current will automatically increase; instruct patient to release handle when he or she feels sensation, or manually increase current dial until patient gives prearranged signal; lift tip from the tooth.

(4) May want to test surrounding teeth (control) or similar tooth for comparison (as discussed previously).

c. Interpretation of test results is generally all or none: scales can range from 1 to 10 or 1 to 50.

(1) Response at low electric stimulus level, tooth is vital; the closer to the 1 reading, the healthier the tooth.

(2) If NO response, tooth is nonvital; the farther from the 1 reading, the poorer the prognosis.

d. Differing response levels do NOT indicate different stages of pulp degeneration.

(1) May give false-positive reading because of stimulation of nerve fibers in periodontium.

(2) Posteriors may give misleading readings because of combination of vital and nonvital root canal pulps.

(3) Does NOT work on teeth with metal crowns (short-circuiting) or ceramic crowns (insulating).

PERIODONTAL EVALUATION

Periodontal evaluation is the examination of the soft and hard tissues surrounding the tooth structure. MAIN role of the dental professional is to educate patient on characteristics of a healthy periodontium and its maintenance so that patient will AVOID periodontal (gum) disease and its complication of tooth loss.

• See Chapters 2, Embryology and Histology: anatomy of periodontium; 4, Head, Neck, and Dental Anatomy: occlusal evaluation; 5, Radiology: radiographic assessment; 13, Periodontology: dental biofilm and calculus, periodontal disease, occlusal trauma; 17, Community Oral Health: dental biofilm and periodontal indices.

A. Clinical description of healthy periodontium:

1. Color: uniform pale to coral pink from mucogingival attachment to the free gingival margin; may be pigmented with melanin (related to complexion and race).

2. Contour and size: include free gingiva margins that fit snugly and follow curved lines around necks of the teeth, interdental papillae are knife edged and pointed and fill the embrasure space.

3. Consistency: firm and resilient.

4. Surface texture of attached gingiva: usually stippled owing to rete pegs, which connect oral epithelium of the oral mucosa to underlying lamina propria.

5. Free (marginal) gingiva: smooth tissue but NOT bound to underlining tissue; position is 1 to 2 mm coronal to the CEJ.

6. Bleeding (either spontaneous or on probing [BoP]) and exudate: NOT present.

B. Clinical description of diseased periodontium:

1. Signs of inflammation:

a. Acute inflammation:

(1) Appears bright red because of dilation of blood vessels and proliferation of blood cells.

(2) Begins in area of the interdental papilla; FIRST site is the col (fragile portion of periodontium).

(3) Tissue is swollen and edematous in early stages.

(4) Consistency is spongy and soft; tissue indents easily when pressed and hangs away from tooth; loss of stippling causes a smooth and shiny look because of increased infiltration of fluid and inflammatory elements into tissue cells.

(5) Bleeds easily because of junctional epithelium (JE) ulceration from damage to lamina propria's blood vessels; BoP is the MOST objective method of assessing active inflammation and can identify patients at risk for disease progression; however, ONLY risk and NOT sign of progression; lack of BoP is a sign of healthy gingiva.

(6) Suppuration (pus) is a sign of acute inflammation and infection; exudate may appear clear, white, or yellow depending on composition of white blood cells (WBCs) and inflammatory debris.

b. Chronic inflammation:

(1) Appears dark red to bluish red magenta; however, when extremely chronic, will appear fibrotic and near normal in color.

(2) Interdental papilla appears flattened, blunted, or cratered; gingival margins may be rolled; clefts and festoons may be present.

(a) Widening interdental embrasures: with recession comes loss of interdental papillae; classified as type I through type III.

(b) Factor to consider when choosing interdental oral care method.

(3) Consistency is tough and fibrotic, with leathery or hard, nodular-like surface texture.

(4) BoP may NOT be present and is NOT as obvious as with acute inflammation (especially with smokers).

C. Dental biofilm (etiological or causative agent): slight, moderate, or severe levels; supragingival or subgingival.

1. Combination of dental biofilm and host response to periodontal pathogens influences initiation and progression of periodontal disease.

2. Mineralization results in development of calculus deposits on tooth enamel and cementum, restorations, prosthetic appliances; acts as attachment mechanism for new colonies of new dental biofilm.

3. Can be made visible by disclosing solution to identify areas continually missed or can be measured using an index; two-tone solution stains new red and old blue.

D. Radiographic examination (has limitations):

1. Healthy periodontium: interproximal alveolar crestal bone is 1 mm apical to CEJ; lamina dura is dense, radiopaque, and continuous; NO furcation involvement.

2. Diseased periodontium: horizontal and/or vertical bone loss, widened PDL space, furcation involvement (radiolucent); thinning or loss of definition in lamina dura (alveolar bone proper); may have pulpal complications as well.

E. Probe depths of epithelial sulcus from the free gingival margin to the base of the pocket:

1. Probing depths (PD): recorded on a periodontal chart and include six readings per tooth (three on facial; three on lingual); note BoP for each reading; note other associated periodontal concerns such as recession, furcation, reduced attached gingiva, mobility.

2. **Gingival pocket** (or pseudopocket): enlargement of the gingiva that causes the margin of the gingiva to proliferate in a coronal direction; there is NO apical migration; pocket is suprabony and reversible with good homecare and professional intervention.

3. **Periodontal pocket:** JE to migrate apically, allowing destruction of epithelial attachment (EA); involves destruction of deeper periodontal structures, cementum, PDL, bone.

a. Suprabony pocket: JE is apical to the CEJ but coronal to crest of the alveolar bone.

b. Infrabony pocket: JE is apical to crest of the alveolar bone (further classified as to three types).

F. **Recession:** level of the marginal gingiva is apical to the CEJ, measured in millimeters using periodontal probe.

G. **Clinical attachment level** (CAL): level from probing from a fixed point such as the distance from CEJ to base of the pocket (EA).

1. When CEJ is covered: to obtain CAL, first measured from gingival margin to CEJ, then subtracted from overall probing depth.

2. When CEJ is level with gingival margin: CAL is measured by probing depth.

3. With recession: CAL is measured from CEJ to EA (some add recession and probing depth).

H. **Mucogingival defects:** loss of the width of attached gingiva (<1 mm or nonexistent); measurement of attached gingiva is found by subtracting probing depth from total width of gingiva (gingival margin to mucogingival junction).

1. Type I defects: pockets extend apically to or beyond mucogingival junction, but a firm keratinized pocket wall exists.

2. Type II defects: alveolar mucosa acts as marginal gingiva, with NO zone of attached gingiva.

I. **Furcation involvement:** loss of interradicular bone on multirooted teeth; suspected when 4-mm probe depth is recorded on a multirooted tooth even with normal gingival contour; classified by extent of bone destruction:

1. Class I: soft tissue suprabony lesion with increased pocket depth; can detect concavity but CANNOT enter; radiographs show NO radiolucency.
2. Class II: probe can enter furcation, since there is a horizontal component and possibly a vertical or infrabony defect, but CANNOT extend through; radiographs may show slight radiolucency or furcation arrow for maxillary proximal furcas; may involve one or more furcations, but there is NO communication between them.
3. Class III: probe can pass (depending on soft tissue location) between facial and lingual, since bone is NOT attached to the roof or dome interdentally of the furca; radiographs show obvious radiolucency or furcation arrow for maxillary proximal furcas; Subdivided into two categories:
   a. Furca covered by tissue, harder to pass probe through.
   b. Furca NOT covered by tissue.
4. Class IV: soft tissue has receded and furcation is clinically visible because interdental bone has been destroyed; probe can easily pass through; radiographs show larger radiolucency.

J. **Mobility:** movement of tooth because of loss of support by periodontium; classified (or graded) by extent of horizontal and vertical movement.

1. Class I: moves 1 mm or less in any direction.
2. Class II: moves more than 1 mm in any direction but CANNOT be depressed.
3. Class III: moves MORE than 1 mm and can be depressed in the socket.

K. Additional diagnostic tests that can be used to assess periodontal health and disease are culture analysis and antibiotic sensitivity, DNA probes, enzyme immunoassays (enzymes tested may be derived from host or periodontal pathogens), immunological tests.

L. Documentation protocol:

1. Record probing depths, bleeding points, recession, furcations, mobility, reduced attachment level, bone level.
2. Determine periodontal status (healthy or American Academy of Periodontology [AAP] periodontal type) and periodontal case type.
3. Explain status to patient and possible recommended treatment options to the patient.
4. Record patient's response and willingness to proceed with treatment.
5. Failure to diagnose and properly treat periodontal disease is the MAIN cause of malpractice lawsuits (see Chapter 18, Ethics and Jurisprudence).

M. Referral protocol: dental hygienist CANNOT make referral to specialist, ONLY supervising dentist can.

1. Establish referral guidelines for the dental office.
2. Explain the need for special care to the patient.
3. Assist the patient in scheduling an appointment with a specialist.
4. Communicate with the specialist and patient to ensure continuity of care.

N. If patient does NOT follow through with treatment:

1. Discuss and document reasons for noncompliance.
2. Answer any additional questions patient may have.
3. Continue to see patient for regular maintenance appointments.
4. Monitor periodontal status and continue to encourage patient to seek additional care.
5. Confirm patient's understanding of consequences of noncompliance.

CLINICAL STUDY

Age	46 YRS	**SCENARIO**
Sex	☒ Male ☐ Female	On completion of the patient's dental exam, it is apparent that he clenches his teeth; has moderate gingivitis with fibrotic, enlarged, and bulbous interdental papilla; and has dental biofilm covering more than 50% of his teeth.
Height	5'10"	
Weight	185 LBS	
BP	110/78	
Chief Complaint	"I can't get floss between my teeth."	
Medical History	Seizure disorder Allergy to penicillin (Pen-Vee K) and diazepam (Valium)	
Current Medications	phenobarbital (Luminal) 30 mg qd phenytoin (Dilantin) 100 mg qd	
Social History	Food bank director	

1. What are common oral side effects of the patient's drugs and disease? Into what category do these drugs fall?
2. Given his history of clenching, what clinical signs could be expected in examination of his mouth?
3. What recommendations can be made for improving the patient's oral hygiene self-care?
4. What should the treatment plan include?

1. Phenytoin (Dilantin) can cause gingival hyperplasia (overgrowth of tissue). Because of injury from seizure trauma, scars on the lips and tongue and possibly fractured teeth may be found. Both drugs, phenytoin (Dilantin) and phenobarbital (Luminal), are anticonvulsants.
2. Clenching frequently results in scalloping of lateral borders of the tongue. Occlusal surface of molars will demonstrate wear (appear shiny), and dentin may become exposed as the enamel is worn away. Wear is also common on the incisal edges of anteriors. Patient may also have mobility, which is the movement of tooth resulting from loss of support by periodontium.
3. The patient could improve his oral self-care by using shred-resistant floss made of polytetrafluoroethylene (PTFE) or thin waxed floss. Powered toothbrush may help improve oral hygiene self-care because of built-in timers, ease of technique, and increased access to hard to reach tooth surfaces.
4. Treatment plan should include thorough assessment of medical history, specifically including most recent seizure, drug regimen, and compliance. Dental exam should include extraoral and intraoral examination, with special evaluation of existing periodontal condition. Complete dental and periodontal chart would be obtained and appropriate radiographs taken. Oral hygiene self-care instructions should involve patient by having him give return demonstration of brushing and flossing to observe technique. The patient will need thorough oral prophylaxis including debridement therapy, as well as a reappointment for evaluation with the supervising dentist in 4 to 6 weeks to consider need for gingivectomy, assess oral hygiene self-care, and determine continued care interval.

PREVENTION OF DENTAL DISEASE AND INJURY

It is IMPORTANT that dental hygienists use evidence-based decisions to support preventive treatment of patients. **Evidence-based decisions** are based on verified research evidence that certain signs or symptoms are predictive of certain outcomes. For instance, the finding of a greater number of *S. mutans* organisms poses a greater risk for future caries development than does a low count. The following devices and materials are designed to preserve the integrity of the natural dentition and protect the teeth and supporting tissues from disease or injury.

Include devices, dentifrices, fluoride, enamel (pit and fissure) sealants, mouth protectors.

Oral Hygiene Devices and Self-Care Practice

Oral hygiene devices include toothbrushes and other devices for self-care practice.
- See Chapter 16, Special Needs Patient Care: special oral care devices.
A. Toothbrushes:
    1. Manual brush selection and brushing technique:
        a. BEST to choose head size that corresponds with size of mouth and tooth accessibility.
        b. Handles SHOULD be easy to grip with minimal slippage and rotation during use; larger handles increase grasp ability with arthritis, other physical disabilities.
        c. Selection of bristle:
            (1) Ends should be rounded nylon filaments (LEAST damaging to gingival tissues).
            (2) Filament diameter determines hardness or softness (thinner filaments are softer and more resilient).
            (3) Nylon filaments are preferred over natural bristles because more resistant to bacterial accumulation, more easily rinsed and dried, durable, maintain form; ends are rounded and closed, which repels water and debris.
            (4) Multitufted bristles support adjacent bristles, allowing more cleaning action while being less traumatic to gingival tissues.
        d. Technique:
            (1) Use light-to-medium pressure to ensure removal of dental biofilm.
            (2) Develop sequence to ensure brushing of ALL teeth and tooth surfaces.
            (3) Brush two to three times per day for 2 to 3 minutes.
        e. Methods:
            (1) Sulcular/Bass method: for removing at gingival margin.
                (a) Filaments are directed apically and angled at 45°, brush is vibrated back and forth with a very short small motion, keeping brush tip engaged in sulci.
                (b) MOST widely accepted technique; BEST method for ALL patients.
            (2) Roll method: for removing at gingival margin and clinical crown.
                (a) Filaments are directed apically, rolled toward occlusal surface, forcing filaments interproximally.
                (b) BEST for children, although easy to miss areas if brush is NOT correctly placed.
            (3) Modified Stillman's method: for removing at gingival margin.

(a) Uses vibratory motion to stimulate tissue addition of the roll stroke, removes from the buccal and lingual surfaces; bristles are directed apically at gingival margin; roll stroke and vibratory motion are used.

(b) Adequate technique for all patients.

(4) Charter's method: MOST useful for around orthodontic bands and brackets, fixed prostheses, recent postsurgical wounds.

(a) Uses vibratory motion with bristles directed occlusally.

(b) Sides of bristles contact gingival margin and tooth surface.

(5) Circular (Fones') method: for removal on clinical crown.

(a) Uses rotational motion on buccal and lingual surfaces.

(b) Good FIRST method for young children, NOT recommended for adults.

(6) Horizontal or scrub method: for removal on buccal, lingual, and occlusal surfaces.

(a) Uses horizontal scrubbing motion.

(b) Detrimental to gingival tissues, causing abrasion and recession.

2. Powered toothbrushes: effective as manual with CORRECT use.

a. Brush motion can be rotational, counterrotational-oscillating, counterrotational-sonic; technique is product dependent and SIMILAR to manual techniques.

b. Bristle placement is angled at 45° to gingival margin; smaller brush heads are site specific and require MORE time to clean all teeth.

c. Automatic timer and audible cues help to brush for specified amount of time (usually 2 minutes); useful in encouraging thorough cleaning.

d. Recommended for orthodontic appliances, malposed teeth, periodontal disease, arthritis and other grasping disabilities, caregivers.

B. Interdental care: IMPORTANT factor is type of interdental embrasure.

1. Floss is available in a variety of textures, thickness, materials and SHOULD be used daily for effective dental biofilm control.

a. Waxed/polytetrafluorethylene (PTE) coated floss: BEST for persons with tight contacts, amalgam overhangs, or rough restorations.

b. Unwaxed floss: can be used by persons with FEW restorations and with normal contact tightness.

c. Tufted floss or yarn: BEST for large embrasure spaces or under orthodontic wires.

d. Technique:

(1) Gently inserting the floss between the teeth, wrapping the floss snugly around each proximal tooth surfaces, and using an up-and-down motion from sulcus to contact to remove dental biofilm.

(2) Floss handle: BEST for those with larger hands or one functional hand; floss-threaders: BEST to get under bridges and orthodontic wires.

2. Interdental brushes: BEST to cleanse wide embrasures (type II to III) or furcations.

a. Conical and tapered brushes fixed to a wire and then inserted on plastic handle.

b. Single tufted brush with tapered or flat groups of filaments inserted on plastic handle (also called end-tuft brush).

(1) For MOST effective cleaning, use brush slightly larger than the embrasure.

(2) Can further enhance effect of antimicrobial agent by delivering chemical into embrasure area with interdental brush.

3. Interdental tip: removes excess debris from embrasure area and slightly apical to the gingival margin.

a. Soft flexible rubber tip is ideal to adapt into embrasure space, LESS likely to cause trauma than plastic tip; trace along gingival margin and move in and out of the embrasure space.

b. Toothpick in a holder (e.g., Perio-aid) is BEST for removing dental biofilm in periodontal pockets and adjacent to orthodontic appliances; round or square-round toothpick is placed in a plastic handle.

(1) Trace along gingival margin and move back and forth in the embrasure space; for periodontal patients, tip is placed on the tooth and traced into the col and furcation area.

(2) Care is taken NOT to place excessive force on gingival tissue; for orthodontic patients, tip is placed on the tooth and traced around orthodontic brackets or bands.

c. Wooden interdental cleaner (e.g., Stimudent): in areas where interdental papillae are missing (type III).

(1) Triangular; flat part of triangle is placed toward the tissue.

(2) Burnishing action is used against one side of the embrasure, then the other side.

C. Tongue cleaning devices: IMPORTANT to reduce dental biofilm accumulation and malodors (halitosis, bad breath) caused by production of volatile sulfur compounds (VSCs) by bacteria on dorsal surface.

1. Plastic scrapers: place on the posterior portion of the tongue and pull forward to "scrape" the dental biofilm coating off.

2. Toothbrushes: also effective tools for removing this coating; placed on the posterior portion of the tongue and "swept" forward (four or five times); brushing without dentifrice (toothpaste) may reduce the gag flex.

D. Oral irrigators: reduce gingivitis, reduce dental biofilm toxicity by altering microflora, deliver antimicrobial agents (controversial use).
   1. Supragingivally, standard tip provides steady, low-pressure, pulsating stream of water or other fluid agent to dislodge loosely adherent dental biofilm at or slightly apical to the gingival margin; tip is directed at a 90° angle to the tooth at the gingival margin.
   2. Subgingivally, sulcus tip (e.g., Pic Pocket) provides pulsating, low-pressure stream of water or chemotherapeutic agent to the sulcus or periodontal pocket; can dislodge unattached or loosely adherent dental biofilm; tip is directed at a 45° angle with the tip directed into sulcus or pocket; gives deeper subgingival penetration of water or antimicrobial agent.

Dentifrices

Dentifrices (toothpastes) are substances used in conjunction with a toothbrush or other applicator to assist in the removal of dental biofilm (dental plaque) and materia alba from the teeth and gingiva. However, mechanical action from brushing is the MAJOR method for removal of soft deposits and NOT the use of dentifrices. SHOULD select products with ADA Seal of Acceptance for demonstrated therapeutic value with safety and efficacy. With acceptance, ALL have safe levels of abrasiveness.

A. Basic ingredients:
   1. Water and glycerine (to keep paste from drying out) and thickeners (to stay on toothbrush and squeeze out of the tube).
   2. Detergents to remove fatty films; water softeners to make the detergents work better.
   3. Surfactants to help remineralization process by improving wetting on enamel and provide foam (love those bubbles in America!); MOST common are either sodium lauryl sulfate (SLS) or ammonium lauryl sulfate.
   4. Abrasives such as calcium pyrophosphate, dibasic calcium phosphate dihydrate, tricalcium phosphate, hydrated alumina, hydrated silica, and sodium metaphosphate.
   5. Binder such as carboxymethylcellulose (gum to keep the solid and liquid components of paste from separating); coloring agents such as food dyes; flavoring agents such as specific oils and extracts.
   6. Sweeteners, preferably nonnutritive such as sodium saccharin, so bacterial growth is NOT encouraged.
   7. Titanium dioxide to make paste opaque and white.

B. Fluoride-containing (for cavity protection, increased remineralization): source of fluoride for the tooth surface; control demineralization and promote remineralization.
   1. Active ingredients for OTC: sodium fluoride (NaF, 0.24%/1100 ppm) or sodium monofluorophosphate (Na_2PO_3F, 0.76%/1000 ppm) or stannous fluoride (SnF_2, 0.45%) (see later discussion).
   2. SHOULD be used at least once daily; those at high risk for caries may use several times per day.
   3. Should NOT be used on small children; digestion of fluoride can affect developing permanent tooth buds, causing white spots (hypocalcification); once the guardian is sure child is NOT swallowing it, it can safely be used. See Table 11-1 for amount suggested per age group of children. Can also cause chronic toxicity; see later discussion under "Fluorides."
   4. Prescription strength products have higher levels (NaF, 1.1%/5000 ppm) (Prevident 5000, Fluoridex); used on developed dentitions for patients with high caries risk.

C. Anticalculus ("tartar" control or prevention): binds to crystals and prevents them from adhering to the tooth surface, thereby reducing rate of crystal growth of supragingival calculus by as much as 40%.
   1. Active ingredients: soluble pyrophosphate (5% to 1.3%) or zinc chloride.
   2. Examples: noted on label.

D. Antigingivitis and antiplaque (see further discussion with oral microbials): reduces gingivitis associated with dental biofilm by antimicrobial action against bacteria.
   1. Active ingredients: stannous fluoride (Sn_2, 0.454%) or triclosan (0.30%).
   2. Examples: Gum Care, Total, ProHealth.
   3. Essential oils may be added (thymol, menthol, eucalyptol, methylsalicylate, 25% alcohol); example: Listerine (see below).

E. Desensitizing: reduce dentinal hypersensitivity, MUST be continually used (see earlier discussion).

Table 11-1 Amount of fluoridated dentifrice (toothpaste) recommended per age group for children

Age	Amount
Under age 1	None
Age 1 to 3	Rice grain-sized amount
Age 4 to 5	Pea-sized amount

From National Maternal and Child Oral Health Resource Center.

1. Active ingredients: potassium nitrate (KNO_3, 0.5%) or sodium fluoride (NaF, 0.243%), or strontium chloride ($SrCl_2$, 10%); casein phosphopeptide; or amorphous calcium phosphate (CPP-ACP).
2. Examples: Sensitivity Protection, Denquel, Sensodyne SC.

F. Whitening: have limited ability; include papain (Citroxain), silica, carbamide peroxide.

G. Other possible ingredients:
   1. Allantoin: relieves the irritation caused by detergents, alkalies, acids.
   2. Casein phosphopeptide–amorphous calcium phosphate (CPP-ACP)(MI paste, MI paste plus with fluoride): can also help with remineralization by depositing on tooth surface, then filling in the enamel surface defects; especially helpful in high caries risk as with xerostomia.
   3. Xylitol: inhibits *Streptococcus mutans* metabolism; may be used in combination with other anti-caries products.
   4. Lauryl sarcosinate: replaces some or all of SLS, since it can irritate oral mucosa.
   5. Poloxamer 407 (nonionic foaming agent): to reduce soft tissue irritation; does NOT resolve inflammation.
   6. Sodium bicarbonate (baking soda): for taste and mouth feel; combines with acids to release carbon dioxide gas, adding to foam produced by brushing; also mild abrasive and may reduce numbers of acid-loving bacteria, although lasts ONLY as long as mouth stays alkaline.

Fluoride Use

Several chemical formulations and delivery agents provide a wide variety of ways to deliver adequate fluoride to the teeth. Fluoride protection from caries is ONLY by way of topical use and NOT systemic; also helps reduce dentinal hypersensitivity. Discussion in this chapter will center on fluoride delivered in the dental office and home use.

- See Chapter 17, Community Oral Health: community fluoride programs and supplementation (water and oral).

A. Topical fluoride is found in dentifrices (toothpastes discussed earlier), gels and foams, mouthrinses, varnishes.

B. Topical application of fluoride to the erupted tooth: works MAINLY on smooth surface remineralization (sealants work MAINLY on pit and fissure surfaces).
   1. Posteruption maturation of the enamel surface.
   2. Prevention of demineralization and remineralization of early caries.
   3. Decreasing enamel solubility and maximizing enamel resistance to decay.

4. Alteration of dental biofilm; inhibits bacterial activity by inhibiting enolase, enzyme needed by bacteria to metabolize carbohydrates.

C. Types: sodium (NaF), acidulated phosphate (APF), stannous (SnF_2).
   1. NaF (2% aqueous; pH 9.2) neutral gel or foam:
      a. If professionally delivered: four appointments, 2 to 7 days apart, to provide MOST topical benefits for caries control and desensitizing therapy.
      b. Active ingredient in MOST mouthrinses sold OTC.
      c. Also used after whitening (since neutral but must be without coloring).
      d. Stable solution; easy to store.
   2. APF (1.23% NaF in 0.1 M orthophosphoric acid; pH 3.0) gel or foam:
      a. If professionally delivered: requires ONLY one application at each recall visit for caries control.
      b. Requires 4-minute application for MOST fluoride uptake into enamel.
      c. Absolute contraindication on composite, porcelain, sealant materials; causes pitting and roughening.
      d. Gels for home use contain 1.1% concentration.
   3. SnF_2 (8% aqueous; pH 2.1 to 2.3) gel or foam:
      a. If professionally delivered: requires ONLY one application for caries control and desensitizing therapy.
      b. Unpleasant taste and can cause extrinsic staining (brown, orange, tan).
      c. Unstable; MUST be mixed for each application.
   4. The ADA has NOT accepted two-part rinses (APF/SnF_2) as effective, and concerns have also been raised regarding the potential of these rinses to be easily ingested, which could lead to toxicity.
   5. Fluoride varnishes contain NaF (e.g., Duraphat, Duraflor), possibly xylitol:
      a. Thin coating of resin (yellow or white) that is applied to the tooth surface; delivered in controlled-release system for caries control and desensitizes; dries immediately upon contact with saliva.
      b. Does NOT require professional oral prophylaxis before application; requires LESS cooperation from patient.
      c. Brushed on; can eat or drink but MUST refrain from brushing, rigorous rinsing, abrasive foods for 3 to 4 hours.
      d. Repeated at 3-month intervals for high risk; 6-month intervals for lower risk.
      e. BEST for primary caries (see earlier discussion); BETTER than other delivery systems in which fluoride is washed away by saliva and eating;

useful for infants, disabled, those with swallowing difficulties.

D. Professional application of topical gel or foam fluoride: does NOT require professional oral prophylaxis before application.

1. Children 4 to 18 years of age need application once or twice a year depending on caries risk.
2. Adults may need fluoride treatment depending on caries incidence, xerostomia, or dentinal hypersensitivity.
3. Tray application: do NOT overfill the tray.
   a. Fit Styrofoam trays to the mouth, and place gel or foam in the trays.
   b. Dry teeth with air syringe; place trays in mouth for 4 minutes.
   c. Control salivary flow with saliva ejector; expectorate fluoride into saliva ejector.
   d. Floss teeth after tray removal; instruct NOT to eat or drink for 30 minutes.
4. Paint-on application:
   a. Isolate teeth with cotton rolls; dry teeth with air syringe.
   b. Paint foam or gel on with cotton-tipped applicator and leave for 4 minutes.
   c. Control salivary flow with saliva ejector; expectorate saliva into saliva ejector.
   d. Floss teeth and instruct NOT to eat or drink for 30 minutes.

E. Self-administered topical fluoride: compliance will affect success of caries reduction.

1. May be in the form of an OTC or prescription mouthrinse or gel, OTC or prescription dentifrice, lozenge (discussed later in section on geriatric patient).
2. Gels are brushed on once a day; mouthrinses are used after brushing and before bedtime if possible; dentifrices used as often as person brushes.
3. SHOULD refrain from rinsing, eating, or drinking after home administration for at least 30 minutes.
4. Supervision of use is necessary until child has demonstrated ability NOT to swallow it; should NOT be swallowed (can lead to chronic toxicity and hypocalcification of permanent teeth).
5. Mouthrinses for home use: daily with 1 teaspoon; swish between teeth for 60 seconds and expectorate.
   a. OTC MAINLY contain NaF (0.05%) (low-potency, high-frequency rinse).
   b. Prescription-strength fluoride mouthrinses (high-potency, low-frequency rinse):
      (1) 0.2% NaF (once a week).
      (2) 0.05% NaF (once daily).
      (3) 0.2% APF (once daily).
6. Fluoride trays (custom or stock): designed to hold fluoride gels in close proximity to teeth.

a. Used with head and neck radiation therapy that would cause subsequent damage to the salivary glands; also for other xerostomic systemic conditions or patients at high risk for dental caries.
b. Formed to cover entire clinical crowns for each arch; filled with neutral sodium fluoride; worn for duration of high-risk period; however, with permanent salivary dysfunction have continual use.

F. Toxicology: concentration of fluoride is regulated by FDA.

1. Calculation of amount of fluoride ingested:
   a. NaF: $(4.5) \times$ (no. mL swallowed) $\times$ (NaF concentration [e.g., 0.05%, 1.1%]) = mgF.
   b. APF: $(10) \times$ (no. mL swallowed) $\times$ (APF concentration [e.g., 1.23%]) = mgF.
   c. SnF$_2$: $(2.4) \times$ (no. mL swallowed) $\times$ (SnF$_2$ concentration [e.g., 0.4%, 8%, 10%]) = mgF.
2. Metabolism of ingested fluoride:
   a. 86% to 97% absorbed in the stomach.
   b. Excess excreted through kidneys, sweat glands, feces.
3. Chronic fluoride toxicity:
   a. Can cause dental fluorosis, skeletal fluorosis, renal damage.
   b. Severity can be influenced by increased intake of naturally fluoridated water, increased intake of food with fluoride, nutritional diseases, diets low in calcium.
4. Acute fluoride toxicity:
   a. Can cause nausea, vomiting, heavy salivary flow, stomach pain, diarrhea.
   b. In severe cases, cramping of extremities, breathing difficulty, heart failure, dilated pupils, hyperkalemia, hypocalcemia.
5. Emergency treatment with excessive ingestion of fluoride:
   a. If fluoride ingestion is <5 mg/kg body weight:
      (1) Give milk orally.
      (2) Observe for several hours.
   b. If fluoride ingestion is >5 mg/kg body weight:
      (1) Induce vomiting.
      (2) Give milk orally.
      (3) Admit to hospital and observe several hours.
   c. If fluoride ingestion is >15 mg/kg body weight:
      (1) Induce vomiting; activate EMS system.
      (2) Admit to hospital immediately; EMS personnel will start calcium gluconate intravenously and monitor for heart dysrhythmias.
6. Certainly lethal dose (CLD): estimated dosage range of a drug that may cause death:

a. Child CLD: 0.5 to 1 g (varies with size and weight).

b. Adult CLD: NaF is 5 to 10 g taken at one time, or 32 to 64 mg/kg.

Oral Antimicrobials

Oral antimicrobials (chemical antibiofilm agents) destroy oral microorganisms within dental biofilm (bactericidal) or prevent growth (bacteriostatic). **Substantivity,** ability to adhere to tooth structure for long periods, enabling slow release, is also IMPORTANT factor. Can be in form of mouthrinses, dentifrices, or other forms; can be delivered with oral irrigation. Includes chlorhexidine, essential oils, quaternary ammonium compounds, triclosan, sanguinarine, SnF_2, oxygenating mouthrinses. Must be kept in mind that most are MORE effective on gingivitis than periodontitis because action is not able to occur deep within periodontal pocket.

- See Chapter 13, Periodontology: subgingival antimicrobials.

A. Basic ingredients in mouthrinses (see earlier discussion on dentifrices):
  1. Water, alcohol, flavoring agents, sweetener.
  2. Active ingredient(s):
     a. Oxygenating (cleansing and antimicrobial) and astringent (shrinks tissue).
     b. Anodynes (relieve pain) and buffering agent (relieves pain, reduces oral acidity, dissolves mucinous film).
     c. Deodorizing agent (reduces malodor) and antimicrobial (reduces oral microbial count and bacterial activity)

B. Chlorhexidine digluconate mouthrinses (at 0.12%, Peridex, PerioGard; can be diluted to 0.06%):
  1. Requires prescription if dispensed; contains alcohol (11.6%) unless noted; contraindicated if alcohol presents further complications.
  2. High substantivity and bactericidal for gram-positive and gram-negative bacteria and fungi; reduces gingivitis (as much as 60%); treatment of aggressive periodontal disease, candidiasis, herpetic stomatitis; also used postsurgically.
  3. Side effects may include exogenous extrinsic brown staining, increased supragingival calculus, poor taste, altered taste sensation, and in some, reversible desquamation with dryness, soreness, ulceration of the oral mucosa; LESS effective in presence of lauryl sulfate, fluoride, blood, protein.
  4. Recommended to rinse with 15 mL twice daily for 30 seconds; SHOULD be used short term.

C. Phenolic compound (essential oils) (e.g., Listerine mouthrinse, dentifrice):
  1. OTC, contains thymol, menthol, eucalyptol, methylsalicylate, 25% alcohol; contraindicated for those who are sensitive to alcohol.

2. Low-substantivity antimicrobial agents used to alter bacterial cell wall, reduce gingivitis (30%).
  3. Strong taste, stains the teeth, may cause burning sensation in some individuals.

D. Quaternary ammonium compound: contains cetylpyridinium chloride; may contain domiphen bromide.
  1. May contain as much as 18% alcohol.
  2. Has slight but NOT substantive antiplaque activity.

E. Triclosan (Total dentifrice) (see earlier discussion):
  1. OTC; second-generation to Listerine.
  2. Low substantivity; reduces gingivitis.

F. Sanguinarine (Viadent dentifrice, mouthrinse):
  1. OTC; originates from bloodroot *(Sanguinaria canadensis)* plant.
  2. Has NO significant effects unless rinse and paste are used together; alcohol (10% to 14%).
  3. Minimal substantivity; interferes with bacterial glycolysis and binds to dental biofilm to reduce microbial adherence; reduces gingivitis.
  4. NOT as effective as chlorhexidine or phenolics.

G. SnF_2: has weak antigingivitis effects, available in dentifrice (0.45%) or mouthrinse (0.4%), but may cause exogenous extrinsic orange-tan stain; contains NO alcohol.

H. Povidone-iodine: used with necrotizing or HIV-associated periodontal disease.

I. Oxygenating mouthrinses (e.g., Amosan, Orthoflur, Oxyfresh, hydrogen peroxide [needs to be diluted]).
  1. NO effect on dental biofilm.
  2. Short-term use intended for oral wound cleansing and soothing effects.
  3. Long-term use has shown serious side effects, including carcinogenesis, tissue damage, mucosal ulcerations, hyperkeratosis, black hairy tongue.

Enamel Sealants

Enamel (pit and fissure) **sealants** are composed of organic polymers that bind to the enamel surface MAINLY by mechanical retention to reduce caries.

- See Chapter 17, Community Oral Health: community sealant programs.

A. Purpose: act as physical barriers to prevent oral bacteria and their nutrients from collecting *within* a pit and fissure on occlusal or facial and lingual surfaces (then creating acid environment essential for caries initiation).
  1. NOT very effective in interproximal spaces and on other smooth tooth surfaces (where topical fluoride is MORE effective).
  2. Can reduce occlusal fillings up to 50% on molars, 10% on premolars for permanents.
  3. Primary teeth are LESS retentive than permanents (difference in enamel structure); success has NOT been shown.

B. Indications:
1. Deep occlusal pits and fissures; *highest* to *lowest* risk for caries:
   a. First and second permanent molars.
   b. First and second primary molars.
   c. First and second premolars.
   d. Third molars.
2. Facial and lingual smooth surface pits; *highest* to *lowest* risk for caries:
   a. Buccal pits of mandibular molars.
   b. Lingual pits of permanent maxillary molars.
   c. Lingual pits of permanent maxillary incisors.
3. With higher rate of decay, needs to have risky areas sealed as soon after eruption as possible.
4. Xerostomic conditions may lead to decay.
C. Relative contraindications:
1. Open occlusal lesions or caries on proximal surfaces.
2. Adult with low caries and restoration rate.
3. Well-coalesced pits and fissures.
4. Behavior that does NOT allow a dry field, if needed for hydrophobic resins.
5. Small percentage of the population is known to have allergic response to acrylate resins.
6. Short life expectancy of the tooth.
D. Composition:
1. Contains organic monomer bisphenol-A diglycidylether methacrylate (bis-GMA), reaction product of bisphenol A and glycidyl methacrylate; ADA considers exposure to bis-GMA an "acute and infrequent event with little relevance to estimating general population exposures."
2. Unfilled types: resin component of dental composites; filled types: filler of inorganic material such as glass for strength to reduce occlusal wear from chewing and to increase opacity for easier visualization.
3. Hydrophobic ("water hating"—must use dry field) or hydrophilic ("water loving"—saliva provides wet environment necessary for activation) resins; hydrophilic are LESS technique sensitive.
4. Fluoride-releasing types (fluoride salt, fluorosilicate glass) or calcium phosphate inclusion may help protect the tooth structure from caries by aiding with remineralization.
E. **Polymerization:** adding together of many molecules to produce larger molecule (polymer), forms highly cross-linked polymer network.
1. Autopolymer (chemical reaction, self-curing, liquid products contained in two bottles):
   a. Activator: bis-GMA and initiator: benzyl peroxide.
   b. Equal drops of each are mixed together; resin liquid hardens in 1½ to 2 minutes.

2. Photopolymer (visible light or light cured): second generation (first generation used UV light, harder to manipulate, more expensive).
   a. One component system; does NOT require mixing; chemical initiator is NOT activated until illuminated by light source.
   b. Unlimited working time; less chance of incorporating air bubbles into materials, causing failure.
   c. However, takes MORE working time to flow into pits and fissures (grooves).
F. Application:
1. Clean enamel surfaces with pumice or air abrasive polisher; ALL types can be placed *after* fluoride treatment and/or professional oral prophylaxis (even with fluoride paste) because of etching of enamel.
2. For hydrophobic resins, isolate area with moisture control if needed (rubber dam, cotton roll holders, moisture-absorbent dry angles [Dri-Angles], cheek pads); MOST common cause of failure is moisture contamination with these types.
3. Dry tooth surface for 30 seconds.
4. Etch with phosphoric acid (30% to 50%) for 15 to 20 seconds for permanents and 20 to 30 seconds for primary teeth, apply to pits and fissures and at least a few millimeters beyond final margin of sealant.
   a. Called "tooth conditioner" by some manufacturers; creates micropores in enamel so that the sealant flows and *mechanically* locks in; some also have chemical bonding.
   b. Use eye protection for clinician, assistant, patient.
   c. May cause burns; avoid contact with oral tissues, eyes, skin; if accidental contact occurs, flush affected area with generous amounts of water; in case of contact with eyes, immediately rinse with water and seek <u>immediate medical attention</u> (see Chapter 10, Medical and Dental Emergencies).
5. Rinse (large amount) for 30 seconds and dry again for 30 seconds; dry tooth is essential for successful retention of sealant material if hydrophobic; tooth is dried until has chalky, frosted appearance.
6. Etch again if tooth does NOT have chalky, frosted appearance, and dry thoroughly again; older permanent and primary teeth may need re-etch.
7. If chemically reactive, mix parts.
8. Apply sealant material into pits and fissures with brush, cannula, or plastic instrument, most posterior tooth FIRST; do NOT apply excessive amount (to AVOID occlusal discrepancies), since taste can be offensive if material touches tongue.

9. If sealant flows onto soft tissue, rinse immediately, then reapply to tooth.
10. If light curing, illuminate according to directions (UV use, shield from eyes).
11. After has set, wipe sealed surface with wet cotton pellet; allows removal of air-inhibited layer of nonpolymerized resin; failure to perform this may leave an objectionable taste.
12. Use of dental floss is recommended to ensure open contacts, especially if a clear sealant is used.

D. After application:
1. Evaluate sealant both visually and tactilely for complete coverage, checking for voids, bubbles, adequate seal; check interproximal surfaces with floss for any excess material.
2. If any deficiencies in the material, MORE material should be applied.
3. IMPORTANT to evaluate occlusion with articulating paper for *filled* resins and make any necessary adjustment; *unfilled* resins will wear down naturally and do NOT require occlusal adjustment.
4. Inform guardian of procedures that have been completed, and instruct that chewing ice, hard candies, or other hard objects can fracture sealant, which causes leakage; leakage can lead to decay.
5. Reevaluate sealants periodically to ensure still intact; replace or add to sealant when necessary.
6. Avoid use of APF forms of fluoride, which can cause roughing and pitting.
7. If material fails, this is MAINLY result of operator error; MOST likely to occur within first 6 months after placement, with greatest loss in first molars, least loss in premolars.

Mouth Protectors

Mouth protectors (mouthguards) are designed to prevent mouth injuries.
• See Chapter 15, Dental Biomaterials: impressions.
A. Used by participants in sporting activities to protect dentition from direct or indirect trauma.
1. MOST sports injuries involve the oral cavity, MAINLY in contact sports.
2. The National Collegiate Athletic Association (NCAA) adopted mouth protector rule; MUST be worn, colored for compliance and ease of finding if lost.
B. Types:
1. Stock: made of rubber, polyvinyl chloride, or polyvinyl acetate–polyethylene copolymer.
   a. Available at retail shops.
   b. Manufactured in limited sizes (small, medium, large).
2. Mouth-formed: have *outer*, harder shell, typically made of polyvinyl chloride, and *inner* liner made of acrylic gel, silicone rubber, or polyvinyl acetate.
   a. Available at retail shops.
   b. Typically are heated and then formed around the teeth.
3. Custom-made: fabricated from thermoplastic resin sheet, heated and vacuum processed onto plaster model of individual's teeth.
   a. Require four basic steps to fabricate: (1) taking impression of arch; (2) pouring model; (3) forming thermoplastic material over model; (4) trimming and finishing.
   b. Fit by a clinician; BEST because of reduction in gagging, irritation of the oral tissues, speech impairment.

CLINICAL STUDY

Age	13 YRS	**SCENARIO**
Sex	☒ Male ☐ Female	The patient is in the dental office for an emergency. Last week, while playing football, he was tackled and suffered another head concussion. Visual examination reveals small incisive fractures on teeth #6 and #7. His 12-year molars are partially erupted.
Chief Complaint	"Wow, I sure got hit hard and my teeth got hurt too."	
Medical History	Broken ribs last year	
Current Medications	Concussion 2 years ago None	
Social History	Grade school student	

1. What preventive dental measures might have been recommended to the patient and his guardians before football season? Give the rationale for these recommendations.

2. What might his pupils have looked like with the concussion?
3. Because of a busy schedule, the dental hygienist left the patient's alginate impression unwrapped on the

laboratory counter until the following day. What result will this have on the final study model?

4. Describe the basic steps for fabricating a custom-made mouth protector.

1. Use of a mouthguard is recommended for prevention of injury to the patient's teeth and mouth. Mandatory mouthguard and facemask regulations for high school and junior college football players were enacted because of the high facial and oral injury rate. Although use of mouthguards is mandated, compliance must be achieved for effectiveness. Mouthguard can protect the dentition from direct or indirect trauma. Clinician should discuss not only fabrication of mouth protector, but also consequences of noncompliance in wearing guard during sporting activities (e.g., chipped and broken teeth, avulsed teeth). Clinician should explain that a custom-made mouth protector is designed by clinician to specifically fit individual's teeth. As a result, custom-made appliance feels more comfortable, reduces gagging and irritation to oral tissues, decreases speech impairment. Advantages over the stock, store-bought, or mouth-formed item may contribute to compliance with use.

2. His pupils would have possibly been different sizes in response to shining a light on them.

3. If alginate impressions are stored for more than 1 hour in air, they lose accuracy because of process called syneresis, or loss of water by evaporation and exuding of fluid. Final study model in this case will be inaccurate, leaving the mouthguard to be possibly ill fitting.

4. First, alginate impression of maxillary arch is needed. Once a good impression is made, study model is fabricated. Maxillary model then must be trimmed and a thermoplastic sheet of material must be vacuum formed over the model, trimmed, and finished by buffing the edges.

PATIENTS WITH SPECIAL CONCERNS

Over a lifetime, patients may present with a number of special oral conditions that must be managed as part of comprehensive dental hygiene care. The following conditions need to be recognized, evaluated, and treated appropriately by the dental hygienist, and patients (or guardians) need to be educated about role in self-care and disease prevention. *These patient groups may be included in the case-based portion of the NBDHE (Component B).*
- See Chapter 16, Special Needs Patient Care: medically disabled patients.

Pediatric Patient

Pediatric patients can benefit MOST from working with the dental hygienist, since there is such an opportunity to get an early start on oral health. Clinician can work with patients as they move from infants in their guardians' arms to children coming for dental visits and then to adolescents.
- See Chapter 7, Nutrition: eating disorders.

A. Infants:
1. Educate guardian about early childhood caries (ECC) (see earlier discussion).
2. Instruct guardian on use of soft toothbrush or gauze to clean oral tissues and teeth of infant.
3. NO dentifrice should be used that contains fluoride (see earlier discussion of dentifrices) to reduce risk of damage to developing permanent teeth ("white spots" or hypocalcification caused by localized fluorosis).
4. FIRST dental appointment is recommended within 6 months of eruption of first tooth or at *1 year of age.*

B. Children:
1. See Table 11-1 for amount of dentifrice per age group at each brushing to minimize fluoride consumption if swallowed.
2. Guardian SHOULD be involved with brushing and flossing until small motor skills develop and child can become proficient with dental biofilm removal.
3. Short attention span of child demands shorter dental appointments; explain procedure and equipment at level a child can understand.
4. Special attention should be given to AVOID swallowing professionally applied fluorides during application, since may cause nausea or cause toxic effects (in large doses).

C. Adolescents:
1. To promote good hygiene practice, appeal to tooth appearance and acceptance from peers; treat as transitioning adults.
2. Puberty gingivitis is prevalent during these years; educate teens on role in self-care; age group can be associated with aggressive periodontitis (especially localized form).
3. Orthodontic appliances common; special tools may include powered toothbrush, oral irrigator, tufted toothbrush, floss threaders, Superfloss, and additional fluoride (daily fluoride mouthrinse, brush-on gel fluoride) or calcium products for remineralization (see later discussion on orthodontic fixed and removal appliance care).
4. Transitional period to adulthood: MUST include discussion of drug usage (including tobacco use), poor dietary habits, eating disorders, oral piercing, STDs, birth control pills, pregnancy, traumatic injury from sports and lifestyle (mouthguards).

Pregnant Patient

Full-term pregnancy is defined as the 40-week-long developmental period of the fetus.

- See Chapters 2, Embryology and Histology: human development; 9, Pharmacology: pregnancy, placental barrier, drug usage; 13, Periodontology: pregnancy-related periodontal disease.

A. Pregnancy is divided into first, second, third trimesters; each has own focus:
  1. During first trimester: embryo becomes a fetus and fetal organ systems develop.
     a. Lips, palate, and tooth buds form, and mineralization of the tooth tissues starts toward the end.
     b. Nearly ALL drugs pass through by way of the placenta to enter the circulation.
     c. Thus is MOST critical period of development, during which birth defects (teratogenic effects) may occur from infection, prescription or illegal drug use, alcohol or tobacco use, or nutritional deficiency.
  2. During second trimester: fetal organ systems mature and fetal growth continues.
  3. During third trimester: fetus becomes fully mature and gains weight; average birth weight is 7 to 8 pounds.
B. Systemic signs: undergoes systemwide changes during pregnancy; NO trimester is without complications.
  1. During first trimester, may have difficulty with nausea and vomiting that predispose patient to malnutrition because of appetite loss.
     a. Caries may result from acid in vomit contacting teeth and oral structures; BEST period for preventive dental examination.
     b. However, if periodontal disease or caries infections are severe and NOT treated, may increase risk of premature low-birth-weight infant; oral pathogens may stimulate uterine contractions and cause premature labor.
     c. Appointments may have to be shorter but scheduled MORE often to accomplish this important reduction of risk to growing fetus.
  2. During second trimester, over morning sickness, risk for developmental disturbances of fetus is lower (SAFEST trimester), fetus is small enough that patient can still sit comfortably in dental chair.
  3. During third trimester, may have difficulty sitting or lying in dental chair for entire appointment.
C. Oral signs:
  1. Erosion of enamel may occur in response to frequent vomiting, which accompanies severe morning sickness.
     a. Small, frequent meals of healthy, noncariogenic foods SHOULD be recommended.
     b. Mouth SHOULD be rinsed thoroughly with water after vomiting, and mineralizing fluoride and calcium products should be applied daily.
     c. Frequent intake of fermentable carbohydrates for nausea puts woman at HIGH risk for caries; gagging and nausea may lead to inadequate performance of homecare.
  2. Many drugs such as tetracycline and its derivatives are contraindicated during pregnancy to AVOID intrinsic staining effects during mineralization of the teeth (see earlier discussion under stains); other antibiotics can be substituted.
  3. Inadequate oral homecare can predispose patient to gingival inflammation; although pregnancy itself does NOT cause the inflammation, elevated hormonal influences of estrogens and progesterone during pregnancy can exaggerate gingival response to microorganisms; inflammation is reduced somewhat after pregnancy is over.
     a. Pregnancy gingivitis: generalized gingival enlargement with overall appearance of sore, reddened, swollen, bleeding tissues; frequently associated with *Prevotella intermedia;* dental biofilm control instruction and thorough instrumentation are essential.
     b. Pyogenic granuloma (pregnancy tumor): localized area of gingival enlargement, typically involving interdental papillae, appears as painless, mushroom-shaped hyperplasia that bleeds easily and typically diminishes after birth (Figure 11-8).
D. Risk factors for oral health:
  1. Need to AVOID radiographs unless necessary to the provision of dental care; if needed for emergency care, limit the number of radiographs, use lead apron with thyroid collar, use paralleling technique that does NOT require angulations toward the abdomen.
  2. Administer local anesthetics that have been specified for pregnancy (category B: lidocaine and prilocaine); general and nitrous oxide sedation use is a relative contraindication, would need <u>medical consult</u> before proceeding.

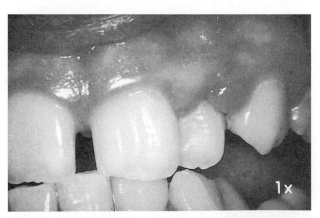

Figure 11-8   Pyogenic granuloma (pregnancy tumor).

3. Restorative, scaling (and root planing) procedures should be performed as needed in light of risk of dangerous infections; however, elective preventive and restorative dental procedures can be performed safely at ANY time but may be delayed for comfort and safety to second and third trimesters.

E. Barriers to care:
   1. During pregnancy: morning sickness (gagging, nausea, lack of appetite); inability to sit comfortably for long periods (backache, frequent urination, fatigue, dizziness); and economic difficulty because of increased medical costs and possible reduction or loss of employment income.
   2. After pregnancy: lack of time (return to work, family obligations) and economic difficulty because of increased costs associated with child rearing and possible reduction or loss of employment income.
   3. Nursing: many drugs are excreted into the breast milk and affect the newborn, SIMILAR to drugs passing through the placental barrier; <u>medical consult</u> indicated.
   4. Postnatal depression can occur; MUST be noted by dental providers and referral made for treatment.

F. Professional dental care: early intervention is KEY to health of both mother and child.
   1. Should be based on needs, in terms of both frequency and level of care; more frequent care (every 3 months) may be necessary for those with less-than-desirable homecare, those with periodontal disease, or those whose morning sickness results in frequent vomiting.
   2. Should include routine oral prophylaxis (and root planing); avoid taking radiographs or giving drugs.
   3. Should be provided in limited, shorter appointments as required for patient comfort.

   a. Allow patient to shift position as needed, preferably to left side when orthostatic hypotension presents.
   b. Supine positioning MUST be avoided if hypotension persists; breaks for restroom use.

G. Patient or caregiver education:
   1. General health and well-being and a well-balanced diet that meets needs of both mother and fetus.
      a. Adequate consumption of protein, calcium, folic acid, and vitamins A, B-complex, C, and D.
      b. Education regarding dental myth "losing a tooth for every child"; explain how adequate calcium intake during pregnancy will prevent loss of calcium from the bones; calcium is removed from bones *before* teeth.
   2. Dental biofilm-induced and hormone-influenced inflammatory effects on gingiva and effect of vomiting on enamel erosion; rinsing with water instead of brushing after vomiting should be recommended.
      a. Meticulous dental biofilm control; includes proper toothbrushing and flossing daily.
      b. Can skip using a dentifrice if causes gagging or use later in evening.
   3. Fluoride application via dentifrices, gels, or rinses as needed, depending on risk for caries.
      a. Topical fluoride supplementation should be provided ONLY for benefit of the mother.
      b. NO studies have found a link between systemic prenatal fluoridation and reduction in rate of caries in offspring.
   4. Reasonable approach is to AVOID radiographs unless diagnosis of oral disease demands attention.
   5. Tobacco cessation if necessary owing to lower risks of reduced birth weight, spontaneous abortions, prenatal deaths, sudden infant death syndrome; also good time to consider quitting because of second-hand smoke effects on offspring.

CLINICAL STUDY

Age	28 YRS	**SCENARIO**
Sex	☐ Male ☒ Female	The patient has come to the dental office because her gums are bleeding and swollen. She does not have routine dental examinations; she prefers to wait until she has a dental problem before making an appointment.
Height	5'3"	
Weight	145 LBS	
BP	115/78	
Chief Complaint	"My mother lost a tooth for every child she had. Is that going to happen to me?"	
Medical History	Five months pregnant, no complications, first child	
Current Medications	Prenatal vitamins	
Social History	Assistant principal at local trade school	

1. In what trimester of pregnancy is the patient? What fetal development occurs during this trimester?
2. What special precautions, if any, are recommended when treating a pregnant patient?
3. What is the most likely cause of the bleeding and swollen gums? What recommendations should be made?
4. Does she need to worry about losing a tooth for every child? Why? Why not?

1. She is in second trimester of pregnancy. During this developmental period, organs of fetus mature and growth continues.
2. Radiographs generally are postponed during pregnancy, unless emergency condition indicates need for them. Use of drugs is not recommended at any time during pregnancy unless emergency condition indicates need for them. If there are any questions regarding either radiographs or drugs prescribed by the dental office, a medical consult with patient's physician would be indicated. Special consideration during dental treatment should be made regarding potential for nausea and/or orthostatic hypotension.
3. Patient appears to be experiencing pregnancy gingivitis, influenced by sex hormones, exaggerated response to dental biofilm. Recommendations should include oral prophylaxis and meticulous homecare, including toothbrushing and flossing.
4. Loss of a tooth for every child is a myth. If inadequate calcium intake occurs during pregnancy, calcium is removed from the mother's skeletal and alveolar bones, not from the teeth. She should be informed of the need for adequate calcium in the diet, and myth should be dispelled. Most teeth are lost because of unrestored caries and/or periodontal disease, most likely explanation for her mother's lost teeth.

Geriatric Patient

There are three generally recognized gerontological stages: (1) "young old" (ages 65 to 74); (2) "old" (ages 75 to 84); (3) "old old" (ages 85+). Occurrence of chronic diseases and multiple disease processes increases with age. Many fall into the category of medically disabled because of these diseases.
- See Chapters 6, General and Oral Pathology: chronic diseases and conditions; 16, Special Needs Patient Care: specific medical and physical disabilities.
A. Common diseases or conditions:
  1. CVD accounts for MORE than half of all deaths.
     a. Oral complications and treatment plan alterations vary based on the type and severity of the disease; MUST determine functional capacity (FC), the patient MUST meet 4 metabolic (MET) equivalents before dental care.
     b. A 4- to 6-week delay before emergency or elective dental care is needed after cardiac surgery or episode such as an MI; will need medical consult before all dental treatment.
     c. MOST serious emergencies in the dental office are related to this disease.
     d. CVA results in coordination and mobility impairments that may require adaptive aids and assistance with personal oral hygiene care.
  2. Dementia and Alzheimer's disease in some form; incidence of senility increases with age.
     a. Ensuring suitable personal daily oral care is MAIN concern.
     b. Oral complications and alterations in dental hygiene care are MORE frequently associated with the drugs that are used to control the disease.
     c. With Alzheimer's disease, may experience seizure disorders and may have phenytoin (Dilantin)-associated gingival hyperplasia.
  3. Arthritis is a common source of discomfort and disability (see later discussion): MOST concerns are with oral care alterations and recommended use of modified oral hygiene aids, such as powered toothbrushes and floss holders.
  4. Individuals with DM are at increased risk for periodontal disease.
     a. Uncontrolled disease may require antibiotic premedication before dental treatment.
     b. Appointments ideally should take place after meal, when blood sugar is stable.
  5. Sensory defects:
     a. Include visual impairment and hearing loss.
     b. Modification of oral hygiene aids and practices is often necessary to accommodate impairment.
  6. Oral adverse drug reactions: SHOULD be advised and educated about oral side effects.
     a. High prescription drug use; MOST take at least one drug with potential adverse reactions.
     b. Xerostomia is MOST common drug-induced oral condition.
     c. Abnormal homeostasis, soft tissue reactions, taste changes, alterations in host responses, gingival overgrowth also occur.
  7. Osteoporosis: MOST common bone disease.
     a. Thinning and weakening of skeletal structure, which leads to loss of bone density and possible fracture.
     b. Women are four times MORE at risk for this condition than men, especially *after* menopause.
     c. Evidence of loss of bone density may be apparent in the bones of the jaw in severe cases (possibly noted on radiographs).
B. Oral signs:
  1. Prevention of dental disease has resulted in increasing number of older adults retaining teeth (dentate).

2. Many oral conditions once believed to be a normal part of aging currently are recognized as sequelae to disease.

3. Age-related oral changes (normal) include darkening of the teeth, attrition, gingival recession.

4. Disease-related oral changes:

   a. Drug-induced oral conditions:

     (1) Xerostomia (dry mouth).

     (2) Gingival hyperplasia, oral candidiasis, stomatitis, glossitis.

     (3) Hairy tongue.

     (4) Trigeminal neuralgia.

   b. Periodontal disease: increases in severity with age because of accumulated lifelong attachment loss.

     (1) Slight gingival recession (1 to 2 mm) is considered a normal part of aging.

     (2) Recession in excess of 1 to 2 mm MOST likely is result of past or present periodontal disease activity.

   c. Caries: especially root surfaces because of gingival recession from periodontal disease and improper brushing; xerostomia is often contributing factor.

   d. Oral cancer:

     (1) MORE cases occur; elderly are majority of related deaths (however, now occurring in younger adults because of human papilloma virus [HPV]).

     (2) MORE common in men than in women, associated with alcohol and/or tobacco use.

   e. Barriers to care:

     (1) Income limitations are an obstacle to dental care.

     (2) Few have dental insurance; Medicare does NOT reimburse dental services.

     (3) Discretionary income is used to cover cost of dental care.

     (4) Education is positively correlated with seeking adequate dental care.

       (a) As general rule, overall have LESS formal education than younger populations.

       (b) Young old are BETTER educated and are MORE likely to demand high-quality healthcare than old old.

   f. Residential status affects ability to seek and receive dental care.

     (1) MAJORITY live in family settings (are homebound).

     (2) Some are homebound but continue to live at home with assistance.

     (3) About one in four can expect to spend some time in assisted living (nursing home).

   g. Use of dental services varies.

     (1) LESS than half visit dentist annually.

     (2) Individuals with natural teeth are MORE than four times as likely to seek dental care.

Edentulous Patient

MAJORITY of alveolar ridge resorption occurs in the first year after extraction, with MORE bone resorption in the mandible. Alveolar ridges continue to change (remodel) throughout life. Patient still needs dental care even if does NOT have any teeth present. Dentures and implants are discussed next.

- See Chapters 6, General and Oral Pathology: denture-associated lesions (denture sore mouth, candidiasis, hyperplasias, angular cheilitis); 15, Dental Biomaterials: denture care.

A. Reasons for an annual dental visit:

   1. Soft tissue examination for early identification of cancer and other oral condition(s).

   2. Cleaning and maintenance of denture and implants, as well as soft tissues.

   3. Evaluation and reinforcement of good oral self-care for BOTH the denture or implant and oral mucosa.

   4. Dentures need to be replaced or relined periodically (7 to 10 years) as supporting alveolar ridge changes.

B. Dentures SHOULD be left out of the mouth for some portion of every day so that the supporting mucosa can have a recovery (rest) period; standard recommendation is to leave them out overnight when patient sleeps.

C. Dentures SHOULD be permanently marked with the wearer's identification; kept in liquid bath when outside oral cavity.

Patient with Dental Prostheses or Appliances

Prosthesis is an artificial replacement for a missing body part. Dental prosthesis typically replaces one or more teeth.

- See Chapter 15, Dental Biomaterials: dental prosthetics and denture care.

A. Removable prostheses: full denture, overdenture with either retained natural teeth or implants, and removable partial denture and obturator.

B. Fixed prostheses: fixed partial denture (bridge), dental implant, and implant-supported complete denture (if it CANNOT be removed); individual crowns are considered in this category.

C. Appliances are special devices designed for specific function or to create specific therapeutic outcome.

   1. Removable appliances: orthodontic appliances, such as head gear, retainers, or occlusal splints.

   2. Fixed appliances: orthodontic appliances, such as bands, brackets, or palatal expander, periodontal splints, space maintainers.

D. Prostheses and appliances are subject to accumulation of dental biofilm, calculus, materia alba, stain; need BOTH daily cleaning by the patient and routine professional maintenance care.
   1. Teeth adjacent to and supporting removable or fixed prosthesis or appliance typically are more dental biofilm retentive and harder to clean; higher risk for caries and gingival inflammation.
   2. Soft tissues under removable prostheses and appliances are MORE prone to irritation and lesions:
      a. To prevent soft tissue damage, removable prostheses and appliances should be kept clean.
      b. Also left out of the mouth for some portion of each day (e.g., leave denture out overnight when sleeping).
E. Professional care of full or partial removable denture and orthodontic retainers:
   1. Goal is removal of dental biofilm, calculus, stain without damaging the acrylic or metal surface.
   2. One or more of the following cleaning methods is used: ultrasonic bath, careful scaling, polishing, use of denture or other toothbrush.

3. Special care is needed to prevent abrasions or wear on acrylic surfaces; avoid bending or breaking partial clasps and retainer wires.
4. Standard precautions are followed to prevent cross-contamination.
F. Professional care for fixed orthodontic appliances:
   1. Principles of debridement are SAME, but brackets, wires, and ligatures require special adaptation and care to prevent disturbing or straining metals.
   2. Patients need MORE personalized and specific instruction in dental biofilm control methods to adapt to all areas of the teeth and appliances.
   3. Regular or special toothbrushes (narrow shape, smaller, powered), oral irrigators, floss threaders, and toothpicks, with or without adapters, are recommended.
   4. Daily self-administered fluoride application or calcium products are highly recommended to prevent decalcification (white spot) and caries around bands and brackets (see earlier discussion).

CLINICAL STUDY

Age	69 YRS	**SCENARIO**
Sex	☐ Male ☒ Female	Patient presents to the dental office with a pain on chewing in the mandibular left molar area. She wears upper denture and lower partial denture.
Height	5'2"	
Weight	155 LBS	
BP	115/70	
Chief Complaint	"My mouth hurts here."	
Medical History	Alzheimer's disease, middle stages Incontinent Congestive heart failure (CHF) 2 years ago	
Current Medications	10 mg nifedipine (Procardia) t.i.d. 20 mg furosemide (Lasix) t.i.d.	
Social History	Retired sociologist	

1. What are the common oral side effects of the patient's drugs?
2. What are the common mental and physical impairments with middle-stage Alzheimer's disease?
3. Describe the procedures for professional cleaning of partial dentures.
4. Describe common oral manifestations seen in Alzheimer's patients.

1. Calcium channel blocker nifedipine (Procardia) can cause gingival hyperplasia, and loop diuretic furosemide (Lasix) may contribute to xerostomia and its sequelae. Diuretics are the first-line intervention for high blood pressure (HBP). Channel blockers vasodilate coronary and peripheral arterioles, lowering blood pressure.
2. Alzheimer's disease, nonreversible dementia, affects thinking, memory, and personality. Patients in middle stage can experience disorientation, loss of coordination, restlessness and anxiety, language difficulties, sleep pattern disturbances, progressive memory loss, catastrophic reactions, and pacing.

3. To professionally clean partial dentures, place them in a zipper-locked plastic bag with solution. Then sonicate the bag with dentures in the ultrasonic bath for 15 minutes. Wash partial dentures thoroughly with soap, and rinse before returning them to the patient. Never use bleach to clean partial dentures because it can corrode the metal framework and clasps.

4. No specific oral signs are present with patients who have Alzheimer's disease; however, oral diseases do develop as disease progresses. In the late stages of disease, oral hygiene neglect, resultant decay, periodontal disease, and tissue trauma are common. Because use of antidepressants is common in this population group, xerostomia can also contribute to oral diseases.

Patient with Implant

Individualized dental biofilm control regimens MUST be developed for patients with implants because each implant system is unique. Depending on whether the prosthesis can be removed, dental biofilm control may present difficult challenges for the patient. Homecare cleaning aids that are effective, safe (must NOT scratch the titanium implant), and easy to use SHOULD be chosen. Patient's understanding of proper methods, frequency of use, and techniques of using cleaning aids and adjuncts SHOULD be evaluated.

• See Chapter 13, Periodontology: implant surgery, peri-implantitis, professional care (instrumentation).

A. If an overdenture is present, MUST be removed daily for cleansing and soaking, SAME as any denture; dental biofilm MUST be removed from around abutments.

B. If the prosthesis is NOT removable, dental biofilm removal becomes MORE difficult; requires use of a variety of oral hygiene aids.

1. Traditional toothbrushes, end-tuft brushes, interproximal brushes with nylon core tips (rather than metal core tips), and powered interproximal brushes (Rotadent).

2. Tufted floss, floss threaders, yarn, gauze folded into a ribbon, floss cords (Postcare) and dental tape or ribbon (G-Floss), plastic elastomeric flange-floss (Proxi-floss).

3. Wooden interdental cleaners, plastic interdental cleaners, rubber-tipped stimulators.

4. Rinsing and swabbing implant interface with 0.12% chlorhexidine is often recommended for short-term use after abutment connection surgery or when inflammation is present.

C. Homecare methods and techniques should be reviewed thoroughly at each recare appointment.

Abused Dependent Patient

Clinicians should be aware of the signs of dependent abuse. Dependents are any persons under the care of another and include children, disabled adults, elderly. Abuse can be physical neglect or abuse, emotional deprivation or abuse, sexual abuse or exploitation.

• See Chapter 18, Ethics and Jurisprudence: reporting abuse.

A. Types of abuse:

1. Physical neglect: failure to provide healthy environment for a dependent includes provision of adequate food, clothing, supervision, healthcare, living environment, personal hygiene; educational neglect can be either deliberate or result of ignorance.

   a. Dental neglect: willful failure of caregiver to provide appropriate treatment for dental disease when disease causes pain, discomfort, or delays in growth and development.

   b. Includes rampant caries, untreated oral or facial trauma, untreated oral infection.

2. Physical abuse: nonaccidental biting, striking, burning, lacerating, or other type of conduct that results in injury.

3. Emotional deprivation: failure to provide for emotional needs of a dependent; includes withholding love, lack of caring, alienation, chronic criticism (common in immature guardians).

4. Emotional abuse: purposeful use of demeaning, vengeful, demanding, or aggressive behaviors to control dependent, includes role-reversal, whereby child or dependent controls caregiver (common in immature guardians).

5. Sexual abuse: purposeful use of dependent for nonconsensual sexual acts, or sexual acts with dependent who is unable to give informed consent.

6. Sexual exploitation: purposeful use of nonconsensual dependent or dependent who is unable to give informed consent to provide some form of sexual act for sexual or monetary gain of caregiver.

B. Signs of physical neglect:

1. Unkempt appearance, including soiled clothing; dirty hair, hands, and skin; poor personal hygiene; inappropriate clothing or clothing in need of repair; lack of dental or medical care.

2. Lack of appropriate supervision, which can include allowing dependent unrestricted freedom to roam the streets, leaving dependent home alone, failing to provide needed assistance in proper oral and personal hygiene.

3. Improper or inadequate nutrition, which includes allowing indiscriminate eating and drinking of junk foods and beverages, restricting dietary choices, or providing too little food to give adequate nutrition.

C. Signs of physical abuse:

1. Bruising: on areas of the body where bruising typically does NOT occur.

   a. Note that accidental bruising (NOT associated with abuse) typically occurs in areas overlying bone (shins, forehead) or areas that protrude (knees, elbows).

   b. Nonaccidental bruising (associated with abuse) tends to occur in areas unlike those mentioned and may take on the shape of the object used to hit or pinch (fingers, hands, paddle, bat, belt buckle, teeth); bruising tends to occur on the buttocks, thighs, face, neck, and upper arms; be suspicious if:

     (1) Exhibits discomfort when sitting or lying in the dental chair.

     (2) Multiple and multistage bruises are evident.

     (3) Bruises are visible ONLY where clothing shifts during movement (e.g., tops of thighs).

     (4) Description of an incident does NOT match the visual evidence.

     (5) Wears clothing that is unseasonable and used to cover bruising (e.g., long-sleeved or legged garments in warm weather).

   c. Bruising can be in various stages of healing; may be a strong indicator of abuse because accidental injury typically does NOT occur frequently enough to cause bruising in different stages:

     (1) New: reddish purple.

     (2) Week-old: greenish.

     (3) Two-week-old: yellowish.

     (4) Two-to-four-week-old: brownish.

2. Lacerations tend to occur on lips, eyes, or face; lacerated maxillary labial frenum can indicate forced feeding.

3. Bites anywhere on the body (unless obviously made by toddler) are signs of abuse:

   a. Greater than 3 cm from canine puncture to canine puncture indicates bites were made by adult.

   b. Useful for identifying the perpetrator; bite marks are very individual.

   c. Bites caused by humans create puncture or pressure-type wounds that leave mark; animal bites typically cause tearing.

4. Burns that appear suspicious and have NO reasonable explanation; often are made by cigarettes, immersion in hot water, or rope (in cases of confinement).

5. Hitting: purposeful delivery of blows:

   a. Associated with bruising, fractures, and internal injuries (brain hemorrhage, retinal hemorrhage, and laceration or rupture of internal organs).

   b. To the face and head can result in fractured jaws, broken or avulsed teeth, lacerated lips.

6. Hair pulling is indicated by bald patches and thinning hair.

7. Head banging may be evidenced by bruising of back of the head, loss of consciousness, and retinal hemorrhage (shaken baby syndrome).

8. Inappropriate behavior is common in the abused:

   a. Inappropriate fearfulness and crying.

   b. Abrupt changes in behavior when separated from a caregiver.

   c. Delays in language and growth development in infants and children.

   d. A withdrawn, unhappy character.

D. Signs of emotional deprivation or abuse:

1. Improper behavior of a caregiver, including displays of anger, a condescending attitude, and criticism of a patient in front of others.

2. Improper behavior of the patient, including extreme displays of fear, dependence, and withdrawal.

E. Signs of sexual abuse and exploitation:

1. Discomfort of the genital-rectal area when walking or upon sitting.

2. Sexually explicit behavior in a child.

3. Refusal to allow clinician to enter mouth.

4. Severe gag reflex.

5. Bruising of the palate NOT associated with accidental injury.

6. Oral lesions of sexually transmitted diseases.

F. Oral signs of abuse:

1. Risk factors include a fear of dental procedures, inappropriate behavior in the dental office, inability to control gagging during procedures.

2. Facial trauma, as evidenced by bruising, lacerations, bite marks, or burns in unlikely locations or associated with an unlikely cause.

3. Palatal bruising, which is associated with forced oral sex.

4. Torn maxillary labial frenum, which is often associated with forced feedings.

5. Severe caries or doral infections that remain untreated after caregiver is notified of need for treatment.

6. Oral lesions associated with sexually transmitted diseases.

G. Barriers to care include communication difficulties with both patient and caregiver: dental professional may feel unprepared or uneasy dealing with abuse situations, patient may be fearful of reporting abuse to anyone, and caregiver may be in denial of any wrongdoing; abusive caregiver who feels threatened with discovery may fail to keep appointments or may switch dental offices.

H. Professional care and homecare:

1. Building trust with patient by explaining all procedures and encouraging appropriate behavior.

2. Immediately reporting suspicion of abuse to supervising dentist or appropriate agency.

3. Discussing superficial treatment of injured areas; refer to physician as needed.

I. Patient or caregiver education: should include discussion of need to reevaluate injured area at a later date.

CLINICAL STUDY

Scenario: Six-year-old male patient is visiting the dental office for his annual examination, oral prophylaxis, and fluoride treatment. His father walks him to the dental chair, kisses the top of his head, and returns to the reception room. His teeth are very clean and show no evidence of caries or gingivitis. During inspection of the oral mucosa, a purplish bruise the size of a quarter is observed along the midline, in the posterior third of the hard palate. When asked about the bruise, the patient indicates that he is unaware of its cause. He is well behaved while his teeth are being cleaned, although he gags whenever the clinician touches his tongue or gingival tissues in the molar regions. Because of his strong gag reflex, taking bitewing radiographs is difficult and giving a fluoride treatment is impossible. At the end of the appointment, when the father is shown the bruised area and asked whether he is aware of its cause, he indicates that he has no idea why the area is bruised.

1. What are possible causes of the purplish bruise on the patient's hard palate? How old is the bruise? What evidence is there to support your theory of the cause?
2. What causes a gag reflex? Identify ways to manage a gag reflex while taking radiographs or giving a fluoride treatment.
3. Is any follow-up of the palate lesion necessary, and if so, why?

1. Palate bruise is caused when a hard object strikes palate with enough force to cause superficial blood vessels to rupture and blood to pool in area. Type of bruise can be caused innocently when person falls with a candy sucker, pen, or other hard object in the mouth, forcing object against palate. However, may indicate sexual abuse, in which penis is forced against hard palate. Because neither child nor father can recall injury to palate, bruising is recent, and strong gag reflex is exhibited, it is prudent to suspect that bruising may be sign of sexual abuse. Guardian and child most likely would recall recent traumatic incident with enough force to cause large area of bruising.
2. Gag reflex is caused when oral tissues, particularly in the posterior regions, are hypersensitive to films, instruments, or fingers that are moved across oral tissues or are retained in place for long periods. May be associated with previous unpleasant experiences, such as poor clinical technique or sexual abuse. Techniques to manage gagging include calming patient by explaining all procedures; working efficiently and confidently; providing distraction by having patient breathe

through the nose, bite on bite block, or concentrate on another object; or, in severe cases, applying a local anesthetic gel, salt, or ice to desensitize the area just before the procedure, as well as using nitrous oxide sedation. Radiograph films should be quickly placed in the mouth, after tubehead is focused, and removed immediately upon exposure. Tray used in fluoride treatment should be left in the mouth for 1 minute only (or less if not tolerated well), and patient should be complimented on the ability to maintain the tray for that long (major benefit of the fluoride is received and tolerance can be increased as patient's confidence rises). Possibly fluoride varnish should be used as an alternative.
3. Palatal lesion should be examined by supervising dentist, photographed if possible (no parental permission is required if abuse is suspected), described and documented in the patient record, and examined 1 week later for signs of resolution. When abuse of any type is suspected, authorities (department of social services, police department, or other such agency) should be notified while child is in operatory, if possible, or immediately afterward, if not; health professional should not attempt to confront caregiver regarding concerns of abuse.

HEALTH PROMOTION AND DISEASE PREVENTION FACTORS

Promoting health and disease prevention is a primary objective of the dental professional and is MOST successful when the patient is involved. Motivation and its related factors, including communication, can work toward this objective.

Motivation

Motivation is defined as the readiness to act, or the driving force behind our actions. Influenced by a patient's perception of responsibility for own health. Internally motivated people believe they can influence their own lives (they are responsible for success or failure), have control over their own health, and will be motivated to change long-term health behaviors. Externally motivated people feel they have little control over life events, tend to believe in fate (feel they are NOT responsible for their health), require MORE supervision and direction, and need an outside source to reinforce positive health beliefs.

Self-Perception of Need

Patient needs are identified through interview and observation; focusing on a patient's expressed chief concern or complaint helps identify patient's motivational force. Needs theories are useful in determining the motivational process. Maslow's Hierarchy of Needs (Figure 11-9) demonstrates that as one need is met, a person is motivated to

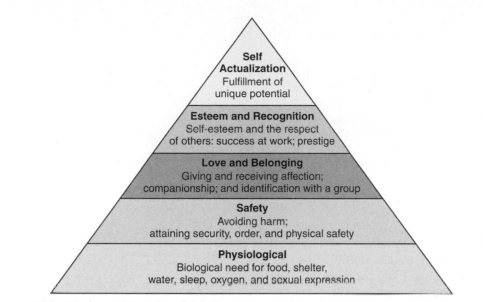

Figure 11-9 Maslow's Hierarchy of Needs. (From Gaylor LJ: The administrative dental assistant, ed 2, St. Louis, 2007, Saunders/Elsevier.)

satisfy the next need higher in the hierarchy; safety, love, and ego are the needs MOST often associated with motivating a patient.

Basic physical safety needs MUST be met first (first two levels). Love and belonging, feeling a part of a group, and being a part of a significant relationship are typically met at the third level. Self-esteem and ego or a belief in one's self is the fourth level. Self-actualization development, fulfillment of one's ambitions and life's goals, and realizing one's potential are at the fifth level. The human needs conceptual model incorporates concerns about the patient and his or her environment, specific health and oral health needs, and dental hygiene actions (Figure 11-10).

Factors That Influence Motivation

Personal and social needs are major factors in motivating change.

A. Unmet needs serve as motivation for change: social acceptance and peer group approval are the MOST common motivating forces and are stronger motivating factors than health promotion:
  1. Stain and dental biofilm or calculus accumulated on teeth affect appearance and serve as motivation for removal.
  2. Malador (halitosis, bad breath) is socially unacceptable and serves as strong motivation for self-care.
B. Pain is ONLY an immediate motivation and does NOT serve as long-term motivation. Dental health is frequently neglected because the nature of the disease is nonthreatening; once disease becomes more threatening, patient will perceive need for action.

C. Sincerity, concern, and rapport with healthcare provider are directly related to level of motivation for self-care by the patient. Age and level of health belief affect action:
  1. Children: gear toward guardian who assists child with oral hygiene tasks.
  2. Adolescents: gear toward social acceptance.
  3. Adults: gear toward social acceptance, health maintenance, tooth retention, cost factors.

Communication

Communication is an essential component of managing oral hygiene care. It is continuous, inevitable, and irreversible; conducted on several levels; influenced by physical setting.

• See Chapter 13, Periodontology: compliance and noncompliance.
A. Nonverbal communication or behavior skills involve body orientation, posture, facial expressions, gestures, touch, distance and space, tone of voice, and hesitation. Expressed message is MOSTLY nonverbal:
  1. Perceived message of nonverbal communication influences relationship-building process between patient and healthcare provider.
  2. Effective nonverbal communication connotes interest and involvement, aids in expression of thoughts and feelings, expresses the level of comfort and relaxation, and can give insight into the patient.
  3. Body gestures:
    a. Hand gestures by the patient that give insight are white-knuckle grasp, finger pointing, and extending the hand as sign of welcome.

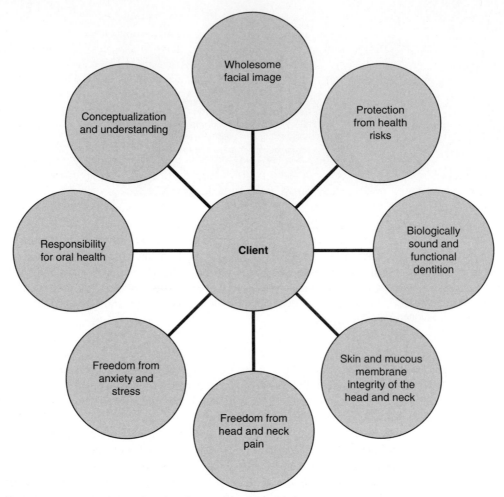

Figure 11-10   Human needs related to oral health and disease. (Modified from Harris and Christensen, 2003. In Darby ML, Walsh M: Dental hygiene theory and practice, ed 2, St. Louis, 2009, Saunders/Elsevier.)

b. Crossed arms may indicate patient feels defensive; arms open and relaxed at side may convey patient's willingness to accept information.

c. Voice signals include loudness, intonation, or inflection and can express anger, fear, excitement, and cooperation level.

B. Verbal communication involves language and listening skills of both healthcare provider and patient:

1. Provider's language SHOULD be kept simple, direct, and nonthreatening; use verbiage with meaning so patient understands the disease process and consequences.

2. Listening skills are necessary to achieve good comprehension of patient's concerns, attitudes, and feelings, as well as specific health beliefs:

a. Eye contact conveys interest by listening and being fully attentive; helps patient relax and feel comfortable; clinician communication is enhanced when eye level is same.

b. Head nodding and verbal "yes" aid in expressing involvement.

c. Feedback involves paraphrasing what the patient has said; enhances open communication and allows expression of thoughts and feelings; also gives the patient an opportunity to validate and/or correct the perception of verbal and nonverbal behavior.

3. Facilitative or cooperative communication is the give *and* take between patient and provider; creates a harmonious relationship, builds rapport, and gives a sense of empathy, respect, warmth, genuineness, and self-disclosure; also enables the patient to be involved in process of care and increases patient compliance.

C. Questioning techniques encourage communication process:

1. Open-ended questions: require an explanation or description; who, what, where, when, why, and how are BEST word choices to begin.

2. Closed questions: require yes, no, or a simple nod of the head; BEST way to move conversation along and to get closure, confirmation, or agreement to an action.
3. Answers to questions should NOT be judged; patient MUST feel that the answers have value.
4. Provider's acceptance of answers will encourage patient openness.

D. Learning principles:
   1. Learning ladder demonstrates the principles of instruction (Figure 11-11):
      a. Present small amounts of information; organize teaching sessions logically and systematically.
      b. Use visual aids to enhance learning; let the patient set the pace for learning.
      c. Present information at an appropriate age level.
      d. Supervise the patient's skill and habit development by involving the patient through return demonstrations.
      e. Provide immediate and specific feedback.
   2. Active participation requires patient to set goals, fit behaviors into daily schedule, and decide which dental cleaning aids patient is willing to use.

a. The fewer dental cleaning aids introduced, the greater the chance for compliance (so do NOT *bling bling bling* the patients with what you have in your operatory!).
b. Use of dental cleaning aids SHOULD be re-evaluated for need, compliance, and skill during maintenance visits.
c. Introducing additional dental cleaning aids should be considered ONLY as skill and compliance are achieved with present aids.

E. Planning individualized instruction:
   1. Assess patient needs:
      a. Ask if patient has any specific concerns or is experiencing any pain; ask what patient considers to be current dental needs.
      b. Evaluate soft and hard tissues for pathological changes and document findings.
      c. Assess radiographs for pathological changes and document findings.
      d. Identify risk factors, such as tobacco use, diabetes mellitus, handicaps or disabilities, immuno-compromised conditions, stress.
      e. Identify patient's health beliefs and dental IQ and apply to treatment planning.
      f. Determine patient's current oral hygiene techniques and effectiveness by looking at tissue health and amount of deposits.
   2. Establish a treatment plan by prioritizing needs and treatment.
      a. Plan strategies that account for the patient's dental IQ, health beliefs, and behavior.
      b. Build in reevaluation steps throughout treatment.
   3. Implement individualized instruction by explaining the rationale and dental techniques to be used; give treatment options; explain needs and answer questions; initiate oral hygiene techniques by the patient; initiate treatment.
   4. Evaluate treatment by observing and recording dental biofilm levels, changes in tissue health, and skill performance of oral hygiene at each appointment; reinforce oral hygiene technique at subsequent appointments, modifying as needed, assess the success of the treatment, and retreat as necessary; document self-care progress or lack of progress in record.

CLINICAL STUDY

Scenario: A 37-year-old woman has been a patient at the dental office for 2 years. She has a high caries risk because of poor dental care as a child. However, she is not very motivated to floss as needed, even though she has been shown how to floss and why she should floss. When it is discussed, she crosses her arms in front of her and says she is not in pain now so why does it matter?

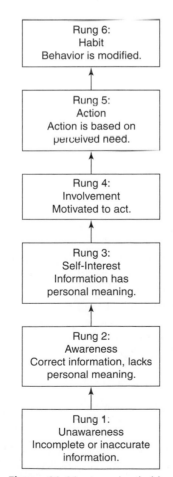

Figure 11-11 Learning ladder.

1. What does it mean when she crosses her arms in front of her?
2. What type of process could help with understanding this patient? What can the dental hygienist do to help motivate the patient? Should the hygienist mention that she could be in pain someday because of caries?

1. It is a nonverbal message. Crossed arms may indicate that patient feels defensive, while arms open and relaxed at side may convey patient's willingness to accept information.
2. Dental hygienist could use concept of the learning ladder to help with motivation of patient. When she first came to the office, the patient was on bottom rung, rung of unawareness. Dental hygienist has the obligation to educate and motivate this patient into daily flossing to achieve optimal oral health, since she has a risk of caries, and move up the ladder to flossing being a habit. It is important to keep in mind that patients typically will not progress to the top rung of the ladder in one or two hygiene visits, but through regular visits and consistent guidance. Clinician needs to remember that sincerity, concern, rapport are directly related to level of motivation for self-care by the patient. Discussion should be geared toward individual needs for the patient such as social acceptance, health maintenance, tooth retention, cost factors to increase motivation as an adult. Pain is only an immediate motivation and does not serve as long-term motivation. Discussion of caries and pain it could bring is not a good idea for motivating the patient.

Review Questions

1 Subjective information is diagnostic. Subjective information is obtained through tests and taking measures.
   A. Both statements are true.
   B. Both statements are false.
   C. The first statement is true, the second is false.
   D. The first statement is false, the second is true.

2 A patient with coronary artery disease will present with all of the following, EXCEPT one. Which one is the EXCEPTION?
   A. Use of nitroglycerin
   B. Chest pain with exertion and anxiety
   C. Valvular defect
   D. Inadequate circulation of blood to the heart

3 Patients with pacemakers may
   A. report taking digitalis or calcium channel blockers.
   B. present with swollen ankles.
   C. report taking warfarin.
   D. present with dilated pupils.

4 Patients with kidney disease experience all of the following, EXCEPT one. Which one is the EXCEPTION?
   A. Need for premedication to prevent IE when a surgical shunt has been placed

   B. Decreased white blood cell formation and function
   C. Longer half-life of medications
   D. Frequent infections and poor healing

5 One of following is NOT used in treating hypertension. Which one is the EXCEPTION?
   A. ACE inhibitors
   B. Nitroglycerin
   C. Beta-blockers
   D. Diuretics
   E. Calcium channel blockers

6 All of the following are examination techniques for evaluating the soft tissues of the head and neck, EXCEPT one. Which one is the EXCEPTION?
   A. Visual observation
   B. Percussion
   C. Palpation
   D. Auscultation
   E. Olfaction

7 All of the following are true of entries made into the dental record, EXCEPT one. Which one is the EXCEPTION?
   A. Entries should be lengthy, with detailed recordings of recommended treatments and patient responses.
   B. Entries should use adequate space to record brief and accurate statements of diagnosis and treatment rendered.
   C. Entries should summarize a patient's response, noting wants, needs, and expectations.
   D. Entries serve as a legal document.

8 Rhinophyma is BEST described as
   A. a butterfly-shaped lesion over the bridge of the nose.
   B. an overgrowth of glands causing a red, bulbous nose.
   C. numerous infected hair follicles surrounding the nasal septum.
   D. a clear drainage from the nose caused by an extended sinus infection.
   E. an obstructed airway caused by a deviated septum.

9 A maxillary torus
   A. is of little significance and need not be recorded as a clinical finding.
   B. may need to be removed or reduced before the fabrication of a full denture.
   C. is often removed to improve the patient's ability to clean the lingual surfaces of the maxillary molars.
   D. can become malignant in 15% of the female population.

10 All of the following are lesions that can be found on the tongue, EXCEPT one. Which one is the EXCEPTION?
   A. Fibroma
   B. Hemangioma
   C. Mucocele
   D. Carcinoma

11 One of the following is NOT associated with mucogingival defects. Which one is the EXCEPTION?
   A. Lack of attached gingiva
   B. Clefting
   C. High frenum attachment
   D. Tissue trauma

12 A pigmented nevus
   A. rarely has hair growing from surface.
   B. is generally isolated to the posterior dorsum of the tongue.
   C. is rarely elevated above the surface of the skin.
   D. may have brown pigmentation.

13 Which of the following is a malignant tumor with etiology directly related to sunlight exposure?
   A. Squamous cell carcinoma
   B. Juvenile melanoma
   C. Basal cell carcinoma
   D. Intradermal nevus

14 What is the MOST common oral site for the appearance of squamous cell carcinoma?
   A. Floor of the mouth
   B. Tongue
   C. Alveolar mucosa
   D. Palate

15 Which of the following lesions has the highest mortality rate of all cancerous lesions?
   A. basal cell carcinoma
   B. squamous cell carcinoma
   C. malignant melanoma
   D. juvenile melanoma

16 Kaposi's sarcoma is MOST commonly found in patients with which one of the following diseases?
   A. Uncontrolled type 2 diabetes
   B. AIDS infection
   C. Tertiary syphilis
   D. Genital herpes

17 A sealant is placed on permanent molars to help prevent
   A. Class I caries.
   B. Class II caries.
   C. Class III caries.
   D. Class IV caries.
   E. Class V caries.

18 A metal casting is a restoration made from which of the following?
   A. Plastic mold
   B. Plaster mold
   C. Metal mold
   D. Plastic pattern
   E. Waxed pattern

19 Hypocalcification is an area on the tooth that
   A. needs to be restored.
   B. has started to demineralize.
   C. has started to remineralize.
   D. has not completely calcified.

20 Attrition is loss of tooth structure caused by which of the following?
   A. Bacterial influences
   B. Excessive horizontal forces
   C. Chemical influences on the cusp tips and incisal edges
   D. Mechanical wearing

21 All of the following are associated with ankylosed teeth, EXCEPT one. Which one is the EXCEPTION?
   A. First and second primary molars
   B. Hollow sound on tapping
   C. Need for extraction
   D. Subocclusal location
   E. Roots fused to underlying bone

22 When an enamel organ is invaginated internally during tooth development, it is referred to as which of the following?
   A. Gemination
   B. Dens-in-dente
   C. Dilaceration
   D. Fusion

23 What is the BEST method for identifying a pulpal condition in a patient?
   A. Comparing results from electric pulp tester to standardized scores for that tooth type
   B. Looking for radiolucent areas at the apex of teeth on periapical films
   C. Testing both the suspected and several control teeth by several methods and comparing the results among teeth
   D. Using the cold test (usually ice sticks, dry ice, or ethyl chloride)

24 All of the following are true of a percussion test, EXCEPT one. Which one is the EXCEPTION?
   A. It can identify a problem of either periodontal or pulpal origin.
   B. If the patient reports a very sensitive tooth, gentle finger pressure is used at first
   C. Teeth are tapped or moved in both a horizontal and a vertical direction.
   D. Positive results indicate inflammation in the pulp chamber.

25 Which of the following tests is MOST widely used in conjunction with electric pulp testing to provide a definitive test for pulp vitality?
   A. Heat test
   B. Cold test
   C. Palpation
   D. Percussion

26 An electric pulp tester can be used on patients with all the following, EXCEPT one. Which is the EXCEPTION?
   A. Congestive heart failure
   B. Angina pectoris
   C. Rheumatic heart disease
   D. Cardiac pacemaker

27 Which of the following is TRUE regarding chronic inflammation?
   A. Bleeds spontaneously when probed
   B. Appears soft and spongy
   C. Appears edematous and bright red
   D. Appears leathery and tough

28 Which one of the following is a limitation of the use of radiographs for the assessment of periodontal disease?
   A. Artifacts that may be mistaken for pathological changes
   B. A three-dimensional object projected on a one-dimensional surface
   C. Interproximal areas that are difficult to see on radiographs
   D. Consideration of age of the patient
   E. Amount of gingival enlargement

29 Which one of the following characteristics would be LEAST desirable in a toothbrush?
   A. Head size that corresponds to mouth size
   B. Handle that is easy to grip
   C. Bristles that are natural
   D. Bristles that are multitufted

30 What is the MOST widely accepted method of toothbrushing?
  A. Roll technique
  B. Modified Stillman's
  C. Charter's
  D. Bass

31 To reduce calculus formation, which one of the following components is added to dentifrice?
  A. Potassium nitrate
  B. Soluble pyrophosphate
  C. Strontium chloride
  D. Sodium citrate

32 All of the following are CORRECT in regard to chlorhexidine mouthrinse, EXCEPT one. Which one is the EXCEPTION?
  A. Active against gram-positive microorganisms
  B. Approved in the United States in a concentration of 0.12%
  C. An antimicrobial agent
  D. To be used on a long-term basis

33 Phenolic compounds do which of the following?
  A. Alter the bacterial cell wall
  B. Reduce caries
  C. Promote oral wound cleansing
  D. Interfere with bacterial glycolysis

34 After application of topical fluoride foam or gel, the patient should be instructed NOT to eat or drink for what period of time?
  A. 10 minutes
  B. 15 minutes
  C. 20 minutes
  D. 30 minutes
  E. 60 minutes

35 Emergency treatment for acute fluoride toxicity if ingestion is >5 mg/kg body weight would include all of the following, EXCEPT one. Which one is the EXCEPTION?
  A. Giving milk orally
  B. Inducing vomiting
  C. Observing patient for several hours
  D. Monitoring patient for irregular heartbeat

36 The acid etching technique used for the placement of pit and fissure sealants involves
  A. 10% to 20% boric acid.
  B. 30% to 50% phosphoric acid.
  C. 40% to 50% maleic acid.
  D. 10% to 20% phosphoric acid.

37 Pit and fissure sealants are MOST effective in preventing caries
  A. on occlusal surfaces.
  B. on interproximal surfaces.
  C. in lingual cingulum.
  D. in buccal pits of molars.

38 Which fluoride is the active ingredient in MOST over-the-counter fluoride rinses?
  A. Stannous fluoride
  B. Acidulated phosphate fluoride
  C. Hydrogen fluoride
  D. Sodium fluoride

39 Which fluoride is contraindicated for use on composite and porcelain restorations?
  A. Sodium fluoride
  B. Hydrogen fluoride
  C. Acidulated phosphate fluoride
  D. Stannous fluoride

40 One of the following is INCORRECT regarding fluoride varnishes. Which one is INCORRECT?
  A. Varnishes are not washed away by saliva or food.
  B. Application of varnish requires less cooperation from the patient.
  C. Sodium fluoride is one of the frequently used fluorides.
  D. Application of varnish requires more cooperation from the patient.

41 One of following is INCORRECT regarding fluoride. Which one is INCORRECT?
  A. Promotes demineralization of the enamel
  B. Inhibits acid production in dental biofilm
  C. Prevents demineralization of the enamel
  D. Decreases adherence of dental biofilm

42 What symptoms might a child exhibit if he or she ingested a toxic dose of fluoride?
  A. Caustic burns on mouth and throat
  B. Nausea, vomiting, diarrhea, increased salivation, and thirst
  C. Sloughing of oral mucosa
  D. Syncope and falling out of chair

43 Externally motivated people
  A. believe in fate.
  B. feel they are responsible for success.
  C. will be motivated to long-term health behavior.
  D. require little supervision and direction.

44 According to Maslow's Needs Hierarchy, which of the following needs is (are) associated with motivating a patient?
  A. Self-actualization and fulfilling one's ambition
  B. Need for freedom
  C. Safety, love, and self-esteem
  D. Need to own space and maintain control

45 Which one of the following influences motivation on a short-term basis?
  A. Esthetics
  B. Malodor
  C. Cost
  D. Pain

46 Which one of the following body gestures may indicate that the patient has become defensive?
  A. Hands gripping the arms of the chair
  B. Arms crossed over the chest
  C. Hands linked behind the neck
  D. Shoulders slumped forward

47 Which one of the following is an example of a "closed question"?
  A. How many times a day do you brush your teeth?
  B. Do you floss your teeth daily?
  C. What kind of toothbrush do you use?
  D. When do you floss your teeth?

48 According to the Learning Ladder Continuum, at what level is behavior modified?
- A. Awareness
- B. Self-interest
- C. Involvement
- D. Habit

49 When planning individual instruction, what is the MOST important question to ask?
- A. What can we do for you today?
- B. How long has it been since you have seen a dentist?
- C. How often do you brush your teeth?
- D. When do you want to schedule your dental treatment?

50 All of the following are true with regard to the aging patient, EXCEPT one. Which one is the EXCEPTION?
- A. Generally has a softer diet
- B. Is more sensitive because of recession
- C. Is more likely to experience dry mouth
- D. Has more interproximal caries than other age group

51 One of the following statements is INCORRECT regarding pregnant women. Which one is INCORRECT?
- A. Oral prophylaxis is an accepted treatment during pregnancy.
- B. Pregnant women may have gingivitis and require multiple cleanings.
- C. Dental treatment is best performed during the first and third trimesters.
- D. Pregnant women should be educated on early childhood dental health.

52 One of the following is NOT a dental prosthesis. Which one is the EXCEPTION?
- A. Single-tooth dental implant
- B. Maxillary denture
- C. Four-unit bridge
- D. Space maintainer

53 All of the following are examples of dental appliances, EXCEPT one. Which one is the EXCEPTION?
- A. Single-tooth crown
- B. Periodontal splint
- C. Orthodontic retainer
- D. Occlusal night guard

54 All of the following are reasons for an edentulous patient to have an annual dental visit, EXCEPT one. Which one is the EXCEPTION?
- A. Soft tissue exam could identify early cancer or other harmful lesions.
- B. Dentures need to be relined or replaced annually.
- C. Dentures need periodic cleaning.
- D. Self-care of denture needs reinforcement.
- E. Underlying mucosa of denture needs evaluation.

55 All of the following diseases or disorders are associated with aging, EXCEPT one. Which one is the EXCEPTION?
- A. Cardiovascular disease
- B. Hypertension
- C. Diabetes mellitus
- D. Senile dementia
- E. Muscular dystrophy

56 Which one of the following oral manifestations is a result of normal aging?
- A. Xerostomia
- B. Attrition
- C. Stomatitis
- D. Glossitis
- E. Periodontitis

57 In older individuals, decay is MOST commonly located on _____ surfaces.
- A. occlusal
- B. proximal
- C. root
- D. lingual

58 The majority of elderly individuals
- A. live in family homes.
- B. live in nursing homes.
- C. have dental insurance.
- D. visit the dentist annually.

59 The failure of a caregiver to provide dental care for a dependent when obvious signs of dental decay are present is considered
- A. physical neglect.
- B. physical abuse.
- C. emotional abuse.
- D. emotional deprivation.
- E. sexual abuse.

60 Which one of the following is commonly associated with physical abuse?
- A. Bruising along the shins
- B. Abrasions on the knees
- C. Tearing of the maxillary frenum
- D. Fracture of the tibia

61 Bruising associated with physical abuse often is
- A. red and purple.
- B. green.
- C. green and yellow.
- D. red, green, yellow, and brown.

62 Morning sickness puts a woman at risk for
- A. caries.
- B. malnutrition.
- C. periodontal disease.
- D. constipation.

63 Which of the following is contraindicated during pregnancy?
- A. Daily flossing
- B. Tetracycline usage
- C. Mouthrinses containing alcohol
- D. Frequent meals

64 All of the following are associated with morning sickness, EXCEPT one. Which one is the EXCEPTION?
- A. Vomiting
- B. Enamel erosion
- C. High-carbohydrate snacks
- D. Nausea
- E. Periodontitis

65 When taking radiographs of a pregnant patient, the clinician must do all of the following, EXCEPT one. Which one is the EXCEPTION?
   A. Use the paralleling technique.
   B. Limit the number of radiographs.
   C. Recline the chair in a supine position.
   D. Have patient hold the radiographs.

66 The "losing a tooth for every child" myth is based on the premise that
   A. calcium needed for the baby's growth is removed from the mother's teeth as needed.
   B. constant vomiting in the first trimester causes demineralization of tooth enamel.
   C. gagging leads to poor oral hygiene and caries.
   D. gingivitis can cause displacement and eventual loss of teeth.

67 The key to a successful dental biofilm control program is
   A. accurate instruction.
   B. an appropriate length of instruction.
   C. patient motivation.
   D. multiple reinforcement appointments.

68 The toothbrushing technique in which the bristles are applied to the sulcular area and moved back and forth with short strokes in a vibratory motion is the
   A. Stillman's technique.
   B. modified Stillman's technique.
   C. Charter's technique.
   D. Bass technique.

69 Furcation areas are BEST cleansed with
   A. dental floss and interdental brushes.
   B. toothpicks with handles and dental floss.
   C. interdental brushes, toothpicks with handles, and end-tuft brushes.
   D. dental floss, interdental brushes, and toothpicks with handles.

70 The mouthrinse that has the highest substantivity and also has been shown to reduce dental biofilm and gingivitis is
   A. chlorhexidine digluconate.
   B. phenolic compounds.
   C. cetylpyridinium chloride.
   D. sanguinarine.
   E. stannous fluoride.

71 Dentifrices that contain soluble pyrophosphates or zinc chloride are labeled
   A. antigingivitis dentifrices.
   B. antibiofilm dentifrices.
   C. antisensitivity dentifrices.
   D. antitartar dentifrices.

72 Xerostomia caused by radiation, medications, or a pathological condition is of concern to the dental hygienist because it places the patient at greatest risk for the development of
   A. oral cancer.
   B. calculus.
   C. periodontal disease.
   D. root caries.

73 Sodium fluoride compounds, calcium hydroxide, potassium oxalate, and ferric oxalate are all agents commonly used in
   A. calculus-softening products.
   B. tooth-desensitizing products.
   C. tartar-control dentifrices.
   D. anticavity products.

74 Dentinal hypersensitivity occurs frequently in periodontal patients. Spontaneous remission without therapeutic intervention can be expected in
   A. 10% to 20% of patients.
   B. 20% to 45% of patients.
   C. 50% to 60% of patients.
   D. 60% to 70% of patients.

75 Agents that have been shown to be effective desensitizers include all of the following, EXCEPT one. Which one is the EXCEPTION?
   A. Strontium chloride
   B. Zinc citrate
   C. Potassium nitrate
   D. Zinc chloride

76 Mary, a 76-year-old woman with osteoarthritis, presents for routine oral care. Her homecare is good, but she is having some difficulty with care of the lingual surfaces of the mandibular molars. Based on this information, how many times a day should Mary brush and with what type of toothbrush?
   A. Two times a day with a manual toothbrush
   B. Two times a day with a powered toothbrush
   C. Once a day with a manual toothbrush
   D. Once a day with a powered toothbrush

77 Harold, a 54-year-old businessman, presents for oral hygiene instruction. He has a three-unit bridge on teeth #13 through #15, tooth #14 is missing, and teeth #13 and #15 are pontics. In addition, large embrasure spaces on all posterior teeth are noted. Deep pockets are noted on DF #30, MF #31, and DF #18. Based on these findings, which of the following interdental dental biofilm removal aids would be the BEST choice for Harold?
   A. Textured floss, rubber tip stimulator, dental tape, and floss threaders
   B. Waxed floss, floss threaders, toothpick tip, and interproximal brush
   C. Unwaxed floss, threaders, interproximal brush, and wood stick (wedge stimulator)
   D. Dental tape, threaders, wood stick, and toothpick tip

78 At a recent recall appointment, 16-year-old Larry has been found to have rampant caries after many years of being caries free. He has always had dry mouth because of using his inhaler for his asthma. Recently he has started to work at a drive-through window at a fast food restaurant, and he can have all the soft drinks he wants. He has begun to sip them to help him keep awake. Based on his history, what would be the BEST protocol for controlling his caries?
   A. Select other snacks from carbohydrate foods.
   B. Use a 0.5% fluoride dentifrice before going to bed.
   C. Use an alcohol-containing mouthwash containing fluoride.
   D. Chew sugar-free gum containing xylitol.

79 Harold, an 82-year-old retired fireman, calls the office and wonders what he should do. He was recently prescribed blood thinners because of a risk of cardiac problems. He states that he is getting bleeding gums sometimes when he brushes and feels maybe he should cancel his appointment next week What should Harold be told?

A. Go off the blood thinners and come into the office for his regularly scheduled appointment.

B. When the blood thinner regimen ends, call the office for an appointment, since the dental care can wait.

C. Stay on blood thinners, and the office will obtain a medical consult before his appointment.

D. Stay on blood thinners, and the office will try to accommodate his situation by not performing invasive procedures.

80 Mary is your morning patient. She is a 28-year-old librarian who has just had a baby. She has no family locally, so she asks many questions about oral care for the newborn. Which of the following would you want to include with your talk with Mary?

A. Use a pea-sized amount of fluoride dentifrice.

B. Place watered juice in baby bottle at night.

C. Green stain is an exogenous intrinsic stain.

D. She also needs to care for her mouth.

Answer Key and Rationale

1 **(A)** Subjective information (feelings, perceptions, and attitudes) is obtained from the patient. Objective information is such items as facts and results of tests and measurements. BOTH objective information and subjective information are useful in making a diagnosis. Some clinicians use SOAP (Subjective, Objective, Assessment, Plan).

2 **(C)** Valvular defects do NOT affect coronary artery disease. Coronary artery disease causes the arteries of the heart muscle to narrow, reducing blood flow to the heart and resulting in chest pain that can be relieved by nitroglycerin.

3 **(A)** Digitalis and calcium channel blockers help to regulate irregular heartbeat and are often prescribed to patients after the pacemaker is inserted. Swollen ankles are a common physical presentation of congestive heart failure. Warfarin (Coumadin) is an anticoagulant taken for chronic heart disease to aid in blood thinning and results in less pressure being exerted against the arterial walls. Patients with dilated pupils may be using cocaine.

4 **(B)** Leukemia is a disease of the white blood cells that causes poor function and a decreased formation of white blood cells. Kidney disease causes frequent infections and a longer half-life of drugs because of the kidney's inability to break down drugs efficiently. Antibiotic premedication is recommended for renal disease patients who have had a surgical shunt placed.

5 **(B)** Nitroglycerin (NTG) is used for the treatment of angina. ACE inhibitors, beta-blockers, diuretics, and calcium channel blockers could ALL be used to treat hypertension.

6 **(B)** Visual observation, palpation, auscultation, and olfaction are all examining techniques to evaluate soft tissues. Percussion can be used to evaluate teeth.

7 **(A)** Dental record entries should be brief and accurate, NOT lengthy, and include detailed statements of diagnosis and treatment rendered. Should summarize patient responses and are considered legal documents.

8 **(B)** Rhinophyma is an overgrowth of sweat and sebaceous glands of the nose, which makes the nose appear red and bulbous. Associated with heavy alcohol consumption. Lupus erythematosus is associated with a butterfly-shaped lesion over the nose.

9 **(B)** Maxillary torus, a benign overgrowth of bone, is NOT of real significance in MOST people. Should fabrication of a denture be needed, a torus may interfere with the patient's ability to successfully wear the denture (rocking or inability to achieve a seal). As a result, surgical removal or reduction of the torus may be needed before denture fabrication.

10 **(C)** Mucocele is a mucus (saliva)-filled cyst that results from blockage of a salivary duct. It is usually associated with the minor salivary glands found in the labial and buccal mucosa, but NOT in the tongue. A mucocele under the tongue is called a ranula.

11 **(D)** Tissue trauma is associated with irritation from a foreign object, NOT mucogingival defects. Lack of attached gingiva, clefting, and a high frenum attachment are associated with mucogingival defects.

12 **(D)** Pigmented nevus lesion may have a brown pigmentation. Often has a hair growing from the surface, may be scattered anywhere over the body, and may be flat or elevated from the surface of the skin.

13 **(C)** Malignant lesion that is associated with the skin exposure to the sun is a basal cell carcinoma. Squamous cell carcinoma is associated with smoking, alcohol, and syphilis. Juvenile melanoma and intradermal nevus are NOT malignant lesions.

14 **(B)** MOST common oral site for a squamous cell carcinoma is the tongue. Less frequently, it may appear on the floor of the mouth, alveolar mucosa, or palate.

15 **(C)** Malignant melanoma has the highest mortality rate of all cancerous lesions. Mortality rate for squamous cell carcinoma is NOT as high. Prognosis for recovery from basal cell carcinoma is good when treated early. Juvenile melanoma is NOT a malignant lesion; benign compound nevus in young people; resembles a malignant melanoma histologically.

16 **(B)** Kaposi's sarcoma is indicative of an AIDS diagnosis. Uncontrolled diabetes, syphilis, and genital

herpes are NOT specifically associated with Kaposi's sarcoma.

17 (A) Enamel sealants are placed to help prevent caries in occlusal pits and fissures (Class I caries) of permanent posterior teeth.

18 (E) Waxed pattern is used in development of a metal casting of a restoration. When heated, it evaporates, leaving room for the heated metal to be forced into the empty space.

19 (D) Areas that are hypocalcified have never completely calcified and may never need to be restored. Decalcified area originally was calcified and at some point started to break down. Remineralized area is tooth structure that has started to break down but has reversed its demineralization process and has hardened.

20 (B) Excessive horizontal forces, such as those caused by bruxism or clenching, can result in attrition of the occlusal or incisal tooth surfaces. Bacterial influences cause caries and periodontal disease. Chemical influences, such as those associated with bulimia, cause erosion (acid destruction of enamel), affecting the lingual of the maxillary anterior teeth. Mechanical wearing is associated with abrasion.

21 (C) MOST common ankylosed teeth are primary first and second molars and may be identified by a hollow sound produced on tapping and by location inferior to the occlusal plane. Many ankylosed teeth have NO permanent teeth present to erupt should the ankylosed tooth be extracted. Primary tooth is usually retained for as long as possible.

22 (B) Dens-in-dente is an invagination of enamel organ during tooth development. Gemination is division of single tooth germ by invagination, resulting in incomplete formation of two teeth. Dilaceration is distortion of a root and crown linear relationship, whereas fusion is the union of two tooth buds.

23 (C) There is NO one BEST test for identifying pulp vitality. ANY individual test can give a false-positive or false-negative result. BEST system is to use several types of clinical data, comparing findings among several of the teeth.

24 (D) Positive results to percussion test indicate inflammation in periodontal ligament that may originate from the pulp or periodontal problem. Moving tooth in both directions (horizontal and vertical) tests all of different fibers that constitute the periodontal ligament.

25 (B) Electric pulp testing (EPT) and thermal testing are the MOST specific tests for pulp vitality. Cold is a more versatile and therefore MORE commonly used thermal test than heat. Percussion and palpation also provide information regarding the status of the pulp but are NOT as definitive as cold and EPT.

26 (D) During use of electric pulp tester (EPT), patient is exposed to a small electrical current that might interfere with the patient's cardiac pacemaker. Use of EPT is a noninvasive test, so a patient with rheumatic heart disease would NOT be exposed to a potential bacteremia. EPT is NOT very painful or stressful, so should NOT pose particular risk for patients with heart conditions without a pacemaker.

27 (D) Chronically inflamed tissue appears tough and fibrotic, often having a leathery appearance. It does NOT bleed easily and often looks nearly normal in color. Acute inflammation appears edematous, soft, spongy, and bright red.

28 (A) Artifacts can be mistaken for pathological changes on radiographs. Assessment limitation may result from three-dimensional object being projected on a two-dimensional surface. Interproximal areas are easiest areas to assess bone loss. Buccal and lingual areas are difficult to assess because of the density of the tooth structure. Periodontal disease can occur in people of all ages. Enlarged soft tissue is NOT a major focus and is difficult to detect in the evaluation of periodontal disease on radiographs.

29 (C) Natural bristles are less desirable than nylon filaments. Nylon filaments cause less damage to the tissues and are rinsed and dried more easily, more durable, and more resistant to bacterial accumulation. When choosing a toothbrush for a patient, consider head size relative to the size of the patient's mouth and handles that are easy to grip.

30 (D) Bass or sulcular method is MOST widely accepted toothbrushing method. Bristles are angled at 45° toward the gingival margin. Efficient in removing dental biofilm and BEST method for ALL types of patients. Roll technique is useful preparatory instruction for modified Stillman's method. Modified Stillman's method incorporates a vibratory stroke followed by a roll stroke. Charter's method, which requires that bristles be angled toward occlusal surface, is BEST for orthodontic patients.

31 (B) Anti-calculus-forming (tartar control) dentifrice contains soluble pyrophosphates. Potassium nitrate, strontium chloride, and sodium citrate are components found in desensitizing dentifrice.

32 (D) Chlorhexidine mouthrinse is intended for short-term use as an antimicrobial agent active against gram-positive and gram-negative microorganisms, as well as fungi. Approved for use in the United States at concentration levels of 0.12%.

33 (A) Phenolic compounds (such as Listerine) alter the bacterial cell wall. Fluorides reduce caries. Oxygenating agents are intended to cleanse wounds, and sanguinarine agents interfere with bacterial glycolysis.

34 (D) Patient should NOT eat or drink for 30 minutes after fluoride application (foam or gel) to avoid disturbing action of the fluoride. A period of 10 or 15 minutes is NOT long enough; 1 hour is excessive.

35 **(D)** Monitoring heartbeat (irregular or arrhythmia) is NOT necessary until fluoride ingestion reaches >15 mg/kg body weight. Drinking milk, inducing vomiting, and observing patient for several hours are all appropriate actions to take for fluoride ingestion >5 mg/kg of body weight.

36 **(B)** Etching process involves the use of 30% to 50% phosphoric acid, applied to the pits and fissures to be sealed. Acid removes inorganic materials and creates tiny crevices and micropores into which sealant material can flow, producing mechanical bonding. Mechanical bonding is force that holds sealant to enamel, although some also have a chemical bond.

37 **(A)** The occlusal surfaces of the teeth are the MOST accessible to acid etching, and therefore the effectiveness of sealants is greatest on these surfaces.

38 **(D)** Sodium fluoride is fluoride MOST commonly used in OTC rinses. Sodium fluoride is a stable solution, which makes it ideal for this type of distribution. Hydrogen fluoride is principal industrial source of fluorine and hence the precursor to many important compounds, including pharmaceuticals and polymers (e.g., Teflon).

39 **(C)** Acidulated phosphate fluoride has been shown to cause pitting and roughening of composite and porcelain materials. Therefore sodium fluoride is indicated for patients with extensive restorative work that involves these materials. Stannous fluoride can cause staining and therefore is also NOT recommended. Hydrogen fluoride is principal industrial source of fluorine and hence the precursor to many important compounds, including pharmaceuticals and polymers (e.g., Teflon).

40 **(D)** One of the major advantages of these varnishes is the fact that they do NOT require patient compliance with oral care instructions. Semiannual applications have been used as an alternative for adopting the regimen of regular rinsing with fluoride.

41 **(A)** Fluoride is effective at preventing caries because of its ability to inhibit the acid production in dental biofilm and decrease the adherence of materials to fluoride-covered surfaces. Fluoride replaces some of the hydroxyl ions in enamel with fluorapatite, which is LESS soluble and MORE resistant to acids. Fluoride ions act as a reservoir of fluoride during demineralization to promote the remineralization of enamel.

42 **(B)** Certainly lethal dose (CLD) of fluoride is the amount that is likely to cause death if ingested (when NO counteragent therapy is applied). The adult dose is 5 to 10 g of NaF taken at one time, and the children's dose is 0.5 to 1 g (depending on the size and weight of the child). Signs and symptoms of acute toxicity include gastrointestinal distress (nausea, vomiting, diarrhea, abdominal pain, increased salivation, thirst). Systemic distress includes hypocalcemia, CNS convulsions, and cardiovascular and respiratory distress. Emergency treatment includes induction of vomiting and ingestion of large volumes of fluoride-binding liquids such as limewater, milk, and antacids that contain aluminum or magnesium hydroxide. Activate (EMS) system for acute toxicity.

43 **(A)** Externally motivated people believe in fate. They are NOT easily motivated to long-term health behavior and require more supervision and direction. Internally motivated people believe they are responsible for their success and will be motivated to long-term health behavior. They require little supervision and direction.

44 **(C)** Safety, love, and self-esteem are generally associated with motivating a patient according to Maslow's Needs Hierarchy. Self-actualization and fulfilling one's ambitions are part of the hierarchy but are NOT associated with motivating patients. Need for freedom, need for one's own space, and need to maintain control are part of the Dental Hygiene Human Needs Conceptual Model (Darby and Walsh.)

45 **(D)** Pain is a short-term motivating factor. Once pain leaves, the motivation diminishes. The way one looks to others (esthetics), smell of one's breath, and cost of treatment may be considered long-term motivators.

46 **(B)** Crossing the arms across the chest indicates that the patient has become defensive. Grasping the arms of the chair may indicate apprehension. Linking the fingers behind the neck shows that the patient is confident. Shoulders slumped forward may indicate uncertainty or lack of confidence.

47 **(B)** The question "Do you floss your teeth daily?" requires a yes or no answer, making it a closed question. Open-ended questions ask the patient who, what, where, when, why, or how and require the patient to give more than a yes or no answer.

48 **(D)** Habit is formed when behavior is modified. Awareness, self-interest, and involvement are all steps in forming a habit.

49 **(A)** The MOST critical question to ask a patient is "What can we do for you today?" Additional questions may also need to be asked, but ONLY after the patient's major concern (chief complaint) has been addressed.

50 **(D)** Aging patient is more likely to experience root caries than any other age group. More likely to experience dry mouth (xerostomia) and sensitivity (dentinal hypersensitivity) because of recession; diet is often of a softer nature.

51 **(C)** If dental treatment (other than oral prophylaxis) is needed, BEST time to provide the treatment is during second trimester. First trimester is NOT the best time because of the rapidly changing fetus; however, treatment would NOT be detrimental during this time; may be necessary to treat periodontal disease to prevent premature low-birth-weight infant. Restorative dental care is generally avoided during the first trimester unless it is emergency care and involves a serious infection. Third trimester is often avoided because the patient may be uncomfortable lying in the dental chair. Multiple recall appointments may be necessary during the pregnancy because of hormonal changes that may cause an inflammatory response of the gingiva. This is also a good time to educate the mother-to-be on early childhood dental care.

52 (D) Space maintainer (fixed or removable) is an appliance designed for a specific function or therapeutic outcome, usually to hold the space of a prematurely lost primary molar, preventing drift of more distal teeth into the open space. When permanent tooth begins to erupt, appliance will be removed or NOT worn. Dental prosthesis is defined as artificial replacement for missing body part; good dental examples are dental implant, denture, or dental bridge.

53 (A) Single-tooth crown is a fixed prosthesis, an artificial replacement for the crown of the tooth. Dental prosthesis replaces single or several teeth. Periodontal splints, orthodontic retainers, and occlusal night guards are all dental appliances. Designed for specific functions or therapeutic outcomes such as stabilizing teeth.

54 (B) Dentures can last many years without replacement or relining, especially once the bone support has stabilized after the extraction of teeth. Immediate dentures, however, may need to be relined after the first year. Annual examinations are IMPORTANT for denture wearers because of the benefits of a soft tissue examination, denture cleaning, and evaluation and reinforcement of good oral self-care.

55 (E) Aging is associated with many disorders and diseases. Cardiovascular disease (CVD), hypertension (HBP), diabetes mellitus (DM), and senile dementia are common among aging individuals. Muscular dystrophy (MD) is an inherited disorder that causes weakness and deterioration of the muscles and is often evident in childhood.

56 (B) Attrition, darkening of the teeth, and gingival recession are the ONLY oral manifestations (signs) that are considered a result of normal aging. Xerostomia, stomatitis, glossitis, and periodontitis are often seen in the aging population but are associated with illness and/or drug use rather than with aging itself.

57 (C) Decayed (carious) root surfaces are especially problematic for older individuals and are directly related to increased incidences of gingival recession, periodontal disease (exposes the roots to oral environment), and xerostomia (often drug induced; reduces salivary flow and pH-neutralizing effects). Caries on occlusal, proximal, and lingual surfaces is NOT specifically related to age unless it is located at or apical to the gingival margin.

58 (A) Majority of elderly individuals live in a family home. Fewer live in assisted living (nursing home),

at least for a while. Few elderly have dental insurance or visit dentist annually.

59 (A) Failure of a caregiver to provide dental care for a dependent with obvious caries (dental decay) is considered dental neglect, a form of physical neglect. Emotional abuse and emotional deprivation are harmful behaviors that affect the emotional needs of a person. Sexual abuse involves nonconsensual sexual acts.

60 (C) Tearing of the maxillary frenum, MOST commonly associated with forced feeding, is a type of physical abuse. Bruising along the shins and abrasions of the knees are common injuries in children, NOT typically associated with abuse. Fractures of the tibia and other long bones can occur from falls and are NOT typically a sign of abuse.

61 (D) When physical abuse occurs frequently, bruising in various stages is apparent. Variations in coloration (red, green, yellow, and brown) may indicate numerous abuse incidents, from days to weeks apart. New bruise is reddish purple, then turns green, then yellow, and finally brown, during the course of 2 weeks.

62 (B) Morning sickness puts a woman at significant risk for malnutrition. Caries can be a result of morning sickness if vomiting is present and frequent. Periodontal disease and constipation are NOT directly associated with morning sickness.

63 (B) Tetracycline, an antibiotic, is contraindicated during pregnancy. Associated with yellow-brown exogenous intrinsic staining of the dentition, and should be avoided during pregnancy and early childhood. Flossing and frequent meals (low in simple carbohydrates) are recommended. Alcohol mouthrinses are acceptable for patient use as long as they are NOT swallowed and patient does not have dry mouth or other sensitivity to alcohol.

64 (E) Periodontitis is NOT associated with morning sickness, unlike vomiting, enamel erosion, ingestion of high-carbohydrate snacks, and nausea.

65 (C) Unnecessary radiographs SHOULD be avoided during pregnancy. If radiographs MUST be taken, a paralleling technique should be used and the number of radiographs taken should be limited to ONLY those that are absolutely necessary for diagnostic purposes. Reclining the chair in a supine position is unnecessary and may be uncomfortable for a pregnant patient.

66 (A) The "losing a tooth for every child" myth is based on the premise that the calcium needed for the baby's growth is removed from the mother's teeth as needed. Skeletal bones (including the alveolar bones) supply calcium for the baby that is NOT provided in the diet. Constant vomiting in first trimester may indeed cause demineralization of tooth enamel, and gagging may lead to poor oral hygiene; both may increase the risk of dental caries, but the effects can be reduced by daily use of fluoride gels or rinses. Gingivitis is associated with raised hormonal levels and inadequate dental biofilm removal and does NOT cause displacement or loss of teeth; inflammation does regress usually at pregnancy's end.

67 (C) Patient motivation is the MOST important key to a successful dental biofilm control program. Although the accuracy of instruction, the amount of time spent, and multiple reinforcement appointments are all important, all efforts will be futile if hygienist is unable to motivate patient to comply with regimen.

68 (D) Bass method of brushing involves placing bristles in the sulcular area and moving them back and forth in a vibratory motion. BOTH Stillman's and modified Stillman's techniques involve placing the bristles on the marginal gingiva and moving them in a vibratory motion. Charter's technique advocates pointing bristles away from the gingiva.

69 (C) Furcation areas are difficult to cleanse with conventional toothbrushes and dental floss. Special disposable interdental brushes, toothpicks attached to the ends of handles, and end-tuft brushes have been shown to be MOST effective in these difficult-to-access areas.

70 (A) Chlorhexidine digluconate significantly reduces dental biofilm and gingivitis and exhibits high substantivity. Phenolic compounds, cetylpyridinium chloride, and sanguinarine have NOT been shown to exhibit substantivity or significant antibiofilm qualities. Stannous fluoride has demonstrated only weak antigingivitis effects.

71 (D) Anticalculus agents and tartar control dentifrices (toothpastes) contain either soluble pyrophosphates or zinc citrate as active ingredient.

72 (D) Xerostomia presents a significant risk for the development of root caries when the preventive washing action of the saliva is diminished. Oral cancer, calculus, and periodontal disease are unaffected by xerostomia.

73 (B) Sodium fluoride, calcium hydroxide, potassium oxalate, and ferric oxalate are compounds that are MOST commonly used for desensitizing root surfaces.

74 (B) Although dentinal hypersensitivity occurs frequently after periodontal therapy, spontaneous remission without further intervention has been shown to occur in approximately 20% to 45% of patients in 4 to 8 weeks, LESS noticeable 2 to 3 weeks after nonsurgical periodontal therapy.

75 (B) Zinc citrate is MOST effective as an anticalculus agent rather than a desensitizing agent. Strontium chloride, potassium nitrate, and zinc chloride have demonstrated effective desensitizing properties.

76 (D) Although toothbrushing traditionally has been recommended after each meal, now it is suggested that thorough dental biofilm removal is needed at least once a day. Because the patient has osteoarthritis, powered toothbrush may be easier for her to manipulate.

77 (B) Waxed (or unwaxed) floss and floss threaders are BEST used to clean the bridge. Textured floss also is BEST used for cleaning under bridges. Toothpick tip can be used for teeth with deeper pockets, and interproximal brush is BEST used for large embrasure spaces. Rubber tip stimulators and wood sticks do NOT remove dental biofilm under gumline or between large spaces. Dental tape is BEST used for contacts that are NOT too tight.

78 (D) Xylitol reduces microbial numbers and helps with remineralization. The patient can use it on the job, and it will promote salivary flow. To reduce caries, the clinician would instead select other snacks from noncarbohydrate foods, recommend prescription of 1.1% fluoride dentifrice (NaS at 5000 ppm), and suggest a non-alcohol-containing mouthrinse (alcohol can promote oral dryness).

79 (C) "Blood thinners" are anticoagulant or antiplatelet agents. Used for treatment of CVD to increase blood flow by suppressing or delaying coagulation of blood. Discontinuation of drug for dental care may be hazardous because of embolus or thrombus formation. Side effects can be prolonged; spontaneous or internal bleeding can occur; hematoma MORE likely with some local anesthesia injections (especially inferior alveolar nerve block). Requires monitoring bleeding by INR levels. However, with CVD it is important to have a healthy periodontium, so patient should NOT wait or have less done than what is needed. Thus he should probably stay on "blood thinners"; office can obtain the medical consult and then see him for his regular appointment and procedures after discussing it with his physician.

80 (D) Discussion should include the patient's need to also take care of her mouth, since decreasing the parent's or guardian's levels of dental biofilm and resultant lowered level of dental disease may decrease the child's risk of dental disease. She should NOT use any dentifrice with fluoride with an infant, since the newborn can swallow it, possibly affecting developing permanent tooth buds, causing "white spots" (hypocalcification from localized fluorosis); once she is sure child is NOT swallowing the toothpaste as it grows older, the toothpaste can safely be used. She should place water in the baby bottle at night; breastfeeding is an alternative that does NOT promote caries. Green stain is an endogenous extrinsic stain from Nasmyth's membrane, and MOST of it can be brushed off.

CHAPTER 12

Instrumentation

PURPOSE OF INSTRUMENTATION

The purpose of clinical instrumentation is to create an oral environment where periodontal health is maintained and tissues can return to health. It is accomplished by debridement (or scaling) of the teeth to remove hard deposits to discourage dental biofilm (dental plaque) attachment, such as calculus and/or stain during an oral prophylaxis or nonsurgical periodontal therapy (NSPT), as well as periodontal maintenance (PM). Manual instruments, power-driven instruments, or combination of the two can be used to effectively debride (scale) the teeth and accomplish this goal. Loupes and a headlight are BOTH useful for improving instrumentation. Use of the dental endoscope (Perioscope) creates further opportunity for successful NSPT or PM by offering a tool to aid in definitive instrumentation.

Any instrument that means removal of endotoxins (altered cementum) or by-products of microorganisms from root surface is controversial, and use of other means for removal of dental biofilm is now stressed. Also controversial is the use of traditional root planing with removal of root structure to produce a smooth, glasslike root surface. In addition, soft tissue curettage with removal of the pocket lining is no longer recommended for health of the tissue. Section on polishing in this chapter covers the selective method. *Discussion of all these issues is included to allow for changes in testing materials over time.* The term "operator" may be used here instead of "clinician" when discussing instrumentation. The Centers for Disease Control and Prevention (CDC) recommends antimicrobial mouthrinse before any instrumentation.

- See CD-ROM for Chapter Terms and WebLinks.
- See Chapter 13, Periodontology: NSPT and PM discussion.

Positioning

The CORRECT positioning of BOTH patient and clinician during instrumentation is critical to long-term comfort and effectiveness of clinician. Takes into account ergonomic principles and incorporation of neutral positioning (see later discussion). Transfer of instruments is not discussed here, except to emphasize that to prevent injury to patient, instruments should NEVER be passed over the patient's face or eyes. Also not discussed is concept of work zones that are set up like a "clock" around the patient (review from class texts).

- See Chapters 6, General and Oral Pathology, and 16, Special Needs Patient Care: medical diseases and disabilities and additional modifications.

A. Advantages of CORRECT patient positioning:
1. Improves visibility and access to treatment area.
2. Increases treatment efficiency.
3. Increases patient comfort during appointment.
4. Reduces clinician discomfort and fatigue.
5. Reduces possibility of occupational injury such as cumulative trauma disorder (repetitive strain injury) to neck, shoulders, wrist, hand (discussed later).

B. Principles of patient positioning for instrumentation:
1. Basic position using supine position from upright position for initial patient seating:
   a. Chair back is almost parallel to floor; parallel to floor for maxillary arch and raised 20° for mandibular arch.
   b. Patient is almost parallel to floor; head, heart, and feet are at approximately same height; patient is NOT upright:
      (1) Reduces possibility that patient could undergo syncope (fainting), especially during invasive procedures such as local anesthetic administration.
      (2) Relative contraindication: congestive heart failure, severe breathing difficulties, advanced pregnancy, back injuries.
2. Patient's head position:
   a. Top of head SHOULD be at top of chair to provide clinician access to the mouth.
   b. Head and neck SHOULD be aligned with the spine and supported by chair and headrest.
3. Adjustments to improve visibility and access:
   a. Treatment of maxillary arch:
      (1) Arch SHOULD be positioned so that occlusal plane is perpendicular to floor.
      (2) Light positioned over chest; shines into mouth at an angle.
   b. Treatment of mandibular arch:
      (1) Arch SHOULD be approximately parallel to floor.
      (2) Light positioned directly over mouth, shines straight down.

C. Principles of clinician positioning:
1. Positioning on stool:
   a. Feet flat on floor and height adjusted so thighs are parallel to floor.
   b. Sit back on stool so that body weight is fully supported and back is against backrest.
   c. Keep knees and legs apart to create tripod effect between two feet on floor and stool base to give stable seated position.
   d. Arms on a stool allow clinician to rest arms and shoulders between procedures.
2. **Ergonomics** (good body mechanics): designing tasks and work areas to maximize the efficiency and quality of work.
   a. Head SHOULD be centered over spine for support; clinician's chin is tilted gently downward for visibility, but head is not tilted to right or left.
   b. Eyestrain is reduced by having mouth at comfortable focal distance, ~15 inches from clinician's eyes to mouth; clinician may need to consider an eye examination and/or loupes if this is NOT comfortable distance.
   c. Back is straight without being rigid, tilting forward from hips rather than curling the back or hyperextending neck when necessary to get closer.
   d. Keep body weight evenly centered on stool.
   e. Shoulders SHOULD be relaxed and even, neither raised toward the ears nor rotated forward (especially if patient is somewhat upright).
   f. Upper arm SHOULD be kept close to sides, elbows bent, forearms parallel to the floor.
   g. Patient's chair height is adjusted to place the mouth at level of clinician's elbows.
   h. Wrist is held straight (neutral position) as much as possible; other bending of wrist such as pronounced flexion, extension, or deviation to side SHOULD be avoided to prevent excessive stress on the nerves in wrist area.
   i. Hands SHOULD be positioned so that palms are facing inward toward clinician's midline as much as possible and in same horizontal plane as forearm (neutral position).
   j. Assistant SHOULD be at higher level than operator.
D. **Cumulative trauma disorders** (repetitive strain injuries):
1. Neuromuscular injuries resulting from the accumulation of chronic small traumas to the same area are a potential occupational hazard for dental personnel.
2. Injuries to neck, shoulders, hand, wrist, and back have ALL been reported (e.g., carpal tunnel syndrome, entrapment of median nerve in carpal tunnel leading to pain and numbness).

3. Preventive behavior:
   a. CORRECT body mechanics or ergonomic considerations MUST always be incorporated, using *neutral* body positions.
   b. BEST positioning of patient for clinician's comfort and access.
   c. BEST instrumentation to minimize repetitious motions; includes using sharp instruments.
   d. Varying the activities and positions during appointment to alternate muscles used.

CLINICAL STUDY

Scenario: A dental hygienist is on the first day of his new position at a large dental clinic. Before taking this new position, he was the only dental hygienist for over 10 years at the same small dental practice after graduating top of his class at age 20. He notices that he is unable to put his feet on the floor when he sits on the stool provided for him. He also has trouble instrumenting the lower arch; it just seems there is not enough overhead light, especially on the lingual of the anteriors. He also wants to get closer to his patients; he has forgotten what the effective distance to a patient's mouth is. At the end of the day he notices that his back hurts. He is worried about what this means to his future in his profession.

1. What factors does the dental hygienist need to consider in order to discover why he is having a backache?
2. What could he have done to help with overhead lighting during instrumentation of the mandibular arch, especially the lingual of the anteriors?
3. What is the distance he should have maintained to his patient's mouths? What can he do if this distance seems too far away?
4. If this situation continues for many years without any changes to his way of practice, what could the outcome be for him?

1. His backache may result from leaning over too close to his patients and not putting his feet flat on the floor with the stool he used. He should be able to sit back on the stool so body weight is fully supported and the back is against backrest. His back should be straight without being rigid, tilting forward from hips rather than curling the back or hyperextending neck when necessary to get closer (see later discussion). In his new employment he needs to locate, request, or adjust a stool that will allow him to practice in a safe and effective ergonomic working position.
2. For treatment of mandibular arch, arch should be approximately parallel to the floor, with overhead light positioned directly over mouth, shining straight down. He may want to see if he can take advantage of more indirect vision and/or illumination with his

mirror when he is instrumenting the linguals of the anteriors.

3. He needs to keep himself at comfortable focal distance, ~15 inches from his eyes to patient's mouth; may need to consider an eye examination and/or loupes if this is not a comfortable distance.

4. If this continues over time, he could be looking at development of a cumulative trauma disorder, a neuromuscular injury resulting from the accumulation of chronic small traumas to the same area (his back), an occupational hazard for him.

Manual Instruments

Manual (hand) **instruments** are classified as either assessment or treatment instruments. However, many treatment instruments can also be used for assessment during treatment. Manual instruments include mirrors, explorers, probes, scalers, curets, hoes, files, chisels; available in BOTH basic designs and types and those for specific functions.

Basic Instrument Design

Basic manual instrument design determines the intended purpose and location of use. Specific selections are also based on personal preference and/or ergonomic concerns. Instrumentation with manually activated instruments, BOTH for assessment and for treatment, requires high degree of precision and control and in some cases power and force. CORRECT use of instruments can BEST be accomplished with consistent application of basic principles of instrumentation.

A. Basic instrument design (Figure 12-1):
1. Handle: can be either single or double ended; varies in composition; either metal or high-density plastic.
   a. Varies in diameter; either narrow or large:
      (1) Larger means BETTER instrument control.
      (2) Larger means BETTER transmission of fine vibrations because of hollowness.
   (3) Larger decreases muscle fatigue and cumulative traumatic disorder.
   (4) Common diameters: ⅜, 5⁄16, ¼, 3⁄16.
   b. Varies in surface texture, ranging from smooth to rough-textured, knurled, or serrated.
      (1) Rough reduces slippage in wet environment.
      (2) Rough decreases muscle fatigue and cumulative trauma disorder.
2. Shank: connects working end to handle.
   a. Functional shank is between working end and handle.
   b. Terminal (lower) shank is between working end and first bend.
   c. Length determines area of access:
      (1) Shorter shanks used in normal sulcus depth and around anteriors.
      (2) Longer shanks have additional length of terminal shank; used in deep, narrower pockets and around posteriors.
   d. Thickness determines shank flexibility, which determines whether instrument is flexible or rigid:
      (1) Thinner, flexible shanks allow greater tactile sensitivity for finer hard deposits.
      (2) Thicker, rigid shanks have greater strength for heavier hard deposits.
   e. Angles and length determine use; angulation is simple or complex:
      (1) Simple, straighter shanks on anteriors.
      (2) Complex, angled, or bent shanks on posteriors.
3. Working end: part that does the work.
   a. Curets and scalers (sickle [Jaquette] scalers) are MOST common sharp instruments; cutting edges formed by junction of face and lateral sides.
   b. Probes and explorers are MOST common assessment instruments; do NOT have cutting edges; probe tip is dull or blunt, explorer tip is sharp; tip of nonsharp instruments is the "nib."

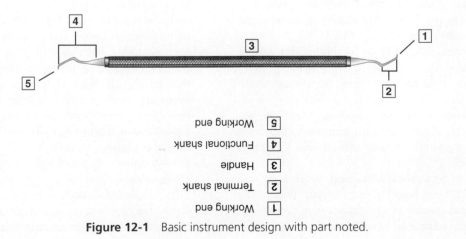

5 Working end
4 Functional shank
3 Handle
2 Terminal shank
1 Working end

Figure 12-1   Basic instrument design with part noted.

c. Mirrors and cotton pliers have special functions and designs.

4. Well-balanced instrument is BEST:
   a. Designed with middle of working end centered on long axis of handle.
   b. Easier to use, more comfortable to hold, provides better leverage.

B. Manual instrument types: functions and area of use are based on design of working end.

1. Mirrors:
   a. Front surface MOST common; reflective coating on face is easily scratched but does NOT produce ghost images.
   b. Plane or flat mirrors cause double or ghost images, and concave mirrors magnify images; may cause some distortion.
   c. Functions are multiple and may be combined:
      (1) Retraction of cheek, lips, or tongue improves access and/or visibility.
      (2) **Indirect vision:** observation of reflected image when direct vision is impaired or impractical; visualization of lingual of mandibular posteriors, distal of maxillary posteriors, etc.
      (3) **Indirect illumination:** provides illumination of dark area by reflected light bounced off mirror face; detection of caries and/or calculus.
      (4) **Transillumination:** light reflected from mirror through tooth to observe shadowing; indication of caries, calculus, pulpal health, especially interproximally.

2. Explorers (Figure 12-2):
   a. Thin, wirelike working ends tapered to a point and circular in cross section.
   b. Shanks are simple (for hard caries detection) or complex (for hard deposit and root surface exploration).

c. Ends are single or paired (mirror-imaged).
d. Function as providers of tactile information; many need more than one for NSPT:
   (1) Assessment of hard deposits (especially calculus) and irregular tooth surface during ALL phases of dental hygiene treatment.
   (2) Identification of complex tooth anatomy and pocket characteristics (e.g., concavities, contours of epithelial attachment).
   (3) Detection of carious lesions; assessment of restorations for irregularities, lack of marginal integrity.
e. Basic types:
   (1) Shepherd's hook (#23): hooked single end, BEST for caries detection and restoration evaluation.
   (2) Pigtail (or cowhorn): curved shank paired ends, BEST for hard deposit and for exploration of healthy sulcular areas.
   (3) The #17: right-angled single end, straight and narrow shank with short 2 mm working end, BETTER for hard deposit and root surface exploration.
   (4) The #3A: long curved shank single end, BEST for hard deposit and root surface exploration.
   (5) The (ODU) #11/12: area-specific for maxillary molars with paired ends and complex shanks (Gracey-like, others available), BEST for hard deposit and root surface exploration.

3. Probes (periodontal probes): calibrated measuring tool, usually single ended but can be combined with explorers or other probes on one end; blunt tip (Figure 12-3):

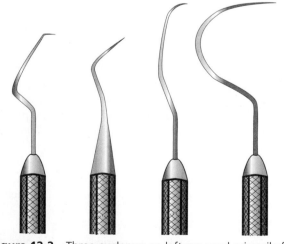

Figure 12-2 Three explorers on left are used primarily for calculus detection; shepherd's hook on right is used for caries detection or evaluation of restorations.

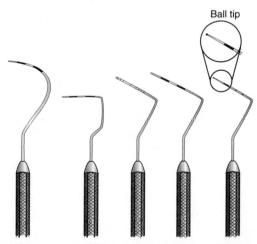

Figure 12-3 Periodontal probes (from left to right): Nabor's is curved for furcations, PCP12 with Marquis markings on modified shank, Williams markings at 1-2-3-5-7-8-9-10, Marquis with 3-6-9 markings, WHO with ball tip used to record PSR.

a. Measurements in millimeters; variations in way increments are displayed; color coding with dark or light bands improves ease of reading (some have yellow bands):
   (1) Marquis: 3-6-9-12 mm markings; Williams: 1-2-3-5-7-8-9-10 mm markings; Michigan O with 3-6-8, also PCP12 with variable markings on modified Novatech shank, easier to align with vertical tooth axis.
   (2) WHO: 0.5-mm ball tip and 3.5-5.5-8.5-11.5 mm markings; used ONLY for periodontal screening and recording (PSR).
   (3) Nabor's (furcation): paired curved design with or without millimeter markings at 3-mm intervals; BEST for identification of furcations and to examine root and/or pocket topography.
   (4) Digital (computer): MORE accurate with repeatable measurements, since uses same amount of force and measures to tenth of millimeter.
   (5) Laser lightbeam (DIAGNOdent): detects new and residual hard deposits on subgingival areas up to 9 mm with up to 80% accuracy (twice that of conventional probe).
b. Functions:
   (1) Periodontal assessment:
       (a) Measures sulcular and pocket probing depth (PD), distance from gingival margin to epithelial attachment (EA) of the junctional epithelium (JE).
       (b) Measures clinical attachment levels (CAL), distance from cementoenamel junction (CEJ) to EA if gingival margin is at or apical to CEJ; distance from gingival margin to EA if gingival margin is coronal to CEJ.
       (c) Measures recession, distance from CEJ to gingival margin (when margin is apical to CEJ).
       (d) Measures width of attached gingiva, distance from gingival margin to mucogingival junction, minus sulcus or pocket depth.
       (e) Assesses gingival characteristics, including bleeding on probing (BoP), with or without indices, presence of suppuration (pus), tissue consistency.
       (f) Detects hard deposits and root surface roughness, root and/or pocket topography.
   (2) Other uses:
       (a) Overjet assessment: distance from maxillary incisal edge to facial of mandibular central; more than 3 mm of overhang.
       (b) Overbite assessment: distance of overlap of anteriors in vertical dimension; more than one-third overlap.

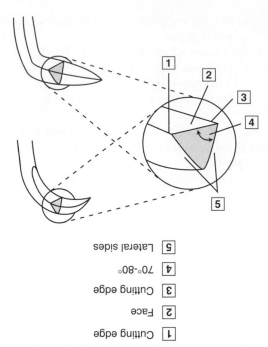

5	Lateral sides
4	70°-80°
3	Cutting edge
2	Face
1	Cutting edge

Figure 12-4 Sickle scaler working ends may be either straight or curved. All are triangular in cross section.

       (c) Measurement of oral lesions for diagnostic purposes.
4. Scalers (sickle scalers, Jacquette scalers, S204) (Figure 12-4):
   a. Working ends may be straight or curved but are always triangular in cross section, with two cutting edges.
   b. Cutting edges converge to form sharp point at the tip.
   c. Lateral sides converge to form pointed back.
   d. Straight shanks for anteriors (single ended) and contra-angled for posterior (paired).
   e. Functions:
       (1) MAINLY for supragingival hard deposits, can be used 1 to 2 mm below free gingival margin.
       (2) BEST for initial debridement of heavier hard deposits because of strength.
       (3) NOT for removal in contacts and tight proximal surfaces, because of thin, pointed tip; pointed tip also increases risk of subgingival laceration or gouging curved tooth surfaces.
5. Curets (Figure 12-5):
   a. Lateral sides that taper to form rounded back on working end, with rounded toe.
   b. Half-moon shape in cross section.
   c. Simple shanks for anteriors and complex for posteriors.
   d. Paired, mirror-imaged working ends (matched sets, e.g., #11/12, #13/14).

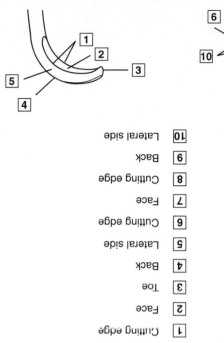

10	Lateral side
9	Back
8	Cutting edge
7	Face
6	Cutting edge
5	Lateral side
4	Back
3	Toe
2	Face
1	Cutting edge

Figure 12-5   The basic design of all curets is rounded toe, rounded back, and a half-moon-shaped cross section.

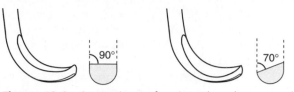

Figure 12-6   Comparison of universal and area-specific curets. Universal curets have a 90° angle between the face and the terminal shank, which gives them two functional cutting edges. Area-specific curets have offset angle with a 70° angle between the face and the terminal shank. This makes lower cutting edge the only one that is used for debridement.

Table 12-1   Gracey area-specific curets

Gracey curet	Designated area of use
Gracey 1-2 and 3-4	Anterior teeth
Gracey 5-6	Anterior or premolar teeth
Gracey 7-8 and 9-10	Posterior teeth buccal and lingual surfaces
Gracey 11-12 and 15-16	Posterior teeth mesial surfaces
Gracey 13-14 and 17-18	Posterior teeth distal surfaces

e. Functions:

(1) MOST versatile; BEST for both supragingival and subgingival hard deposits, depending on thickness, length, angulation of shank, working end.

(2) BEST promotion of tissue safety because of rounded toe and back; BEST manual instrument for safe and effective subgingival adaptation.

(3) Controversially: excellent cutting and smoothing abilities for traditional root planing, removal of altered cementum, as well as hard deposits; produces smoothest root surface but removes MOST root structure.

f. Two design types: universal and area specific (Figure 12-6):

(1) Universal curets:

(a) Blade face at 90° to terminal (lower) shank.

(b) Has two parallel cutting edges per working end.

(c) Treat ALL surfaces with just one instrument by use of ALL four cutting edges (two cutting edges per working end and two working ends per curet).

(2) Area-specific curets: Gracey curet MAINLY used (Table 12-1):

(a) Blade face "offset" to 60° to 70° to terminal (lower) shank.

(b) Has one cutting edge per working end (on longer, lower side of blade).

(c) Long shanks and offset angles allow MOST effectiveness in deep, narrower pockets (after fives with about 3 mm longer shanks and also narrower blades; even smaller with micro mini and mini-fives).

(d) Designed to adapt to specific surfaces and teeth; treatment of ALL surfaces of posteriors requires MORE than one instrument.

(3) Turgeon curet: adaptation of Gracey curet with narrower working end and modified triangular blade in cross section that is easier to sharpen.

(4) Langer curets: hybrid of universals with area-specific specifics; long, complex shank design, with blade face that is 90° to lower shank, with two parallel working and cutting edges; must be used in set to access entire dentition, and adaptation is difficult in the posterior with poor access.

(5) O'Hehir area-specific curets: have circular discs at working end with extended lower shank; used with push/pull strokes in deep periodontal pockets and furcations.

6. Hoes (hoe scalers) (Figure 12-7):

a. Bulky working end that gives great strength but makes subgingival access and adaptation difficult; careful adaptation and instrument control are critical to prevent damage.

b. Straight cutting edge with two sharp corners that can gouge a root surface if poorly adapted;

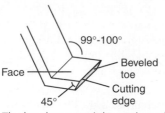

Figure 12-7 The hoe has a straight cutting edge. Since it is a bulky instrument, used mainly supragingivally.

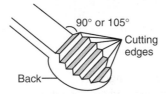

Figure 12-8 Periodontal file has multiple cutting edges. It is a thin instrument that may be used subgingivally when it fits.

straight cutting edge makes adaptation to curved areas difficult; angulation of blade to shank is 99° to 100°.
   c. Function:
      (1) BEST for removal of heavy supragingival; primarily on lingual of mandibular anteriors and distal of MOST posteriors.
      (2) Interproximal removal ONLY if adjacent tooth is missing.
      (3) Vertical pull strokes and two-point instrument contact with BOTH cutting edge and shank adapted to tooth for increased control.
      (4) Rarely used, replaced by others such as ultrasonics (still used when ultrasonics contraindicated).
7. Files (periodontal files) (Figure 12-8):
   a. Multibladed hoes that are thin and rounded; thick shank gives strength; angulation of blade to shank is 99° to 105°.
   b. Recommended technique includes vertical pull stroke with as many blades as possible adapted to tooth and root surface.
   c. Careful adaptation of flat blade is needed when working subgingivally to avoid gouging and root damage.
   d. Requires special sharpening instrument, either tanged or triangular file sharpener.
      (1) Rarely used, replaced by others such as ultrasonics (used when ultrasonics contraindicated).
   e. Functions:
      (1) Best for crushing calculus, especially on burnished calculus.
      (2) Best for smoothing CEJs and overhangs.
      (3) Best for removal in areas of limited access such as deep, narrow pockets because of small size and flat shape.

8. Chisels (chisel scalers):
   a. Straight cutting edge continuous with shank; single or paired ends; blade is flat and beveled at 45°.
   b. Use of push stroke (ONLY push instrument EXCEPT for O'Hehir curets).
   c. Function:
      (1) Best for supragingival use on heavy interproximal; mainly on anteriors; there must NOT be any interdental papilla.
      (2) Pushing from facial surface through interproximal surface toward lingual.
      (3) Rarely used, replaced by others such as ultrasonics (used when ultrasonics contraindicated).
9. Implant maintenance instruments (see Chapter 13, Periodontology):
   a. Made of material that will NOT scratch smooth surface of implants; working ends made of various forms of plastic, graphite, resin, or titanium instruments; ultrasonic tips can use fixed or disposable plastic covers.
   b. Shapes vary; some resemble familiar curets and others are uniquely shaped to adapt to round implant shapes.
   c. Functions:
      (1) Removal from surfaces without scratching; very light, lateral force is ALL that is normally needed.
      (2) Recommended technique is SIMILAR to curet.

Principles of Manual Instrument Use

Principles of manual instrument use include grasp, fulcrum, adaption, angulation, stroke.
A. Grasp:
   1. Pen grasp: SAME way you would hold a pen when writing, grasping handle with thumb and first finger while middle finger supports instrument from underneath; used with mouth mirror.
   2. Modified pen grasp: BEST grasp with manual instruments for BOTH assessment and treatment.
      a. Technique:
         (1) Thumb and index finger are placed opposite each other and have primary grasp and control.
         (2) Handle rests on hand between second joint of the index finger and webbed area formed between thumb and rest of the hand.
         (3) Pad of middle finger, usually toward side, but NOT on fingernail, rests lightly at junction of shank and handle below thumb and index finger.
         (4) Thumb and index finger are usually placed on the handle near the shank when using a traditional intraoral fulcrum (tooth surface).

(5) Ring finger rests against middle finger and is used as fulcrum finger.
   (a) For extraoral fulcrum, ALL fingers may be moved farther up handle, away from working end.
   (b) Variation of grasp: index finger is bent more and moved higher on handle, giving tripod finger placement.

b. Advantages:
   (1) Stable grasp with control.
   (2) Allows instrument to be rolled in fingers easily.

c. Used during assessment:
   (1) Minimum finger pressure SHOULD be exerted against instrument.
   (2) BEST to use light grasp that allows information, especially vibrations, to be sensed by fingertips (e.g., feeling explorer bumping over hard deposit, into furcations, or probe reaching EA).
   (3) Pad of middle finger is MOST important in sensing vibrations transmitted up shank.

d. Used during treatment:
   (1) Grasp should be light during exploratory strokes made with curets and during placement phase of working stroke.
   (2) Grasp should be moderate to firm during activation phase of working stroke.
   (3) Close correlation between pressure of grasp and amount of lateral pressure against tooth surface.

3. Palm thumb grasp: rarely used with debridement instruments; limits mobility and tactile sensitivity.
   a. Technique:
      (1) Handle is wrapped in palm with ALL four fingers around it.
      (2) Working end is toward thumb, and thumb is left free to act as fulcrum or for special function.
   b. Uses:
      (1) Air-water syringe and rubber dam clamp holder.
      (2) Porte polisher for selected areas (see later discussion).
      (3) Instrument sharpening with Neivert Whittler sharpener or handpiece mounted stone (see later discussion).

B. **Fulcrum** (finger rest): mechanical leverage point that allows greater force to be exerted at working end without increased effort.
   1. Purpose:
      a. Both MORE force and MORE lateral pressure can be exerted.
      b. Provides point of stabilization.
      c. Allows greater control over instrument and working stroke, MAINLY stroke length.
      d. Allows greater patient safety and comfort.
      e. Reduces clinician strain and fatigue.
      f. Traditional intraoral fulcrum: effective and comfortable for patient in MOST cases: fulcrum finger (ring finger) is placed on tooth surface and remains in contact with middle finger; rocking or pivoting motion is used.
      g. Alternative intraoral fulcrums: BEST when used to increase adaptation, improve angulation, or create more effective fulcrum (leverage) location or to create more physiologically sound wrist position: opposite-arch, cross-arch, finger-on-finger.
      h. However, when forced to separate fulcrum from instrument grasp fingers (considered split fulcrum), clinician has a loss of stability and strength in working stroke, even with palm-up intraoral rest.
      i. Extraoral fulcrums: BEST to increase access and effectiveness by improving adaptation and angulation, especially for posteriors, in small mouths, and in deep pockets of periodontally involved teeth; used MAINLY to increase power and control during working stroke, since whole hand activated:
         (1) MUST be at 9 o'clock position and use extended grasp farther down handle.
         (2) Palm or back of fingers or hand is rested against the face and reinforced finger rest.
         (3) Finger or thumb of noninstrumenting hand is pressed against shank.
         (4) Gracey curet's lower shank MUST be parallel to surface before starting stroke.
         (5) Can also be used with ultrasonics.

C. **Adaptation:** relationship of working end to the tooth surface.
   1. Evaluating adaptation:
      a. Cutting end SHOULD be positioned so that one third of working end closest to tip is against the tooth (toe third).
      b. Point SHOULD be adapted to the tooth as portion of toe third; if point is adapted off of the tooth, can cause soft tissue laceration and discomfort.
      c. Heel of working end SHOULD be kept close to the tooth to prevent excessive distention of pocket tissue.
      d. SAME guidelines for adaptation are used with both assessment and treatment instruments.
   2. Analyze adaptation difficulties:
      a. Worst adaption on curved areas (e.g., line angles) or convex (e.g., mesial surface of maxillary first premolars) or narrow roots (e.g., lingual

mandibular anteriors), with poor access (e.g., third molars) or deep pockets.

b. Common solutions to adaptation difficulties:
   (1) Rolling instrument in fingers.
   (2) Moving fulcrum.
   (3) Adjusting hand orientation on fulcrum.
   (4) Changing instruments.
   (5) Altering stroke direction and orientation of instrument on tooth (e.g., for line angle, use oblique stroke with toe toward apex).

D. **Angulation:** angle formed between working end and the tooth surface.
   1. Assessment instruments (explorers, probes):
      a. For caries detection, point of explorer is pressed into tooth surface with terminal portion meeting tooth at 90°.
      b. For hard deposit and root surface exploration, working end of explorer is angled about 15° from tooth surface with ONLY toe (terminal) third lightly touching.
      c. Periodontal probe is positioned close (almost parallel) to tooth surface with end in contact with the root surface (also considered adaptation).
      d. When probing proximal surface where there is adjacent tooth, probe MUST be angled 20° to 30° into col (see Chapter 4, Head, Neck, and Dental Anatomy).
   2. Treatment instruments (scalers, curets): angle formed between face of blade and tooth surface (see discussion next on strokes).
      a. For insertion into sulcus or pocket: angle is NOT present; as flat against tooth surface as possible.
      b. For scaling and working stroke: angle is 70° to 80°; LESSER angle such as <45° results in burnished hard deposits.
      c. For curets ONLY:
         (1) For root planing stroke: angle becomes MORE closed at 60° to 45° (controversial).
         (2) For soft tissue curettage stroke: angle becomes >90° so that cutting edge is directed toward epithelial lining of diseased pocket wall; digitally support tissues (NOT recommended).

E. Stroke: types differ by amount of pressure applied to tooth (lateral pressure) and by length and direction of movement; goal is to cover ALL tooth surfaces.
   1. **Exploratory stroke:** used with ALL instruments for assessment.
      a. Grasp and lateral pressure SHOULD remain light throughout, SHOULD be overlapping and multidirectional.
   2. **Walking strokes:** use of up-and-down motion while moving forward around tooth in small steps; used with probes since EA varies in depth and contour.

3. **Working stroke** (scaling stroke; activation phase): used with treatment instruments.
   a. Tight and controlled grasp with moderate to heavy lateral pressure, dictated by hard deposit tenacity; lightest grasp and pressure that will remove deposit is BEST.
   b. Overlapping, with various stroke directions.
4. Root planing stroke (controversial):
   a. Grasp is moderate to light.
   b. Length becomes progressively longer and lateral pressure becomes lighter as root is smoothed (can be followed by root debridement stroke, even lighter pressure to remove dental biofilm on previously planed root).
   c. Direction is multidirectional, with cross-hatching.
5. Stroke parts:
   a. Insertion:
      (1) Position working end at base of sulcus or pocket apical to hard deposit.
      (2) For bladed instrument, angle for insertion of scalers and curets SHOULD be as close to flat against tooth surface as possible; NO angle.
      (3) BEST if grasp and lateral pressure are light.
   b. Preparation for activation varies depending on type of stroke intended; for working or scaling stroke: grasp is tightened, desired angulation is established, lateral pressure is increased.
   c. Activation:
      (1) Movement to accomplish purpose of the stroke (wrist-rock) (e.g., exploration, probing, scaling, root planing).
      (2) Stroke length and direction will vary.
      (3) Hard deposit removal is from MOST subgingival to MOST coronal.
6. Stroke direction:
   a. Selection of stroke direction is based on anatomy of individual tooth, access to tooth and surface, instrument selection, type of hard deposit.
   b. Options in stroke direction: vertical, horizontal or circumferential, oblique, cross-hatching (combination vertical, horizontal, oblique).
7. Stroke length:
   a. Shorter strokes give more control and used for hard deposit removal.
   b. Longer strokes typically used for assessment (exploring and probing) and root planing.
   c. SHOULD overlap strokes to ensure that all areas of tooth surface are instrumented.
   d. BEST to treat each root as a separate tooth, if access permits, with combination of horizontal, vertical, and oblique strokes.

INSTRUMENT SHARPENING

Manual instruments become dull with use. **Sharpening** is technique of grinding one or both surfaces that join to form the cutting edge of manual instrument blade until a fine, sharp edge is produced.

A. Objectives:
1. Preserves original instrument shape, maintains sharp edge, maintains effectiveness of instrument design, extends useful life of instrument, and reduces instrument replacement costs.
2. Increases ease and quality of instrumentation by decreasing hand fatigue and potential for occupational injury.
3. Increases patient comfort because of decreased scaling pressure and reduced number of working strokes needed.

B. Need and frequency of sharpening:
1. ALL instruments with a cutting edge need sharpening on a regular basis:
   a. Cutting edge of instrument is formed by junction of face and lateral side; has length but should NOT have width.
   b. With use, sharp cutting edge is worn away, becomes rounded and dull, needs to be sharpened.
2. Rate at which instrument becomes dull is determined by:
   a. Number of working strokes taken since last sharpening.
   b. Amount of lateral pressure used.
   c. Nature of the deposit.
   d. Composition of metal instrument; carbon steel holds edge longer than stainless steel.
   e. When instrument was previously sharpened; sterilization in autoclaves (steam) can dull sharp instruments.
3. Sharpen at FIRST sign of dullness:
   a. Amount of work or scaling done since last sharpening; the more working strokes and heavier the deposits, the sooner sharpening is needed.
   b. "Feel" of the instrument on the teeth or deposit; dull instruments have LESS grab (slip easily), tend to burnish hard deposits, and have reduced tactile sensitivity during exploring and light scaling.
   c. Sharpness test shows instrument to be dull (see assessment discussion below).
   d. Instruments may need sharpening periodically during a debridement procedure.

C. Mechanical sharpeners (Sidekick, Periostar): can be used for ease and MOST consistent results, with various stones available.

D. Hand sharpening with stones and lubricants:
1. Arkansas stone: natural stone with fine grit.
   a. Lubricated with a fine oil or petroleum jelly before each use to prevent glazing (metal particles clogging pores of stone).
   b. May be sterilized by ALL sterilization methods but may become dry and more brittle with repeated exposure to high heat.
2. Ceramic stone: hard, synthetic stone with fine to medium grit (abrasive particle size).
   a. Lubricated with water or used dry (useful for maintaining sterile stone).
   b. Tolerates ALL sterilization methods.
3. India stone: synthetic stone with medium grit.
   a. Recommended lubricants include oil and water to prevent glazing.
   b. Can remove large amount of instrument in short amount of time because of increased abrasiveness.
   c. Tends to groove and show wear with extended use.
   d. Tolerates ALL sterilization methods.
4. Shapes of stones: vary; includes wedge-shaped, cylindrical, conical stones (use on the instrument face).
5. Stone maintenance:
   a. Protect the stone and use lubricant matched to the stone type.
   b. Use entire surface of stone to prevent grooving.
   c. Clean stone before sterilization; remove lubricant and metal particles from stone (glazing) using soap and a brush or ultrasonic bath (if already contaminated).
   d. Sterilize stone between patients.

E. Technique: two methods, instrument stable or stone stable.
1. General principles:
   a. Shape of each new instrument SHOULD be studied so that it can be preserved.
   b. Each working end has either one cutting edge or two parallel cutting edges that need to be sharpened.
   c. Appropriate angles SHOULD be maintained:
      (1) Internal angle of 70° to 80° MUST be preserved in BOTH curets and scalers for maximum effect of cutting edge.
      (2) Angle from face of the curet or scaler to stone SHOULD be 100° to 110° (Figure 12-9).

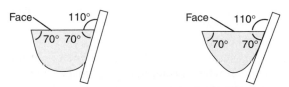

Figure 12-9 Instrument sharpening angles. Angulations for sharpening both curets and sickle scalers (left to right) are the same. Angle between the instrument face and the stone should be 110° with an internal angle of 70°.

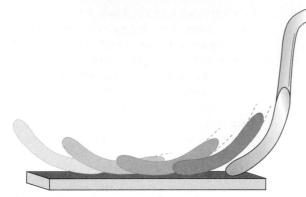

Figure 12-10 Instrument sharpening: stone movement from heel to toe. The entire lateral side of the instrument should be sharpened. This may require a dramatic change in position as the instrument is sharpened from the heel to the toe, as shown with this posterior Gracey curet, or it may be a very slight shift from heel to toe in a universal curet. This adjustment of the stone to instrument relationship is critical for maintaining the original shape of the instrument.

    d. Selected surfaces are sharpened:
      (1) Lateral side is the MAIN surface to sharpen.
      (2) Face may also be sharpened, usually to remove wire edge or to maintain or recover original shape.
    e. **Wire edge:** irregular projection that may form from burnished metal particles that extend beyond the surface being sharpened (e.g., when sharpening lateral surface, wire edge will project above face).
      (1) Prevention or removal:
        (a) Prevented by ending on a stroke away from cutting edge (usually downstroke).
        (b) **Honing:** removing wire edge by taking one or two light sharpening strokes on adjacent surface (on face when the lateral surface is sharpened).
  2. Instrument stable; MOST widely used technique:
    a. Instrument is held steady, either suspended in front of clinician or supported against a counter edge.
    b. Stone is moved up and down over lateral sides; stone is moved over face, from heel to tip or toe.
  3. Stone stable; LESS used technique (Figure 12-10):
    a. Involves flat stone that is laid on instrument tray or used with honing machines and sharpening devices.
    b. Instrument is moved across surface to sharpen lateral sides; may also still move stone over face.
F. Assessment (evaluation) for sharpness:
  1. Accumulation of metal filings:
    a. During actual sharpening process, metal removed from instrument collects on face and is used as general indication that blade is sharp.

    b. **Sludge:** when oil used as lubricant, accumulation of oil and metal; when water used as lubricant, ONLY metal particles collect.
  2. Use of test stick:
    a. Apply instrument at same angle for scaling; press cutting edge into stick and release; however, shaving stick will dull blade.
    b. Sharp instrument SHOULD bite or grab stick surface when lightly pressed into surface and released; test entire cutting edge.
    c. May be used to evaluate instrument for sharpness or dullness; can be part of standard instrument setup, sterilized between patients.
  3. Light reflection (glare) test:
    a. Using lighting, hold cutting edge to be evaluated so that it is directed toward evaluator's eye.
    b. Sharp cutting edge becomes a fine line and will NOT reflect light; dull cutting edge has width and will reflect light.
  4. Magnification (hand or loupes):
    a. May assist in assessment of blade for sharpness and contour.
    b. Especially helpful with the light reflection test and when recontouring instrument.
G. Instrument recontouring and replacement:
  1. **Recontouring:**
    a. Used for instrument that NO longer has its original shape but still has sufficient metal bulk in the blade.
    b. Goal is to recreate the original shape of the blade using same principles and techniques as for regular sharpening; metal is usually removed from BOTH the lateral sides and the face.
  2. Replacement:
    a. Replace an instrument when blade width or length has been so reduced that the blade is at increased risk of fracture during use.
    b. Also recommended when instrument blade effectiveness has been decreased by loss of original or intended shape.
    c. Variables for lifespan: frequency of use (number of setups etc.), difficulty of patients, use of ultrasonics, type of metal in instrument.

Power-Driven Scaling Instruments

Use of **power-driven scaling instruments,** combined *with* manual instruments, may give BETTER results in most cases than either one alone.
A. Indications for use:
  1. Prophylaxis (includes deplaquing for dental biofilm and stain removal).
  2. Periodontal debridement (includes scaling and root planing [controversial—see earlier discussion]) and/or NSPT, possibly before surgical therapy.

3. Supportive periodontal therapy (periodontal maintenance [PM]).
4. Overhang and orthodontic cement removal.

B. **Sonic scalers:** frequency range of 2500 to 7000 cycles/sec (cps).
1. ALL sides are active and MOST effective; elliptical motion.
2. Power sources: compressed air, attaches to high-speed handpiece position on dental unit.
3. Advantages:
   a. Does NOT generate heat, therefore does NOT require fluid lavage as coolant (although lavage is desirable for other reasons).
   b. Inexpensive, highly portable; small, light.
4. Disadvantages: noisy and poor deposit removal because of LOW power.

C. **Ultrasonic scalers:** frequency range of 18,000 to 50,000 cps.
1. Power source: electrical energy that connects to standard electrical outlet.
2. Two types divided on manner of converting electrical power to mechanical movement (vibrations) at working end:
   a. **Magnetostrictive scaler** (18,000 to 45,000 cps): uses magnetic oscillations within metal stack or rod; elliptical pattern with ALL surfaces of the tip active (Cavitron, Odontoson).
   b. **Piezoelectric scaler** (35,000 to 50,000 cps): uses crystal oscillations; linear pattern with two sides of the tip active, limiting adaptation (Satelec, EMS, Symmetry).
3. Unit controls:
   a. Power setting selection:
      (1) Controls amplitude and size of tip movement; high power gives high amplitude or large tip movement.
      (2) Based on treatment needs and tip used:
         (a) Low to medium: used for light or finishing debridement, root planing, or deplaquing, sensitive root surfaces, light and thin tips.
         (b) Medium to high: used for removal of heaver deposits, heavy or thicker tips.
   b. Tuning controls frequency of the tip movement:
      (1) Autotune: majority have built-in control.
      (2) Manual tune: allows clinician to adjust, giving greater control and thus potentially increasing patient comfort.
   c. Fluid: functions as coolant for machines that generate heat during operation and provides therapeutic benefits.
      (1) Fluid volume: may vary by manufacturers' recommendations, typically, set to give fast drip of water from the tip and halo of fine droplets.
      (2) Fluid source and type:
         (a) Water from dental unit SHOULD be purged through dental unit and powered-scaler for 2 to 5 minutes at start of the day; from 30 seconds to 2 minutes between patients (SIMILAR to time used for air-water syringe).
         (b) External fluid supplies using sterile water, antimicrobial solutions, or temperature-controlled water can have advantages for patient treatment.
      (3) Suction: high-speed (high-volume evacuator [HVE]) is BEST, slow-speed used if patient is compliant.
      (4) O-ring (if present): provides rubber seal for handpiece coolant.

D. Ultrasonic instrument tips/inserts:
1. Technique:
   a. Tip parallel to long axis of the tooth with point pointing toward apical direction.
   b. Last few millimeters of tip are MOST effective and SHOULD be positioned against the tooth.
   c. Point of working end should never be directed toward the tooth surface, especially the root surface (can cause gouging).
   d. BEST to use light grasp to encourage use of light pressure; heavy grasp (pressure) reduces effectiveness of tip, also causes increased discomfort to patient, possibility of root damage, and unnecessary wear.
   e. If patient is sensitive for one tooth, BEST to move on to next tooth and use manual scaling on sensitive tooth.
   f. If whole dentition is sensitive, may need to check warmth of water, pressure of tip on teeth, need for local anesthetics and/or manual scaling (plus files, hoes, chisels).
   g. Replace tip with loss of 2 mm from working end.
2. Standard (conventional, universal) tips:
   a. Thick, strong, shaped like anterior curet or probe.
   b. BEST used to remove heavier deposits and for initial debridement.
   c. May be used for supragingival and subgingival debridement but NOT to base of deeper pockets; possibly in shallow pockets.
   d. Often used at higher power setting; heavier metal tip does NOT move as much as a thin tip at the same power setting.
   e. Important to usually use manual instrumentation afterward if using ONLY standard tips.
3. Periodontal or thin (slim, narrow-profile) tips:
   a. Longer and thinner than standard, shaped like probe in terminal portion, may be diamond coated, beveled, or bladed.

b. Often in sets with right and left contra-angled tips and straight tip.

c. Used at low power to prevent patient discomfort and damage to tip for magnetostrictive, EXCEPT can use high power for piezoelectric.

d. BEST for removing light deposits or following initial debridement *after* use of standard tip.

e. May be used to base of deep pockets, giving extensive coverage.

f. Portions of root that CANNOT be accessed must be instrumented manually with curets because of better adaption.

g. Manual instrumentation produces smear layer when debris is moved over subgingival root surface, so after curet is used, ultrasonic SHOULD be used on low setting with a thinner insert to provide final smoothing stroke and remove smear layer.

4. Furcation tips: small ball-like projection at the very end of the tip.

a. May prevent damage to root when working in tight furcation areas, use *after* manual instrumentation, since may burnish hard deposits.

b. Available in right and left, and straight thin and slim style tips.

5. Diamond calculus removal tips: specially designed to cut through tenacious calculus while protecting the root surface.

E. Therapeutic effect:

1. Deposit removal:

a. For calculus, is effective as with manual in MOST cases except in deep, narrow pockets (see earlier discussion).

b. For extrinsic stains, very effective (less need for polishing).

2. Pattern for treatment:

a. Treatment begins at MOST coronal areas of deposit and moves to MOST apical or subgingival deposits in contrast to manual instruments, which move from MOST subgingival to MOST coronal.

b. LESS root structure is removed than with manual instruments.

3. **Fluid lavage:** fluid associated with power-driven scalers reaches base of the pocket.

a. Serves as oral irrigator, flushing away the unattached dental biofilm, fractured calculus, hemorrhage products (controversial endotoxin detoxicification of root surfaces).

b. **Cavitation:** fine mist around the tip of power-driven scaler, which consists of small bubbles.

(1) From the bubbles bursting to produce the mist.

(2) When occurs near microorganisms, causes small shock wave that can disrupt or lyse bacterial cell walls.

c. Acoustic (micro) streaming: fluid flow exerts considerable force and turbulence.

(1) Can disrupt cell walls and kill microorganisms.

(2) MOST effective on highly motile organisms.

4. SIMILAR action as ultrasonic bath for instrument processing; healing is comparable between power-driven and manual instrumentation.

5. Furcations at Class II and III can be MORE effectively treated with power-driven instruments than with manual instruments.

F. Comparison of power-driven to manual instrumentation:

1. Advantages of power-driven instruments:

a. Faster than manual debridement.

b. Require light (featherlike) touch SIMILAR to probing:

(1) Easier to establish finger rest (fulcrum), but it is NOT used for leverage or increased power of working stroke.

(2) Less clinician fatigue and possibly less cumulative trauma disorder.

c. NO cutting edges unlike other instruments:

(1) Less soft tissue trauma, creating less discomfort and bleeding.

(2) NO need to achieve effective scaling angulation; effective in stationary position.

(3) Effective on ALL sides (less true for piezoelectric, since active mainly on lateral sides, and sonic instruments) and in any stroke direction.

(4) NO need for instrument sharpening.

d. Thinner and longer than curets in some cases to provide BETTER access to deep pockets and furcations.

e. Provides oral irrigation:

(1) Reduces microorganisms.

(2) Washes field for visibility.

(3) Improves patient comfort in many cases (warm water).

2. Disadvantages of power-driven instruments:

a. Constant water management (to control heat and clear areas difficult to access or view because of debris) and evacuation required in most cases.

b. Aerosol if produced carries microorganisms and hemorrhage products; may be health risk to certain patients.

c. Access is NOT always achievable, e.g., contact areas of mandibular anteriors.

3. Relative contraindications:

a. Respiratory and immunocompromised risk patients:

(1) Oral microorganisms will be incorporated into aerosol if produced and will be inhaled by patient.

(2) Potential for development of respiratory infection exists in susceptible patients.

b. Restorations:

(1) NOT for use on porcelain or composite restorations and implants unless implant tips are used (either fixed or with disposable plastic covers).

(2) May be used on adjacent tooth structure, but all margins of restorations SHOULD be avoided unless purpose is to remove amalgam overhang.

c. NOT for use on demineralized areas: may remove or damage weakened tooth structure.

d. MORE uncomfortable for patients with pronounced gag reflex and obligatory mouth breathers.

e. Vibrations may be uncomfortable on sensitive roots; may remove smear layer over dentinal tubules, creating dentinal hypersensitivity.

f. Children:

(1) Newly erupted teeth MORE susceptible to damage from vibrations.

(2) Large pulp chambers of primary teeth may be MORE heat sensitive.

g. BEST to discontinue use if patient reports discomfort; substitute manual instrumentation; have deaf patient turn off hearing aids.

4. NO contraindication for cardiac pacemakers; older ones that were unshielded presented problem, but now ALL shielded; if any questions, obtain medical consult.

5. Patient and insert preparation:

a. Provide information to patient about the procedure; drape patient to protect from aerosol spray.

b. Follow standard precautions; use preprocedural antimicrobial rinse.

c. Lubricate O-ring (if present) with water; seat tip or insert into handpiece with gentle push-twist motion.

d. Adjust power for effective debris removal, tip selected, and patient comfort.

CLINICAL STUDY

Age	44 YRS	SCENARIO
Sex	☒ Male ☐ Female	Patient presents with generalized pocket depths of 4 to 5 mm and slight vertical bone loss. There is a large band of heavy stained calculus on the lingual of his mandibular anterior teeth. Radiographs reveal amalgam overhangs on #3 and #14. The dental hygienist is debating whether to use an ultrasonic scaler on him but then decides to use it, at least for the initial debridement of the scheduled quadrant of nonsurgical periodontal therapy. The patient also told the dental hygienist that he does not have a lot of time to sit in the dental chair today as he is due in court. When tooth #7 was instrumented, the patient felt very sensitive.
Height	5'10"	
Weight	235 LBS	
BP	120/82	
Chief Complaint	"I am sorry I am bleeding so much."	
Medical History	Cardiovascular disease Prehypertension	
Current Medications	Low-dose aspirin 86 mg qd	
Social History	Superior court judge Son works as a barista in a popular coffee stand, so he gets free espresso	

1. Was the ultrasonic the instrument of choice for scaling the patient's teeth? What tips should be used?
2. What type of stain does this patient have?
3. Is the ultrasonic scaler contraindicated because of medical history? Why is he bleeding? Why is he taking aspirin?
4. What should the dental hygienist do if the patient has sensitivity when the ultrasonic is used?

1. The instrument of choice for this patient was the ultrasonic scaler, since it will keep bleeding down with its less traumatic force and flush the area as it is used. It is also quicker than manual instruments and effective for removing overhangs and heavy deposits of calculus and stain, reducing time needed for polishing the stain. Using the piezoelectric with high-speed suction is best; it is the fastest of the power-driven at 25,000 to 50,000 cps. Universal or standard tips, best for higher settings, would be best for heavy deposits. Hygienist must remember that two sides of the tip are active with this ultrasonic. Should be followed up with manual scaling, if needed.

2. This patient has exogenous extrinsic stain from drinking black coffee; can become intrinsic into the dentin with wearing of tooth enamel such as with attrition or with exposure of root surface.

3. The patient's medical history does not present a contraindication for the use of the ultrasonic scaler, even with presence of cardiovascular disease (CVD). Certain older pacemakers that are unshielded were a contraindication, but now all pacemakers are shielded and do not present a problem. He is bleeding because he is on antiplatelet (low-dose [LD] aspirin) therapy for his cardiac history, thus reducing risk of thrombosis and embolism formation. American Dental Association has stated that drug therapy rarely needs to be discontinued before most dental procedures because of adverse reactions; there is a greater risk of thromboembolic events than uncontrollable bleeding if temporarily stopped. These events could increase risk that an emergency situation can occur with patient care.

4. If the patient is sensitive on one tooth, the hygienist should continue scaling unless he experiences sensitivity elsewhere. If this is the case, manual instruments should be used instead.

SELECTIVE POLISHING

Selective polishing is polishing ONLY those surfaces of the teeth that have extrinsic stain that has NOT been removed by ultrasonic or manual instrumentation when esthetics is valued by patient. Currently MOST accepted approach to polishing. Important to AVOID iatrogenic damage, which is especially important for root surfaces and restorations. This can BEST be accomplished by applying fine **grit** (particle-size) agent with cup attached to prophy angle on slow-speed handpiece and/or with air-driven polishing system. Polishing should NOT be considered routine part of the oral prophylaxis, according to the "Position Paper on Polishing" by ADHA (see CD-ROM). Many clinicians are considering polishing first *before* other instrumentation to remove loose debris and staining so as to provide a clearer field of vision while working.

• See Chapters 6, General and Oral Pathology: intrinsic stain development; 11, Clinical Treatment: extrinsic stain evaluation.

A. Purposes:
1. Improve esthetics by removal of extrinsic stain (MAIN purpose; of questionable therapeutic value).
2. Prepare tooth to receive sealants (NOT used before all sealants).
3. Meet patient's expectations and increase patient satisfaction.

B. Relative contraindication:
1. Removal of tooth structure that CANNOT be replaced:
   a. Ditching can occur when pressure on the cup is applied unevenly or excessively.

b. Repeated polishings can remove cementum, exposed dentin, and even enamel, especially interproximally, which can change dynamics of oral clearance.

c. Decalcified areas (white and/or brown spot lesions) are more rapidly abraded than intact teeth and should be NOT be polished with abrasive pastes.

d. Outermost layer of the tooth is the MOST fluoride-rich layer; if part of this layer is removed, SHOULD follow up with topical fluoride treatment.

e. Recently erupted teeth are less mineralized, making structure MORE easily removed.

2. Increased roughness to promote dental biofilm reattachment:
   a. Use of coarse agent and/or excessive pressure or use of brush attachment can cause grooving or roughening of tooth surface; especially true of the root, but even enamel can be affected.
   b. Some restorative materials, such as gold, composite, or esthetic restorations, can be scratched or dulled or even suffer loss of material with rubber-cup or brush; air-powder abrasives have been shown to damage ALL restorative materials, especially composites and other esthetic materials.

3. Polishing can cause frictional heat:
   a. Teeth with large pulp chambers, such as primary teeth, are susceptible to heat.
   b. Metal restorations can transmit heat to the pulp.
   c. Frictional heat can be reduced by:
      (1) Using light pressure against the tooth.
      (2) Rotating cup or brush at slower speed.
      (3) Decreasing duration of time of contact between the tooth and cup or brush.
      (4) Using agent with sufficient wetness to slide over the tooth surface.

4. Contamination from microorganisms:
   a. Bacteremia (bacteria in blood) may lead to gingival inflammation.
   b. Aerosol containing microorganisms is created by ALL rotary instruments, especially by air-powered abrasive system.
   c. To reduce contamination:
      (1) Use of safety glasses by patient and clinician; preprocedural antimicrobial mouthrinse.
      (2) Complete coverage of clinical surfaces; posttreatment surface decontamination.

5. Effect of the abrasive agent: abrasive particles can be forced into the pocket or even into the tissue itself.
   a. When treating patients who have deep pockets or need extensive instrumentation, polishing

precedes scaling or takes place later at reevaluation appointment to prevent agent from being introduced into the tissue and causing further inflammation.

    b. Few individuals have negative reaction either to the fluoride in commercial pastes or to abrasive particles or other components of agent.

C. Polishing methods (older method was by porte polisher, a wooden stick held in metal handle that was rubbed on tooth with agent; may be able to pick one up on eBay or see on "Antiques Roadshow"!):

  1. Rubber cup or brush is attached to prophy angle on slow-speed handpiece.

    a. Advantage: BEST method of working agent over the tooth surface.

    b. Disadvantages (see earlier discussion):

      (1) Greater speed can cause excessive abrasion to tooth surface, resulting in loss of tooth structure and ditching if the force on cup is applied unevenly.

      (2) Frictional heat can be generated and can cause discomfort to patient.

      (3) Care must be taken NOT to traumatize gingival tissues or pulp.

    c. Equipment:

      (1) Slow-speed handpiece provides rotational energy to power movement of angle.

      (2) Prophy angle:

        (a) Right-angled or contra-angled attachment that attaches to the handpiece and holds agent, usually a rubber cup, bristle brush, or rubber polishing point.

        (b) Available as either disposable product or reusable product that can be sterilized between uses.

      (3) Polishing device moves agent over the tooth surface.

        (a) Rubber cup has hollow center to hold agent and thin edges that flare to adapt to various smooth tooth surfaces; flexes slightly to conform interproximally.

        (b) Bristle brush and agent are used for occlusal surfaces and concave areas of the tooth; must NOT be used near the gingiva (controversial).

        (c) Rubber polishing points can apply polishing abrasive to interproximal surfaces if there is adequate space (controversial).

        (d) Dental floss or tape can work the abrasive over interproximal surfaces (controversial).

      (4) Abrasive agent:

        (a) Abrasive quality is controlled by size of abrasive particle, with smallest particles the least abrasive, and chemical and physical properties of the abrasive being used (e.g., hardness, particle shape, fracture, wear characteristics).

        (b) Pumice and silicone dioxide are COMMON agents.

        (c) Agent must always be used in a moist paste form, NOT dry.

        (d) Some rubber cups are already impregnated with silica pumice granules.

    d. Technique for rubber cup or brush:

      (1) Use LEAST abrasive agent that will remove stain; do NOT use anything coarser than medium grit; fine grit is BEST (Plus-type is very coarse).

      (2) Use slowly rotating cup to apply the agent; use light pressure; do NOT allow the cup to remain on the same area of the tooth.

      (3) Keep the cup parallel to the tooth surface to avoid grooving the surface, especially at the cervical area.

      (4) Keep the duration of contact between tooth and cup to a minimum; flex the cup to adapt the cup edges into the interproximals.

      (5) Rinse (irrigate) and suction (high-speed, high-volume evacuator [HVE] BEST) the patient frequently.

      (6) Adapt brush bristles to work the polishing agent into the grooves of the occlusal surfaces.

      (7) Use dental floss and polishing agent to clean interproximals (controversial).

  2. **Air-powder polish** (air-abrasive polish, air polishing [AP]): system that uses special air-powered machine to deliver slurry that contains abrasive sodium bicarbonate powder, water, and air; powder products of aluminum trihydroxide or calcium carbonate are also available, as well as glycine powder air polishing (GPAP) with LESS abrasive qualities.

    a. Advantages:

      (1) BEST for removing extrinsic stain quickly and effectively.

      (2) Places LESS stress on clinician's hand and wrist (less pressure and manipulation) than rubber cup or porte polishing.

      (3) Possible LESS damage to tooth surface than is caused by manual instruments or rubber-cup polish.

      (4) BETTER than rubber-cup polish to prepare occlusal surfaces for some types of sealants.

      (5) May use GPAP within periodontal pockets up to 4 mm to remove subgingival biofilm during PM.

b. Disadvantages:
   (1) Causes transient irritation to gingiva NOT lasting more than few days (not dissimilar to rubber cup polishing if accidentally contacting soft tissue) if using more abrasive powders.
   (2) Produces aerosol that contains BOTH sodium bicarbonate (if used) or other powder ingredients and oral microorganisms with potential to be inhaled by both patient and clinician and spread to clinical surfaces (up to 6 feet).
   (3) See earlier discussion on contraindications and precautions for list of specific medical conditions.
   (4) More abrasive powders have been shown to alter or damage restorative materials, especially composites and porcelain; may want to use less abrasive powders (need to check with manufacturers).
   (5) Still does NOT remove calculus; need other forms of hard deposit removal; many use AP, especially GPAP, at start of PM to provide a clearer field of vision while working.
c. Equipment (Prophy-jet, Cavijet-combined Cavitron):
   (1) Uses air pressure from dental unit to propel slurry of water, sodium bicarbonate, air through small nozzlelike opening.
   (2) Disposable aerosol reduction device is attached to evacuation system at one end and fits over the nozzle of device at the other end; adapted to the tooth surface and captures aerosol so it can be suctioned away (BEST to use high-speed suction, high-volume evacuator [HVE]).
d. Technique: BOTH patient and clinician wear protective eyewear and drapes or garments (personal protective equipment [PPE]).
   (1) Patients SHOULD remove contact lenses and protect lips with application of lubricant.
   (2) CORRECT tip angulation decreases aerosol creation; incorrect angulation is MOST common cause of excess aerosol production:
       (a) For anteriors, tip is directed at 60° toward facial and lingual surfaces.
       (b) For posteriors, tip is directed at 80° toward facial and lingual surfaces.
       (c) For occlusal surfaces, tip is directed at 90° to occlusal plane.
   (3) Rapid, sweeping strokes are used with the tip held about 4 to 5 mm from tooth surface.
       (4) Spray is angled away from gingival margin.
       (5) Polishing for 5 seconds or less per tooth is usually adequate for stain removal.
3. Absolute contraindication:
   a. Because of possible systemic absorption of sodium bicarbonate powder (if used) for patients with a medical history of:
      (1) Hypertension (high blood pressure [HBP]), need for low-sodium diet, renal insufficiency.
      (2) Addison's disease, Cushing's syndrome, metabolic alkalosis.
      (3) Taking mineralocorticoid steroids, antidiuretics, or potassium supplements.
   b. Because of inhalation of abrasive particles (if used) and/or microbially contaminated aerosol for a patient with a history of:
      (1) Respiratory and infectious diseases.
      (2) Immunological diseases and immunosuppression therapy.
   c. Because of damage inflicted by abrasives (if used), NOT on unhealthy periodontium and/or restorative materials, especially composites and other esthetic materials; abrasion may be reduced by use of LESS abrasive powders.

Instrument Processing

Care MUST be taken during instrument processing to ensure that reusable instruments are safely cleaned and sterilized. Instruments MUST be exposed to all three parameters of sterilization: time, temperature, and presence of steam, as well as weekly spore testing to ensure effective sterilization.
- See Chapter 8, Microbiology and Immunology: infection control procedures, standard precautions, surface disinfection, sharps, and waste handling.
A. Cleaning instruments:
   1. Manual cleaning (hand scrubbing): BEST for instruments that would be damaged if exposed to ultrasonic cleaner (i.e., some handpieces); with multiple-use utility (heavy rubber or neoprene) and personal protective equipment (PPE).
   2. Ultrasonic cleaner (bath) should MAINLY be used, safer than manual cleaning, and instruments SHOULD be handled with multiple-use utility (heavy rubber or neoprene) gloves and PPE.
      a. Sonicating for time recommended by manufacturer (1 to 10 minutes); cassettes take longer (15 minutes).
      b. Acts MAINLY by physical agitation (cavitation with tiny bubbles forming and collapsing, SAME as ultrasonic scaler) and chemical action (solution helps dissolve organic residue).

c. Overloading SHOULD be prevented; solution MUST contact all surfaces.

d. Instruments with detachable parts SHOULD be disassembled; hinged instruments MUST be opened.

3. Instruments SHOULD be rinsed and allowed to air dry (if towel drying, carefully pat dry).

B. Packaging instruments: using bags or wrapped cassettes, BOTH sealed with indicator tape (chemical monitoring) designed for type of sterilization process, steam or heat, being used; improper packaging can melt, char, or even prevent sterilizing agent from reaching instrument pack contents, or may release unwanted chemicals into sterilizer chamber.

C. Sterilizing instruments (Table 12-2):

1. Instruments SHOULD be sterilized if they can be (includes new instruments); otherwise disposable SHOULD be used; weekly spore testing (biological monitoring) SHOULD be done as indicated, ONLY way to determine whether sterilization has occurred (see discussion next).

2. Moist heat (steam under pressure) using autoclave: at 15 lb/in^2, generates temperature of 121° C at 15 to 20 minutes.

a. Requires that instruments have space around them to enable steam to reach ALL surfaces and tight seal against the outside to provide necessary pressure and temperature.

b. Advantages: any item can be sterilized, depending on nature of materials and load.

c. Disadvantages: inability of some instruments to withstand the heat (plastics melt); possibility of corroding and pitting high-carbon steel instruments, slightly dulling sharp instruments; inability to penetrate oils or powders; distilled water SHOULD be used instead of tap water, which often contains minerals and impurities; this can minimize corrosion and pitting.

d. Quick turnover steam (flash) sterilization (e.g., Statim, Kwikclave sterilizer):
   (1) Uses GREATER pressure and heat than traditional steam sterilizers.
   (2) Sterilizes unwrapped instruments in 3 to 12 minutes; should be used ONLY for instruments that are to be used promptly on removal.

3. Chemical vapor (chemiclave, MDT): uses combination of chemicals (alcohol, formaldehyde, ketone, acetone, water) instead of water to create vapor for sterilizing in 20 minutes.

a. Gas vapors MUST penetrate instrument packaging; requires purchasing manufacturer's chemical solution; increases sterilization costs.

b. Advantages: BEST for corrosion- and rust-free operation and keeps instruments sharp; ease of operation; quick drying of instruments.

c. Disadvantages: use of hazardous chemicals; MUST have adequate ventilation because of chemicals.

4. Dry heat (oxidation) (dryclave): electric dry air oven requires materials to be exposed to a temperature of 180° C for 1 to 2 hours.

a. Used for instruments that CANNOT be sterilized safely by steam autoclave and is BEST for oils and powders if stable at temperatures reached during sterilization and for sharp instruments such as for surgery.

b. Depends on rapid heat transfer from circulating air to instruments (similar to cooking oven).

c. Advantages: maintenance of sharp edges on instruments, noncorrosiveness, and usefulness on materials unable to withstand steam under pressure.

d. Disadvantages: LESS efficient than moist heat, requires longer exposure and higher

Table 12-2 Methods of sterilization and related spore testing agents

Method	Time	Temperature	Pressure (psi)	Weekly spore testing
Moist heat (steam autoclave): standard	15-20 min	250° F 121° C	15	*Bacillus stearothermophilus*
Moist heat (steam autoclave): quick	3-12 min	270° F 130° C	30	
Chemical vapor (chemiclave)	20 min	270° F 130° C	20-40	*Bacillus stearothermophilus*
Dry heat (oven): standard	1-2 hr	320° F 160° C	—	*Bacillus subtilis*
Dry heat (oven): quick	8-12 min	375° F 190° C	—	
Ethylene oxide	10-16 hr to 24-48 hr	Room temperature	—	*Bacillus subtilis*

temperatures, careful loading to ensure sterilization, inability of unwrapped instruments to stay sterile for long.
  e. Quick sterilization using dry heat (e.g., Cox):
    (1) Maintains internal heat at 375° F.
    (2) Sterilizes wrapped instruments in 12 minutes, dental handpieces in 8 minutes.
    (3) Continuously ready; requires NO warm-up time.
  5. Ethylene oxide (toxic gas): major gaseous sterilant for sterilizing nonbiological materials at room temperature, metal 10 to 16 hours, nonmetal 24 to 48 hours.
    a. Primarily in hospitals and larger clinics; is NOT used in dental offices.
    b. Advantages: effectiveness without damaging MOST instruments, use of low temperatures for effective sterilization, and ability to penetrate different wrapping materials.
    c. Disadvantages: longer processing times, high cost of equipment, use of hazardous chemicals.
  6. Chemical sterilants and disinfectants (cold sterilization):
    a. MUST be approved by Environmental Protection Agency (EPA) as a high-level disinfectant to be used for semicritical items.
    b. Reserved ONLY for items (noncritical, semicritical) that CANNOT withstand heat sterilization; are NOT a substitute for sterilization by steam, dry heat, chemical vapor, or ethylene oxide.
    c. To achieve high-level disinfection, items MUST be immersed for long periods, 6 to 10 hours; may be used ONLY for 28 to 30 days.
    d. LEAST used because of inability to verify sterilization of instruments.
    e. CANNOT be used on packaged instruments; thus maintaining "sterile" state is difficult; after immersion, instruments MUST be rinsed with sterile water, dried, and stored in sterile containers.
    f. Contain chemicals that are toxic to patients and dental healthcare personnel (DHCP).
D. Specific dental equipment processing: note that specific areas of instrument processing area need to be specifically laid out to ensure effective processing such as demarcating contaminated and sterile areas.
  1. Handpieces:
    a. MUST be appropriately sterilized for patient protection.
    b. Some handpieces can be heat sterilized; this SHOULD be a priority when purchasing.
    c. Handpieces that CANNOT be adequately sterilized require a compromise in the office infection control plan.
    d. May be damaged by disinfectants used in the dental office (i.e., fiberoptic handpieces).

    e. MUST be maintained and sterilized according to the manufacturer's instructions to maximize the life of the handpiece.
  2. Prophy angles, contra-angles, air-water syringes:
    a. MUST be sterilized to prevent transmission of infectious agents from patient to patient.
    b. SHOULD be kept in sufficient supply; treatment areas SHOULD contain several replacement pieces to facilitate sterilization of contaminated handpieces and air-water syringes.
    c. MUST be maintained and sterilized according to manufacturer's instructions to maximize life of the equipment.
    d. Consideration SHOULD be given to use of disposables:
      (1) Reusable prophy angles:
        (a) MUST be taken apart before sterilization.
        (b) Lubricated according to manufacturer's recommendations, before and after sterilization.
      (2) Reusable air-water syringes:
        (a) MUST be thoroughly flushed before sterilization.
        (b) Some types are autoclavable (BOTH syringe and tips).
    e. May have interchangeable tips that can be sterilized.
  3. Ultrasonic tips: when sterilized in dryclave and NOT with steam, the rubber O-ring (if present) dries out, becomes ineffective, and needs replacing or leakage will occur.
E. Storing instruments:
  1. Instruments SHOULD be cooled before being stored.
  2. Instruments SHOULD be stored in coverings such as bags or wrapped cassettes to preserve sterility for future procedures and NOT free and uncovered.
  3. Instruments MUST be stored in a clean, dry drawer or shelf, with door to promote instrument sterility.
F. Contamination events: moisture exposure, holes in packaging, even dust on pouch may contaminate instruments when pouch is opened; any event requires repackaging and resterilizing instruments before use.

Biological Monitoring of Sterilization Process

Weekly biological monitoring of the sterilization process MUST be performed to ensure that the process is effective. The CDC requires dental offices to verify proper functioning of sterilization cycles on weekly basis, using biological indicators.
A. Indicator types:
  1. Chemical (heat-sensitive) indicators verify ONLY that sterilizing conditions of correct temperature have been reached, NOT that sterilization has been

achieved; used with indicator tapes on paper sterilization bags or wrapped cassettes when packaging instruments (indicated by lines turning black).

2. Biological indicators containing specific organisms are the ONLY way to verify that sterilization of the chamber contents has been achieved when spores contained in the biological indicator are destroyed; used because they can withstand chemical and mechanical forces but NOT sterilization.
   a. *Bacillus stearothermophilus* spores: autoclave and chemiclave sterilizers.
   b. *Bacillus subtilis* spores: dry heat and ethylene oxide sterilizers.

B. Spore testing (using biological indicators discussed above):
   1. Indicated once a week or during the training of new instrument processing staff.
   2. Whenever new packaging material is tried, when new sterilizer is used, after a sterilizer has been repaired.
   3. When different method of loading the sterilizer is employed.
   4. Vary placement of spore test in sterilizer chamber to confirm that sterilization occurs in all areas.

C. Records of the process and results of biological monitoring MUST be kept to comply with federal regulations and to provide documentation in case of a liability suit.

CLINICAL STUDY

Scenario: A dental hygienist is working as a temporary employee through an agency. When she goes to get instruments out of the drawer, she finds that the autoclave bag markings have turned color but some instruments have been stored without coverings. She goes to use the instruments and notices that there are dried-on blood deposits on some of the tips. She also notices that the disposable air-water syringe tips are in the cold solution but are being used frequently all day long. All this disturbs her. When she goes to sterilize her instruments in the autoclave, the other dental hygienist tells her to put them on top of the autoclave, next to the dryclave, and they will be taken care of later. The dental hygienist has a problem with this but follows instructions. She also notices that the O-rings on the Cavitron tips are wearing out and there is leakage when she uses it. Update: she is very disappointed in this office, will not work there again, and will let the temporary agency know of her concerns.

1. Is the fact that the autoclave bag has changed color proof of proper autoclaving? Why does it bother her that the instruments are stored without coverings?
2. What should she do with the air-water tips to ensure that they are in fact sterile?
3. What should she do to ensure that there is no dried blood left on instruments that she uses?

4. What could be the cause for the O-ring of the ultrasonic showing wear?
5. Her ethical principle of wanting sterile instruments for her patients demonstrates what type of ethical principle?

1. Bag color change (black stripes) indicates only that instruments were exposed to heat such as being laid on top of the autoclave; it is a type of chemical indicator only (like instrument tape) and not a biological indicator (such as a spore indicator) that indicates sterilization. Instrument processing areas should be carefully laid out, and there should be specified areas where contaminated instruments are placed to ensure proper handling. Instruments should be stored in coverings such as bags and wrapped cassettes to preserve sterility for future procedures and should not be kept free and uncovered.

2. She should keep them in the cold sterile (chemical disinfectant) for at least 6 to 10 hours to achieve disinfection, depending on the manufacturer's instructions, or ask if they can be disposed of; such methods cannot be used on critical instruments. Since the tips are disposable, that means that they are plastic and cannot be put into the autoclave or dryclave because they will melt.

3. She should be sure to use ultrasonic cleaner for all instruments for 1 to 10 minutes (or 15 minutes for cassettes). This will ensure that debris (such as blood) is loosened up and will not dry on instruments when they are put in autoclave or dryclave, preventing the instrument from being fully sterilized.

4. Appears that these were sterilized in dryclave, not one with steam, thus drying out the O-rings; if this continues, the instrument tips will be ineffective and need replacement of the rubber O-rings or leakage will occur during use.

5. She is demonstrating nonmaleficence; this is the belief that the action is wrong if harm is inflicted on others.

Review Questions

1 Correct clinician and patient positioning should have all of the following advantages for the clinician, EXCEPT one. Which one is the EXCEPTION?
   A. Reduces the chance of upper body pain and/or injury for the clinician
   B. Reduces the number of instruments needed to complete a full-mouth debridement
   C. Improves visibility of the treatment area
   D. Reduces the possibility that the patient might faint during treatment

2 A well-positioned patient should present with which of the following situations?

A. Top of the head at the top of the dental chair

B. Feet higher than head and heart

C. Head turned to the right for a right-handed clinician

D. Chair back at about a 45° angle, if the patient has a strong gag reflex

3 When the maxillary arch is treated, the patient is typically asked to tilt the chin downward (or chair back is slightly raised) to improve access and visibility. When the mandibular arch is treated, the patient is positioned with the maxilla perpendicular to the floor for maximum access and visibility.

A. Both statements are true.

B. Both statements are false.

C. The first statement is true, the second is false.

D. The first statement is false, the second is true.

4 All of the following are true of the principles of correct clinician positioning, EXCEPT one. Which one is the EXCEPTION?

A. Both feet are kept on the floor except when seated at 7 or 8 o'clock position, and the inside leg is crossed over the outside leg to allow seating closer to the patient for improved access.

B. The feet and legs are kept apart to create a more stable seated position on the stool.

C. The stool height is adjusted so that the clinician's thighs are parallel to the floor.

D. The body is seated to the back of the stool so that the spine is supported by the back rest.

5 The incidence of occupational injury can be reduced by the use of good body mechanics. Which one of the following is NOT good use of body mechanics?

A. Keeping the shoulders relaxed and even

B. Keeping the upper arms near the body and the forearms parallel to the floor

C. Tilting forward and hyperextending the neck to improve visibility

D. Keeping the patient's mouth at a comfortable focal distance of about 15 inches from the clinician's eye

6 Curet Q has a shank with complex angles and is designed for use in periodontal pockets. Curet Q is excellent for removal of light deposits. Which design characteristic would need to be changed for instrument Q to be effective in removing moderate deposits?

A. Thickness of the shank

B. Length of the lower (terminal) shank

C. Toe of the blade

D. Length of the blade

E. Back of the blade

7 A well-balanced instrument MUST be designed with which of the following?

A. Two cutting edges

B. Two mirror-imaged working ends, one on each end of the handle

C. Straight or simple shank

D. Middle of the working end centered on the long axis of the instrument handle

8 Mirrors are used for many purposes, including soft tissue retraction, indirect vision, indirect illumination, and transillumination. Transillumination is the illumination of a dark area of the mouth by bouncing light off the mirror face.

A. Both statements are true.

B. Both statements are false.

C. The first statement is true, the second is false.

D. The first statement is false, the second is true.

9 The cross-sectional shape of the working end of various instruments helps define the category and function of the instrument. All are correctly matched between instrument type and cross-sectional shape, EXCEPT one. Which one is the EXCEPTION?

A. Explorer—circle

B. Universal curet—half moon

C. Sickle—triangle

D. Area-specific curet—ellipse

10 The primary instruments for assessment of the periodontal status and dental hygiene treatment needs of a patient are various explorers and probes. A Nabor's probe is designed specifically for identifying and determining the characteristics of furcations.

A. Both statements are true.

B. Both statements are false.

C. The first statement is true, the second is false.

D. The first statement is false, the second is true.

11 Which of the following would be the BEST choice for removal of calculus around the contacts and adjacent interproximal areas of the mandibular anterior teeth?

A. Sickle scaler

B. Universal curet

C. Area-specific curet

D. Chisel

12 Universal curets and area-specific curets share a number of design features, EXCEPT one. Which of the ones below is the EXCEPTION?

A. Rounded toe and rounded back

B. Two cutting edges per working end

C. Simple shanks for anterior teeth and complex shanks for posterior teeth

D. Paired, mirror-imaged working ends

13 Which of the following area-specific curets was designed to treat the mesial surfaces of posterior teeth?

A. Gracey 5-6

B. Gracey 11-12

C. Gracey 13-14

D. Gracey 17-18

14 Instruments designed for the debridement of implants usually

A. should be made of plastic.

B. are standard metal instruments.

C. have unique shapes.

D. cause light scratches on the surface.

15 All of the following are true of the modified pen grasp EXCEPT one. Which one is the EXCEPTION?
   A. Thumb and middle finger are placed opposite each other on the handle.
   B. Handle rests between the thumb and the second joint of the index finger.
   C. Ring finger rests against the middle finger and is used as the fulcrum finger.
   D. Pad of the middle finger rests on the instrument.

16 All of the following are true of fulcrums, EXCEPT one. Which one is the EXCEPTION?
   A. Effective use of a fulcrum can increase control over the working stroke.
   B. Ring finger is also called the fulcrum finger.
   C. Extraoral fulcrum should be used whenever possible.
   D. Fulcrum is a mechanical leverage.

17 The optimum angle of the instrument face to the tooth surface for scaling is between 45° and 60°. The optimum angle for root planing is 70° to 80°.
   A. Both statements are true.
   B. Both statements are false.
   C. First statement is true, the second is false.
   D. First statement is false, the second is true.

18 What is the range of movement at the tip of the working end for MOST sonic scalers?
   A. 2500 to 7000 cycles/sec
   B. 18,000 to 45,000 cycles/sec
   C. 35,000 to 50,000 cycles/sec
   D. 18,000 to 50,000 cycles/sec

19 The two types of machines for ultrasonic scaling are the magnetostrictive and piezoelectric. Magnetostrictive ultrasonics convert electrical power to tip movement through magnetic oscillations and have a generally elliptical pattern of tip movement, whereas piezoelectric units use a crystal to convert electricity to movement and generally have a linear pattern of tip movement.
   A. Both statements are true.
   B. Both statements are false.
   C. First statement is true, the second is false.
   D. First statement is false, the second is true.

20 Slim- or thin-style ultrasonic tips are the BEST choice for which kinds of deposits?
   A. Heavy and light calculus
   B. Heavy calculus
   C. Light calculus
   D. All deposits

21 When beginning ultrasonic instrumentation on a tooth with both supragingival and subgingival calculus, one would typically begin on the more apical calculus and end with the more coronal. Subgingival calculus removal is at least as effective with ultrasonic instruments as with manual instruments if one is thorough with both.
   A. Both statements are true.
   B. Both statements are false.
   C. First statement is true, the second is false.
   D. First statement is false, the second is true.

22 In deep, narrower pockets and hard to reach subgingival areas, curets are the instrument of choice. Because ultrasonic tips do NOT have a specific cutting edge, there is no need to achieve a specific face to tooth working angle as with a curet or sickle scaler.
   A. Both statements are true.
   B. Both statements are false.
   C. First statement is true, the second is false.
   D. First statement is false, the second is true.

23 While NOT essential for successful treatment, both a standard pen grasp and a soft tissue fulcrum are recommended for use with ultrasonic instrumentation because they
   A. foster a lighter working stroke.
   B. improve penetration of fluid to the base of the pocket.
   C. are gentler to the soft tissue.
   D. prevent clinician fatigue.

24 Why is it critical that the point of the ultrasonic tip never be adapted to the root surface?
   A. Can gouge and permanently damage the root surface
   B. Generates too much heat
   C. Not effective in deposit removal
   D. Uncomfortable for the clinician

25 What is the MAIN reason instrumentation with an ultrasonic scaler takes less time than manual instrumentation?
   A. Fewer strokes are needed.
   B. Clinician tires less easily.
   C. Less pressure is needed.
   D. Strokes are performed more quickly.

26 All of the following may be considered a contraindication to the use of an ultrasonic scaler, EXCEPT one. Which one is the EXCEPTION?
   A. Decalcified tooth surface
   B. Obligatory mouth breather
   C. Shielded pacemaker
   D. Newly erupted teeth

27 During ultrasonic scaling, the clinician should wear
   A. eye protection and a facial mask.
   B. eye protection and a facial shield.
   C. a facial shield and a facial mask.
   D. a facial shield, eye protection, and a facial mask.

28 When the instrument is used with reasonable skill and care, which of the following is generally considered acceptable to treat with an ultrasonic scaler?
   A. Amalgam
   B. Composite
   C. Porcelain-fused-to-metal crown
   D. Esthetic veneer

29 Which of the following is the BEST rationale for polishing?
   A. Brightening the patient's teeth and smile
   B. Removing extrinsic stain
   C. Removing calculus accumulations
   D. Giving the patient's mouth a clean, fresh feeling

30 As a regular part of oral prophylaxis, selective polishing has replaced full-mouth polishing for all of the following reasons, EXCEPT one. Which one is the EXCEPTION?
  A. Repeated polishing can remove cementum, dentin, and even enamel.
  B. Dental biofilm can be removed by other, less damaging means.
  C. Fluoride-rich layer is removed.
  D. Treatment time is reduced.

31 Which of the following is a potential problem caused by polishing?
  A. Creation of a bacteremia as a result of abrasive particles being absorbed systemically
  B. Allergy to ingredients of commercial polishing pastes, which is more common than is generally believed
  C. Creation of a microbial-laden aerosol that is inhaled by the patient and spread to surrounding surfaces
  D. Vaporization of mercury during amalgam polishing procedures, even when correct technique is used

32 In a rubber-cup polishing system, the slow-speed handpiece causes the shaft to rotate in the prophy angle, which causes the rubber cup to turn and move the polishing abrasive over the tooth surface. Regardless of the polishing system used, it is the abrasive agent that produces the polishing action.
  A. Both statements are true.
  B. Both statements are false.
  C. First statement is true, the second is false.
  D. First statement is false, the second is true.

33 In an air-powder polishing system, polishing is produced by a mixture containing abrasive particles to clean the tooth, water to prevent heating and to dilute the abrasive, and air to provide force to deliver the abrasive to the tooth surface. This system causes more damage to composites and to tooth surfaces than other methods of stain removal.
  A. Both statements are true.
  B. Both statements are false.
  C. First statement is true, the second is false.
  D. First statement is false, the second is true.

34 To make air-powder polishing MORE effective and comfortable, the angle of the tip to the tooth is important. What are the recommended angles?
  A. Anterior teeth 40° and posterior teeth 60°
  B. Anterior teeth 60° and posterior teeth 80°
  C. Anterior teeth 80° and posterior teeth 40°
  D. Anterior teeth 45° and posterior teeth 15°

35 All of the following are true of sharpened instruments, EXCEPT one. Which is the EXCEPTION?
  A. Less pressure needed to remove the deposit
  B. More likely to slip during instrumentation
  C. Less chance of occupational injury
  D. More likely to produce a clean tooth surface

36 The cutting edges of scaling instruments dull with use. Dull cutting edges are less effective in removing deposits than are sharp cutting edges.
  A. Both statements are true.
  B. Both statements are false.
  C. First statement is true, the second is false.
  D. First statement is false, the second is true.

37 Which of the following BEST indicates that an instrument is dull?
  A. The instrument grabs at the root surface.
  B. Light does not reflect off the cutting edge.
  C. Over 10 working strokes have been taken.
  D. Calculus is being burnished.

38 Which of the following is CORRECT statement describing an Arkansas stone?
  A. Natural stone that should be lubricated with oil before use and can only be chemically sterilized
  B. Synthetic stone that does not need to be lubricated before use and can be sterilized by any means
  C. Natural stone that should be lubricated with oil before use and can be sterilized by any means
  D. Synthetic stone that should be lubricated with water before use and can be sterilized by any means

39 Which of the following is the MOST abrasive sharpening stone?
  A. Ceramic stone
  B. Arkansas stone
  C. India stone
  D. All have similar abrasive grit

40 Which one of the following is NOT a general principle of instrument sharpening?
  A. The angle between the instrument face and the stone is about 110°.
  B. The original shape of the instrument should be preserved.
  C. Metal is removed equally from the lateral surface and the face.
  D. The internal angle of the cutting blade of a curet or a sickle scaler MUST be maintained at about 70°.

41 A wire edge is a projection that forms as metal particles are burnished to form an extension beyond the surface being sharpened. It is important to prevent the formation of a wire edge because it is difficult to remove after it is created.
  A. Both statements are true.
  B. Both statements are false.
  C. First statement is true, the second is false.
  D. First statement is false, the second is true.

42 When the lateral sides of a sickle are sharpened with an instrument-stable technique,
  A. the face of the instrument is positioned so that it is parallel with the floor or countertop.
  B. a face-to-stone angle of about 70° is established.
  C. the stone is moved in an up-and-down motion ending on the upstroke.
  D. the stone should not rotate or move in any way except up and down.

43 When comparing sharpening technique between a universal and a Gracey curet for an instrument-stable technique, which of the following remains the same?
  A. Rotation of the stone on its long axis is usually the same.
  B. Stone position or angulation is the same.
  C. Terminal shank position is the same.
  D. Number of cutting edges sharpened is the same.

44 The rule of thumb for working on the maxillary arch is that the
   A. arch should be approximately parallel to the floor.
   B. light is positioned over the chest and shines into the mouth at an angle.
   C. arch should be positioned so that the occlusal plane is perpendicular to floor.
   D. light is positioned directly over the nose and shines onto the chin at an angle.

45 For BEST control of infection in the dental office, dental handpieces used for coronal polishing procedures should be
   A. heat sterilized.
   B. disinfected with chemical agents.
   C. sonicated in general purpose cleaner.
   D. wiped with alcohol.

46 What is the FIRST step in the process of sterilizing instruments?
   A. Storing instruments to preserve their sterility for future procedures
   B. Packaging instruments in appropriate sterilizer bags
   C. Steam-sterilizing instruments to kill bacteria, fungi, and viruses
   D. Placing instruments in the ultrasonic bath to remove debris

47 When moving instruments from the ultrasonic bath to the sink for rinsing, what type of gloves should be worn?
   A. Multiple-use utility gloves
   B. Sterile examination gloves
   C. Nonsterile examination gloves
   D. Plastic overgloves

48 After prophylaxis of an HIV-positive individual has been completed, the instruments should be
   A. soaked in household bleach.
   B. sterilized for 10 minutes longer than the standard sterilization time.
   C. sterilized using the same techniques as for all other sterilizable instruments.
   D. placed in double sterilizer bags to avoid the cross-contamination of other instruments.

49 The biological indicator *Bacillus stearothermophilus* is used to determine effective sterilization in which of the following sterilizers?
   A. Moist heat and chemical vapor
   B. Chemical vapor and dry heat
   C. Ethylene oxide and moist heat
   D. Dry heat and ethylene oxide

50 Moist heat sterilization
   A uses steam under pressure.
   B. is safe for all instruments.
   C. prevents corrosion of instruments.
   D. penetrates oils and powders.

51 Of the following methods of sterilization, which one requires the longest cycle?
   A. Moist heat
   B. Dry heat
   C. Chemical vapor
   D. Ethylene oxide

52 Biological testing during the sterilization process MUST be accomplished _____ to ensure the effectiveness of the process.
   A. daily
   B. weekly
   C. biweekly
   D. monthly

53 Shorter strokes with a scaling instrument give more control and are used for assessment (exploring). Longer strokes are typically used for deposit removal.
   A. Both statements are true.
   B. Both statements are false.
   C. The first statement is true, the second is false.
   D. The first statement is false, the second is true.

54 Cold sterilization is widely used because of its ability to verify sterilization of instruments.
   A. Both the statement and reason are correct and related.
   B. Both the statement and reason are correct but NOT related.
   C. The statement is correct, but the reason is NOT.
   D. The statement is NOT correct, but the reason is correct.
   E. NEITHER the statement NOR the reason is correct.

55 Which of the following explorers is considered BEST for caries detection?
   A. Shepherd's hook
   B. The #17 style
   C. The ODU 11/12
   D. Pigtail or cowhorn

Answer Key and Rationale

1 **(B)** Correct (good) patient and clinician positioning may improve efficiency by providing better visibility and reducing chance for upper body pain and injury to clinician. Does NOT change number of instruments needed to treat all surfaces of the teeth. Correct patient positioning reduces possibility that patient might undergo syncope (fainting) during treatment, mainly placement in supine position. Other special instances include semiupright (45° for respiratory disorders) and Trendelenburg positions (subsupine, with feet higher level than head, when syncope has occurred).

2 **(A)** Well-positioned patient SHOULD have head at the top of chair to give clinician optimum access to the mouth from all clock or zone positions. SHOULD be in a supine position MOST of the time with the head, heart, and feet at about the same level. SHOULD turn the head as needed for the clinician to have the best access. Patients with a strong gag reflex will do best in a full supine or fully upright position.

3 **(B)** Both statements are false. First statement describes CORRECT (good) patient positioning for mandibular arch, and second statement describes CORRECT (good) patient positioning for maxillary arch.

4 **(A)** Sitting with legs crossed causes stress along spine and reduces circulation to the legs. LESS stable

seated position than having the weight evenly distributed, with legs apart and back supported.

5 **(C)** BEST body position allows support by the skeletal and muscular system. Includes keeping head centered over the spine, although the chin may be tilted down slightly to look into mouth from comfortable distance away. SHOULD keep shoulders and arms down in relaxed positioned. SHOULD consider moving patient, before stressing their own bodies by awkward positioning.

6 **(A)** Thickness and rigidity of shank MOST directly influence quality of deposits (tenacity, volume) the instrument will remove. Thicker shank makes instrument more rigid and better able to remove bulky and dense deposits.

7 **(D)** Instrument is considered well balanced if relationship of working end to the handle makes the instrument comfortable to hold and easy to use. Occurs when middle of working end is centered on an imaginary line that also runs through the handle.

8 **(C)** Four functions of a mirror are soft tissue retraction, indirect vision, indirect illumination (reflected lighting), and transillumination. Illumination of a dark area of the mouth with light bounced off mirror face is indirect illumination. For transillumination, light is reflected off mirror and directed through the teeth to observe shadows caused by caries and calculus.

9 **(D)** ALL curets, whether universal or area specific, are half-moon shaped in cross section. Difference between the two is the relationship of the face to the terminal shank. Cross-sectional shape of explorer is a circle, and (sickle) scaler is a triangle.

10 **(A)** Explorers and probes are used as primary instruments of assessment. Probes, with a variety of numerical demarcations, are used to measure pocket depth, clinical attachment levels (CAL), recession, and width of attached gingiva and to determine a variety of tissue and root characteristics such as bleeding on probing (BoP) and root anatomy. Nabor's probes have a curved design that BETTER fits into furcation areas. Explorers are BEST used to identify calculus and other deposits, root texture and anatomy, pocket contours, also to identify caries and marginal status of restorations.

11 **(A)** (Sickle) scalers taper to a thin point at working end. This fits BEST the tight areas around contacts and the interproximal. BOTH types of curets have difficulty fitting into tight contact areas. Chisels (rarely used) are BEST for gross debridement of anteriors; NOT suitable for fine scaling around either contact or gingiva.

12 **(B)** Universal curets do have two cutting edges per working end; however, area-specific curets have ONLY one cutting edge per working end.

13 **(B)** Individual area-specific curets are designed to instrument a particular type of tooth, or in posteriors, even a particular tooth surface. Gracey 11-12 and 15-16 are for mesial surfaces of posteriors. Gracey 13-14 and 17-18 are for distals of same teeth. Gracey 5-6 is for any of the surfaces of anteriors and premolar teeth.

14 **(A)** It is critical that implants NOT be scratched or damaged. Plastic debridement instruments have been shown NOT to scratch, whereas standard metal instruments do scratch, May be shaped like curets or scalers (sickle scalers) or have unique shapes that specifically fit around implant surfaces.

15 **(A)** Thumb and index finger are usually placed opposite each other on the instrument handle with the middle finger placed below them on or near the instrument shank.

16 **(C)** BEST fulcrum is intraoral fulcrum placed on tooth surface near working area. Fulcrum is mechanical leverage when used for instrumentation; increases the control over working stroke. Ring finger is known as the fulcrum finger.

17 **(B)** Angles have been reversed between these statements. MORE open angle is needed for scaling of larger deposits. BEST is in range of 70° to 80°. Root planing is a finishing procedure (controversial), and the blade angle becomes progressively more closed. Optimum is 45° to 60°.

18 **(A)** MOST sonic scalers operate in the 2500 to 7000 cycles/sec range (cps). MOST magnetostrictive ultrasonics operate at 18,000 to 45,000 cps, and piezoelectric operate at 35,000 to 50,000 cps. Range of ultrasonics is from as low as 18,000 cps to high limit of 50,000 cps.

19 **(A)** All of this information is accurate and highlights MAIN difference between the two types of ultrasonics.

20 **(C)** Slim- or thin-style tips are very effective in removing light calculus, NOT as effective for heavy calculus removal as thicker tips.

21 **(D)** Ultrasonic debridement is begun at MOST coronal deposits and progresses toward more apical deposits. BOTH manual and ultrasonic instrumentation is effective in removing calculus from subgingival areas.

22 **(D)** In deep, narrower pockets and hard-to-reach areas like furcations, ultrasonics are generally considered superior instrument. Long, thin, probelike tips will reach into deep, narrow pockets easily. More advanced furcations have been shown to have lower bacterial count after ultrasonics than after manual instruments. Without a cutting edge, angulation of the face of the blade to the tooth is NOT possible, and this makes it easier to use the ultrasonic instruments. Good tip-to-tooth adaptation is still important. Treating each root as a separate tooth, if access permits, with a combination of horizontal, vertical, and oblique strokes is recommended.

23 (A) Lighter, more relaxed pen grasp and use of a soft tissue fulcrum place less pressure of the instrument tip on the tooth, and that results in therapy that is more effective and more comfortable. Each of the other answers may occur as a coincidental benefit, but improved therapy is the driving rationale. Increased options in fulcrums may lead to BETTER adaptation and therefore deeper instrumentation, which will result in deeper fluid penetration because the fluid follows the tip. Softer, lighter working stroke will be more comfortable to the patient's soft tissue, and the clinician will be more relaxed and less fatigued.

24 (A) Adapting the tip of ultrasonic against the root can result in damage to the root surface. Use of point is NOT as effective as adapting the side of the tip. Heat generation is NOT affected, and discomfort is caused to the patient but NOT the clinician.

25 (D) Comparable number of working strokes is needed to completely treat the root surface but can be taken more quickly and easily because there is NO need to establish a working angle or lateral pressure and also the strokes are effective in BOTH directions. Action of an ultrasonic stroke is easy and uniform like an eraser motion. Statements that the clinician is less tired and pressure is lighter are true but NOT the main reasons for the difference.

26 (C) Shielded pacemaker is shielded (protected) from ultrasonic action and is considered safe for treatment. Older ones were NOT shielded; ALL pacemakers today are shielded. In demineralized areas, may remove or damage weakened tooth structure. Individual who always breathes through the mouth will have difficult time breathing with the water spray in the mouth. Newly erupted teeth have large pulps that may be heat sensitive and enamel that is NOT fully mineralized.

27 (C) Ultrasonic scaling, even with high-speed suction, produces tiny, contaminated droplets in the air around the patient's mouth. Clinician MUST use barrier techniques for protection. Face shield provides the BEST eye protection but has an opening in the chin and neck area that allows aerosols access to the clinician's respiratory system. Thus facial mask is needed also to complete barrier protection for clinician.

28 (A) Amalgams can be debrided with an ultrasonic scaler if care is used. It is TRUE that amalgam can be removed; in fact, power-driven scalers are BEST instrument to use for overhang removal, but the same could be said of a scaler (sickle scaler). Composites have shown surface damage from ultrasonic instrumentation. Porcelain-fused-to-metal crowns and esthetic veneers can be fractured or loosened with ultrasonic use.

29 (B) Polishing is an option for removing extrinsic stain. Will brighten the teeth ONLY, if stain is present.

Polishing will BOTH remove dental biofilm (dental plaque) and give the mouth a clean feeling; however, potentially damaging to the teeth if repeated too often and there are other LESS potentially harmful methods of accomplishing these tasks, such as demonstration of toothbrushing and other oral hygiene methods, use of ultrasonics, and light manual instrumentation.

30 (D) Time is NOT reduced because dental biofilm MUST be removed by alternative means. Selective polishing is BETTER than general polish because it is more protective of the tooth surface. Repeated polishing can remove tooth structure, especially fluoride-rich surface layer. Biofilm removal, traditional reason for polish, can be accomplished by other methods that have less potential to damage the tooth, such as demonstration of toothbrushing and other oral hygiene methods, use of ultrasonics, and light manual instrumentation.

31 (C) Polishing always creates microbial-containing aerosol. Bacteremia may be caused when inflamed gingiva is polished, and oral bacteria, NOT abrasive particles, are introduced into the body. Allergy to commercial pastes is possible but rare. With CORRECT (good) polishing technique, including NO frictional heat, mercury should NOT be released from amalgam restorations.

32 (A) Polishing action is accomplished by the abrasive particles. Rubber cup, brush, wood stick, and force of the air in air-powder polish are ONLY a means of applying abrasive for polishing, NOT cause of the polishing. LESS abrasive powders are available for all techniques.

33 (C) First statement regarding the components and roles of the ingredients of the polishing slurry is correct. Air-powder polishing systems usually do cause MORE damage to composites because the "blasting action" removes some component of the composite material; less abrasion is possible with LESS abrasive powders. However, regarding tooth structure, air-powder polishing, no matter what powder is used, removes LESS tooth structure than curets when used to remove stain on root surfaces and causes less abrasion on enamel than rubber-cup polishing.

34 (B) For anteriors, tip of the nozzle is directed at 60° toward the tooth and at 80° toward posteriors.

35 (B) Dull, NOT sharpened, instruments are MORE likely to slip during instrumentation. Sharpening improves quality of debridement and makes treatment more comfortable and effective for BOTH patient and clinician.

36 (A) With use, metal is worn away from cutting edge, making the shape rounded at the junction of the face and lateral side where once they formed a sharp edge. Rounded cutting edge is NOT as effective in engaging and removing deposits, since it is dull.

37 (D) Dull instrument is MORE likely to slide over deposit, causing burnishing. As it dulls, will tend to slide on the tooth surface and have less bite or grab than sharp instrument. Dull or rounded surface will reflect light. Standard rule CANNOT be made about number of strokes to take before sharpening because it varies by the amount of lateral pressure being applied, nature of deposit, metal composition.

38 (C) Arkansas stone is a natural quarried stone. SHOULD be lubricated with fine oil before use and may be sterilized by any of the conventional methods, although may become MORE brittle with repeated exposures to high heat.

39 (C) India stone is MOST abrasive, with its medium grit. Although Arkansas and ceramic stones may vary somewhat, are less abrasive.

40 (C) Typically, MORE metal is removed from the lateral surface, rather than the lateral surface and the face equally, when sharpening. Besides making instrument thinner so that is fits into the sulcus more easily, it is believed that preserving the face-to-back dimension maintains instrument strength BEST for the pressures and stresses created by scaling.

41 (C) First statement is true, the second is false. First statement is accurate description of how wire edge is made. Important NOT to have wire edge when instrument is applied to a tooth because wire edge fractures easily and metal can become embedded in gingiva or root surface. Easy and equally acceptable to prevent or remove wire edge during sharpening procedures.

42 (A) Scaler (sickle scaler) is held stable with face parallel to the floor (terminal shank is perpendicular to floor). Internal angel of the curet is 70°, but visible angle that is formed between instrument face and stone is 110°. To prevent wire edge, important to end sharpening of each area with downstroke so that NO metal is burnished above the face.

43 (B) Position and the movement of stone are the same. Several other aspects are NOT the same because of differences in instrument design. Gracey curets are typically MORE curved from heel to toe, necessitating more rotation of stone on long axis. Also, because blade of Gracey is offset at 70°, the terminal shank is NOT perpendicular to floor during sharpening and ONLY one cutting edge is used (or sharpened) on each working end.

44 (C) With treatment of maxillary arch, arch SHOULD be positioned so that occlusal plane is perpendicular to floor and light is positioned over chest; light shines into mouth at an angle. With treatment of mandibular arch, the arch SHOULD be approximately parallel to floor and light positioned directly over mouth; light shines straight down.

45 (A) Dental handpieces SHOULD be heat sterilized between patients to prevent spread of infectious disease; older handpieces that CANNOT be sterilized compromise infection control procedures in dental office.

46 (D) FIRST step in sterilization of instruments is to remove debris by placing in ultrasonic cleaner (NOT manually cleaning). Instruments are then packaged in appropriate sterilization bags or wrapped cassettes after being rinsed and dried, then sterilized, allowed to cool, and stored to preserve sterility.

47 (A) Multiple-use utility gloves provide maximum clinician protection against inadvertent occupational exposures. Examination gloves and overgloves do NOT provide adequate protection for handling contaminated instruments during sonication and sterilization procedures.

48 (C) Standard Precautions (from CDC), including autoclaving instruments, are designed to protect dental healthcare personnel and patients from blood-borne pathogens and infective agents (these latter regulations and guidelines are regulated instead by OSHA). Instruments used for HIV-infected individual SHOULD be handled as ALL other autoclavable instruments are handled. NO extra time is needed, and double bagging is NOT necessary. Soaking instruments in bleach will corrode them and NOT significantly improve sterilization results.

49 (A) Moist heat (autoclave) and chemical vapor sterilizers (chemiclave) use spores of *B. stearothermophilus*. Ethylene oxide and dry heat sterilizers use spores of *B. subtilis*. BOTH are biological indicators of sterilization.

50 (A) Moist heat sterilization (autoclave) uses steam under pressure. NOT all instruments can withstand conditions in steam autoclave (e.g., metal instruments can corrode and plastics melt); does NOT penetrate oils or powders.

51 (D) Ethylene oxide requires 10 to 16 hours to be effective on metal instruments. Dry heat cycle MUST last 1 to 2 hours, and moist heat cycle MUST last 15 to 20 minutes (flash sterilization occurs in 3.4 to 12 minutes). Chemical vapor cycles require 20 minutes for effective sterilization.

52 (B) Biological testing (using spores) SHOULD occur on weekly basis to monitor effectiveness of sterilization process as required by CDC.

53 (B) Both statements are false. Shorter strokes during scaling give MORE control and deposit removal. Longer strokes are used MAINLY for assessment (exploring).

54 (E) Neither statement nor reason is correct. Cold sterilization is used less because of inability to verify sterilization of instruments.

55 (A) Shepherd's hook explorer is BEST for caries detection and restoration evaluation; the others are BEST for deposit and root surface exploration.

CHAPTER 13

Periodontology

PERIODONTIUM

Periodontium consists of gingival tissues, periodontal ligament (PDL), cementum, alveolar bone. Functions as attachment mechanism, shock absorber, line of defense against external agents; attaches the tooth to its bony housing (alveolus), provides resistance to forces of mastication, speech, and deglutition, maintains body surface integrity by separating the external and internal environment, adjusts for structural changes associated with wear and aging through continuous remodeling and regeneration, and defends against external harmful factors.

- See CD-ROM for Chapter Terms and WebLinks.
- See Chapters 2, Embryology and Histology: healthy periodontium; 6, General and Oral Pathology: periodontal lesions; 8, Microbiology and Immunology: background information; 11, Clinical Treatment: periodontal evaluation and charting; 17, Community Oral Health: epidemiology of periodontal disease.

Periodontal Diseases and Risk Factors

Periodontal (gum) diseases, including gingivitis and periodontitis, are serious infections that, left untreated, can lead to tooth loss. Periodontal pathogens alone may NOT lead to development of disease. Degree of destruction varies greatly from one individual to another, which suggests that other factors may alter host's resistance. These factors have been labeled risk factors.

Risk factors affect prevalence, incidence, severity, development of a disease—periodontal disease in this case. Some of these factors, such as genetics and age, are beyond individual's control but others, such as tobacco use or stress factors, can be modified. Even endocrine disorders, nutritional deficiencies, drug reactions, HIV status can somewhat be modified. Increased incidence of periodontal disease may in turn represent a risk factor for cardiovascular disease (CVD) or birth of preterm, low-birth-weight baby, as well as pose a serious threat to people whose health is compromised by diabetes mellitus, respiratory diseases, or osteoporosis.

A. Major background risk factors: most NOT able to modify.
  1. Age: prevalence increases directly with increasing age as a result of repeated inflammatory episodes during lifetime.
  2. Gender: men tend to have higher incidence than women.
  3. Race: African Americans have consistently demonstrated higher prevalence than Caucasians.
  4. Education: *inversely* related to increasing levels of education.
  5. Income: *inversely* related to increasing levels of income.
  6. Residence: slightly MORE prevalent in rural than in urban areas.
  7. Geography: NO significant differences have been noted in the United States.
B. Major systemic risk factors: MOST able to modify somewhat.
  1. Tobacco use.
  2. Endocrine disorders:
    a. Diabetes mellitus.
    b. Hyperparathyroidism.
    c. Hormonal factors.
  3. Nutritional deficiencies.
  4. Adverse drug reactions.
  5. Stress or psychosocial.
  6. HIV/AIDS.
  7. Neutrophil (polymorphonucleocyte [PMN]) abnormalities.
  8. Genetics: genetic predisposition has been related to inherited systemic diseases and to familial occurrences with some forms (e.g., Down syndrome); NOT able to modify at this time.

Tobacco Use Risk

Tobacco is the MOST important risk factor involved in periodontal disease. Nicotine and other chemicals embed on the root surface and act as toxic irritants, in addition to causing constriction of area blood vessels. Result is that tobacco users are at greater risk for periodontal disease and LEAST likely to heal after treatment. Thus it is the MOST traumatic habit for periodontium and the hardest to modify, but when tobacco ceases to be a risk factor, it is the MOST effective part of the overall therapy for periodontal disease.

- See Chapter 9, Pharmacology: tobacco cessation.
A. Tobacco smokers: always double amount the patient reports smoking and one cigar is equal to one pack of cigarettes.
  1. Tend to exhibit MORE severe levels of disease: deeper pockets, higher periodontal index scores, greater bone loss, higher rates of attachment loss,

more calculus (serves as contributing factor in dental biofilm accumulation, prevents pocket healing) than nonsmokers.

2. Increased prevalence of moderate to severe periodontal disease, directly related to number of cigarettes or cigars smoked per day, number of years, current smoking status.

3. May have altered host response to various forms of periodontal therapy.

   a. Carbon monoxide in smoking reduces oxygen concentrations, consequently inhibiting movement of WBCs in gingival sulcus into periodontium (chemokinesis, chemotaxis) and depleting capacity to engulf and destroy bacteria (phagocytosis).

   b. Smokers also have decreased levels of salivary antibodies (IgA) and serum IgG and IgM antibodies to *P. intermedia* and *F. nucleatum,* two periodontal pathogens.

4. Increased risk for recurrent/refractory periodontitis because of failure to respond to treatment (discussed later).

B. Smokeless (spit) tobacco users:

1. Have LOCAL exposure to high concentrations of tobacco products; may play role in localized attachment loss.

2. At higher risk for various forms of periodontal disease, as well as caries and oral cancer.

Endocrine Disorder Risk

Endocrine glands secrete hormones that regulate cellular metabolism and maintain physiological homeostasis. Endocrine diseases, such as diabetes mellitus and hyperparathyroidism, have been associated with greater risk of periodontitis; MOST can be modified with treatment. Fluctuations in hormones (through puberty, menstruation, pregnancy, oral contraceptives, perimenopause or menopause) have also been shown to alter tissue response to local factors and therefore are risk factors for development of gingivitis and periodontitis, although MOST changes are temporary.

- See Chapters 6, General and Oral Pathology: endocrine diseases; 11, Clinical Treatment: pregnant patient.

A. Diabetes mellitus (DM): genetically associated, debilitating endocrine disorder characterized by glucose intolerance.

1. Types:

   a. Type 1: develops before age 30; MUST be controlled with insulin therapy.

   b. Type 2: MOST common form occurs after age 40; may be controlled by diet, oral hypoglycemic agents, or LESS frequently, insulin therapy.

2. Associated with high blood glucose levels that result from decreased insulin levels and create variety of systemic effects, including vascular disease,

reduced host resistance, increased incidence of periodontal disease.

3. Defective polymorphonucleocytes (PMNs), PMN chemotaxis, microangiopathy of periodontal tissues, increased collagen breakdown, microbial alterations have been cited as rationales for periodontal disease prevalence.

4. Oral manifestations: xerostomia, candidiasis, increased caries, burning mouth, altered taste.

5. Second major risk factor *after* tobacco use, MAINLY type 1; type 2 with insulin therapy shows a SIMILAR risk.

6. In patients with uncontrolled DM, oral manifestations include multiple periodontal abscesses, velvety red gingival tissues, marginal proliferation of periodontal tissues.

B. Hypothyroidism: associated with occasional gingival hyperplasia.

C. Hyperparathyroidism: excessive production of parathyroid hormone (PT), which helps control calcium metabolism.

1. Caused by benign adenoma or malignancy and results in osteoporosis, multilocular radiolucent jaw lesions, loss of lamina dura, "ground glass" appearance of alveolar bone.

2. Results in MORE rapidly demineralized alveolar bone when occurs in presence of periodontitis.

D. Alterations in hormones: puberty, pregnancy, oral contraceptives, infertility treatments, perimenopause and menopause ALL affect periodontium (but ALL are temporary because hormonal levels change).

1. Puberty: involves increased levels of hormones, which alter capillary permeability and increase fluid accumulation in the gingiva, resulting in increased risk for gingivitis in presence of dental biofilm.

2. Menstruation: even with normal, cyclical hormonal fluctuations has NOT been shown to increase risk of gingivitis; gingivitis has been shown to be actually lower than during ovulation and premenstruation, when hormones may peak.

3. Pregnancy:

   a. Strong correlation with development of gingival changes such as gingivitis, gingival enlargement, pyogenic granuloma (pregnancy tumor).

   b. Results in increased levels of progesterone, altering capillary permeability and tissue metabolism, making tissues MORE at risk for inflammatory changes in presence of possibly minimal levels of dental biofilm.

   c. Associated with high levels of anaerobes, such as *Prevotella intermedia* (Pi).

4. Oral contraceptives (birth control pills [BCPs]):

   a. Drugs that have been shown to elevate hormone levels and thus mimic pregnancy.

b. Therefore affect gingival tissues in manner SIMILAR to pregnancy; place at risk for gingivitis.

c. However, lower doses generally used may NOT affect periodontium.

5. Infertility treatments: women with MORE than three cycles had higher levels of gingival inflammation, bleeding, and gingival crevicular fluid (GFC); severity strongly associated with duration of drugs.

6. Perimenopause and menopause:

a. Related to mucocutaneous disorders such as erosive lichen planus and mucous membrane pemphigoid.

b. Risk for osteopenia and osteoporosis (discussed later).

c. May affect periodontium if on hormone replacement therapy (SIMILAR to pregnancy or BCPs).

CLINICAL STUDY

Age	25 YRS	**SCENARIO**
Sex	☐ Male ☒ Female	The patient, whom the dental office has been seeing regularly every 6 months for oral prophylaxis, presents with pocket depths that have increased from 3 to 4 mm and a bleeding score of 60%, according to the Ainamo and Bay bleeding index. Signs of gingival inflammation are present in the form of marginal erythema, generalized bulbous interdental papillae, and rolled margins. This finding is unusual for the patient because she has always exhibited meticulous oral hygiene. Moreover, dental biofilm and calculus are not present in noticeable quantities during this visit.
Height	5'10"	
Weight	220 LBS	
BP	120/82	
Chief Complaint	"I gave up smoking and still my gums are a mess. Is it my being pregnant?"	
Medical History	4 months pregnant Quit smoking 4 months ago	
Current Medications	None	
Social History	Student nurse	

1. What is the most likely American Academy of Periodontology (AAP) classification of the patient's condition?

2. What factors are contributing to her condition? Discuss bleeding index used.

3. How should this condition be treated?

4. What information can be given to the patient to help prepare her for other possible complications?

1. Dental plaque (biofilm)-induced gingivitis caused by endocrine system changes. Her pocket depths are no greater than 4 mm and most likely are pseudopockets because signs of inflammation include gingival edema, which causes tissue enlargement.

2. Predominant factor contributing to the patient's condition is pregnancy. During pregnancy, increased levels of progesterone have been associated with increased risk for gingivitis. Also frequently associated with high levels of anaerobes, such as *Prevotella intermedia* (Pi). Gingival bleeding index assesses bleeding of the gingival margin in response to gentle probing, used as indicator of gingival health or disease. To score it, divide the total number of areas that bleed by the number of gingival margins examined, then multiply the result by 100 to arrive at a score (percentage).

3. Thorough professional debridement, elevated dental biofilm control measures, and education regarding correlation between the pregnancy and contributing factors will keep the disease under control.

4. Gingivitis associated with pregnancy begins in second or third month and is most severe in second and third trimesters. Moreover, in pregnant women localized enlargements in interdental papillae may form bleeding growths, referred to as pyogenic granulomas (pregnancy tumors). If these lesions occur, most will disappear at end of the pregnancy as hormones become more regulated. The patient should be congratulated for quitting smoking for own health and that of unborn child. Tobacco use is number one factor in periodontal disease; also affects health of child, now during pregnancy and later with presence of second-hand smoke. However, continued gingivitis can still put patient at risk for a preterm low-birth-weight child.

Nutritional Deficiency Risk

Poor nutrition lowers resistance to periodontal disease, which makes deficient individuals MORE at risk for infection and severe forms of periodontitis. In United States, nutritional deficiencies are found MOST commonly among elderly, lower socioeconomic groups, drug and alcohol abusers. Food consistency also has been recognized as contributing factor to accumulation of dental biofilm and thus development of periodontal disease. Poor nutrition can be modified with proper diet.

• See Chapter 7, Nutrition: diet counseling.

A. Vitamin A deficiency: effect of deficiency NOT known even though involved in synthesis of epithelial cells, proteoglycans, fibronectin, procollagen.

B. Vitamin B_2 (riboflavin) deficiency: may affect the oral cavity, causing angular cheilitis, glossitis, oral ulcerations.

C. Vitamin B_6 (pyridoxine) deficiency: since involved in carbohydrate metabolism; may induce generalized stomatitis, glossitis, gingivitis, and other oral symptoms.

D. Vitamin B_{12} (cobalamin) deficiency:
1. May result from diet or may be caused by altered absorption (pernicious anemia).
2. May make gingival tissues MORE at risk for epithelial dysplasia and malignant transformation.
3. Generally accompanied by folic acid deficiency; folic acid is of interest because may reduce gingivitis or phenytoin (Dilantin)-induced gingival hyperplasia.

E. Vitamin C (ascorbic acid) deficiency:
1. Adversely affects periodontal connective tissue, capillary integrity, and wound healing because vitamin C is essential to collagen biosynthesis.
2. When prolonged, may cause scurvy, which induces severe periodontal changes.

F. Vitamin D deficiency:
1. Results in altered levels of plasma calcium and phosphorus, which interferes with mineralization of organic bone matrix; leads to rickets in children and osteomalacia in adults.
2. Results in loss of lamina dura and thinning of cortical plates (radiographically).
3. May cause common dental anomalies, such as delayed development of the permanent dentition, enamel hypoplasia, cemental resorption, open apical foramina, enlarged pulp chambers, and frequent pulp stones.
4. In adults may lead to osteomalacia, which destroys PDL and resorbs alveolar bone; causes replacement fibrous dysplasia.

G. Antioxidants such as beta-carotene; vitamins A, C, E; selenium may be involved in reducing or preventing diseases caused by free oxygen radicals; thus may play role in treating some forms of oral cancer and have been shown to be involved in tissue destruction associated with periodontitis and chronic inflammatory osteoarthritis.

H. Other nutritional disorders:
1. Osteoporosis:
a. Loss of bone mass caused by imbalance of plasma calcium and phosphorus levels; EARLY loss of bone density with osteopenia.
b. Severity of bone loss increases if periodontitis is superimposed on osteoporosis.
2. Protein deficiency (undernutrition): when severe, significantly reduces host defenses and wound healing.
a. In MOST severe forms (kwashiorkor, marasmus, cachexia) exhibits oral changes such as glossitis, angular cheilitis, xerostomia, increased gingival inflammation, periodontal bone loss.
b. Kwashiorkor is also associated with increased incidence and severity of necrotizing periodontal disease, resulting in cancrum oris (noma or oral gangrene).
c. LESS severe forms still affect oral health among alcoholics, anorexics (self-starvation), long-term bedridden and hospital patients, those taking drugs that depress appetite or increase metabolism.

Stress and Psychosocial Risk

Increased risk for and severity of periodontal disease have been reported during stressful life events such as death, divorce, war. Plasma corticosteroid levels become higher during exposure to stressful stimuli and act to suppress protective portions of immune response. Strongest example of correlation between stress and periodontal disease is necrotizing periodontal disease (discussed later). Stress can be minimized and controlled and in MOST cases is temporary in nature.

Adverse Drug Reaction Risk

Drugs may have a variety of adverse effects in the oral cavity, ranging from allergic to toxic reactions, including gingival hyperplasia and xerostomia. Although drugs themselves do NOT cause periodontal disease, may provide locally irritating conditions that place individual at risk. Unless a drug is taken indefinitely, MOST side effects would be temporary and able to be modified by time.

• See Chapters 9, Pharmacology: drugs and side effects; 11, Clinical Treatment: management of xerostomia.

A. Gingival hyperplasia (see later discussion for more specifics and for surgical treatment; Figure 13-1):
1. Associated with anticonvulsants (phenytoin), immunosuppressants for organ and bone marrow transplants (cyclosporin); calcium channel blockers (nifedipine, diltiazem, verapamil); cannabis.
2. Decreases effectiveness of dental biofilm removal during oral hygiene care; hyperplasia is increased with poor oral hygiene.

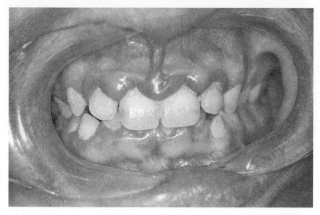

Figure 13-1 Gingival hyperplasia associated with anticonvulsant drug therapy (phenytoin [Dilantin]). (From Bath-Balogh M, Fehrenbach MJ: Illustrated dental embryology and anatomy, ed 2, Philadelphia, 2006, Saunders/Elsevier.)

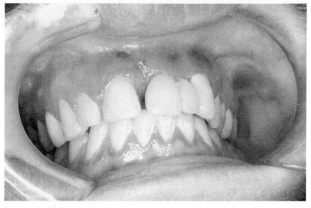

Figure 13-2 HIV-associated periodontitis with linear gingival erythema (note gingival Kaposi's sarcoma [KS]).

B. Xerostomia (see later discussion of benefits): side effect of many drugs.

HIV/AIDS Status Risk

Oral manifestations of HIV infection often are first signs of AIDS. Dental hygienist may be the first person to identify such manifestations because of seeing patients often over time. Prevalence of periodontal disease and other oral manifestations in patients with HIV/AIDS varies significantly, depending on decline of immune system, lifestyle, early recognition, treatment, ALL of which can modify it as a risk factor.
- See Chapter 8, Microbiology and Immunology: HIV/AIDS.

A. HIV- associated gingivitis:
  1. Linear gingival erythema (LGE): well-defined red band along free gingival margin, with NO bleeding on probing (BoP).
  2. Punctate or diffuse erythema of attached gingiva.
B. HIV-associated periodontitis (Figure 13-2):
  1. Defined by presence of LGE, attachment loss, cratering in area of interdental col, severe clefting, which often accompanies recession.
  2. Treated by conventional nonsurgical periodontal therapy (NSPT) in conjunction with meticulous homecare.
C. AIDS-associated necrotizing ulcerative periodontitis (NUP): see later discussion.

CLINICAL STUDY

Age	38 YRS	**SCENARIO**
Sex	☒ Male ☐ Female	Patient has a chronic cough that he notes has persisted for several months. The extraoral examination reveals bilateral generalized lymphadenopathy. Intraorally, several large ulcerations that are red and raw are noted on the hard palate. Additionally, a thick white coating appears on portions of the hard palate and all of the soft palate, extending into the pharynx; when the coating is wiped off with gauze, raw inflamed tissue is exposed. The gingival tissues have a definite red band along the facial gingival margins of the maxillary arch; however, no bleeding is detected.
Height	6'4"	
Weight	185 LBS	
BP	105/68	
Chief Complaint	"My mouth hurts so bad that I can't eat. And I have not been feeling well lately."	
Medical History	Tuberculosis 5 years ago Epstein-Barr infection 2 years ago	
Current Medications	OTC ginseng qd	
Social History	Unemployed graphic designer	

1. What systemic condition is the patient likely to have?
2. What might be causing the severe pain in his mouth?
3. What is the significance of the palatal ulcerations?
4. What treatment for the patient's oral condition should be discussed?
5. What periodontal maintenance interval is recommended, after his acute problems have subsided?

1. This patient is likely to have HIV/AIDS, based on generalized lymphadenopathy, generalized malaise, linear gingival erythema (LGE; classic sign of HIV), probable candidiasis, oral ulcerations.
2. Severe pain is most likely caused by the open palatal ulcerations. Candidiasis and LGE typically are not painful.
3. Palatal ulcerations are most likely herpetic lesions, since they are on tissue overlying bone; aphthous ulcers are on tissues that do not cover bone.
4. Tactful discussion should include immediate referral to a physician if patient does not reveal his HIV status. His oral condition requires prescriptions for antiviral drug, such as acyclovir, for herpetic lesions and antifungal agent, such as nystatin (Mycostatin), clotrimazole (Mycelex), ketoconazole (Nizoral), for the candidiasis. In addition, povidone-iodine and chlorhexidine rinses (without alcohol because of open sores) would reduce pain and discomfort the patient is experiencing. May need a lidocaine oral rinse to help with eating.
5. All patients with HIV/AIDS should be seen monthly for periodontal maintenance because oral manifestations of the disease, including those of the periodontium, often occur rapidly and are extremely destructive.

Neutrophil Abnormality Risk

The MAIN etiological factor in development of gingivitis and periodontitis is dental biofilm. Also recognized that bacteria and host response MUST be in balance to avoid disease. One of the MAIN players in active host response is the PMN. When PMN response is impaired, bacteria flourish and disease often becomes MORE severe. Most cases of altered host response are NOT able to be modified at this time as risk factors, unless resulting from treatment and drug use.

- See Chapters 6, General and Oral Pathology: neutropenias; 8, Microbiology and Immunology: PMN structure and function.
A. Neutropenias:
  1. Associated with decrease in circulating PMNs.
  2. Manifested as skin infections, upper respiratory infections, otitis media, stomatitis, early exfoliation of the teeth, severe gingivitis with ulceration.
  3. May be caused by drugs, radiation, Down syndrome, leukemia, DM, tuberculosis, autoimmune disorders.
  4. Oral manifestations include gingivitis, aggressive periodontitis, oral ulcerations.
  5. When systemic, MOST often are idiopathic.
     a. Cyclic neutropenia is a rare condition characterized by neutropenic episodes that persist for 1 week, occur every 3 weeks, and result in sore gingiva, aphthous ulcers, aggressive periodontitis.

B. PMN dysfunctions:
  1. Adherence defects: include leukocyte adherence defect (LAD), genetic autosomal recessive defect:
     a. Impair successful margination of PMNs, preventing migration to sites of infection.
     b. Clinical condition characterized by recurrent bacterial infections, diminished pus formation, prolonged wound healing, leukocytosis.
     c. Dental manifestations are characterized by aggressive periodontitis, progressive alveolar bone loss, premature exfoliation of primary and permanent teeth, severe gingival inflammation.
  2. Chemotaxis defects: involve impairment of directional migration of PMNs toward attracting molecules such as bacteria.
     a. Include several rare diseases and syndromes that involve defects in PMN locomotion and chemotaxis, such as DM, Down syndrome, ulcerative colitis, Job's syndrome, Chédiak-Higashi syndrome, lazy leukocyte syndrome, Papillon-Lefèvre syndrome (these rare ones discussed later).
     b. Associated with aggressive periodontitis.

ETIOLOGY OF PERIODONTAL DISEASE

Many factors are involved in the etiology of periodontal disease, including host response, microbiology, oral contributing factors, occlusal trauma.

Etiology: Host Response

Bacteria interact with host in MOST cases of periodontal disease. In healthy individuals, active host response quickly results in slight inflammation, which destroys the antigens (bacteria). However, periodontal health depends on balance between BOTH protective and destructive systems. When host response is impaired, MORE rapid destruction of periodontium results. Included in host response are the defense mechanisms of the oral cavity, inflammatory response, immune response, all discussed next. See also later discussion of pathogenesis of periodontal disease for host response to etiological factors over time.

- See Chapter 8, Microbiology and Immunology, for related discussion.

Defense Mechanisms of Oral Cavity

Natural defense mechanisms that exist in the oral cavity include intact epithelium, saliva, gingival crevicular fluid. Mechanisms work together to defend against mechanical, bacterial, chemical aggression.
A. Intact epithelium provides physical barrier between external noxious substances (e.g., bacterial enzymes such as collagenase and other by-products) and deeper lamina propria.

B. Saliva:
   1. Functions to mechanically cleanse oral cavity.
   2. Buffers acids produced by bacteria from the dental biofilm.
   3. Controls bacterial activity.
   4. Contains antibacterial components such as lysosomes and lactoperoxidase.
   5. Contains secretory IgA for immune resistance against bacteria, food residues, fungi, parasites, viruses.
C. Gingival crevicular fluid (GCF):
   1. Increased amount correlated with severity of gingival inflammation.
   2. Provides antibacterial action by bringing white blood cells (WBCs, leukocytes) and antibodies into close proximity with bacteria from dental biofilm.
   3. Supplies complement factors that serve to initiate BOTH vascular and cellular inflammatory responses that can damage the periodontium.
   4. Provides sticky plasma proteins in the sulcus that serve as adhesive for junctional epithelium (JE), keeping it intact.
   5. Contains BOTH cellular and organic elements:
      a. Cellular elements include bacteria, desquamated epithelial cells, PMNs, lymphocytes, monocytes.
      b. Organic components:
         (1) C3 and C5a: play role in release of histamine; also facilitate chemotaxis and phagocytosis.
         (2) IgG and IgM: function in activation of complement system.
         (3) IgG: facilitates phagocytosis.
         (4) IgG, IgA, IgM: prevent tissue destruction by neutralizing bacterial endotoxin.
         (5) Serum IgA: prevents penetration of antigens across epithelial barriers.

Inflammatory Response

Inflammation is the natural response to insult; divided into three phases that include acute, chronic, repair. NOT only does inflammation seek to fight the insult, it also adds insult to injury against the periodontium.
A. Acute phase of inflammation, "FIRST line" of defense; subdivided into vascular response and cellular responses:
   1. Vascular response: develops rapidly following initial insult.
      a. Provides plasma proteins and fluid necessary for rapid isolation of irritant.
      b. Fluid produced is responsible for associated tissue edema.
      c. Vascular dilation causes increased blood volume and decreased velocity, resulting in hyperemia.
      d. Initial vasoactive response is produced by release of histamine and serotonin by mast cells located in lamina propria.
   2. Vascular permeability is sustained by additional chemical mediators:
      a. Kinins.
      b. Prostaglandins.
      c. C3 and C5a from complement system.
      d. Lysosomal enzymes released from leukocytes.
B. Cellular response:
   1. MAIN defense cell released in acute phase of inflammation is PMN.
      a. PMNs leave central stream of blood vessel (margination) and adhere to endothelial walls (pavementing).
      b. PMNs escape through endothelial walls by emigration (diapedesis).
      c. PMNs move to injured area (migration) by chemotaxis (directed movement).
      d. Main function of PMN is phagocytosis (engulfment of foreign objects such as debris and bacteria).
         (1) Mature PMNs are capable of living for ONLY few hours in highly acidic environment.
         (2) After PMNs die, release enzymatic contents of lysosomes, causing MORE damage.
   2. Considerable debris accumulates, requiring addition of defense cells that are capable of living in acid environment.
   3. Appearance of macrophages and histiocytes (both are related blood monocytes in connective tissue) signals beginning of next stage of inflammation, chronic phase.
C. Chronic phase of inflammation, "second line" of defense:
   1. MAINLY involves chronic inflammatory cells, attracted to area of inflammation by active proteins called lymphokines that are released by lymphocytes to do MORE containment of inflammation.
   2. Involves macrophages (within tissue), which function to phagocytose or debride area.
   3. Lymphocytes become MAIN cells, in the form of either T cells or B cells.
      a. B cells are concerned with humoral immunity; differentiate into plasma cells, which produce specific antibodies (immunoglobulins [Ig]) targeted at immobilizing specific antigens.
      b. B cells also produce memory cells that are capable of producing MORE antibodies on demand.
      c. T cells are concerned with cellular immunity and are classified as T4 activator cells, T8 suppressor cells, killer (cytolytic) cells.
   4. Elevated plasma C-reactive protein (CRP) is noted with periodontal disease; may be future predictor (inflammatory marker) for *activity* of disease (similar to cardiovascular disease); periodontal therapy would then seek to modify levels of CRP. However, it is NOT considered specific enough for use during diagnostic procedures.

D. Repair phase of inflammation:
1. Begins when macrophages debride site.
2. Involves fibroblasts from surrounding connective tissue that migrate to injured area and begin to secrete tropocollagen (precursor to collagen) to produce fibrotic (scar) tissue.
3. Involves endothelial cells that proliferate and provide MORE oxygen tension.
4. Involves development of granulation tissue, composed of fibroblasts, new immature collagen, new capillaries.

Clinical Signs of Inflammation

Inflammation is identified by several clinical (cardinal) signs, including gingival bleeding and changes in gingival color, contour, position.

A. Gingival bleeding on probing (BoP):
1. Characteristic of the tissue destruction that occurs during acute inflammation.
2. Results from vascular engorgement, increased blood flow, loss of vascular wall integrity, and microulceration of the sulcular epithelium (SE) initially and then later also JE, which exposes deeper lamina propria.
3. May be spontaneous or may follow provocation.
4. MOST reliable sign of acute inflammation, although late sign; lack indicates gingival health.
B. Gingival color changes:
1. Occur during BOTH destructive and proliferative stages of inflammation.
2. Result from thinning of epithelial layers, decrease in keratinization, engorgement of subepithelial blood vessels, capillary proliferation.
3. Bright red color occurs during acute stage of inflammation and is associated with vascular hyperemia.
4. Bluish color is associated with chronic inflammation and venous stasis.
C. Changes in gingival consistency:
1. Occur during either destructive or proliferative stage of inflammation.
2. Include edema, softness, friability during acute inflammation.
3. Caused MAINLY by accumulation of tissue fluid during acute stage of inflammation, thinning of the epithelial layers, loss of keratin.
4. Result in increases in density of tissues during chronic and repair stages of inflammation; these occur because of proliferation of fibroblasts, which produce collagen in the form of scar tissue, giving firm, fibrotic consistency.
D. Changes in surface texture:
1. May include loss of stippling if stippling was present during gingival health.
2. Loss of stippling appears as shiny surface; caused by loss of keratin, thinning of epithelium, accumulation of connective tissue fluid.

3. Loss of stippling is LEAST reliable sign of inflammation.
4. Also changes in gingival contour occur as result of either increased tissue fluid (edema) or increased cellular elements (fibrosis); result in rolled margins and blunted interdental papillae.
E. Changes in gingival position:
1. ALL relative to CEJ; result in increased height of gingival margin because of edema and tissue proliferation.
2. Result in recessed margins, which have numerous causes ranging from edema, to toothbrush abrasion, to malposed teeth.

Immune Response

Immune response is a complex entity that consists of BOTH nonspecific and specific components. Because of large numbers of bacteria that inhabit the oral cavity, effective host response is required to minimize disease and tissue destruction. Important to recognize that majority of tissue damage produced during periodontal inflammation is caused by the host's response to bacteria. Evidence now suggests that periodontal disease is possibly an autoimmune disorder, in which immune factors in the body attack the person's own cells and tissue—in this case, those in the gingival tissues.

A. Nonspecific host responses (innate host defense mechanisms):
1. Inflammatory response:
   a. Arachidonic acid cascade: produces several biologically active products, including prostaglandins, leukotrienes, thromboxane.
   b. MOST notable effects are vascular permeability and attraction of phagocytic cells.
   c. Also attract antibodies and complement that aid in destruction of bacteria and their by-products.
   d. Products of arachidonic acid cascade are potentially harmful to periodontal tissues and are part of the pathogenesis of periodontal disease.
2. Complement system:
   a. More than 20 serum proteins become activated during inflammation and exhibit potent biological activity.
   b. Activated through classical pathway or alternate pathway.
   c. Effects of activation (by either pathway):
      (1) Production of opsonins that enhance phagocytosis (see below).
      (2) Mast cell release of histamine that causes vasodilation.
      (3) Release of chemotactic factors that causes migration from the blood system of PMNs and macrophages to specific sites.
      (4) Production of factors capable of destroying bacterial cell walls.

3. Phagocytic system:
   a. Consists primarily of PMNs and macrophages.
   b. Phagocytes kill bacteria in two different ways:
      (1) Oxygen-dependent system: bacteria are destroyed in phagolysosome in the cell itself, by lysosomal enzyme called myeloperoxidase.
      (2) Non-oxygen-dependent system: enzymes and other cationic proteins (e.g., neutral proteases, acid hydrolases) in lysosomes of PMNs and macrophages degrade bacteria after they have been ingested.

B. Specific host responses mediated by lymphocytes:
   1. T cells provide cellular immune response:
      a. Release of cytokines that include potent products, such as tumor necrosis factor-alpha (TNF-alpha) and interleukin-1-beta, that are capable of inducing bone resorption.
   2. B cells provide humoral immune responses by producing plasma cells that in turn produce specific antibodies and immunoglobulins (Igs):
      a. Prevent bacterial cell walls from attaching to oral surfaces.
      b. Trigger activation of complement system.
      c. Neutralize toxins and enzymes released by bacteria.
   3. In addition, white blood cells (WBCs) produced by immune response to bacteria release a family of enzymes called matrix metalloproteinases (MMPs), which break down connective tissue, such as that within the periodontium.

Etiology: Microbiology

Strong relationship exists between microbial dental biofilm and periodontal disease. However, constant presence of microorganisms in the oral cavity and its relationship to disease is a complex issue that involves MANY factors, including host response, microbial virulence, genetics. Periodontal disease is essentially a disease caused by bacteria. However, mere presence of bacteria does NOT preordain disease. Host defense mechanism of the individual is the balancing factor in maintenance of health. If BOTH bacterial load and host response are in balance, NO disease occurs. If either a critical mass of bacteria is reached or host response is somehow impaired, disease occurs. Etiology therefore should be discussed from perspective of BOTH host response and bacteria.

Dental Biofilm

Dental biofilm (dental plaque) is a living, highly organized, and complex microbial ecosystem composed of more than 300 species of bacteria embedded in a gelatinous matrix. Classified as either supragingival or subgingival. Microflora associated with each type of periodontal disease classification as noted in the Human Oral Microbiome Database (HOMD) are listed in each subcategory, as well as Table 13-1. Presence of dental biofilm (and associated calculus) is the MOST common reason for gingivitis (NOT more obscure causes such as vitamin C deficiency).

- See Chapter 8, Microbiology and Immunology: microbiology overview.

A. Types:
   1. **Supragingival dental biofilm:**
      a. Found coronal to the margins on clinical crowns of teeth or within sulcus or pseudopocket:
         (1) With healthy gingiva:
            (a) Composed MOSTLY of cocci and rods that are gram positive and aerobic.
            (b) Equal percentages of gram positive cocci and *Actinomyces;* LESS than 15% are anaerobic.
         (2) With early gingivitis: increased numbers of anaerobic, gram-negative cocci and rods.

Table 13-1 Main periodontal pathogens

Microorganism	Gram stain reaction, motility	Associations
Aggregibacter (previously *Actinobacillus*) *actinomycetemcomitans* (Aa)	Gram negative, nonmotile	Chronic periodontitis (less than with Pg) and aggressive periodontitis, both localized and generalized; can invade tissue
Tannerella forsythensis (Tf) (previously *Bacteroides forsythus* [Bf])	Gram negative, nonmotile	Early stages of gingivitis and chronic periodontitis
Campylobacter rectus (Cr)	Gram negative, motile	Chronic periodontitis
Porphyromonas gingivalis (Pg)	Gram negative, nonmotile	Chronic periodontitis (most prevalent) and generalized aggressive periodontitis
Prevotella intermedia (Pi)	Gram negative, nonmotile	Gingivitis with pregnancy and chronic periodontitis
Treponema denticola (Td)	NA, motile	Chronic periodontitis; can invade tissue

(3) With chronic gingivitis: increased numbers of anaerobic, gram-negative, filamentous organisms, fusobacteria, spirochetes.

(4) Microbial microcosm increases in complexity by means of progressive, sequential colonization on clean tooth:

(a) Formation of acquired pellicle from salivary proteins on tooth surface.

(b) Attachment by microorganisms (via specific mechanisms), which colonize over time: first, gram-positive aerobic cocci, then gram-negative anaerobic rods, then motile organisms (i.e., spirochetes).

b. Within pits and fissures: morphology allows growth; MOSTLY *Streptococcus mutans, Actinomyces naeslundii.*

2. **Subgingival dental biofilm:** located in pockets apical to the crest of marginal gingiva within periodontal pocket.

a. Diseased periodontium: MORE anaerobic because subgingival area provides LESS oxygen tension, which is MORE conducive to anaerobic growth.

b. During active periodontal disease: MOSTLY anaerobes at ≥90% of organisms present, typically with 75% of them gram-negative organisms; there are also large numbers of gram-negative, facultative anaerobic organisms.

c. Divided into three zones (LOCATION LOCATION LOCATION—hey, real estate is real estate):

(1) Tooth-attached: attached along tooth surface from gingival margin almost to the JE at base of pocket.

(a) MOSTLY gram positive, although gram-negative cocci and rods present.

(b) Associated with calculus formation, root caries, root resorption.

(2) Epithelium-attached: loosely attached to inner lining.

(a) Layers closest to pocket lining have large numbers of motile, gram-negative, anaerobic microorganisms and spirochetes.

(b) Microorganisms are seen invading ulcerated inner pocket lining into lamina propria and have been found on outer portions of alveolar bone; MAINLY involves *Aggregatibacter* (previously *Actinobacillus*) *actinomycetemcomitans* (Aa) and *Treponema denticola* (Td).

(c) Relative proportions are related to nature of disease activity; MOSTLY

associated with gingivitis and periodontal disease.

(d) MOST virulent and detrimental portion of dental biofilm to periodontium.

(3) Unattached: free-floating in pocket; since pocket has LESS mechanical stress, attachment is NOT vital; at base of pocket is MAINLY unorganized gram-negative rods and spirochetes, separated from inner pocket lining by WBCs.

d. The pH is regulated MAINLY by saliva; from 6.75 to 7.25 (see more information in Chapter 11, Clinical Treatment).

e. There is a consistent distance from dental biofilm to alveolar bone that is never <0.05 mm and never >2.7 mm; microorganisms can cause destruction of alveolar bone crest only when it is <3 mm away from dental biofilm.

Bacteria-Mediated Tissue Destruction

Tissue destruction mediated by bacteria is caused by release of toxins and enzymes from these microorganisms.

A. **Bacterial enzymes** (hyaluronidase, collagenase, ribonuclease) affect host cells and intercellular (ground) substance; proteolytic and hydrolytic enzymes destroy cells and increase permeability of epithelial and connective tissues.

B. Bacterial cell walls of microorganisms that are released at the time of their destruction:

1. Gram-negative: **lipopolysaccharides** (LPS, endotoxin):

a. Activate alternate pathway of immune complex fixation process (via complement).

b. Side reaction proteins are BOTH chemotactic and cytolytic (C3, C5, C5a).

2. Gram-positive: **lymphotoxins** (LT, exotoxin):

a. Inhibit the chemotactic response of the host cells.

b. Inhibit host cell phagocytosis.

c. Create resistance to killing and digestion within phagolysosomes of host cells.

d. Release toxins that are cytolytic and/or cytotoxic.

Etiology: Oral Contributing Factors

Although dental biofilm has been recognized as MAIN etiological factor in initiation and progression of gingivitis and periodontitis, other oral contributing factors play a role in retention of dental biofilm. These factors may be divided into local functional factors and local predisposing factors.

A. **Local functional factors:** weaken the PDL, widening the PDL space and thus promoting dental biofilm accumulation; include missing teeth, malocclusions, tongue thrusting and mouth breathing habits, parafunctional habits such as chewing on pencils or other foreign objects, traumatic occlusion (discussed next).

B. **Local predisposing factors:** harbor dental biofilm microorganisms, responsible for promoting oral disease.

1. Include calculus, materia alba, dental stains, faulty restorations and overhangs, food impaction, untreated caries, tooth anatomy (e.g., furcas).
2. Supragingival and/or subgingival calculus is the MOST significant among this group of factors because it BOTH harbors dental biofilm and consists MAINLY of mineralized dental biofilm.
   a. **Supragingival calculus:** mineralized supragingival dental biofilm from salivary minerals.
      (1) Found coronal to margins on clinical crowns of teeth, typically yellowish white; may darken with age or dietary staining.
      (2) Found MOST commonly on lingual surfaces of mandibular anteriors and on buccal surfaces of maxillary first and second molars; BOTH adjacent to salivary gland ducts that promote mineralization of dental biofilm.
      (3) Found LEAST on occlusal surfaces because of mastication.
      (4) Composed of MAINLY inorganic (70% to 90%) and some organic (10% to 30%) content.
         (a) Inorganic mineral component is made up MAINLY of calcium phosphate (75.9%) and calcium carbonate (3.1%), with traces of magnesium, sodium, potassium, fluoride, zinc, strontium.
         (b) Organic component is mixture of protein-polysaccharide complexes, desquamated epithelial cells, leukocytes, carbohydrates, lipids, glycosaminoglycans, various types of microorganisms.
      (5) Primary crystalline structure is MAINLY calcium hydroxyapatite, $Ca^{10}(PO_4)^6(OH)_2$; includes smaller amounts of octocalcium phosphate, whitlockite, brushite.
   b. **Subgingival calculus:** mineralized subgingival dental biofilm from GCF's minerals, which are originally from associated gingival tissue blood supply.
      (1) Located in sulcus and pockets apical to the crest of marginal gingiva; typically is dense, hard, dark brown or black, firmly attached to root surface.
      (2) Composition differs slightly from that of supragingival calculus, MAINLY by higher ratio of calcium to phosphate and increased sodium.
      (3) Normal mode of attachment to the tooth is by means of salivary acquired pellicle; mineralization occurs within 24 to 72 hours, and maturation occurs in an average of 12 days.
      (4) May form MORE tenacious attachment by penetrating cementum and/or mechanically locking into surface irregularities, making removal difficult (YES!).
   c. Rate of calculus formation varies among individuals, may also vary among teeth; calculus may be light, moderate, or heavy.
3. **Food impaction:** forceful wedging of food into periodontium by occlusal forces, which leads to dental biofilm retention.
4. Food debris:
   a. Although rapidly cleared away from oral cavity, tends remains on the teeth and oral mucosa.
   b. Cleared from mouth by salivary flow and mechanical action of tongue, cheeks, and teeth.
   c. Adherence varies with food composition.
5. **Materia alba:**
   a. Yellow or grayish white acquired bacterial coating; soft, sticky, LESS adherent than dental biofilm; can be flushed away with water.
   b. Composed of microorganisms, desquamated epithelial cells, leukocytes, salivary proteins, lipids.
6. Dental stains include a variety of extrinsic stains produced by foods, tobacco products, poor oral hygiene; may attach to external tooth surfaces, creating rough surface for retention of dental biofilm (see Chapter 11, Clinical Treatment).
7. Faulty dentistry (iatrogenic factor) plays IMPORTANT role in dental biofilm retention; includes poorly fitted margins of dental prostheses, overcontoured crowns, rough crown margins, faulty or overhanging restorations, clasps of partial dentures.

Etiology: Occlusal Trauma

It is important for the dental hygienist to recognize BOTH normal and abnormal occlusal form and function in progression of periodontal disease. Occlusal disharmonies can have a profound influence on periodontal disease risk and are considered local contributing factors. Recognizing and recording signs and symptoms of occlusal dysfunction and then providing referrals for diagnosis and treatment are important components of dental hygiene care.

- See Chapters 4, Head, Neck, and Dental Anatomy: occlusion discussion; 6, General and Oral Pathology: temporomandibular joint disorder (TMD).

A. **Hyperfunction:** slightly increased forces that result in nonpathological form of adaptation.
   1. Associated histological changes characterized by increase in number of fiber bundles in PDL; result in increased width of PDL and increased thickness of alveolar bone.
   2. CANNOT be noted clinically; NOT associated with tooth mobility.
B. **Occlusal trauma:** pathological alterations or adaptive changes that develop in periodontium as result of undue forces generated by muscles of mastication.
   1. Defined in two ways:
      a. Damage to the periodontium caused *directly* by stress.
      b. Damage caused *indirectly* by the teeth of the opposing jaw.
   2. Effect of occlusal forces on periodontium is dependent on magnitude, direction, duration, frequency.
C. Injury results when occlusal forces exceed adaptive capacity of the periodontium.
   1. Associated histopathological features result from areas of pressure and tension between the tooth root and the alveolar bone; MORE severe level of changes as noted in hyperfunction.
   2. Can be noted clinically.
D. Clinical signs and symptoms of occlusal trauma:
   1. Evidence of wear facets and/or a history of bruxism or clenching; possibly abfraction; MAINLY premolars.
   2. Tilted or missing teeth and tooth mobility.
   3. Occlusal interferences in excursive mandibular movements.
   4. Radiographic evidence of widened PDL space of involved teeth, with loss of continuity of lamina dura.
   5. Radiographic evidence of increased cementum at apices of involved teeth (hypercementosis) and/or root resorption.
E. Types of occlusal trauma: either primary or secondary; may result from hypofunction or disuse atrophy.
   1. **Primary occlusal trauma:** excessive occlusal forces applied to teeth with healthy periodontium; alveolar bone levels are supportive.
   2. **Secondary occlusal trauma:**
      a. Excessive occlusal forces applied to teeth with diseased periodontium; alveolar bone levels are already deficient in support.
      b. MOST common in cases of chronic periodontitis in which alveolar bone support may be inadequate to withstand forces of occlusion (whether normal or excessive).
F. Hypofunction and disuse atrophy: occlusal forces are either decreased or removed entirely; decrease in collagen fiber production in PDL and in alveolar bone formation.

1. **Hypofunction:** nonpathological form of adaptation characterized by slight decrease in occlusal forces; slight reduction in BOTH collagen fibers and bone deposition occurs, with narrower PDL, but is NOT seen on radiographs.
2. **Disuse atrophy:** pathological process when ALL occlusal forces are removed; involves extreme weakening of the supporting structures.
   a. Requires absence of occlusal antagonist; results in obvious reduction in BOTH fibers and bone, with radiographically detectable narrowed PDL space.
   b. Also radiographic evidence of decreased bone trabeculation in cancellous bone.
   c. Always accompanied by increased tooth mobility; tooth supererupts into space of opposing arch.

Pathogenesis of Periodontal Disease

Although gingivitis does NOT necessarily progress to periodontitis, periodontitis is always preceded by gingivitis. Unknown when transition occurs clinically. Diagnosis of periodontitis is made when inflammation extends into epithelial attachment (EA, attachment apparatus), resulting in attachment loss and subsequent periodontal pocket formation. Progression of disease occurs in four distinct histological stages; first three result in gingivitis, and fourth manifests as periodontitis. This progression has certain clinical pathogenic ramifications.

A. Histological pathogenesis:
   1. Initial lesion (stage I):
      a. Response of tissues to dental biofilm occurs in FIRST 2 to 4 days after biofilm invasion; considered subclinical.
      b. Involves initial vasoconstriction followed by subsequent vasodilation and margination; emigration and migration of PMNs into lamina propria result in slight alteration of JE and increase in GCF.
   2. Early lesion (stage II): acute gingivitis stage, which occurs within 4 to 7 days after insult.
      a. Results in further invasion of JE, causing ulceration of SE and JE, destruction of connective tissue fibers.
      b. Involves appearance of chronic inflammatory cells, such as macrophages and lymphocytes.
   3. Established lesion (stage III): chronic stage of inflammation, which occurs 14 days after initial insult.
      a. MOSTLY plasma cells, bacterial enzymes, and cell by-products such as collagenase that are destructive to the collagen in periodontal tissues.
      b. May persist from weeks to years and remain stable or may progress to advanced lesion.
   4. Advanced lesion (stage IV): occurs ONLY when inflammation invades supporting periodontium (PDL and alveolar bone); marks conversion of gingivitis to periodontitis.

a. Depends on host response and presence of specific bacterial species.

b. Coronal portion of JE becomes detached and migrates along root surface.

c. Cementum is altered as it becomes exposed by inflammatory bacterial products, and superficial layer contains LPS.

d. FIRST PDL fibers involved are alveolar crest fibers, then later deeper fibers become involved; transseptal (interdental) fibers are NOT involved until the tooth is almost lost, they realign more apically as inflammation occurs, protecting the deeper tissues (noted in SAME levels of mobility that are affected first).

e. Involves bone destruction initially in the alveolar crest that then spreads by blood vessels and bone marrow deeper into the alveolar bone.

f. Destruction results in the response of the periodontium by forming either fibrotic tissue or granulation tissue.

    (1) Fibrous tissue (scar or cicatricial tissue) with its excess collagen formation.

    (2) Granulation tissue is young collagen tissue that bleeds easily.

B. Clinical pathogenesis:

1. Gingivitis: inflammation of the gingival tissues.

    a. Caused by invasion of JE and SE by dental biofilm; with vasostagnation, retained tissue fluids and eventual fibrosis produce gingival enlargement or edema.

    b. Results in gingival pocket (pseudopocket) where pocket formation is NOT accompanied by apical migration.

2. Periodontitis: inflammation of the periodontium.

    a. Occurs with apical migration, results in periodontal pocket.

    b. As inflammatory process destroys gingival and PDL fibers, apical proliferation and migration of JE and SE occur.

    c. Disease becomes self-perpetuating with formation of deeper pockets because dental biofilm, primary etiological agent, can grow and mature in MORE anaerobic environment of the deeper pocket.

    d. Growth of periodontal pathogens is encouraged as removal by patient becomes increasingly difficult because of depth of pocket; if allowed to persist, chronic infection causes severe destruction and eventual tooth loss.

    e. Pocket continues its progression apically; stimulation of alveolar bone resorption is part of the inflammatory process.

        (1) Classifications of periodontal pockets:

            (a) **Suprabony pocket:** base of pocket is coronal to level of alveolar bone, with horizontal bone loss.

            (b) **Infrabony pocket:** base of pocket is apical to level of alveolar bone, with vertical bone loss; three distinct types: one-walled, two-walled, three-walled defects (Figure 13-3).

f. Superficial gingival tissues range from inflamed with its fragility, bleeding, redness to fibrotic with its whitened and hardened appearance.

g. Periods of inactivity (remission) alternating with periods of activity (exacerbation).

CLASSIFICATION OF PERIODONTAL DISEASES ▬

Although numerous classification systems exist for periodontal diseases, MOST commonly used system was developed by the 1999 International Workshop for Classification of Periodontal Diseases and Conditions sponsored by AAP (see CD-ROM). Classification has numerous subcategories (especially for gingivitis); only major categories are discussed here (Table 13-2). **Refractory** is NOT a separate entity from other forms of periodontitis; term is applied in

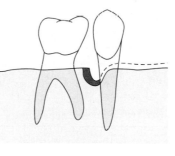

One-walled

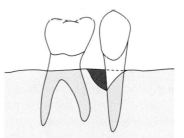

Two-walled

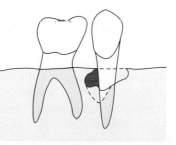

Three-walled

Figure 13-3 Infrabony pocket with a one-walled, two-walled, and three-walled defect.

Table 13-2 American Academy of Periodontology (AAP) classification of periodontal diseases and conditions *(abbreviated version)*

Classification	Conditions
Periodontal health	None
Gingival diseases	A. Dental plaque (biofilm)-induced gingival diseases B. Nonplaque (biofilm)-induced gingival lesions
Chronic periodontitis* (slight: 1-2 mm attachment loss; moderate: 3-4 mm attachment loss; severe: >5 mm attachment loss)	A. Localized B. Generalized (>30% of sites are involved)
Aggressive periodontitis* (slight: 1-2 mm attachment loss; moderate: 3-4 mm attachment loss; severe: >5 mm attachment loss)	A. Localized B. Generalized (>30% of sites are involved)
Periodontitis as manifestation of systemic diseases	A. Associated with hematological disorders B. Associated with genetic disorders C. Not otherwise specified
Necrotizing periodontal diseases	A. Necrotizing ulcerative gingivitis B. Necrotizing ulcerative periodontitis
Abscesses of the periodontium	A. Gingival abscess B. Periodontal abscess C. Pericoronal abscess
Periodontitis associated with endodontic lesions	Combined periodontic-endodontic lesions
Developmental or acquired deformities and conditions	A. Localized tooth-related factors that modify or predispose to plaque (biofilm)-induced gingival diseases and periodontitis B. Mucogingival deformities and conditions around teeth C. Mucogingival deformities and conditions on edentulous ridges D. Occlusal trauma

*Attachment loss and not probe readings determines the clinical attachment levels (CAL) with/without recession and edema.

conjunction with other forms to mean that the case does NOT readily respond to treatment (e.g., refractory chronic periodontitis, refractory aggressive periodontitis).

Gingival Diseases

Forms of gingival diseases include dental plaque (biofilm)-induced and nonplaque (biofilm)-induced gingivitis. Common examples are discussed.

A. Dental plaque (biofilm)-induced gingivitis (management is discussed later):
  1. Characteristics:
     a. MOST common form of gingivitis and found to some extent in MAJORITY of population.
     b. Exhibits bleeding on probing (BoP); MOST significant feature.
     c. Painless condition; also typically manifested as redness and swelling of gingival margins and interdental papillae (i.e., rolled margins, rounded interdental papillae, flabby tissues, loss of stippling), presence of gingival pockets (pseudopockets) possible.
  2. Subcategories:
     a. Gingival diseases modified by systemic factors: endocrine and systemic and blood dyscrasias.

(1) Gingivitis MAINLY associated with puberty and pregnancy:
  (a) Caused by dental biofilm; hormonal alterations tend to exaggerate inflammatory response.
  (b) During puberty: poor diet and poor oral hygiene may also exaggerate response; affects BOTH males and females.
  (c) During pregnancy: increased levels of progesterone have been attributed to increased risk for gingivitis and presence of *Prevotella intermedia* (Pi).
     (i) Begins in second to third month and MOST severe in second and third trimesters.
     (ii) With localized interdental papillae enlargements, pyogenic granulomas (pregnancy tumors); red or magenta, smooth, shiny; disappear at the end of pregnancy.
  (d) Clinical characteristics:
     (i) Red to bluish red gingiva caused by increased vascularity.

(ii) Enlarged, edematous gingiva (especially with pregnancy), with increased tendency to bleed.

(2) Gingivitis associated with leukemia: disease of blood-forming tissues characterized by production of excessive numbers of immature WBCs.

(a) Regardless of the form, dental biofilm is primary etiological agent; histological changes associated with leukemia modify and aggravate inflammatory response to local irritants.

(b) Clinical characteristics:

(i) Purplish blue color caused by blood stagnation, with enlargement of marginal and interdental papillae in form of tumorlike masses.

(ii) Moderately firm to friable tissues, with shiny surfaces that may have ulcerations, necrosis, and pseudomembrane.

(iii) Spontaneous bleeding (in MOST cases), with gingival pockets (pseudopockets).

b. Gingival diseases modified by medications and malnutrition.

(1) Gingivitis associated with vitamin C deficiency: severe cases result in scurvy (scorbutic gums); however, this vitamin deficiency alone CANNOT cause inflammation (take that, Captain Jack Sparrow!).

(a) Exaggerated because a deficiency of this vitamin creates increased tendency for gingival hemorrhage, degeneration of collagen fibers, edema of gingival tissues.

(b) Clinical characteristics:

(i) Bluish red gingiva, with enlargement of marginal gingiva.

(ii) Soft, friable, smooth, and shiny gingival surfaces, with possible pseudomembrane, if necrosis has occurred.

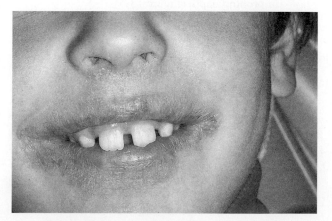

Figure 13-4 Acute herpetic gingivostomatitis.

(iii) Tendency to bleed spontaneously, with gingival pockets (pseudopockets).

B. Nonplaque (NOT biofilm)-induced gingivitis:

1. Gingival diseases of bacterial, viral, or fungal origin:

a. Primary herpetic gingivostomatitis: oral manifetation of a primary infection with HSV-1; occasionally HSV-2 (genital herpes) (see Chapter 8, Microbiology and Immunology) (Figure 13-4).

b. Mainly present in infants and children; however, becoming MORE common among young adults infected with HSV-2; symptomatic in ONLY 10% to 20% of persons infected with HSV-1.

c. Characteristics: fever, malaise, headache, irritability, lymphadenopathy.

(1) Oral lesions that begin as small, yellow vesicles and coalesce to form larger, round ulcers with gray centers and bright red borders

(2) Lesions may appear on any keratinized oral mucous membranes, including lips, tongue, gingival tissues, buccal mucosa, palate.

(3) Serious to extreme pain that restricts eating and drinking and may threaten the patient's health.

d. Treatment: palliative because disease is viral and typically runs course in 7 to 10 days.

(1) Extremely infectious disease; poses major risk to clinician because transmission of virus through inadvertent puncture results in herpetic whitlow and eye infection (result can be blindness); MUST follow all infection protocols with standard precautions.

(2) Involves patient and parent education in gentle dental biofilm removal and proper diet; fluid intake to prevent dehydration is IMPORTANT.

2. Gingival diseases of genetic origin:

a. Familial (hereditary) gingival enlargement (idiopathic gingival hyperplasia): rare hyperplastic disease with unknown etiology.

(1) Enlarged marginal, interdental, attached gingival tissues; affects facial and lingual surfaces of BOTH arches.

(a) Affected tissues are pink, firm, resilient, bulbous, and fibrotic without bleeding; tissues may obscure occlusion.

(b) May exhibit inflammatory changes in response to local irritants.

3. Gingival manifestations of systemic condition:

a. Allergic gingivitis: hypersensitivity or abnormal response of tissues to specific agents.

(1) May be oral manifestation of systemic allergic response, if sensitivity is to food or drug.

(2) Also may manifest as localized contact allergy to dentifrices, mouthwashes, topical anesthetics, or other dental therapeutic agents.

(3) Antigen (and NOT dental biofilm) is MAIN etiological agent.

(4) Redness, soreness, gingival necrosis, edema, ulceration, possible vesicle formation.

b. Desquamative gingivitis, gingivitis associated with dermatoses: rare chronic condition that involves interdental, marginal, and attached gingival tissues.

   (1) Recently linked to several dermatological diseases and drugs, although exact nature unknown.

   (a) Diseases include pemphigus, pemphigoid, benign mucous membrane pemphigoid, lichen planus; MAINLY affects older woman. but so do these other disorders (however, NOT direct result of menopause).

   (b) Associated drugs (stomatitis medicamentosa) include sulfonamides, gold salts, arsphenamine, aminopyrine, antibiotics, barbiturates, salicylates.

   (2) Slight, moderate, or severe; redness of marginal and attached gingival tissues, with periods of exacerbation and remission.

   (a) As severity increases, localized areas of epithelium begin to peel away, exposing painful connective tissues.

   (b) In MOST severe form, irregular areas of gingiva are fiery red, smooth, shiny; exposed connective tissues contain blisters that bleed and are extremely painful.

   (3) Degenerative condition (NOT associated with dental biofilm) with ONLY secondary inflammatory reaction.

4. Gingival diseases modified by medications:

a. Noninflammatory gingival enlargement: may be produced by certain drugs, with or without presence of inflammatory condition; NOT associated with dental biofilm, although inflammation exists (see earlier discussion).

   (1) Phenytoin (Dilantin), anticonvulsant drug: causes enlargements in over half of prescriptions given to patients (Figure 13-1); other anticonvulsants rarely cause it.

   (a) Clinical characteristics: generalized enlargement of marginal and interdental gingiva, which causes increased sulcular depths (gingival pockets, pseudopockets); interdental areas become MORE enlarged and often obscure occlusion.

   (b) Enlarged tissues appear firm, fibrotic, pale pink, and resilient and have less tendency to bleed.

   (c) Tissues also appear lobed, and although enlargement is generalized, frequently MORE pronounced in anteriors.

   (d) MORE common in younger patients, rarely affects edentulous spaces; however, increased levels with poor oral hygiene and with increased dental biofilm.

   (2) Cyclosporine, immunosuppressive drug used to prevent organ transplant rejection and to treat type 1 DM and other autoimmune disorders; drug causes enlargements in one third of adults and in even MORE children.

   (3) Calcium channel blocking drugs, such as diltiazem (Cardizem), nifedipine (Procardia), and verapamil (Isoptin), treatment of angina pectoris; produce gingival enlargements SIMILAR to phenytoin (Dilantin) in some individuals; MORE uncommon with amlodipine (Norvasc).

Chronic Periodontitis

Chronic periodontitis is the MOST common form of periodontitis ("garden variety," that is why we pick at it!). Although may begin subclinically in adolescence, does NOT become evident until *after* age 35. Because of chronic nature, progresses slowly; management is discussed later.

A. Characteristics: severity is *directly* related to amount of hard and soft deposits on tooth surfaces.

1. NOT associated with abnormal host or systemic diseases.

2. Presence of periodontal pockets, bone loss, eventual tooth mobility.

3. MOST commonly exhibits horizontal interdental bone loss, eventually progresses to interradicular areas (furcations), possibly with a FEW areas of vertical interproximal bone loss.

4. Degree of periodontal disease activity is *directly* related to amount of bone and PDL destruction; determined MORE accurately by measures of clinical attachment level (CAL) than by measures of probing depth (Figure 13-5).

B. Considered mixed infection, since involves several bacterial species (Table 13-1): *Porphyromonas gingivalis* (Pg) typically MOST prevalent; with *Aggregatibacter* (previously *Actinobacillus*) *actinomycetemcomitans* (Aa); *Tannerella forsythensis* (Tf) (previously *Bacteroides forsythus* [Bf]); *Prevotella intermedia* (Pi); *Fusobacterium nucleatum* (Fn); *Campylobacter rectus* (Cr); *Treponema denticola* (Td) (Bad boys, bad boys, whacha you gonna do?).

C. Clinical signs, with periods of BOTH exacerbation and remission:

1. Chronically inflamed gingiva, with color that varies from red to bluish to normal.

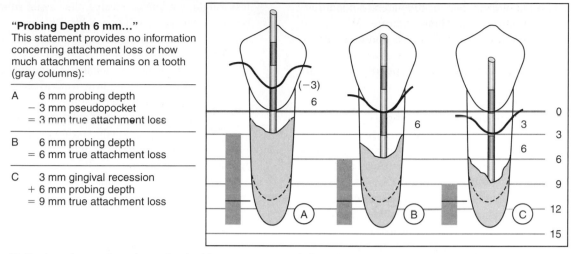

"Probing Depth 6 mm..."
This statement provides no information concerning attachment loss or how much attachment remains on a tooth (gray columns):

A   6 mm probing depth
     − 3 mm pseudopocket
     = 3 mm true attachment loss

B   6 mm probing depth
     = 6 mm true attachment loss

C   3 mm gingival recession
     + 6 mm probing depth
     = 9 mm true attachment loss

Figure 13-5 Attachment loss determined with measurement of clinical attachment levels with differing gingival margin levels.

2. Gingiva that varies in consistency from edematous to fibrotic, with enlarged appearance.
3. Contour that is rounded at the margins and typically blunted interdentally, exhibiting a loss of stippling.
4. Evidence of attachment loss and periodontal pockets, with tendency for BoP.
5. Radiographic signs of bone loss that may include lack of definition of the lamina dura, fuzzy crestal lamina, horizontal or angular (vertical) bone loss, or radiolucencies of bifurcations and trifurcations (furcation involvement).
6. Rough root surfaces, calculus, exudate that may be purulent (pus).
7. Tooth mobility, which varies from none to extensive.

D. Categorized into three MAIN categories based on severity, then subcategorized again as localized or generalized, which indicates more or less than >30% involvement:
1. Slight: slight loss of bone (involving ONLY alveolar crest) and PDL, with 1 to 2 mm of attachment loss.
2. Moderate: more advanced loss of bone and PDL, with 3 to 4 mm of attachment loss; may be accompanied by tooth mobility and furcation involvement.
3. Severe: further progression of disease; results in advanced loss of bone and PDL, with >5 mm of attachment loss; accompanied by increased tooth mobility and furcation involvement.

CLINICAL STUDY

		SCENARIO
Age	44 YRS	A full-mouth series (FMX) of radiographs is taken in addition to a complete periodontal evaluation. Examination reveals moderate levels of dental biofilm at the gingival margins, moderate gingivitis, heavy subgingival and supragingival calculus, tobacco staining. Molars #3, #19, #30, and #31 are badly decayed but are no longer painful. Radiographs indicate a loss of crestal bone throughout posterior areas of the mouth. Probe readings are 3 to 4 mm in anterior sextants and 4 to 6 mm in posterior areas (with attachment loss at 3 to 4 mm). No recession is noted.
Sex	☐ Male ☒ Female	
Height	5'8"	
Weight	275 LBS	
BP	115/75	
Chief Complaint	"I am afraid of the dentist but I am so embarrassed about my teeth."	
Medical History	Two caesarean sections Past cigarette smoker, quit 2 years ago	
Current Medications	None	
Social History	Waitress, employed after being full-time mom for 15 years Restaurant employer offers dental insurance	

1. Identify a likely diagnosis for the patient's condition. What does loss of crestal bone indicate? What AAP classification fits this case? How do you measure attachment loss?
2. Identify factors contributing to her periodontal condition.
3. Discuss treatment options.
4. What is the prognosis for this disease?

1. MOST likely diagnosis for patient's condition is periodontitis, based on loss of crestal bone, age, amount of deposits, lack of routine dental care. The AAP classification is generalized (>30% of sites involved) moderate chronic periodontitis because attachment loss is at 3 to 4 mm, with slight horizontal bone loss evident on radiographs in the posterior sextants. With no recession, attachment loss can be determined by clinical attachment levels, through measuring pocket depth and then subtracting measurement of gingival margin to CEJ.
2. Factors contributing to periodontal condition include tobacco use (smoking), inadequate oral hygiene, lack of professional dental care.
3. Appropriate treatment should include thorough periodontal debridement with local anesthetic coverage (preferably by quadrant), oral hygiene instruction, tobacco cessation, extraction or restoration of decayed teeth. Patient should return in 4 to 6 weeks for reevaluation of periodontal health. Any areas with continued bleeding should be evaluated and undergo debridement if needed to promote healing. Homecare should be assessed, and additional instruction should be given as needed.
4. Prognosis is the prediction of the duration, course, and termination of a disease and the likelihood of its response to treatment. Prognosis for chronic periodontitis is good, if patient refrains from smoking, practices good homecare, and complies with appropriate supportive periodontal therapy (typically involving oral prophylaxis every 3 months).

Aggressive Periodontitis

Diagnosis of **aggressive periodontitis** is made on clinical, radiographic, and historical findings that show rapid attachment loss and bone destruction, possible familial aggregation of disease as described in APP "Parameter on Aggressive Periodontitis" (2000) (see CD-ROM).
A. Characteristics: systemically healthy, EXCEPT for periodontal disease.
   1. Periodontal tissue destruction greater than would be expected given level of local factors.
   2. MORE periodontal pathogens (see below), as well as phagocyte abnormalities and increased production of prostaglandin E_2 and interleukin-1b.
B. Categories are SIMILAR to chronic periodontitis in number of teeth involved and severity of attachment loss (slight, moderate, severe); then again subcategorized into localized and generalized forms:
   1. Localized (LAP): circumpubertal onset (Figure 13-6).
      a. Periodontal damage localized to permanent first molars and incisors; however, atypical patterns of affected teeth are possible.
      b. Associated with periodontal pathogen *Aggregatibacter* (previously *Actinobacillus*) *actinomycetemcomitans* (Aa), with PMN dysfunction (function abnormalities).
      c. HIGH serum antibody response to infecting agents.
   2. Generalized (GAP): usually affects people under 30 years of age, but may be older (Figure 13-7).
      a. Generalized interproximal attachment loss affecting at least three permanent teeth other than first molars and incisors; occurs in pronounced episodic periods of destruction.
      b. Associated with periodontal pathogens *Aggregatibacter* (previously *Actinobacillus*) *actinomycetemcomitans* (Aa) and *Porphyromonas gingivalis* (Pg), with PMN dysfunctions; MORE similar to the microflora of chronic periodontitis.
      c. LOW serum antibody response to infecting agents.
C. Management: given its rapid course and serious consequences, patients (or guardians, as appropriate) SHOULD be informed of the disease process, therapeutic alternatives, potential complications, expected results, responsibility in treatment.

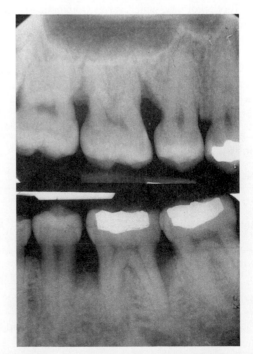

Figure 13-6 Localized aggressive periodontitis (LAP).

1. Consequences of NO treatment should be explained; failure to treat appropriately can result in progressive and often rapid loss of periodontal supporting tissues, may have adverse effect on the prognosis, and could result in tooth loss.
2. Given this information, patients (or guardians, as appropriate) should then be able to make informed decisions regarding periodontal therapy.
3. Therapy consists of <u>medical consult</u> for systemic factors and 2-week regimen of antibiotics in conjunction with conventional nonsurgical periodontal therapy; periodontal surgery may be required to restore periodontal health.

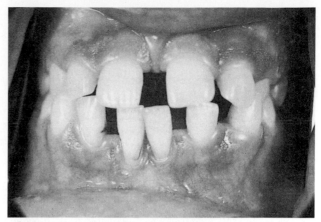

Figure 13-7   Generalized aggressive periodontitis (GAP).

CLINICAL STUDY

Age	14 YRS	SCENARIO
Sex	☐ Male ☒ Female	Patient of record who is scheduled on time for her 6-month oral prophylaxis. Her gingival tissues continue to appear healthy, and her mouth is dental biofilm free. She brushes her teeth twice daily and flosses four to five times a week. Probing depths are 2 to 3 mm throughout her mouth, with the exceptions of teeth #3, #14, and #8, which have readings of 6, 6, and 9, respectively. Bleeding on probing (boP) is noted in the pockets only.
Height	5'6"	
Weight	124 LBS	
BP	98/58	
Chief Complaint	"I never had deep pockets like these before. What should I do?"	
Medical History	Parents both have dentures Always seems to have a cold or flu	
Current Medications	None	
Social History	High school student who is interested in a dental career	

1. Identify a likely diagnosis for the patient's condition. How might radiographs assist in the diagnosis?
2. Identify factors that might have contributed to her periodontal condition.
3. Discuss treatment options.
4. What is the prognosis for this disease?

1. Most likely diagnosis for the patient's condition is localized aggressive periodontitis, which may be indicated by the presentation of vertical bone loss on radiographs of teeth #3, #14, and #8 and probing depths of these teeth. Diagnosis of aggressive periodontitis is based on clinical, radiographic, and historical findings that show rapid attachment loss and bone destruction, possible familial aggregation of disease. Except for periodontal disease, patients are systemically healthy. The other feature that may be present is periodontal tissue destruction greater than would be expected given level of local factors (healthy patient and mouth, with no dental biofilm).

2. Contributing factors to periodontal condition could include elevated levels of *Aggregatibacter* (previously *Actinobacillus*) *actinomycetemcomitans* (Aa) or *Porphyromonas gingivalis* (Pg), phagocyte abnormalities, increased production of prostaglandin E_2 and interleukin-1b.
3. Condition typically is treated with a 2-week regimen of antibiotics in conjunction with conventional nonsurgical periodontal therapy; medical consult is imperative. Periodontal surgery may be required to restore periodontal health.
4. Prognosis is the prediction of the duration, course, and termination of a disease and the likelihood of its response to treatment. Prognosis good throughout most of the mouth, except for teeth #3, #14, and #8, because no bleeding is noted and sulcus depths are normal in the rest of the mouth. Prognosis for the areas with pocketing is fair because significant amounts of bone loss already have occurred and there is BoP, showing

active inflammation. However, compliance with home-care and professional dental care should contain bone loss indefinitely.

Periodontitis as Manifestation of Systemic Diseases

Systemic diseases that affect immune function, inflammatory response, and tissue organization can modify the onset and progression of all forms of periodontal disease. See earlier discussion of systemic factors with DM, HIV/AIDS, neutrophil abnormalities.

- See Chapter 6, General and Oral Pathology: Down syndrome, neutropenias, diabetes mellitus.
A. Includes subcategories for hematological disorders (acquired neutropenia, leukemias, and other), genetic disorders (familial and cyclic neutropenia, Down syndrome, leukocyte adhesion deficiency syndromes, Papillon-Lefèvre syndrome, Chédiak-Higashi syndrome, histiocytosis syndromes, glycogen storage disease, infantile genetic agranulocytosis, Cohen syndrome, Ehlers-Danlos syndrome types IV and VIII, hypophosphatasia, and other disorders not otherwise specified (NOS).
   1. Papillon-Lefèvre syndrome: inherited autosomal recessive disease characterized by hyperkeratotic skin lesions of palms, soles, knees, elbows; may cause severe destruction of periodontium; onset occurs after age 4.
   2. Chédiak-Higashi syndrome: rare disease that affects production of cellular organelles; produces partial albinism, slight bleeding disorders, recurrent bacterial infections, including periodontitis.
   3. Hypophosphatasia: rare familial skeletal condition characterized by rickets, poor cranial bone formation, premature loss of both primary and permanent dentitions.
B. Category acknowledges that management of periodontal disease should be carried out in conjunction with management of associated systemic disease; it is expected that other diseases will eventually be listed as more is known about systemic diseases and their relationship to periodontal disease.

Necrotizing Periodontal Diseases

Necrotizing periodontal diseases (NPD) include necrotizing ulcerative gingivitis (NUG) and necrotizing ulcerative periodontitis (NUP). BOTH appear to be opportunistic infections resulting from diminished systemic resistance to bacterial infection and may differ ONLY in terms of tissue, with NUP extending deeper into periodontium. NOT communicable.

A. NUG: associated with specific bacterial accumulations occurring with LOWERED host resistance (immunocompromised, such as with PMN chemotaxis and phagocytic defects), as well as in undernourished children (kwashiorkor).
   1. Characteristics: sudden onset, fetid metallic breath (fetor oris), cratered (punched-in) interdental papillae, ulcerative necrotic gingival sloughing (pseudomembrane), with spontaneous gingival bleeding; possible lymphadenopathy, fever.
   2. Has been associated with preexisting gingival inflammation, severe nutritional deficiency, smoking, preexisting systemic disease (e.g., Down syndrome, leukemia, HIV/AIDS, leukopenia, anemia, ulcerative colitis), stress, fatigue.
   3. Associated with specific combinations of microbes that appear to become pathogenic ONLY when the host defenses are diminished; also, spirochetes and fusiform bacillus may be present.
   4. Management: USUALLY responds rapidly to reduction of oral bacteria by a combination of personal dental biofilm control and professional debridement.
      a. If lymphadenopathy and/or fever accompanies oral symptoms, systemic antibiotics may be indicated.
      b. Use of chemotherapeutic rinses by the patient may be beneficial during initial treatment stages.
      c. Patient counseling should include instruction on proper nutrition, oral care, appropriate fluid intake, tobacco cessation, if needed.
      d. Comprehensive periodontal evaluation should follow resolution of acute condition.
      e. After acute inflammation of lesion is resolved, additional intervention may be indicated to prevent disease recurrence or to correct resultant soft tissue deformities; needs 3-month PM appointment.
B. NUP: rapid necrosis and destruction of the gingiva, PDL, alveolar bone (Figure 13-8).
   1. Usually represents extension of NUG with lowered host resistance; overall superficial appearance SIMILAR to NUG but MORE severe involvement of the interdental papillae (punched out).

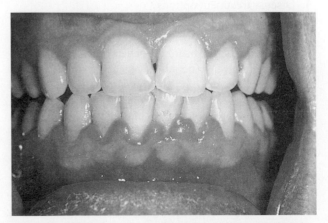

Figure 13-8 Necrotizing ulcerative periodontitis (NUP).

2. LACK of conventional periodontal pockets because of removal of tissue by ulcerative necrosis.

3. Has been reported among BOTH HIV-positive and HIV-negative individuals, but true prevalence is unknown.

   a. With HIV/AIDS-related NUP, presence of necrotizing stomatitis involving vestibules and palate, with infection extending into bone, producing deep, craterlike lesions (stoma), with sequestra (bone fragments).

   b. May become gangrenous stomatitis (noma).

   c. Antibiotic therapy should be used with caution in HIV-positive patients because of possibility of inducing opportunistic infections; SHOULD be seen monthly because oral manifestations often develop rapidly and are extremely destructive; need <u>medical consult</u>.

4. MAIN microorganisms are spirochetes and gram-negative organisms.

5. Management:

   a. Involves debridement, which may be combined with irrigation with antiseptics (e.g., povidone-iodine or diluted 3% hydrogen peroxide) to be used twice daily, antimicrobial oral rinses (e.g., chlorhexidine), administration of systemic antibiotics (such as metronidazole [Flagyl]).

   b. Later appointments can occur within 1 to 2 days, and with significant improvement MORE thorough deposit removal can begin; need to stop chlorhexidine rinses because of staining and calculus buildup and to stop hydrogen peroxide rinses because of development of black hairy tongue.

6. Patient counseling should include instruction on proper nutrition, oral care, appropriate fluid intake, tobacco cessation, if needed.

7. Comprehensive periodontal evaluation should follow resolution of the acute condition; need to set up periodontal maintenance (PM, recare) appointments to prevent recurrence.

CLINICAL STUDY

Age	19 YRS	SCENARIO
Sex	☒ Male ☐ Female	The patient arrived for an emergency appointment at his general dentist. After questioning, he indicates that he has had a fever and has been feeling run down since he completed his final exams 2 days ago and he is back to smoking again instead of eating. During visual examination, his gingiva appears fiery red and swollen. The interdental papillae are grayish white and ulcerated. A strong malodor is noted when he opens his mouth.
Height	6'2"	
Weight	175 LBS	
BP	105/68	
Chief Complaint	"My mouth is so sore and I am beat."	
Medical History	Cigarette smoking, one pack	
Current Medications	None	
Social History	College student, runs track	

1. Identify factors that have contributed to the patient's periodontal condition.
2. Identify a likely diagnosis for his condition.
3. Discuss treatment options.
4. What is the prognosis for this disease?

1. Factors that have contributed to oral disease include stress and inadequate oral hygiene (spirochetes and gram-negative organisms). Other contributing factors may include his smoking, fatigue, inadequate nutrition.

2. The patient most likely has necrotizing ulcerative gingivitis (NUG). It is an opportunistic bacterial infection that often occurs in young people who are under stress and have not been taking good physical care of themselves. Inadequate care may include smoking and drinking, as well as inadequate nutrition and dental biofilm removal and lack of sleep.

3. He needs a series of treatments. Immediate concern should be to gently debride affected areas. Accomplished with ultrasonic and/or sonic scalers to gently flush the area with oxygenated water. Topical and/or local anesthetics may be needed if debridement causes discomfort. If fever and/or lymphadenopathy is present, systemic antibiotics may be prescribed by the supervising dentist. A 0.12% chlorhexidine rinse should be prescribed (for use twice daily for a short time until the infection has subsided). Dental biofilm control methods and need for adequate sleep and nutrition should be discussed with patient. He should be seen within a few days to assess the gingival healing, remove more dental biofilm and calculus, and reinforce homecare. At a third

appointment, scheduled 3 to 5 days later, an assessment of healing, removal of remaining dental biofilm and calculus, and reinforcement of oral hygiene instructions should take place. Referral to a periodontist is recommended if gingival architecture requires correction as noted on reevaluation appointment.

4. Prognosis for NUG is good. After the patient completes therapy and begins to take better care of his health, his condition will improve. In a few cases surgery is required to repair gingival contour.

Abscesses of Periodontium

Abscess of the periodontium includes gingival, periodontal, pericoronal (pericoronitis), combined. **Abscess** is a localized collection of suppuration (pus) in a cavity formed by disintegration of tissues.

- See Chapter 6, General and Oral Pathology: periapical and developmental abscesses.

A. Gingival abscess: typically occurs as a result of injury caused by forceful occlusion of foreign object in the gingiva.
   1. Characteristics:
      a. Tends to occur on marginal gingiva; NOT associated with deeper periodontal pockets or with disease.
      b. Raised, painful area of acute inflammation accompanied by pus (suppuration).
   2. Treatment consists of:
      a. Incision, drainage, and irrigation with antimicrobials.
      b. Warm salt water rinses after surgery.
      c. Scaling of the teeth in the adjacent area.
B. Periodontal abscess: caused by entrapment of bacteria in periodontal pocket through occlusion of the pocket by foreign debris, such as popcorn kernel or incomplete scaling (calculus).
   1. Characteristics: may be acute or chronic, associated with preexisting periodontal disease.
      a. Initially an acute inflammatory reaction that results in pus (suppuration), with redness, localized swelling, throbbing or pulsating pain, rapid onset, rapid bone loss, vital pulp that rules out a pulpal origin.
      b. Acute abscess sometimes stabilizes by draining through sulcus and/or fistula in adjacent tissues, then becomes chronic abscess that is often painless.
   2. Treatment:
      a. Drainage, typically through the pocket, then irrigation with antimicrobial agent such as povidone-iodine or chlorhexidine.
      b. Antibiotics may be required if fever and/or lymphadenopathy is present.
      c. If diagnosed and treated early, prognosis is excellent and lost bone typically regenerates.

3. Pericoronal abscess (pericoronitis): direct result of entrapment of food and bacteria under operculum (flap of gingival tissue), which ultimately becomes inflamed and painful.
4. Characteristics:
   a. Occurs MOST commonly in distal region of partially or fully erupted mandibular third molars that are covered, partially or fully, by operculum.
   b. MOST commonly occurs in young adults between the ages of 17 and 26.
   c. Exhibits as pain, fever, pus (purulent exudate); trismus may also be present (MAIN cause).
   d. If NOT taken care of promptly (especially in immunocompromised patient), may lead to Ludwig's angina (see Chapter 6, General and Oral Pathology).
5. Treatment:
   a. Initially gently debride and irrigate the area under the operculum with antimicrobial such as diluted hydrogen peroxide.
   b. If fever is present, antibiotics may be prescribed.
   c. Recommend plenty of rest, fluid intake to avoid dehydration, warm salt water rinses.
   d. Later, if area should show signs of improvement, can be flushed again and MORE thoroughly debrided.
   e. Educate patient regarding dental biofilm control in location; may need to have tooth extracted and/or operculum surgically removed.

Periodontitis Associated with Endodontic Lesions

Lesions are called combination abscesses or combined periodontal-endodontic lesions. Difficult to diagnose; may involve a pulpal abscess that spreads through accessory canals to the periodontium or vice-versa. Causes severe damage and may cause tooth loss if left untreated.

- See Chapters 6, General and Oral Pathology: endodontic lesions; 15, Dental Biomaterials: endodontic therapy.

DEVELOPMENTAL OR ACQUIRED DEFORMITIES AND CONDITIONS

Category includes local factors associated with teeth and restorations, mucogingival deformities around teeth and on edentulous ridges, and occlusal trauma (see earlier discussion).

CLINICAL ASSESSMENT

Clinical assessment is a crucial component of periodontal therapy because it forms the foundation on which an appropriate plan of care can be developed. During clinical assessment, information about patient's past and present health from the medical and dental histories and dialogue, personal habits, and clinical findings are compiled to identify all risk factors that affect BOTH patient care and disease etiology. Assists in identifying nondental risk factors, such as tobacco use, diet, stress, that may play a role in the patient's periodontal condition. Supplemental methods to determine risk factors, including dental biofilm tests and software programs, can help with the process.

- See Chapters 6, General and Oral Pathology: medical conditions related to systemic factors; 11, Clinical Treatment: recording history, patient assessment, charting.

Periodontal Assessment

Periodontal assessment includes an evaluation of topography of the gingiva and related structures that change from periodontal health to periodontal disease conditions. Includes collecting data on surrogate measurements such as color, contour, texture.

- See Chapter 11, Clinical Treatment: periodontal evaluation.

A. Involves identifying presence of inflammation in gingiva:
  1. Color: changes from "coral pink," indicating health (with pigmentation differences), to overt signs of redness, indicating gingival ulceration and engorgement of blood vessels that occur during inflammatory process.
  2. Contour: in health follows the contour of the teeth; margins are knife edged (in normal tooth arrangement) and interdental papillae appear pointed; rolled marginal tissues and rounded interdental papillae suggestive of inflammation.
     a. Other changes in contour related to hyperplastic tissues:
        (1) **McCall's festoons:** lifesaver-like enlargements around free gingival margins.
        (2) **Stillman's clefts:** narrow, slitlike clefts where marginal gingiva has receded; produced by atrophy of facial gingiva and extensions of adjacent hyperplastic tissue.
  3. Texture: LEAST reliable sign of inflammation; may appear as loss of stippling during inflammation.
  4. Consistency: in health is firm and resilient; when inflamed, marginal and interdental papillae become bulbous and flabby, if edematous; bulky and firm from scar tissue accumulation, if fibrotic.
  5. Bleeding on probing (BoP):
     a. Although late sign of inflammation, MOST reliable and widely accepted sign of active inflammation.
     b. Record of bleeding indices establishes baseline measure from which goals can be established and serves as powerful motivational tool.

c. Poor positive predictor of periodontal disease, but conversely a very strong negative predictor; may NOT indicate periodontal disease; continued absence is a strong predictor of continued periodontal health.

6. GCF: increases during inflammation because of edema; in MORE severe cases of inflammation becomes milky, contains numerous PMNs and by-products, referred to as suppuration (pus).

7. Periodontal tissue destruction with attachment loss and periodontal pockets:
   a. Periodontal probing performed to measure depth of periodontal pockets and amount of CAL; considered "gold standard" for determining extent of periodontal tissue destruction.
   b. While probing, CAL is the probing depth measured from a fixed point such as the distance from cementoenamel junction (CEJ) to base of the pocket (EA) to determine attachment loss (Figure 13-5).
      (1) When CEJ is covered: to obtain CAL, first measure from gingival margin to CEJ, then subtract from overall probing depth; probing depth > CAL.
      (2) When CEJ is level with gingival margin: CAL is measured by probing depth; CAL = probing depth.
      (3) With recession: CAL is measured from CEJ to EA (some add recession and probing depth); CAL > probing depth.
      (4) Either manual or automated probes; typically involve measurements at six sites per tooth.
      (5) Even though measurements of probing depth are repeatable to within 1 mm >90% of the time, standard deviation of repeated CAL measurements of the same site by experienced examiner with a manual probe is BETTER at around 0.8 mm.
   c. To encourage all dental practitioners to include routine probing in patient care, periodontal screening and recording (PSR) system was developed.
      (1) Modification of the Community Periodontal Index of Treatment Needs (CPITN) developed by World Health Organization (WHO).
      (2) System involves probing each of six routine sites per tooth but recording ONLY highest reading per sextant and interpreting findings with code that determines whether full-mouth recording of all probing depths is required; uses WHO probe.
   d. Presence and distribution of dental biofilm, calculus, stain are identified and recorded to assist in setting goals with the patient.

(1) Dental biofilm is the MAIN etiological agent in development of periodontal disease; extent and distribution must be determined to facilitate removal.

(2) Several epidemiological indices assist in recording dental biofilm (see Chapter 17, Community Oral Health).

(3) Calculus and stain are contributing factors for periodontal disease owing to involvement in biofilm retention, and treatment planning needs to include removal.

(4) Extent and tenacity of calculus deposits and stains determine length of therapy, thus important components of treatment planning.

e. Proximal contact relationships of teeth should be evaluated; open contacts encourage food impaction, and tight contacts prevent effective interproximal cleansing.

f. Determining extent of mobility of teeth and dental implants indicates extent of damage to supporting structures of periodontium; considered predictor of attachment loss and thus risk factor for continued progression of periodontal disease.

(1) Mobility is BEST tested with handles of two instruments (or with automated mobility tester, Periotest).

(2) Several mobility scales exist.

(3) Teeth with moderate to advanced mobility are MORE likely to be lost than teeth without mobility; labeled a risk factor in prediction of periodontal breakdown.

g. Determining presence and degree of furcation involvement; prognosis is poor for teeth with extensive furcation involvement because homecare is almost impossible and accessibility during therapy becomes a major obstacle.

(1) Several scales classify furcation involvement.

(2) Curved, calibrated Nabor's probe is BEST instrument for detection of furcations.

(3) Teeth with moderate to advanced furcation involvement are MORE likely to be lost than teeth without furcations; labeled a risk factor in prediction of periodontal breakdown.

h. Presence of malocclusion and occlusal pathological changes should be assessed routinely; BOTH considered risk factors for periodontal breakdown.

i. Status of dental restorations and prosthetic appliances should be evaluated to determine whether overhanging margins and poorly contoured crowns exist; considered risk factors for periodontal breakdown.

Radiographic Assessment

Radiographic assessment includes evaluation of interdental septa, amount and pattern of bone loss, furcation involvement that may be present with periodontal disease.

• See Chapter 5, Radiology: radiographic interpretation.

A. Satisfactory number of diagnostic-quality radiographs must be interpreted to determine extent of bone loss, includes full-mouth periapical (FMX) radiographs, vertical bitewings, and possibly panoramic radiographs to accurately assess periodontal status:

1. Fuzziness of alveolar crests and breaks in continuity of lamina dura (alveolar bone proper) are the FIRST sign of periodontal breakdown.

2. With further periodontal breakdown, slight to moderate bone loss can be seen as horizontal or MORE extensive loss as vertical or angular; dependent on pathway of inflammation and disease (Figure 13-9).

3. Loss of interradicular bone in furcation areas on multirooted teeth shows further disease progression.

4. Widening of PDL space (location of PDL) and hypercementosis at apices indicate occlusal trauma.

5. Overhanging margins, interproximal calculus spears, root caries may also be present and associated with periodontal breakdown.

B. Limitations in the diagnosis of periodontal disease:

1. Destruction of alveolar bone typically is greater than it appears in radiographs (SIMILAR to calculus, which is also much worse than indicated!).

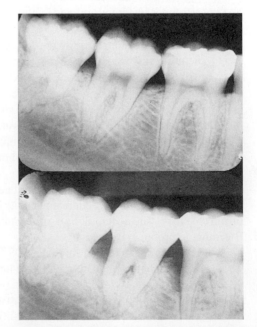

Figure 13-9 Horizontal *(top)* and vertical bone loss *(bottom)*.

2. Destruction of facial and lingual cortical plates is often NOT fully detectable in radiographs.

Supplemental Risk Factor Methods

These supplemental risk factor methods play IMPORTANT role in the identification of risk factors and coupled with clinical parameters (surrogate measurements), such as BoP and attachment loss, can be strong predictors of future disease progression.

A. Classified by four categories: physical, microbiological, biochemical, or immunological.
   1. Physical assessment tests include measures of subgingival temperature and GCF flow rates as they relate to inflammation.
      a. Higher subgingival temperature correlated to presence of inflammation can be measured by an automated, computerized, temperature-sensitive probe (Periotemp System).
      b. Higher flow rate of GCF correlated to gingival inflammation and useful adjunct for monitoring response to periodontal therapy can be measured (Periotron 6000).
   2. Microbiological tests are ONLY adjuncts for identification of bacterial species and are used MAINLY to determine risk for aggressive forms of periodontal disease but can be used for chronic forms; however, important to recognize that these tests are NOT diagnostic; SHOULD be used solely for identification and monitoring purposes.
      a. Culturing of possible periodontal pathogens has been considered "gold standard" for identification and quantification of bacterial species.
      b. Enzymatic methods (BANA test) for identifying presence of periodontal pathogens such as *T. denticola, P. gingivalis, T. forsythensis.*
      c. Immunological assays (such as enzyme-linked immunosorbent assay [ELISA]) for the identification of specific microbes.
      d. DNA probes for accurate identification and quantification of microbial pathogens have advantage of NOT requiring a living specimen; include *A. actinomycetemcomitans, P. gingivalis, P. intermedia.*
   3. Biochemical assessments are MORE sophisticated laboratory tests to identify various biochemical markers found in GCF and are involved in host response.
   4. Immunological assessment tests identify antibodies to specific periodontal pathogens in either blood serum or GCF. Correlations have been found between higher antibody levels and active disease; however, relationship to disease progression has NOT been established.

B. Software programs can help measure and communicate an individual patient's risk of periodontal disease from a database.

INTERPRETATION OF EVIDENCE, PRESUMPTIVE DIAGNOSIS, TREATMENT PLANNING, AND PROGNOSIS

Dental hygiene diagnosis involves interpreting data into coherent description of condition or disease in terms that can be addressed by dental hygienist. These data include the medical and dental history and clinical, radiographic, and adjunctive evidence. Then data must be interpreted to determine a differential diagnosis by the supervising dentist. ONLY after the differential diagnosis has been established can an appropriate plan of care be devised. ALL evidence collected during the initial assessment MUST be considered in developing a differential diagnosis, which is then used to determine patient's prognosis and treatment.

With diagnosis the patient is classified into one of the four periodontal case types (see later discussion). Noted in the reports "Risk Management Series, Diagnosing and Managing the Periodontal Patient" (ADA) and "Current Procedural Terminology for Periodontics and Insurance Reporting Manual" (AAP); recommendations for treatment are available for each case type (see CD-ROM).

A. Developing the diagnosis involves:
   1. Prioritizing immediate extraoral and intraoral problems.
   2. Identifying any systemic component of the disease process.
   3. Reviewing the patient's clinical signs and symptoms.
   4. Looking for radiographic signs of disease.
   5. Evaluating the human needs deficits of the patient.
B. Establishing the differential diagnosis includes:
   1. Determining the health status of the periodontium.
   2. Determining whether the gingivitis, if present, is associated with dental biofilm.
   3. Identifying whether condition is chronic periodontitis or more aggressive form.
   4. Making presumptive diagnosis, which is the BEST possibility after examining all the evidence.
C. Possible diagnostic categories include health, gingivitis, and periodontitis; then a more specific diagnosis can be identified (presumptive diagnosis), which is used to guide the development of the treatment plan.
D. Final diagnosis can be made ONLY after completion of initial therapy (phase I) and reevaluation of clinical response to therapy; this response guides further treatment planning.

Prognosis

Prognosis is prediction of the duration, course, and termination of a disease and the likelihood of its response to treatment.

A. Overall prognosis strongly influenced by patient's attitude.
B. For gingivitis, is dependent on:
   1. Other pathological changes besides inflammation.
   2. Presence of systemic risk factors.
   3. Patient compliance with oral hygiene.
C. For periodontitis:
   1. Is dependent on:
      a. Assessment of past bone response.
      b. Height of remaining bone.
      c. Periodontal attachment loss.
      d. Patient age.
      e. Presence of malocclusion.
      f. Presence of systemic risk factors.
   2. Is NOT related to compliance with oral hygiene.
D. For individual teeth, is dependent on:
   1. Loss of attachment, depth of periodontal pockets, width of attached gingiva.
   2. Mobility, furcation involvement, tooth morphology.

Determining Appropriate Plan of Action

Determining appropriate plan of action for each patient involves treatment planning, phases of treatment, and dental hygiene plan of care.
A. Treatment planning goals:
   1. Developing individualized plans based on the specific needs of each patient.
   2. Incorporating "evidence" in the development of the plan.
   3. Developing evidence-based, patient-specific treatment protocols.
   4. Determining methods and the sequence for delivering appropriate treatment.
   5. Eliminating and controlling etiological and predisposing factors.
   6. Emphasizing the maintenance of health and preventing disease recurrence.
B. Phases of treatment are divided into five groups:
   1. Preliminary phase: addresses any dental or periodontal emergencies and MAINLY involves treatment of all acute and painful oral conditions (see Chapter 6, General and Oral Pathology).
   2. Phase I (initial) therapy: etiological phase that deals MAINLY with control or elimination of etiological factors and includes dental hygiene plan of care.
      a. Patient education, dental biofilm control instruction, risk factor counseling (see Chapter 11, Clinical Treatment).
      b. Periodontal debridement (including scaling) (see Chapter 12, Instrumentation).
      c. Margination: recontouring of defective margins of restorations (see Chapter 15, Dental Biomaterials).
   3. Phase II therapy: surgical phase; involves procedures designed to reduce effects of disease and also includes regenerative techniques (discussed later).
   4. Phase III therapy: includes all restorative procedures, orthodontics, splinting, occlusal therapy (see Chapter 15, Dental Biomaterials).
   5. Phase IV therapy: recare or periodontal maintenance (PM) or maintenance phase (involves dental hygiene plan of care); patient usually remains in this phase for life (discussed later).
      a. Occasional relapses may require patient to repeat initial therapy, but patient ALWAYS returns to PM procedures.
      b. Appropriate PM intervals are determined individually; based on tissue response and home-care efforts of the patient.

Dental Hygiene Plan of Care

Dental hygiene plan of care is developed by dental hygienist *after* diagnosis and prognosis of the case. Typically involves phases I and IV of the comprehensive treatment plan of periodontal therapy.
• See Chapter 18, Ethics and Jurisprudence: informed consent.
A. Plan of care:
   1. MUST meet individual patient needs and MUST follow an orderly sequence.
   2. Involves determining number of appointments and time required for each, depending on needs.
   3. Always requires reevaluation 4 to 6 weeks (1 month) after initial therapy (for all periodontal patients) to assess tissue response, determine appropriate periodontal maintenance (PM, recare) interval (discussed later), evaluate need for referral to a periodontist, if not the treating dentist.
B. May follow a suggested guideline for determining number of appointments for various periodontal case types; however, individual needs may alter model and MUST always take precedence over any suggested protocols:
   1. Case type I (gingival disease): typically is completed in one appointment; recare (recall) interval is established at that time.
   2. Case type II (early periodontitis): often requires more than one appointment, may require use of local anesthetics; is followed by reevaluation appointment.
   3. Case type III (moderate periodontitis): typically is divided into quadrants; requires local anesthesia and several appointments, including reevaluation appointment.
   4. Case type IV (advanced periodontitis): typically is divided into quadrants or sextants; may require treatment of individual teeth, depending on extent and tenacity of the deposits; local anesthetics are routinely used and reevaluation appointment is planned.

5. Case type V (severe periodontitis): may require single or multiple visits with local anesthesia, depending on amount of debridement necessary with adjunctive therapy (see later discussion); more frequent recare (recall) appointments are often required.

NONSURGICAL PERIODONTAL THERAPY

Nonsurgical periodontal therapy (NSPT) is initial treatment of gingival and periodontal diseases, involves eliminating pathogenic microorganisms through definitive instrumentation procedures, dental biofilm control instruction, other adjunctive procedures. Also called phase I periodontal therapy (initial therapy). With oral-systemic disease links that have been established, BETTER clinical outcomes of NSPT are MORE important than ever.

- See Chapters 11, Clinical Treatment: patient motivation and dental biofilm removal methods; 12, Instrumentation: deposit removal including selective polishing.

A. Goals of NSPT: can be divided into short- and long-term goals:
   1. Short-term goals:
      a. Removal of hard and soft deposits through instrumentation.
      b. Definitive dental biofilm control instruction.
      c. Control of systemic and other risk factors.
   2. Long-term goals:
      a. Reduction or elimination of gingival inflammation.
      b. Elimination of pockets caused by edema.
      c. Restoration of periodontal health.

B. Rationales for NSPT:
   1. Removal of primary etiological agent, dental biofilm, other local irritants.
   2. Initiation of dental biofilm control measures.
   3. Modification of risk factors, BOTH local and systemic, wherever possible (e.g., overhang removal).
   4. Reduction or elimination of inflammation.
   5. Evaluation of tissue response.
   6. Establishment of periodontal maintenance (PM, recare) procedures (discussed later).

C. Procedures and techniques of NSPT:
   1. Oral hygiene instruction, which is comprehensive and individualized, to facilitate daily dental biofilm removal (can be instituted as separate appointment for tissue conditioning before scaling appointment).
   2. Scaling for purpose of supragingival and subgingival calculus removal.
   3. Preprocedural mouthwash to lower bacterial count in aerosols and decrease the potential for bacteremia.
   4. Periodontal debridement; includes scaling together with subgingival dental biofilm removal and identification of dental biofilm retentive factors; may include adjunctive chemotherapeutic agents.
      a. Treat the areas that have discomfort FIRST, unless tissue health is a factor.
      b. Treat either the quadrant with the fewest teeth or the one with least severe periodontal disease.
         (1) Makes first appointment less complicated.
         (2) Helps orient the anxious patient to clinical procedures.
      c. Use local anesthesia and/or nitrous oxide sedation based on patient's previous pain control experiences, severity of infection, type of calculus, potential for discomfort, and present sensitivity of hard and soft tissues.
      d. When two quadrants are treated at the same time, selecting maxillary and mandibular quadrants minimizes patient posttreatment discomfort.
   5. Root planing, targeted toward removal of cementum or surface dentin impregnated with calculus, endotoxins, or bacteria; current evidence has led to MORE conservative approach to this procedure; thus a glassy, smooth root surface is NO longer goal of NSPT; questionable procedure.
   6. Closed gingival curettage techniques to remove diseased soft tissues from within the pocket wall; currently is believed to have limited value in NSPT and is used ONLY in selected cases.
   7. Selective coronal polishing to remove retentive supragingival dental biofilm and stains for cosmetic reasons.
   8. Occlusal evaluation for identification of related contributing factors.

D. Effectiveness of NSPT:
   1. Effectiveness, whether performed by manual or powered instrumentation, has been well documented.
   2. Decreased probing depths and reduction in BoP are expected outcomes of therapy.
   3. Gains in attachment in deeper pockets are reasonable expectations.
   4. Generally healthier oral environment typically results.
   5. Close monitoring of all clinical parameters is necessary to prevent or arrest progression of disease after therapy.

Adjunctive Therapies

Because of highly infective microbial population present in diseased periodontal pocket, other therapies, used concomitantly with periodontal debridement, may be useful adjuncts to NSPT. Include chemical and antibiotic adjunctive therapies.

A. Chemical adjuncts:
   1. Include antimicrobial rinses that are given before NSPT; NOT shown to have significant benefits.

2. Include subgingival irrigation, which, when combined with scaling, may enhance success of NSPT (controversy regarding benefits).
   a. Irrigation is considered elective part of therapy.
      (1) To be effective, must meet the following requirements:
         (a) Must reach base of pocket.
         (b) Bactericidal concentration of agents must be employed.
         (c) Must exhibit substantivity.
      (2) Methods of delivery
         (a) Use of hand syringe with cannula tip.
         (b) Use of pulsated irrigation devices, with either rubber tip or cannula.
   b. Commonly used irrigants:
      (1) 0.12% chlorhexidine digluconate.
      (2) 0.4% stannous fluoride.
      (3) 0.05% povidone-iodine.
   c. Include desensitizing agents for dentinal hypersensitivity, used as adjuncts to NSPT (also postsurgery); recommended because sensitivity after therapy is a commonly reported problem (see Chapter 11, Clinical Treatment).
B. Antibiotics:
   1. Systemic antibiotics:
      a. Sometimes necessary in treatment of MORE serious forms of periodontal disease because MOST of these conditions exhibit host impairment.
      b. In all cases, is BEST if the pathogens are identified (by culture and sensitivity, by DNA probing, or by immunofluorescent testing) to determine which antibiotic agent should be prescribed (see earlier discussion).
      c. Commonly prescribed adjuncts to NSPT include amoxicillin, ampicillin, Augmentin, tetracyclines, metronidazole, ciprofloxacin, clindamycin.
      d. Doxycycline hyclate (20 mg capsule bid) (Periostat): use of low-dose (LD) antibiotic at subantimicrobial dose (SDD) to suppress destructive enzymes such as collagenase produced during inflammatory process *rather* than to reduce bacterial numbers by blocking matrix metalloproteinases (MMPs); used twice daily for up to 9 months; results in decreased pocket depths and attachment loss; taking a common nonsteroidal antiinflammatory drug, such as aspirin or ibuprofen (Advil) along with doxycycline, may enhance the effectiveness of this treatment.
   2. Local delivery of antibiotics (controlled release):
      a. Used in cases that do NOT respond to conventional NSPT.
      b. When used concomitantly with scaling, has been shown to decrease probing depth and reduce BoP and microbes.
   c. FDA-approved examples:
      (1) Tetracycline fibers (Actisite, no longer available in United States): controlled-release impregnated fibers are placed in pockets greater than 5 mm for 10 days; placed in pocket in successive layers, with gingival retraction cord packing instrument, then sealed with cyanoacrylate adhesive; cord is removed after 10 days.
      (2) Doxycycline hyclate, 50 mg (Atridox): bioabsorbable, two-part formulation is mixed and placed by syringe in a periodontal pocket, where hardens on contact with saliva and slowly releases drug for a week; suppresses bacteria by inhibiting protein synthesis, thus bacteriostatic.
      (3) Chlorhexidinegluconate, 2.5 mg (PerioChip): biodegradable, rectangular chip placed in periodontal pockets greater than 5 mm, releases drug biphasically (40% initially; remainder over 7 to 10 days); bactericidal.
      (4) Minocycline hydrochloride, 1 mg (Arestin): powder (microspheres) gives extended release for up to 21 days, with no interdental cleaning for 10 days, no probing for 30 days, no retreatment for 3 months; bactericidal.
   d. Other controlled-release agents include chlorhexidine gels (1% and 2%), metronidazole gels, clindamycin HCl gel.

SURGICAL PERIODONTAL THERAPY

After completion of NSPT, tissue response is evaluated and need for surgical intervention is determined. IMPORTANT for the dental hygienist to understand indications and contraindications for basic surgical procedures to reinforce significance to the patient.
A. Rationale: reduction of disease progression when nonsurgical interventions have failed.
B. Goals:
   1. Pocket reduction for BETTER access to homecare procedures and professional debridement (MOST important).
   2. Correction of mucogingival defects and removal of inflamed tissues.
   3. Drainage of periodontal abscesses.
   4. Providing access for restorative dental procedures.
   5. Regeneration of tissue lost to disease.
   6. Placement of dental implants.
   7. Improved esthetics.
C. Considerations: several factors must be taken into consideration before surgical procedure is recommended; include probing depths, bone loss, value of affected tooth, patient factors.

1. Pocket probing depths (PD):
   a. Must be >5 mm.
   b. Typically difficult to debride professionally.
   c. Typically make performance of homecare by patient difficult.
2. Bone loss:
   a. If MORE than half of the bone remains, osseous surgery is viable option.
   b. If LESS than half of bone remains, grafting or regenerative techniques may be required.
   c. Choice of procedure depends on type of bone loss and bony defects (e.g., horizontal, vertical, one walled, two walled).
3. Value of the tooth: some LESS valuable than others, may NOT be worth saving (e.g., third molar).
4. Dental biofilm control: demonstration of adequate dental biofilm control measures is necessary.
5. Age of the patient:
   a. NOT significant, except in determining the speed of disease progression.
   b. Healing is similar in BOTH young and old patients.
   c. Relationship of surgery to quality of life SHOULD be considered for geriatric patients.
6. Health of the patient:
   a. Poor health contraindicates surgery.
   b. If periodontal disease is contributing to poor health, surgery may be indicated after medical consult.
7. Patient preference:
   a. Patients MUST be informed of all risks and benefits of surgery.
   b. Patients must understand the ramifications of NOT having surgery.
   c. Patients MUST be willing to increase frequency of PM appointments and perform MORE difficult dental biofilm removal procedures if opt NOT to have surgery.
D. Presurgical drug notations: NO drugs related to bleeding 2 weeks before surgery, including over-the-counter (OTC) drugs; for MOST healthy patients reduction of postsurgical swelling starts with taking 600 to 800 mg of ibuprofen (Motrin, Advil) 1 hour before treatment; effective analgesic (pain killer) and antiinflammatory.

Periodontal Surgical Procedures

Basic periodontal surgical procedures include gingivectomy, periodontal flap procedures, osseous surgery, and regeneration procedures. Implant surgery discussed later. Based on review of the literature, AAP concludes that there is a great need to develop an evidence-based approach to the use of lasers for the treatment of chronic periodontitis and insufficient evidence to suggest that any specific laser-based treatment is superior to the traditional modalities of therapy.
• See Chapter 7, Nutrition: presurgery and postsurgery diets.
A. **Gingivectomy:** to reduce pocket depths by removal of the soft tissue pocket wall.
   1. Indicated in deep gingival pockets that have fibrotic tissue and deep periodontal suprabony pockets.
   2. Example: removal of excess tissue with gingival hyperplasia as result of drug therapy (see earlier discussions).
B. **Periodontal flap procedures:** used during procedures that correct mucogingival defects (discussed later).
   1. Provide access to and visibility of the root surfaces, reduce pocket depths surgically, stimulate regeneration of lost periodontal attachment in periodontal pockets.
   2. Indicated in periodontal pockets that extend to or beyond mucogingival junction and for infrabony pockets.
      a. **Modified Widman flap technique:** repositioning of reflected gingival tissues against the tooth at approximately the preoperative position.
      b. **Apically positioned flap technique:** repositioning the reflected flap MORE apically, compared with original position, to reduce pocket depth.
C. **Crown lengthening:** used when tooth needs to be restored but there is NOT enough tooth structure coronal to the free gingival margin to support direct or indirect restoration (crown).
   1. Can occur when tooth breaks off at margin or restoration that has extensive caries underneath is lost, thus exposing MORE of tooth by removing some soft tissue and bone after flap procedure.
   2. Allowed to heal with temporary crown for at least 3 months before tooth is prepared for final crown; to allow gingival tissues to recede.
   3. Also used for removal of soft tissue with "gummy" smile; unusually large amount of attached gingiva around maxillary anterior teeth.
D. **Osseous surgery:**
   1. Used to reduce bony walls of infrabony pockets and to reshape abnormal alveolar contours.
      a. **Ostectomy:** removal of alveolar bone that is directly attached to the tooth via PDL fibers.
      b. **Osteoplasty:** recontouring of alveolar bone that is NOT directly supporting the tooth.
   2. Performed in conjunction with periodontal flap procedure to treat defects including:
      a. One-walled and two-walled infrabony pockets.
      b. Interdental osseous craters.
      c. Broad three-walled infrabony pockets.
      d. Reversed alveolar bone architecture.

    e. Bulbous facial and lingual bony contours:
      (1) Buttressing bone: abnormal thickening of bone in areas where trabeculae have been weakened by resorption.
      (2) Festoons: wavy contours of bone found between the teeth.

E. Periodontal regenerative procedures in infrabony pockets and class II furcations; includes regeneration procedures and/or bone grafting:
  1. **Guided tissue regeneration** (GTR): placement of various materials to form a barrier that prevents JE downgrowth and encourages connective tissue reattachment.
    a. Thorough debridement of the area, with flaps reflected.
    b. Placement of barrier material (e.g., Gortex or collagen) over defect; flap is closed coronally to the material.
  2. **Bone grafts:** placement of various materials in osseous defects before flap closure to encourage regeneration of lost tissue (see also later discussion with implants).
    a. Autografts: taken from the patient's hip (iliac crest) or jawbone.
    b. Allografts: taken from another person (e.g., freeze-dried from cadavers).
    c. Xenografts: taken from another species (e.g., bovine, coral).
    d. Alloplasts: synthetic bone minerals (e.g., hydroxyapatite [MAIN form of calcium found in bone], calcium sulfate, or ceramics).

F. Soft tissue grafting for correction of mucogingival defects:
  1. Type I defects: pockets extend apically to or beyond mucogingival junction, but a firm keratinized pocket wall exists; apically positioned flap is BEST treatment.
  2. Type II defects: alveolar mucosa acts as marginal gingiva, with NO zone of attached gingiva.
    a. Treatment consists of transfer of masticatory mucosa from an *adjacent area* of the mouth.
      (1) Lateral sliding pedicle graft: moving keratinized tissue from area immediately adjacent to defect without completely detaching from original spot, sliding it over defect, then attaching with sutures.
      (2) Double papillae flap: taking equal amounts of tissue from the two adjacent interdental papillae, sliding them over to cover the defective area, and joining the tissues with sutures.
    b. Free autogenous soft tissue graft: removing a piece of keratinized gingiva from *another area* of the mouth, such as palate, and suturing it to defective region to completely cover defect.

      (1) Dehiscence: bursting through bone of a root as the tooth continues to erupt so that the bone does not extend to its normal proximity to the CEJ; fenestration: circumscribed defect that creates a "window" through the bone over the prominent root.
      (2) Defects NOT present on radiographs and probing are limited; sounding (pushing probe through anesthetized soft tissue over the root) may be used.

G. Healing after surgery:
  1. Healing of surgical wound commences immediately after surgery with formation of a blood clot to protect the wound and allow healing to begin.
  2. Epithelial healing is accomplished within 7 days, at which time sutures, if NOT resorbable, and dressing, if placed, may be removed.
  3. Gingivectomy wounds take longer to heal than flap procedures because healing is by secondary intention rather than by primary intention.
  4. Osseous healing does NOT begin until 1 month after surgery; complete healing and remodeling do NOT take place until 4 to 6 months after surgery.

H. Effectiveness is dependent on patient's long-term thoroughness in dental biofilm control.
  1. Thoroughness should be reinforced at each PM appointment.
  2. Compliance with ongoing PM therapy is single MOST important factor in success of surgical and nonsurgical therapy.

I. Dental hygienist's role in periodontal surgery:
  1. When surgery is discussed, explained, and performed for patient, discussing advantages and disadvantages.
  2. Acting as patient advocate by asking questions and providing answers to concerns that patient may NOT be able to verbalize.
  3. Participating in postoperative suture and dressing removal (see next section).
  4. Removing postsurgical dental biofilm, following up with wound care, providing homecare instructions.
  5. Motivating patient to engage in long-term maintenance of dental biofilm control.
  6. Providing PM procedures at regular recare intervals.

Postsurgical Procedures

Postsurgical procedures include placement of sutures by supervising dentist, periodontal dressings, and provision of postoperative instructions. *See state laws for more information on local practice acts for dental hygienists concerning these duties.*

A. Sutures: placed at the end of surgical procedure to hold the tissues in place or close (proximate) so the wound can heal by primary intention.

1. Made of surgical silk, resorbable gut, or synthetic material.
2. Removed between 7 and 14 days after placement, if NOT resorbable, when tissues have undergone healing.
3. May be interrupted or uninterrupted, but knot always faces buccal surface.

B. **Periodontal** (surgical) **dressing** (pack): includes several types of dressing materials.
   1. Placed over surgical area to protect wound and increase patient comfort.
   2. SHOULD remain in place for approximately 1 week.
   3. Materials: zinc oxide–eugenol or zinc oxide–noneugenol (metallic oxide and fatty acids).
      a. Eugenol was used to help with adhesiveness of the dressing (Coe-pak, Periocare) but made the removal challenging, so dressing without eugenol is used MORE commonly (nothing to do with any other characteristics of eugenol).
      b. Clear, translucent, light-cured dressings (Barricaid VLC) are used for esthetic concerns.
   4. Mixing and application of the dressing:
      a. Lubricate lips to prevent moist and sticky dressing material from adhering during placement.
      b. Mix together equal lengths of each component paste until well blended and color is homogeneous; create two rolls that approximate length of surgical area.
      c. Using sterile gauze, gently dry area to be covered.
      d. Control bleeding before placing by applying pressure to area with sterile gauze sponge until bleeding subsides; if this does NOT work, hemostatic agents may be necessary.
      e. Dressing should be adapted far enough into interproximal areas that facial and lingual surfaces of the dressing are joined together to form mechanical lock between the dressing and the teeth; extend NO further occlusally than middle third of the teeth and do NOT allow to interfere with normal occlusion.
   5. Patient instructions:
      a. Avoid eating, drinking, rinsing for FIRST hour after placement to allow dressing to harden.
      b. Rest of instructions are SIMILAR to those for postoperative (see next).
   6. Removing the dressing:
      a. Gently loosen from the soft tissues with pair of cotton pliers and curet; lift away from wound site.
      b. Rinse area gently with sterile saline to cleanse it of surface debris.
      c. If the dressing was placed over sutures, suture material may be incorporated into the hardened dressing material, special care in removal required.

C. Postoperative instructions can include:
   1. Directions for mouthrinses, antibiotics, analgesic medications.
   2. Instructions to eliminate strenuous activity.
   3. Directions regarding continued bleeding (both oral and written).
   4. Recommendation of soft diet; AVOID spicy foods.
   5. Directions regarding periodontal dressing, if placed.
   6. Inform that swelling may occur, can be minimized with use of ice; 30 minutes on, then 60 minutes off, for 48 to 72 hours.
   7. Directions for homecare, including brushing with soft-bristled toothbrush and gently debriding dressing area.
   8. Reminder to return for suture removal, if needed.

PERIODONTAL MAINTENANCE

Success of periodontal therapy depends on successful maintenance of health and prevention of recurring disease. To accomplish this healthy state for any length of time, regular **periodontal maintenance** (PM, recare, continuing care) appointments and procedures are required. These are at relatively short intervals to reinforce homecare, control accumulation of dental biofilm–retentive deposits, and deal with such problems as root caries and dentinal hypersensitivity with postsurgical exposure of dentin. Usually patient is seen every 3 months or four times a year by the dental hygienist.

• See Chapter 11, Clinical Treatment: health promotion, disease prevention factors, dentinal hypersensitivity, root caries.

A. Role of the dental hygienist:
   1. MAIN provider of PM procedures; role is critical to the success of periodontal therapy.
   2. MUST work in collaboration with supervising dentist and/or periodontist in provision of high-quality oral healthcare.
   3. MUST function as cotherapist; must encourage patient to assume ultimate responsibility for maintenance of periodontal health.

B. Rationale: preservation of stability achieved during active NSPT can be accomplished ONLY through repeated PM visits.

C. Objectives: preservation of CAL, maintenance of bone height, control of inflammation, control of dental biofilm.
   1. Preservation of CAL:
      a. Monitoring probing depths at PM appointments, which can predict attachment loss, signaling return of disease, or can indicate stability.
      b. Recording of CAL, which SHOULD take place periodically at PM appointments for baseline comparison.

2. Maintenance of alveolar bone height:
   a. Periodic radiographic evaluations of bone levels are necessary for comparison with baseline levels.
   b. Radiographs do NOT indicate active disease; ONLY illustrate historical bone loss.
   c. Evidence of continued bone loss is indicative of disease progression.
   d. MAIN goal is to prevent further bone loss, which can lead to eventual tooth loss.
3. Control of inflammation:
   a. To halt disease progression, inflammation MUST be eliminated.
   b. Repeated evaluation of the gingival tissues for signs of inflammation at PM appointments enables the dental hygienist and patient to effectively control disease progression. All BoP sites MUST be recorded, since BoP has been shown to be the MOST reliable sign of inflammation.
4. All aspects of oral health MUST be evaluated at each PM appointment; includes identification of new hard and soft tissue lesions, significant systemic disease that might affect oral health, any other disharmonies or discrepancies that may affect oral health.
5. Evaluation and reinforcement of oral hygiene:
   a. Compliance with oral hygiene procedures requires frequent reinforcement.
   b. Regular observation and recording of dental biofilm scores assist in motivating the patient.
   c. Direct observation of homecare techniques can assist in behavior modification.
   d. Dental biofilm control education is as IMPORTANT and as difficult as the technical aspects of therapy.

D. Effectiveness:
   1. BOTH surgical and nonsurgical periodontal therapies have been shown to be effective in eliminating active disease but ONLY if routine PM is performed at regular intervals.
   2. Periodontal therapy without regular PM may result in increased attachment and alveolar bone loss.
   3. Meticulous dental biofilm control and professional debridement control disease in MOST cases.

E. Compliance is KEY to successful therapy.
   1. Major challenge for the dental hygienist, since there can be LOW compliance rates; MUST spend time explaining significance of PM appointments to maintenance of oral health.
   2. Reasons for noncompliance are complex:
      a. Failure to understand significance.
      b. Interpretation of chronic disease as NOT life threatening.
      c. Economic issues; value of care to patient; socioeconomic status (SES) of patient.
      d. Fear.
      e. Influence of friends and family.
      f. Perceived indifference on part of dental hygienist.
   3. Success of periodontal therapy rests on performance of adequate daily dental biofilm control.
      a. Dental hygienist is responsible for educating and motivating patient to perform these procedures routinely.
      b. Compliance with oral hygiene has been shown to diminish within 30 days of commencement.
      c. The MORE aids that are introduced, the LESS compliant a patient is likely to be.
      d. Interproximal aids are difficult to use and lead to LACK of compliance.
      e. Powered toothbrushes have been shown to increase patient compliance.
   4. Noncompliance with either PM appointments or maintenance of oral hygiene results in continued disease progression.

F. Techniques for enhancing compliance:
   1. Simplify explanations.
   2. Accommodate program to suit needs; satisfied patients are MORE compliant.
   3. Write down oral hygiene regimens to serve as reminders.
   4. Provide positive reinforcement.
   5. Remind patients of appointments.
   6. Identify noncompliers before commencement of initial therapy and discuss consequences of noncompliance.
   7. Keep compliance records to guide behavior modification and for legal purposes.

G. Components of appointment:
   1. MAIN aims of the PM appointment are to evaluate stability of the results of initial therapy; to thoroughly debride all tooth surfaces; to eliminate any factors that may support persistence of disease-producing microorganisms; to evaluate and reinforce dental biofilm control.
   2. Procedures performed at the PM appointment:
      a. Medical and dental history updates.
      b. Oral and dental examinations.
      c. Evaluation of:
         (1) Pocket probing depths and CAL to ascertain attachment loss and gingival recession.
         (2) BoP and suppuration.
         (3) Tooth mobility and furcations.
         (4) Mucogingival involvement.
         (5) Root caries and dentinal hypersensitivity.
      d. Radiographic examination as necessary.
      e. Dental biofilm control evaluation, which involves:
         (1) Dental (dental biofilm) index score.
         (2) Education, motivation, and reinforcement regarding dental biofilm control.

(3) Provision of oral hygiene instructions, including:

    (a) Review of toothbrushing and interdental cleansing techniques.

    (b) Reinforcement of significance of daily homecare.

f. Periodontal debridement.

  (1) Removal of all supragingival and subgingival dental biofilm and calculus.

  (2) Selective polishing, if rationale exists.

  (3) Fluoride and calcium therapy, if warranted.

  (4) Desensitization, as needed.

g. Referral to an appropriate specialist, if warranted.

h. Establishment of appropriate PM intervals that meet individual's needs.

H. Recurrence of disease is common.

  1. Causes of recurrence:

    a. Insufficient dental biofilm control; incomplete removal of deposits during therapy.

    b. Faulty restorations and/or prostheses that foster dental biofilm accumulation; LACK of compliance with regular PM appointment intervals.

    c. Systemic conditions that affect the host response.

  2. Sometimes, despite appropriate therapy and compliance, disease remains active or refractory (occurs in 10% of all periodontal patients).

  3. Return of disease requires that initial therapy be repeated, results be reevaluated, and decisions be made regarding surgical alternatives; also requires referral to a specialist.

  4. Other treatment modalities may include microbiological monitoring and/or antibiotic therapy.

DENTAL IMPLANTS ▰▰▰▰▰▰▰▰▰

Because dental implants are vulnerable to bacterial invasion and subsequent failure, dental hygienist can play important role in BOTH patient education and professional maintenance.

- See Chapters 11, Clinical Treatment: implant charting and homecare; 12, Instrumentation: professional care.

A. Implants are designed for several uses:

  1. To support dentures in edentulous mouths.

  2. As abutments in partially edentulous mouths to support fixed bridgework.

  3. To replace single teeth.

B. Types include endosseous, subperiosteal, transosteal implants:

  1. **Endosseous implant:** placed directly in the bone; may be either root form or blade form; MOST commonly used system.

    a. Root form is MORE common than blade form; may be conical, cylindrical, threaded-screw, perforated, or hollow baskets.

    b. Made MOSTLY of titanium; however, polymers, ceramics, and other metals are used.

    c. May be sprayed or coated with plasma of titanium, aluminum oxide, hydroxyapatite, or single-crystal sapphire.

  2. **Subperiosteal implant:** positioned over the bone; consists of cast framework with projections protruding through the mucosa that are designed to support complete removable denture.

  3. **Transosteal** (staple) **implant:** surgically placed through the mandible; provides anchorage for removable mandibular denture; often made of gold or Vitallium instead of titanium.

  4. Mini implants: smaller, LESS invasive implant fixtures used in immediate-loading surgery (discussed next).

C. Relative contraindications:

  1. Uncontrolled type 1 DM and/or smoking because healing after any type of surgical procedure is delayed owing to poor peripheral blood circulation.

  2. Poor volume and height of bone available (often the complementary procedures sinus augmentation and block graft are needed to provide enough bone, discussed later).

Implant Surgery

Traditional implant surgery typically can take place either 2 weeks or 3 months after extraction (delayed immediate postextraction implant placement) or 3 months after tooth extraction (late implantation). Consists of two surgeries, and typically takes 2 to 6 months before final permanent replacements are placed. During this time patients can wear removable temporary tooth replacements over the implant sites.

However, technology affords some patients ability to have immediate-loading dental implants; immediately placed after tooth extraction, and temporary fixed tooth replacement is attached. MOST patients need the longer treatment plan, which has an excellent history going back many years. Only traditional method is discussed here.

A. Traditional surgical method:

  1. First surgery:

    a. Osteotomy performed by drilling a hole through the bone to place the implant in the jaw.

    b. Covering implant with gingiva and allowing 2 to 6 months for healing and osseointegration.

  2. Second surgery:

    a. Implant is exposed, and placement of the abutment fixture, which protrudes coronal to the gingiva, is made.

    b. Final "loading" is performed, which involves placement of the prosthesis onto the abutment.

      (1) Early loading (1 week to 12 weeks).

      (2) Staged loading (3 to 6 months).

      (3) Late loading (more than 6 months).

B. Success is dependent on:
1. Careful selection of the candidate; relative contra-indications may compromise success:
   a. History of blood dyscrasias, DM, smoking, or other diseases that compromise health.
   b. Poor oral health (e.g., gingivitis, periodontitis).
   c. Poor oral hygiene practices.
   d. Poor quality and quantity of bone.
2. Careful preparation of the implant site:
   a. Overheating of the bone should be avoided.
   b. If bone overheats, necrosis may occur, which may result in fibrointegration rather than osseointegration.
3. Accurate sizing of the placement site:
   a. Preserving ample keratinized tissue around implant.
   b. Parallel placement of multiple implants, which allows prostheses to be attached with screws.
4. Allowing time for BOTH healing and osseointegration (2 to 6 months) before loading the implant.
C. **Osseointegration:**
1. Direct contact or integration of the bone to implant; provides MOST stable attachment.
2. **Fibrointegration:** connective tissue grows between bone and implant; LESS likely to exhibit long-term success in contrast to osseointegration.
D. Tissue interface:
1. Consists of gingiva surrounding implant, SIMILAR to that which surrounds a normal tooth except there are NO gingival or PDL fibers between gingiva and bone.
2. Area between JE and the bone is composed of connective tissue, which touches the implant surface directly and contains collagen fibers that run parallel (rather than perpendicular) to the implant surface.
   a. The SE is nonkeratinized, and cells at the base of the sulcus form a JE that attaches to the implant by means of a basal lamina and hemidesmosomes.
   b. Implant sulcus depths range from 1.3 to 3.8 mm.
   c. This interface or biological seal prevents penetration of bacteria and their toxins to osseointegrated implant surface.
E. Complementary procedures:
1. **Sinus lifting:** thickens inadequate part of atrophic maxilla toward the sinus with assistance of bone grafting, creates a BETTER quality bone site.
2. Bone grafting is necessary in patients who have a LACK of adequate maxillary or mandibular bone in terms of front to back (lip to tongue) depth or thickness, top to bottom height, and left to right width; sufficient bone is needed in three dimensions to securely integrate with the rootlike implant (see earlier discussion).
   a. Typically, implants are placed at least as deeply into bone as crown or tooth will be coronal to the bone, a 1:1 crown to root ratio.
   b. This ratio establishes target for bone grafting in MOST cases; if 1:1 or better cannot be achieved, the patient is usually advised that only short implant can be placed and NOT to expect a long period of usability.
   c. Improved bone height, difficult to achieve, is particularly important to ensure ample anchorage of the implant's rootlike shape because it has to support mechanical stress of chewing, just like a natural tooth.
   d. If an implant is too shallow, chewing may cause dangerous jawbone crack or full fracture.
   e. Wide range of grafting materials and substances may be used (see earlier discussion).

Professional Implant Maintenance

Professional maintenance procedures for implants include assessing tissues, probing implant sulcus depths, checking for BoP and mobility, assessing dental biofilm and calculus deposits, removing deposits, obtaining annual radiographs, and discussing homecare with patient.
- See Chapters 11, Clinical Treatment: implant homecare; 12, Instrumentation: implant scaling, manual and ultrasonics.
A. ONLY instruments made specifically for implants should be used for removal of hard and soft deposits and for probing; conventional metal instruments can scratch the surface, making them LESS biocompatible with the surrounding tissues and MORE conducive to dental biofilm accumulation.
B. Sonic and ultrasonic instrumentation and air-powder polishing should be avoided, unless implant plastic tips with ultrasonic scaler, either fixed or disposable, are used.
C. Rubber-cup polishing with fine powder, such as tin oxide, or with fine-grit commercial polishing paste may be performed selectively, as with natural teeth.
D. Implant-supported prosthesis should be removed yearly to permit thorough debridement and to check for stability.
E. A 3-month recare (recall) interval should be established for at least first year after implant placement.

Implant Failure and Periimplantitis

Failure of a dental implant is MOST often related to failure to osseointegrate correctly. Affected implants have **periimplantitis** rather than periodontitis. Dental hygienist SHOULD be able to recognize a failing implant. Treatment requires removal of implant. Considered a failure if lost or mobile or shows postimplant bone loss of greater than 1.0 mm in the first year, greater than 0.2 mm a year thereafter.

A. Characterized by mobility (MOST important), pocketing, BoP, exudate, progression of bone loss, dull sound on percussion, radiographic evidence of peri-implant radiolucency.
B. Periimplant tissues are at risk for invasion by microorganisms the SAME as natural periodontium.
   1. Microbiota found in implant sulcus are SIMILAR to those in natural sulcus, in BOTH health and disease.
   2. Because of risk for infection, maintenance of implants is a MAIN concern.
   3. Prevention of infection includes excellent maintenance education with antibiotics before and after surgery, along with mouthrinses such as chlorhexidine.
C. Risk of failure occurs MAINLY with smokers; MORE rarely implant may fail because of poor positioning at the time of surgery or may be overloaded initially, causing failure to integrate.
   1. For this reason, frequently placed ONLY after patient has stopped smoking.
   2. If BOTH smoking and positioning problems exist before implant surgery, clinicians often advise patients that a bridge or partial denture may be a BETTER solution than an implant.

Review Questions

1 Which of the following groups of risk factors for periodontal disease have the MOST capacity to be modified?
   A. Age, genetics, and race
   B. Smoking, gender, and HIV
   C. Diabetes, nutritional deficiencies, and neutrophil abnormalities
   D. Stress, smoking, and pregnancy
2 Nutritional deficiencies are considered risk factors for periodontal disease because they
   A. contribute to accumulation of dental biofilm.
   B. promote bone loss.
   C. lower the host response.
   D. are associated with lower socioeconomic groups.
3 Oral side effects of a deficiency in vitamin B_6 (pyridoxine) include all of the following, EXCEPT one. Which one is the EXCEPTION?
   A. Gingivitis
   B. Glossitis
   C. Stomatitis
   D. Candidiasis
4 A deficiency of which vitamin, responsible for the biosynthesis of collagen, will adversely affect periodontal connective tissue and wound healing?
   A. Vitamin A
   B. Vitamin B
   C. Vitamin C
   D. Vitamin D

5 When vitamin D deficiency occurs in adults, the resulting effects on the periodontium include all of the following, EXCEPT one. Which one is the EXCEPTION?
   A. Resorption of the alveolar bone
   B. Destruction of the PDL
   C. Fibrous dysplasia of the bone
   D. Hyperplasia of the gingiva
6 Which of the following nutritional deficiencies has been associated with an increased incidence of necrotizing gingivitis?
   A. Osteoporosis
   B. Osteomalacia
   C. Marasmus
   D. Kwashiorkor
7 Multilocular radiolucent jaw lesions, the loss of lamina dura, and a ground glass appearance of the alveolar bone are MOST characteristic of
   A. a vitamin D deficiency.
   B. hyperparathyroidism.
   C. osteomalacia.
   D. Paget's disease.
8 During puberty, an adolescent is MOST susceptible to the development of gingivitis because of
   A. poor oral hygiene habits.
   B. altered capillary permeability.
   C. decreased levels of hormones.
   D. altered chemotactic response.
9 Recent evidence indicates that desquamative gingivitis is MOST likely a feature of all of the following, EXCEPT one. Which one is the EXCEPTON?
   A. Menopause
   B. Erosive lichen planus
   C. Mucous membrane pemphigoid
   D. Pemphigus
10 The rationale for the prevalence of periodontal disease in patients with diabetes mellitus includes all of the following, EXCEPT one. Which one is the EXCEPTION?
   A. Defective PMN chemotaxis
   B. Microangiopathy of the periodontal tissues
   C. Increased collagen breakdown
   D. Increased fibrosis of the periodontal tissues
   E. Microbial alterations
11 Multiple periodontal abscesses, velvety red gingivae, and marginal proliferation of the gingivae are common oral manifestations of
   A. type 1 diabetes.
   B. type 2 diabetes.
   C. uncontrolled diabetes.
   D. controlled diabetes.
12 A decrease in circulating neutrophils results in
   A. spontaneous gingival hemorrhage.
   B. oral herpetic lesions.
   C. an impaired host response.
   D. leukemia.
13 Neutropenia is present in all of the following, EXCEPT one. Which one is the EXCEPTION?
   A. Down syndrome.
   B. Diabetes mellitus.
   C. Autoimmune disorders.
   D. CNS dysfunction.

14 Cyclosporine, diltiazem, phenobarbital, and nifedipine are drugs that
   A. belong to the beta-blocker category.
   B. cause xerostomia.
   C. cause gingival enlargement.
   D. suppress the immune system.

15 The primary etiological factor in periodontal disease is
   A. bacteria.
   B. host response.
   C. bacteria and host response.
   D. poor oral hygiene.

16 Dental biofilm associated with gingival health is typically composed of
   A. gram-positive aerobic cocci and rods.
   B. gram-negative aerobic cocci and rods.
   C. gram-positive rods and spirochetes.
   D. gram-negative rods and spirochetes.

17 With a diagnosis of localized aggressive periodontitis, which of the following microorganisms would be present in large levels?
   A. *P. gingivalis*
   B. *A. actinomycetemcomitans*
   C. *T. forsythensis*
   D. *P. intermedia*

18 Bacterial enzymes that can affect host cells and ground substance include all of the following, EXCEPT one. Which one is the EXCEPTION?
   A. Hyaluronidase
   B. Collagenase
   C. Ribonuclease
   D. Lipase

19 Bacterial endotoxins are responsible primarily for
   A. destroying host cells.
   B. activating the complement cascade.
   C. releasing enzymes.
   D. killing bacteria.

20 All of the following are antibacterial components found in saliva, EXCEPT one. Which one is the EXCEPTION?
   A. Lysozyme
   B. Lactoperoxidase
   C. Macrophages
   D. Secretory IgA

21 One of the following is NOT a chemical mediator of vascular permeability. Which one is the EXCEPTION?
   A. Histamine and serotonin
   B. Kinins and prostaglandins
   C. Thyroxine
   D. C3 and C5
   E. Lysosomal enzymes

22 When PMNs begin to adhere to endothelial walls during the period of vascular dilation, this is referred to as
   A. margination.
   B. emigration.
   C. migration.
   D. chemotaxis.

23 The FIRST cell to appear in chronic inflammation that constitutes the body's second line of defense is the
   A. neutrophil.
   B. macrophage.
   C. lymphocyte.
   D. basophil.

24 All of the following types of lymphocytes are responsible for cellular immunity, EXCEPT one. Which one is the EXCEPTION?
   A. T4 activator cells
   B. T8 suppressor cells
   C. Killer cells
   D. B cells

25 The chronic inflammatory cells responsible for humoral immunity are
   A. macrophages.
   B. B lymphocytes.
   C. T lymphocytes.
   D. monocytes.

26 The appearance of fibroblasts and new capillaries is characteristic of which stage of inflammation?
   A. Acute stage
   B. Chronic stage
   C. Remission stage
   D. Repair stage

27 The primary tissue destruction that occurs during the inflammatory phase of periodontal disease is produced by the by-products of
   A. bacterial cell walls.
   B. complement proteins.
   C. antibodies.
   D. arachidonic acid cascade.

28 The release of chemotactic factors that cause the migration of neutrophils and macrophages to specific sites is controlled by the
   A. phagocytic system.
   B. complement system.
   C. arachidonic acid cascade.
   D. kinin system.

29 The cytokine released by T cells that is capable of inducing bone resorption is
   A. arachidonic acid.
   B. prostaglandin.
   C. interleukin-1.
   D. myeloperoxidase.

30 Within 4 to 7 days after dental biofilm accumulation, what histopathological lesion occurs?
   A. Initial lesion
   B. Early lesion
   C. Established lesion
   D. Advanced lesion

31 When a lesion extends into the periodontal ligament and alveolar bone, it is classified histologically as an
   A. initial lesion.
   B. early lesion.
   C. established lesion.
   D. advanced lesion.

32 The clinical signs and symptoms of occlusal trauma include radiographic evidence of a
  A. narrowed periodontal ligament space and clinical evidence of tooth mobility.
  B. narrowed periodontal ligament space and clinical evidence of tooth extrusion.
  C. widened periodontal ligament space and clinical evidence of tooth mobility.
  D. widened periodontal ligament space and clinical evidence of tooth extrusion.

33 Damage that occurs when the amount of alveolar bone is normal but excessive occlusal forces are present is referred to as
  A. primary occlusal trauma.
  B. secondary occlusal trauma.
  C. hyperfunction.
  D. hypofunction.

34 During inspection of the patient's mouth, several wear facets on the teeth are noted and determined to be nonfunctional. This sign is indicative of
  A. decay.
  B. TMJ disorder.
  C. trismus
  D. bruxism.

35 Subgingival calculus, in the etiology of periodontal disease, is a
  A. primary etiological factor.
  B. local predisposing factor.
  C. local functional factor.
  D. systemic contributing factor.

36 Calculus is composed primarily of
  A. inorganic matter.
  B. organic matter.
  C. microorganisms.
  D. protein polysaccharide complexes.

37 A soft, sticky, yellow or grayish white substance that partially adheres to the teeth is referred to as
  A. bacterial dental.
  B. materia alba.
  C. food debris.
  D. acquired pellicle.

38 The MOST commonly occurring form of periodontal disease is
  A. gingivitis.
  B. chronic periodontitis.
  C. aggressive periodontitis.
  D. periodontal abscess.

39 The MOST significant feature of chronic gingivitis is
  A. marginal redness.
  B. edema of the gingival margins.
  C. bleeding on probing (BoP).
  D. a loss of stippling.

40 A deficiency in vitamin C causes all of the following, EXCEPT one. Which one is the EXCEPTION?
  A. Gingival inflammation
  B. An increased tendency for hemorrhage
  C. The degeneration of collagen fibers
  D. Poor wound healing

41 A 17-year-old male patient presents with purplish blue gingiva, tumorlike masses around several interdental papillae, shiny gingival surfaces with ulcerations, and spontaneous bleeding. The patient looks pale and says that he has been tired, has not felt well for a while, and is undergoing some medical tests. A possible diagnosis might be
  A. necrotizing ulcerative gingivitis.
  B. primary herpetic gingivostomatitis.
  C. leukemia.
  D. puberty gingivitis.

42 Localized, enlarged interdental gingiva that form tumorlike growths may accompany
  A. leukemic or pregnancy gingivitis.
  B. pregnancy gingivitis or necrotizing ulcerative gingivitis.
  C. necrotizing ulcerative gingivitis or diabetic gingivitis.
  D. diabetic gingivitis or AIDS-associated gingivitis.

43 A patient complains that the gums are very sore in the lower right posterior region of her mouth. Her oral hygiene is meticulous, and there is no visible dental biofilm. Her tissues appear very healthy, except for the region surrounding her first molar, which appears red and edematous and has several small vesicles on the marginal gingiva surrounding the full nonprecious metal crown. A diagnosis of this condition might be
  A. desquamative gingivitis.
  B. menopausal gingivitis.
  C. allergic gingivitis.
  D. aphthous ulcers.

44 Desquamative gingivitis is frequently linked with all of the following EXCEPT one. Which one is the EXCEPTION?
  A. Pemphigus
  B. Pemphigoid
  C. Lichen planus
  D. Drugs
  E. Pregnancy

45 Inflammatory gingival overgrowth is associated with all of the following, EXCEPT one. Which one is the EXCEPTION?
  A. Bacterial dental biofilm
  B. Phenytoin
  C. Cyclosporine
  D. Calcium channel blockers
  E. Bulimia

46 Severe enlargement of the entire gingiva, including both facial and lingual surfaces, occasionally occurs with no apparent explanation. This condition is MOST likely caused by
  A. the use of cyclosporine.
  B. the presence of type 1 diabetes mellitus.
  C. a rare hereditary or familial condition.
  D. the presence of epilepsy.

47 A 19-year-old college student presents for emergency care complaining of pain in the gingiva, spontaneous bleeding, and a bad metallic taste in his mouth. During inspection a fetid odor, punched-in interdental papillae covered with a gray pseudomembrane, and the spontaneous bleeding are noted. This patient MOST likely has
  A. primary herpetic gingivostomatitis.
  B. leukemia.
  C. necrotizing ulcerative gingivitis.
  D. AIDS-associated gingivitis.

48 A periodontal pocket whose base is coronal to the level of the alveolar bone is referred to as a(n)
  A. pseudopocket.
  B. relative pocket.
  C. suprabony pocket.
  D. infrabony pocket.

49 A patient with generalized moderate chronic periodontitis received scaling of the maxillary right arch 2 weeks ago. The patient returns for treatment of the mandibular right quadrant but complains of a dull, throbbing pain around the maxillary right molar area. During inspection, an 11-mm pocket depth and accompanying suppuration on the mesial facial surface of tooth #2 are found. The chart indicates that the pocket depth before scaling was 6 mm. This patient MOST likely has developed
  A. a periodontal abscess.
  B. a periapical abscess.
  C. an endo/perio lesion.
  D. pericoronitis.

50 A systemic condition characterized by hyperkeratotic skin lesions of the palms, soles, knees, and elbows, severe destruction of the periodontium, and onset before age 4 is
  A. Chédiak-Higashi syndrome.
  B. hypophosphatasia.
  C. Papillon-Lefèvre syndrome.
  D. Down syndrome.

51 LGE is associated with
  A. diabetic gingivitis.
  B. leukemic gingivitis.
  C. AIDS-associated gingivitis.
  D. chronic gingivitis.

52 You learn at his appointment that thyroid cancer has been diagnosed in your patient and he must undergo radiation therapy. How should you plan his periodontal therapy?
  A. Perform all necessary periodontal therapy immediately, before his radiation therapy.
  B. Wait until after his radiation therapy has been completed and the cancer has been eliminated before proceeding with his periodontal therapy.
  C. Ask the patient whether he wishes to have his periodontal therapy before or after radiation therapy.
  D. Do noninvasive therapy before his radiation treatments and complete the more invasive care after he is feeling better.

53 The personal history is important for the identification of all of the following nondentally related risk factors for periodontal disease, EXCEPT one. Which one is the EXCEPTION?
  A. Smoking
  B. Alcohol consumption
  C. Diet
  D. Stress
  E. Social status

54 Lifesaver-like enlargements surrounding the free gingival margins are BEST referred to as
  A. rolled margins.
  B. Stillman's clefts.
  C. McCall's festoons.
  D. marginal hyperplasia.

55 The "gold standard" for determining the extent of periodontal tissue destruction is the measurement of
  A. clinical attachment level.
  B. periodontal pockets.
  C. bleeding in response to probing.
  D. bone loss through radiographic analysis.

56 The periodontal screening and recording (PSR) system is a modification of the
  A. Ramfjord index.
  B. Russell index.
  C. CPITN (WHO).
  D. Loe and Silness index.

57 It is important for a dental hygienist to examine the condition of tooth proximal contact areas because
  A. drifting may occur if contacts are not tight.
  B. contact areas affect a patient's homecare abilities.
  C. contact areas affect a patient's occlusion.
  D. extrusion may change a contact point.

58 Tooth mobility, furcation involvement, malocclusions, overhanging margins of restorations, and the status of prosthetic appliances are all important because they are classified as
  A. etiological factors for periodontal disease.
  B. systemic risk factors for periodontal disease.
  C. local risk factors for periodontal disease.
  D. primary risk factors for periodontal disease.

59 The use of supplemental periodontal diagnostic tests should be reserved exclusively for
  A. the identification of risk factors.
  B. definitive periodontal diagnosis.
  C. treatment planning purposes.
  D. identifying unusual periodontal diseases.

60 The BANA test, ELISA test, and DNA probe are all used for the measurement of
  A. biochemical markers in gingival crevicular fluid.
  B. bacterial enzymes.
  C. bacterial species.
  D. bacterial antibodies.

61 The phase of periodontal treatment that involves the elimination of etiological factors is
  A. phase I therapy.
  B. phase II therapy.
  C. phase III therapy.
  D. phase IV therapy.

62 All periodontal patients who have received initial therapy require an evaluation after
A. 1 to 2 weeks.
B. 4 to 6 weeks.
C. 2 to 3 months.
D. 4 to 6 months.

63 An assessment of Mr. Forbes identifies his condition as ADA case type III, with average pocket depths of 5 to 6 mm and moderate to heavy subgingival calculus in MOST areas. His initial therapy should MOST closely resemble which of the following nonsurgical periodontal therapy treatment plans?
A. One appointment for completion of all debridement
B. Two appointments without any local anesthesia
C. Two appointments with local anesthesia
D. Four appointments with local anesthesia

64 Rationales for nonsurgical periodontal therapy include all of the following, EXCEPT one. Which one is the EXCEPTION?
A. The need for surgical access
B. The modification of risk factors
C. The removal of bacterial dental (etiological agent) and other local irritants
D. The initiation of dental control measures
E. The evaluation of tissue response

65 Which one of the following is NOT a goal of periodontal surgery?
A. Reducing pocket depths for better access to homecare
B. Correcting mucogingival defects
C. Retaining inflamed tissues
D. Regenerating tissues lost to disease

66 A surgical procedure that reduces pocket depths by removing the soft tissue pocket wall in supragingival pockets is referred to as a
A. gingivectomy.
B. modified Widman flap.
C. guided tissue regeneration.
D. ostectomy.

67 One-walled and two-walled infrabony pockets are BEST treated surgically with which of the following procedures?
A. Ostectomy
B. Osteoplasty
C. Osteotomy
D. Ostectomy and osteoplasty
E. Osteoplasty and osteotomy

68 Bone grafting material that is taken from another person (freeze-dried from cadavers) is referred to as a(n)
A. allograft.
B. autograft.
C. xenograft.
D. alloplast.

69 Which of the following is a description of a type II mucogingival defect?
A. Alveolar mucosa acts as marginal gingiva, without a zone of attached gingiva.
B. Pockets extend to or beyond the mucogingival junction.
C. Gingiva is recessed beyond the mucogingival junction.
D. Port-hole defect is present in the alveolar mucosa.

70 Periodontal surgical dressings are placed over a surgical wound for protection and should remain in place for
A. 3 to 5 days.
B. 7 to 10 days.
C. 12 to 14 days.
D. 18 to 21 days.

71 Which one of the following is NOT a goal of periodontal maintenance therapy?
A. Preservation of clinical attachment levels
B. Maintenance of alveolar bone height
C. Control of inflammation
D. Evaluation and reinforcement of the patient's oral hygiene
E. Correction of mucogingival defects

72 Compliance with oral hygiene measures decreases within
A. 1 month.
B. 2 months.
C. 3 months.
D. 4 months.

73 Which of the following procedures is NOT a part of the recare appointment?
A. Complete periodontal evaluation
B. Quadrant scaling with anesthesia
C. Oral hygiene instructions
D. Tooth desensitization as needed

74 During one of Mrs. Smith's routine recare appointments, increases in pocket depths in several areas, multiple areas of bleeding in response to probing, and moderate to heavy calculus deposits in several molar areas are detected. The BEST approach would be to
A. review oral hygiene more thoroughly, emphasizing the effects of noncompliance.
B. treat the areas that exhibit breakdown.
C. repeat initial therapy by quadrant and reevaluate after 4 weeks.
D. refer Mrs. Smith to a periodontist for surgical intervention.

75 The acute periodontal abscess initially is BEST treated with
A. drainage of the abscess.
B. antibiotics.
C. tooth extraction.
D. tetracycline fiber placement.

76 A raised, painful area of acute inflammation on the marginal gingiva, with no accompanying periodontal pockets and no radiographically visible bone loss, MOST likely is a(n)
A. acute periodontal abscess.
B. periapical abscess.
C. gingival abscess.
D. combination abscess.

77 If a patient presents with pericoronitis, the dental hygienist's role in caring for the patient may include all of the following, EXCEPT one. Which is the EXCEPTION?
A. Irrigation of the area under the operculum
B. Gentle debridement under the operculum
C. Providing a prescription for antibiotics
D. Providing oral hygiene instruction

78 The MOST important instruction that a dental hygienist can provide to the parents of a patient with primary herpetic gingivostomatitis is
A. to keep the child isolated because the virus is contagious.
B. to engage in gentle, daily dental biofilm removal.
C. to strictly follow diet instructions.
D. to encourage daily fluid intake.

79 If a patient with necrotizing ulcerative gingivitis (NUG) or a patient with pericoronitis has been prescribed a hydrogen peroxide rinse, the patient should discontinue the rinse after
A. 3 days.
B. 7 days.
C. 14 days.
D. 21 days.

80 A root-form or blade-form implant placed directly into the bone is classified as a(n)
A. endosseous implant.
B. subperiosteal implant.
C. transosteal implant.
D. staple implant.

81 The MAIN purpose of two-step implant surgery is to allow
A. fibrointegration.
B. osseointegration.
C. bone regeneration.
D. settling to occur.

82 The interface or biological seal found around an implant is created by the formation of a long junctional epithelium that is attached to the implant surface by
A. glycosaminoglycans.
B. connective tissue.
C. hemidesmosomes.
D. gap junctions.

83 Dental biofilm in a recently cleaned mouth contains
A. leukocytes, epithelial cells, and a few gram-positive cocci.
B. leukocytes, cocci with filaments increasing, and newly formed rods.
C. gram-negative anaerobic bacteria, white blood cells, and spirochetes.
D. gram-negative aerobic bacteria, gram-positive cocci, and spirochetes.

84 Which statement is CORRECT regarding calculus?
A. By itself, can cause disease
B. Attachment mechanism for oral biofilm
C. Easily removed with a sharp curet
D. Supragingivally appears darker because of blood pigments

85 Approximately 2 weeks ago, four quadrants of periodontal debridement were completed on Catherine, a 34-year-old woman with diabetes and the mother of two young children. She presents for her reevaluation, during which an appropriate maintenance (recare) interval will be determined. Catherine is removing dental biofilm fairly well and her gingival tissue has improved, as evidenced by decreased bleeding, inflammation, and pocketing. Slight marginal redness remains on the lingual surface of the mandibular molars. A 3-month maintenance interval is recommended. What factor was the PRIMARY reason for this recommendation?
A. Response to the individualized debridement
B. Dental biofilm removal ability
C. Current oral health or disease state
D. Periodontal disease risk factors

Answer Key and Rationales

1 **(D)** Although age, gender, genetics, and neutrophil (PMN) abnormalities are NOT modifiable, possible to minimize or control stress and quit smoking (HARDEST modifiable factor). Because pregnancy is a temporary condition, it is considered modifiable.

2 **(C)** Poor nutrition results in lowered resistance (host response) to infections, including periodontal diseases. Individuals with nutritional deficiencies are therefore MORE at risk for severe forms of periodontal disease; however, such deficiencies have NOT been shown to contribute to dental biofilm accumulation, bone loss, or lower socioeconomic status (SES).

3 **(D)** Vitamin B_6 (pyridoxine) deficiency is NOT associated with the development of candidiasis. Vitamin B_6 is involved in carbohydrate metabolism, and deprivation may result in generalized stomatitis, gingivitis, glossitis, and other oral symptoms.

4 **(C)** Vitamin C is essential to collagen biosynthesis; deficiency adversely affects periodontal connective tissue integrity and wound healing. Vitamin A is associated with the synthesis of epithelial cells. Vitamin B is a group of vitamins with multiple roles. Vitamin D is involved in maintaining calcium and phosphorus levels.

5 **(D)** Vitamin D deficiency is NOT associated with development of gingival hyperplasia. In adults, is called osteomalacia and is characterized by destruction of PDL, resorption of alveolar bone, replacement fibrous dysplasia.

6 **(D)** Severe protein deficiency, or kwashiorkor, has been associated with increased incidence and severity of necrotizing gingivitis. Marasmus (general starvation), osteoporosis, and osteomalacia have NOT been linked with necrotizing gingivitis.

7 **(B)** Multilocular radiolucent jaw lesions, loss of lamina dura, and ground glass appearance of the alveolar bone are characteristics of excessive production of parathyroid hormone and hyperparathyroidism. This combination of lesions is NOT characteristic of the others.

8 (B) Increased, rather than decreased, levels of hormones alter capillary permeability and increase tissue fluid accumulation in the gingiva, resulting in an increased risk for gingivitis in presence of dental biofilm. Altered chemotactic response has NOT been demonstrated in cases of puberty gingivitis.

9 (A) Desquamative gingivitis is NOT associated with menopause, but MORE likely a feature of mucocutaneous disorders, such as lichen planus, mucous membrane pemphigoid, pemphigus.

10 (D) Increased fibrosis of the periodontal tissues is NOT a common occurrence in diabetic patients and is NOT related to prevalence. Defective PMN chemotaxis, microangiopathy of periodontal tissues, increased collagen breakdown, microbial alterations have been cited as rationales for prevalence of periodontal disease in individuals with diabetes mellitus.

11 (C) In uncontrolled diabetes mellitus, oral manifestations include multiple periodontal abscesses, velvety red gingivae, and marginal proliferation of the periodontal tissues. Although risk for periodontal breakdown exists in controlled cases of type 1 and type 2 diabetes mellitus, oral manifestations can be controlled with frequent periodontal maintenance (PM, recare) appointments.

12 (C) Although it is well established that periodontal disease is caused by dental biofilm, it is also recognized that impairment in host response increases risk for periodontal breakdown. Because neutrophils (PMNs) are KEY players in the host response, shortage results in increased risk for periodontal infections.

13 (D) Cause of neutropenia is multifactorial but is NOT associated with CNS dysfunction. Because term neutropenia refers to reductions in the neutrophil (PMN) count, conditions such as Down syndrome, diabetes mellitus, and a variety of autoimmune disorders are all capable of producing neutropenic states.

14 (C) ONLY thing that cyclosporine (immunosuppressant), phenobarbital (an anticonvulsant), and diltiazem and nifedipine (calcium channel blockers) have in common is ability to produce gingival overgrowth by hyperplasia.

15 (A) MAIN etiological agent in the development of periodontal disease is dental biofilm, which contains pathogenic bacteria. However, host response is recognized as a balancing factor because mere presence of bacteria does NOT preclude disease.

16 (A) Dental biofilm associated with gingival health typically is composed of gram-positive aerobic cocci and rods. Gram-negative microorganisms increase in numbers as gingivitis and periodontitis progress. Spirochetes are gram-negative organisms.

17 (B) Elevated levels of *Aggregatibacter* (previously *Actinobacillus*) *actinomycetemcomitans* (Aa) have been associated with localized aggressive periodontal disease. Note also that *Tannerella forsythensis* (TF) was previously *Bacteroides forsythus* (Bf).

18 (D) Lipase is an enzyme that aids fat metabolism, NOT a bacterial enzyme. Proteolytic enzymes such as hyaluronidase, collagenase, and ribonuclease affect host cells and intercellular substance (ground substance) by increasing permeability of epithelial and connective tissues and outwardly destroying cells.

19 (B) Bacterial endotoxins are responsible for activating alternate pathway of the immune complex fixation process known as the complement cascade. Side reaction proteins of this process are BOTH chemotactic and cytolytic.

20 (C) Macrophages are large defense cells that appear in larger numbers during chronic inflammation, typically NOT found in saliva. Saliva contains antibacterial components such as lysosomes and lactoperoxidase, as well as secretory IgA.

21 (C) Histamine, serotonin, kinins, prostaglandins, C3 and C5, and lysosomal enzymes are ALL mediators of vascular permeability, unlike thyroxine (T_4) from the thyroid gland, which is involved in controlling rate of metabolic processes in the body and influencing physical development.

22 (A) Process by which PMNs leave the central stream and adhere to the endothelial cell walls of blood vessels is called pavementing or margination. Emigration, migration, and chemotaxis follow as cells escape through endothelial walls into the connective tissues and move along chemical gradients to the attracting microorganisms.

23 (B) Monocyte and connective tissue macrophage signal the beginning of chronic stage of inflammation. Soon afterward, lymphocytes arrive at scene and eventually become the predominant cell. Basophils typically are present ONLY in allergic conditions. The neutrophil (PMN) is the predominant cell in acute inflammation and is first cell on scene.

24 (D) B cells are responsible for humoral immunity. Cells that are responsible for cellular immunity are T4 activator cells, T8 suppressor cells, cytotoxic (killer) cells.

25 (B) The B-cell lymphocyte is responsible for humoral immunity, and the T-cell lymphocyte is responsible for cellular immunity. Macrophage and/or monocyte is a phagocytic cell that appears first during chronic inflammation.

26 (D) Combination of fibroblasts, new immature collagen, new capillaries constitute granulation tissue that is formed during repair stage of inflammation.

27 (D) Products of the arachidonic acid cascade are potentially harmful to periodontal tissues and are part of the pathogenesis of periodontal disease. BOTH antibodies and complement proteins are later attracted and assist in the destruction.

28 (B) Complement system is responsible for the release of chemotactic factors that cause the migration of neutrophils (PMNs) and macrophages to specific sites. Phagocytic system is composed of PMNs and macrophages. Arachidonic acid cascade and kinin system are responsible for other aspects of the immune response.

29 (C) As part of the process of cellular immunity, T cells release potent cytokines, such as interleukin-1, that are capable of causing bone resorption. Arachidonic acid has the potential for tissue destruction, and prostaglandin is a mediator of vascular permeability. Myeloperoxidase is found in the saliva and is a protective enzyme.

30 (B) Initial lesion occurs in the first 2 to 4 days, early lesion occurs in 4 to 7 days, established lesion occurs after 14 days, and advanced lesion occurs ONLY after inflammation invades supporting periodontal tissues.

31 (D) Advanced lesion is characterized by invasion of periodontal tissues, PDL and alveolar bone. Initial, early, and established lesions do NOT typically involve PDL and alveolar bone.

32 (C) Clinical signs and symptoms of occlusal trauma always include radiographic evidence of a widening of periodontal (PDL) space and clinical evidence of tooth mobility. Tooth extrusion typically is related to the LACK of opposing tooth. Narrowed PDL space is associated with a LACK of occlusal contact.

33 (A) Primary occlusal trauma is defined as damage that occurs when the amount of alveolar bone is normal but there is an INCREASE in occlusal forces. Secondary occlusal trauma occurs when there is a deficiency in the amount of alveolar bone support. Neither hyperfunction NOR hypofunction results in irreversible damage.

34 (D) Bruxism is MOST common oral habit; involves grinding and can be recognized by presence of nonfunctional wear facets. Wear facets are NOT associated with decay, TMJ disorder (TMD), or trismus.

35 (B) Dental biofilm is considered MAIN etiological factor in development of periodontal disease; however, several contributing factors have been identified that make individual MORE prone to oral biofilm retention and thus disease risk. One such factor is subgingival calculus, considered a local predisposing factor. Missing teeth, malocclusions, and traumatogenic occlusion are considered local functional factors. Systemic contributing factors include those conditions that lower host response and raise the risk of disease.

36 (A) Calculus is composed of approximately 70% to 90% inorganic matter and 10% to 30% organic matter. Organic component is a mixture of protein polysaccharide complexes, desquamated epithelial cells, leukocytes, carbohydrates, lipids, glycosaminoglycans, various types of microorganisms. Primary crystalline structure is calcium hydroxyapatite, $Ca^{10}(PO_4)^6(OH)_2$; includes trace amounts of octocalcium phosphate, whitlockite, brushite.

37 (B) Materia alba is a yellow-gray acquired bacterial coating, soft, sticky, LESS adherent than dental biofilm. BOTH dental biofilm and salivary acquired pellicle are usually visible ONLY if stained with a dye (disclosing solution). Food debris may be any color or texture, depending on retained food.

38 (A) MOST commonly occurring form of periodontal disease is gingivitis, inflammation of the gingival tissues. Chronic periodontitis is the second MOST common form of periodontal disease; aggressive periodontitis and periodontal abscess are LESS common.

39 (C) MOST significant feature of chronic gingivitis is marginal bleeding on probing (BoP); marginal redness, edema, loss of stippling may or may NOT be found.

40 (A) Vitamin C deficiency alone CANNOT cause inflammation; however, deficiency in vitamin C causes increased tendency for gingival hemorrhage, degeneration of the collagen fibers, poor wound healing.

41 (C) Clinical characteristics of leukemia include purplish blue gingiva, interdental tumorlike masses, and shiny gingival surfaces that may have ulcerations and spontaneous bleeding. A case of necrotizing ulcerative gingivitis (NUG) should be ruled out because purplish blue gingival tissues and tumorlike masses are NOT common characteristics. Puberty gingivitis must be ruled out because the patient is older. Because of his age, primary herpetic gingivostomatitis, which typically occurs during the first 5 years of life and is NOT associated with tumorlike masses, also should NOT be a consideration.

42 (A) Localized tumorlike growths on the interdental gingiva are commonly found in BOTH leukemic gingivitis and pregnancy gingivitis (pyogenic granuloma). However, these enlargements are NOT characteristic of NUG, diabetic gingivitis, or AIDS-associated gingivitis.

43 (C) Allergic hypersensitivity involves an abnormal response of the tissues to specific agents, which typically manifests as redness, pain, edema, ulceration, and possible vesicle formation. Patient has an allergy to nonprecious metal crown on #30. No mention was made of desquamating tissues or tissues that were peeling away, which rules out desquamative gingivitis. Menopausal gingivitis has NOT been established as an acceptable term, and aphthous ulcers should be ruled out because they occur ONLY in the soft tissues (nonkeratinized), NOT on tissues overlying bone (keratinized).

44 **(E)** Pregnancy is associated with pyogenic granuloma (pregnancy tumor) rather than desquamative gingivitis. Although the exact nature of desquamative gingivitis is unknown, recent links have been made to several drugs and dermatological diseases, including pemphigus, pemphigoid, and lichen planus.

45 **(E)** Eating disorder, bulimia, is associated with enamel erosion rather than gingival overgrowth. Drugs such as phenytoin (Dilantin), cyclosporine, and calcium channel blockers initially cause gingival overgrowth by hyperplasia. When dental biofilm accumulates on the enlarged gingival tissues, inflammatory response ensues and results in inflammatory gingival overgrowth.

46 **(C)** Rare hyperplastic disease with unknown etiology, idiopathic gingival hyperplasia, believed to be familial or hereditary. NO association has been established between this condition and diabetes, epilepsy, or use of drugs.

47 **(C)** Spontaneous bleeding, metallic taste, fetid odor, punched-in interdental papillae, gray pseudomembrane are ALL typical characteristics of necrotizing ulcerative gingivitis (NUG). Primary herpetic gingivostomatitis and leukemia do NOT exhibit the characteristic punched-in interdental papillae.

48 **(C)** Periodontal pockets are classified as either suprabony or infrabony. If the base of the pocket is coronal to the alveolar bone, it is a suprabony pocket. However, if the base of the pocket is apical to the alveolar bone crest, it is infrabony. BOTH pseudopockets and relative pockets are gingival and NOT periodontal pockets.

49 **(A)** Rapid pocket destruction (from 6 mm to 11 mm within a few weeks) and presence of suppuration are suggestive of periodontal abscess. Entrapment of virulent microorganisms after an incomplete scaling procedure results in pus formation and rapid tissue destruction. Periapical abscess results in intermittent sharp pain with localized swelling. The combination (endodontic-periodontal) lesion has characteristics of BOTH periapical and periodontal abscesses; pericoronitis (pericoronal abscess) is a severe, localized infection associated with third molars.

50 **(C)** Papillon-Lefèvre syndrome is characterized by hyperkeratotic skin lesions of the palms, soles, knees, and elbows; involves severe destruction of the periodontium before age 4. Chédiak-Higashi syndrome produces partial albinism, slight bleeding disorders, and periodontal diseases. Hypophosphatasia is characterized by poor bone formation, rickets, and the premature loss of the dentition. Down syndrome (trisomy 21) manifests as mental and growth retardation and is characterized by a high prevalence of aggressive periodontal disease.

51 **(C)** LGE is typically associated with patients who have HIV/AIDS. Characteristic red band of marginal gingiva that rarely bleeds has NOT been demonstrated in diabetic or leukemia-associated gingivitis or even chronic gingivitis.

52 **(A)** Individuals undergoing cancer radiation therapy are at risk for development of osteoradionecrosis and should have any significant periodontal disease eliminated and teeth extracted before radiation therapy. Continuing periodontal therapy after radiation treatment begins is extremely risky.

53 **(E)** Social status is NOT an important characteristic to gather from the personal history, unlike other nondental risk factors such as stress, smoking, diet, alcohol consumption, which may play a role in patient's periodontal condition.

54 **(C)** Lifesaver-like enlargements surrounding free gingival margins are McCall's festoons. Stillman's clefts are narrow, slitlike areas where marginal gingiva has receded. Rolled margins are LESS enlarged than McCall's festoons, and marginal hyperplasia demonstrates greater overall enlargement.

55 **(A)** Clinical attachment level (CAL) is considered "gold standard" for determining the extent of periodontal tissue destruction. Pocket depths may vary according to amount of edema and hyperplasia. Bleeding on probing (BoP) is indicator of active disease but does NOT indicate extent of damage. Bone loss through radiographic analysis is less reliable because of associated distortion and magnification issues and extent of visualization.

56 **(C)** The PSR was developed to encourage general practitioners to probe routinely. System is modification of the CPITN, which was developed by the World Health Organization (WHO). Other indices are measurements of dental biofilm, debris, calculus, gingivitis.

57 **(B)** Condition of tooth proximal contact areas should be evaluated because open contacts encourage food impaction and tight contacts prevent effective interproximal cleaning. This is of MAJOR concern to dental hygienists, who develop homecare strategies for patients to facilitate cleansing of these difficult areas.

58 **(C)** Tooth mobility, furcation involvement, malocclusions, overhanging margins of restorations, and status of prosthetic appliances are considered local risk factors for the development of periodontal disease. Dental biofilm is considered the MAIN etiological factor; systemic diseases, host response factors, genetic predispositions are considered systemic risk factors.

59 **(A)** Although supplemental diagnostic tests were developed to diagnose specific periodontal diseases, none is truly diagnostic. However, these tests play important role in identification of risk factors and, coupled with clinical evidence, can be strong predictors of future disease progression.

60 **(C)** All tests measure bacterial species. The BANA test measures presence of *T. forsythensis* (previously *B. forsythus*), *T. denticola,* and *P. gingivalis.* The ELISA and DNA tests measure quantities of *P. gingivalis, P. intermedia, A. actinomycetemcomitans.*

61 **(A)** Phase I therapy is initial stage, deals with elimination of etiological factors. Phase II is surgical phase, phase III is restorative and orthodontic phase, phase IV is periodontal maintenance (PM, recare) procedures.

62 **(B)** All periodontal patients require a 1-month (4 to 6 weeks) reevaluation after initial therapy to assess tissue response and to establish appropriate periodontal maintenance (PM, recare) interval or determine whether referral to a periodontist for further treatment is necessary.

63 **(D)** For moderate to heavy calculus deposits and 5- to 6-mm pocket depths, quadrant scaling with local anesthesia would be the BEST possible treatment option (case type IV).

64 **(A)** Need for surgical access is a rationale for surgical therapy. Rationales for nonsurgical periodontal therapy (NSPT) include modification (control) of risk factors, removal of etiological agents, initiation of dental biofilm control, evaluation of tissue response.

65 **(C)** Retaining inflamed tissues is NOT a goal of periodontal surgery; goals are to reduce pocket depths, provide BETTER access for homecare, correct mucogingival defects, remove inflamed tissues, regenerate tissues lost to illness.

66 **(A)** Gingivectomy procedure is designed to reduce pocket depths by removing the soft tissue pocket wall in suprabony pockets. Modified Widman flap exposes the periodontium to provide access for other procedures. Guided tissue regeneration involves placement of barrier materials to prevent downgrowth of JE and stimulate MORE coronal reattachment of connective tissues. Ostectomy involves removal of alveolar bone.

67 **(D)** Ostectomy and osteoplasty are used to treat one-walled and two-walled defects in infrabony pockets. Osteotomy refers to the sectioning and repositioning of bone and is employed during mandibular advancement surgery.

68 **(A)** Freeze-dried bone from cadavers that is used as grafting material is an allograft. Autografts involve donor bone taken from the patient's own body, and xenografts are bone specimens obtained from other species (e.g., cows). Alloplast materials are synthetic substances that are used for bone grafting procedures.

69 **(A)** A type II mucogingival defect refers to a defect in which the alveolar mucosa acts as marginal gingiva without a zone of attached gingiva. Type I defects occur when pockets extend to or beyond the mucogingival junction but have a firm keratinized pocket wall.

70 **(B)** Periodontal surgical dressings are placed over the surgical wound for protection and should remain in place for at LEAST 7 days to allow for adequate healing. Dressing and suture removal typically are performed concomitantly.

71 **(E)** Correcting mucogingival defects is NOT a goal of recare or periodontal maintenance (PM) therapy. Such therapy is performed to maintain optimal oral health through preservation of clinical attachment levels (CAL), maintenance of alveolar bone height, control of inflammation, as well as the evaluation and reinforcement of patient oral hygiene.

72 **(A)** Compliance studies have shown that oral hygiene decreases within 30 days of instruction (1 month), which suggests a MAJOR challenge for the dental hygienist regarding patient motivation.

73 **(B)** Quadrant scaling with anesthesia is performed during initial therapy, NOT during recare (periodontal maintenance [PM]) appointments. Complete periodontal examination, oral hygiene instructions, and periodontal debridement are routinely performed at recare appointments. Tooth desensitization is typically performed based on need during recare appointments.

74 **(C)** With the return of active disease, initial therapy should be repeated by quadrant with anesthesia, followed by a reevaluation in 4 weeks. At the reevaluation appointment, appropriate course of action should be determined and may include referral to a specialist, return to recare (periodontal maintenance [PM]) intervals, or other treatment options such as antibiotics and surgery.

75 **(A)** Treatment of a periodontal abscess includes drainage and antimicrobial irrigation. Antibiotics are prescribed ONLY if lymphadenopathy and/or fever is present. Tooth extraction and tetracycline fiber placement are rarely considered.

76 **(C)** Gingival abscesses are NOT associated with bone loss or deeper periodontal pockets, but periodontal abscesses are always associated with BOTH. Periapical and combination abscesses involve periapical bone loss; combination abscesses may also be characterized by deeper periodontal pockets.

77 **(C)** If fever and lymphadenopathy are present, supervising dentist may decide to prescribe an antibiotic. Dental hygienist's role would involve gentle debridement, irrigation of the area under operculum with antimicrobial agent, and provision of oral hygiene instruction.

78 **(D)** Painful lesions associated with this condition often prevent the child from eating and drinking. Dehydration in a child may be life threatening, therefore IMPORTANT that daily fluid intake be stressed to the parent.

79 **(B)** Use of hydrogen peroxide intraorally MUST be discontinued in 7 to 10 days to prevent the development of black hairy tongue.

80 **(A)** Endosseous implants are shaped in the form of roots and blades and are directly implanted into the bone. Subperiosteal implants are in the form of a metal framework that is placed over the alveolar bone to provide support for complete and removable dentures. Transosteal (staple) implants are surgically placed through the mandible to provide anchor for a removable lower denture.

81 **(B)** After the initial placement of implant, surgical site is covered for approximately 3 to 6 months to allow osseointegration (implant to bone integration) to take place; this process leads to MOST stable attachment in most cases. Fibrointegration should be avoided because implant failure typically follows. Bone regeneration and settling are NOT related factors.

82 **(C)** Cells at the base of the implant sulcus form a junctional epithelium (JE) that attaches to the implant by means of a basal lamina and hemidesmosomes. Glycosaminoglycans constitute intercellular "glue."

Hemidesmosomes are part of the basal lamina and basement membrane that forms between the tooth and the epithelium and therefore are NOT part of the connective tissue. Gap junctions are cell-to-cell attachment mechanisms that typically are found in epithelial tissues.

83 **(A)** Dental biofilm in a recently cleaned mouth contains leukocytes, epithelial cells, few gram-positive cocci. Biofilm that is 2 to 14 days old will contain leukocytes, filamentous cocci, rods, gram-negative anaerobic bacteria, gram-positive cocci, white blood cells, spirochetes.

84 **(B)** Calculus acts as an attachment mechanism for dental biofilm; by itself, does NOT cause disease. May be hard to remove regardless of sharpness of the instrument. Subgingival calculus may appear darker because of blood pigments.

85 **(D)** A patient with insulin-dependent diabetes has a compromised immune system, especially if glucose levels are unstable. A 3-month recare or periodontal maintenance (PM) interval is recommended because diabetes is a risk factor for periodontal disease. Further periodontal destruction may result if therapy is NOT provided at frequent intervals. Catherine's response to treatment will be short-term, depending on dental biofilm removal ability, length of appointment, and control of diabetes. Her risk factors play the MOST important role in determining a PM phase.

CHAPTER 14

Pain Management

DENTAL PAIN

Pain is sum total of responses (behavioral, emotional, motivational, psychological) to actual or impending tissue damage from noxious stimulus.

• See CD-ROM for Chapter Terms and WebLinks.

A. Types of *dental* pain:
1. Caused by dental disease or trauma.
2. As result of dental treatment (iatrogenic).
3. After dental treatment.

B. Pain perception:
1. Physioanatomical process by which pain is received and transmitted by neural structures from end organs and pain receptors, through conductive and perceptive mechanisms.
2. Does NOT differ much from person to person, same in MOST healthy persons, but can be affected by both disease and toxic states.

C. Pain reaction:
1. Manifestation of perception of pain that has been perceived by the brain.
2. Determines what a patient will do about the unpleasant experience of pain.
3. Differs a great deal from person to person because of past dental experiences and various factors such as fatigue, stress, fear, apprehension, age, emotional state, education.

D. **Pain threshold:** tolerance shown to pain; there are differing levels:
1. Hyporeactive: high pain threshold, tolerates pain well, shows little reaction to pain.
2. Hyperreactive: low pain threshold, does NOT tolerate pain well, shows more reaction to pain.
3. However, MOST patients vary between two types depending on factors (discussed earlier).

E. Gate control theory of pain (GCT):
1. Explains unusual phenomenon of pain past specific neural pathway of pain sensation.
2. Specific neuroanatomical pathway carries impulse from site of stimulus to cortex of the brain where it is perceived as pain and then person receives a painful sensation.
3. Thus perception of physical pain is NOT direct result of activation of pain receptor neurons, but instead is modulated by interaction between different neurons.
4. Before pain messages can reach the brain, messages encounter "nerve gates" in spinal cord

(sympathetic ganglion [SG]) that open and close depending on a number of factors:
   a. When gates are opening, MORE pain messages get through and pain can be intense.
   b. When gates close, pain messages are prevented from reaching the brain and pain may NOT even be experienced.

F. Responses to pain:
1. Physiological: increased respiratory rate, increased heart rate (HR), increased blood pressure (BP).
2. Physical: crying out, tapping feet, cold sweat, altered facial expression, white knuckles, inability to sit still.

G. Pain control and dental office:
1. Pain is a major factor that brings patients to dental office, while fear and anxiety about pain are MOST common reasons patients fail to seek dental care; many AVOID dental treatment until forced into office with an emergency.
2. Control of pain and anxiety is therefore essential part of dental practice:
   a. To accomplish this objective, various techniques are used, including psychological approaches, local anesthetics of various types, and combinations of sedative and general anesthetic agents.
   b. Choice of MOST appropriate modality for particular situation is based on training, knowledge, and experience of clinician; nature, severity, duration of procedure; age and physical and psychological status of patient; level of fear and anxiety; previous responses to pain control procedures.
   c. MUST keep "gates closed" to pain messages to control dental pain (see earlier discussion) (No pain, lots of gain!).
3. Important part of stress control protocol, especially in management of patients with cardiovascular disease (CVD).

Anxiety Management

Anxiety is the feeling of apprehension and fear characterized by physical symptoms such as palpitations, sweating, feelings of stress. Anxiety keeps many people from receiving necessary dental treatment because of fear of pain or discomfort. **Fear** is excessive apprehension or anxiety. Understanding dental fear can help in selecting appropriate methods for alleviating patient discomfort. Anxiety and fear are common occurrences in the dental office and can be managed by a variety of techniques. Sometimes fear can become excessive and involve a **phobia,** which promotes inaction (failure to seek necessary dental treatment).

A. Etiology of *dental* anxiety and fear:
1. Anxiety and fear are typically based on past dental experiences.
2. May be based on fearful experiences related by others (friends or family) or portrayed by media.
3. Iatrogenic causes arise from personal experiences with dental situations and personnel (typically during childhood); two greatest dental fears are needles and dental drill.
4. Feeling a loss of control can increase dental anxiety and fear.

B. Treatment of dental anxiety, fear, phobias:
1. Using systemic desensitization (small doses of positive experiences) for highly anxious patients increases tolerance for dental encounters.
2. Explaining procedures thoroughly decreases fear of unknown.
3. Increasing patient control during each treatment session decreases fear of helplessness and increases sense of trust (allow patient to help with suction by holding patient saliva ejector or pick out favorite flavor of topical).
4. Using relaxation techniques in dental environment, includes headphones or other distracters, calming voice, biofeedback, adhering to time schedule.
5. Using pharmacological control of anxiety:
   a. Antianxiety premedication, either orally or IV, with benzodiazepines (BZDs), diazepam (Valium), or alprazolam (Xanax); patient will have LESS memory of stressful dental procedures (see Chapter 9, Pharmacology).
   b. Topical and/or injected local anesthesia agents can remove pain during dental procedures (discussed later).
   c. Sedation with nitrous oxide can give MORE relaxation, increase pain threshold, decrease awareness of time and procedures, increase sense of well-being (discussed later).
   d. Posttreatment with antiinflammatories (such as ibuprofen) can reduce inflammation and thus pain, helping with healing (see Chapter 9, Pharmacology).

CLINICAL STUDY

Scenario: A 35-year-old woman has not been to the dentist's office for 10 years. During her last dental experience, she had two third molars extracted and the local anesthetic initially used did not provide pulpal anesthesia. Repeated injections did not improve the situation but did make her more anxious and uncomfortable, and the extraction proceeded without anesthesia for the patient. Lately her gums have been bleeding and sore. Her husband persuaded her to have a thorough exam and cleaning. After diagnosis of generalized chronic periodontitis, her treatment plan suggests nonsurgical periodontal therapy by quadrant dental hygiene using local anesthesia of the involved regions. On the day of her appointment with the dental hygienist, the patient calls and cancels.

1. What is the major problem confronting the patient?
2. Identify the most effective methods for treating the patient's condition.
3. What is the difference between fear and a phobia?

1. Anxiety related to past dental experiences is the problem the patient is most likely confronting.
2. First, the patient must visit the dental office to be fully informed about the necessary dental procedures. Next, for site-specific soft tissue anesthesia the hygienist should help patient identify problems that occurred before and explain choices that will decrease likelihood of similar occurrences during dental hygiene treatment. Patient needs to feel in control of situation.
3. Phobia is excessive fear that leads to inaction, such as failure to seek necessary dental treatment, which can be detrimental to a person's health and well-being.

Sensory Innervation

Peripheral nervous system (PNS) comprises sensory *(afferent)* nerves that carry sensations of pain to central nervous system (CNS), and motor *(efferent)* nerves that transmit messages from CNS to muscles and glands. Understanding of sensory nerve anatomy and physiology and action of local anesthetics is essential to pain management. Sensory nerves are *afferent* nerves that carry sensations of pain to the CNS.

- See Chapters 3, Anatomy, Biochemistry, and Physiology: nervous system anatomy and physiology; 4, Head, Neck, and Dental Anatomy: trigeminal nerve.

A. Anatomy of a nerve:
1. **Myelinated nerves** (comprise MOST nerves in the body), divided into three zones:
   a. **Dendrite** (free nerve endings): reacts to stimuli in the surrounding tissues.
   b. **Axon:** pipeline that delivers impulses to CNS.
   c. **Terminal nerve endings** (arborization): synapse with CNS nerves.
2. Structure of single nerve fiber: myelin sheath covers axon, composed MAINLY of lipid layers (75%) and protein (20%) (Figure 14-1):
   a. Lipid layers: act as barriers to some molecules and as binding sites for lipophilic components of local anesthetics.

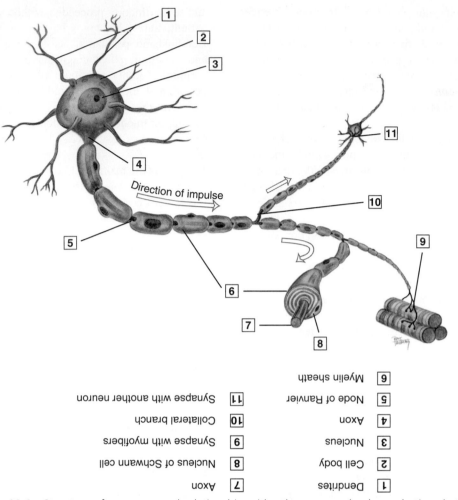

Figure 14-1 Structure of a neuron and relationship with other neuron (and muscle tissue). (From Bath-Balogh M, Fehrenbach MJ: Illustrated dental embryology and anatomy, ed 2, Philadelphia, 2006, Saunders/Elsevier.)

1 Dendrites		
2 Cell body		8 Nucleus of Schwann cell
3 Nucleus		9 Synapse with myofibers
4 Axon		10 Collateral branch
5 Node of Ranvier		11 Synapse with another neuron
6 Myelin sheath		7 Axon

b. Proteins: act as channels to allow some ions (Na⁺, K⁺) to pass through nerve membrane.

3. Layers of a nerve:
   a. Epineural sheath: outermost layer; NOT a barrier to anesthetics.
   b. Epineurium: connective tissue layer; carries fasciculi, blood vessels, and lymphatic vessels; as anesthetic diffuses through epineural sheath and blood vessels, begins to eliminate anesthetic.
   c. Perineurium: surrounds the fasciculi; greatest barrier to local anesthetic.

4. **Nodes of Ranvier:** constrictions 0.5 to 3 mm apart; nerve impulses travel from node to node.

B. Structure of a nerve bundle: MANY peripheral nerves have hundreds to thousands of tightly packed axons in bundles called **fasciculi** (Figure 14-1).

1. Mantle bundles: outside of nerve bundle, receive anesthetic FIRST; innervate proximal areas (posteriors) and lose anesthetic properties FIRST.

2. Core bundles: inside of a nerve bundle; receive anesthetic last and in lower concentration because of distance from anesthetic source and presence of more blood vessels; innervate distal areas (anterior) and lose anesthetic properties last.

C. Physiology of a nerve:

1. Nonstimulated nerve has Na⁺ ions *outside* the membrane, K⁺ ions and negative ions *inside,* and resting potential of −70 mV.

2. Stimulation of nerve is caused by mechanical (instrument in the soft tissue), chemical, thermal, or electrical means; starts depolarization process; permits movement of ions across nerve membrane; electrical potential changes from 50 to 60 mV to +40 mV; as electrical potentials change, impulse moves along nerve from node to node.

3. Repolarization occurs when Na⁺ ions begin to move back across nerve membrane to increase negative potential inside nerve; from stimulation to repolarization, process takes ~1 msec.

LOCAL ANESTHESIA

Dental patients can benefit from removal of pain during dental procedure with **local anesthesia,** as well as hemorrhage control from use of a **vasoconstrictor,** along with use of **topical anesthesia.** Can be used alone or with a combination of nitrous oxide sedation, which alone does NOT replace local anesthesia for pain control, since it is an analgesic and not an anesthetic. *Local anesthesia administration by dental hygienists is allowed in only some states and usually under the supervision of a dentist.*

The CORRECT administration of local anesthesia involves understanding nerve anatomy and physiology, pharmacology, armamentarium, technique, and possible complications. Action of local anesthetic agent depends on chemical structure and pH of the solution and body tissues.

A. Mode of action: a local anesthetic prevents or blocks Na^+ channel function in neurons.
   1. Stabilizes the nerve membrane so that the membrane threshold is elevated to point where depolarization does NOT occur.
   2. Thus, Na^+ channels do NOT open and Na^+ ion will NOT enter the axon.
   3. Depresses all unmyelinated fiber FIRST and larger myelinated fibers last.
   4. General order of loss of function (first *to* last): pain, temperature, touch, proprioception, motor nerve function.
B. Chemical formula of agent (Figure 14-2):
   1. Aromatic group (lipophilic [hydro*phobic*] component): affinity for the lipid portion of the myelin sheath, which helps local anesthetic agent attach to the nerve membrane and block the nerve impulse.
   2. Intermediate chain: either ester (−COO−R) or amide (NHCO−R) group; determines mode of biotransformation or metabolism (see later discussion).
   3. Amino end (hydro*philic* component): makes anesthetic agent injectable; amides dissolve poorly in water and are unstable on exposure to air; therefore hydrochloride (HCl) is added to produce a salt that is MORE soluble and stable.

C. Discussion of pH: mathematical measure of acidity and alkalinity, expressed as negative logarithm:
   1. Acidic substances have higher concentrations of hydrogen (H^+) ions and therefore can give up more H^+ ions; alkaline (base) substances have lower concentrations of H^+ ions and can accept more H^+ ions.
   2. The pH of normal tissue is 7.4; pH of inflamed tissue is lower, between 5 and 6 (more acidic).
   3. Decreased extracellular pH does NOT decrease nerve action; internal pH of a nerve is constant; decreased extracellular pH does decrease action of an anesthetic.
   4. The pH of anesthetic without epinephrine (vasoconstrictor) is 5.5; anesthetic with epinephrine is ~3.3 pH.
      a. Manufacturers acidify anesthetic to inhibit oxidation (breakdown) of epinephrine.
      b. Anesthetic may burn slightly on deposition because of difference *between* pH of anesthetic and pH of tissues.
      c. MORE acidic the anesthetic, slower its onset; using cartridge warmers, can break down pH of local anesthetic, increasing the burning during deposition (also destroys the vasoconstrictor).
D. Dissociation of local anesthetics: ability of a local anesthetic to dissociate, indicated by pK_a number.
   1. The pK_a number is a constant that characterizes equilibrium of a particular compound; also measures molecule's affinity for H^+ ions:
      a. Equilibrium equation is the pK_a equation: $RNH^+ \rightleftharpoons RN + H^+$
      b. Cation: RNH^+ is a positively charged molecule that is responsible for binding at the receptor site and decreasing the Na^+ that enters the nerve.
      c. Free base: RN is an uncharged molecule that is responsible for the diffusion of anesthetic through surrounding tissues and the nerve sheath.
   2. Clinical implications of the pK_a number, since each anesthetic has pK_a number:
      a. Lower the pK_a number (below 7.5), the MORE lipophilic free base molecules (creates greater diffusion, quicker onset, longer duration), but the LESS cations available to bind the anesthetic.
      b. When the pH of anesthetic is same as the pK_a number, equal amounts of BOTH base and cation exist.
      c. Equilibrium shifts:
         (1) Shifts *left* (cation state) when there are MORE hydrogen ions (low pH).
         (2) Shifts *right* (free base state) when there are FEWER hydrogen ions (high pH).

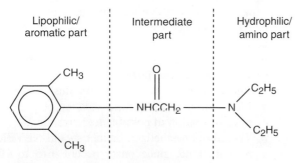

Lipophilic/ aromatic part	Intermediate part	Hydrophilic/ amino part

Figure 14-2 Chemical formula for a local anesthetic.

d. The MORE free base molecules available, the greater the diffusion of anesthetic through tissues and membrane, and therefore the faster the onset of action.

3. The pH of anesthetic is lowered with addition of epinephrine (pH 3.3):
   a. When MORE cations exist, more Na^+ is bound at the nerve receptor, which creates greater binding power.
   b. LESS free base leads to less diffusion and slower onset.
   c. Surrounding tissues buffer MORE acidic solutions.

4. The pH of inflamed tissues is low (5 to 6), so MORE cations exist; therefore MORE Na^+ is bound at nerve receptor site:
   a. LESS diffusion of anesthetic into surrounding tissues causes slower onset and leads to ineffective anesthesia.
   b. Surrounding tissues are NOT able to buffer more acidic solutions because of lower pH.
   c. Patient may need MORE local anesthetic agent because of acidic conditions; block may be MORE effective than infiltration, since agent is NOT near inflamed tissues.

Pharmacology of Local Anesthetics and Vasoconstrictors

Understanding the metabolism, action, dosage calculations, and specific functions of topical and local anesthetic agents and vasoconstrictors helps the clinician to request and use these agents more safely and efficiently. Clinician MUST prevent an **overdose** (OD) situation, which is an accidental or intentional use of a drug in an amount higher than is normally used.

- See Chapter 9, Pharmacology: local anesthetic and vasoconstrictor pharmacology.

A. Types of agents:
   1. Ester agents: NO longer available as injectables, ONLY topicals (usually 20% benzocaine):
      a. Biotransformed to paraaminobenzoic acid (PABA) in blood plasma by enzyme pseudocholinesterase.
      b. Half-life (rate at which 50% of the anesthetic is eliminated from the blood) is 2 to 8 minutes.
      c. Have lower potential for OD (toxicity).
      d. MORE likely to cause allergic reaction (to PABA).
   2. Amide agents: BOTH injectables and topicals (NOT as useful at 5%) available:
      a. LESS likely to cause allergic reaction because methylparaben, which can cause allergic reactions, has been eliminated as preservative.
      b. Biotransformed MAINLY in liver (MUST have healthy liver tissue).
      c. Have greater potential for OD (alone, without vasoconstrictor) because higher blood levels occur until agent reaches liver for biotransformation.
      d. Half-life is 50 to 120 minutes.
         (1) EXCEPTION: Articaine's half-life is different from other amides.
            (a) Falls under amide class, but its associated ester group also allows plasma metabolism via pseudocholinesterase, purportedly increasing rate of breakdown and reducing its toxicity.
            (b) Difference in metabolism gives advantage of having a 30-minute half-life, in contrast to lidocaine, which has a 90-minute half-life.

B. Distribution and elimination of agents:
   1. After entering blood, agents permeate ALL body tissues.
   2. Are vasodilators; thus vasoconstrictors are added in MOST cases to decrease vasodilation.
   3. Esters and amide agents are BOTH eliminated mostly through the kidneys.

C. Phentolamine mesylate (Oraverse): injection via syringe, which accelerates return of normal soft tissue sensation (i.e., sensation of lip and tongue), as well as function following restorative and periodontal procedures, and helps prevent any self-inflicted oral trauma that may occur with a long-lasting injection of local anesthetic containing a vasoconstrictor; contains an alpha-adrenergic antagonist that acts as a vasodilator, resulting in faster diffusion of anesthetic into the cardiovascular system and away from site.

Local Anesthetic Agent Action

Local anesthetic is an anesthetic drug that induces local anesthesia by inhibiting nerve excitation or conduction. These agents also have effects on central nervous system (CNS), cardiovascular system (CVS), respiratory system.

- See Chapter 10, Medical and Dental Emergencies: local anesthesia emergency protocol in a dental setting.

A. CNS effects:
   1. Low levels have NO effect but can provide anticonvulsive properties by raising seizure threshold; used to treat epileptic seizures.
   2. Preconvulsive levels can cause slurred speech, shivering, twitching, flushed feeling, dream state, lightheadedness, blurred vision, tinnitus.
      a. Lidocaine may cause mild sedation or drowsiness, indication of possible toxic reaction.
      b. Therefore anesthetized patient should NEVER be left alone, since onset occurs in 5 to 10 minutes.

3. Convulsive levels cause convulsions, CNS depression, respiratory depression and arrest.

B. CVS effects:
1. Low levels produce NO effects.
2. High (non-OD) levels cause mild hypotension (low blood pressure) by relaxing smooth muscles.
3. At OD levels, can produce profound hypotension, which causes decreased myocardial contractions, decreased cardiac output, decreased peripheral resistance.
4. Lethal levels lead to CVS collapse caused by massive peripheral vasodilation, decreased heart contractions, and decreased heart rate (bradycardia).

C. Respiratory system effects:
1. Non-OD levels relax action of bronchial smooth muscles.
2. OD levels can lead to respiratory arrest as result of CNS depression.

Vasoconstrictor Action

Vasoconstrictors if used in local areas cause constriction of the arterioles and capillaries. Vasoconstrictors act on alpha (α) and/or beta (β) receptors, depending on the body tissues.

A. Chemical structure of a vasoconstrictor (Figure 14-3):
1. Benzene ring with two OH groups in the third and fourth positions is a catechol.
2. Benzene ring with an amine group in another position is a catecholamine.
3. MOST vasoconstrictors are catecholamines:
   a. Epinephrine, norepinephrine, dopamine: ALL occur in nature.
   b. Levonordefrin and isoproterenol: BOTH synthetics.
4. Do NOT use cartridge warmers, since inactivate vasoconstrictors.

B. Adrenergic receptors: present naturally in MOST body tissues.
1. Includes two types of receptors:
   a. Alpha (α) activation causes contraction of smooth muscles in blood vessels.
   b. Beta (β) activation:
      (1) β_1 activation in heart and small intestine, responsible for cardiac stimulation and lipolysis.
      (2) β_2 activation in bronchi, vascular beds, uterus produces bronchodilation and vasodilation.
2. MOST vasoconstrictors used in dentistry exert action on adrenergic receptors:
   a. Epinephrine: acts on both α and β receptors, but MAINLY on β receptors.
   b. Norepinephrine: acts on both α and β receptors, but MAINLY on α receptors.
   c. Levonordefrin (synthetic): acts on both α and β receptors, but MAINLY on α receptors.

C. Types of vasoconstrictors:
1. Epinephrine (adrenalin): one MOST commonly used in United States:
   a. MORE potent; found in BOTH natural and synthetic forms.
   b. In skeletal muscle and blood vessels, produces both vasodilation (*small* amounts act on β_2 sites) and vasoconstriction (*large* amounts act on α receptors).
   c. MAINLY used at 1:100,000 for nerve blocks and not 1:50,000 concentrations (usually only infiltrations and intraseptal injections); use of additional dosage does NOT increase duration and/or effectiveness, ONLY hemorrhage control.
2. Norepinephrine (Levarterenol): NOT used in United States, but used in other countries:
   a. LESS potent than epinephrine (one fourth as potent) and demonstrates LESS systemic action.
   b. Activation of α receptors in the smooth muscles of palatal blood vessels can cause ischemia and then tissue necrosis.
3. Levonordefrin (Neo-Cobefrin): NOT as commonly used in United States:
   a. LESS potent than epinephrine (one fifth as potent); demonstrates LESS systemic action so used at higher concentration (1:20,000) when used with agents such as 2% mepivacaine; has same onset, depth, duration of anesthesia in both pulpal and soft tissue as lidocaine with epinephrine.
   b. NOT as strong in hemorrhage control as epinephrine (IMPORTANT in dental procedures involving bleeding and need for hemorrhage control, such as dental hygiene procedures).

D. Inclusion of vasoconstrictors:
1. Medical considerations for use of vasoconstrictors:
   a. <u>Absolute contraindications</u>:
      (1) Cardiovascular disease (CVD): acute incident (myocardial infarction [MI, heart attack] or cerebrovascular accident [CVA, stroke]) *within* last 4 to 6 weeks or unable to meet 4 METs (metabolic equivalents); high blood pressure (HBP) ≥140/90 mm Hg; unstable or severe angina pectoris that is relieved by rest.

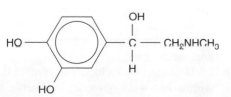

Figure 14-3 Chemical structure of a vasoconstrictor.

(2) With uncontrolled or undiagnosed hyperthyroidism, may cause thyroid storm.

(3) Recreational cocaine (crack) user (within 24 hours); could be fatal.

b. Relative contraindications:

(1) Reduced levels needed with MOST other chronic CVD histories; however, still may need to use a limited amount to ensure pain control (reduces endogenous [own] epinephrine of patient with CVD); see next section.

(2) Patients taking tricyclic antidepressants (TCAs): NEITHER norepinephrine NOR levonordefrin (Neo-Cobefrin) should be used; substitute epinephrine if needed.

2. Consideration for duration of appointment:

a. Addition increases duration of anesthetic effects.

b. Concentration and type affect duration of a local anesthetic.

3. Consideration for hemostasis during appointment:

a. Epinephrine in large quantities acts as a vasoconstrictor; in smaller quantities becomes vasodilator that has potential to increase bleeding postoperatively.

b. Injection SHOULD be close to the area of bleeding to be effective; may want to add epinephrine 1:50,000 levels (available with lidocaine agent) as interseptal injection *after* other injections.

c. Epinephrine has BETTER hemostatic control levels than levonordefrin (Neo-Cobefrin), which is important with bleeding that may occur with nonsurgical periodontal maintenance.

E. Vasoconstrictor use causes slight burning upon injection (MORE than with plain) because of presence of preservative (sodium metabisulfate), since it is acidic to increase agent's shelf-life (discussed later) but this side effect does not preclude use or add need for plain preinjection.

Dosage Calculations

Dosage calculations for local anesthetics are based on the size and general health of patient and on type and concentration of the anesthetic agent and vasoconstrictor. The **maximum recommended dose** (MRD) is the dose established by manufacturer (in milligrams per pound).

A. MRD for each anesthetic agent (Box 14-1).

B. Concentration of vasoconstrictors: ratio of vasoconstrictor to milliliters of solution (Box 14-2).

1. MRD of epinephrine:

a. MRD for healthy patient is 0.2 mg per appointment.

b. MRD for patient with CVD is HALF as much: 0.04 mg per appointment.

2. MRD of levonordefrin (Neo-Cobefrin) for all patients is 1.0 mg per appointment.

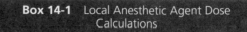

Box 14-1   Local Anesthetic Agent Dose Calculations

QUESTIONS/ANSWERS

A. How many milligrams/milliliter of agent are there in solution per percentage concentration of anesthetic agent?

B. How many milligrams of agent are there per cartridge?

C. What is the MRD in number of cartridges of agent allowed per individual patient?

1. To change % concentration of agent to mg/mL, first divide by 100, then multiply by 1000.

2. To find mg of agent per cartridge, multiply mg/mL by 1.8 mL/cartridge.

3. To find MRD of agent for patient, multiply patient's weight by established MRD in mg/pound.

4. To find mL of agent, divide MRD in mg of agent by mg/mL of agent.

5. To find MRD in number of cartridges for patient, divide mL of agent by 1.8 mL/cartridge.

EXAMPLE: LOCAL ANESTHETIC AGENT DOSE CALCULATION USING 2% LIDOCAINE FOR 150 LB PATIENT

1. **Percentage grams to milligrams/milliliter:** 2% ÷ 100 = .02 g/mL x 1000 mg/g = 20 mg/mL.

2. **Milligrams per cartridge:** 20 mg/mL x 1.8 mL/cartridge = 36 mg/cartridge.

3. **Patient MRD:** 2 mg/lb (MRD) x patient's weight (e.g., 150 lb) = 300 mg.

4. **Milliliters of solution:** 300 mg ÷ 20 mg/mL = 15 mL.

5. **Number of cartridges per patient:** 15 mL ÷ 1.8 mL/cartridge = 8.3 cartridges.

Fast Tip: **Eliminate steps 4 and 5 by dividing mg MRD/patient by 36 mg/cartridge:** 300 mg ÷ 36 mg/cartridge = 8.3 cartridges.

MRD, Maximum recommended dosage by manufacturer.

Local Anesthetic Agents and Vasoconstrictors

Vasoconstrictors and local anesthetic agents must be chosen carefully, based on the medical concerns and type of dental procedure to be performed. Anesthetic is selected based on whether its duration is appropriate to procedure being performed.

A. Selection considerations:

1. Medical concerns (if vasoconstrictor used, see earlier discussion):

a. True allergy to local anesthetic agent is rare (past history may be to esters, usually NOT to amides); may be allergic to preservative for vasoconstrictor (sodium metabisulfite); try plain anesthetic agent.

b. CVD concerns include incident (MI, CVA) within last 4 to 6 weeks or unable to meet 4 METs, HBP ≥140/90 mm Hg, unstable or

---

Box 14-2 Calculation of Vasoconstrictor Concentration

1. To change grams to milligrams, multiply by 1000, since ratio equals 1 gram of drug per milliliters of solution.
2. To find mg of vasoconstrictor drug per mL of solution (mg/mL), divide mg of drug by mL of solution.
3. To find mL of solution, divide MRD* of vasoconstrictor in mg by mg/mL.
4. To find number of cartridges, divide MRD mL of solution by 1.8 mL/cartridges.

EXAMPLE: CALCULATION OF CONCENTRATION OF VASOCONSTRICTORS USING 1:100,000 EPINEPHRINE/ML OF SOLUTION
1. Ratio: 1:100,000 = 1 g of drug per 100,000 mL of solution.
2. 1 g = 1000 mg of drug per 100,000 mL of solution.
3. 1000 mg ÷ 100,000 mL = 0.01 mg/mL.

EXAMPLE: VASOCONSTRICTOR DOSE CALCULATION FOR HEALTHY ADULTS AND CVD PATIENTS USING EPINEPHRINE
MRD for healthy adult patient: 0.2 mg per 1:100,000 epinephrine.
MRD for patient with CVD: 0.04 mg per 1:100,000 epinephrine.
How many cartridges of anesthetic with epinephrine can a healthy adult have?
0.2 mg of drug ÷ 0.01 mg/mL = 20 mL; then 20 mL ÷ 1.8 mL/cartridge – **11.11 cartridges.**
How many cartridges of anesthetic with epinephrine can a patient with CVD have?
0.04 mg of drug ÷ 0.01 mg/mL = 4 mL; then 4 mL ÷ 1.8 mL/cartridge = **2.2 cartridges.**
Note: Levonordefrin [Neo-Cobefrin] allows 1 mg vasoconstrictor/any patient/visit.

MRD, Maximum recommended dosage *by manufacturer;* clinicians may be more conservative in use.

severe angina pectoris, uncontrolled or undiagnosed hyperthyroidism.
   c. Pregnant patients (use category B: lidocaine and prilocaine, NOT category C: mepivacaine, articaine, bupivacaine).
2. Onset and duration:
   a. Onset is determined by properties of local anesthetic agent, including its dissociation.
   b. Duration (short, medium, or long acting) is determined by site of injection, type of anesthetic agent, addition of vasoconstrictor, patient's idiosyncrasies (Tables 14-1, 14-2, and 14-3).
B. Local anesthetic agents with and without vasoconstrictors (plain):
   1. Lidocaine, mepivacaine, prilocaine are available BOTH with vasoconstrictor and without (plain).

2. Bupivacaine, articaine, etidocaine are available with vasoconstrictor.

Topical Anesthetics

Topical anesthetics are useful for providing light, localized anesthesia to the first 2 to 3 mm of the oral mucosa as a preinjection agent. May also be used alone before procedures involving soft tissues (nonsurgical periodontal therapy). Must be placed on oral mucosa for 2 to 3 minutes per Materials Safety Data Sheet (MSDS).
• See Chapter 9, Pharmacology: discussion of topical anesthesia using gel or patch.
A. Action:
   1. MOST are higher concentrations than injectable anesthetics (20% benzocaine) and thereby increase diffusion of the active ingredients through oral mucosa and open wounds.
      a. Efficient diffusion leads to faster onset.
      b. Increased water solubility increases diffusion and onset; water insolubility decreases diffusion and onset but increases duration by retaining topical anesthetic at the site.
   2. Do NOT contain vasoconstrictors.
      a. Without vasoconstrictors, duration is decreased but potential for OD is increased because of the faster uptake of agent into blood.
      b. Higher concentrations increase potential for OD and toxicity because uptake of agent into vascular system is greater.
      c. Controlled use is optimum for safety; NOT to be used for more than one or two quadrants per appointment.
B. Concern for allergenic potential (see earlier discussion).

Local Anesthesia Armamentarium

Preparing the armamentarium for delivery of local anesthetic involves knowledge of the syringe, needle, cartridge, proper setup procedures, care of equipment, safe handling, and prevention and management of associated problems. **Aspiration** is the process of removing fluids (or gases) from the body with a suction device (syringe with piston). It allows the clinician to know if the needle tip is in a blood vessel to prevent an intravascular injection.
A. Syringe:
   1. **Syringe** types:
      a. Harpoon syringe: MOST commonly used one (Figure 14-4):
      b. Self-aspirating syringe (Figure 14-5):
         (1) Metal projection presses on rubber diaphragm of the cartridge; pushing on the thumb ring increases the pressure of projection on the diaphragm.
         (2) Thereby increases pressure inside the cartridge, aspiration occurs, then pressure is released.

Table 14-1 Short-acting local anesthetics

Local anesthetic	Onset (min)	Duration: pulp (min)	Duration: soft tissue (hr)	Dose/ cartridge (mg)	MRD/Body weight (mg/lb)	MRD for healthy adult (mg)	Maximum cartridges for 150 lb patient
2% lidocaine HCl (Xylocaine)	2-3	5-10	1-2	36	2	300	8.3
3% mepivacaine HCl (Carbocaine)	1.5-2	20-40	2-3	54	3*	400*	7.4*
4% prilocaine HCl (Citanest Plain)	2-4	10-20	1.5-2	72	2.7	400	5.5

Data from Malamed SF: Handbook of local anesthesia, ed 5, St. Louis, 2004, Mosby/Elsevier.
MRD, Maximum recommended dose.
*Manufacturer's recommendation.

Table 14-2 Medium-acting local anesthetics

Local anesthetic	Onset (min)	Duration: pulp (hr)	Duration: soft tissue (hr)	Dose/ cartridge (mg)	MRD/Body weight (mg/lb)	MRD for healthy adult (mg)	Maximum cartridges for 150 lb patient
2% lidocaine HCl, 1:50,00/100,000 epi-nephrine (Xylocaine)	2-3	1	3-5	36	3*	500*	13.8*
2% mepivacaine HCl, 1:20,000 levonorde-frin (Carbocaine with Neo-Cobefrin)	1.5-2	1-1.5	3-5	36	3*	400*	11*
4% prilocaine HCl, 1:200,000 epineph-rine (Citanest Forte)	2	1-1.5	3-8	72	2.7	400	5.5
4% articaine HCl, 1:100,000/200,000 epinephrine (Septocaine)	1-9	1	3-5	72	3.2	476	7

Data from Malamed SF: Handbook of local anesthesia, ed 5, St. Louis, 2004, Mosby/Elsevier.
MRD, Maximum recommended dose.
*Manufacturer's recommendation.

c. High-pressure syringe (Ligmaject):
  (1) Used MAINLY for periodontal ligament (PDL) (intraligamentous) injection (type of intraosseous injection), which permits measured dose of solution and overcomes tissue resistance; for other PDL injection with traditional syringe, see Table 14-4.
  (2) May cause trauma to surrounding tissues if increased solution (under pressure) is forced into PDL space; if this situation occurs with primary teeth, can also cause trauma to developing permanent teeth.
d. Safety syringes (UltraSafe, Safety Plus): LESS risk of needlestick injury (see later discussion).

2. Handling of syringes: should be checked for rust, harpoon sharpness, working piston.
  a. Leakage during injection: caused by offset needle placement into rubber diaphragm or by loose needle.
  b. Broken cartridge: caused by too much pressure when engaging harpoon or by bent harpoon.
  c. Disengagement of harpoon during aspiration: caused by dirty, dull, or broken harpoon or NOT securely engaging rubber stopper in cartridge.
B. Needles: stainless steel, disposable, presterilized, sharp to decrease potential for cross-contamination (Figure 14-6):

Table 14-3 Long-acting local anesthetics

Local anesthetic	Onset (min)	Duration: pulp (hr)	Duration: soft tissue (hr)	Dose/ cartridge (mg)	MRD/Body weight (mg/lb)	MRD for healthy adult (mg)	Maximum cartridges for 150 lb patient
0.5% bupivacaine HCL, 1:200,000 epinephrine (Marcaine)	3-10	1-2	5-9	9	0.6	90	10
1.5% etidocaine HCL, 1:100,000 epinephrine (Duranest)	1.5-3	1.5-2	4-9	27	3.6	400	14.8

Data from Malamed SF: Handbook of local anesthesia, ed 5, St. Louis, 2004, Mosby/Elsevier.
MRD, Maximum recommended dose.

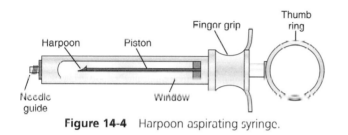

Figure 14-4 Harpoon aspirating syringe.

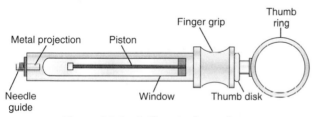

Figure 14-5 Self-aspirating syringe.

1. **Bevel:** oblique surface to penetrate soft tissue without resistance; placed toward bone to prevent trauma to overlying periosteum (bone's surface).
2. **Shank:** length is measured from bevel tip to the hub:
   a. Short shank: ~1 inch/~25 mm.
   b. Long shank: ~1.58 inches/~40 mm.
3. **Gauge:** measure of inside diameter of lumen; larger the number, smaller the needle; thus smaller *to* larger: 30, 27, 25-gauge.
   a. *Smaller* gauge needles (30-gauge) with smaller lumen are NOT recommended for less pain:
      (1) Deflect MORE when penetrating tissues, reduces accuracy because solution is deposited away from intended site.
      (2) Smaller lumen increases possibility of clogging needle with blood cells, MORE likely to show false-negative aspiration.

Table 14-4 Periodontal ligament injection technique*

Anatomy anesthetized	Pulpal and soft tissue and nerve endings in area of injection
Needle gauge and length	27-gauge, short, extra short, or ultra short or CLAD
Depth of penetration	Base of pocket until resistance is met
Landmarks	Pocket area, mesial of distal root
Site of penetration	Long axis of root on mesial or distal with bevel toward root
Deposition site	Base of pocket
Cartridge amount (1.8 mL/cartridge)	0.2 mL
Complications	Pain
Advantages	Minimal dose required; no unnecessary structures anesthetized; works better with CLAD
Disadvantages	Leakage of anesthetic; difficult to deposit with non-pressure syringe; not with inflammation or primary teeth present

*See manufacturer's directions for use of pressure syringe (Ligmaject); dental hygienists may not be allowed to perform intraosseous injections in some states.

   b. *Larger* gauge needles (27- to 25-gauge) with larger lumen are BEST, with long shank with 25 gauge and short shank with 27 gauge.
      (1) Deflect LESS when penetrating tissues, increasing accuracy because solution is deposited close to intended site.

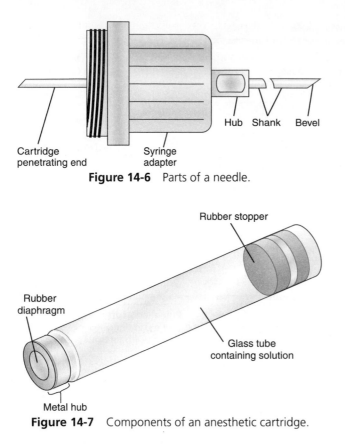

Figure 14-6 Parts of a needle.

Cartridge penetrating end · Syringe adapter · Hub · Shank · Bevel

Rubber stopper · Rubber diaphragm · Glass tube containing solution · Metal hub

Figure 14-7 Components of an anesthetic cartridge.

(2) Easier to aspirate, since increases true-negative aspiration, LESS likely to show false-negative aspiration.

(3) Short shank needles with 27-gauge are used on MOST commonly administered injections, EXCEPT inferior alveolar nerve block (and thus buccal nerve block done immediately after) uses long shank with 25-gauge.

4. Hub or needle adapter: some have bevel indicator dots.

5. Cartridge-penetrating end: sharp to penetrate rubber diaphragm of cartridge.

6. Needle cap/sheath.

C. **Cartridges:** cylindrical tube of agent, color-coded by manufacturer to distinguish types, holds 1.8 mL of anesthetic (Figure 14-7):

1. Rubber stopper: coated with silicone to ease movement, engaged by harpoon, then pushed by piston to dispel solution; may/may not have rubber latex.

2. Aluminum cap: holds rubber diaphragm in place.

3. Rubber diaphragm: acts as seal to prevent anesthetic from leaking around needle, as long as needle penetrates the diaphragm squarely and NOT on an angle, does NOT have rubber latex.

4. Contents besides agent and vasoconstrictor (additives):

a. Hydrochloride (HCl): added to agent to create acidic salt for BETTER water solubility; increases diffusion of agent to nerve; makes anesthetic injectable.

b. Sodium chloride: added to make solution MORE isotonic with soft tissues.

c. Sodium metabisulfite: antioxidant that is added to preserve vasoconstrictor (if present) by reacting with oxygen to produce sodium bisulfate (more acidic, slight increase in burning during injection [MORE than plain]); can act as allergen.

d. Distilled water: provides remaining volume.

5. Handling of cartridges:

a. SHOULD be checked before use for clear solution without large bubbles, normal stopper, noncorroded/rusty cap.

(1) Bubbles that are small (1 to 2 mm): acceptable; however, larger bubbles mean that solution was frozen, which causes chemical changes.

(2) Extruded stopper: caused by freezing cartridge or by storing in disinfectant.

(3) Corroded/rusty cap: caused by cartridge breakage in round tin container (10-cartridge blister packs decrease breakage) or by immersion in disinfectant (metal cap).

b. With vasoconstrictors, shelf-life is shorter at 18 months; without vasoconstrictors, shelf-life is longer at 24 months.

c. Burning during injection: normal response to pH of agent; however, those containing disinfectant or vasoconstrictors and overheating (by cartridge warmer) can cause increased burning during injection.

d. To maintain viable anesthetic: do NOT autoclave, soak in disinfectant, or keep in direct sunlight or in warmers; wipe ends with 70% alcohol solution if NOT used.

D. Computer-controlled local anesthesia delivery (CLAD) system (CompuDent/Wand, Comfort Control):

1. BOTH use traditional cartridges and either traditional needles or safety (Luer-Lok) needles; provides MORE controlled amounts of anesthetic solution delivered for ALL types of injection techniques.

2. Handpiece is held with a pen grasp and is lighter than traditional syringes; as needle penetrates, clinician steps on a pedal/uses finger-touch control to activate flow of anesthetic solution ahead of needle path.

3. Has auto-aspiration feature that can be used for any type of injection; amount deposited for MOST injections is 0.6 to 0.9 mL.

4. MUST be used to perform AMSA block injection (discussed later).

CLINICAL STUDY

Scenario: During an initial dental hygiene appointment with new patient, the dental hygienist observes blood in a cartridge (positive aspiration) during administration of an inferior alveolar nerve (IA) nerve block (2% lidocaine with 1:100,000 epinephrine). A 25-gauge long needle is being used. A large amount of blood fills the cartridge quickly. The patient with generalized moderate chronic periodontitis reports no medical conditions and exhibits no significant need for dental restoration.

1. What is the most likely cause of the positive aspiration?
2. How should the clinician handle this situation?
3. Are positive aspirations preventable? Was the needle used appropriate one for this injection?

1. If tip of the needle is located in large artery during aspiration, blood will quickly flow into cartridge. Artery that is most likely to be penetrated is inferior alveolar (IA) artery. Veins are more passive and typically cause blood to enter the cartridge more slowly and in smaller amounts.
2. Clinician should stop the injection and remove the syringe from the patient's mouth. Cartridge and needle should be changed and the injection should be repeated until there is negative aspiration. Later, both the cartridge and needle should be placed in the biohazardous waste.
3. No, the purpose of choosing a needle with appropriate lumen size is for very purpose of getting positive aspiration when needle inadvertently enters a blood vessel. For patient safety, there must not be deposition of solution in a blood vessel while administering anesthetic. Accomplished by aspirating and checking for blood in cartridge before injection, and possibly again in different plane (adjusting bevel) during injection process in highly vascular areas (IA artery with IA nerve block). Needle used (gauge and length) was appropriate for injection, since both lumen size (gauge) and length (must contact bone) are important to achieve safety with injection of IA nerve block.

Local Anesthesia Preparation

It is important for the clinician to properly prepare for the local anesthesia procedure. Includes patient preparation, proper selection of equipment, anesthetic and vasoconstricting agents, proper assembly of syringe and needle, preparation of injection site. MUST follow standard precautions. Aspiration MUST be performed to prevent an intravascular injection.
A. Preinjection: review medical history for contraindications, determine appropriate anesthetics, record blood pressure reading.
   1. Review treatment plan for injections to be performed to determine appropriate needle lengths/gauges and anesthetic.
   2. Have patient rinse with preprocedural antimicrobial mouthrinse.
B. Armamentarium setup:
   1. Select appropriate syringe (harpoon, self-aspirating, or pressure).
   2. Select appropriate cartridge:
      a. According to patient treatment and medical needs.
      b. According to date and physical appearance; should have no large bubbles, clear color, rust/corrosion-free cap, rubber stopper without needle punctures.
   3. Select appropriate needle according to scheduled injections.
   4. Place hemostat/locking cotton pliers on tray for potential retrieval of a broken needle (NOT recommended as much).
   5. Select appropriate topical anesthetic and amount (larger doses can produce toxicity).
   6. Prepare for needle recapping (device/method).
C. Syringe setup:
   1. Place cartridge in syringe; then place needle in syringe so that cartridge penetrating end passes through the diaphragm and into anesthetic, squarely and NOT at angle.
   2. Engage harpoon in rubber stopper with firm, gentle motions so as to not break glass cartridges (self-aspirating syringe has NO harpoon).
   3. Rotate needle bevel so that on penetration faces the bone (so do NOT scrape periosteum).
   4. Dispel some solution to ensure correct needle placement in cartridge.
   5. Make sure that harpoon is engaged (for harpoon syringe only) by pulling on the thumb ring with negative pressure.
D. Site preparation:
   1. Inspect site for lesions (do NOT inject with abscess formation).
   2. Dry tissues to decrease microbial levels with patting motion to decrease abrasions.

Local Anesthesia Delivery

Safe delivery of local anesthetics depends on thorough knowledge of proper injection techniques, signs of OD or allergy, proper handling and disposal of equipment.
- See Chapter 8, Microbiology and Immunology: standard precautions, sharps/waste handling (needle and cartridge); 10, Medical and Dental Emergencies: needlestick injury, emergency protocol in a dental setting.
A. During treatment: keep syringe out of view; patient in supine position to avoid syncope (MOST common reaction).
   1. Larger window should face clinician to ensure ability to see positive aspirations.

2. Ensure correct point and depth of penetration; to prevent loss of broken needle, do NOT bury hub in soft tissue.
3. Aspirate harpoon syringe by retracting piston and harpoon; aspirate self-aspirating syringe by pushing forward and then releasing pressure.
   a. Aspirate in two planes in MORE vascular areas to ensure that needle has NOT entered a blood vessel and drawn up the vessel wall during aspiration; may lead to false-negative aspiration.
      (1) Highly vascular areas with higher risk of positive aspiration and hematoma (in order): inferior alveolar, mental and incisive, posterior superior alveolar blocks.
   b. Blood that enters the cartridge may indicate that the needle has entered blood vessel or is in hematoma-induced, blood-filled tissue; change needle and cartridge and try again at different site or angle.
4. Inject slowly, at rate of ~1 minute per cartridge, to decrease potential for OD and for patient comfort.
5. Deposit appropriate amount of anesthetic, according to patient's treatment plan.
6. Change needle when barbed, or after several injections because the needle becomes dull.
7. Evaluate success of the injection; if necessary, repeat the injection with appropriate adjustments.

8. Observe standard precautions:
   a. Do NOT inject in presence of abscess or severe infection (needletrack infection).
   b. Avoid touching nonsterile surfaces (patient napkin) or picking up debris (gauze) on needle.
   c. Use device or method to recap needle to decrease potential for needlestick injuries.
B. Monitor patient during and after injection for signs of adverse reactions.
   1. Allergic reactions MUST be handled immediately, according to emergency protocol.
   2. OD (toxicity) reactions MUST be handled according to emergency protocol.
   3. For treatment or prevention of vasodepressor syncope (fainting, MOST common adverse reaction), patient should be placed in subsupine position (Trendelenburg position).
C. Dispose of needle and cartridge in an appropriate sharps container (BOTH needles and cartridges are biohazardous waste because they contain aspirated body fluids, including blood).
D. Posttreatment chart entry:
   1. Record vital signs, BP, and HR.
   2. Record type of injection, including type and amount of anesthetic (NOT expiration date of cartridge).
   3. Record any complications that need immediate or delayed attention (e.g., hematoma, trismus).

CLINICAL STUDY

Age	34 YRS	SCENARIO
Sex	☐ Male ☒ Female	The patient is in the dental office for his first oral prophylaxis appointment in 7 years. He appears apprehensive at the beginning of the appointment. After the treatment procedures for the appointment are explained, the patient asks the dental hygienist to stop because he feels hot and dizzy. Perspiration is apparent on his forehead.
BP	121/84	
Chief Complaint	"I really hate the drill and needles that you all seem to like using!"	
Medical History	None	
Current Medications	None	
Social History	Policeman	

1. What type of situation is the patient probably experiencing?
2. What emergency management or protocol should be initiated at this time?
3. If the patient loses consciousness, what steps should be followed?
4. What has caused this situation to occur?

1. The patient is most likely is experiencing syncope (fainting), most common emergency in dental office. Dizziness indicates that he is still in presyncope stage;

in this stage lowered blood pressure (hypotension), increased pulse rate, tachycardia (>100 beats per minute for adult) would be present. If this continues, syncope may occur, which is characterized by loss of consciousness, shallow breathing, dilated pupils, lowered blood pressure (hypotension), thready pulse.
2. At this time, he should be positioned in Trendelenburg position, subsupine with feet elevated higher than head.
3. If becomes unconscious, essential to open airway using head-tilt chin-lift technique. Prevents tongue from obstructing the airway and is indicated for any patient

(without a history of cervical spine injury) who is losing consciousness. Ammonia inhalant can be used to stimulate breathing, if necessary. Oxygen (5 liters/min with a nasal cannula) may also be administered. Careful monitoring until vital signs return to baseline is essential because syncope is likely to recur soon after recovery; vomiting most commonly occurs after unconsciousness, so turning the patient on his left side and having high-speed suction (high-volume evacuation) available will minimize aspiration. No further dental treatment should be performed at this time (need to wait 24 hours), and patient should be released. Later in the day, patient should be called at home to ensure well-being.

4. Stress indicated by apprehension about appointment, causing decreased oxygen flow to the brain, is the likely psychogenic cause of his syncope. His discussion about the drill and needle may have brought up issues from past dental experiences. Future appointments will have to deal with his apprehension by education and stress control.

INJECTION PROCEDURES

Appropriate injections are based on teeth that need to be anesthetized and anatomical landmarks. Maxillary and mandibular divisions of fifth (V) cranial nerve (trigeminal nerve) are targets for local dental anesthesia. Maxillary cortical plate is thin; allows local anesthetic to penetrate through cortical plate to anesthetize maxillary nerves, so injections, both infiltrations (Table 14-5) and blocks, are

Table 14-5 Infiltration technique

Anatomy anesthetized	Single tooth: pulpal and facial or lingual soft tissue
Needle gauge and length	27-gauge; short
Depth of penetration	Depth to above apex
Landmarks	MB fold, long axis of tooth, apex of tooth
Site of penetration	Superior to apex at depth of MB fold or lingual/palatal
Site of deposition	Apex of tooth
Cartridge amount (1.8 mL cartridge)	0.45 mL (¼ cartridge)
Complications	Inadequate pulpal anesthesia if below apex of tooth or too far away from cortical plate
Advantages	Easy technique; anesthetizes only one tooth
Disadvantages	No substitute for block anesthesia of quadrant; many injections; short duration; increased volume

very successful. Mandibular cortical plate is thicker than maxillary cortical plate, especially in posterior region; block injections are more successful than infiltrations in this region. Note that intraseptal injection (type of intraosseous injection) interproximally into interdental bone is not discussed.

- See CD-ROM for related figure demonstrating common local anesthesia in the oral cavity.
- See Chapter 4, Head, Neck, and Dental Anatomy: anatomy related to each local anesthetic procedure.

Maxillary Injection Procedures

Maxillary nerve block injections include posterior superior alveolar (PSA), middle superior alveolar (MSA), anterior superior alveolar (ASA), infraorbital (IO), greater palatine (GP), nasopalatine (NP), anterior middle superior alveolar (AMSA). See Table 14-6 for a guide to maxillary injections. This section discusses specific complications for each block.

A. Complications with PSA nerve block:
1. Deposition site that is too shallow decreases pulpal anesthetic effect.
2. Pain occurs when needle contacts bony alveolar process.
3. Mandibular anesthesia occurs when vertical angle (45° to the occlusal plane) is too close to 0° (flat).
4. Deposition site that is too deep increases potential for hematoma caused by entering pterygoid plexus of veins and/or maxillary artery.

B. Complications with MSA, ASA, IO nerve blocks:
1. Pain occurs when needle contacts bony zygomatic arch, nasal spine, or alveolar process.
2. May cause ONLY soft tissue anesthesia without pulpal anesthesia when deposition sites are either too coronal or too far away from cortical plate.

C. Complications with GP, NP, AMSA nerve blocks:
1. Since palatal tissue is very tightly adapted to underlying bone, may be difficult or painful.
2. Solution that drips from site of injection has bad taste.
3. GP may cause soft palate anesthesia when lesser palatine nerve is inadvertently anesthetized.
4. NP (ONLY block that anesthetizes both right and left sides) may fail to anesthetize canines.

Mandibular Injection Procedures

Mandibular nerve block injections include inferior alveolar (IA), buccal, mental/incisive (M/I), Gow-Gates (G-G), Akinosi (AK). See Table 14-7 for a guide to mandibular injections. This section discusses specific complications for each block.

A. Complications of IA block:
1. May include failure of anesthesia:
   a. Deposition sites that are too low (inferior to mandibular foramen) decrease anesthetic effect.

Table 14-6 Guide to maxillary block injections

Injection technique	Posterior superior alveolar (PSA)	Middle superior alveolar (MSA)	Anterior superior alveolar (ASA)	Infraorbital (IO)	Greater palatine (GP)	Nasopalatine (NP)	Anterior middle superior alveolar (AMSA)
Anatomy anesthetized	Molars (all but MB root first molar*); pulpal and buccal soft tissue	Premolars, pulpal and buccal soft tissue, and MB root first molars*	Canine, lateral, central; pulpal and facial soft tissue	Area that covers ASA and MSA	Premolars and molars; lingual soft tissue only	Canines, laterals, centrals, bilaterally; lingual soft tissue only	Area that covers ASA, MSA, NP, GP
Needle gauge and length	27-gauge; short	27-gauge; short	27-gauge; short	27-gauge; long	27-gauge; short	27-gauge; short	CLAD only
Depth of penetration	4-8 mm up to 10-16 mm, no bony contact	4-6 mm, no bony contact	4-6 mm, no bony contact	16 mm (half length); bony contact in fraorbital foramen roof	<5 mm, bony contact	<5 mm, bony contact	<5 mm, bony contact
Landmarks	DB root of second molar, MB fold	Second premolar, MB fold	Lateral, canine, canine eminence, MB fold	Infraorbital notch, depression of infraorbital foramen (finger pressure maintained), MB fold	Median palatine suture, gingival margin, first and second molars	Incisive papilla, marginal gingival of centrals	Median palatine suture, gingival margin, first and second premolars
Site of penetration	Distal buccal second molar, 45° to occlusal plane and 45° to midsagittal plane, depth of MB fold	Superior to second premolar at depth of MB fold	Superior to lateral, angled toward canine fossa, depth of MB fold	Infraorbital foramen where ASA and MSA nerves join IO nerve; preinjection depth can be made by estimating extraorally using infraorbital notch, at depth of MB fold	Between first and second molar and halfway between gingival margin and median palatine suture, with pressure anesthesia*	Base of incisive papilla, 10 mm from marginal gingiva of centrals, with pressure anesthesia	Halfway between first and second premolar on palate and halfway between gingival margin and median palatine suture, with pressure anesthesia*
Site of deposition	Posterior surface of maxilla	Apex of second premolar	In canine fossa	Apex of first premolar	Just anterior to GP foramen	Just anterior to NP foramen	Between first and second premolars on palate

Continued

Table 14-6   Guide to maxillary block injections—cont'd

Injection technique	Posterior superior alveolar (PSA)	Middle superior alveolar (MSA)	Anterior superior alveolar (ASA)	Infraorbital (IO)	Greater palatine (GP)	Nasopalatine (NP)	Anterior middle superior alveolar (AMSA)
Cartridge amount (1.8 mL cartridge)†	1.3 mL (¾ cartridge)	0.45 mL (¼ cartridge)	0.45 mL (¼ cartridge)	0.9 to 1.2 mL (½ to ⅔ cartridge)	0.45 mL (¼ cartridge) or until blanching	0.3 mL or until blanching	>0.3 mL or until blanching
Advantages	Atraumatic, high rate of success; fewer injections than infiltration	Covers premolar area and MB root of first molar*	Easy technique	Covers area of both ASA and MSA with just one injection, less volume	Less volume and less needle penetration	Less volume and less needle penetration	Less pain, more volume, no soft tissue anesthesia, covers large area of quadrant
Disadvantages	Hematoma; trismus, infection	Nerve not present in 28% of population*	Ballooning of tissues	Fear of eye damage (unfounded)	Soft palate may be anesthetized; swallowing is difficult; discomfort	Discomfort; solution is difficult to place	Need CLAD, delayed onset, short duration, still need PSA to complete quadrant

*Anatomy can vary among patients.
†Amount can vary per patient; amount given is average for 2% agents (usually half as much for 4% agents).

Table 14-7 Guide to mandibular block injections

Injection technique	Inferior alveolar (IA)	Buccal	Incisive/mental (I/M)	Gow-Gates (G-G)	Akinosi (AK)
Anatomy anesthetized	IAN: Molars to midline; pulpal, buccal soft tissue; premolars to incisors; LN: lingual soft tissue included by diffusion	Molars: buccal soft tissue only	(I): Premolars to midline, pulpal with M included; (M): facial soft tissue, lower lip and chin only	Molars to midline, pulpal and buccal/lingual soft tissue, mylohyoid, auriculotemporal	Molars to midline, pulpal buccal/lingual soft tissue, mylohyoid nerve
Needle gauge and length	25- or 27-gauge; long	27-gauge; mostly long	27-gauge; short	27-gauge; long	27-gauge; long
Depth of penetration	25 mm (¾ long needle), bony contact	2-5 mm, bony contact	2-5 mm	25-30 mm (¾ long needle to before hub)	25 mm (¾ long needle)
Landmarks	Contralateral premolar, pterygomandibular fold and space, coronoid notch	Occlusal plane, buccal cusps of most distal molar	Mental foramen, height of MB fold	ML cusp of second maxillary molar, tragus of ear, head and neck of condyle	MG junction, external oblique ridge
Site of penetration	Pterygomandibular space, lateral to the pterygomandibular fold, medial of anterior border of ramus*	Lateral to ramus, just inferior to occlusal level of buccal cusps of most distal molar	Between first premolar and second premolar, slightly distal to mental foramen	Distal to terminal molar at height of ML cusp of second molar	Distal to terminal molar at height of MG junction
Deposition site	At mandibular foramen	Lateral to ramus	Distal to mental foramen	Lateral region of condylar neck	Medial of ramus, higher than IAN and lower than G-G
Cartridge amount (1.8 mL cartridge)†	1.5 to 3.6 mL (just less than 1 up to 2 cartridges)	0.45 mL (¼ cartridge)	0.9 mL (½ cartridge)	1.8 to 3.6 mL (1 to 2 cartridges)	1.5 to 1.8 mL (just less than 1 up to 1 cartridge)
Advantages	Single penetration permits most quadrant treatment	Easy technique; many methods of injection; high success rate	High success rate; good for crossover innervation	Single injection for IAN, L, and LB; used for accessory nerve innervation; lasts longer	Single injection for IAN, L, LB; useful when mouth cannot open
Disadvantages	Hematoma; low success rate (85%); may require two injections†	Uncomfortable when bone is contacted	May balloon tissue or cause hematoma	Difficult to see landmarks, delayed onset	Difficult to see penetration site

*Anatomy can vary among patients.
†Amount can vary per patient; amount given is average for 2% agents (usually half as much for 4% agents).

b. Deposition sites that are too shallow (shallow to pterygomandibular space) decrease anesthetic effect to the IA nerve but may anesthetize lingual nerve.

c. May be successful except for mandibular first molar; may receive accessory innervation from mylohyoid nerves; corrected with G-G, lingual infiltration, or PDL injection.

d. Crossover innervation from opposite side involving the mandibular anteriors can be eliminated by means of PDL injection or contralateral mental/incisive injection.

e. If bone is contacted after penetration of less than half of long needle, clinician needs to reposition syringe barrel more over anteriors; needle tip will now be more posterior.

f. If bone is NOT contacted after penetration of more than half to three quarters of long needle, clinician to withdraw needle and reposition syringe barrel more over posteriors; needle tip will now be more anterior.

2. Touching the shallower lingual nerve during penetration causes patient to react (sudden movement); clinician should reassure patient about "tingling sensation" or lingual shock and continue injection unless movement is too great to control injection.

3. Bone should be contacted after penetration of three quarters or more of the long needle to ensure NOT injecting into the parotid gland, which contains the seventh (VII) cranial nerve (facial nerve); may cause transient facial paralysis lasting 2 hours or less.

4. If trismus of medial pterygoid muscle (mastication) is present and patient CANNOT open mouth, AK is recommended.

B. Complications of buccal block:
   1. May have ballooning of solution.
   2. Pain upon contacting bone.

C. Complications of mental or incisive blocks:
   1. May have ballooning of solution.
   2. Patient may feel mental nerve shock.
   3. May have hematoma from piercing mental blood vessels.

D. G-G: failure to connect with condylar neck; deposition of solution in masseter muscle.

E. AK: pain when contacting ramus or alveolar bone.

CLINICAL STUDY

Age	30 YRS	**SCENARIO**
Sex	☐ Male ☒ Female	The patient presents in the dental office for nonsurgical periodontal therapy. Her periodontal evaluation reveals generalized severe chronic periodontitis, with moderate inflammation and generalized 5- to 6-mm pocket depths. Only three small caries noted. The dental hygienist begins after the patient has been administered the right inferior alveolar and buccal (long) nerve blocks. When she proceeds with debridement in the lower right quadrant, tooth #30 is sensitive to both manual and ultrasonic instrumentation. All other teeth in the quadrant exhibit profound anesthesia.
Height	5'6"	
Weight	135 LBS	
BP	112/78	
Chief Complaint	"I haven't been to the dentist very much."	
Medical History	None	
Current Medications	None	
Social History	Daycare director, recently divorced	

1. What is the most likely cause of the sensitivity in tooth #30?
2. Identify the most effective ways to handle this sensitivity.
3. What should the dental hygienist do to prevent this situation in the future?
4. Identify other major causes of mandibular anesthesia failure.

1. Most likely cause is accessory sensory nerve innervation (mylohyoid nerve). Mylohyoid nerve branches off V3 superior to mandibular foramen. Nerve runs down and forward along mylohyoid groove on medial surface of mandible. Terminal branches may penetrate the ramus to innervate posterior mandibular teeth, especially the mesial root of the mandibular first molar.

2. Alternative mandibular block, such as the Gow-Gates (G-G) technique, may be used to anesthetize mylohyoid nerve, which can give accessory innervation to the mandibular molars, especially mesial root of the mandibular first molar. Possibly infiltration of the lingual tissues on the medial of the mandible of the involved mandibular first molar or PDL injection of the tooth would also accomplish anesthesia.

3. Prevention includes taking thorough dental history of past anesthesia and recording sensitivity in patient treatment record for subsequent appointments, since this accessory sensory innervation may be bilateral.

4. Other major causes of mandibular anesthesia failure include anatomical variations, infections, needle deviation, and improper type, placement, or amount of anesthetic.

Systemic Complications with Local Anesthesia

Systemic complications can occur with administration of local anesthetics, and others are local, such as needle breakage or trismus. MOST concern is with systemic complications; however, they rarely occur in comparison with local ones. Specific systemic complications for this procedure include OD and allergy.

- See Chapter 10, Medical and Dental Emergencies: syncope, allergic emergencies in a dental setting.
A. Types of adverse drug reactions:
  1. Caused directly by effects of drugs; include side effects and OD.
  2. Caused by sensitivity that is unique to the patient because of:
     a. Disease (e.g., methemoglobinemia).
     b. Emotional disturbance (e.g., psychogenic syncope).
     c. Allergy to the local anesthetic (rare).
B. Factors in OD (toxicity) of local anesthetic:
  1. Patient factors include age, weight, sex (e.g., pregnancy), disease, genetics (e.g., deficient pseudocholinesterase).
  2. Drug factors include vasoactivity, concentration of the anesthetic, dose, route of administration, rate of injection, vascularity of site, vasoconstrictor use.
C. Causes of OD of local anesthetic:
  1. Total dose that is too large; dose is determined by weight, physical status, age.
  2. Rapid absorption into blood; rate of absorption is decreased by vasoconstrictor use.
  3. Intravascular injection; occurs MOST often (in both veins and arteries) with IA, M/I, PSA nerve blocks (areas also with highest positive aspirations); clinician MUST be sure to aspirate and inject slowly (60 sec/mL); may want to aspirate twice and in different plane.
  4. Slow biotransformation (greater than 30 minutes); caused by systemic diseases such as atypical pseudocholinesterase and liver disorders.
  5. Slow elimination (greater than 30 minutes); caused by renal disease.
D. Mild to moderate OD of local anesthetic:
  1. Signs and symptoms include talkativeness, excitedness, slurred speech, apprehension, stutter, muscle twitching, increased blood pressure, increased heart rate, increased respiration, lightheadedness, dizziness, inability to focus, tinnitus, drowsiness, disorientation.
  2. Treatment includes reassuring patient, administering oxygen (prevents acidosis), and monitoring vital signs; supervising dentist may administer diazepam (Valium, anticonvulsant) slowly (5 mg/min); if reaction is delayed, hepatic and renal functions should be checked; cause should be determined before anesthetics are given again.
E. Moderate to high OD of local anesthetic:
  1. Signs and symptoms include seizures, decreased blood pressure, decreased heart rate, unconsciousness with or without convulsive seizures, CNS depression that leads to respiratory depression.
  2. MOST likely cause is intravascular injection of local anesthetic.

3. Treatment includes placing patient in supine position, protecting patient from convulsive injury, providing basic life support (BLS) and activating EMS system, administering oxygen; supervising dentist may inject anticonvulsants (see earlier discussion).
F. Epinephrine (vasoconstrictor) OD (LESS common than agent OD because epinephrine is normally in the body):
  1. Signs and symptoms:
     a. Fear, anxiety, tenseness, restlessness, headache, tremor, perspiration, weakness, dizziness, pallor, respiratory difficulty.
     b. Increased blood pressure and heart rate, possible cardiac dysrhythmias, including tachycardia and fibrillation.
  2. Likely causes:
     a. Concentration of epinephrine that is too high (optimum safe concentration is 1:100,000 or lower).
     b. Administering too much epinephrine at one time (in addition to embedded gingival retraction cord).
     c. Injecting anesthetic with epinephrine directly into a blood vessel; prevented by aspiration.
  3. Treatment:
     a. No treatment is necessary if brief in duration.
     b. If prolonged, terminate procedure, seat patient upright to decrease CVS effects, reassure patient, give oxygen (unless hyperventilating), provide BLS, activate EMS system.
G. Allergy to local anesthetics (LESS common now because of exclusive use of amide injectables):
  1. Signs and symptoms:
     a. Dermatological: urticaria, including wheals (smooth patches), itching, angioedema (i.e., localized swelling).
     b. Respiratory:
        (1) Bronchial asthma is a classic sign; includes respiratory distress, dyspnea, wheezing, flushing, cyanosis, perspiration, tachycardia, anxiety.
        (2) Laryngeal edema; associated swelling can block upper airway.
  2. Causes: allergy is a hypersensitive state caused by exposure and subsequent reexposure to allergen.
     a. MORE likely to experience allergic reactions to esters than to amides because esters break down into PABA; includes topicals (mainly esters such as 20% benzocaine).
     b. MOST likely allergic reaction now is to sodium metabisulfite, used as antioxidant to preserve vasoconstrictor.
  3. Management of allergy history:
     a. Assume presence of allergy until it is disproved; postpone routine elective care until cause is known, refer to allergist if necessary.

b. After <u>medical consult</u> that allows amide injection, avoid use of topical esters (20% benzocaine), instead use amides (lidocaine, prilocaine) for topical administration (although not as strong at 5% or less); use plain local anesthetic agents without vasoconstrictor such as 2% lidocaine (Xylocaine), 3% plain mepivacaine (Carbocaine), or 4% prilocaine (Citanest) (not same duration levels).

CLINICAL STUDY

Age	78 YRS		SCENARIO
Sex	☐ Male ☒ Female		The patient is in the dental office to have tooth #31 extracted. The tooth crown is badly decayed. Root resection before removal is anticipated. During a previous dental office visit, the patient experienced swollen lips and oral mucosa, with difficulty breathing after receiving an injection.
Height	5'4"		
Weight	125 LBS		
BP	105/58		
Chief Complaint	"I am worried about the injection because of the last time!"		
Medical History	Allergy to local anesthesia		
Current Medications	None		
Social History	Retired manager of girls' softball team Widow		

1. Did the patient have an allergic reaction to a local anesthetic, or was her reaction psychosomatic? Explain.
2. Identify the common types of local anesthetic agents used in dentistry. Which agent(s) are least likely to cause an allergic reaction? Which are most likely to cause an allergic reaction?
3. Before the patient is given a local anesthetic, what precautions should be taken?
4. Discuss the type of injection(s) that are needed to anesthetize tooth #31 for extraction. Identify the intraoral clinical anatomical landmarks associated with the area.

1. Patient showed signs of delayed allergic reaction to local anesthetic agent, namely swelling of oral tissues and respiratory difficulty. Allergy to anesthetic agents is rare. However, emergency protocol in the dental setting must be instituted.
2. Common local dental anesthetic agents include amides, least likely to cause allergic reaction and used only for injectables, and esters, which are most likely to cause an allergic reaction but are no longer used for injectables. She probably has an allergenic history based on past use of ester agent because of her age. However, local anesthetic allergic reactions are usually related to the presence of the preservative sodium metabisulfite used as an antioxidant for vasoconstrictor. Using plain local anesthetic without vasconstrictor such as 2% lidocaine (Xylocaine), 3% mepivacaine (Carbocaine), or 4% prilocaine (Citanest) will prevent most local anesthetic–related allergic reactions. This means that the appointments will have to be brief, since there is little duration (or hemorrhage control) with these plain agents. In addition, articaine contains sulfites; may want to avoid this agent for patients with allergies, especially asthmatic population. Note that topical agents used should not contain ester agents such as 20% benzocaine but lidocaine and/or prilocaine instead, even if at lower percentage. In any case, both medical and dental consult is indicated.
3. Following precautions should be taken: (a) consult with former dentist about type of anesthetic that was given when patient experienced reaction or refer her for allergy testing; (b) avoid use of topical and/or local agents that contain offending agent (probably ester or sodium metabisulfite or possibly use of articaine); (c) consider medical and dental consult information.
4. For extraction of tooth #31, 25-gauge long needle should be used. Injections should include inferior alveolar (IA) nerve block (also anesthetizes lingual nerve by diffusion) and buccal (long) nerve block. Intraoral clinical anatomical landmarks associated with area include retromolar pad, coronoid notch, pterygomandibular fold (raphe), pterygomandibular space (triangle), medial surface of anterior border of ramus.

Local Complications with Local Anesthesia

MOST local complications from local anesthetic administration are short term and are basic risks to local anesthesia administration.

A. Pain or burning during administration:
1. Causes: careless technique or callous attitude, dull needle with multiple injections, rapid deposition of the anesthetic, difference between pH of tissues and agent, contamination of cartridges with alcohol or sterilants; use of cartridge warmer because anesthetic is colder than room temperature,
2. Prevention: employ proper technique; inject slowly; use preinjection topical anesthesia; replace barbed needles; use sharp needles; handle unused cartridges properly; use local anesthetics at room temperature.

B. Hematoma: blood into extravascular spaces, especially noted on PSA nerve block injection.
1. Cause: nicking a blood vessel; if artery, tissue vessel will rapidly increase in size; if vein, perhaps nothing.
2. Management if large:
   a. Apply direct pressure, possibly with ice for at least 2 minutes.
   b. Inform patient of possible side effects, including cosmetic effects, soreness, limited movement.
3. Prevention:
   a. Review knowledge of anatomy, strive for CORRECT technique, minimize penetrations.
   b. Use short needle for PSA nerve block with proper depth and angulations.
   c. NEVER probe with needle and penetrate slowly.

C. Tongue, lips, and cheek trauma (chewing tissue):
1. Cause: long-acting anesthetics, MAINLY with children or mentally disabled or with use of long-acting agent.
2. Management: place cotton roll between the lips and teeth, then warn patient or caregiver about need to AVOID hot foods and chewing until anesthesia wears off.
3. Prevention: using sticker; informing guardians or caregivers of effects: remind NOT to burn or chew anesthetized tissues.

D. Trismus: motor disturbances of trigeminal nerve, MOSTLY spasms of masseter muscle, cause difficulty in opening mouth.
1. Causes:
   a. Trauma to muscles and vessels caused by repeated penetrations or hitting a nerve.
   b. Infection from contaminated cartridges.
   c. Increased hemorrhage from a hematoma.
   d. Excessive volumes of anesthetic injected into tissue.
2. Management:
   a. Use of heat therapy, analgesics, muscle relaxants.
   b. Encourage to exercise muscles by chewing gum (sugarless).

   c. If improvement does NOT occur in 48 hours, supervising dentist can prescribe antibiotics for 7 days.
   d. If improvement does NOT occur after antibiotics, refer patient to oral surgeon.

E. Transient facial nerve paralysis: temporary paralysis on side of injection, inability to open and close eyes, mouth droops on same side.
1. Cause: inadvertent injection into posteriorly located parotid gland during administration of IA nerve block because of anesthesia of fifth (V) cranial nerve (facial nerve), contained in gland.
2. Management:
   a. Instruct patient to close eyelid manually to keep eye moist (take off contacts).
   b. Reassure patient that paralysis is temporary and will disappear when anesthetic effects wear off (within 2 hours).
3. Prevention: use CORRECT technique for block by contacting bone before injecting.

F. Persistent anesthesia (paresthesia): MAINLY in mandible, especially with IA nerve block (affects lingual nerve MORE than IA nerve).
1. Causes: trauma from contaminated (e.g., with alcohol) cartridge or by needles; pressure caused by excessive bleeding at site of injection; anatomy of site; associated with 4% agents in mandible.
2. Management:
   a. Reassure patient and explain that affected area can require 2 to 12 months to regenerate nerves.
   b. Have patient examined every 2 months; if lasts longer than 1 year, refer to oral surgeon and/or neurologist.
3. Prevention: proper handling of cartridges and proper technique; many also recommend using ONLY 2% type of agents in mandible.

G. Needle breakage (rare):
1. Causes: sudden movement, smaller gauge needles (30-gauge); up to hub in tissue; bent needles.
2. Management: includes use of hemostat or locking cotton pliers to remove broken needle from tissue; radiographs of embedded needle may be needed and referral to oral surgeon is required (see Chapter 6, General and Oral Pathology).
3. Prevention: use larger gauge (27- or 25-gauge) needles; do NOT bury the hub or bend needles; do NOT redirect inside tissue.

NITROUS OXIDE

Fearful dental patients can benefit from the relaxing effects of sedation with **nitrous oxide**. This sedative can be used alone and in combination with local dental anesthesia. However, nitrous oxide sedation does NOT replace local anesthesia for pain control, since is an analgesic and NOT an anesthetic.

Pharmacology of Nitrous Oxide

Nitrous oxide is a colorless, tasteless, sweet-smelling inorganic gas that is NOT flammable but does support combustion. Commercially prepared by heating ammonium nitrate crystals in an iron retort at 240° C, then storing as a liquid at 750 pounds pressure per square inch (psi). As inhaled gas, does NOT combine chemically with body tissues but MAINLY affects the CNS. Works by stimulating the release of inhibitory neurotransmitters at the neuropathway junction located within the brain.

It is exchanged in the lungs, beginning with the respiratory bronchioles and ending at the pulmonary alveolus. It is NOT metabolized in the body but is eliminated by diffusion properties from the lungs. Highly soluble in blood plasma, therefore has analgesic properties in concentrations as LOW as 20%. Note that higher altitudes increase demand for higher concentrations of use because of increased need for oxygen in blood.

- See Chapters 3, Anatomy, Biochemistry, and Physiology: respiratory system; 9, Pharmacology: nitrous oxide pharmacology.

Patient Selection for Nitrous Oxide

Effective administration of nitrous oxide sedation involves both CORRECT patient selection and CORRECT management of the sedation unit. *Nitrous oxide administration by dental hygienists is allowed in only some states and usually under the supervision of a dentist.*

- See Chapter 10, Medical and Dental Emergencies: physical classification system using ASA designations.

A. Patient selection using American Society of Anesthesiologists (ASA) physical classification system:
  1. ASA I and II: considered appropriate candidates.
  2. ASA III: greater risk but may be used after <u>medical consult</u>.
  3. ASA IV: high risk; must seek <u>medical consult</u>; usually NOT appropriate to use with this patient.
B. <u>Absolute contraindications</u>:
  1. Recent ophthalmic surgery during which gas was administered to protect eye after surgery for up to 3 months; can disrupt the bubble and cause blindness.
  2. Cystic fibrosis.
  3. Lack of patient cooperation or existence of communication barrier (such as differing language).
  4. Patients with head trauma or shock.
  5. Middle ear infection (can experience ear pain because of increased pressure).
  6. Fear of nitrous oxide or need to always be in control (NEVER talk anyone into use).
C. Relative contraindications:
  1. Respiratory infection such as with sinus or tonsils; cold; active allergies; active tuberculosis (TB).
    a. Gas enters lungs through nasopharyngeal passages, so MUST be clear for gas to work.
    b. With TB, difficult to sterilize contaminated items; postpone until infection resolved.
  2. Chronic obstructive pulmonary disease (COPD), such as emphysema, chronic bronchitis, or lung cancer.
    a. Depend on lowered blood oxygen level to stimulate respiration, and with increased oxygen saturation may go into apnea and stop breathing; match test to check for pulmonary health.
    b. Physician discretion for hypoxic drive, <u>medical consult</u> recommended.
  3. Pregnancy: sedation of choice for short-term use, <u>medical consult</u> recommended.
  4. Epilepsy: hyperventilation may occur, inducing epileptic fit, <u>medical consult</u> recommended.
  5. Other mental disabilities: intellectual disability (mental retardation), autism, Alzheimer's disease, chemical dependency (alcohol or substance abuse): care MUST also be exercised, <u>medical consult</u> recommended.
  6. Psychiatric patients and patients taking mood-altering drugs: care MUST be exercised, <u>medical consult</u> recommended.
  7. Emotional instability (death, divorce, job loss): care MUST also be exercised.
  8. Children:
    a. Safe, but NOT all are candidates.
    b. May NOT be effective for children with behavioral problems or other special needs; sedatives administered orally or IV may work BETTER.

Procedures for Administration of Nitrous Oxide

For the safe administration of nitrous oxide sedation, patient must be screened and monitored for contraindications (see earlier discussion) and sedation unit MUST be checked for safety. National Institute for Occupational Safety and Health (NIOSH) has shown that controls can allow LOWER nitrous oxide concentrations in dental operatories (see CD-ROM). MUST follow <u>standard precautions</u>.

A. Patient considerations:
  1. Take thorough medical history.
  2. Monitor during administration of gas to determine consciousness and intolerance.
  3. Instruct patient NOT to talk to decrease exhalation of gas into the room air and keep sedation constant.
B. Nitrous oxide–oxygen unit:
  1. Thoroughly check unit for leaks and unsafe equipment.
  2. Monitor MAIN "fail-safe" features:
    a. Universal color scheme: used for tanks (blue for nitrous oxide; green for oxygen); tanks for the two gases are NOT interchangeable.

b. **Flowmeter:** measures how much of BOTH oxygen and nitrous oxide is delivered in liters per minute (Lpm)
   (1) Minimum flow of oxygen is 2 Lpm and nitrous oxide flow is 0.5 Lpm.
   (2) Nitrous oxide shuts off when oxygen quits; also, clinician can turn off nitrous oxide at any time.
c. **Scavenger system:** removes exhaled gases from mask (nasal hood) and room air.
d. **Flush system:** available to provide 8 or more liters of 100% oxygen to patient if there are signs of intolerance.
e. **Reservoir bag:** used to assist or control respiration during procedure and in the event of an emergency.
f. Nitrous tank: remains at 750 psi until it is MOSTLY empty; meter CANNOT be used to tell how much is left in the tank, UNLIKE the tank of oxygen, which can tell amount left.

C. Preprocedural steps:
1. Look at chart for last entry involving use and pain control issues for patient.
2. Have patient use restroom, take off contacts (eyes can get dry from air from mask).
3. Obtain preprocedure vital signs.
4. Have patient supine with legs uncrossed to prevent changes in circulation and paresthesia (numbness).
5. Explain procedure to patient; also explain potential sensations associated with gas.
   a. Percentage noted is ONLY somewhat relevant for current appointment.
   b. MOST common mistake is to automatically deliver a preset percentage to ALL patients.
6. Look for any changes in emotional state and listen for any similar verbal cues.

D. Procedural steps:
1. Turn on unit and push in flush valve to allow air for first breaths.
2. Adjust mask for proper secure fit and turn on scavenger system.
3. Determine and administer to patient the CORRECT liter flow using 100% oxygen:
   a. Considered **minimum flow rate** (tidal volume [TV]) when patient is breathing comfortably:
      (1) Average adults breathe 4 to 6 Lpm.
      (2) Athletes and large adults breathe 7 to 8 Lpm.
      (3) Children and small adults breathe 4 to 5 Lpm.
   b. Make sure reservoir bag is NOT overinflated or underinflated while patient is breathing; SHOULD fluctuate as patient breathes.

c. Some units automatically determine oxygen level when gas level is adjusted.
4. At 1-minute intervals, decrease oxygen flow by same amount that nitrous oxide flow is increased until patient acknowledges appropriate effects:
   a. Process allows nitrous oxide to be titrated (given incremental amounts); current standard of care.
   b. Limits amount of drug that is required; allows variety and safe performance of prolonged procedure.
   c. Takes 30 to 60 seconds for changes in gas levels to be felt by patient.
5. Once flow is at level where patient is comfortable, start procedure.
6. Increase level of nitrous oxide during painful or stressful portions of treatment by 5% Lpm from present levels to ensure pain control.
7. Continue to monitor patient for signs of intolerance, including nausea, diaphoresis (perspiration), unconsciousness, or changes in behavior (see later discussion).
   a. Patients must NEVER be left unattended; otherwise they may feel that they have been left alone and may panic, become agitated, or remove mask; also, oversedation and toxicity could occur.
   b. Once baseline is achieved, level of nitrous oxide SHOULD be dropped back 0.5 to 1.0 Lpm and oxygen turned up by same amount; can also be decreased near end of appointment.
8. When nitrous oxide is NO longer needed, have patient breathe 100% oxygen for at least 5 minutes or until effects of sedation disappear (see later discussion on importance).

E. Postprocedural steps:
1. Always evaluate recovery: verbal should be same as if nothing happened.
2. Obtain postprocedure vital signs.
3. Document use in records.
4. Thank patient for cooperation, and reinforce success of appointment.
5. Have patient wait 15 minutes before leaving if driving:
   a. Motor skills and attention can be affected for as long as 15 minutes after patient stops breathing gas.
   b. Offense for person to drive while under influence of drugs; office can be held liable.

Signs and Symptoms Associated with Nitrous Oxide Use

There are signs and symptoms associated with nitrous oxide use. However, response varies under sedation. Never liken it to alcohol, since that may upset the patient.

Table 14-8 Signs and symptoms in response to nitrous oxide sedation

Concentration of N$_2$O (%)	Possible response*
10-20	Body warmth, tingling of hands and feet
20-30	Numbness of thighs
20-40	Numbness of hands, feet, and tongue, droning sounds present, dissociation begins and reaches peak, mild sleepiness, analgesia (minimum at 30%), euphoria
30-50	Sweating, nausea, increased sleepiness
40-60	Dreaming (possibly sexual), laughing, further increase in sleepiness, tending toward unconsciousness, increased nausea and vomiting
50 and over	Loss of consciousness and light general anesthesia

*Standard of care states that N$_2$O should be used at <50% for most dental procedures because higher levels increase risk of complicating signs and symptoms.

Since MOST nonsurgical dental procedures (such as those performed by a dental hygienist) use minimal levels of sedation (less than 50% of gas, standard of care), patient remains awake and aware while breathing and can participate in treatment. Patient will still be able to respond to requests and answer questions, but speech may be slightly slurred and responses may be slower than usual. Will be relaxed and cooperative, probably will NOT feel any injections or other discomforting parts of dentistry, and will lose track of time. Effective sedation occurs in MOST patients. This level of gas keeps complications from occurring and maintains safety (Table 14-8). See later discussion of complications.

A. Signs:
   1. Patient awake, drowsy, relaxed appearance.
   2. Eye reaction and pupil size, BP, HR, and RR normal.
   3. Flushing of skin with slight perspiration and lacrimation.
   4. Little or no gagging or coughing; speech infrequent and slow.
   5. Minimal movement of arms and legs.
   6. Lessened pain reaction.
B. Symptoms:
   1. Sense of security, feeling of warmth, pleasant floating sensation.
   2. Tingling in hands and feet.
   3. Feeling of heaviness or lightness.
   4. Changes in way sounds are heard (everything sounds far away).

Nitrous Oxide Complications

Nitrous oxide is very safe. However, about 15% of patient experience side effects, including headache, nausea, vomiting. Other possible side effects are excessive sweating and shivering. Behavioral problems (possibly sexual dreaming) may occur. If patient experiences side effects, gas can be turned off and patient can breathe 100% oxygen for up to 5 minutes. Patient SHOULD tell immediately about any discomfort or other concerns. MOST complications result from excessive levels of gas (more than 50%) or NOT monitoring patients while they are under influence of gas.

• See Chapter 10, Medical and Dental Emergencies: dental emergencies.
A. Nausea: MORE common than vomiting.
   1. With prompt recognition, can be eliminated; unrecognized, it can lead to vomiting.
   2. Patient monitoring is major means of preventing.
      a. Watching face, arms, and body for any unusual expression or movements.
      b. Looking for pained features and other signs such as pallor, sweating, hands over abdomen.
   3. Causes:
      a. Increased depth or length of sedation; concentration of gas.
      b. Overwrought patient.
      c. If patient has inherent tendency to become nauseated, may be premedicated with prescription or OTC antiemetic drugs (dimenhydrinate [Dramamine]); some should be avoided during pregnancy.
      d. Presence or absence of food in stomach; heavy meal is NOT recommended but does not require empty stomach.
      e. Changes in patient's position; mouth breathing and prolonged conversation reduce sedation level; once patient is resedated with reminder to nose breathe, may revert to mouth breathing ("roller coaster").
   4. Management: by decreasing gas concentration by ~5% to 10% until patient feels comfortable.
B. Vomiting (emesis): prevented by prompt recognition and management of nausea; LESS common than nausea.
   1. MORE common in children; may vomit without warning.
   2. Caused by oversedation; higher risk during induction when communication is harder and patient is more likely to mouth breathe.
   3. Vomitus may be aspirated because of position of head in dental chair; potential to produce obstructed airway and its complications.
   4. Warning signs are nausea, pallor, cold sweat, cold and clammy hands, increased salivation, active swallowing.

5. Immediately turn off gas flow, permitting patient to breathe 100% oxygen.
   a. Remove delivery apparatus from face and removable dental equipment from mouth.
   b. Turn head and body to side to allow vomitus to pool in cheek and NOT pharynx.
   c. Use basin and/or high-speed suction (high-volume evacuator) to remove vomitus.
6. After incident, have patient breathe 100% O_2 again to reduce further vomiting.
   a. Patient may NOT want to have delivery apparatus on again for fear of becoming sick again, so explain need for oxygen.
   b. Explain that vomiting was an unusual occurrence and is UNLIKELY to occur again, to avoid discouraging patient from future use.

C. Excessive sweating:
   1. May normally become flushed by the peripheral vasodilating properties of gas; minor perspiration is usually noted on forehead, arms, or hands.
   2. If severe, concentration of gas is slowly reduced by ~5% per in attempt to make patient comfortable.
   3. If unable to stop patient's perspiring, procedure is aborted.
   4. However, if accompanied by pallor, drop in BP, and/or increased HR, give patient 100% oxygen, provide BLS, activate EMS system.
D. Shivering: NOT uncommon but can be uncomfortable; usually develops at end of procedure.
   1. With the flushing and sweating that occur with use, core, temperature can be reduced.
   2. Reassure that everything is fine; place blanket over patient to speed warming process.

CLINICAL STUDY

		SCENARIO
Age	37 YRS	The patient has an appointment today for a crown lengthening on a maxillary molar tooth before the final restoration is placed. To reduce her gag reflex, the clinician would like to use nitrous oxide sedation during the appointment. Near the end of the appointment, the patient becomes pale, starts to sweat on her forehead, and places her hands on her abdomen.
Sex	☐ Male ☒ Female	
Height	6'2"	
Weight	185 LBS	
BP	102/56	
Chief Complaint	"I am really nervous about the needle!"	
Medical History	Knee replacement surgery twice Back surgery last year	
Current Medications	OTC vitamin preparations qd	
Social History	Marathon runner	

1. What is a crown lengthening procedure?
2. How does the patient's being an athlete change the treatment using nitrous oxide sedation?
3. How does nitrous oxide sedation help the patient with the gag reflex?
4. How will the clinician respond to her fear of needles when using nitrous oxide sedation?
5. What does it mean when the patient places her hands over her abdomen and becomes pale and sweaty?

1. Crown lengthening is used when tooth needs to be restored but there is not enough tooth structure above the free gingival margin to support direct or indirect restoration (crown).
2. As an athlete, the patient may need greater volume of air for her breathing than the average, nonathletic adult, who would receive 5 to 6 Lpm, so her minimum flow rate (tidal volume [TV]) during nitrous oxide sedation should be increased if desired by patient.

Athletes and large persons can be at 7 to 8 Lpm; children and small adults are at 4 to 5 Lpm.
3. Nitrous oxide sedation calms gag reflex, which is especially noted when working on the maxillary molar teeth as in this patient's case.
4. Clinician needs to increase nitrous oxide by 5% (0.5 Lpm) and decrease same amount of oxygen to make her more comfortable during the injection of local anesthetic or any other painful, invasive procedure. After injection, amount of gas can be reduced to original base levels or less and same amount of oxygen can be increased.
5. Patient is becoming nauseated (pale and sweaty with hands on abdomen and sweating forehead) because higher levels of gas are present during last part of the appointment. To possibly prevent this, clinician needs to reduce amount of gas and increase level of oxygen until patient feels comfortable. To avoid this situation, the clinician should have begun to reduce the nitrous oxide levels near the end of the appointment.

Nitrous Oxide Abuse

Nitrous oxide can be abused by dental personnel for recreational use (acute) or because of psychological dependence (chronic).

- See Chapter 9, Pharmacology: substance abuse patient.
A. Short-term effects:
   1. May have slurred speech; difficulty maintaining balance when walking; delay in responding to questions; no response to stimulus such as pain, loud noise, or speech; may lapse into unconsciousness.
   2. Person who is rendered unconscious is likely to stop breathing within seconds as result of depressed nervous system; if remains conscious and stops breathing gas, recovery can occur within a few minutes.
   3. Person who remains unconscious and continues to inhale pure gas is likely to die.
   4. Death also occurs when users, in attempt to reach higher state of euphoria, breathe gas in confined space (small room, inside automobile) or by placing head in plastic bag.
   5. Long-term exposure (several minutes) is NOT necessary before death occurs.
B. Effects of chronic use: unusual but can occur, may cause vitamin B_{12} (cobalamin) deficiency.
   1. Red blood cell count is lowered, resulting in anemia and nerve degeneration.
   2. Painful and/or numbing sensations, unsteady walk, or irritated appearance.
   3. May also result in depression of heart muscular functioning and cardiac disturbances.
C. Dental personnel recommendations:
   1. Exposures SHOULD be minimized to prevent short-term behavioral and long-term reproductive health effects.
   2. Under OSHA guidelines, accepted level of nitrous oxide in the dental operatory should NOT exceed 50 ppm (parts per million).
   3. *Chronic* exposure should be avoided by women in first trimester of pregnancy and infertile individuals using in vitro fertilization procedures (linked to spontaneous abortions in surgical nurses), also those with neurological complaints and immunocompromised persons because of bone marrow suppression.

Review Questions

1 In a sensory neuron, the dendrite zone functions to
   A. synapse with CNS nerves.
   B. support metabolism.
   C. receive a stimulus.
   D. direct ion movement.

2 Which of the following local anesthetic agents is MOST appropriate if severe and prolonged postoperative surgical dental pain is expected?
   A. With 3% mepivacaine (Carbocaine)
   B. With 4% prilocaine with epinephrine (Citanest Forte)
   C. With 2% bupivacaine (Marcaine) with epinephrine
   D. With 2% lidocaine (Xylocaine) with epinephrine
   E. With 2% mepivacaine with levonordefrin (Carbocaine with Neo-Cobefrin)

3 Which of the following statements concerning nitrous oxide use is CORRECT?
   A. Requires a long time for recovery
   B. Used to induce stage III anesthesia quickly
   C. Both flammable and explosive
   D. The safest of all analgesics

4 Which descriptions can be used in relation to trismus and local anesthesia procedure?
   A. Extremely rare
   B. Total lack of sensation
   C. Motor disturbance of the trigeminal nerve
   D. Sensory disturbance of the trigeminal nerve

5 Which of the following is an immediate treatment for injection-induced hematoma?
   A. Ice and pressure
   B. Surgical removal
   C. Heat placement
   D. Aspirin injection

6 Which of the following situations is CORRECT in regard to the dissociation of local anesthetics?
   A. The more base molecules $(RN + H^+)$ available, the better the diffusion properties.
   B. The more cation molecules (RNH^+) available, the better the diffusion properties.
   C. The fewer base molecules $(RN + H^+)$ available, the weaker the binding properties.
   D. The fewer cation molecules (RNH^+) available, the greater the binding properties.

7 What is the BEST response when a patient experiences vasodepressor syncope with local anesthetic administration?
   A. Activate emergency medical system.
   B. Begin cardiopulmonary resuscitation.
   C. Place the patient in a subsupine position.
   D. Administer 1:1000 injectable epinephrine.

8 Which of the following explains why, when a vasoconstrictor is added, the pH of a local anesthetic (2% lidocaine), which was approximately 6.8, drops to approximately 4.2?
   A. Epinephrine (vasoconstrictor) is acidic.
   B. Epinephrine (vasoconstrictor) is basic.
   C. Preservative (sodium metabisulfite) is acidic.
   D. Preservative (sodium metabisulfite) is basic.
   E. Tissue has a pH of 5.5.

9 Which of the following describes the half-life of a local anesthetic agent?
   A. Rate at which the local anesthetic is eliminated from the blood
   B. Rate at which the local anesthetic effects the blockage of the nerve impulse
   C. Length of time an anesthetic can be stored before it is no longer effective
   D. Average length of time it takes for anesthesia to wear off

10 Positive aspiration indicates all of the following situations, EXCEPT one. Which one is the EXCEPTION?
A. Needle is in a blood vessel.
B. Hematoma developed.
C. Poor technique was employed.
D. Appropriate needle gauge was used.

11 What is the MOST likely cause of an overdose reaction when a patient receives 2% lidocaine with 1:100,000 epinephrine and experiences symptoms of overdose approximately 30 minutes after the injection?
A. Excessive dose of lidocaine
B. Injection of the solution into a blood vessel
C. Liver dysfunction or renal impairment
D. Rapid injection of the solution

12 What part of the chemical structure makes a local anesthetic agent hydrophilic?
A. Amino group
B. Aromatic ring
C. Intermediate chain
D. Benzene ring

13 A local anesthetic solution must form a salt to
A. enable the anesthetic to penetrate the nerve membrane.
B. enable the anesthetic to diffuse through the tissue to the nerve.
C. decrease the acidic properties of the solution.
D. increase the shelf-life of the solution.

14 All injectable local anesthetic drugs used in dentistry are
A. vasoconstrictors.
B. vasodilators.
C. neither vasoconstrictors nor vasodilators.
D. both vasoconstrictors and vasodilators.

15 What is the MOST likely cause of a patient giving a sudden jump and complaining of a tingling sensation shooting downward in the jaw during an inferior alveolar nerve block?
A. Injecting too rapidly for the situation
B. Injecting into the inferior alveolar artery
C. Contacting the lingual nerve
D. Contacting the inferior alveolar nerve

16 Which of the following situations would MOST likely cause a leaky anesthetic cartridge?
A. Piercing the cartridge diaphragm on an angle
B. Failing to screw the needle tightly onto the syringe
C. Air bubbles in the cartridge
D. Moderate corrosion on the metal cap

17 Performing aspiration in two planes during administration of a local anesthetic is necessary to
A. prevent the needle from entering a blood vessel and causing trauma.
B. ensure that the bevel is facing the bone to prevent trauma.
C. reduce the internal pressure of the cartridge
D. ensure that a blood vessel wall is not drawn against the bevel during aspiration

18 An inferior alveolar nerve block does NOT provide anesthesia if the solution is deposited too
A. medially.
B. laterally.
C. superiorly.
D. inferiorly.

19 Which determines the depth of penetration for a maxillary infiltration local anesthetic injection?
A. Length of the needle
B. Root length of the tooth
C. Gauge of the needle
D. Location of the zygomatic bone

20 During the administration of an inferior alveolar nerve block, resistance is met after 25 mm. The resistance is MOST likely caused by which anatomical structure?
A. Medial pterygoid muscle
B. Internal oblique ridge
C. Pterygomandibular raphe
D. Medial surface of the ramus

21 During the administration of an inferior alveolar nerve block, resistance is met after 25 mm. Which of the following is the BEST way to proceed?
A. Continue to penetrate tissue until the needle insertion depth reaches the hub.
B. Aspirate and then slowly deposit the solution.
C. Withdraw the needle, reinsert the needle superiorly, and penetrate until bone is recontacted.
D. Back off slightly, redirect the needle laterally, and penetrate until bone is recontacted.

22 Which of the following muscles may be involved in trismus during the administration of an inferior alveolar nerve block?
A. Buccinator
B. Lateral pterygoid
C. Masseter
D. Medial pterygoid

23 In which of the following situations is the Akinosi technique for local anesthesia indicated?
A. Alternative to the posterior superior alveolar nerve block
B. When trismus decreases the ability to open the mouth
C. For young children or mentally disabled adults
D. When bilateral mandibular anesthesia is required

24 What is the deposition site for the anterior superior alveolar nerve block?
A. Apical to the lateral incisor
B. At the apex of the canine
C. In the canine fossa
D. Over the central incisor

25 For which of the following nerve block injections does tissue blanching indicate an adequate deposition of local anesthetic agent?
A. Posterior superior alveolar
B. Anterior superior alveolar
C. Nasopalatine
D. Mental
E. Inferior alveolar

26 To determine the maximum recommended dose of a local anesthetic for a particular patient, the clinician MUST do which of the following?
A. Multiply the age of the patient by the dose per cartridge.
B. Multiply the manufacturer's number for milligrams per pound by the weight of the patient.
C. Divide the milligrams per cartridge of the local anesthetic by the weight of the patient.
D. Divide the maximum cartridges allowed by the milligrams per cartridge of the local anesthetic.

27 The BEST way to approach a fearful dental patient about to undergo extensive dental hygiene treatment is to
A. perform treatment quickly to reduce the time that the patient is stressed.
B. tell the patient that nitrous oxide–oxygen sedation is available.
C. give little information about the procedures to avoid frightening the patient.
D. increase the patient's control of the treatment session.

28 All of the following are fail-safe components of the nitrous oxide unit, EXCEPT one. Which one is the EXCEPTION?
A. Minimum flow of nitrous oxide is 2 Lpm.
B. Different universal colors are used to label oxygen and nitrous oxide.
C. Oxygen and nitrous oxide tanks cannot be interchanged.
D. Scavenger system is used to decrease exhaled gases.

29 The MAIN goal of nitrous oxide sedation of the dental patient is
A. decreased chair time for patient care.
B. stress and anxiety reduction.
C. compliance for opening the mouth.
D. to put the patient to sleep.

30 The PRIMARY safety factor for the patient with nitrous oxide administration is use of
A. oxygen flush button.
B. disposable masks only.
C. titration technique.
D. infection control standards.

31 Patient indications for nitrous oxide sedation include
A. mild anxiety.
B. emotionally unstable.
C. severe mental retardation.
D. severe cerebral palsy.

32 Patient contraindications for nitrous oxide sedation can include
A. language barrier.
B. asthma patient.
C. overactive gagger.
D. cardiac patient.

33 For BEST sedation appointment results, the patient should usually receive oxygen alone for _____ at the end of the nitrous oxide administration.
A. 1 to 2 minutes
B. 3 to 5 minutes
C. 6 to 10 minutes
D. 10 to 20 minutes

34 Chronic exposure to nitrous oxide by the dental staff can BEST be prevented by use of
A. titration methods.
B. a pin-index system.
C. a scavenging mask system.
D. infection control standards.

35 A scavenging system is designed to
A. collect exhaled nitrous oxide and return it to the tank.
B. collect exhaled nitrous oxide and vent it out through the suction system.
C. control the source of infection in the mask from the patient.
D. control costs of the nitrous oxide gas.

36 Which of the following is the primary site of action for nitrous oxide?
A. Central nervous system
B. Urinary system
C. Respiratory system
D. Cardiovascular system

37 About how long does it usually take for the patient to feel the changes to the level of the flow of the gases when nitrous oxide is administered?
A. 5 to 10 seconds
B. 20 seconds
C. 30 to 60 seconds
D. 2 minutes

38 Which of the following is a common mistake when using nitrous oxide in dentistry?
A. Individualizing the amount of nitrous oxide the patient receives
B. Using the O_2 flush button to remove mixture of gases from bag
C. Once baseline is achieved, dropping back the level of nitrous oxide
D. Allowing patients to let the dental staff know how they feel

39 Which of the following signs should be present during general dental treatment levels of sedation with nitrous oxide?
A. Patient is asleep
B. Lessened pain reaction
C. Extra movement of arms and legs
D. Speech frequent and rapid

40 Which of the following should be done when introducing the patient to the nitrous oxide procedure?
A. Ask the patient to refrain from mouth breathing
B. Allow only the patient to choose mask fit.
C. Liken the feeling to use of alcohol.
D. Have the patient sit upright with legs crossed.

41 Which of the following is a pharmacological property of nitrous oxide?
A. Sour smelling
B. Amber colored
C. Explosive
D. Inorganic

42 The reservoir bag while using nitrous oxide in the dental office should remain
A. overinflated.
B. deflated.
C. partially inflated.
D. stored in the drawer.

43 Which of the following can happen to a patient who feels the symptoms of nausea?
A. Hands over stomach
B. Feels fine
C. Smiling face
D. Red complexion

44 What needs to be done before you begin nitrous oxide administration on a patient in a dental office?
A. Have patient use the restroom.
B. Have patient put contact lenses in.
C. Only take pulse reading.
D. Have patient wait to use restroom.

45 Which of the following statements concerning nitrous oxide sedation is CORRECT?
   A. A dental patient can be left unattended for a short time if the patient has had this sedation before.
   B. The fail-safe system does not permit the flow of nitrous oxide if the flow of oxygen is interrupted.
   C. All child patients are excellent candidates for sedation.
   D. Patients who are highly anxious about dentistry are excellent candidates for sedation.

46 Which of the following describes an action potential in a neuron?
   A. Local event
   B. Small in amplitude
   C. Travels down an axon toward the synapse
   D. Caused by an influx of negative ions

47 Which of the following four types of nerve fibers has the fastest conduction velocity?
   A. Unmyelinated small fiber
   B. Unmyelinated large fiber
   C. Myelinated small fiber
   D. Myelinated large fiber

48 When local anesthesia is used to anesthetize the inferior alveolar nerve, which nerve is secondarily anesthetized?
   A. Posterior superior alveolar
   B. Anterior superior alveolar
   C. Lingual
   D. Infraorbital

49 What should a dental professional do immediately if a patient shivers when under nitrous oxide sedation?
   A. Have the patient use the restroom.
   B. Cover the patient with a blanket.
   C. Increase tidal volume.
   D. Give the patient 100% oxygen.
   E. Abort the procedure.

50 All of the following should be done immediately after the administration of nitrous oxide, EXCEPT one. Which one is the EXCEPTION?
   A. Administer 100% oxygen to clear the patient.
   B. Take blood pressure reading.
   C. Allow the patient to drive.
   D. Thank the patient for cooperation.

Answer Key and Rationales

1 **(C)** Dendrite zone is composed of small nerve endings at the terminal ends of nerves. These free nerve endings receive stimuli from tissues. When clinician places a curet in a pocket and nerve endings of dendrite zone receive the stimulus, this sends the impulse along the nerve to the CNS, which interprets the sensation as pain.

2 **(A)** The 2% bupivacaine (Marcaine) is a long-acting local anesthetic agent that lasts 1 to 2 hours as an infiltration and 5 to 9 hours as a nerve block for pulpal anesthesia, with vasoconstrictor epinephrine concentration at 1:200,000. Others are shorter acting even with vasoconstrictors epinephrine and levonordefrin added, and shorter still without epinephrine. Bupivacaine is generally NOT used for dental hygiene care because of its long action.

3 **(D)** Inhaled nitrous oxide–oxygen does NOT combine chemically with body tissues and thus is safest of all analgesics. Gas is taken in and eliminated in the same state, and recovery is quick; nitrous oxide supports combustion but is NOT flammable or explosive. In the dental office setting, nitrous oxide should NOT be used to induce stage III anesthesia.

4 **(C)** Trismus is a motor, NOT sensory, disturbance of the fifth (V) cranial (trigeminal). It disturbs motor nerves that affect the muscles of mastication and increases difficulty in mastication and in opening and closing the mouth. Trismus is common and seldom involves a complete loss of sensation.

5 **(A)** Tearing a blood vessel causes a hematoma. Initial treatment includes applying ice to the area with direct pressure for 2 minutes to decrease blood flow. Hematoma does NOT need surgical removal because it will dissipate with time. Initially, heat and aspirin should NOT be used because they may increase bleeding in the area. Heat may be applied after 4 to 6 hours or the next day to increase healing.

6 **(A)** Base molecules (RN) are uncharged ions and are responsible for the diffusion properties of the local anesthetic; the more free base molecules available, the BETTER the diffusion properties. Number of cation molecules (RNH) determines the anesthetic's binding ability; the more cations, the longer the anesthetic agent remains in the targeted area.

7 **(C)** Vasopressor syncope is fainting that is caused by a pooling of blood in the muscles, which decreases the blood flow to the brain. Performing procedures with patient in a supine position helps prevent syncope. If syncope does occur, patient should be placed in a subsupine position (Trendelenburg position), with feet higher than head to the floor; this increases the blood flow to the brain. Activating the emergency medical service (EMS) system, beginning cardiopulmonary resuscitation (CPR), and administering epinephrine are NOT appropriate choices for this common emergency.

8 **(C)** Agents with vasoconstrictors require preservatives to extend shelf-life to between 18 and 24 months (level for plain agents). The manufacturer adds preservative (sodium metabisulfite) to make the local anesthetic MORE acidic so it will last longer.

9 **(A)** Half-life is defined as the rate at which half of agent is eliminated from blood. For example, lidocaine has half-life of 90 minutes, which means that 50% of agent is eliminated in 90 minutes.

10 (C) Careful technique is important but does NOT eliminate chance of positive aspiration. Aspiration is act of drawing fluids into a syringe. If needle tip is in a blood vessel, blood will flow into the cartridge. If needle tip is NOT in a blood vessel, interstitial fluids will flow into the cartridge. However, if blood flows into tissues from a hematoma (tearing of the blood vessel) and clinician aspirates, blood will flow into the cartridge, giving a positive aspiration. Positive aspiration is indication that needle lumen size was inadequate for aspiration.

11 (C) Slow rise (30 minutes or more) in blood levels of lidocaine indicates that amide is NOT undergoing proper elimination, typically because of liver dysfunction or renal impairment. Rapid rise in blood levels of lidocaine can be caused by excessive dose of local anesthetic, by injecting too quickly, or by injecting anesthetics into blood vessel.

12 (A) Hydrophilic portion of local anesthetic is amino group, which determines diffusion properties of anesthetic. If amino group does NOT exist, anesthetic CANNOT be injected into tissues. Aromatic and benzene rings provide lipophilic portion, which increases nerve penetration. Intermediate chain determines whether anesthetic is ester or amide.

13 (B) Local anesthetic agents must be combined with hydrochloride to form a salt, which makes anesthetic more soluble in water (diffuses through tissue) and thus more injectable. Does NOT increase anesthetic agent's shelf-life, affect acidic properties, or enable anesthetic to penetrate nerve membrane.

14 (B) Local anesthetic agents used in dentistry act as vasodilators of the blood vessels in surrounding areas. Vasoconstrictors are added to INCREASE duration of agent and to decrease the potential toxic effects of too much anesthetic in blood.

15 (C) One major complication of the inferior alveolar (IA) nerve block is caused by the close proximity of the more superficial lingual nerve and the potential for contacting this nerve during penetration. When the lingual nerve is contacted, patient feels tingling (lingual shock) along the nerve that enters ramus at the mandibular foramen. Injecting TOO rapidly will cause discomfort during the injection, NOT tingling. Injecting into IA artery may cause an overdose reaction.

16 (A) Needle must pierce the diaphragm so that it is able to make a tight seal around the needle. If needle pierces the diaphragm on an angle, making oval hole, faulty seal will result and cause leakage of anesthetic. Loosely tightened needle may cause needle to fall off but will NOT cause leakage of solution. Cartridges exposed to freezing temperatures may exhibit bubbles and SHOULD be discarded. Corrosion of metal cap, even when moderate, indicates that its outer surface has been exposed to disinfectant or anesthetic and thus should be discarded.

17 (D) If the needle is in a blood vessel during aspiration, blood vessel wall can be drawn in against the bevel, giving false-negative aspiration. Rotating needle and aspirating again increases likelihood of accurately determining needle location. Injecting local anesthetic into a blood vessel greatly increases potential for overdose reactions. Aspiration will alert the operator of (NOT prevent) possibility of entering a blood vessel. Observation of needle bevel before insertion is necessary to prevent scraping of periosteum. Aspiration *increases* rather than *decreases* internal pressure of cartridge.

18 (D) If the anesthetic is deposited inferior to mandibular foramen, inferior alveolar nerve will NOT be anesthetized. Deposition of the anesthetic at superior deposition site will provide anesthesia. Deposition superiorly, medially, and laterally may slow the speed of onset but will result in anesthesia.

19 (B) To anesthetize a single tooth using infiltration, anesthetic must be deposited at or above root apex. Important to know length of root to provide adequate anesthesia to individual tooth. NEITHER length or gauge of needle NOR location of zygomatic bone is necessary to determine depth of penetration for infiltration anesthesia.

20 (B) One of the first bony landmarks for the inferior alveolar nerve (IAN) block is the internal oblique ridge. If positioning is too low, this landmark will be contacted ALMOST immediately during insertion, or as soon as approximately half of the needle progresses through the tissue (less than 16 mm). Contact with the medial pterygoid muscle may occur but offers little resistance. Pterygomandibular fold (raphe) is another landmark used for insertion during the IAN block, which would be lateral to this structure but medial to the target site. Contact with the medial surface of the ramus should occur when bone is contacted after penetration of three fourths or more of the needle, usually 25 mm in depth, for an average adult.

21 (D) Depth of penetration for the inferior alveolar nerve block is approximately three quarters of long needle, usually 25 mm in depth. Medial surface of the ramus should be contacted before any solution is deposited to prevent deposition into the posterior-placed parotid salivary gland with a resultant transient facial paralysis (temporary anesthesia of the facial nerve contained in gland).

22 (D) On the medial surface of the ramus, the medial pterygoid muscle, muscle of mastication, runs superiorly from the posterior, inferior angle of the ramus and covers the mandibular foramen and inferior alveolar nerve. Penetration of this muscle may cause trismus. Buccinator is NOT a muscle of mastication, whereas pterygoid and masseter muscles are NOT located near the site of inferior alveolar nerve injection.

23 **(B)** Akinosi technique, used as an alternative mandibular block, is indicated when the patient CANNOT open mouth. This technique is NOT specifically indicated for young children, mentally disabled adults, or bilateral mandibular injections.

24 **(C)** The ASA nerve is a branch of the maxillary division of the fifth (V) cranial (trigeminal). Terminal nerve endings are located within alveolar process in the area of the canine fossa.

25 **(C)** For NP nerve block injection, amount of anesthetic deposited should be just enough to blanch tissues. Other injections listed require deposition of solution in milliliters.

26 **(B)** For each type of local anesthetic, manufacturer establishes a maximum recommended dose (MRD) (in milligrams per pound). To determine MRD for a patient, clinician should multiply MRD per pound by weight of patient. The MRD for 2% lidocaine is 2 mg/lb; thus a 140 lb patient could safely receive 280 mg of lidocaine.

27 **(D)** Increasing fearful patient's control decreases fear by allowing patient to determine comfort level. Fearful dental patients require more than quick appointments and limited information about procedures and pain control methods.

28 **(A)** Minimum flow for oxygen (NOT for nitrous oxide) is 2 Lpm. This fail-safe component ensures that patient does NOT inhale nitrous oxide without oxygen. Color-coding, noninterchangeable tanks, and scavenger systems are ALL fail-safe components.

29 **(B)** Main goal of nitrous oxide sedation is stress and anxiety reduction; clinician does NOT want to put the patient to sleep but to make patient feel drowsy. Patient's ability to open mouth does allow clinician to know that patient is NOT oversedated. May NOT want to use mouth blocks for this reason.

30 **(C)** MAIN safety factor for patient with nitrous oxide is use of titration technique, current standard of care. Nitrous oxide is added to oxygen flow in small, incremental amounts. Limits amount of drug that is required, allows variety and the safe performance of a prolonged procedure. Oxygen flush button allows patient to have air to breathe at first part of administration. Infection control, possibly with use of disposable masks, does add to safety by reducing possibility of transfer of infectious material, but it is NOT as important as reducing toxicity in patient with titration.

31 **(A)** Mild anxiety is an indication for nitrous oxide sedation. Patients' emotional instability and severe intellectual disability (mental retardation) are relative contraindications for its use; depends on individual case as well as medical consult if desired. Absolute

contraindication is cerebral palsy, especially if severe.

32 **(A)** Patient (relative) contraindications do include language barrier, since patient should be able to communicate immediately if experiencing any complications that might be serious. Important indications for use of gas include asthma (more oxygen), strong gag reflex (controls it), and cardiac disease (relaxes patient).

33 **(B)** For best sedation appointment results, the patient SHOULD usually receive oxygen alone for 3 to 5 minutes at the end of the nitrous oxide administration, which allows the gas to be removed from the body. However, it may be longer for some patients. In addition, patient needs to wait 15 minutes or longer before driving.

34 **(C)** Chronic exposure to nitrous oxide by dental staff can be prevented by use of scavenging system, which removes excess gas from operatory. Titration methods are for safety, but for the patient, as is use of infection control standards.

35 **(B)** Scavenging system is designed to collect exhaled nitrous oxide and vent it out through the suction system.

36 **(A)** MAIN site of action for nitrous oxide is the central nervous system, causing sedation (depression of system).

37 **(C)** Takes 30 to 60 seconds for patient to feel changes to the level of flow of the gases when nitrous oxide is administered. Patience is IMPORTANT when dealing with changes made to level until patient feels the difference, especially if any less serious side effects such as nausea are encountered.

38 **(B)** Using the oxygen flush button to remove mixture of gases from bag is a COMMON mistake when using nitrous oxide in dentistry; oxygen flush button is used for giving the patient the first breaths. Others help to reduce complications such as nausea and vomiting that can occur with NOT individualizing amount, NOT reducing amount near end of appointment (prevents oversedation), and NOT allowing patient to let staff know about discomfort.

39 **(B)** Lessened pain reaction is the MOST important sign present during general dental treatment levels of sedation with nitrous oxide. Patient should NEVER be asleep (could go into deeper stages of sedation), and with good sedation there is less movement of arms and legs and speech is infrequent and slow.

40 **(A)** Patient must NOT mouth breathe, since this contaminates the operatory, reduces sedation, and gives uneven levels of sedation, which can lead to nausea and then vomiting. Staff must help patient choose the mask for a good, comfortable fit. They must NEVER liken sedation to alcohol or it may NOT be desired by the patient. Legs should be uncrossed to allow circulation and even blood pressure, and patient should be supine to prevent syncope.

41 (D) Nitrous oxide is sweet smelling with NO color, is NOT explosive, and is inorganic (metal) (this can present a problem when discussing issue with patients who love the green, organic way of living; NOT the same meaning as sprouts and such).

42 (C) Reservoir bag while using nitrous oxide in the dental office should remain partially inflated and then changes with each breath. This means the patient has the CORRECT tidal volume (TV, minimum flow rate) for breathing comfortably and the seal of the system is tight. TV is set with oxygen before nitrous oxide is titrated in; this is a standard of care. An overinflated bag so that patient complains of breathing against the rapid flow of air means that TV is too high; if bag is deflated and patient feels air blowing in eyes, mask should be checked for leaks, which may or may NOT be corrected by a 2 × 2 gauze square, the mask should be adjusted, or a smaller mask should be provided. However, if patient complains of NOT receiving enough air with deflated bag, scavenging unit may need to be adjusted, TV may need to be increased, or hoses may have become kinked.

43 (A) Hands over stomach indicate that the patient is experiencing nausea. Pallor, NOT redness, would indicate a serious complication, and there is also a change in the patient's blood pressure, heart rate, and respiration. Clinician needs to abort the procedure with gas turned off and oxygen placed at 100% and provide BLS and institute EMS system.

44 (A) Patient should use restroom before procedure, since this can give a feeling of warmth. Blood pressure, NOT just pulse, should be taken beforehand, and patient should take out contact lenses, since air from mask can be drying to eyes.

45 (B) Fail-safe system does NOT permit the flow of nitrous oxide if the flow of oxygen is interrupted. Thus if the unit has been adjusted to allow ONLY nitrous oxide, the persons involved may be abusing it. Others are NOT correct; a patient should NEVER be left when gas is being administered, NOT all children are candidates, and the highly anxious are also NOT candidates.

46 (C) Action potentials travel down an axon toward the synapse. Action potentials relative to graded potentials are large in amplitude, travel, do NOT decrement, and are caused by a relatively large flux of positive ions such as Na^+ or Ca^{+2}. An action potential is a "spike" of positive and negative ionic discharge that travels along the membrane of a cell.

47 (D) Myelinated fiber is large, is insulated by myelin, and allows saltatory conduction. Type and size of fiber both result in an increased conduction velocity. Myelin is an electrically insulating phospholipid layer that surrounds the axons of many neurons. It is an outgrowth of glial cells; Schwann cells supply myelin for peripheral neurons, whereas oligodendro cytes supply it to central nervous system.

48 (C) At the base of the tongue, lingual nerve ascends and runs between the medial pterygoid muscle and mandible, anterior and slightly medial to the inferior alveolar nerve. Thus lingual nerve is anesthetized FIRST by diffusion during inferior alveolar (IA) anesthetic nerve block. Others ALL innervate structures of maxilla.

49 (B) If patient shivers, cover with a blanket. Have patient use restroom before, since voiding can bring a feeling of warmth.

50 (C) Must NOT allow patients to drive until they are completely removed from the effects of sedation, usually after 15 minutes or more.

CHAPTER 15

Dental Biomaterials

CHARACTERISTICS OF DENTAL MATERIALS

Understanding of mechanical, physical, electrical, surface, biological properties of dental materials enables clinician to determine proper use and care of dental materials.

• See CD-ROM for Chapter Terms and WebLinks.

Mechanical Properties

Mechanical properties include reactions of materials to application of external forces, such as the magnitude of biting forces.

A. Forces:
1. Tensile force: tends to pull object apart or elongate object.
2. Compressive force: downward application on object, compressing (pushing or crushing) structure (i.e., biting by teeth).
3. Shear force: rotation, twisting, or sliding of one portion of material by another portion.
4. Bending combination of ALL types of force.

B. **Stress:** reaction with which object resists external force (Figure 15-1). Example: stretching of orthodontic band causes stress because wire is being pulled in tension; can resist this external force up to point of fracture.
1. Stress = Force kg per mo^m/Area inches/meters.
2. Thus the smaller the area over which a force is applied, the larger the value of the stress.
3. Stress-related properties:

a. Ultimate strength: highest stress reached before fracture.
b. Fracture strength: point at which a material breaks.
c. Tensile strength: breaking strength when tested in tension.
d. Compression strength: breaking strength when tested in compression.

C. **Strain:** deformation; change in length or dimension of a dental material because of applied stress.
1. Deformation or change in length (inches per meter)/ Original length (inches per meter). Example: dental waxes exhibit strain much MORE quickly than amalgam because of differences in stiffness.
2. The MORE stiff an object, the greater its ability to resist dimensional change.
3. Strain-related properties:
a. **Elastic deformation:** when material recovers after load is released or after material breaks.
b. **Plastic deformation:** permanent strain or change in shape of object that results when stressed beyond elastic limit.
c. **Elongation:** percentage of change in length up to point of fracture.
d. **Ductility:** ability of a material to withstand significant plastic or permanent deformation under stress before fracturing (e.g., gold), opposite of brittleness.
e. **Brittleness:** ability of material to fracture before undergoing significant amount of plastic or permanent deformation when placed under stress (e.g., glass fiber), opposite of ductility.
f. **Malleability:** ability of material to be compressed without fracturing; SIMILAR to ductility but specifically refers to compressive force applications.

D. **Elasticity:** permits material to be deformed by applied load and then assume original shape when load is removed (just like Gumby and Pokey). Examples: orthodontic wires resist fracture upon manipulation by clinician; adjustment of clasps on partial dentures; ability of fixed partial denture (dental bridge) to withstand forces of mastication.
1. **Modulus of elasticity:** measure of stiffness of material and ability to resist bending or change in shape.

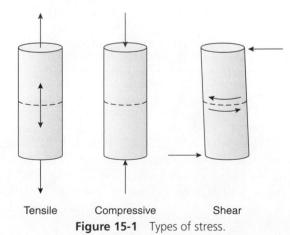

Tensile   Compressive   Shear

Figure 15-1 Types of stress.

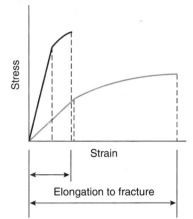

Figure 15-2 Diagram of the stress/strain curve.

Table 15-1 Hardness of restorative materials

Dental material	KHN
Acrylic	20
Dentin	70
Calculus on teeth	86
Enamel	350
Porcelain	400-500

KHN, Knoop hardness number.

2. **Stress/strain curve:** graphically shows change in dimension for given application and identifies important points such as elastic limit, proportional limit, and permanent deformation; used in dental research (Figure 15-2).
3. **Elastic limit** (proportional limit): maximum stress that material can withstand without being permanently deformed.
4. **Inelasticity:** permanent deformation as result of applied force.

E. **Hardness:** resistance of a solid to penetration. Example: clinician must instruct denture patients NOT to use abrasive cleansing materials, such as a paste with grit having higher hardness than denture, to prevent excessive abrasion of denture because of its low abrasion resistance.
   1. Hardness tests:
      a. Knoop: diamond indenter; ONLY one used in dentistry to produce value (Knoop hardness number [KHN]).
      b. Vickers: square-based diamond point.
      c. Rockwell: diamond cone and hardened steel ball indenter.
      d. Brinell: steel ball (oldest test).
   2. The higher the hardness number, the harder the material. Example: porcelain has high resistance to abrasion with high hardness number; conversely, it has ability to abrade opposing materials with lower hardness numbers such as tooth enamel and amalgams (Table 15-1).

CLINICAL STUDY

Age	59 YRS	SCENARIO
Sex	☐ Male ☒ Female	The patient is in the dental office because of a fractured tooth. Visual examination of tooth #18 reveals a fracture of the ML cusp. The remainder of the tooth holds a large MOD (mesio-occlusal-distal) amalgam restoration. After the dentist removes all of the old amalgam, some caries is discovered that will result in a near pulpal exposure. Patient also has amalgam restorations in teeth #2, #14, #19, and #31, and full gold crowns on teeth #3 and #30.
Chief Complaint	"I bit down on a popcorn kernel and my tooth broke."	
Medical History	Pancreatitis last year Past alcoholic, sober for 15 years	
Current Medications	None	
Social History	Animal groomer Likes gardening	

1. What mechanical properties were involved in the fracture of tooth #18?
2. The dentist decides to place a cavity liner before restoring this tooth. Explain what material would be appropriate and why.
3. How should this tooth be restored? Select an appropriate restorative material, and include indications and contraindications for different restorative materials.

1. Stress from biting on the popcorn kernel created both compressive and tensile forces on the tooth; smaller the area over which a force is applied, the larger the value of stress. In this instance, occlusal surface of #18, from contact with the kernel, magnified the stress. Second property involved was strain (reaction of tooth #18 to biting stress), which resulted in fracture of ML cusp.

2. Calcium hydroxide is appropriate material for lining the cavity. Advantages of material: (1) encourages recovery of the pulp by stimulation of secondary and reparative dentin; (2) protects pulp; (3) sufficiently strong. Mineral trioxide aggregate (MTA) may also be effective for lining the cavity.
3. Tooth #18 will probably require full-coverage restoration because of extensive loss of tooth structure. Because the tooth that opposes #18 has never been restored, full gold crown is indicated; gold would cause minimal abrasion of #15. Porcelain would be contraindicated in this circumstance because has high hardness number (KHN 400-500) compared with enamel (KHN 350) and would therefore result in the eventual abrasion of tooth #15.

Physical Properties

Physical properties depend primarily on the type of atoms and bonding that is present in a material. Allows clinician to understand how given material will withstand oral environment (i.e., temperature fluctuations, biting forces, moisture).

A. Thermal properties: reaction to temperature changes within oral cavity and subsequent expansion and contraction. Example: rapid change in oral temperature would occur when eating ice cream cone immediately before drinking cup of hot coffee and affect restorations by expansion.
   1. **Coefficient of thermal expansion:** value or measurement of change in length per unit length for each degree of temperature change (change in volume in relationship to change in temperature).
      a. The higher the coefficient of expansion, the greater the degree of contraction and expansion involved when material is exposed to temperature changes.
      b. Because of differences in expansion and contraction rates of restorative materials and tooth structures, microleakage of oral fluids between the restoration and tooth can occur (Table 15-2).
B. **Thermal conductivity:** ability of dental material to transmit heat.

Table 15-2 Expansion of tooth and dental materials: linear thermal coefficients of expansion

Material	Coefficient ($\times 10^{-6}$/°C)
Tooth	11.4
Amalgam	25.0
Acrylic resin	81.0
Composite resin	35.0
Silicone impression material	210.0

1. Enamel and dentin are poor thermal conductors, compared with gold alloys and amalgam.
2. Cements overlie and insulate inner pulp in areas of deep cavity preparations covered by metal restorations.

C. Electrical properties: generation of electrical currents through a variety of means.
   1. **Galvanism:** small electrical currents that result from opposing of dissimilar metals across dental arches (Figure 15-3).
      a. Have potential to create tooth hypersensitivity by irritating the pulp.
      b. Roughness and pitting can also occur as result of galvanic action.
   2. **Corrosion:** deterioration of metal by chemical or electrochemical reaction.
      a. Can be result of adjacent restorations that are composed of dissimilar metals.
      b. Also may result from chemical attack of metals by components in saliva and food; considered **tarnish.**

D. Color properties: give restorations and prosthetic appliances appearance of natural teeth and soft tissues (esthetics); important in selecting tooth-colored restorations and calibrating whitening procedures (digital machines available).
   1. Hue: dominant color of object (i.e., red, yellow, blue).
   2. Value: lightness or brightness of color; amount of gray present; MOST important color property.
   3. Chroma: intensity of color.

E. Translucency: how light enters the tooth; affected in several ways:
   1. Part of the light may be transmitted completely *through* the tooth (the MORE light that is transmitted through, the MORE translucent the material).
   2. Part of the light may be reflected *from* the surface of the tooth and thus may NOT penetrate at all.

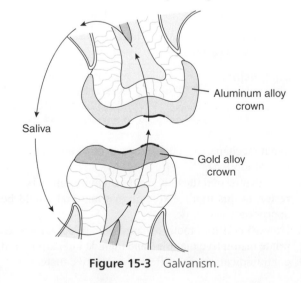

Figure 15-3 Galvanism.

3. Part of the light may *enter* the tooth and then scatter and be absorbed (refraction).
   a. Composites and ceramics (glass) can be made with varying degrees of translucency by adding opaquing agents to block light penetration; common problem with older anterior restorations, especially when photographed.
   b. Anterior teeth can be very translucent at the incisal edge; extreme or excessive whitening procedures can actually increase this, creating the appearance of gray teeth.

Surface Properties

Surface properties are associated with surface of dental materials and include surface tension and absorbability.
A. Solids: MOST materials in dentistry.
   1. Have regular arrangement of atoms and molecules; crystalline or rigid at all temperatures below its melting point.
   2. In contrast, **amorphous** structures have NO regularity or form; they possess many characteristics of solids but are noncrystalline; those such as glass do NOT possess a definite melting or freezing point. Example: dental waxes are amorphous and gradually soften without definite melting point.
B. Liquids: some dental materials are liquids at some point and then change to solids by cooling or chemical reactions.
   1. Irregular arrangement of atoms and molecules.
   2. Includes reversible hydrocolloid materials heated to liquefaction.
C. Attaching solid structures to each other: by mechanical bonding, cohesion, adhesion.
   1. Mechanical bonding:
      a. Does NOT require intimate attraction between atoms and molecules of the substances involved.
      b. Examples:
         (1) Dental cements with crown: liquid cement penetrates into irregularities on internal surface of crown and into porosities in tooth structure, thus creating locking mechanism.
         (2) Acid etch technique for most enamel sealants and resin materials: minute pores are produced in enamel and dentin when acid is applied, allowing spaces for interlocking of materials.
   2. **Cohesion:** force of attraction between *like* kinds of atoms and molecules within material, resulting in tenacious bond. Example: cohesive forces that hold cement together and prevent fracture within cement.
   3. **Adhesion:** force of attraction between *unlike* atoms and molecules on two different surfaces when brought into contact.
      a. MORE tenacious bond than mechanical bonding.
         (1) Primary bond: chemical bond between atoms and molecules; example: dyeing cloth.
         (2) Secondary bond (MOST common): van der Waals forces, or physical attraction between atoms and molecules that does NOT provide as strong a bond as chemical bonding. Example: materials with polyacrylic acid, such as glass ionomer cements and polycarboxylate cements.
      b. Adhesion helps control the problem of microleakage around dental restorations.
      c. Effectiveness of adhesion is determined as follows (Figure 15-4):
         (1) **Wetting:** degree to which an adhesive will spread out on a surface.
         (2) Contact angle: angle between the adhesive and surface that is measured to give a value for wetting; the larger the contact area, the BETTER the chance of adhesion.
         (3) Surface energy: the higher the surface energy, the greater the attraction of atoms to the surface, resulting in better adhesion (e.g., metals have high surface energy).
      d. Inhibition or failure of adhesion is affected by:
         (1) Dirty or contaminated surfaces: result in reduced surface energy of adherent, thus reducing ability to attract other atoms and molecules.
         (2) Viscosity: adhesives with high viscosity have high resistance to flow, are less likely

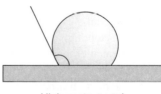

High contact angle

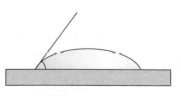

Moderate contact angle

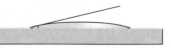

Low contact angle

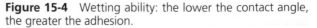

Figure 15-4 Wetting ability: the lower the contact angle, the greater the adhesion.

to spread out on a surface; if viscosity is too low, though, may be hard to control placement of the adhesive.

(3) Shrinkage of adhesives during hardening: causes adhesive to pull away from tooth/restoration, thus compromising adhesion.

Biological Properties

Biological properties refer to the biological response of the human body to various materials and the continued examination of the host–foreign body response. Response of both patients and clinicians can involve allergy, microleakage, and toxicity factors.

- See Chapter 8, Microbiology and Immunology: allergic reactions, including rubber latex allergy.
A. Allergic response (immediate or delayed contact allergic reaction type):
    1. Elicited in patients who are sensitized to nickel-containing materials; occurs infrequently.
    2. Possibly also rubber latex allergy for both patient and clinician from rubber latex rubber dam and gloves; may be associated with placement of restorative materials; other restorative, rubber dam (silicone), and glove (vinyl) materials are available.
    3. Higher percentage of women are sensitive or allergic to nickel and/or rubber latex.
B. **Microleakage:**
    1. Inability of materials to adequately seal margins by adhesion, allows leakage of saliva, dental biofilm (dental plaque), and by-products into the area, which can lead to secondary caries, pulpitis, pain, necrosis.
    2. LESS potential with polyacrylic acid, currently ONLY material able to adhere sufficiently to avoid microleakage.
C. Toxic effects of materials: can occur during and after restoration of carious tooth, may subject pulp to injury.
    1. Includes microleakage, thermal shock, galvanism, chemical irritation.
    2. Can be minimized or eliminated by taking proper steps (e.g., using insulating bases, tooth isolation with rubber dam).

IMPRESSION MATERIALS

Function of impression and replication materials is to accurately record hard and soft tissues in the oral cavity. **Impressions** produce *negative* reproduction, which then can be used by clinician for construction of restorations to replace missing tooth structure and for fabrication of preventive devices. Vary in accuracy and ease of use, especially in removal from the mouth, such as around tooth **undercuts,** portion of tooth that lies between its height of contour and attached gingiva. Replication materials to preserve the impressions are discussed in next section.

A. Classification of impression materials:
    1. Inelastic materials: rigid impression materials are restricted to applications in which NO undercuts exist.
        a. Compound (modeling plastic): tray compound and impression compound.
        b. Zinc oxide–eugenol (ZOE) impression paste: LESS use, replaced by rubber impression materials.
        c. Impression plaster: LESS use because of rigidity and ease of fracture; used primarily to mount casts on articulator.
    2. Elastomeric materials: aqueous elastomeric materials (hydrocolloid): largely replaced by BOTH alginate and rubber base impression materials:
        a. **Hydrocolloid** is a suspension of fine particles dispersed in water to produce a viscous solution.
        b. Irreversible hydrocolloid, such as alginate, and reversible hydrocolloid, such as agar-agar.
    3. Nonaqueous elastomeric materials (rubber):
        a. Polysulfide (mercaptan rubber).
        b. Silicone rubber; BOTH condensation and addition (polyvinylsiloxane) types.
        c. Polyether.
B. Composition and chemistry:
    1. Compound (modeling plastic): 40% resin, 7% wax, 3% organic acid, 50% filler, coloring agent.
        a. Thermoplastic (material will reversibly soften on heating and harden on cooling).
        b. Tray compound is in shape of a tray; impression compound is in form of sticks and cones.
    2. ZOE impression paste: supplied as two-paste system: zinc oxide, eugenol, oils (such as oil of cloves), resin, additives.
    3. Irreversible hydrocolloid (alginate) (Table 15-3).

Table 15-3 Composition of irreversible hydrocolloid alginate impression material

Ingredient	Percentage (%)	Function
Diatomaceous earth	60	Filler
Calcium sulfate	16	Reacts with potassium alginate to create gelation
Potassium alginate	15	Reacts with calcium sulfate to create gelation
Zinc oxide	4	Filler
Potassium titanium fluoride	3	Accelerates setting of gypsum
Trisodium phosphate	2	Retardant

Table 15-4 Composition of reversible hydrocolloid

Ingredient	Percentage (%)	Function
Agar-agar	8-15	Substance is extracted from a type of seaweed whose fibrils form a colloid that results in a partially rigid but elastic gel
Water	80-85	Main component that occupies the spaces between the agar-agar fibrils
Borax	Trace amounts	Increases the strength of the gel (also can retard the setting of gypsum; requires the addition of an accelerator)
Potassium sulfate	2	Accelerates the setting of gypsum

4. Reversible hydrocolloid (agar) (Table 15-4).
5. Polysulfide: supplied as two-paste system:
  a. Base: 80% organic polymer-containing reactive mercaptan groups and 20% reinforcing agents.
  b. Catalyst: MOST often is lead dioxide.
6. Silicone rubber:
  a. Condensation type: supplied as base and accelerator; available in light, regular, heavy-bodied consistency and as putty:
    (1) Base: silicone liquid, dimethylsiloxane.
    (2) Accelerator: tin organic ester suspension and alkyl silicate.
  b. Addition: type (polyvinylsiloxane): supplied as two-paste or putty system, with silicone and silane hydrogens.
7. Polyether: supplied as BOTH base and catalyst; base is polyether and catalyst is sulfonic acid ester.
C. Characteristics, properties, manipulation of each:
1. Compound:
  a. Flow is 85% at 113° F and 6% at mouth temperature (98.6° F); hardens in mouth.
  b. Tray compound is stiffer and has less flow than impression compound.
  c. Thermoplastic; does NOT involve chemical change.
  d. LOW thermal conductivity.
2. ZOE:
  a. Soft-set ZOE is tougher than and NOT as brittle as hard-set ZOE.
  b. BOTH types are classified as rigid; CANNOT be used to record undercut areas.
  c. Setting time that is shortened by presence of water, high humidity, high temperatures.

  d. Accurate; has low dimensional change during setting of ~0.1%.
  e. Adheres to tray compound or acrylic tray material, eliminating need for tray adhesive.
3. Irreversible hydrocolloid (alginate):
  a. Suspension of molecules (colloid) in some type of dispersion medium (water); a liquid colloid is a sol.
    (1) Liquid sol is changed into a gel by chemical means, which is an irreversible process.
    (2) Normal-set alginate sets in not less than 2 minutes, not more than 4½ minutes (mixing time, 1 minute).
    (3) Fast-set alginate sets in 1 to 2 minutes (mixing time, 30 to 45 seconds).
    (4) Water/powder (W/P) ratio affects setting time; thinner mixes increase time required for material to set; increased powder decreases setting time.
  b. Has 1.5% permanent deformation.
    (1) Increased strength if thick rather than thin mixes are used.
    (2) Results in increased tear and compressive strength if impression is left in mouth until fully set.
    (3) Less accurate impression material than agar/rubber impression materials.
    (4) Loses accuracy (dimensional change) if stored for MORE than 10 minutes in air because of syneresis (loss of water by evaporation and by exuding fluid); wrap in moist paper towel or keep in 100% humidity and pour as soon as removed.
    (5) If stored in contact with water, will absorb water (imbibition), leading to dimensional change.
  c. Procedure for use:
    (1) Mixing:
      (a) Fluff alginate powder container or package; measure appropriate amount of cool water for required number of scoops of alginate; place water in plastic bowl.
      (b) Add alginate powder to water in bowl, thus helping to eliminate entrapped air in final mix.
      (c) Stir powder and water vigorously to wet powder completely, strop (wipe) mix against side of the bowl for 60 seconds to homogenize and remove bubbles.
      (d) Visually inspect mixture for a creamy, thick consistency.
    (2) Filling and seating the tray:
      (a) Spray tray with adhesive, then fill with mixture by spatula, from posterior regions forward.

(b) Smooth alginate surface with moistened finger; precoat the occlusal and other anatomical areas (e.g., vaulted palate, frenums) for BETTER impression.

(c) Seat tray in a posterior to anterior direction.

(d) Border mold by pulling lips and cheeks over tray and hold tray in place until alginate sets.

(3) Removing and pouring impression:

(a) Lift lips and cheeks away with fingers to break seal.

(b) Grasp handle and pull tray away from teeth with quick (thrust or snap) motion for less distortion.

(c) Wash impression under cool water to eliminate saliva and blood.

(d) Spray impression with disinfectant and seal in plastic bag for 10 minutes.

(e) Rinse thoroughly and pour impression as soon as possible or store in 100% humidity, 15 minutes maximum.

4. Reversible hydrocolloid (agar): sol is changed into gel by physical (cooling) reaction and therefore is reversible; gives highly accurate impression; MUST be poured immediately to avoid dimensional changes.

5. Polysulfide: provides MOST reproduction of surface detail.

a. Demonstrates shrinkage of impression material during first 24 hours; therefore models and dies SHOULD be poured within 1 hour.

b. Highly compatible with model plaster and stone; long shelf-life, improved by refrigeration.

6. Silicone rubber:

a. Condensation type:

(1) LESS working and setting time than polysulfides.

(2) LESS viscosity than polysulfides, making them easier to mix.

(3) Greater dimension change than polysulfides; reproduces fine details.

(4) Compatible with model plaster and stone.

(5) Known to cause allergic reactions.

b. Addition (polyvinylsiloxane) type:

(1) Low dimension change of 0.1%; does NOT require immediate pouring, can be delayed for up to 7 days.

(2) Lowest level of permanent deformation of ALL elastomeric impression materials on removal from mouth.

(3) MORE stiff than polysulfides and condensation silicones; makes removal from undercuts MORE difficult; NOT as stiff as polyethers.

(4) Causes LESS tissue reaction than condensation silicones.

(5) Very hydrophobic material, can cause problems with trapped air bubbles on the surface when pouring gypsum casts or dies; surfactants added to make MORE hydrophilic.

7. Polyether:

a. LESS working time than any of the rubber impression materials.

b. Permanent deformation greater than that of polysulfides, but NOT as low as that of silicones.

c. High stiffness and low flexibility, thus can cause problems during removal from mouth; trays must be made short of tissue undercuts, NOT for removable appliances.

d. Lower dimension change than any other rubber material, EXCEPT for polyvinylsiloxane.

e. Can cause tissue irritation because of aromatic sulfonic acid ester catalyst.

D. Clinical uses:

1. Compound:

a. Tray compound: primary impression for dentures; another impression material, such as rubber base, put into tray to make secondary or corrective impression.

b. Impression compounds: border molding for denture impressions.

2. ZOE impression paste: cementing media; also is used for surgical dressings (after periodontal surgery), temporary restorations, root canal filling material, bite registration paste, impression material for dentures.

3. Irreversible hydrocolloid:

a. Diagnostic (study) cast for educational purposes, fabrication of fluoride trays and mouth protectors, orthodontic appliance construction.

b. Preliminary cast for development of complete and partial dentures (to make trays and diagnoses).

4. Reversible hydrocolloid: SAME uses as irreversible hydrocolloid but produces MORE accurate detail.

5. Polysulfide:

a. Inlay and crown impressions.

b. Development of fixed partial dentures (bridge) and secondary (final) impressions for dentures.

6. Silicone:

a. Polyvinylsiloxane (addition silicone): same uses as polysulfide.

b. Condensation silicone: used for inlay and crown impressions as well as fixed partial dentures.

7. Polyether: SAME uses as condensation silicone.

Table 15-5 Water/powder (W/P) ratios of gypsum materials*

Gypsum	Water (mL/100 g powder)
Model plaster (type II)	37-50
Dental stone (type III)	28-32
High-strength dental stone (type IV-V)	19-24

*Recommended W/P ratios vary among products and manufacturers.

Replication Materials

Impression plaster and stone are examples of **replication materials** that are used to produce *positive* reproduction of impressions. Standard precautions for lab discussed later.

A. Composition: gypsum is calcium sulfate hemihydrate ($CaSO_4 \cdot 2\ H_2O$).

B. Types:
1. Model plaster (type II): heating gypsum under atmospheric pressure results in a porous, irregularly shaped material.
2. Dental stone (type III): heating gypsum under steam pressure results in hemihydrate particles that are less porous and MORE uniform in shape.
3. High-strength dental (die) stone (type IV [low expansion], V [high expansion]): dehydrating gypsum in 30% solution of calcium chloride results in LEAST porous hemihydrate particles.

C. Characteristics and properties:
1. Hemihydrate: physical differences in hemihydrate particles determine manipulative properties for mixing particles and use of each.
   a. Mixing (Table 15-5):
      (1) Amount of water needed depends on size, shape, porosity of the particles.
      (2) Porous, irregularly shaped hemihydrate crystals require MORE water to facilitate wetting and mixing.
      (3) High-strength stone requires LEAST amount of water.
      (4) Too *much* water prolongs setting time and creates weaker cast or die.
      (5) Too *little* water results in increased expansion.
   b. Setting:
      (1) When mixed with water, forms hard substance.
      (2) Produces heat (exothermic reaction) through chemical reaction of hemihydrate with water.
      (3) Allow 45 to 60 minutes to set before removing impression from the cast or die.
2. Accelerators and retarders: more practical method of controlling setting time than varying W/P ratio (added by manufacturer).
   a. Accelerator is potassium sulfate (salt solution); reduces setting time from ~10 minutes to 4 minutes.
   b. Retarder is borax; increases setting time (blood, saliva, agar, alginate also retard setting).
   c. Impressions thoroughly rinsed and disinfected using infection control protocol (remove traces of blood, saliva).
3. Temperature and humidity:
   a. Higher water temperatures (during mixing) decrease setting times.
   b. High humidity results in decreased setting time.

D. Types and uses of gypsum:
1. Impression gypsum (type I): mount casts on articulators or as interocclusal record.
2. Model plaster (type II): weakest; lowest compressive strength because of excess water, higher W/P ratio; NOT used intraorally; makes study casts (models) for documentation:
   a. To permit clinicians to examine conditions in the mouth from all views; allows study of relationships between adjacent and opposing teeth and permits dentist to examine, measure, and analyze without discomfort to the patient.
   b. Beginning of treatment and progress of involved or long-term treatment; for drawing, completing diagnostic waxing, or performing proposed treatment on models.
   c. To illustrate existing conditions to the patient during case presentation.
   d. To examine occlusal relationships and chart existing factors such as wear facets, open contacts, rotated teeth, and tissue recession.
   e. To demonstrate individualized homecare procedures; allows practice of techniques on models.
   f. Forensic cases.
3. Dental stone (type III):
   a. Used to make casts of impressions for fabrication of dentures and to produce study casts.
   b. Harder, stronger, MORE durable than model plaster (type II); greater strength result of lower W/P ratio.
4. High-strength dental (die) stone (type IV [low expansion] or V [high expansion]).
   a. Type IV: used as die material on which wax patterns of inlays, crowns, and other castings are produced.
      (1) Four times greater compression strength than model plaster (type II) because excess water has been minimized.
      (2) Lowest W/P ratio.
   b. Type V: used as die material with higher expansion to compensate for greater shrinkage that occurs in higher-melting alloys.

E. Procedure for use:
1. Dispensing: weigh powder and vacuum mix; water should be measured in graduated cylinder to get consistent results; dimensional accuracy increased when gypsum is weighed and water is measured.
2. Mixing: performed in a rubber bowl, using a stiff metal spatula, with room-temperature water.
   a. Place water in bowl first and then add powder, sift into water slowly.
   b. Spatulate vigorously for 30 to 60 seconds to break up clumps and enhance wetting of powder, strop (wipe) against side of the bowl.
   c. Vibrate to remove remaining air bubbles; presence of air bubbles results in porosities in cast, reducing strength.
   d. When complete, mix looks very glossy on the surface and has smooth, creamy texture (if sandy, grainy, or watery, incorrect W/P ration has been used and mixing is incomplete); can be BEST accomplished using vacuum mixer technique.
3. Pouring:
   a. Surface of the impression is dried, excess water removed.
   b. Plaster or stone is dripped into one corner of the impression and gently vibrated to slowly move the mix around the arch and express any air to coat impression.
   c. Second increment is added and vibrated; excessive vibration SHOULD be avoided because it creates air bubbles in the material.
   d. Process is repeated until entire surface of impression is coated and teeth imprints are completely filled; larger increments can be added to fill the impression completely.
   e. *One-pour* technique involves initial mix of plaster or stone that is large enough to fill impression and form base; *two-pour* technique involves second mix of plaster or stone, used to form a base after first pour is set.
F. Cast trimming: excess gypsum is removed with lab knife after loss of gloss.

RESTORATIONS

A **restoration** restores or replaces lost tooth structure, teeth, or oral tissues. Includes any filling, inlay, crown, bridge, partial denture, or complete denture.

DIRECT RESTORATIVE MATERIALS

Direct restorative materials can be placed directly in or on a prepared tooth. Advantageous because of immediate results and timesaving benefits. Can be either temporary or permanent restorations.
• See Chapter 11, Clinical Treatment: enamel (pit and fissure) sealants.

Temporary Restoratives

Many procedures cannot be completed in one appointment because of need for lab work or because of complications of infections. In these instances, **temporary** (provisional) **restoration** that is placed over preparation is indicated. Materials such as acrylics, stainless steel, composites, or cements are used in preparation to maintain relationship in occlusion until permanent restoration can be placed.
A. Acrylics with compositions similar to denture bases.
B. Stainless steel or aluminum:
   1. Stiff enough to bear occlusal forces when cemented to prepared tooth with temporary cement.
   2. Easy to cut and adjust; has poor esthetic qualities.
C. Composite-type material:
   1. Of intermediate rigidity, somewhat flexible after light curing.
   2. Flexibility allows easy cutting and removal when permanent restoration is ready for insertion.
D. ZOE (type III) (Fynal):
   1. Designed for use as temporary filling when mixed to base or puttylike consistency.
   2. Protects the pulp; reduces pulpal inflammation.

Permanent Restorations

Permanent restorations are composed of dental materials whose properties allow them to function in the oral cavity for a greater length of service than that of temporary restorations. Include both esthetic and amalgam restorations.
• See Chapter 11, Clinical Treatment: caries classification and dental charting.

Esthetic Restorations

Esthetic (tooth-colored) restorations include ceramics, porcelains, composites.
A. Ceramics: compounds formed by union of metallic oxides and minerals.
   1. Include glass, fine crystal, gypsum.
   2. Glass ceramics are used MAINLY as reinforcing agents and fillers for dental composites and routinely as coatings and veneers to improve esthetics of metallic dental restorations; also in several dental cements and temporary restorations.
   3. Generally considered very brittle materials; CANNOT be bent or deformed without cracking or breaking.
   4. Characterized by high melting points and low thermal and electrical conductivity.
   5. Inert, NOT chemically reactive, biocompatible.
B. Porcelains: specific type of ceramic that is used extensively in dentistry; fabricated by dental technician.
   1. Chosen because of esthetic qualities; matches adjacent tooth structure in color, intensity, translucence.

2. Unique ability to transmit light when illuminated; gives natural and vital appearance.
3. Contains three main components: quartz, feldspar (75% to 80%), kaolin clay (aluminum silicate).
4. High hardness number (Mohs 6 to 7, KHN 400-500); may cause rapid abrasion of opposing enamel, which has lower hardness number (Mohs 5 to 6; KHN 350).
5. Used in restorative dentistry to produce denture teeth, jacket crowns, porcelain-fused-to-metal (PFM) crowns and bridgework, veneers, inlays.
6. Sensitive to acidic preparations, which can cause pitting and roughening; thus MUST use neutral sodium fluoride therapy, also NOT stannous because of staining properties; radiolucent.

C. Composites: used in ALL classes of restorations, as veneers to cover teeth stained by drugs and chemicals such as fluoride or tetracyclines, to fill spaces between teeth (diastemas), to enhance contour of misshapen teeth.
   1. Composed of three MAJOR constituents:
      a. Organic resin matrix: monomers called dimethylacrylates (bis-GMA).
      b. Inorganic filler: quartz, glasses, colloidal silica particles.
      c. Coupling agent: chemically bonds filler to resin matrix (silane).
   2. Composite materials are classified by particle amount and/or size:
      a. Amount of filler resin:
         (1) The greater the amount of filler content, the stronger the restoration.
         (2) The greater the amount of filler content, the LESS wearing away of the restoration.
      b. Size of filler particles:
         (1) Smaller size of the filler particles: MORE polishable restoration.
         (2) Larger size of the filler particles: MORE difficult to achieve smoothly polished finish; however, larger filler particles result in stronger restoration able to tolerate MORE abrasion.
   3. **Polymerization:** chemical reaction that converts small, individual monomer molecules into long, giant polymer molecules.
      a. Consists of activated two containers of composite paste: one contains a benzoyl peroxide initiator, other contains tertiary amine activator.
      b. When mixed, amine reacts with benzoyl peroxide and initiates polymerization.
         (1) Visible light-activated resins: supplied as a single paste that contains both the photo initiator and amine activator.
         (2) Dual-activated resins: contain activation chemicals for both chemical and light-activated resins; when two pastes are mixed, slow chemical activation begins, then exposure to curing light results in rapid photoactivation.
   4. **Polymerization shrinkage:** contraction that accompanies polymerization reaction.
      a. MOST problematic property; even with acid etching of enamel and bonding agents, stresses from shrinkage can exceed strength of bond between restoration and tooth structure, resulting in marginal leakage.
      b. Two techniques for minimizing shrinkage:
         (1) Insertion and polymerization of composite in layers.
         (2) Fabrication of composite inlays.
      c. Composite can be cured more fully in a lab.
         (1) Produces restoration with superior physical and mechanical properties compared with those cured intraorally.
         (2) Extraoral processing eliminates concerns about shrinkage away from the tooth structure; space between the tooth and inlay is filled by composite cement (after lab fabrication, inlay is cemented at second appointment, with dual-cure composite cement).
   5. Thermal conductivity:
      a. Values closely match those of enamel and dentin.
      b. Provide good thermal insulation for dental pulp.
   6. Thermal expansion:
      a. The more organic the matrix, the higher the linear coefficient of thermal expansion.
      b. Microfilled composites have highest values, resulting in greatest dimension changes in response to oral temperature changes.
      c. Hybrid composites have the lowest values because of high filler content.
   7. Water absorption:
      a. Determined by the organic matrix and results in discoloration by water-soluble stains.
      b. Greatest for microfilled composites because of its high organic matrix content.
   8. Radiopacity:
      a. Caused by heavy metal glasses such as those found in some fine-particle composites and *older* hybrid composites.
      b. NOT present in *newer* microfilled composites that are filled with silica or in some fine-particle composites that are filled with quartz.
   9. Compression and tensile strength:
      a. Higher in value when the volume of filler is increased.
      b. Lower in value in microfilled composites because of the percentage of fillers.
      c. Bond strengths between composites and acid-etched enamel are BETTER (about twice as

great) than the bond strengths between composites and acid-etched dentin.

10. Enamel and dentin adhesives with composites:
   a. Enamel adhesives: unfilled resins that are used to enhance the adaptation and bond of composites to etched enamel surfaces.
      (1) Have BEST flow properties that allow them to coat and fill acid-etched enamel (enamel tubules) in a MORE efficient manner than the viscous (thick) composite materials.
      (2) Rely on mechanical interlocking of unfilled resin into enamel rods for adhesion.
   b. Dentin adhesives: necessary for preparations that extend into the dentin.
      (1) Developed with regard for the following composition differences between dentin and enamel:
         (a) In etched dentin ONLY 4% of the dentin surface near the DEJ may contain tubules; near the pulp about 30% of the surface area of dentin may contain tubules.
         (b) Enamel is composed almost entirely of inorganic mineral; in contrast, 30% of weight of dentin is organic.
         (c) Large amount of water exists in dentin tubules; presence of water and organic components lowers surface energy of dentin, making bonding MORE difficult.
      (2) Attachment to dentin requires removal of **smear layer,** layer of loosely adhered debris that remains on the dentinal tubules as a result of the cutting action of a dental drill (or other means).
         (a) Object of adhesion is to remove smear layer while leaving tubules blocked with debris from cavity preparation.
         (b) Removal technique is accomplished with *milder* acid (10% vs. 30%) than that used for enamel etching.

11. Basic principles of bonding: provide mechanical retention in cavity preparations where NO enamel is available for etching and retention:
   a. Isolate (rubber dam is BEST) surface to be bonded; maintain a clean surface.
   b. Follow manufacturer's directions carefully and use a fresh bonding agent; close bottle as soon as possible to prevent evaporation.
   c. Use a protective liner for deep cavities.

12. Sensitive to acidic preparations, which can cause pitting and roughening; MUST use neutral sodium fluoride therapy, NOT stannous because of staining properties.

13. May need to be replaced because of material loss and staining; diet may need to be changed to reduce staining (eat or drink less chromogenic agents).

14. American Dental Association (ADA) considers exposure to materials (bis-GMA) to be "an acute and infrequent event with little relevance to estimating general population exposures" (companies state there is no bisphenol-A [BPA] impurity).

CLINICAL STUDY

Age	47 YRS		**SCENARIO**
Sex	☐ Male ☒ Female		A new patient examination reveals porcelain veneers on the maxillary anterior teeth, several posterior amalgams that are fractured, and mandibular anterior composites that show signs of microleakage. Patient states that she is ready for comprehensive treatment that will protect her oral investment.
Height	5'9"		
Weight	177 LBS		
BP	118/69		
Chief Complaint	"I really have not gone to the dentist a lot lately since my husband was unemployed and without insurance and we kept moving all the time."		
Medical History	Breast cancer survivor		
Current Medications	None		
Social History	Administrative assistant Likes scrapbooking		

1. What would be the value of fabricating study casts for this patient?
2. Would finishing and polishing her amalgams be appropriate care? Explain.
3. What properties of composite dental materials lend themselves to microleakage?
4. Which topical fluoride would be appropriate for this patient? Explain.

1. Study casts would allow demonstration of oral conditions (i.e., fractured amalgams, open margins on composites). In addition, casts could be used to demonstrate homecare techniques and allow the patient to practice those techniques on the models.
2. Fractured amalgams are a contraindication to finishing and polishing procedures. Appropriate care would involve replacement of the worn amalgams. Polishing of amalgam must be done within the first week after placement in most cases.
3. Polymerization shrinkage and thermal expansion. Even with acid etching and the use of bonding agents, stresses from polymerization shrinkage can exceed the strength of the bond between composite materials and tooth structure and fail to prevent marginal leakage. Thermal expansion of composite materials does not match that of tooth structure; therefore a differential expansion occurs that results in the microleakage of fluids between the restoration and the tooth.
4. Neutral sodium fluoride. Acidulated phosphate fluoride can cause pitting and roughening of porcelain and composite materials. Because patient has porcelain veneers on her maxillary anteriors, acidulated phosphate fluoride is contraindicated. Stannous fluoride can result in extrinsic staining (orange, brown, or tan) and thus is also contraindicated.

Amalgam Restorations

Amalgam is an **alloy** (combination of two or more metals) composed of mercury (ONLY pure metal liquid at room temperature) mixed with powder of mainly silver and tin, with other trace elements.

A. Has physical properties suitable for dental restoratives:
  1. Silver: increases setting expansion and strength.
  2. Tin: high solubility in mercury, facilitates amalgamation, decreases setting expansion.
  3. Copper: acts much the same as silver; increases strength, hardness, setting expansion:
     a. Alloys that contain ≤6% copper are low-copper alloys.
     b. Alloys that contain >6% copper are called high-copper alloys, MORE superior and perform BETTER clinically.
  4. Zinc: is often included to minimize oxidation of other metals in alloy.
B. Types of amalgam:
  1. Low-copper: LESS use because of inferior performance.
  2. High-copper: produce alloys with greater strength, higher corrosion resistance, less marginal breakdown, lower creep; MOST accepted and used amalgam alloys; can be made from lathe-cut or spherical particles or may be admixture.
     a. Lathe-cut: powders composed of small shavings or filings produced by a cutting lathe; final powder is blend of various-size particles.
     b. Spherical: contain alloy particles in the form of small spheres, result in easier amalgamation (combining of mercury and other alloys); accomplished with less mercury than lathe-cut; do NOT resist condensation forces and therefore require less condensation force and use of larger diameter condensers.
     c. Admixed alloys (mixture of lathe-cut and spherical alloys):
        (1) Have total copper content that ranges from 9% to 20%.
        (2) Adapt better to cavity walls and produce better contacts with adjacent teeth.
     d. Single composition (ONLY high-copper alloys) contains powder particles of ONLY one composition (high-copper).
C. Setting reactions:
  1. Gamma phases:
     a. Two main types of amalgam alloy composition are silver-tin alloys with or without significant amounts of copper; difference between two alloys is setting reactions with mercury; reaction that occurs between mercury and amalgam alloy is called amalgamation.
        (1) Silver-tin phase/gamma (γ) phase: composed of unreacted alloy particles, strongest phase.
        (2) Silver-mercury phase/gamma 1 (γ_1) phase.
        (3) Tin-mercury phase/gamma 2 (γ_2) phase: weakest component, MORE susceptible to corrosion than either gamma or gamma 1.
           (a) Low-copper: form weak tin-mercury phase, resulting in weaker amalgam with inferior properties.
           (b) High-copper: eliminate tin-mercury phase by forming copper-tin phase, resulting in stronger, MORE superior restoration.
  2. Copper content of alloys:
     a. Low-copper alloys:
        (1) Silver and tin (Ag_3Sn) combination in alloy particle reacts with mercury during trituration (mixing) in the gamma phase, strongest component and phase.
        (2) As mercury becomes saturated with silver and tin, following compounds precipitate out: silver-mercury (Ag_2Hg_3) compound (gamma 1) and tin-mercury (Sn_8Hg) compound (gamma 2).
     b. High-copper alloys:
        (1) Tin has a greater affinity for copper than for mercury, thus a copper-tin compound is formed (eta phase) instead of tin-mercury compound (gamma 2).

(2) Contains enough copper to suppress formation of gamma 2 phase; results in superior properties.

D. Characteristics and properties:
 1. Dimensional changes:
  a. Shrinkage: initially is caused by mercury and alloy particles mixing together:
   (1) Results in a slight gap between amalgam and tooth; allows some leakage of fluids between amalgam and wall of the cavity preparation.
   (2) Eventually leads to formation of corrosion products; seals tooth from oral environment.
   (3) Results in postoperative sensitivity, often because of fluid movement in unsealed dentin tubules; gap allows fluids in.
  b. **Creep:** flow/dimensional change produced in a material under a constant stress:
   (1) Can affect marginal integrity because of chewing forces; creeps or flows into open areas, such as margins, and then fractures.
   (2) Influenced by gamma 2 because is weak, easily deformed; high-copper are STRONGER because gamma 2 does NOT form.
 2. Strength and stiffness:
  a. Strong, especially during compression.
  b. Stiff because it has relatively high modulus of elasticity.
  c. Lower tensile strength; should NOT be placed in thin layers exposed to tensile stress.
 3. Studies show that children who receive dental restorative treatment with amalgam do NOT score significantly better or worse on neurobehavioral and neuropsychological assessments than children who receive resin composite material (concerns about mercury content); however, children who receive restoration with resin may be MORE likely to need additional treatment. However, the FDA has noted that amalgam restorations contain mercury that may cause health problems in pregnant women, children, fetuses.

E. Mixing: goal is to ensure that mercury and alloy are sufficiently mixed to allow the chemical reaction to proceed, thus producing amalgam that condenses and adapts to cavity preparation with minimal porosity.
 1. Requires mechanical amalgamators to triturate alloy and mercury.
 2. Quality is controlled by:
  a. Time, which ranges from 6 to 20 seconds; manufacturer's instructions should be followed.
  b. Speed and force, which can be controlled on variable-speed units (medium setting is MOST often used); efficiency of unit must be periodically checked to ensure quality.
 3. *Undermixed* (undertriturated): dull appearance, grainy texture (difficult to manipulate); quick

hardening; excess mercury left in restoration, which leads to reduced strength.
 4. *Overmixed* (overtriturated): soupy appearance, inability to hold form, difficult removal from capsule.
 5. CORRECT mix: shiny appearance, cohesive form, easy manipulation for condensation.

F. Handling:
 1. Condensation: adaptation to prepared cavity walls, matrix, and margins; forms uniform, compact mass with minimum voids and reduction of excess mercury content.
  a. Removal of excess mercury during condensation results in LESS creep from chewing forces, stronger and LESS dimensional change during setting.
  b. Longer time lapse between trituration and condensation, weaker because of fracturing of crystal formation.
  c. Builds up amalgam in increments to avoid porosities and express excess mercury at each step.
  d. FIRST with smaller-tipped condenser because greater compacting stress can be generated, MOST effective in the depth and corners of the preparation; later use of condensers with larger heads as preparation becomes filled.
  e. Requires overpacking of restoration; slight excess ensures complete filling.
  f. When performed correctly, has a top layer slightly rich in mercury that is removed during carving.
  g. Moisture contamination MUST be avoided because it results in excessive expansion.
 2. Carving: produces CORRECT anatomy; is performed after the amalgam is placed.
 3. Burnishing: smoothing the surface and margins, using *light* pressure; follows carving.
 4. Polishing: performed at least 24 hours after placement; can be performed up to 1 week later; for spherical high-copper alloys may be performed during same appointment.
  a. MUST avoid heat generation during finishing and polishing to prevent release of mercury and subsequent reduction in strength.
  b. MUST use water spray to avoid overheating and damaging or causing discomfort to the pulp (odontoblasts, dentinal tubules).

G. Bonding amalgam to tooth: performed with specially developed adhesives that bond the amalgam to the tooth structure.
 1. Advantages: used for MORE conservative preparations, fracture resistance, increased strength and wear resistant.
 2. Disadvantages: MORE technique sensitivity, increased time for placement, increased cost as a result of increased chair time and practitioner

training for new technique, also delayed expansion if contaminated by saliva, fracturable by excessive occlusion, dimensionally unstable creep (breakdown of margin), and high thermal conductivity.

H. Amalgam safety: involves controlling mercury exposure:
1. Mercury vapor: colorless, odorless, tasteless; makes it a hazard for dental personnel; thus recommended exposure limit (REL) of 0.05 mg/m^3 up to 10-hour workday and 40-hour workweek from National Institute for Occupational Safety and Health (NIOSH).
2. Recommended safety precautions:
   a. Well-ventilated operatories without carpet; collection and storage of amalgam scraps in a well-sealed container that is kept cool; monitoring of actual exposure to mercury vapors.
   b. Preportioned capsules of amalgam reduce the risk of mercury exposure; when cutting amalgam, SHOULD use water spray and high-speed suction (high-volume evacuation); if mercury contacts skin, SHOULD be washed immediately with soap and water.
   c. Amalgam and mercury waste SHOULD be disposed of responsibly in accordance with EPA regulations for the area in which the practice is located.

Cements, Bases, Liners, and Varnishes

Dental cements are used for a variety of applications in dentistry. Depending on how mixed, can serve as luting agents, base materials, or temporary restorations. Liners are applied in thin layer to seal dentin, and varnishes serve as liners under amalgam restorations to seal dentinal tubules and prevent migration of metallic ions from amalgam to tooth.

A. General uses (Table 15-6):
1. Cements:
   a. Luting agents (adhere one surface to another) for inlays, onlays, crowns, bridges, and other structures.
   b. Adhere orthodontic bands to teeth.
   c. Cement pins and posts to teeth for purpose of retaining restorations (temporary or permanent).
2. Bases:
   a. Placed in thick layers to provide thermal insulation under deep metallic restorations.
   b. Have therapeutic benefit for the pulp (are soothing).
3. Liners:
   a. Seal tooth structures against leakage of irritants present in saliva and restorative materials.
   b. Provide protective covering to the pulp in deep cavity preparations (pulp capping) and with pulp exposure.

Table 15-6 Uses of cement, bases, liners, and varnishes

Material	Product	Functions
Zinc phosphate	Flecks	Cement, base
ZOE (type II)	SuperEBA	Cement
ZOE reinforced (type III)	Fynal	Temporary restoration
Glass ionomer	Ketac-Cem	Cement, base, permanent restoration
Polycarboxylate	Durelon	Cement, base
Calcium hydroxide	Dycal	Base, liner
Copal resin varnish	Copalite	Varnish

ZOE, Zinc oxide eugenol.

4. Varnishes:
   a. Seal dentin tubules and prevent migration of agents into the tooth resulting from marginal leakage of a newly placed amalgam.
   b. Prevent the outward migration of metallic ions from the amalgam to the tooth (leads to darkening of tooth structure adjacent to the amalgam); older amalgams are MORE likely to corrode and cause staining than the more modern amalgams.
   c. Use of varnish under amalgams is not being done; instead varnishes are being used with fluoride as preventive measure on outer portion of the dentition.

B. Types and characteristics of cements, bases, liners, varnishes:
1. Zinc phosphate cement (Flecks):
   a. Composition and chemistry:
      (1) Primarily zinc oxide (57%) and magnesium oxide (10%) in powder form.
      (2) Phosphoric acid buffered by alumina in liquid form (acidic).
      (3) Water (33%) controls rate at which the powder and liquid react.
   b. Uses:
      (1) Type I cement (luting agent for crowns, bridges, orthodontic bands) mixed thin and creamy.
      (2) Bases are mixed thick and quickly, with higher powder-to-liquid ratio to obtain maximum strength that will enable material to withstand forces of condensation; results in MORE rapid setting time.
   c. Manipulation techniques:
      (1) Mixing on a *cool* slab over a wide area to allow escape of heat (exothermic reaction) and control setting time, slowing down chemical reaction.

(2) Adding powder in small amounts, with thorough mixing of each increment; extends setting time; mixing with as much powder as possible to reduce acid irritation to pulp.

(3) Reducing any moisture on mixing slab; moisture accelerates setting time and has negative effects on the properties of the cement.

d. Advantages: longest clinical history; useful for multiple restorative procedures; low film thickness, which facilitates easy insertion of restorative work; inexpensive; easy to use; radiopaque.

e. Disadvantages: low pH of 3.5; can irritate pulp; unable to adhere to tooth structure; requires mechanical retention; lacks anticariogenic properties.

2. Zinc oxide–eugenol (ZOE) cements:

a. Composition and chemistry:

(1) Zinc oxide powder and eugenol liquid (oil of cloves), can irritate connective tissue; pH between 7 and 8; may have allergy to oil of cloves so allergic reaction can occur.

(2) Cleanup with water unless set, alcohol or orange solvent on instruments will remove set materials.

(3) Type II (reinforced cements) may contain EBA (orthoethoxybenzoic acid and alumina).

b. Uses:

(1) Type I cements: temporary cementation (Temp-Bond); tensile strength is weaker than that of type II, allows temporary restorative work to be easily removed at second appointment so that permanent restoration can be placed.

(2) Type II cements (alumina EBA): permanent cementation (SuperEBA).

(3) Type III: temporary fillings and thermal insulating bases (IRM).

(4) Type IV: cavity liners.

c. Advantages: multiple uses, LEAST irritating of dental materials, with pH of 7.0 are sedative and palliative to pulp, radiopaque.

d. Disadvantages: lack strength, inadequate for use under composite restorations because they interfere with polymerization process, difficult to remove from tissues and mixing surfaces once they are set, cause sensitivity in some individuals because of eugenol (alternative: noneugenol products, such as Nogenol).

3. Polycarboxylate cement (Durelon):

a. Composition and chemistry:

(1) Zinc oxide in powder form.

(2) Polyacrylic acid in water or viscous liquid solution, LESS irritating to dentin than phosphoric acid in zinc phosphate cement.

b. Uses:

(1) Luting agent in pediatric dentistry for cementation of stainless steel crowns because of gentleness (kindness) to pulp.

(2) Nonirritating base, liner, or temporary cement.

c. Advantages: bonds to the tooth (directly to enamel), gently to pulp, useful in pediatric dentistry because of its gentleness to pulp and ability to bond to stainless steel crowns, useful under composites because does NOT interfere with polymerization.

d. Disadvantages: LESS working time, limited use because does NOT adhere to porcelain, resins, or gold alloys.

4. Glass ionomer cement (Ketac-Cem):

a. Composition and chemistry:

(1) Aluminosilicate glass in finely ground powder.

(2) Polycarboxylate copolymer in water.

(3) Chemical adhesion to tooth structure (similar to that of polycarboxylate cements).

(4) Releases fluoride, gentle (kind) to pulp, translucent, radiolucent.

b. Uses:

(1) Final cementation of crowns and bridges (type I).

(2) High strength base.

(3) Class V restoration because of fluoride release (type II); preferred for geriatric patients with root caries in alternative (atraumatic) restorative therapy (ART).

c. Manipulation:

(1) Mixing time of 30 to 60 seconds, working time of ~2 minutes after mixing.

(2) Must NOT contact water or saliva; moisture causes cement to set too fast.

(3) Once hardened, sensitive to becoming dried out, which results in surface and interior cracks; two methods to alleviate problem:

(a) Coating with varnish immediately after initial hardening has taken place.

(b) Placing layer of unfilled bonding resin over surface and curing it (MORE permanent alternative).

d. Advantages: strong (strength is comparable to zinc phosphate cements), causes LESS irritation than zinc phosphate, contains fluoride, results in anticariogenic property, easy to mix, adheres to tooth structure.

e. Disadvantages: high solubility, complete setting takes about 1 day, thus margins (exposed cement) MUST be protected for the first 24 hours, water causes retardation of the set (requires dry field), requires the use of a base in deep lesions.

5. Calcium hydroxide (Dycal):
  a. Composition and chemistry:
    (1) Base paste: calcium tungstate, calcium phosphate, zinc oxide in glycol salicylate.
    (2) Catalyst paste: calcium hydroxide, zinc oxide, zinc stearate in ethylene toluene sulfonamide.
    (3) Together form amorphous calcium disalicylate when set; pH that varies from 11 to 12; radiopaque.
  b. Uses:
    (1) Direct and indirect pulp capping.
    (2) Protective barrier under composite restorations (does NOT interfere with polymerization).
  c. Manipulation:
    (1) Two-paste system, dispensing of equal lengths of catalyst and base onto a mixing pad; mixed to a uniform color.
    (2) Light-cured cements should be cured by visible light for 20 seconds for each 1-mm layer.
  d. Advantages: encourages pulp recovery by stimulation of reparative dentin, protects the pulp, has sufficient strength (stronger than type IV ZOE cement).
  e. Disadvantages: CANNOT be placed if tooth surface is wet, proportion is difficult to control with an instrument.

6. Varnish (e.g., Copalite):
  a. Composition and chemistry: natural gum, copal resin dissolved in organic solvent.
  b. Uses:
    (1) Assists in sealing cavity preparation, thereby reducing microleakage around the restoration.
    (2) Seals dentinal tubules.
    (3) Serves as protective barrier; reduces possibility of postoperative sensitivity.
  c. Manipulation: application to cavity walls in thin layer with a brush, wire loop, or cotton applicator.
  d. Advantages: seals cavity, reducing microleakage; acts as a barrier to cementing material, reducing postoperative sensitivity.
  e. Disadvantages: NOT required with nonirritating cements (ZOE and polycarboxylates); NOT used under composite resins because resin will soften; NOT used with glass ionomer cement because interferes with bonding to tooth and uptake of fluoride; requires base in deep cavities, since does NOT provide ample protection because of low film thickness.

7. Mineral trioxide aggregate (MTA, ProRoot):
  a. Composition and chemistry: mainly calcium and phosphorus (SIMILAR to dentin), tricalcium aluminate, tricalcium oxide, tricalcium silicate, and others, with bismuth oxide added for radiopacity; biocompatible, providing biological seal.
  b. Uses: medicament for various pulpal procedures such as pulp capping with reversible pulpitis, apexification, repair of root perforations.
  c. Manipulation: mixed with sterile water to provide grainy, sandy mixture; requires moisture to set (hydrophilic), making absolute dryness NOT only unnecessary but contraindicated; takes 4 hours to completely solidify.
  d. Advantages:
    (1) Compressive strength SAME as ZOE type II and III cements but LESS than amalgam.
    (2) Induces deposition of cementum and bone for healing SIMILAR to calcium hydroxide; bacteriostatic properties.
    (3) Sealing ability BETTER than amalgam and SAME as or BETTER than ZOE type II cements; LESS cytotoxic than ZOE type II or III cements.
  e. Disadvantages: once mixed, difficult to manipulate; long setting time.

Finishing and Polishing Materials

Intent of finishing and polishing procedures is to create restorations that fit and maintain occlusal harmony and to produce smooth surface that results in less irritation to intraoral tissues, less dental biofilm and calculus adherence, and decreased potential for the corrosion of metal restorations. Even smallest amount of excess material, **flash,** should be removed.

- See Chapter 12, Instrumentation: selective polishing of dentition.

A. Abrasive procedures:
  1. Abrasion: wearing away or removal of material by rubbing, cutting, or scraping; abrading done by abrasive.
  2. Finishing and polishing: BOTH are wear processes but differ in intent and degree.
    a. Finishing: FIRST restoration or appliance contoured to remove excess material, produce reasonably smooth surface.
    b. Polishing: follows finishing; refers to removal of materials from restoration or appliance with intent of producing smooth, reflective surface that does NOT contain scratches; surface should resemble natural surface.

B. Factors affecting finishing:
  1. Hardness: abrasive's ability to cut.

2. Size of abrasive: influences speed of cut:
   a. Larger particles abrade surface MORE rapidly.
   b. Particles classified by size in micrometers (μm); coarse: 100 μm, medium: 10 to 100 μm, fine: 0 to 10 μm.
   c. Finishing and polishing involves sequential reduction in size of abrasive particles.
3. Pressure:
   a. Pressure of the force, when greater, results in MORE rapid removal of material; creates increased temperature and heat.
   b. Under higher temperatures can lead to distortion or physical changes within appliance or restoration; may cause discomfort for patient because of transmission of heat to pulp.
4. Speed:
   a. When faster, results in faster cutting rates and creates higher temperatures, causing damage to pulp, odontoblasts, and/or dentinal tubules.
   b. When faster, creates greater danger of overcutting the appliance or restoration.
5. Lubrication:
   a. Used MAINLY for less heat buildup.
   b. Facilitates movement of the cutting edge into the surface of the appliance or restoration.
   c. Carries away debris so that the cutting edge does NOT become clogged.
C. Types and composition of abrasives:
   1. Diamond: composed of carbon:
      a. Hardest substance; efficient abrasive because does NOT wear down or lose sharpness as easily as other abrasives.
      b. Chips (natural and synthetic) of various sizes are bonded to metal shanks (i.e., to create diamond burs).
   2. Carbides: include silicon carbide, boron carbide, and tungsten carbide:
      a. Silicon and boron for finishing instruments supplied as particles pressed with binder into discs or wheels for use on handpiece.
      b. Attached to steel shanks as burs or stones (i.e., green stones).
   3. Aluminum oxide: produced as particles bonded to paper discs and strips or impregnated into rubber wheels and points:
      a. Abrasive used for white stones, has fine particles of aluminum oxide and diamond.
      b. Can be mixed into a paste to produce smooth, polished surfaces on many types of restorations, including acrylics and composites.
   4. Zirconium silicate: natural mineral:
      a. Used as polishing agent in strips or discs.
      b. Often is used in prophylactic pastes.
   5. Cuttle: fine particle form of quartz or sand:
      a. Particles are attached to paper discs for use.
      b. In form of beige-colored discs, used in handpieces to finish gold alloys, acrylics, composites.
   6. Tin oxide: used as polishing agent for metallic restorations, especially amalgams and gold in the mouth; produces BEST polishing agent for enamel.
   7. Pumice: natural glass rich in silica; polishes acrylics and enamel.
   8. Rouge: iron oxide powder formed into block or cake; used on rag wheel in dental lathe or handpiece to polish gold in the lab.
D. Finishing and polishing composites:
   1. Finishing composites: with use of plastic matrix strip *before* polymerization, LESS required to produce smooth, regularly contoured surface.
      a. Indications: roughness, discoloration, flash or overhang, overfilled.
      b. Contraindications: open margins, fractured, undercontoured proximal contacts, large overhangs, recurrent caries.
      c. During initial contouring, water is used to avoid heat buildup and damage to the surface; performed with either a carbide bur (12 flutes) or diamond bur (medium-fine) in high-speed handpiece, using light pressure to avoid overcontouring.
      d. Final finishing can be performed dry to facilitate view of margins, may need further finishing with sandpaper discs, using either slow- or high-speed handpiece.
   2. Polishing: use of abrasive sandpaper discs in descending order (coarse to fine); alternative technique uses rubber points (containing abrasives) on a slow-speed handpiece.
      a. Accomplished with aluminum oxide and diamond pastes.
      b. Contain particles as small as 1 μm in diameter to create smooth, reflective surfaces.
E. Finishing and polishing amalgam:
   1. Indications: newly placed, irregular margins such as flash, creep, and minor ditching, overcontoured, poorly defined anatomy, with surface irregularities such as pits, scratches, tarnish, and corrosion.
   2. Contraindications: fractured, open margins (deep ditching), flat proximal contour, open contacts, recurrent caries, large and broad overhangs.
   3. Finishing should be performed 24 to 48 hours after placement because of slow setting of amalgam; in order of use (burs and stones always move from the restoration to the tooth):
      a. FIRST large round finishing bur is used to define gross anatomical features.
      b. Then green stone removes gross surface irregularities from old restorations.

c. Then white stone is used to refine anatomy of older amalgams.

d. Then small round bur is used to define occlusal anatomy; MUST be followed with a large round bur to smooth out scratches from the small bur.

e. Flame-shaped bur is used on interproximal and gingival margins; sandpaper discs are helpful for smoothing (coarse to fine).

4. Polishing is performed with rubber points containing abrasive particles; interproximal strips are available; alternative method uses pumice slurry, followed by slurry of tin oxide.

INDIRECT RESTORATIVES

Many dental procedures require that restoration be fabricated outside of the mouth and cementing media be used for attachment of restoration to appropriate oral structures. Inlays, onlays, veneers, crowns, and bridges (fixed, permanent, permanent fixed denture) are **indirect restoratives** that must be cemented to the teeth. Retention pins may be used with cast restorations for increased retention.

A Restorations:

1. Inlay: used when the portion of the tooth that must be replaced is within the cusps.

2. Onlay: used when one or more cusps are included but entire crown is NOT being replaced.

3. Veneer: cosmetic facing that is bonded to facial surface of anteriors to improve appearance; porcelain veneers have superior resistance to wear and staining.

4. Crowns: two types:

a. Jacket (older term): constructed of all nonmetal components; limitation includes low strength; brittle and CANNOT withstand posterior occlusal stresses without breaking.

b. Porcelain-fused-to-metal (PFM): outer layer of porcelain bonded to inner alloy casting; greater strength.

c. Ceramic: some can be used in the posterior area; have a zirconia core that allows for greater forces.

B. Materials:

1. Dental casting alloys:

a. Metals used for inlays and onlays because of strength and durability.

b. Most metals are classified as noble elements based on lack of chemical reactivity; include gold, platinum, palladium, and other inert ones.

c. Range in amount of gold present in alloy (Table 15-7):

2. Ceramics:

a. Strong and have been used successfully as inlays and onlays.

b. Hard but NOT as abrasive as porcelains, gentler (kinder) to opposing dentition.

Table 15-7 Revised ADA classification system for alloys for fixed prosthodontics (2003)

Classification	Requirement
High noble alloys	Noble metal content >60% (gold + platinum group*) and gold >40%
Titanium and titanium alloys	Titanium >85%
Noble alloys	Noble metal content >25% (gold + platinum group*)
Predominantly base alloys	Noble metal content <25% (gold + platinum group*)

*Metals of the platinum group are platinum, palladium, rhodium, iridium, osmium, and ruthenium.

c. Demonstrate superb esthetic results.

d. The CEREC technique of computer-assisted design (CAD) and computer-assisted machining (CAM) designs and cuts restorations such as inlays, onlays, and veneers at chairside.

(1) Used because ceramics do NOT crack like other glasses and porcelains.

(2) Produces final restoration that is designed, polished, cemented in one appointment.

(3) Equipment is expensive; long-term studies are needed to evaluate longevity.

3. Composites:

a. Two techniques are used:

(1) Indirect technique: requires two appointments, one to make an impression and make a die and second to cement inlay onto prepared tooth.

(2) Direct technique: composite is placed and cured; cured inlay is removed and given a secondary cure, using heat to maximize properties, then cemented onto prepared tooth.

b. Curing causes polymerization shrinkage.

(1) Both inlay techniques complete curing process outside mouth, thus providing BETTER fit than composite restoration, in which curing is accomplished in mouth, which results in shrinkage while composite is bonding to cavity wall.

(2) Marginal integrity is greater for inlays than for direct composites.

(3) Curing in lab allows use of high temperatures, BETTER degree of cure and mechanical properties, resulting in stronger restoration.

4. Porcelain:

a. MAIN advantage is greater resistance to wear and staining.

b. Advantage of natural appearance.

c. Strong during compression but weak when tensile stresses are applied.

d. Can cause abrasion to opposing enamel; MUST be considered when determining appropriate materials for restorations.

PROSTHETICS

For patients in whom some or all of the teeth have been removed, dentures are fabricated to provide an appliance that will not ONLY facilitate the speaking and chewing processes, but also provide esthetic qualities.

• See Chapter 13, Periodontology: implant placement and concerns; 12, Instrumentation: implant care.

Dentures

Complete or full denture is prosthetic device used when all the natural teeth in an arch are lost. Removable partial denture is used when only a few teeth are missing; clasps are used to attach partial denture to remaining teeth. Dentures must be made of materials that are gentle (kind) to soft tissues of the oral cavity, strong enough to withstand forces of mastication, and yet esthetic in appearance.

• See Chapter 6, General and Oral Pathology: denture-related pathology.

A. Parts and materials:

1. Base (rests directly on the soft tissues): consists of acrylic resins, polymethylmethacrylate (PMMA); radiolucent and easily subject to abrasion.

2. Teeth: made of acrylic resin and porcelain; acrylic resin is LESS brittle but LESS resistant to wear; porcelain is MORE resistant to wear but is MORE brittle; BOTH are radiolucent.

3. Clasps (on removables): silver-colored metals, composed primarily of nickel, cobalt, and chromium; strong and highly corrosion resistant (unless placed in bleach for cleaning); radiopaque.

B. Retention: do NOT require use of adhesives if properly fit.

1. Retention is determined by:

a. Size of the area between tissue and denture; retention problems with loss of alveolar process because of age, tooth loss, and/or weight loss.

b. Surface tension of saliva between tissue and denture; thin, ropy saliva with low surface tension causes retention problems.

c. Ability of the saliva to wet the denture; xerostomia can cause retention problem and trauma to the oral tissue.

d. Normal suction qualities of oral tissues: maxillary arch with broad palate has BETTER retentive suction than narrow mandibular arch with its highly attached muscles.

2. Adhesives: increase confidence of denture wearers, NOT needed if well fitting.

C. Patient denture care at home:

1. MUST be placed in liquid bath when taken out for extended periods to prevent dehydration of resin; AVOID hot water because of risk of distortion to base.

2. Brushed after each meal or at LEAST once daily (both base and teeth), BEST to use denture brush made for purpose.

a. Should be instructed NOT to use abrasive dentifrices; acrylic plastic can be easily scratched and worn away.

b. Clasps on partial denture can be brushed with tufted end of brush.

c. To avoid potential breakage, brush over sink lined with towel and/or filled with water.

3. Variety of cleansing and soaking agents can be used, including nonabrasive dentifrices, commercial denture cleansers, soap and water, bleaches; MUST educate on proper use to avoid allergies and toxicities.

4. Homecare solution: using 1 teaspoon of bleach (alkaline hypochlorite) and 2 teaspoons of powdered water softener in glass of water for occasional overnight cleansing; to prevent corrosion, NOT for dentures with metal portions; helps reduce bacterial and fungal growth from *Candida albicans*.

5. MUST still brush and take care of oral tissues in area of prosthesis; recommended prosthesis removal during sleep to allow oral tissue rest.

D. Professional office care:

1. Placing in a 10% bleach solution (stain removal solutions are available) and vibrating in ultrasonic unit in zip-locked bag; brushing after to remove debris and residues.

2. Remaining calculus on non-tissue-bearing surfaces is carefully scaled.

3. Dental biofilm (dental plaque) control should be stressed for both prosthesis and oral tissues, especially with partial dentures, because of caries and because periodontal disease risk for abutment (natural) teeth still exists.

E. Denture liners and conditioners: improve the comfort and retention of dentures.

1. For patients who cannot tolerate hard dental acrylic on oral mucosa, those with thin alveolar ridges who lack supporting structures for dentures, and/or those with permanent weight loss.

2. Materials for lining and conditioning include resilient substances such as acrylics, silicones, and polymers.

3. Cleaning of liners with SAME method that is used for acrylic dentures; care MUST be taken because of softness and poor abrasion resistance.

4. Homemade liner use SHOULD be discouraged; can degrade denture base material, leading to possible improper occlusion and subsequent damage to the oral structures that support denture.

CLINICAL STUDY

Age	68 YRS	**SCENARIO**
Sex	☐ Male ☒ Female	The patient is in the dental office for an examination. She has not seen a dentist for more than 3 years, since she does not have any teeth. Visual inspection reveals that her hard palate is very red. Her dentures have a heavy buildup of dental biofilm and materia alba. The patient also sleeps with her dentures in place and takes them out only after meals to clean them.
Height	5'5"	
Weight	120 LBS	
BP	113/70	
Chief Complaint	"My dentures do not fit really well."	
Medical History	Peptic ulcer, treated with antibiotics	
Current Medications	Lost weight (20 lbs) but is trying to regain it	
Social History	Librarian Pageant winner at age 22	

1. Considering this brief history, what is one possible cause for the patient's red hard palate? What recommendations would you have for this condition?
2. What recommendations should be made regarding the fit of her dentures? Should her weight loss and gain be a significant factor in immediate recommendations?
3. What homecare should the dental hygienist suggest for her dentures?

1. The patient could have denture stomatitis (denture sore mouth) resulting from infection with *Candida albicans*. Use of antifungal agent is indicated to alleviate fungal overgrowth. In addition, soaking dentures nightly in a 10:1 water-to-bleach solution can eliminate fungus on the dentures and maintain a surface compatible with the health of the oral tissues. Patient should be instructed to rinse the dentures thoroughly before placing them in her mouth.
2. When denture fit has been compromised because of weight fluctuation, appropriate to recommend denture adhesive to increase retention. Denture adhesives work by forming viscous paste with the saliva; viscosity of the paste between the denture and tissue results in better retention. Her weight loss and gain is significant factor in immediate recommendations; a more permanent solution would be to add a professional denture liner, but because patient is regaining her lost weight, this should not be recommended.
3. Because the patient sleeps wearing her dentures, she should be instructed to remove her dentures nightly and soak them in a diluted bleach solution (as per answer #1); other soaking solutions are commercially available, but because she is suffering from fungal overgrowth, use of diluted bleach is indicated. In addition, denture brush and instructions on how to brush after each meal can be provided to avoid heavy

buildup of dental biofilm (plaque) and materia alba that is not removed with rinsing or soaking. Should be instructed not to use abrasive dentifrices because can easily scratch acrylic plastic of the dentures. To avoid potential breakage, should be instructed to brush dentures over sink filled with water and/or lined with towel.

Endodontic Therapy and Materials

Endodontic therapy and treatment (root canal) allows a tooth to be saved. Before endodontic therapy is performed, however, it MUST be determined first that the tooth is able to be restored to adequate form and function and has sufficient support by the periodontium. Increased risk with tobacco use.

- See Chapters 2, Embryology and Histology: pulp structure; 6, General and Oral Pathology: endodontic lesions; 11, Clinical Treatment: pulpal evaluation.
- A. Endodontic therapy: sequence of treatment for necrotic pulp.
  1. End result is elimination of infection and protection of decontaminated tooth from future microbial invasion.
  2. Subsequent cleaning and shaping (debridement), then decontamination (sterilization) of the pulp chamber.
     a. Use of files and irrigating solutions; MUST use rubber dam for isolation.
     b. Obturation and filling of decontaminated root canals with inert filling, such as gutta-percha and usually eugenol-based cement; gutta-percha is natural thermoplastic polymer of isoprene, melted and injected; barium is added to make radiopaque.
     c. Radiopaque silver points are NOT deformable (condensable), so cannot create a complete fill or force sealer paste into lateral canals, thus

NO longer used and even are extracted before refill because of long-term failure problems of microleakage and corrosion (with release of toxic products).

3. Tooth is now NO longer vital (does NOT respond to pulp vitality tests).

B. Root end surgery (apicoectomy): removal of apex is performed if infection is spreading, then filled with calcium silicate–based filling materials.

C. Restoration after therapy: teeth tend to be MORE brittle because of loss of blood supply to the teeth, which nourished and hydrated the tooth.

   1. Placement of crown- and cusp-protecting cast gold covering, especially in posterior, has BEST ability to seal and protect.
   2. Anterior teeth may receive just simple restoration.
   3. May need core buildup (amalgam and/or composite) to fill if large amount of tooth is lost; posts (made of stainless steel or casting alloy) added to retain (NOT strengthen) core and cemented into canal to support core buildup.

OTHER SUPPORTIVE PROCEDURES AND TECHNIQUES

Many patients are requesting tooth whitening (bleaching) procedures. Placement of rubber dams and matrices is important supportive technique that is useful in isolating a tooth or the dentition during restorative procedures. Another supportive technique, margination, is the removal of excessive amalgam in a restoration.

Tooth Whitening

External tooth whitening (bleaching) often is the MAIN treatment for lightening vital teeth with extrinsic discolorations as well as intrinsic stains (fluorosis, tetracycline). Results for extrinsic stains are BETTER than for intrinsic stains that may require repeated procedures to obtain even slight to moderate results; yellow teeth have BETTER results than gray teeth. Effectiveness is dependent on application, time, and dose. In all cases of vital whitening, agent is applied to the tooth surface. This is in contrast to internal whitening (bleaching) that places agent inside pulpless or endodontically treated tooth. Temporary post-whitening dentinal hypersensitivity and/or gingival trauma may result from procedure.

• See Chapters 6, General and Oral Pathology: intrinsic stains; 11, Clinical Treatment: evaluation of extrinsic stains.

A. In-office vital procedure:
   1. Preoperative photographs and tooth shades are recorded; need for restorative treatment to complement whitening is discussed.
   2. With 30% to 35% hydrogen peroxide; different techniques involve heat, light, microabrasion; MOST agents are gels.
      a. Microabrasive compounds can remove discolored enamel by use of slow-speed handpiece with special mandrel before procedure.
      b. Gel is placed on enamel 2 mm thick; can be performed with or without heat and light systems; gingival tissues are protected by various methods.
      c. Heat and light systems use powerful light or wand that is calibrated to control temperatures; NO evidence that this provides any benefit.

B. Office-dispensed in-home vital procedure:
   1. Preoperative photographs and tooth shades are recorded; need for restorative treatment to complement whitening is discussed.
   2. With 10% carbamide peroxide solution (equivalent to a 3% hydrogen peroxide solution).
      a. Alginate impression is made, and vacuum-formed mouth trays are fabricated to hold agent against the teeth; tray is worn at prescribed times per day and then per week.
      b. Patient is instructed to report any tissue or tooth sensitivity (critical).
      c. Patient must be seen postoperatively to document changes in tooth shade.
   3. Retreatment may be necessary, depending on patient's habits and chromogenic agents (e.g., tobacco, red wine, coffee, tea); patient SHOULD be informed of this before initial treatment.

C. Over-the-counter (OTC) whitening products: drops, strips, trays are available; may have ONLY slight results, and acidity may cause enamel damage.

Rubber Dams

Rubber dams are sheets of material that attach to clamps, which then are clamped onto teeth for retention in working area. Thin sheets of rubber latex, although silicone is available for patients with rubber latex allergies. When inverted, dam prevents leakage and toxicity to surrounding tissues. A MUST for endodontic therapy, placement of glass ionomers, adhesive procedures such as bonding composites. However, communication is limited during use.

A. Indications:
   1. Used to isolate clinical crowns of teeth for restorative procedures, especially with toxic substances and/or endodontic therapy.
   2. Retracts and controls soft tissues, including lips, cheeks, tongue, with limited gingival retraction.
   3. Prevents moisture contamination of the teeth and optimum visibility of operative site.
   4. Protects patient against swallowing or aspirating dental instruments and restorative materials.
   5. Prevents patient from choking on excess water spray; decreases clinician contact with saliva and blood; decreases aerosol in treatment area.

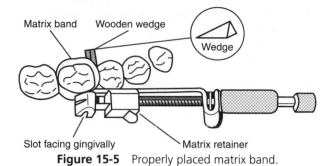

Figure 15-5 Properly placed matrix band.

B. Contraindications:
1. Patients with severe breathing and psychological problems.
2. If used on patient with chronic obstructive pulmonary disease (COPD), must have continuous slow flow of oxygen.
3. Partially erupted teeth (clamp will NOT fit).
4. Patients with behavioral problems (e.g., small children).

Matrices

Matrices are materials used in the restoration of teeth to replace missing components of teeth. Allow dental materials to be formed into the shape of the original component or portion of the tooth (proximal or axial). When matrix is NOT placed properly, there can be leakage of materials, causing overhang (Figure 15-5).
A. Anterior composite restorations:
1. Plastic strips (i.e., Mylar strips) are used to place anterior composites; MUST be clear to allow transmission of light when polymerizing composite material.
2. Composite is placed FIRST and then the matrix is placed, polymerized, and then removed.
a. Oxygen inhibits polymerization; covering with plastic, nonporous matrix keeps oxygen out and allows maximum hardness.
b. Provides smooth, regularly contoured surface, thus LESS time required for finishing restoration.
B. Amalgam restorations:
1. Metal matrix bands are used for amalgam restorations that involve walls of a tooth.
a. Tofflemire matrix retainer and band (Figure 15-5):
(1) Small opening of the band MUST always point toward the cervical portion or root of the tooth.
(2) Slotted side of the retainer MUST always point toward the root of the tooth to allow removal of the retainer after the restorative material has partially set or crystallized.

(3) Retainer is usually positioned on the facial side of the tooth being worked on (in the vestibule).
2. Matrix is placed FIRST and then amalgam; wedge may be used to hold the matrix in place. Afterward, the matrix is carefully removed so as to not disturb the restoration.

Margination

Margination (recontouring) is the process of removing excess restorative material to establish a smooth margin, to smooth the surfaces of the restorative material, and to recontour functional tooth anatomy. See earlier discussion of finishing composites and amalgam restorations.
A. Consequence of overhanging margins:
1. Retention of dental biofilm (dental plaque) and other deposits:
a. Can result in recurrent caries.
b. Can cause periodontal problems such as gingival bleeding and bone loss.
D. Manual techniques.
1. Amalgam knives are used with short, overlapping, shaving strokes to remove amalgam in small increments and to prevent fracture of the margin (anterior or posterior).
2. Files include coarse files for removing the bulk of the amalgam and fine files for smoothing the margins.
3. Finishing strips are used after gross amalgam has been removed by an amalgam knife or file.
C. Power-driven techniques:
1. Finishing burs and stones MUST be kept in constant motion with light, sweeping movement to decrease possibility of leaving marks and grooves.
2. Discs have different abrasivities and are used in overlapping strokes diagonally across cavosurface margins; disc is rotated from tooth to amalgam to avoid ditching restoration.
3. Ultrasonic scalers are BEST for removing overhangs; some models have special tips for removal.

Dental Lab Infection Control

Dental lab infection control SHOULD follow the guidelines of standard precautions, including that ALL patient items are treated the same, NO matter what the health history indicates. Items that ultimately will come into contact with the oral cavity MUST be sterilized. Lab items that can withstand the heat of sterilization SHOULD be sterilized to increase overall level of infection control in the dental lab. High-level disinfection of lab products (prostheses) that contact oral mucosa often is sufficient if infection control protocols prevent cross-contamination. Routine cleaning and disinfection of lab equipment and environmental surfaces should be accomplished with the SAME regularity as in the dental office.

- See Chapter 8, Microbiology and Immunology: infection control protocol, standard precautions.
A. Lab area:
    1. Disposable paper should be placed on countertops.
    2. Disposable plastic coverings should be placed over areas that are likely to be touched.
    3. Shielding device and high-volume suction used during polishing and grinding to minimize aerosolization of microorganisms and grinding products.
    4. Counters should be regularly wiped down with hospital-level disinfectant approved by the Environmental Protection Agency (EPA).
B. Personal protective equipment (PPE) is worn during work with contaminated lab materials.
C. Dental impressions: carry saliva, blood, and microorganisms, must be decontaminated.
    1. Rinsed with tap water right after impression is made.
    2. Soaked in disinfectant that is recommended for impression material, for period recommended by manufacturer; different disinfectants may be needed for different impression materials.
    3. Rinsed again with tap water to remove disinfectant before impression is poured.
D. Complete, fixed, and removable partial dentures are disinfected (see earlier discussion under dentures).
E. Fixed and removable prosthetic devices are disinfected after being returned from the lab, after placement in the mouth, and after in-office adjustment.
    1. Disinfectant is checked for compatibility with materials used in prosthetic device.
    2. Prosthetic device is rinsed with tap water.
    3. Prosthetic device is disinfected for the time recommended for tuberculocidal disinfection.
    4. Device is rinsed again with tap water and allowed to dry.
    5. Professional cleaning of removable prosthetic devices in the dental office: same as for dentures, but do NOT use solutions that would cause corrosion on metal portions.

Review Questions

1 The proportional limit of a material is the stress
   A. beyond which elasticity first begins to occur.
   B. at which strain hardening ceases to occur.
   C. beyond which plastic deformation begins to occur.
   D. at which fracture occurs.
2 The amount of deformation or change in the length of a dental material is called
   A. stress.
   B. yield point.
   C. strain.
   D. galvanism.

3 The modulus of elasticity is the measure of a material's
   A. hardness.
   B. stiffness.
   C. percentage of elongation.
   D. ductility.
4 The hardness of a material is defined as the resistance of its surface to
   A. elastic deformation.
   B. strain.
   C. scratching.
   D. indentation.
5 What is the definition of adhesion?
   A. Type of bonding that does not require intimate attraction between the atoms and molecules of two substances
   B. Reaction with which an object resists an external force
   C. Attraction between like atoms and molecules on two different surfaces as they are brought into contact
   D. Attraction between unlike atoms and molecules within a given material
6 Van der Waals forces refer to which type of bond?
   A. Cohesion
   B. Primary
   C. Secondary
   D. Chemical
7 Before adhesion can occur between a liquid and a solid, it is essential that the solid surface
   A. provide some mechanical interlocking with the liquid.
   B. be wetted by the liquid.
   C. exhibit a large contact angle with the liquid.
   D. enter into some form of chemical reaction with the liquid.
8 Which of the following materials is considered an elastic impression material?
   A. ZOE impression paste
   B. Reversible hydrocolloid
   C. Impression plaster
   D. Tray compound
9 The clinician can reduce the potential for permanent deformation when removing an alginate impression from the mouth by removing it
   A. slowly and carefully.
   B. before it is fully set.
   C. with patient assistance.
   D. with a quick snap.
10 Why do manufacturers include calcium sulfate as a component of alginate impression material?
   A. Reacts with potassium alginate to create gelation
   B. Serves as a filler
   C. Acts as a retardant
   D. Accelerates the setting of gypsum
11 Which of the following statements concerning agar impression material is CORRECT?
   A. Composed primarily of diatomaceous earth
   B. Changed into a gel by a physical reaction
   C. Changed into a gel by a chemical reaction
   D. Also known as irreversible hydrocolloid

12 What is a disadvantage for the use of polysulfide rubber impression material?
  A. Lacks accuracy in recording detail
  B. Has a poor shelf-life
  C. Lacks compatibility with model plaster and stone
  D. Has strong odor and stains clothing

13 Which of the following is NOT considered true for polyether rubber impression material?
  A. Has the longest working time of any of the rubber impression materials
  B. Stiffest of any of the rubber impression materials
  C. Can cause tissue irritation because of the aromatic sulfonic acid ester catalyst
  D. Has great flexibility, which may result in problems when it is removed from the mouth

14 The chemical composition of both plaster and dental stone is
  A. calcium sulfate dihydrate (2 $CaSO_4 \cdot 2\ H_2O$).
  B. potassium sulfate.
  C. calcium sulfate hemihydrate [$(CaSO_4)_2 \cdot \frac{1}{2}\ H_2O$].
  D. potassium alginate.

15 Increasing the water/powder ratio of any of the gypsum materials results in
  A. decreased setting time.
  B. stronger cast or die.
  C. increased setting expansion.
  D. increased setting time.

16 What is the reason plaster requires more water for mixing than stone?
  A. Hemihydrate crystals are more porous and irregularly shaped.
  B. Its particles are formed by heating gypsum under steam pressure.
  C. It has the least porous hemihydrate particles of all of the gypsum materials.
  D. Hemihydrate crystals are more regular in shape and have a smoother surface.

17 Which of the following could lead to the corrosion of restorative materials?
  A. Adjacent restorations constructed of similar metals
  B. Amalgam in close contact with a ceramic restoration
  C. Adjacent restorations constructed of dissimilar metals
  D. Close contact of a gold onlay and a gold crown

18 Which of the following restorative materials has a thermal expansion closest to that of tooth structure?
  A. Acrylic resin
  B. Amalgam
  C. Gold
  D. Composite resin

19 The organic resin matrix used in composite restoration is composed of
  A. polymethyl methacrylate (PMM).
  B. vinyl silane.
  C. polystyrene.
  D. bisphenol-A glycidyl methacrylate (bis-GMA).

20 Polymerization shrinkage, the MOST serious problem associated with dental composites, leads to
  A. pitting of the composite surface.
  B. marginal leakage.
  C. wear of the composite.
  D. water absorption.

21 For dentin adhesives, acid etching is accomplished with
  A. 30% phosphoric acid.
  B. 40% maleic acid.
  C. 10% phosphoric acid.
  D. 37% EDTA.

22 The higher content of which metal increases amalgam strength and superiority?
  A. Zinc
  B. Silver
  C. Tin
  D. Copper

23 For a cavity preparation in which there has been a near pulp exposure, which of the following materials would be the BEST to use to protect the tooth?
  A. Polycarboxylate
  B. Zinc phosphate
  C. Glass ionomer
  D. Calcium hydroxide

24 Which of the following is CORRECT statement about the use of zinc phosphate cements?
  A. The powder is added to the liquid all at once.
  B. Moisture on the slab will accelerate the setting time.
  C. The cement is mixed over a small area of the slab.
  D. Cooling the mixing slab decreases the setting time.

25 In a clinical situation in which a patient requires a deep cavity preparation and an amalgam restoration must be placed, which of the following would be the BEST choice for a base?
  A. Zinc oxide–eugenol
  B. Glass ionomer
  C. Polycarboxylate
  D. Cavity varnish

26 When using a dental cement mixed for use as a base, which of the following is CORRECT?
  A. The final mix should be thin and creamy.
  B. A low powder-to-liquid ratio should be employed.
  C. It will have a slow setting time.
  D. A high powder-to-liquid ratio should be employed.

27 Which of the following cements actually bonds to tooth structure?
  A. Zinc phosphate cement (Flecks)
  B. Glass ionomer cement (Ketac-Cem)
  C. Calcium hydroxide (Dycal)
  D. Polycarboxylate cements (Durelon)

28 The finishing and polishing of amalgam restorations are indicated for which of the following listed circumstances?
  A. Open contacts
  B. Fractured amalgams
  C. Open margins between tooth and amalgam
  D. Surface irregularities

29 When should the polishing of a newly placed amalgam generally be performed?
  A. Immediately after placement
  B. 24 to 48 hours after placement
  C. 12 hours after placement
  D. 1 month after placement

30 Which of the following is a polishing abrasive?
A. Tin oxide
B. Sand
C. Diamond
D. Alumina

31 A restoration that is used when one or more cusps of a tooth are in need of replacement but a full crown is NOT indicated is a(n)
A. veneer.
B. inlay.
C. jacket.
D. onlay.

32 Which of the following is a disadvantage of using gold for restorative procedures?
A. Lack of esthetic qualities
B. Susceptibility to corrosion and tarnish
C. Poor biocompatibility with oral tissues
D. High strength and durability

33 Which of the following statements is CORRECT regarding the use of porcelain in indirect restorations?
A. Does not create a natural appearance for the restoration
B. Can cause abrasion to opposing teeth
C. Weak in compression
D. Stains easily

34 Patients who wear dentures should be instructed to
A. use an abrasive dentifrice to remove debris.
B. soak dentures in full-strength household bleach.
C. use hot water to cleanse dentures.
D. keep dentures in water when not in the mouth.

35 What is the major etiological factor of denture stomatitis?
A. *S. mutans*
B. Papillomavirus
C. *S. salivarius*
D. *C. albicans*

36 For BEST results in casting procedures, water and investment powders should be
A. cooled.
B. aerated.
C. vacuum mixed.
D. measured.

37 Which of the following will cause delayed expansion in an amalgam restoration containing zinc?
A. Heavy condensation
B. Excess mercury in the mix
C. Overtrituration of the amalgam
D. Contamination by moisture during manipulation

38 Brinell and Knoop tests both measure
A. hardness.
B. ductility.
C. elasticity.
D. malleability.

39 Orange solvent is BEST used to clean the instrument after mixing which of the following?
A. Amalgam
B. Polycarboxylate
C. Zinc oxide and eugenol
D. Bis-GMA

40 Dental alloys become amalgam when mixed with which metal?
A. Silver
B. Lead
C. Mercury
D. Magnesium

41 What is the preferred consistency of ZOE cement used for a temporary restoration?
A. Fluid and creamy
B. Firm and brittle
C. Puttylike
D. Watery

42 One of the following metals is NOT found in an amalgam. Which one is the EXCEPTION?
A. Tin
B. Silver
C. Copper
D. Magnesium
E. Zinc

43 Alginates must be removed with a quick thrust or snap because if NOT they will cause irregularities in the impression.
A. Both the statement and reason are correct and related.
B. Both the statement and reason are correct but NOT related.
C. The statement is correct, but the reason is NOT.
D. The statement is NOT correct, but the reason is correct.
E. NEITHER the statement NOR the reason is correct.

44 Overhangs can be caused if the _____ is NOT placed properly.
A. wooden wedge
B. matrix band
C. rubber dam
D. anesthetic block

45 Which of the following is a contraindication for the use of a rubber dam?
A. A patient with severe breathing or psychological problems
B. Prevention of moisture contamination
C. Decreased operator contact with saliva and blood
D. Decreased aerosol in the treatment area

Answer Key and Rationales

1 **(C)** Proportional limit is the point on the stress/strain diagram at which stress and strain are directly proportionate to one another. If stress is removed at this point, strain recovers and there is NO deformation. Permanent deformation occurs above the proportional limit, when stress and strain are NO longer in proportion to one another and stress is greater than material can withstand (like your head after studying; feels like it is going to explode).

2 (B) Strain is defined as deformation or change in length and dimension of dental material that results from applied stress. Stiffness of object determines ability to resist dimensional change and strain.

3 (B) Modulus of elasticity is a measure of a material's stiffness. Stiffness is an IMPORTANT issue in selection of restorative materials because large deflections are undesirable under conditions such as biting forces. When materials MUST withstand the forces of mastication, preferable to have high modulus of elasticity.

4 (D) Hardness is material's resistance to indentation. Hardness of dental materials is MOST commonly reported in Knoop hardness numbers (KHN). Knoop hardness test uses diamond indenter and calculations to create hardness number. The larger the indentation, the smaller the hardness number. Enamel (350) and porcelain (400-500) are two of hardest materials and therefore have two of highest numbers; however, porcelain crown will abrade enamel because of differences in hardness if contact in opposing dental arches.

5 (C) Adhesion is force of attraction between the molecules and atoms on two different surfaces when brought into contact with one another. For instance, when orthodontic bracket is cemented to a tooth, adhesion between cement and the tooth surface holds bracket in place.

6 (C) Van der Waals forces refer to secondary bonds, which involve physical attraction between atoms and molecules of adhesive and adherend. Physical attraction does NOT provide as strong a bond as primary bonds in which a chemical union occurs. MOST common type of adhesion involves secondary bonding, which occurs with zinc phosphate cement. This cement does NOT involve chemical union between the cement and the tooth.

7 (B) For chemical and physical adhesion to occur, it is essential that adhesive and adherend be in intimate contact. Therefore adhesive is typically liquid that can easily flow over entire surface and then come into contact with all of small roughness on that surface. Adhesive is said to "wet" the adherend.

8 (B) Impression materials can be classified as either elastic or inelastic. Reversible hydrocolloid (agar) is elastic material with sufficient flexibility to allow removal from undercuts without permanent deformation.

9 (D) BEST to remove elastomeric impression materials with a quick snap that decreases the stress placed on the impression. Reduction of stress decreases likelihood of permanent deformation.

10 (A) Calcium sulfate reacts with potassium alginate to initiate the gelation of alginate impression material. Alginate is placed in the mouth in liquid state and through chemical reaction is changed into gel. This property allows the material to flow around the oral structures when initially placed in the mouth and to harden into a gel for easy removal without deformation.

11 (B) Agar impression material is changed into a gel by a physical reaction that involves water-cooled impression trays. Agar gel is converted to a sol when heated in water (212° F) and then becomes a gel when cooled to 110° F. For this reason, agar impression material is also known as reversible hydrocolloid.

12 (D) Polysulfide was the first rubber impression material developed. Although polysulfide has many useful properties, such as accuracy of detail, lead dioxide in catalyst gives off a strong odor and causes permanent staining of clothing.

13 (D) Polyether impression materials are stiffer than polysulfides and silicones. This stiffness can present problems in removing impression from undercuts. One way to compensate is to increase thickness of material between impression area and tray.

14 (C) Chemical composition of both plaster and dental stone is calcium sulfate hemihydrate. Gypsum, rock from which plaster and stone are formed, occurs widely as calcium sulfate dihydrate. In manufacturing process, water is driven off to form calcium sulfate hemihydrate. Plaster is made by heating gypsum at atmospheric pressure; use of steam pressure results in dental stone.

15 (D) Increasing water/powder (W/P) ratio of gypsum materials produces thinner mix that takes longer to set. Thinner mix results in weaker cast or die.

16 (A) The MORE porous and irregularly shaped the hemihydrate crystals, the MORE water required for mixing. Plaster is MOST porous and irregularly shaped of all of gypsums. Dental stone is LESS porous than plaster and also has MORE regularly shaped particles. High-strength dental stone particles are nonporous, dense, and smooth.

17 (C) Corrosion is result of a chemical or electrochemical reaction. Electrical current is created by close proximity of dissimilar metals, resulting in dissolution of metals. Dissolution of metals causes roughness and pitting of restoration.

18 (C) Thermal expansion of tooth structure is 11.4, and thermal expansion of gold is 15 ($\times 10^{-6}$/°C). Thermal expansion of restorative materials often does NOT match that of the tooth. For example, thermal expansion of composite resin is ~35. This differential expansion becomes problematic in dentistry because it results in microleakage of oral fluids between the tooth and restoration, which can lead to decay and discomfort.

19 (D) The bis-GMA is a liquid resin to which inorganic component, such as silicate or glass particles, is added, forming paste or composite material.

20 (B) Stresses from polymerization shrinkage can exceed the bond strength and cause a pulling away of the material from the tooth structure, resulting in marginal leakage. Two clinical problems that result from leakage are secondary caries and staining or discoloration of restoration.

21 (C) Weaker solution of acid etch is used on dentin than that used for enamel because of concern for pulpal damage.

22 (D) Tin-mercury compound that is formed when amalgam is mixed results in gamma 2, weakest of the phases in the setting reaction process. Tin has a greater affinity for copper than mercury; thus higher copper alloys form a copper-tin compound instead of the tin-mercury compound. Copper-tin compound is sufficient to suppress gamma 2 formation, resulting in stronger restoration.

23 (D) Calcium hydroxide cement is used for BOTH direct and indirect pulp capping and as protective barrier beneath composite restorations. One of unique properties of this cement is that it stimulates formation of reparative dentin. The pH of cement is basic.

24 (B) Any moisture on slab or from condensation results in accelerated setting times and adverse effects on properties of cement.

25 (A) Zinc oxide–eugenol cements, because of neutral pH, have sedative effect on the pulp. For this reason, especially useful when deep cavity preparations might lead to posttreatment sensitivity.

26 (D) High powder-to-liquid ratio is employed to produce a mix having a thick, puttylike consistency that can be applied to the floor of cavity preparation with amalgam condenser. In addition, high powder-to-liquid ratio results in quicker setting time and a stronger product.

27 (D) One advantage of the polycarboxylate cements is ability to bond chemically to tooth structure. Cement adheres through an ionic interaction between negatively charged molecules in the cement and positively charged atoms, such as calcium in tooth structure.

28 (D) Finishing and polishing are indicated when surface irregularities might serve as dental biofilm (dental plaque) traps or cause irritation to the tissue because of roughness of surface. In instances of fractured amalgams, open margins, or open contacts, new amalgam restoration SHOULD be placed.

29 (B) MOST amalgams are ready for polishing 1 day (24 hours) after placement. This time lag between placement and polishing allows the amalgam to finish hardening fully.

30 (A) Tin oxide (SnO_2) is a pure white powder that is used extensively as final finishing and polishing agent for teeth and metallic restorations. Intent of polishing is to create smooth surface on restoration or appliance that does NOT contain scratches. Tin oxide is mixed with water, alcohol, or glycerin and used as paste. Finishing abrasives are coarse, hard particles, and polishing abrasives are fine particles.

31 (D) Onlay is often desirable when full coverage of tooth by crown is NOT necessary. Traditionally, only metals were used as restorative materials in production of onlays because of high strength and durability. As demand for esthetics has increased, dentistry has begun to use materials such as ceramics in production of these restorations.

32 (A) Gold traditionally has been used in dentistry because of superior properties, including ease with which it can be worked, resistance to tarnish and corrosion, ability to withstand the oral environment, and strength. Demand for MORE esthetic dentistry has resulted in restorations in which porcelain is fused to metal (PFM) to give patient MORE natural-looking replacement restoration.

33 (B) Porcelains (KHN 400-500) have a greater hardness than enamel (KHN 350), which presents potential problem when they are placed in opposition to one another in the dental arches. Because porcelain can abrade enamel, often is used ONLY on buccal and facial surfaces.

34 (D) Acrylic material used in the fabrication of dentures can shrink if it is left in a dry environment. Resulting dimensional change is corrected when water is again absorbed by denture; however, dentures will feel tight when first replaced.

35 (D) Major etiological factor of denture stomatitis is poor oral hygiene, which results in formation of mature dental biofilm (dental plaque). Contains microorganisms that cause tissue inflammation along with pathogenic yeast microorganisms, primarily *Candida albicans*. Condition can be provoked or worsened by constant wearing of denture. Candidiasis can be treated as localized infection with antifungal preparations and improved hygiene. May be necessary to soak denture in antifungal solution or bleach.

36 (D) For BEST results in casting procedures, water and investment powders of gypsum should be measured so that W/P ratio is CORRECT. Gypsum products are used MAINLY for positive reproductions and replicas of oral structures, casts, dies, or models.

37 (D) Delayed expansion in amalgam restoration containing zinc will occur because of contamination by moisture during manipulation. During manufacture, zinc reduces oxidation of the other metals in alloy. Zinc reacts with water to produce hydrogen gas, causing amalgam restoration to expand and seem to push out of the preparation (delayed expansion). Should NOT even be handled with fingers to reduce moisture contamination (current standards do NOT allow this anyway). Zinc-containing amalgams have longer clinical life.

38 (A) Brinell and Knoop (KHN) both test hardness, resistance of a solid to penetration. The higher the hardness number, the harder the material.

39 (C) Orange solvent (love that tropical smell!) is BEST used to clean instrument that was used to mix zinc oxide–eugenol (ZOE). Thus set ZOE materials can be dissolved with a variety of organic solvents, such as alcohol and orange solvent. Can also use alcohol to clean instrument.

40 (C) Dental alloys become amalgam when mixed with the metal mercury, ONLY pure metal that is liquid at room temperature. When liquid mercury is mixed with amalgam alloy, mercury both is absorbed by particles and dissolves surface of the particles. Mercury toxicity is concern in dentistry because mercury and its chemical compounds are toxic to kidneys and central nervous system.

41 (C) Preferred consistency of ZOE cement to be used for a temporary restoration is puttylike. When zinc oxide is mixed with eugenol, zinc oxide–eugenol (ZOE) cement is result.

42 (D) Magnesium is NOT found in an amalgam; is a metal alloy of tin, silver, copper, zinc. Dental amalgam is made by mixing approximately equal parts of powdered metal alloy with mercury.

43 (A) Both the statement and the reason are correct and related. Alginates MUST be removed with quick thrust (snap) because if NOT will cause irregularities in the impression.

44 (B) Overhanging margins on restorations result in retention of dental biofilm (dental plaque), which can result in recurrent caries and periodontal problems. Matrix band MUST be placed properly to prevent this.

45 (A) Use of rubber dam is contraindicated for patients with severe breathing and/or psychological problems, for patients who have behavior problems, and also when teeth are only partially erupted and clamp will NOT fit securely onto them.

CHAPTER 16

Special Needs Patient Care

BASIC PRINCIPLES OF CARE FOR SPECIAL NEEDS PATIENTS

Disability is a permanent or long-term condition, including physical, medical, psychological, and/or mental limitations, that requires individual consideration in planning treatment. Risk factors for NOT achieving oral health are listed when involved.

- See CD-ROM for Chapter Terms and WebLinks.
- See Chapters 6, General and Oral Pathology: common medical diseases and disorders; 10, Medical and Dental Emergencies: emergency protocol; 11, Clinical Treatment: modifications of dental treatment; 9, Pharmacology: drug therapies and antibiotic premedication, substance abuse.

A. Types of disabilities:
1. **Developmental disabilities:** may be present at birth (result of a genetic defect, brain damage, or nutritional or other deficiency during prenatal development) or may occur before adulthood; considered permanent conditions (e.g., chromosomal abnormalities, autism, cerebral palsy, fetal alcohol syndrome, postnatal infections, birth anoxia, epilepsy).
2. **Acquired disabilities:** obtained from external forces during adulthood, related to illness or injury (e.g., traumatic head injury, spinal cord injury, multiple sclerosis, arthritis).

B. Classifications:
1. **Medical disabilities:**
   a. Medically compromised, associated with conditions that affect major organs of the body (discussed in other chapters).
2. **Communication disabilities:**
   a. Related to neurological damage to parts of the brain responsible for language and speech development.
   b. Include aphasia, apraxia, dysarthria.
3. **Sensory disabilities:**
   a. Conditions associated with the senses.
   b. Include varying degrees of blindness and hearing loss.
4. **Cognitive disabilities:**
   a. Associated with reduced mental capabilities.
   b. Include intellectual disability (mental retardation), Alzheimer's disease, mental illness.
5. **Orthopedic disabilities:**
   a. Conditions associated with use of the legs and arms.
   b. Include loss of limbs, paralysis, arthritis, cerebrovascular accident (CVA, stroke), myasthenia gravis, Parkinson's disease, multiple sclerosis.

Levels of Function

Assessment of functional level involves evaluation of ability to perform **activities of daily living** (ADLs) such as bathing, eating, dressing, speaking, walking. The higher the functional level, the greater the ability to take care of themselves. ADL assessments have different rating scales and four levels. First level (I) refers to highest level of function, and last refers to lowest level (IV). If guide dog is being used, do not pet or interfere with dog; ask how to handle the dog.

- See Chapter 18, Ethics and Jurisprudence: informed consents and those who have lower functioning levels.

A. ***High*** **function category** (levels I and II):
1. Able to attend to MOST of ADL needs with some supervision and encouragement.
2. Require daily reminder for oral care and encouragement to go slowly and thoroughly; may require assistance with transportation.
3. Capable of giving informed consent.

B. ***Moderate*** **function category** (level III):
1. Need supervision and assistance with some ADLs.
2. May require use of gestures, demonstration, or adaptive equipment for communication.
3. NOT able to give informed consent; power of attorney or guardianship documentation MUST be obtained to determine with whom to discuss treatment.

C. ***Low*** **function category** (level IV):
1. Little or NO ability to perform ADLs themselves.
2. Require second or third party to provide daily care; usually homebound.
3. NOT able to give informed consent; power of attorney or guardianship documentation MUST be obtained to determine with whom to discuss treatment.

Common Barriers to Healthcare

Americans with Disabilities Act (ADA) helped improve access to healthcare. Includes laws that govern wheelchair access to public buildings and restrooms, barrier-free public buildings, improved telecommunications for hearing- and vision-impaired individuals. Prohibits discrimination on basis of disability in employment, government, public accommodations, education, commercial facilities, telecommunications, and transportation. Dental offices are viewed as places of public accommodation. Special needs patients still face many barriers.

A. Communication barriers:
1. Include attitudes of healthcare workers about treating and communicating with disabled individuals, and patient and family attitudes toward dental care.
2. Forms that are readily understood by employees and patients; may include obligation to provide translators at no cost.
3. Involve hearing and visual losses and speaking difficulties:
   a. Always talk directly *to* patient, even when caregiver is present, unless patient is NOT able to communicate.
   b. Patient informed consent is required (when patient is cognizant) *before* patient care can be discussed with caregivers and others.

B. Physical barriers:
1. Include stairs, narrow doorways, heavy doors, distant parking, area rugs or other floor coverings that could cause tripping, lack of elevators, narrow restroom stalls, restricted access to drinking fountains, telephones, and restrooms.
2. Proper design of office spaces to accommodate needs of employees and patients in case of new offices and some remodeling projects (Box 16-1).
   a. Remove access barriers, where such removal is "readily achievable."
   b. Defines readily achievable to mean easily accomplishable without much difficulty or expense.

Box 16-1 American Dental Association Standards for Accessible Design

After handicapped parking space, route of travel must be free of obstruction and at LEAST 36 inches wide.
Minimum 32-inch door opening is needed with at least 18 inches of clear wall space on pull side of door next to the handle.
Door handle must be NO higher than 48 inches above floor and of lever type, able to be operated with closed fist.
Greeting desk may be required to be NO more than 36 inches high at some point to accommodate someone in wheelchair.
Hook for coats NO higher than 48 inches above the floor.
Circulation paths through public areas, all obstacles cane-detectable (located within 27 inches of floor or higher than 80 inches, or protruding less than 4 inches from wall).
A 5-foot circle for turning wheelchair completely.
Cabinets must be between 28 and 34 inches in height.

C. Transport barriers:
1. MOST common; many prefer safety of the home to problems associated with public or private transportation.
2. Can influence ability to reach important destinations such as the dental office.

D. Economic barriers:
1. Greatest limitations to receiving necessary dental care:
   a. Have only Social Security and other governmental programs as means of economic support.
   b. Those who are employed typically earn low wages.
      (1) Any money received is required for primary needs such as shelter and food.
      (2) Medical and dental care is many times relegated to the bottom of list of needs.
   c. Those on Medicaid and Medicare CANNOT find providers who are willing to accept less than customary fees for services.
2. Paying for dental services difficult because most are paid out of pocket and are not covered by insurance.

E. Motivational barriers:
1. MOST common for those who rely on others for partial care.
2. May be complicated by communication difficulties.
   a. Although cognizant, may be NOT able to communicate needs to caregivers.
   b. Some may also be forgetful; written instructions *in addition* to verbal instructions should be given to BOTH patient and caregiver.

F. Employment barriers: responsible practices that prohibit discrimination against those with physical or mental impairment coupled with reasonable accommodations for employees.

Patient with Communication Disorders

Patients with communication disorders are *either* NOT able to make speech sounds because of structural disease or damage, or NOT able to understand language or form thoughts into words. Related in discussion to disabilities in later sections.

A. Types:
1. **Aphasia:**
   a. NOT able to put thoughts into words or to understand language.
   b. Caused by neurological damage or organic brain disorder such as dementia.
2. **Apraxia:**
   a. NOT able to form speech sounds properly.
   b. Caused by central nervous system (CNS) lesion or organic brain disorder such as dementia.
3. **Dysarthria:**
   a. NO clear speech pattern, slurring, as result of damage to the CNS or peripheral nervous system (PNS).

b. Motor speech disorder associated with cerebrovascular accident (CVA, stroke), cerebral palsy, Parkinson disease.

B. Oral signs:
   1. Depend on severity of condition and loss of muscle control.
   2. Difficulty in clearing food and inability to clean the teeth adequately may cause increased risk of caries and periodontal disease.
   3. Difficulty swallowing and NOT being able to perform or understand need for good oral hygiene may also complicate oral health.

C. Risk factors: choking when swallowing is difficult; inadequate nutrition.

D. Barriers to care:
   1. Economic cost if the disability affects employment.
   2. Transportation if not able to drive.
   3. Communication when speech production or comprehension is difficult.

E. Professional and homecare: maintenance of adequate homecare, with assistance as needed.

F. Patient or caregiver education: discussion about oral health and need for excellent oral care; caregivers who provide oral care SHOULD hear instructions.

CLINICAL STUDY

Age	17 YRS	SCENARIO
Sex	☒ Male ☐ Female	During an intraoral examination of a new patient, generalized moderate gingivitis is noted. The patient has not had dental radiographs taken for 2 years. He is unable to keep his mouth open, and communication with him is difficult.
Chief Complaint	Unknown	
Medical History	Developmentally disabled Wheelchair bound Spastic movements	
Current Medications	diazepam (Valium) 10 mg tid	
Social History	Lives with his family on weekends Lives at special school during the week	

1. What disability does the patient have?
2. What barriers or risks does the patient face in receiving adequate professional dental care? What radius for turning around a wheelchair does the dental office need to provide if it is being newly designed or remodeled?
3. Recommend homecare products and procedures for this patient.
4. What specific procedures should the dental office prepare to provide while treating him?

1. The patient has cerebral palsy (CP), developmental disability present since birth, possibly caused by exposure to virus prenatally or lack of adequate oxygen intake immediately after birth.
2. Physical barriers the patient may face include lack of wheelchair access. Communication barriers are also likely with spasticity because speech production is difficult. Risks associated with provision of professional oral care include accidental injury from involuntary movement. A 5-foot circle for turning a wheelchair completely around is needed in a new or remodeled dental office.
3. Recommendations for homecare should include as much emphasis on self-care as possible. If patient is not able to adequately clean his mouth or if brushing causes trauma because of spasticity, caregivers must perform toothbrushing procedures. Adaptive aids, such as lengthened toothbrush handle and fixed toothpaste cap, in addition to powered toothbrushes and oral irrigators, may be helpful.
4. Communication difficulties may be present and may affect interaction between clinician and patient. Parent or caregiver can provide useful link when communications are ineffective. Clinicians should be prepared to safely handle a wheelchair transfer to dental chair. Relaxed atmosphere and good rapport will help reduce spastic movements associated with emotional distress. Spastic movements can be risky for both patient and clinician, so solid instrumentation fulcrums are required. Mouth props, body wraps, and head restraints may be needed. Extra cushioning and/or frequent repositioning can reduce discomfort. Because of his age, panoramic radiograph may be indicated to check development of third molars and other oral structures. Bitewing radiographs can be taken by having parent or caregiver stabilize his head with one arm and hold film and holder in his mouth with the other hand.

Patient with Sensory Impairment

Patient with sensory impairment has loss of sight or hearing that makes communication and other daily living issues difficult. Sensory impairments often occur as result of infection, trauma, or disease, but some may be inherited.

A. Types:
1. Hearing impairment:
   a. Severity can range from *slight* to *total* deafness.
      (1) Conductive: outer or middle ear involvement of conduction pathways to inner ear.
      (2) Sensorineural: damage to sensory hair cells of inner ear or its nerves.
      (3) Mixed: combination of both.
      (4) Central: damage to the CNS or pathways.
   b. Can occur as result of infection, trauma, disease, drugs, or heredity.
      (1) In adults: commonly noise induced or side effect of streptomycin as a child.
      (2) In children: heredity, pregnancy, birth complications, meningitis.
   c. May be indicated by inappropriate responses to questions or lack of interest in verbal communication.
   d. Hearing aids may help restore some hearing acuity (in-the-ear or canal); may involve a cochlear implant.
2. Visual loss or blindness:
   a. Many affected individuals are NOT able to read with correction.
   b. FEW legally blind individuals are completely blind.
   c. Blind individuals may exhibit sensitivity to light.
B. Oral signs NOT directly associated with visual or hearing impairment:
   1. Poor oral hygiene and accompanying oral disease are common.
   2. May occur because of inadequate presentation of oral hygiene instruction.
C. Factors that reduce effectiveness of oral care in the dental office:
   1. For visually impaired, NOT able to see objects in path or to visualize instructions or procedures being done.
   2. For hearing impaired:
      a. NOT able to understand instructions; fear or shock in response to unexplained procedures.
      b. May feel discomfort when hearing aids are on during noisy procedures.
      c. SHOULD be asked to turn off or take off hearing aids or unhook implants when noisy powered devices such as high-speed handpiece or ultrasonic or sonic scaling instruments are being used.
      d. Conduction of vibrations from dental equipment via teeth and bone can also be disturbing and such equipment should be used ONLY if necessary.
      e. Moisture is a consideration for hearing aids and cochlear implants; moisture-proof surgical bonnet or small shower cap can be used to cover patient's ears.
D. Barriers to care:
   1. Physical obstacles such as doorways and stairs; finding their way in new surroundings is difficult for blind.
   2. Lack of transportation; arranging transportation and/or relying on caregiver for scheduling and transportation is cumbersome.
   3. Lack of communication; MORE challenging for sensory-impaired individuals; can sometimes cause healthcare providers to be apprehensive about communicating with them.
   4. Economic issues; good employment opportunities may be MORE limited for sensory-impaired person.
E. Professional and homecare:
   1. For visually impaired:
      a. Positioning of caregivers and others to visual advantage of patient (directly in front of patient).
      b. Verbally oriented approach; explain procedures before performing them; always use "tell, touch, feel" approach; do NOT leave the room without advising patient.
      c. Use of large visual aids and materials and/or provision of tape-recorded homecare instructions.
      d. AVOID shining operatory lamp in patient's eyes and yelling loudly.
   2. For hearing impaired:
      a. Elimination of loud or background noises when attempting to communicate, such as high- or low-speed suction (high-volume evacuator [HVE]), radio, or piped-in music.
      b. If patient has some hearing, direct speech to the hearing ear; do NOT wear mask.
      c. Positioning of caregivers and others so patient can see facial features (particularly lips and tongue) of person speaking; do NOT wear mask.
      d. Use of sign language (manual communication that includes finger spelling), message board, or interpreter if patient NOT able to read lips (speech); provide written homecare instructions; MUST ask patient which means of communication is preferred and how communication can be improved.
F. Patient or caregiver education:
   1. For visually impaired:
      a. Extremely descriptive explanations are IMPORTANT because they make use of other senses (particularly hearing), which are better developed.
      b. Use appropriate changes in tone of voice when providing information, since facial expressions may NOT be seen.
      c. Involves explanation and demonstration (on the hand) of each procedure; patient should handle

visual aids to improve understanding; caregiver should be involved as needed.

2. For hearing impaired:
   a. Use of demonstration is particularly effective when explaining techniques of oral care.
   b. May use mirror, interpreter, sign language, or message board to explain things that are NOT easily demonstrated.
   c. Includes take-home written instructions for effective reinforcement.

CLINICAL STUDY

Age	70 YRS	SCENARIO
Sex	☒ Male ☐ Female	Patient has kept regular dental visits and was seen 3 months ago for his routine maintenance appointment. On intraoral examination the newly hired dental hygienist finds that he has a very red marginal gingiva around #20, which is a full crown.
Chief Complaint	"My gums are really bleeding on this tooth!"	
Medical History	Hearing impaired, hearing aids in both ears Streptomycin toxicity as child	
Current Medications	None	
Social History	Post office employee	

1. What should the dental hygienist do about the patient's hearing device? Where should the hygienist stand when speaking to him?
2. Of what significance is the fact that he has bleeding gums?
3. What is the significance of the redness around #20?
4. To whom should the hygienist refer the patient to for #20?

1. The dental hygienist should face the patient without wearing the mask when speaking to him and have him turn off the hearing device during noisy procedures.
2. Bleeding gingiva could be indicative of a change in his oral hygiene care level, and the hygienist must find out what the patient is doing and how to help him with this problem.
3. Marginal redness around #20 could indicate that the crown is invading the biological width of the tissues.
4. The dental hygienist can only refer patients to the general dentist, although it is known that this patient may need to see a periodontist. However, the supervising general dentist must make that referral.

Cognitive Disabilities

Common cognitive disabilities include intellectual disability (mental retardation), cerebral palsy, autism, attention deficit–hyperactivity disorder or attention deficit disorder, learning disorder, Alzheimer's disease. Mental illness is considered separately in the next section.

A. **Intellectual disability** (mental retardation): MOST common developmental disability (Box 16-2).
   1. Below-average intellectual functioning (IQ below 70 to 75) caused by chromosomal disturbances;

> **Box 16-2** Intellectual Disability Defined by Intelligence Quotient (IQ) Scores*
>
> Normal intellectual functioning, IQ = 100
> Mild mental retardation, IQ = 55-70 (educable)
> Moderate mental retardation, IQ = 40-55 (trainable)
> Severe mental retardation, IQ = 25-40 (some training possible)
> Profound mental retardation, IQ <25 (total care is required)

*Because of variability in testing, these classifications are NOT always appropriate and an individualized approach is always indicated.

by infection, trauma, or disturbance during fetal development; by trauma or infection during birth; or by trauma or nutritional deficiencies during childhood.
   a. Down syndrome (trisomy 21): form particularly IMPORTANT in dentistry because of associated intraoral anomalies (short, narrow palate; large, fissured tongue) and risk factors for periodontal disease (Figure 16-1). Usually walk with a "waddle" and have dexterity problems, so homecare can be a problem.
   b. Fetal alcohol syndrome (FAS): disorder associated with prenatal exposure to alcohol. Intellectual disability (mental retardation), poor coordination, behavioral disorders, growth disturbances, and abnormal facial features (epicanthal folds, low nasal bridge, small head, and small mouth [micrognathia]) (Figure 16-2).
   2. Systemic concerns tend to be MORE extensive in more severely intellectually disabled (mentally retarded) individuals.

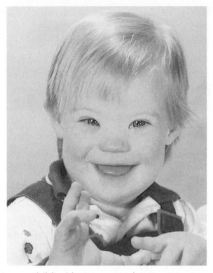

Figure 16-1 Child with Down syndrome (From Bath-Balogh M, Fehrenbach MJ: Illustrated dental embryology and anatomy, ed 2, Philadelphia, 2006, Saunders/Elsevier.)

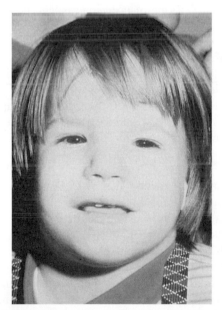

Figure 16-2 Child with fetal alcohol syndrome. (From Bath-Balogh M, Fehrenbach MJ: Illustrated dental embryology and anatomy, ed 2, Philadelphia, 2006, Saunders/Elsevier.)

    a. Affected individuals tend to have characteristic physical traits and body stature; head, face, eyelids, ears, nose may be malformed, depending on syndrome and severity.

    b. Other medical problems commonly associated with intellectual disability (mental retardation):
       (1) Leukemia.
       (2) Congenital heart abnormalities.
       (3) Infectious hepatitis and respiratory infections.
       (4) Epilepsy and neuromuscular disorders.

3. Oral signs:
    a. Delayed or irregular tooth eruption; small, cone-shaped, fused, or missing teeth; malocclusion.
    b. Repercussions of mouth breathing and tongue thrusting, with drooling (sialorrhea) possible; cracked lips.
    c. Increased risk of periodontal disease.
4. Risk factors:
    a. At risk for systemic and local infections because of weakened immune system.
    b. Increased risk of hepatitis B infection if has been institutionalized.
    c. Difficulty modifying behavior.
    d. Poor coordination.
5. Barriers to care:
    a. Dependence on caretaker to make and keep dental appointments.
    b. Cost of dental care.
    c. Mental limitations:
       (1) Build trust; communicate at developmental level; speak simply.
       (2) Reward good behavior; restraints and sedation to manage behavior are recommended ONLY when necessary.
6. Professional and homecare:
    a. Frequent oral prophylaxis to reduce risk of periodontal disease.
    b. Lubrication of lips to reduce risk of cracking.
    c. Awareness that gag reflex may be strong.
    d. Use of anticholinergic drugs for reducing excess salivation during intraoral procedures.
7. Patient or caregiver education:
    a. Repetition of simple, demonstrable homecare procedures with patient and caregiver.
    b. Caregiver supervises and/or performs oral hygiene procedures depending on abilities.
    c. Discussion of periodontal risk and need for excellent daily homecare, frequent progressive oral prophylaxis and examination.

B. Cerebral palsy (CP): limitation ranges from mild *to* severe.
1. Developmental, neuromuscular disorder that results in NO ability to control muscular movement (spasticity).
2. Caused by variety of injuries to the brain (e.g., infection, trauma, poisoning, anoxia), before, during, or not long after birth.
3. Systemic concerns: chronic contraction of muscles, poor coordination and dexterity, intellectual disability (mental retardation) in LESS than half, learning disabilities caused by sensory impairment (hearing and vision), possibly respiratory impairment.
    a. Affected individuals who have seizure disorders take appropriate drugs, antiepileptics.

    b. Communication is often difficult because of motor difficulties (see earlier discussion).

4. Oral signs:

    a. Lack of control of facial muscles; causes difficulties in speech (dysarthria), chewing, and swallowing (dysphagia); may have drooling (sialorrhea).

    b. Difficulty keeping mouth open during dental appointments.

    c. Temporomandibular joint disorder (TMD), tongue thrusting, mouth breathing, bruxism, attrition.

    d. Caries and periodontal disease related to inability to practice good oral hygiene measures because of limited coordination.

    e. Gingival hyperplasia if taking phenytoin (Dilantin); degree of hyperplasia is related to level of oral care (i.e., as dental biofilm increases, so does hyperplasia).

5. Risk factors: inadequate fluoride intake, soft diet, poor motor control, with NO ability to properly maintain own oral care.

6. Barriers to care:

    a. Communication difficulties between patient and dental professional; low self-esteem may also influence desire to communicate.

    b. Unfamiliarity of dental office; causes emotional distress, thereby increasing spastic movement.

    c. Dependence on caregiver, lack of mobility.

    d. Lowered ability of dental professional to provide thorough treatment because of patient's physical limitations.

7. Professional and homecare:

    a. Building trust, desensitizing patient to dental routines, encouraging complete communication.

    b. Realizing that communication barriers do NOT indicate incomprehension.

    c. Avoiding injury to patient or clinician from uncontrolled movements during instrumentation (fulcrums are a must); do NOT move chair without notice; padding or restraints may be necessary to provide assistance in cooperating for the procedure; may need wheelchair transfer (discussed later).

    d. Preventing aspiration of water or other materials placed in the oral cavity.

    e. Using anticholinergic drugs to reduce excess salivation during intraoral procedures.

    f. Involving caretaker and/or assistant during treatment to prevent injury and expedite treatment.

    g. Assisting during seizures (during seizure activity, patient should NOT be moved; area should be cleared of items that may cause injury during convulsive movement).

    h. Using muscle relaxants, sedation, and general anesthesia when they will be of benefit.

    i. Using sheet, blanket, bean-bag chair to make patient feel secure.

8. Patient or caregiver education:

    a. Adaptations of toothbrushes and floss handles as needed.

    b. Evaluation of need for powered cleaning devices (toothbrushes and oral irrigators).

    c. Explanation and demonstration of all homecare procedures; great patience may be necessary, but many patients are willing to learn.

    d. Daily disclosing of dental biofilm and assistance with removal if patient NOT able to thoroughly cleanse own mouth.

    e. Use of mineralizing fluoride and calcium products and chlorhexidine to control disease as needed; used twice daily, chlorhexidine gluconate sprays effectively reduce dental biofilm.

    f. Explanation of need for frequent oral prophylaxis.

C. Autism: lifelong, behavioral developmental disability of unknown etiology.

1. Affects many MORE males than females, becomes evident during first 3 years of life.

2. Identified by NO ability to communicate appropriately; does NOT interact or communicate at age-appropriate level, making behavior management quite difficult.

3. MOST have some degree of intellectual disability (mental retardation).

4. Can be present alone, but many also have intellectual disability (mental retardation), seizures, and other problems.

5. MOST prefer routine (e.g., same foods, same way of doing things), and MOST perform repetitive motions (e.g., hand wringing, head banging).

6. Treated by behavior modification, speech and play therapy, drugs, psychotherapy.

7. Systemic concerns:

    a. Injuries caused by repetitive motions such as head banging and biting.

    b. Metabolic disorders.

    c. Nutritional deficiencies (because diet typically limited to foods that are familiar).

8. Oral signs:

    a. NO difference noted, unless has received insufficient care.

    b. May have tendency for oral trauma because of being aggressive or injuring themselves when brushing.

    c. May have increased risk of caries if has high-carbohydrate diet.

9. Risk factors:
   a. Fear of procedures and NOT understanding need to sit still.
   b. Inadequate nutrition because of strong food preferences.
10. Barriers to care:
    a. Stress of the dental visit.
    b. Communication difficulties because of poor behavior control (caregivers may be embarrassed about child's behavior).
    c. Managing behavior:
       (1) Desensitization over multiple appointments, reinforcement of good behaviors.
       (2) Using physical restraint when safety is concern (see later discussion).
       (3) Sedation and/or general anesthesia (if other methods fail).
    d. Reliance on the caregiver to make and keep appointments.
    e. Likes structure; keep procedures same or similar.
11. Professional and homecare:
    a. Consistency in care and among care providers; preference for routine dictates that SAME dental team members should see patient at each visit.
    b. Shorter, MORE frequent appointments in a quiet, calm environment are preferable to longer, infrequent visits; noises, movement, and other changes are disconcerting and SHOULD be avoided/introduced slowly as needed.
    c. Caregiver should be involved in preparing child for dental visit.
    d. Procedures should be explained to caregiver so that some can be practiced at home in preparation for dental visit.
    e. Homecare instructions SHOULD be performed consistently on daily schedule.
12. Patient or caregiver education:
    a. Short appointments.
    b. Use of BOTH verbal and nonverbal techniques of communication to demonstrate simple oral care instructions.
    c. Discussion with caregiver about need to eat less cariogenic foods.
    d. Need for frequent preventive dental visits to create routine and avoid need for extensive treatment.
D. Attention deficit–hyperactivity disorder (ADHD) or attention deficit disorder (ADD): persistent pattern of severe problems with attention, concentration, restlessness, distractibility, and/or hyperactivity and impulsivity.
   1. Interferes with a person's ability to function at school, at work, or in relationships.
   2. May experience difficulty in performing tasks that require sustained attention; keep appointments short.
   3. See at BEST time of day for patient when "meds are peaking."
   4. Drugs can make person crave sugar, so increased risk of caries.
   5. SAME general considerations as other cognitive disabilities.
E. Specific learning disability (SLD): disorder in one or more of the basic psychological or neurological processes involved in understanding or in using spoken or written language.
   1. Disorders may be manifested in listening, thinking, reading, writing,
   2. Examples: dyslexia, dysgraphia, dysphasia, dyscalculia, and other specific learning disabilities in the basic psychological and neurological processes.
   3. Such disorders do NOT include learning problems resulting primarily from visual, hearing, or motor disabilities, intellectual disability (mental retardation), psychological disabilities, or environmental deprivation.
   4. SAME general considerations as other cognitive disabilities.
F. Alzheimer's disease: causes increasing loss of mental function, affects >65 years of age.
   1. Cause is unknown, but genetics, virus, brain injury, metal toxicity are suspect.
   2. Have difficulty with cognition, depression, bladder and bowel control, tiredness, emotional control, weight loss, other medical conditions.
   3. May take antipsychotic (neuroleptic) drugs that increase risk of bleeding, *Candida* infections, and other infections.
   4. Oral signs: speech difficulties and poor oral hygiene because of loss of cognitive abilities; may include trauma from falls or elder abuse.
   5. Risk factors:
      a. Emotional stress and generalized depression; easily confused and function better in quiet, familiar environment.
      b. Behavior may be uncooperative; dental providers SHOULD speak in short, simple sentences and move slowly.
      c. Change in vasoconstrictors with local anesthesia may be needed because of prescribed drugs.
   6. Barriers to care:
      a. Difficult communication because of cognitive difficulties.
      b. Lack of transportation; must rely on others when not able to transport self.
      c. Caregiver is NOT present to offer homecare instructions for patient.

7. Professional and homecare:
   a. Scheduling short, relaxed appointments during MOST alert times.
   b. Reintroducing staff and procedures to enhance familiarity.
   c. Providing concrete homecare instructions; MUST be repeated because of memory and behavior difficulties.
   d. Reminders to brush and/or assistance with oral care tasks as dementia increases.
8. Patient or caregiver education:
   a. Gaining assistance of caregivers when NOT able to maintain appropriate oral cleanliness.
   b. Importance of frequent dental recalls.
   c. Empathy with difficulties family caregiver faces in caring for loved one.

CLINICAL STUDY

Scenario: A 9-year-old patient with Down syndrome, with the developmental level of 6-year-old, communicates by sign language but communicates orally with people with whom she is comfortable. This is her first dental appointment.

1. Down syndrome is known by another name. What is it? Identify several physical characteristics of this syndrome.
2. What significance does this syndrome have in dentistry?
3. Down syndrome and other forms of intellectual disability (mental retardation) are associated with a number of systemic concerns. Identify several of these.
4. Describe how to provide brushing instructions to the patient.

1. Trisomy 21 is another name for Down syndrome. Individuals inherited extra copy (or portion) of chromosome 21. Common physical characteristics include small skull, flattened nose, large protruding tongue, extra skin folds under eyelids.
2. Often, have delayed tooth eruption, have small and irregularly shaped teeth, are mouth breathers and tongue thrusters, have cracked lips, and are at increased risk for gingivitis and periodontal diseases. Most have a small oral cavity and enlarged fissured tongue. May be at risk for caries (if crave sugar).
3. Systemic concerns and manifestations (signs) associated with intellectual disability (mental retardation) include unusual physical appearance, increased risk of leukemia, congenital heart abnormalities, infectious hepatitis B (in institutionalized individuals), neuromuscular disorders, respiratory infections.
4. The patient is able to comprehend simple, repetitive brushing instructions. Demonstration of technique is particularly important means of communication. She understands the difference between good health and poor health.

Mentally Ill Patient

Clinicians should be aware of the signs, symptoms, and clinical treatment of common mental illnesses or mental disabilities so CORRECT dental management can be followed. MANY patients may be reluctant to talk about problem. MOST patients whose emotional problems affect oral health can be helped by clinicians who are knowledgeable and sensitive. Thorough discussion and medical consult are recommended in cases where complex dental treatment is required; MUST be compliant with drug therapy recommended by their health professionals.

MOST drugs taken will have xerostomia as a side effect. Illness will produce reduced rates of compliance for preventive oral healthcare, as well as reduced ability to obtain or tolerate needed dental treatment. May have atypical odontalgia (AO) in which chronic throbbing and burning pain in oral cavity or temporomandibular joint is present without clear cause, sometimes with severe bruxism. History of substance abuse is quite common; may try to use drugs or alcohol to self-medicate; tobacco use is also common. Substance abuse may induce or amplify symptoms.

A. Anxiety disorders: even MORE likely to fear dental treatment; include phobia, generalized anxiety disorder, social anxiety disorder, agoraphobia, posttraumatic stress disorder, panic disorder, obsessive-compulsive disorder.
   1. Panic disorder: chronic, debilitating condition that can have a devastating impact.
      a. Typically, first attack strikes without warning; affected person worries that another one may occur at any time.
      b. During attack: pounding heart, sweating palms, overwhelming feeling of impending doom; may last only seconds or minutes; experience can be profoundly disturbing.
      c. In severe cases refuses to leave the house for fear of having attack; can lead to fear of being in exposed places (agoraphobia).
      d. May be taking selective serotonin reuptake inhibitors (SSRIs).
   2. Obsessive-compulsive disorder (OCD):
      a. Occurs with equal frequency in men and women; may have familial tendencies; has two components as the name implies:
         (1) Obsessive component: recurrent thoughts, ideas, or images that are disruptive force in sufferer's life; involuntary and result in the compulsive response.
         (2) Compulsive component: response to obsessions in attempt to relieve subsequent mounting anxiety; may be aware of performing these rituals but are unable to stop themselves.
      b. May be taking SSRIs.

B. Mood disorders: includes clinical depression:
1. Clinical depression: unusually intense and sustained sadness, melancholia, or despair.
   a. Accompanied by preoccupation over past minor failings, complaints of bodily aches and pains without physiological basis, social withdrawal.
   b. Increasing prevalence among elderly: MOST common emotional disorder in those >65 years old.
   c. Higher levels of attachment loss and alveolar bone loss (MOST likely related to stress and smoking factors).
   d. May be taking tricyclic antidepressants, MAO inhibitors.
2. Bipolar (affective mood) disorder (manic-depressive illness): may cycle between depression and mania (abnormally elevated mood); similar drugs as noted above for depression as well as drugs termed "mood stabilizers" such as lithium and sodium valproate.
C. Psychotic disorders: thoughts and sensations that do NOT always accurately represent the world around them, such as schizophrenia and delusional disorder.

Orthopedic Disabled Patient

Patients may have orthopedic disability, including loss of limbs, paralysis, cerebrovascular accident (CVA, stroke), arthritis, muscular dystrophy, multiple sclerosis, Parkinson's disease, myasthenia gravis, amyotrophic lateral sclerosis. Cerebral palsy was discussed earlier.

May be fitted for **palatal augmentation prosthesis** (PAP), provided to assist with feeding and swallowing functions with impaired tongue function by reshaping of the hard palate to improve tongue-palate contact. May also have drooling (sialorrhea); anticholinergic drugs are used to reduce excess salivation during intraoral procedures. To protect breathing for some, rubber dam may work if can breathe through nose; patient should NOT be positioned supine but more upright (45°). MOST have transportation difficulties to the dental office because of ambulatory problems; MOST need to use canes, walkers, or wheelchairs; eventually must rely on others; wheelchair transfer will need to be done in the dental office (see discussion next).

A. Amputation: removal of limb or appendage through accidental injury or surgical procedure; amount of functional disability is dependent on type and extent of amputation.
1. May have diabetes mellitus and/or vascular disease; SHOULD have <u>medical consult</u> before dental care, including review of drug therapy.
2. With upper limb amputations may have difficulty with removable prostheses and oral hygiene.
3. May be taking antidepressants and have xerostomia.

B. Paralysis: loss of motor, sensory, and autonomic function of parts of body located below area of spinal cord injury (Christopher Reeve will always be Superman to us!).
1. May be caused by trauma, congenital defect, infection, hemorrhage, or infarction.
   a. Spinal cord injuries typically result in partial or complete paralysis from trauma to spinal cord; many occur in children and young adults.
      (1) MOST common causes include auto accidents, violent crime, sporting accidents.
      (2) Traumatic injury results from physical trauma that causes compression, fracture, or severing of the spinal column; example is compression neck injury suffered during diving accident.
      (3) Amount of injury is related to location and extent of injury; generally, ALL motor, sensory, and autonomic function is lost *below* the point of injury.
         (a) Quadriplegia (tetraplegia): injury is in cervical (neck) region, with loss of sensation and movement in all four limbs and the trunk; loss of sensation and movement may not be complete, with some sensation and movement retained in parts of arms and legs.
         (b) Paraplegia: injury is in thoracic, lumbar, or sacral region; loss of sensation and movement in the legs and in part or all of the trunk, varies according to the level of the injury; generally, the lower the injury, the less the loss of movement and sensation.
         (c) Hemiplegia: total or partial paralysis of one side of the body that results from disease or injury to the motor centers of the brain.
      (4) Spina bifida (myelomeningocele): congenital defect of the spinal column in which some of spinal cord is displaced through opening in spinal column; mother might have been deficient in folic acid.
         (a) Addition of partial or full paralysis is MORE common.
         (b) May have hydrocephalus, excessive accumulation of spinal fluid in the brain that causes excessive skull growth and brain compression in infants; may have shunt for drainage.
         (c) Seizure may occur.
   b. Oral signs: related to ability to care for own oral health; may include dental caries and periodontal disease if oral hygiene is poor and diet or motor function is restricted.

c. Risk factors:
(1) Respiratory difficulty from having NO ability to cough, spasms.
(2) Pressure (decubitus) sores, infection.
(3) NO ability to maintain body temperature.
(4) Autonomic dysreflexia, serious increase in blood pressure from bowel and bladder irritation; can lead to emergency; provide basic life support (BLS) and activate EMS system.

2. Barriers to care:
a. Lack of communication when learning disabilities (spina bifida), depression, and poor self-image (paralysis) are present.
b. Economic loss from reduction in or loss of employment because of severe disability.

3. Professional and homecare:
a. Antibiotic premedication because of shunt for draining excessive fluid from brain.
b. Providing thorough dental hygiene care in a comfortable, relaxed environment.
c. Awareness of the risk for respiratory difficulty from accidental airway blockage when motor dysfunction such as spasticity and tremor occurs.
d. Maintenance of good oral hygiene and use of fluorides and calcium products to prevent dental caries.
e. Encouragement and empathy; extremely IMPORTANT to develop rapport.

4. Patient or caregiver education:
a. Emphasis on self-care, although assistance of caregivers may be sought when efforts to maintain good oral hygiene are not feasible.
b. Adaptive equipment and aids, including powered toothbrushes and oral irrigators.
c. Need for mineralizing fluoride and calcium products.

C. Cerebrovascular accident (CVA, stroke): loss of brain function.
1. Caused by loss of blood flow to the brain via clot, constriction, or rupture of blood vessel supplying the brain.
2. Underlying diseases (e.g., hypertension, diabetes mellitus, drug abuse, atherosclerosis) typically are cause of constriction or tear.
3. Can have temporary or permanent loss of thought, memory, speech, sensation, motion.
4. Side of brain affected is opposite to that of brain injury; *right* hemiplegia (one sided) has to do with verbal loss and *left* with physical loss.
5. Oral signs of CVD: NO greater, unless severely debilitated; may have difficulty with mouth closure and drooling (sialorrhea); can result in tongue being deviated to one side.

6. Risk factors: continued high blood pressure; 4 to 6 weeks delay of emergency and elective dental care after episode; MUST meet 4 METs to determine FC; may be taking anticoagulants and nonsteroidal antiinflammatory agents (NSAIAs) (risk for bleeding; know patient's international normalized ratio [INR]) (see Chapter 9, Pharmacology).
7. Barriers to care: communication if speech and memory affected (see earlier discussion); economic problems if income is restricted because of disability or fixed income.
8. Professional and homecare:
a. Medical consult for antibiotic premedication if valvular replacement, congenital cardiac disease, or heart transplantation involving valves; careful documentation of drug needs.
b. See above discussion of delay of treatment after episode.
c. Caution when administering local anesthetics because of possible interactions with prescribed drugs; may need to lower vasoconstrictor amount .
9. Patient or caregiver education: emphasis on daily meticulous homecare, frequent dental recall, and need to take antibiotic premedication *before* appointment if needed and cardiac drugs *as* prescribed.

D. Arthritis, COMMON disorder of musculoskeletal system that causes painful swelling of the body joints; may have joint replacement.
1. May be caused by infection, allergy, trauma, drug reactions, or heredity; results in fatigue and loss of mobility and hand strength.
2. MORE common forms: rheumatoid arthritis (RA), juvenile rheumatoid arthritis, degenerative joint diseases (osteoarthritis).
3. RA with synovitis of peripheral joints: MOST commonly occurs at 20 to 60 years of age; morning stiffness; symmetrical joint swelling and pain with motion; clinical and radiographic findings include soft tissue swelling (nodules) and erosions, usually at proximal interphalangeal joints, ulnar deviation in phalanges, and joint space narrowing (Figure 16-3).
4. Arthrogryposis: LESS common form caused by decreased fetal movements in the womb; fetus needs to move his or her limbs to develop muscle and joints; if the joints do not move, extra connective tissue develops around the joint and fixes it in place (talonlike appendages).
5. Oral signs: increase in bleeding and oral infection from antiinflammatory drugs (NSAIAs, corticosteroids); TMD may be present (use of heat, exercise, antiinflammatory drugs, analgesics, surgery, prosthodontic rehabilitation); patients with RA may also suffer from Sjögren's syndrome,

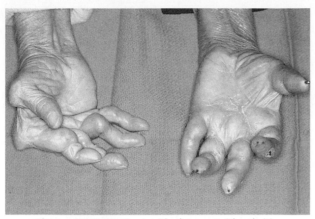

Figure 16-3 Patient with rheumatoid arthritis.

decreased saliva production that requires aggressive preventive care.

6. Barriers to care: long appointments; keeping mouth opened can be uncomfortable; irritability is COMMON in those with chronic pain.

7. Risk factors: side effects of drugs and difficulty with motor activities.

8. Professional and homecare: assessing need for <u>antibiotic premedication</u> in cases of joint replacement by <u>medical consult</u>, need for short appointments with frequent opportunities to close the mouth and need to shift positions in the chair to relieve discomfort.

9. Patient or caregiver education: discussion of oral side effects of arthritis drugs; recommendation for powered toothbrushes and other adaptive aids (enlarged toothbrush handles, floss holders) as needed; recommendation for frequent recall so that appointments are quicker and easier.

E. Muscular dystrophy (MD): inherited, progressive skeletal muscular disorder.

1. Duchenne (severe) MD: begins in early childhood and results in death by age 25; affects MAINLY males.

2. Becker (mild) MD: begins in middle to late childhood and does NOT result in early, premature death; affects BOTH males and females.

3. Systemic concerns: muscle weakness caused by replacement of skeletal (eventually heart and lung) muscle; may have difficulty walking, standing, speaking, eating as disease progresses.

4. Oral signs: related to loss of muscle control, may include injury or infection; irritated gingiva may be caused by open mouth; poor oral hygiene may occur because of reduced ability to provide self-care.

5. Risk factors: trauma from injury (e.g., falling, difficulty swallowing, choking) because of loss of muscle control; oral infection may be caused by inadequate dental biofilm removal.

6. Barriers to care:
   a. Lack of communication; speech difficulties occur as muscle weakness affects muscles of head and neck.
   b. Immobility and difficulty controlling movement.
   c. Economic issues; caregivers are needed to provide full care as disorder progresses.
   d. Dependence on caregiver to make and keep dental appointments.

7. Professional and homecare:
   a. Frequent oral prophylaxis to reduce risk of infection.
   b. Short dental appointments.
   c. Use of bite block to keep mouth open after muscle loss prevents it (see later discussion).

8. Patient or caregiver education:
   a. Supervision and/or performance of oral hygiene procedures by caregiver, if patient is not able.
   b. Adaptive aids to accommodate muscle weakness.
   c. Power-assisted devices to enable self-care.
   d. Discussion with patient and/or caregiver about risk of infection and need for excellent daily homecare and frequent professional oral prophylaxis and examination.
   e. Use of lubricant on lips and oral tissues irritated by open mouth.

F. Multiple sclerosis (MS): incurable, chronic, progressive disease distinguished by demyelination of CNS nerve sheaths; can go into remission for years, then undergo exacerbation and relapse and resurface.

1. Sclerotic plaques replace myelin nerve sheaths; affects 20- to 40-year-olds.

2. Cause is unknown, although autoimmune disease and virus infection are suspected.

3. Normal or near normal life expectancy can be expected; symptoms include general fatigue, weakness, and numbness of body parts during periods of activity; heat sensitivity may occur.

4. Treated with drugs; may be taking corticosteroids, muscle relaxants, antidepressants, immunosuppressants.

5. Oral signs: facial pain, speech disorders (see earlier discussion), facial paralysis in severe cases.

6. Risk factors:
   a. Physical and emotional stresses, such as infections, emotional stress, inadequate rest, excessive exercise, depression.
   b. Side effects of drugs; diet restrictions caused by muscle dysfunction.

7. Barriers to care:
   a. Communication difficulties from dysfunction of speech muscles.
   b. Economic issues when income is restricted because of reduction in or loss of employment.

8. Professional and homecare:
   a. Scheduling short, relaxed appointments, preferably during times of remission.
   b. Keeping at comfortable temperature.
   c. Sedation, general anesthesia, or hospitalization may be required before treatment is provided.
   d. Attention to proper cleansing when facial paralysis and weakness reduce ability to cleanse cheeks and tongue.
   e. Homecare instructions related to frequent cleansing of the oral cavity; powered toothbrushes, adaptive aids, and oral irrigators may be recommended for those who have difficulty cleaning manually.
9. Patient or caregiver education:
   a. Family assistance in maintaining good daily oral hygiene when no longer able to do so.
   b. Daily fluoride supplementation.
   c. Maintenance of adequate diet.
G. Myasthenia gravis (MG): autoimmune disease that affects neuromusculature.
   1. Decrease in number of acetylcholine receptors results in decreased transmission of nerve impulses.
   2. Causes generalized feeling of exhaustion from muscle fatigue and weakness.
   3. Causes paralysis in its MOST severe form, MAINLY affects younger women and older men.
   4. Treated by anticholinesterase drug, surgical removal of thymus, or steroidal hormones.
   5. Oral signs: effects on facial and cervical musculature; leads to loss of control of facial muscles and results in difficulties with smiling, eating, swallowing, speaking, vision; when severe, can cause respiratory distress.
   6. Crisis can occur because of infection (oral included), emotional stress, and surgery; two types of crises:
      a. Myasthenic crisis: causes loss of swallowing and speaking ability and difficulty breathing and seeing; caused by undermedication, underlying illness, risk factors, or worsening of disease.
      b. Cholinergic crisis: related to overmedication with anticholinesterase, occurs within hour of drug use, causes increased muscle weakness, gastrointestinal upset, respiratory difficulties.
      c. For BOTH crises, <u>provide BLS and activate EMS system</u>.
   7. Barriers to care:
      a. Communication difficulties, if experiences facial weakness and paralysis (patient may hold chin with hand to speak).
      b. Generalized fatigue affects ability to get to the dental office.
      c. Economic issues for those on fixed incomes.

8. Professional and homecare:
   a. Scheduling appointments during MOST active periods of the day, soon after drugs are taken and after good night's sleep.
   b. Availability of emergency equipment for respiratory distress during appointments.
   c. Homecare instructions related to preventing oral infections, which are risk factors for crisis development.
   d. Powered toothbrushes and oral irrigators are recommended for those who have difficulty manually cleaning the oral cavity.
   e. Careful attention to proper nutrition, which becomes MORE important when food selections are limited by LESS ability to chew or swallow some foods.
9. Patient or caregiver education: keeping oral cavity in excellent condition to reduce risk of crisis; family members may be enlisted to assist in frequent or daily oral care procedures and transport patient to the dental clinic when no longer able.
H. Amyotrophic lateral sclerosis (ALS, Lou Gehrig's disease): progressive, fatal, neurodegenerative disease.
   1. Unknown etiology; degeneration of motor neurons, nerve cells in CNS that control voluntary muscle movement.
   2. Begins with muscle weakness and atrophy throughout the body, as BOTH upper and lower motor neurons degenerate and die, ceasing to send messages to muscles.
   3. Then NOT able to function, muscles gradually weaken, atrophy, develop fasciculations (twitches) as result of denervation.
   4. Treatment: palliative; patient may be taking muscle relaxants and antiepileptics.
   5. Barriers to care:
      a. Communication difficulties if patient experiences facial weakness and paralysis.
      b. Economic issues for those on fixed incomes.
   6. Professional and homecare:
      a. Short appointments.
      b. Powered toothbrushes and oral irrigators are recommended for those who have difficulty manually cleaning the oral cavity.
      c. Careful attention to proper nutrition, which becomes MORE important when food selections are limited by LESS ability to chew and swallow some foods.
   7. Patient or caregiver education: keeping oral cavity in excellent condition; family members may be enlisted to assist in frequent or daily oral care procedures.
I. Parkinson's disease: slow, progressive degeneration of basal ganglion neurons; results in loss of control of voluntary musculature.

1. Inability to produce adequate levels of dopamine, brain chemical, related to degeneration, although exact cause is unknown; possible causes are exposure to environmental toxins, such as pesticides and mercury, or head injury.
2. Affects MORE men than women, tends to occur during middle to later years of life (ages 50 to 65).
3. Pill-rolling motion of the fingers, masked facial appearance, muscle rigidity, but understands clinician, UNLIKE patients with Alzheimer's.
4. Oral signs: drooling (sialorrhea), difficulty swallowing, tremors, reduced ability or inability to care properly for mouth because of motor dysfunction, which may result in oral infection; speech may be stammering and monotone (see earlier discussion); xerostomia is COMMON side effect of drugs.
5. Treatment: drugs such as levodopa (L-dopa, Madopar, Sinemet) transformed into dopamine or surgery to provide relief from symptoms.
   a. However, long-term use of L-dopa often leads to motor complications that can be difficult to manage.
   b. Dopamine agonists are used early, such as bromocriptine mesylate (Parlodel), pergolide mesylate (Permax), pramipexole (Mirapex), ropinirole hydrochloride (Requip).
      (1) Helps put off need for levodopa and improve motor function.
      (2) Side effects include orthostatic hypotension, irregular heartbeat, and chest pain just as with L-dopa.
6. Risk factors: difficulty with swallowing with restricted diet because of eating difficulties, difficulty walking.
7. Barriers to care:
   a. Communication difficulties because of embarrassment about condition; slurred speech from motor dysfunction occurs later in course of disease.
   b. Economic difficulties associated with loss of employment and reliance on fixed income during later years.
8. Professional and homecare:
   a. Short appointments.
   b. Making patient comfortable during appointments, use of stable instrumentation to deal with tremors, and active listening and encouragement, which are IMPORTANT to sense of well-being.
9. Patient or caregiver education: frequent and proper care of oral cavity, with emphasis on use of adaptive aids as needed; as disease progresses, family assistance should be requested to maintain oral health; frequent dental recall is recommended; emphasize use of larger handled powered toothbrushes.

POSITIONING AND STABILIZATION

Effective patient positioning and stabilization provide for the well-being of patient and efficiency of clinician by offering comfortable, safe environment. However, use of preventive measures SHOULD be considered for elective dental care needs or even treatment deferral if patient's behavior is uncontrollable and/or hysterical.

- See Chapter 16, Special Needs Patient Care: modifications for medical disabilities.
A. Includes stabilization and positioning of patient chair and patient's head and body.
   1. Requires knowing when a patient is MORE comfortable, either sitting upright *or* lying supine for proper care.
      a. Patients prone to decubitus ulcers, such as paraplegics, require careful readjustment of body position and additional cushioning during long appointments.
      b. See earlier discussion for each patient's health concern.
   2. Support and restraint devices; MOST commonly used with neuromuscular disorders or extreme behavioral problems that put patient and/or clinician at physical risk from movement during instrumentation; should NOT be used routinely; sedation is another option but is used as a last resort.
      a. **Mouth props** (blocks): rubber materials that are used to hold the mouth open for patients who are NOT able; some are placed in a closed position and gradually opened as needed; others place the jaws in an open position at all times.
      b. **Head stabilization:** use of clinician's arm to surround patient's head, cup the chin, and hold it still during procedures.
      c. **Body wraps:** sheets and blankets used to wrap and secure the patient with straps; used MAINLY for young children when full-body restraint is necessary.
      d. **Papoose boards:** boards with padded straps that are used to secure patients of ANY age or size during operatory procedures.
B. Wheelchair transfer to dental chair: depending on severity of disability:
   1. Know patient's abilities; may be able to do it alone or with assistance.
      a. **Sliding board:** board is made of hardwood with smooth tapered ends.
      b. Used when patient can transfer alone and ONLY needs assistance, such as with paraplegics.
   2. Use body and NOT back to move patient, pivoting from hips; lift patient, do NOT slide patient into chair.
   3. Single-provider wheelchair transfer (Figure 16-4):

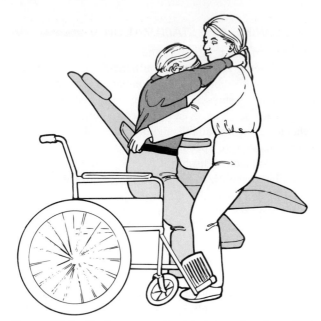

Figure 16-4 Single-person wheelchair transfer of a patient to the dental chair.

    a. Determine whether special padding should be transferred.

    b. Determine whether urine-collecting device is present.

    c. Determine whether there is need to secure limbs because of spastic movements.

    d. Clear the area, and position wheelchair at same or lower height and in direction of and slight angle to dental chair.

    e. Secure transfer belt around waist and remove or release dental chair and wheelchair armrests; set the brake.

    f. Determine whether any special equipment must be transferred or might be in the way and lift the footrests.

    g. While facing the patient, place your feet on either side of the patient's feet.

    h. With your knees holding patient's legs stable, grasp patient under the arms and around the back to grasp the transfer belt.

    i. Place the patient in a standing position.

    j. Rotate patient into the dental chair in a smooth movement.

    k. Position patient on the dental chair; place padding as needed and straighten clothing.

    l. Thank patient for assistance.

  4. Two-provider wheelchair transfer: for heavier and/or more fragile patient.

    a. First clinician: stand behind the patient; help the patient cross his or her arms across chest; place your arms under the patient's upper arms and grasp the patient's wrists.

    b. Second clinician: place both hands under the patient's lower thighs; initiate and lead the lift at a prearranged count (1-2-3-lift).

    c. Both clinicians: using your leg and arm muscles while bending your back as little as possible, gently lift the patient's torso and legs at the same time.

C. Behavior management:

  1. Involves familiarity with special characteristics and needs of patient.

    a. Patience with and empathy for the patient.

    b. Dental visits are MORE successful if the patient is familiarized with the office by frequent, short visits during which procedures are demonstrated.

  2. Inclusion of caretakers in discussions of behavior management.

Review Questions

1 Aphasia, apraxia, and dysarthria are examples of _____ disabilities.
  A. communication
  B. developmental
  C. cognitive
  D. sensory
  E. nervous system

2 Patients who can bathe, feed, and dress themselves but may need to be reminded to brush their teeth and hair are considered _____ functioning.
  A. high
  B. moderate
  C. low
  D. not

3 When discussing homecare procedures with the mildly mentally retarded individual,
  A. speak directly to the caregiver.
  B. use simple demonstrations.
  C. send home printed materials.
  D. discuss the risk of periodontitis.

4 The patient with cerebral palsy is likely to have difficulty with all of the following, EXCEPT one. Which one is the EXCEPTION?
  A. Controlling movement
  B. Communicating
  C. Caries risk
  D. Oral hygiene
  E. Comprehension

5 When treating a patient with autism,
  A. use nonverbal instructions.
  B. follow a consistent routine.
  C. speak in a louder tone of voice.
  D. schedule longer visits.

6 The inability to properly form speech sounds is termed
A. apraxia.
B. aphasia.
C. dysarthria.
D. ataxia.

7 When providing oral healthcare instructions to a visually impaired individual, it is MOST important to
A. talk more loudly.
B. speak more slowly.
C. face the patient.
D. use visual aids.

8 All of the following are oral manifestations associated with arthritis, EXCEPT one. Which one is the EXCEPTION?
A. Angular cheilitis
B. Gingival bleeding
C. Oral infections
D. TMJ discomfort

9 Which one of the following adaptive aids would MOST benefit the patient with arthritic joints of the hands?
A. Extended-handle toothbrush
B. Textured-handle toothbrush
C. Enlarged-handle toothbrush
D. Curved-handle toothbrush

10 Which of the following is noted with a cerebrovascular accident?
A. Sudden loss of blood flow to the heart
B. Caused by restriction in or rupture of a blood vessel
C. Often preceded by rheumatic heart disease
D. Requires NO modification of dental procedures after incident

11 Patients who have suffered spinal cord injuries may have difficulty performing oral care. When teaching oral health-care measures, the clinician should emphasize
A. self-care.
B. proper nutrition.
C. good oral hygiene.
D. caregiver assistance.

12 The level of paralysis or dysfunction associated with a spinal cord injury is MOST closely related to the
A. type of traumatic injury.
B. severity of traumatic injury.
C. location of the traumatic injury.
D. cause of traumatic injury.

13 Which of the following statements regarding the patient with Alzheimer's disease is CORRECT?
A. Alzheimer's disease is a form of dementia that tends to affect the oldest of the old.
B. Patients are confused by change and prefer quiet surroundings.
C. A single long appointment is preferable to several short appointments.
D. Most patients can take care of their oral health needs without the assistance of a caregiver.

14 The disease that affects the myelin sheath and results in fatigue and numbness is
A. muscular dystrophy.
B. multiple sclerosis.
C. Parkinson's disease.
D. Bell's palsy.
E. myasthenia gravis.

15 All of the following disorders may result in facial paralysis, EXCEPT one. Which one is the EXCEPTION?
A. Multiple sclerosis
B. Alzheimer's disease
C. Bell's palsy
D. Myasthenia gravis

16 Which of the following conditions may indicate the need for a patient to be repositioned frequently during a dental appointment?
A. Spina bifida
B. Multiple sclerosis
C. Down syndrome
D. Parkinson's disease

17 Which of the following is a device used specifically for the full-body restraint of young children?
A. Mouth prop
B. Head stabilization
C. Wraps
D. Papoose boards

18 When performing a wheelchair transfer, the dental professional must do all of the following, EXCEPT one. Which one is the EXCEPTION?
A. Clear the area of any obstacles
B. Secure a transfer belt to the patient
C. Raise the chair above wheelchair height
D. Stabilize the patient's legs
E. Grasp the patient under the arms and around back

19 The LEAST likely oral manifestation of Down syndrome is
A. early tooth eruption.
B. fusion of teeth.
C. malocclusion.
D. tongue thrust.
E. missing teeth.

20 All of the following are moderate level of function (level III), EXCEPT one. Which one is the EXCEPTION?
A. The person may need supervision or assistance with some of the activities of daily living.
B. The person may require use of gestures or demonstration or use of adaptive equipment for communication.
C. The person is able to give informed consent.
D. The person is unable to give informed consent.

21 Education by the dental hygienist for a disabled patient should emphasize discussion about oral health and need for excellent oral care, and the caregivers should hear the instructions at the same time as the patient.
A. Both statements are true.
B. Both statements are false.
C. The first statement is true, the second is false.
D. The first statement is false, the second is true.

22 The ultrasonic scaler should never be used on a hearing-impaired person because the conduction of vibrations from dental equipment via teeth and bone can be very disturbing.
A. Both the statement and reason are correct and related.
B. Both the statement and reason are correct but NOT related.
C. The statement is correct, but the reason is NOT.
D. The statement is NOT correct, but the reason is correct.
E. NEITHER the statement NOR the reason is correct.

23 All of the following are cognitive disabilities, EXCEPT one. Which one is the EXCEPTION?
   A. Mental retardation
   B. Cerebral palsy
   C. Autism
   D. Parkinson's disease

24 Lack of folic acid in pregnancy can result in
   A. spina bifida.
   B. cerebral palsy.
   C. deafness.
   D. short attention span.

25 When an adult patient is a paraplegic, clinicians should always assess what the patient can do himself or herself before helping the patient get into the dental chair. The patient will always need to be wrapped in sheets or blankets during dental appointments.
   A. Both statements are true.
   B. Both statements are false.
   C. The first statement is true, the second is false.
   D. The first statement is false, the second is true.

26 Levodopa (L-dopa, Madopar, Sinemet) is used to treat
   A. Parkinson's disease.
   B. Alzheimer's disease.
   C. specific learning disability.
   D. depression.

27 Pill-rolling motion of the fingers has to do with which of the following diseases?
   A. Multiple sclerosis
   B. Rubeola
   C. Parkinson's disease
   D. Cerebral palsy

28 Aphasia is noted for being a(n)
   A. inability to put thoughts into words or to understand language.
   B. inability to properly form speech sounds.
   C. motor speech disorder.
   D. loss of memory or thought.

29 Athetosis, ataxia, and rigidity are associated with which of the following illnesses or conditions?
   A. Parkinson's disease
   B. Cerebral palsy
   C. ADD
   D. Paraplegia

30 Hydrocephalus
   A. is fluid around the heart and lungs.
   B. is fluid in the spinal column.
   C. is fluid in the brain.
   D. has nothing to do with fluid, is just an enlarged head.

Answer Key and Rationales

1 **(A)** Communication disabilities are those related to neurological brain damage that disturbs language and speech development. Aphasia is inability to put thoughts into words or to understand language; apraxia is inability to form speech sounds; and dysarthria results in slurred speech patterns.

2 **(A)** Assessment of functional levels is from *high* (requires little assistance with ADLs) to *low* (caretaker provides MOST or all ADLs). High-functioning patient can bathe, dress, eat, communicate, ambulate well enough to function with ONLY minimal assistance. Patient may require reminders to perform tasks.

3 **(B)** When discussing homecare procedures with a mildly intellectually disabled (mentally retarded) individual, make sure to use simple and demonstrable instructions. Include caregiver so that the caregiver can repeat the instructions as needed. Sending home printed materials and discussing risks for periodontal disease may be beneficial to the caregiver but are NOT appropriate for educating the patient.

4 **(E)** Individuals with cerebral palsy typically are able to comprehend instructions; LESS than half are mentally retarded (intellectually disabled) and in need of simpler instructions. Have difficulty with motor control, speaking, performing homecare procedures, which often results in increased caries risk.

5 **(B)** MOST patients with autism prefer routine and familiar procedures and surroundings. Instructions should be BOTH nonverbal and verbal and kept simple. Tone and loudness of the voice SHOULD be normal. Shorter dental visits are preferred.

6 **(A)** Apraxia is inability to properly form speech sounds. Aphasia is inability to understand language or put thoughts into words, and dysarthria is slurring of speech patterns. All are considered communication disorders. Ataxia is NOT a communication disorder but is a motor disorder that affects ambulation.

7 **(C)** Always face a visually impaired patient when providing oral healthcare instructions to individual. Speaking more loudly or more slowly is MORE appropriate for dealing with hearing impairment. Visual aids may be used but MUST be enlarged to be of benefit.

8 **(A)** Gingival bleeding and oral infections are associated with drugs that are used to treat arthritis. TMJ discomfort occurs when the disease has affected the joint; may even be associated with TMD, disorder of the joint. Angular cheilitis is associated with denture wearing, malnutrition, and candidal infection but NOT with arthritis.

9 **(C)** Toothbrush with larger handle would be MORE beneficial for patient with arthritic joints of the hands. Many arthritics have difficulty with grip strength. Larger brush handle would allow greater control. Extended-handle toothbrush is unnecessary unless the patient has difficulty raising the arms. Textured-handle toothbrush is helpful to prevent slipping but ONLY if on a larger handle that improves the gripping ability of the arthritic. Curved-handle toothbrush is appropriate for reaching molar areas for patients with limited arm movement.

10 (B) Restriction in or rupture of a blood vessel causes cerebrovascular accident (CVA, stroke). Involves sudden loss of blood flow to the brain, NOT to the heart. NOT associated with rheumatic heart disease, and often preceded by underlying diseases such as hypertension, diabetes, drug abuse, or atherosclerosis. Medical consult with patient's primary care physician is important because some modification of dental procedures may be necessary, particularly within the 4 to 6 weeks after the incident, since there may need to be a delay of emergency and elective dental care.

11 (A) Patients who have suffered spinal cord injury should be taught oral self-care. Depression and low self-esteem often accompany this disorder. Use of adaptive aids, powered toothbrushes, and oral irrigators gives patients some control over their own care. Discussion of proper nutrition and good oral hygiene also is important. When necessary, caregiver can offer assistance to the disabled patient.

12 (C) Location of traumatic injury to the spine is MOST closely related to the degree of paralysis or dysfunction associated with the spinal cord injury. Type, severity, cause of injury influence injury in location (vertebral level).

13 (B) Alzheimer's disease, form of dementia, often affects individuals in their middle-to-later years. Individuals often are confused by change and prefer quiet surroundings. For this reason, shorter, MORE frequent appointments are preferable to single, longer appointments. Appointments should be relaxed and involve familiar routines. Oral healthcare instructions should be repetitious and simple. During the early stages of disease, MOST patients can take care of own oral health needs with just a reminder from caregiver. During later stages, caregiver will need to take over MORE of care.

14 (B) Multiple sclerosis (MD) affects myelin sheath and results in fatigue and numbness. Inherited disease in which muscles atrophy and death may result. Myasthenia gravis (MG) and Parkinson's disease are disorders of the nervous system. Bell's palsy is a disease involving facial paralysis and typically is of unknown cause, although any trauma to the facial nerve may result in this paralysis.

15 (B) Alzheimer's disease affects cognition and is NOT associated with paralysis. Multiple sclerosis, Bell's palsy, and myasthenia gravis are disorders that may result in facial paralysis.

16 (A) Spina bifida, defect of neural tube development, often results in paralysis below point of defect. Paraplegics, and others with paralysis, need to be repositioned frequently during a dental appointment. Additional cushioning also helps prevent decubitus (pressure) ulcers. Patients with multiple sclerosis (MS), Down syndrome, or Parkinson's disease typically do NOT suffer from pressure ulcers unless bedridden or confined to wheelchair for long periods.

17 (C) Wraps are devices used specifically for full-body restraint of young children. Often sheets and blankets are wrapped around the child, from neck to toes. Mouth props and head stabilization secure ONLY the jaws and head. Papoose boards are another method of full-body restraint and can be used to secure patients of any age.

18 (C) When performing a wheelchair transfer, clinician must clear the area of any obstacles, secure a transfer belt to the patient, and lower the chair at or below wheelchair height. While facing the patient, the clinician stabilizes the patient's feet with clinician's feet and legs on either side of patient's knees, grasps the patient under the arms and around the back, lifts, and rotates the patient to the dental chair.

19 (A) Individuals with intellectual disability (mental retardation) often exhibit delayed (NOT early) tooth eruption; fused, pegged, or missing teeth; malocclusion; tongue thrusting; mouth breathing.

20 (C) When the person is able to give consent, this is considered a high level of function (level I to II). Answers A and B are moderate levels of function, and answer D is both moderate and low.

21 (A) Both statements are true and also related. Important for the caregiver for a disabled patient giving oral care to the patient to hear what is being advised by the dental hygienist and for the patient to know the type of care that the caregiver will be giving.

22 (D) Statement is not correct, but reason is correct. Conduction of vibrations from dental equipment such as ultrasonic scaler via teeth and bone can be very disturbing to the hearing impaired and such scalers are used ONLY if necessary.

23 (D) All are cognitive disabilities EXCEPT Parkinson's disease. UNLIKE patient with Alzheimer's, patient with Parkinson's can understand the clinician.

24 (A) Spina bifida (myelomeningocele) may be caused by a lack (deficiency) of folic acid in pregnant woman's diet. Cerebral palsy is usually caused by variety of injuries to the brain (e.g., infection, trauma, poisoning, anoxia) before, during, or not long after birth. Deafness can be side effect and result of the use of antibiotic streptomycin (NO longer used) and/or exposure of the pregnant woman to rubella (German measles). Short attention span has to do with attention deficit disorder (ADD).

25 (C) First statement is true and the second is false. With paraplegic adult patients, SHOULD always assess what they can do themselves before helping into the dental chair. This is because paraplegia is an injury in the thoracic, lumbar, or sacral region, with loss of sensation and movement in the legs and in part or all of the trunk, which varies according to the level of the injury. Generally, the lower the injury, the less the loss of movement and sensation. Wraps used MAINLY for young children when full-body restraint is necessary; sheets and blankets are similarly used to wrap and secure the patient with straps.

26 (A) Levodopa (L-dopa, Madopar, Sinemet) is used to treat Parkinson's disease. Alzheimer's is NOT treated by specific medications; ADD is usually treated with methylphenidate (Ritalin) or pemoline (Cylert); depression is treated with antidepressants.

27 (C) Pill-rolling motion of the fingers has to do with Parkinson's disease. Myelin sheath and Schwann's cells are related to multiple sclerosis; Koplik's spots are related to rubeola (measles); spastic movements are related to cerebral palsy.

28 (A) Aphasia is an inability to put thoughts into words or to understand language. Apraxia is the inability to properly form speech sounds. Dysarthria is a motor speech disorder. Alzheimer's disease has the loss of memory or thought.

29 (B) Cerebral palsy is associated with athetosis, ataxia, and rigidity. Pill-rolling motion of the fingers is associated with Parkinson's disease; short attention span is associated with ADD; paralysis is associated with paraplegia.

30 (C) Hydrocephalus is fluid in the brain, associated frequently with spina bifida, although it can also lead to an enlarged head.

CHAPTER 17

Community Oral Health

UTILIZATION OF DENTAL SERVICES

Use of dental services is defined as the proportion of the population who receive dental care services within given period. Factors that affect frequency include age, gender, economics, ethnicity, geographical location, general health status, acquisition of dental insurance. Factors influence and affect each other, interrelationship makes it difficult to determine exact influence of each component.
- See CD-ROM for Chapter Terms and WebLinks.
A. Needs: perceived vs. normative:
  1. Younger children with perceived needs (needs perceived by child or responsible adult) were MORE likely to be episodic users of dental care than children without perceived needs.
  2. Younger children with normative needs (defined by presence of untreated caries diagnosed by dentist) were less likely to be regular users.
  3. Older children with perceived or normative needs were MORE likely to be episodic users, less likely to have had previous-year visit than children with no needs.
B. National dental visits (need to know only approximate values when given for dental health concepts):
  1. Only 76% of children ages 2 to 17 with dental visit in past year.
  2. Only 64% of adults ages 18 to 64 with dental visit in past year.
  3. Only 56% of adults ages ≥65 with dental visit in past year.
C. Use of dental services is disproportionate among population group (factors noted above):
  1. Dental visits have been found to be scarcer among children with lower family incomes.
  2. Access to a dental examination for Medicaid-eligible children has been improved by federal and state programs but remains worse than for those whose family incomes are above poverty (family income ≥201% of Federal Poverty Level [FPL]) (discussed later).
  3. Fewer than 1 in 5 Medicaid-covered children received at least one preventive dental service in recent year; many states provide only emergency dental services to Medicaid-eligible adults.
  4. BOTH groups, poor and near-poor, are considered to be at high risk for poor oral health and are similar in terms of having had "any" dental visit—visit for routine dental examinations, restorative procedures, emergency care, preventive services, or combination.
  5. Poor children have ~12 times MORE restricted-activity days because of dental-related illness than children from higher income families.
D. Currently, individual who MOST regularly uses dental services can be described as a white, college-educated woman with a higher than average income, lives in suburban area, has dental insurance, possesses the characteristics related to good to excellent general and oral health.

Payment for Dental Care

Dental services are paid for by several means, including fee-for-service; third-party plans; usual, customary, reasonable (UCR) fees; capitation plans; dental service corporation plans (e.g., Delta Dental); indemnity plans; direct reimbursement; managed care plans; public financing.
A. Fee-for-service payment: two-party plan whereby the individual who receives dental services pays the fee directly out of pocket to the provider (dentist).
B. Third-party plans:
  1. Include BOTH not-for-profit and for-profit plans.
     a. Involve a contract between dental office (first party), patient (second party), insurance company (third party).
     b. Involve collection of premiums from patient by the third party, which in turn pays dental provider for services rendered.
     c. Regard third party as the insurance company, carrier, insurer, underwriter, or administrative agent.
     d. Insurance holder may be patient's employer, union group, government agency, or welfare fund.
C. UCR fees:
  1. Method of reimbursement used in prepayment plan.
  2. Usual fee: fee most frequently charged by dentists for particular dental service.
  3. Customary fee: maximum benefit payable under particular plan for a specific procedure; is determined by the administrator of the dental insurance benefit plan and based on submitted fees; may or may NOT correlate with patient's submitted fee.

4. Reasonable fee: actual fee charged by dental provider for particular procedure; modified according to each patient's specific circumstances; may or may NOT differ from dentist's usual fee or insurance company's customary fee.

D. Capitation plans: dentist contracts with an insurance program to provide most or all dental services covered by dental benefit program; dentist is given payment on per-capita basis.
   1. Characteristics:
      a. Involve fixed, monthly payments to providing dentist.
      b. Payments based on the number of patients assigned to dentist by benefit program.
      c. Patients are assigned to dentist to receive care.
      d. Monthly payments are received by dentist whether or not patients assigned require treatment.
      e. Co-payments and yearly maximums are features of these plans.
   2. Insurance benefit program assumes that some members will require a significant amount of care and that others will NOT seek care.

E. Dental service corporations (include Delta Dental Plans, MOST common example).
   1. Provided by a dental service corporation, not-for-profit organization that negotiates and provides dental care contracts.
   2. Incorporated state by state and is sponsored by each state's constituent dental society, governed by the insurance laws of each participating state.
   3. Provides dental treatment for clients in private practice facilities.
   4. Assists dentists in providing group purchase of dental care through traditional practice.
   5. Quality assurance is provided by a committee of nonparticipating dentists who conduct posttreatment evaluations to ensure acceptable quality.
   6. Payments to dentists are made through the customary fee structure.

F. Indemnity plans (commercial): operate for profit.
   1. Traditional insurance plans that operate by means of a submittal and reimbursement method.
   2. Require NO filing of UCR fees by dentists.
   3. Based on insurance company-generated "fee profile" that reflects the fees most often charged.

G. Direct reimbursement: occurs when an employer agrees to pay for a portion of an employee's dental treatment.
   1. Allows employee to seek dental care with dentist of choice.
   2. Involves direct payment of fees to dentist by employee/patient.
   3. Employee/patient pays for dental service and submits record of treatment to employer.
   4. Employer reimburses employee/patient according to agreed on reimbursement schedule.

H. Managed care or health maintenance organization (HMO):
   1. Was designed MAINLY to help lower cost of healthcare, participants prepay "fixed" premium for healthcare services.
   2. Curtails choice of providers; participants choose providers from approved list.
   3. Currently operated by BOTH for- and not-for-profit organizations; NO longer has federal constraints or funding.

I. Preferred provider organization (PPO): contracts between practitioners and their insurers to provide healthcare services for lower-than-average fees (fee-for-service plan).
   1. Patients may choose a participating provider to render a covered service.
   2. Service subsequently is paid for by the PPO.

J. Public financing: federal, state, and tribal government provides healthcare for groups such as the military, the Coast Guard, American Indians, Native Alaskans, federal penitentiary inmates.

GOVERNMENT'S ROLE IN ORAL HEALTHCARE

Philosophy of U.S. government gives responsibility for seeking and receiving oral healthcare services to each individual. MOST health-related programs administered by federal government are conducted through Department of Health and Human Services (HHS). Federal government developed two programs for express purpose of improving nation's capacity to provide oral health protection and oral healthcare services.

A. Group I: programs to provide improved oral health protection.
   1. Biological research.
   2. Disease prevention and control.
   3. Planning and development of oral health programs.
   4. Education and services research.
   5. Regulation and compliance functions such as quality assurance and assessment.

B. Group II: programs concerned with provision of oral healthcare services.
   1. Oral healthcare services rendered to specific groups by U.S. Public Health Service (PHS).
   2. The PHS are commissioned officers of Dental Corps who provide services to Indian Health Service (IHS), prisoners in federal penitentiaries, personnel of the Coast Guard and U.S. Merchant Marine, and underserved populations.

C. The PHS also administers research, prevention, resource planning, and development programs by National Institutes of Health (NIH).

1. Largest single source of monetary support for health research and development.
2. Dental component of the NIH is National Institute of Dental and Craniofacial Research (NIDCR), chief sponsor of oral health research.

Federally Funded Services

Federally funded services include services for maternal and child health, Head Start programs, Medicaid, Medicare, and the National Health Service Corps.

A. Maternal and Child Health Services (MCH):
   1. For women of childbearing age.
   2. For children less than 21 years of age.
   3. For individuals with low incomes.
   4. Through grants to improve healthcare for mothers and children.
   5. Dental component of MCH:
      a. Maternity and infant care projects.
      b. Children and youth projects.
      c. Dental health projects for children.
      d. Crippled children services.
      e. Women, Infant, and Children (WIC) program.
B. Head Start developed by Office of Economic Opportunity:
   1. Provides educational, health, and social services to low-income preschool children; enables them to enter school on a level equal to that of their peers from higher income families.
   2. Required to provide dental services to all enrolled children:
      a. Oral health screening.
      b. Oral health education programs.
      c. Sealant programs.
C. Medicaid (Title 19 of Social Security Act): federal program that distributes funds to states for provision of healthcare services to indigent.
   1. States vary on provisions; for most, dental care is option but NOT required; dental benefits, if included, typically are limited; may be limited by age and SES.
   2. Early periodic screening, diagnosis, treatment program (EPSDT):
      a. Oral healthcare services for individuals who are <21 years.
      b. Periodic screening for health defects.
      c. Any necessary diagnosis and treatment determined by screening.
D. Medicare (Title 18 of the Social Security Act): covers individuals >65 years, some disabled individuals:
   1. Provides insurance protection against cost of healthcare.
   2. Consists of two main parts:
      a. Part A:
         (1) Basic plan for hospital and related care.
         (2) Dental payments for routine dental care are *excluded.*

b. Part B:
   (1) Voluntary supplementary plan for physician services and other healthcare services.
   (2) Dental payments for routine dental care are *excluded.*
3. Dental services are limited to those medically necessary, such as oral/maxillofacial needs related to medical condition.
E. National Health Service Corps:
   1. Federal health labor deployment program.
   2. Deploys commissioned officers and civil service employees of PHS to render health services in geographical areas that are underserved because of healthcare shortages.
F. State health agencies (agencies or departments headed by a state or territorial office):
   1. Preventive services for children <18 years.
   2. Restorative and emergency services, screening.
   3. Very small number of states provide specialty services such as orthodontics, prosthetics, or correction and repair of cleft palate.

BIOSTATISTICS

Biostatistics is the tool by which research data are analyzed and results are defined.

A. **Sampling:** provides representation of general population, used in research to manage time and cost involved in conducting research.
   1. Random sampling: every member in population has individual and equal chance of being selected.
      a. Table of random numbers may be used to select sample, or participants may be chosen by lottery.
      b. Prevents researcher bias.
   2. Stratified sampling: modification of random selection.
      a. Divides population into subgroups before selection to ensure that all subgroups are sampled.
      b. Typically involves random selection within each subgroup (stratified random sampling).
      c. Prevents bias because eliminates possibility that members of a subgroup will NOT be selected.
   3. Convenience sampling: simplest method.
      a. Involves selecting convenient group (e.g., classroom, church, club members).
      b. May encourage bias because of sampling of select group; results may NOT be applicable to general population.
   4. Systematic sampling: similar to, but is NOT truly, random sampling because all members of a population do NOT have the same chance of being selected.
      a. Typically begins by determining that every *n*th member on a list will be selected.

b. Starting number is drawn and every *n*th member that follows starting number is selected; another method involves systematically choosing every even-numbered individual and excluding all odd-numbered individuals.

B. **Descriptive statistics:** used to make inferences about a population; involve frequency distribution, graphs, central tendency, and variability.

1. **Frequency distribution:** group of scores arranged from *lowest* to *highest* that contains frequency with which each score occurs; scores can be grouped, ungrouped, or cumulative.

a. Relative frequency: expressed as the frequency with which a specific score is earned (e.g., 15 students scored an 80 on an exam); can be expressed as a percentage.

b. Relative percent: expressed as the percentage of students who receive a particular score (e.g., three students scored 77, or 9.1% of the 33 students who took the exam).

c. Cumulative frequency: expressed as the frequency of occurrence of scores, up to and including any value in the data set; MAINLY used for data grouped by class intervals (e.g., 88 students scored in the range of 75% to 79% or below).

d. Cumulative percent: expressed as the percent frequency of occurrence of scores, up to and including any value in a data set (e.g., 96% of students scored 90 or below on the exam).

2. MOST commonly expressed as a normal (bell) curve (DING DONG, I GET IT!).

a. Exhibits a symmetrical grouping of scores around the mean or center of the curve.

b. Assumptions are made regarding the focal center of the curve.

c. Has a total area of 1 (100%); its mean, median, and mode are equal and are located in the center of the distribution.

(1) The total area is divided into segments called standard deviations.

(2) The area between the mean and one standard deviation to the right is 34.13%, and to the left is 34.13% (the total is approximately 68.26% of the total distribution).

(3) The area between the first and second standard deviations on the right is 13.59%, and on the left is 13.59% (the total is approximately 27.18% of the total distribution).

(4) The area between the second and third standard deviations on the right is 2.15%, and on the left is 2.15% (total is approximately 4.30% of the total distribution).

C. Graphs: visually represent distribution of scores along the *Y*- and *X*-axes.

1. The *Y*-axis typically represents the frequency of scores and typically is vertical.

2. The *X*-axis typically represents the scale that measures a specific variable.

3. Types (see CD-ROM for discussion):

a. Bar graph: two-dimensional representation of discrete data.

b. Histograph: representation formed directly from a frequency distribution.

D. **Central tendency:** measure of the average score; summary or typical score of a distribution.

1. **Mean:** arithmetic value that is computed by dividing the total by its members (e.g., 450 students/3 schools = 150; the mean is 150 students per school); can be influenced by extreme scores.

2. **Median:** point that divides a score distribution into two equal parts, with 50% of the scores falling *below* and 50% of the scores falling *above* that point (e.g., 22, 56, 57, 78, 79, 80, 83, 84, 85, 90, 100; the median is 80 because 5 scores fall below it and 5 fall above it); is LEAST influenced by extreme scores.

3. **Mode:** value that occurs with the MOST frequency in a distribution (e.g., 1, 1, 3, 3, 3, 3, 3, 4, 5, 6, 7, 7, 7, 7, 8, 9; the mode is 3); MORE than one mode can occur; used MAINLY for quick computation.

E. **Variability:** BEST used for describing the spread, range, or distribution of scores.

1. **Range:** difference or distance between *highest* and *lowest* scores (e.g., range is 4 when scores range from 8 to 12); is NOT stable with extreme scores because ONLY uses the highest and lowest scores.

2. **Variance:** measure of average spread of scores around the mean; the greater the dispersion around the mean, the greater the variance; MORE useful than the range because considers all scores.

3. **Standard deviation:** positive square root of variance; the greater dispersion around the mean, the greater the standard deviation; MOST useful measure of variability in descriptive statistics; considers all scores in a distribution.

F. **Inferential statistics:** used to make generalizations from the statistical sample to the general population; effective sampling techniques make the inferences MORE accurate.

1. Student's t-test: procedure that is used MAINLY to make comparisons between the means of two different studies; determines the probability that the differences in the two means are real, and NOT caused by chance.

2. ANOVA: used in place of the t-test whenever more than two means MUST be compared.

3. **Chi-square test:** compares the observed measurement of a given characteristic with the expected measurement for a sample; chi-square statistic is a measure of the difference between the observed and expected measurements; used MAINLY when studying categorical information.
4. **Correlation analysis:** involves the study of two variables and their effects on each other; MOST useful when the number of pairs of variables is large (>30); correlation coefficient is the number that summarizes the strength of the relationship between two variables; is denoted as $r = +1$ or -1; the closer the correlation coefficient is to 1, the stronger the relationship between two variables.

COMMUNITY HEALTH STUDY

Scenario: A junior high school counselor contacted local dental and medical professionals regarding a perceived increase in the number of girls with eating disorders in her school. Several local dental hygienists decided to develop a program for raising the awareness of the dangers of eating disorders for this population of students. To determine the current level of awareness, the dental hygienists developed a pretest that elicited information regarding facts and fallacies related to eating disorders; it also asked students whether they had an eating disorder and whether they knew of a classmate with an eating disorder.

The pretest was voluntarily taken by 410 girls in grades 7 through 9. One week later, the participants gathered in an auditorium, where they listened to information about different eating disorders, their treatment, and the dental and medical effects of the disorders. The participants subsequently watched a 20-minute video of personal accounts of battles against anorexia and bulimia. One week after the presentation, the 410 participants were given a posttest that covered the information on the pretest. Participants scored significantly higher on the facts and fallacies section of the posttest than they did on the pretest.

1. What type of sampling was used in this study?
2. What type of research does this project involve?
3. What are the oral signs of eating disorders?
4. The results of the study showed that students scored much higher on the posttest than on the pretest. What does this indicate?

1. This study used convenience sample (all female students in a school were chosen). Random study is one in which every element in a population has an equal chance of selection. Stratified sample involves selecting members from the subpopulations of a group. Single-subject sampling involves one or a few subjects who exhibit a special condition.

2. This study is an example of educational or behavioral research because it (a) assesses and evaluates the application of an educational or behavioral technique in dentistry or dental hygiene to an individual or group; (b) focuses on knowledge, attitudes, behaviors regarding oral health and disease; (c) was conducted during a short period of time. Unlike this study, educational or behavioral studies typically involve smaller populations than experimental studies.
3. Oral signs or manifestations of eating disorders include enamel erosion (perimolysis), cheilitis, parotid gland enlargement, palatal bruising, thermal sensitivity, enlarged interdental papillae.
4. Fact that students scored much higher on posttest than on pretest indicates that learning occurred as a result of the information presented. However, increase in knowledge may not always lead to a change in behavior.

EPIDEMIOLOGY AND PREVALENCE

Epidemiology is the study of disease prevalence. It is conducted through systematic observation and is used in medicine, social and computer science, biology, and statistics. Epidemiological methods can be applied in dentistry to evaluate the specific disease patterns and needs of a community. Comparisons can be made between groups of a defined population.

A. **Incidence:** rate at which a disease occurs.
   1. Expressed as the number of *new* cases during a specific time.
   2. Incidence rate = The number of cases divided by individuals and time.
   3. I_r = Cases/Individuals and time
   4. Example: 50 individuals in a community of 250,000 died of oral cancer during 2008; I_r = 50 deaths/250,000 individuals per year for the incidence of oral cancer in that community.
B. **Prevalence:** total number of cases of disease in existence in a given population at a given time.
   1. Prevalence = The number of cases divided by population multiplied by 100.
   2. P = Cases/Population × 100
   3. Example: in 2008 there were 300 reported cases of gingivitis among 1000 20-year-old students examined; 300 gingivitis cases/1000 students × 100% = 30% prevalence of gingivitis among the student population.
C. Rate of disease: expressed as a ratio (fraction, numerator/denominator).
   1. Numerator is occurrences of a disease; denominator is possible occurrences of a disease.
   2. Rate = Actual occurrences/Possible occurrences
   3. Example: in 2008 there were 25 cases of gingivitis among 250 teenagers examined; 25 actual/250 possible = 10% rate of gingivitis among the student population (must be very good brushers!).

D. Morbidity (disease) can be expressed as a rate: **morbidity rate** is number of actual diseases divided by number of possible diseases.

E. Mortality (death) can be expressed as a rate: **mortality rate** is number of actual deaths divided by number of possible deaths.

F. **Epidemic:** significantly greater-than-normal incidence of disease.
   1. Describes a disease that spreads rapidly through particular segment of the population.
   2. Describes a disease with MORE cases than expected.

G. **Endemic:** disease with expected (typical) number of cases that continues over time; may be specific to particular geographical area or population.

H. **Pandemic:** disease that occurs throughout population of a country, people, or the world.

I. **Index** (plural, **indices**): systematic way of collecting and arranging data gathered from observations so that they can be quantified, analyzed, understood (specific dental indices discussed later).
   1. Accomplished under specifically defined criteria and conditions.
   2. Example: record of data collected from periodontal probing.
   3. Characteristics of effective index: reliable; reproducible; valid; easily understood and explained.

Epidemiology of Caries

A 2005 report, "The Centers for Disease Control Surveillance for Dental Caries, Dental Sealants, Tooth Retention, Edentulism, and Enamel Fluorosis—United States, 1988-1994 and 1999-2002," used the National Health and Nutrition Examination Survey (NHANES), ongoing survey of representative samples of population.

A. Background concerning caries:
   1. Common chronic disease that causes pain and disability across ALL age groups.
   2. Although dental caries (tooth decay) is LARGELY preventable, remains MOST common chronic disease of children aged 5 to 17 years, four times MORE common than asthma (42% versus 9.5%).
   3. If left untreated, dental caries can lead to pain and infection, tooth loss, edentulism (total tooth loss); pain and suffering resulting from untreated tooth decay can lead to problems in eating, speaking, and attending to learning.
   4. Enamel (dental) sealants are effective in preventing dental caries in occlusal (chewing) and other pitted and fissured surfaces of teeth.
   5. Enamel fluorosis is hypomineralization of enamel related to fluoride exposure during tooth formation (first 6 years for MOST permanent teeth); exposure to fluoride throughout life is effective in preventing dental caries.

B. Trends in caries:
   1. NO change in prevalence of dental caries in primary teeth among children aged 2 to 11 years.
   2. Reduction in prevalence of caries in permanent teeth of up to 10% among persons aged 6 to 19 years and up to 6% among dentate adults aged >20 years.
   3. Increase of 13% in dental sealants among persons aged 6 to 19 years.
   4. A 6% reduction in total tooth loss (edentulism) among persons >60 years.

C. Statistic on caries in United States:
   1. Among children aged 2 to 11 years, 41% had dental caries in primary teeth.
   2. Among children and adolescents aged 6 to 19 years, 42% had dental caries in permanent teeth, and ~90% of adults did.
   3. Among children aged 6 to 19 years, 32% had received enamel sealants.
   4. Adults aged ≥20 years retained a mean of 24/28 natural teeth and 8% were edentulous.
   5. Among persons aged 6 to 39 years, 23% had enamel fluorosis (very mild or greater).
   6. Disparities were noticed across ALL age groups; MAINLY among racial and ethnic groups, in persons with lower education and income, and by smoking status.

Epidemiology of Periodontal Disease

The American Academy of Periodontology (AAP) Research, Science and Therapy Committee (2005) reviewed evidence concerning periodontal disease and formed conclusions. National prevalence of moderate and severe periodontal diseases among dentate adults aged 20 years and older was estimated from the 1999-2004 National Health and Nutrition Examination Survey conducted by NHANES.

- See Chapters 11, Clinical Treatment: charting and assessment of periodontal disease; 13, Periodontology: risk factors for periodontal disease.

A. Background concerning periodontal disease:
   1. Interpreting results of epidemiological studies of gingivitis, and particularly those of periodontitis, is extremely difficult.
   2. Prevalence of disease must be measured in terms of specific definition of each disease and age group affected.
      a. Example: although periodontitis may be defined in one study as an attachment loss of 2 mm, it may be defined in another study as attachment loss of 4 mm.
      b. Therefore describing prevalence of periodontal disease in statistical terms can be difficult and misleading.
      c. Definition of disease must be determined before statistics are interpreted.

B. Trends concerning gingivitis:
1. Dental biofilm (dental plaque) is closely correlated with gingivitis, relationship long considered one of cause and effect.
2. Gingivitis is found in early childhood, is MORE prevalent and severe in adolescence, then tends to level off in older age groups.
3. Gingivitis, associated with widespread dental biofilm and calculus deposits, is standard in adults.
4. Relatively FEW sites with gingivitis go on to develop periodontitis; even so, prevention of gingivitis, in individual patients and in populations, is still FIRST step toward preventing periodontitis.

C. Trends concerning periodontitis:
1. Periodontitis results from a complex interplay between bacterial infection and host response, often modified by behavioral factors.
2. Host response is KEY factor in clinical expression of periodontitis, with only some 20% of periodontal diseases now attributed to bacterial variance.
3. Some 50% of periodontal diseases have been attributed to genetic variance and >20% to tobacco use.
4. While there is a clear causal relationship between poor oral hygiene and gingivitis, relationship of oral hygiene to periodontitis is LESS straightforward; in populations with poor oral hygiene, dental biofilm and supragingival calculus accumulations correlate poorly with severe periodontitis.
5. Oral hygiene can favorably influence ecology of microbial flora in shallow-to-moderate pockets but does NOT affect host response; oral hygiene alone has little effect on subgingival microflora in deep pockets.
6. Some 5% to 20% of any population suffers from generalized severe periodontitis, although slight to moderate periodontitis affects majority of adults; for those who are MOST susceptible, periodontitis becomes MOST evident in teenage and early adult years rather than the later years.

D. Statistics for periodontal disease in United States:
1. Overall, prevalence of moderate and severe periodontal disease ranged from 0.82% to 18.3% for adults aged 20 to 34 years and 0.06% to 2.9% for adults aged 75 years and older.
2. Moderate disease was MOST prevalent in males, non-Hispanic blacks, group with lowest family poverty ratio (<100%), persons with less than high school education.
3. Severe disease was MOST prevalent among males for all age groups (EXCEPT those aged 75 years and older), persons with a family poverty income ratio between 100% to 200%, those with less than high school education.

4. Overall, moderate and severe periodontitis was still prevalent; moderate disease, which is MOST open to preventive measures, was MOST prevalent in non-Hispanic black males, the poorest, and the least educated.

Dental Indices

Dental indices are used in studying BOTH caries and periodontal disease and helping to create preventive programs or to understand individual needs for oral health.

A. O'Leary plaque index: does NOT quantify dental biofilm; monitors oral hygiene performance, indicates location of dental biofilm.
1. Assists in visualization of homecare progress, thus assisting clinicians in emphasizing specific areas of need and tailoring homecare with alternative dental biofilm control aids.
2. Directions for use:
   a. Cross out all missing teeth; divide the teeth into four parts (facial, lingual, distal, mesial) and the mouth into four quadrants; apply disclosing solution and have patient rinse; evaluate presence of dental biofilm using air, mouth mirror, explorer.
   b. Number of dental biofilm surfaces present/Total number of tooth surfaces examined × 100 = % dental biofilm.

B. Oral hygiene index, simplified (OHI-S): developed by Greene and Vermillion, used MAINLY for large populations.
1. Two components, debris index (dental biofilm, materia alba, food) and calculus index, BOTH added together to obtain single score.
2. ONLY facial and lingual surfaces are scored; includes facial surfaces of teeth #3, #8, #14, and #24, and lingual surfaces of teeth #19 and #30.
3. Scoring criteria:
   a. 0 = No debris or stain present.
   b. 1 = Soft debris covering not more than one third of tooth surface.
   c. 2 = Soft debris covering more than one third but not more than two thirds of tooth surface.
   d. 3 = Soft debris covering more than two thirds of tooth surface.
   e. Debris and calculus scores are combined, and total is divided by number of surfaces examined to obtain average OHI-S.

C. Personal hygiene performance index–modified (PHP-M): developed by Podshadley and Haley, modified by Martens and Meskin; used MAINLY to provide patients with information about dental biofilm that will assist in improvement of oral health.
1. Teeth that are selected during the initial visit are used for comparison during subsequent visits.

2. Criteria for use:
   a. Select six teeth, divide each of them into five areas, and label areas a, b, c, d, and e on BOTH facial and lingual surfaces.
   b. Record presence of dental biofilm in each of lettered areas and give one point for each area of dental biofilm; scores range from 0 to 60 (best to worst).

D. Plaque index (PI): developed by Silness and Loe, used MAINLY in conjunction with gingival index (GI) by same authors; assesses thickness of dental biofilm on teeth at gingival margin.
   1. Specific teeth and entire dentition can be assessed using the distal, mesial, facial, lingual surfaces.
   2. Scoring criteria: visually examine dental biofilm or probe to swipe along cervical third; disclosing agent can be used.
      a. 0 = no dental biofilm adheres or visible at gingival third.
      b. 1 = dental biofilm adheres at gingival third; visible with explorer.
      c. 2 = moderate amounts of dental biofilm visible in sulcus or at gingival margin.
      d. 3 = heavy amounts of dental biofilm visible in sulcus or at gingival margin.
   3. Criteria for use:
      a. For individual teeth: total the score for each of the four surfaces and divide by four; for groups of teeth, total individual scores for all teeth in the group and divide by number of teeth in the group; used MAINLY for comparing areas of the mouth.
      b. For individual dentition: total the individual scores for all teeth and divide by the number of teeth; for groups of individuals, total individual dentition scores and divide by number of members in the group.

E. Gingival index (GI; Loe and Silness): index MOST frequently used to evaluate gingivitis; bleeding is MOST critical factor; also assesses tissue bleeding, color, contour, ulceration.
   1. Scoring: use on all or six selected teeth; divide the teeth into four areas (facial, lingual, distal, and mesial).
      a. Total scores from these four areas and divide by number of surfaces examined.
      b. 0 = Normal gingiva.
      c. 1 = Mild inflammation, slight change in color, slight edema, and no bleeding on probing.
      d. 2 = Moderate inflammation, redness, edema, glazing, and bleeding on probing.
      e. 3 = Severe inflammation, marked redness, edema, ulceration, and a tendency toward spontaneous bleeding.

F. Gingival bleeding index (Ainamo and Bay): assesses bleeding of gingival margin in response to probing.
   1. Used MAINLY as indicator of gingival health and disease.
   2. Scoring: positive score indicates percentage of all gingival areas explored that bleed in response to probing.
      a. Divide the total number of areas that bleed by the number of gingival margins examined; then multiply the result by 100 to arrive at a score (percentage).
      b. (+) = bleeding *within* 10 seconds after gentle probing.
      c. (−) = absence of bleeding *after* 10 seconds following probing.

G. Russell's periodontal index (PI): assesses progressive stages of periodontal disease and amount of attachment loss.
   1. Easy to use and understand; results are comparative, used MAINLY for major population groups.
   2. Criteria for use:
      a. Tissues are examined for gingival inflammation, pocket formation (with noncalibrated probe), and masticatory function and given a score.
   3. Scoring:
      a. 0 = Negative: no overt inflammation in investing tissues or loss of function from destruction of supporting tissues.
      b. 1 = Mild gingivitis: overt area of inflammation is present in free gingiva but the area does not circumscribe the tooth.
      c. 2 = Gingivitis: inflammation completely circumscribes tooth; no apparent break in epithelial attachment.
      d. 6 = Gingivitis with pocket formation: epithelial attachment has been breached and pocketing exists; no interference with normal masticatory function; tooth is firm in its socket, no drifting is discernible.
      e. 8 = Advanced destruction with loss of masticatory function: tooth may be loose, drifting, or dull on percussion or may be depressed in its socket.
   4. Findings:
      a. For individuals: PI = Sum of individual scores/ Number of teeth scored
      b. For groups: Group PI = Total of individual scores/Number of individuals examined
   5. Clinical conditions and group PI score ranges:
      a. Indicates clinically normal tissues (0.0 to 0.2).
      b. Indicates simple gingivitis (0.3 to 0.9).
      c. Indicates incipient destructive periodontal disease (0.7 to 1.9).
      d. Indicates established destructive periodontal disease (1.6 to 5.0).

e. Indicates terminal stages of periodontal disease (3.8 to 8.0).

H. Ramfjord's periodontal disease index (PDI): evaluates gingival health, probing depths, dental biofilm and calculus deposits.

1. Used for the Ramfjord teeth (#3, #9, #12, #19, #25, and #28); MOST often are used in clinical studies as a representative sample of the entire dentition.
2. Gingiva is given a score between 0 and 3, depending on the severity of inflammation; pockets are probed on the mesial and facial surfaces and are given a score between 4 and 6.
3. Critical measurement is the distance from the CEJ to the base of the sulcus.
4. Scoring:
   a. 0 = Absence of inflammatory signs.
   b. 1 = Mild to moderate inflammatory gingival change that does not extend around the tooth.
   c. 2 = Mild to moderately severe gingivitis that extends around the tooth.
   d. 3 = Severe gingivitis characterized by marked redness, swelling, and the tendency to bleed and ulcerate.
   e. 4 = Gingival crevice extends apically past the CEJ but not more than 3 mm.
   f. 5 = Gingival crevice extends apically 3 to 6 mm past the CEJ.
   g. 6 = Gingival crevice extends apically more than 6 mm from the CEJ.
   h. Combined gingival and pocket scores reflect an individual's periodontal status.

I. Plaque Assessment Scoring System (PASS): evaluates subgingival dental biofilm, UNLIKE O'Leary plaque index, which only evaluates supragingival dental biofilm.

1. Selects five teeth for examination: four first molars and maxillary incisor; if not available, teeth near the lost molars are used, first distal, then mesial, then mandibular incisor is used.
2. Each tooth selected is divided into areas (mesial, distal, buccal, lingual) and a periodontal probe is swept around 1 mm into the sulcus; if dental biofilm is visible on the probe, recorded as positive score.
3. There are 20 possible sites for dental biofilm surfaces to be evaluated per mouth; score is percentage of surfaces positive for subgingival dental biofilm accumulation.
4. Ideal for the solo clinician and statistically reliable compared to the O'Leary PI.

J. Community periodontal index of treatment needs (CPITN): evaluates pockets, bleeding, and dental biofilm retention factors; developed by Fédération Dentaire Internationale and World Health Organization to assess treatment needs of specific groups.

1. Evaluates six sextants; one score from each sextant is used; excludes third molars unless function as second molars.
2. Probing is performed with the CPITN-E probe.
   a. First and second molars in posterior sextants are examined and only worse of the two scores is recorded; one maxillary tooth and one mandibular anterior tooth are also scored for a total of six scores.
   b. Scoring uses a five-point Likert scale (0 = no signs of periodontal disease and 4 = periodontal pockets of 6 mm or more).
3. Scores are converted to a 4-point treatment needs (TN) classification.
   a. TN 0 = No treatment is needed.
   b. TN 1 = Requires improved oral hygiene.
   c. TN2 = Requires improved oral hygiene and scaling.
   d. TN3 = Requires improved oral hygiene, scaling, and complex treatment.

K. Specific caries indices:

1. DMFT/dmft indices: provide broad picture of caries activity in specific population for BOTH permanent and primary dentitions.
   a. Various components may be used to evaluate specific information that is needed.
   b. Examples for permanent dentition: DMFT = decayed, missing, filled *teeth* and DMFS = decayed, missing, filled *surfaces;* DEFT = decayed, extracted, filled *teeth* and DEFS = decayed, extracted, filled *surfaces;* SIMILAR methods used for primary dentition.
   c. Also available are the df/def indices, which indicate decayed (d), indicated for extraction (e), and filled (f) in the primary dentition.
   d. Data collected from these indices can be used to determine community needs.
2. Unmet treatment needs (UTN) index of particular population:
   a. UTN = Mean number of decayed teeth/Mean number of decayed and filled teeth multiplied by 100.
   b. Can be used to compare treatment needs of one population with those of another (e.g., UTN of a community *with* fluoridated water may be compared with UTN of a community that does *not* have water fluoridation).
3. ECC and S-ECC (early childhood caries and severe-early childhood caries) index: each erupted primary tooth is examined and every surface.
   a. ECC: 1 or more decayed (noncavitated or cavitated lesions), missing (because of caries), or filled tooth surfaces in any primary tooth in a child 71 months of age or younger.

b. S-ECC: younger than 3 years of age, any sign of smooth-surface caries; ages 3 through 5, 1 or more cavitated, missing (because of caries), or filled smooth surface in primary maxillary anterior teeth, or a decayed, missing, or filled score of >4 (age 3), >5 (age 4), or >6 (age 5) surfaces.

4. RCI (root caries) index: evaluates extent of root caries and risk for root caries disease.

a. Includes only those root surfaces exposed to the oral environment by gingival recession.

b. RCI = $(R - D) + (R - F)/(R - D) + (R - F) + (R - N)$; where R = root surface, D = decayed root surface, F = filled root surface, N = intact, sound root surface.

L. Indices that measure fluorosis:

1. Dean's fluorosis index: MOST used in community studies even if less sensitive than other index; individual's fluorosis score is based on the most severe form of fluorosis found on two or more teeth.

2. Tooth surface index of fluorosis (TSIF): MORE sensitive than Dean's; each tooth is examined for signs and assigned a numerical score.

COMMUNITY HEALTH STUDY

Scenario: Children of a Native American tribe between the ages of 12 and 14 were assessed for the need for sealants. The children live in a rural nonfluoridated community. An alphabetized list of names of school-aged children was used to select participants. Of the 980 children on the list, every twentieth child was selected for the study. Among the 49 youths examined, 155 tooth surfaces had restorations, 42 surfaces had decay, and no teeth required extraction.

1. What method of sampling was used in this study?
2. Identify the best index to use for assessing the sealant needs of this population.
3. What do the results of the study indicate?
4. Is fluoridation of the school water supply an example of primary, secondary, or tertiary prevention?
5. Identify the best way to promote the sealant project. Should professional fluoride treatments be a part of the project? If so, when should they be given?

1. Systematic method of sampling was used in this study because every twentieth child was selected from an alphabetized list. Other methods of sampling include random sampling, in which every element in a population has an equal chance of selection; convenience sampling, in which a selection is made for convenience that may not be representative of the general population; stratified sampling, in which members are randomly selected within subgroups; and single-subject sampling, in which the study is of one or a few subjects who exhibit a special condition.

2. Best index to use for assessing the sealant needs of this population is the DMFS because it assesses the decayed, missing, and filled surfaces of teeth. This index would be helpful in identifying pit and fissure surfaces in need of sealants. DEFT and DEFS are indices that identify decayed, extracted, and filled teeth or surfaces of deciduous teeth; they would not be appropriate for studying decayed pits and fissures in the teeth of elementary school-aged children because sealants are not routinely placed on deciduous teeth.

3. Study results indicate that there is a need for both sealant placement and school water fluoridation because the DMFS is 4.1 (D = 0.9, M = 0, and F = 3.2). Water fluoridation would decrease the number of smooth surface caries, and sealants placed on remaining caries-free surfaces would reduce the number of pit and fissure caries.

4. Fluoridation of the school water supply is an example of primary preventive dentistry. It can prevent the onset of disease (caries), reverse the initial stages of disease (demineralization), and arrest the process before treatment is indicated. Secondary and tertiary prevention, respectively, are associated with restoring tissues to near normal function and with replacing lost tissue and providing rehabilitation.

5. Best way to promote the sealant project is to involve community leaders. Involving community leaders allows the project to take on value and priority. Other methods of promoting the project include informational meetings for parents, teacher-student discussions, radio advertising, and informational flyers. Professional fluoride treatment should be given immediately after sealant placement such as with a fluoride varnish.

Epidemiology of Oral Cancer

The "SEER Cancer Statistics Review," a report by the National Cancer Institute, gives rates that are based on cases diagnosed in 2000 to 2004.

• See Chapters 6, General and Oral Pathology: oral cancer and risk factors; 11, Clinical Treatment: examination for oral cancer.

A. Background on oral cancer:

1. Death rate associated with this cancer is particularly high but NOT because it is hard to discover and/or diagnose, rather because it is routinely discovered late in development.

2. Often discovered only when has metastasized to another location, MOST likely cervical lymph nodes; prognosis at this stage of discovery is significantly worse than when caught while still in a localized intraoral area; at these later stages, primary tumor has had time to invade deep into local structures.

3. Patients who survive first encounter with disease have up to a 20 times higher risk of developing second cancer; heightened risk factor can last for 5 to 10 years after first occurrence.

B. Trends on oral cancer:

1. Number of cases and associated levels of mortality have NOT significantly improved in decades.

2. Death rate for oral cancer is higher than that of cancers widely discussed in the media (such as ovarian).

3. Worldwide, problem is much greater, with >400,000 new cases being found each year.

C. Statistics on oral cancer in United States:

1. Incidence:

    a. Median age at diagnosis for oral and pharyngeal cancer was 62 years of age.

    b. Age-adjusted incidence rate was 10.5 per 100,000 men and women per year.

2. Prevalence: in 2004, ~235,856 men and women alive who had oral and pharyngeal cancer history, 150,946 men and 84,910 women.

3. Mortality:

    a. Median age at death for cancer of the oral cavity and pharynx was 68 years of age.

    b. Age-adjusted death rate was 2.7 per 100,000 men and women per year.

PREVENTION OF DENTAL DISEASE

There are different levels of prevention or health promotion. **Health promotion** facilitates a voluntary adaptation of health-seeking behaviors through any combination of learning opportunities; involves behavior changes produced by advice and counseling. **Primary prevention** includes techniques designed to prevent the onset of disease, reverse the initial stages of disease, or arrest a disease process before treatment is needed. **Secondary prevention** includes techniques designed to terminate disease and restore tissues to near normal function. **Tertiary prevention** includes techniques designed to replace lost tissues and rehabilitate to near normal function. ALL discussed can be considered primary preventive oral care services.

Prevention and Control of Caries

Caries can be controlled though use of fluorides, enamel (pit and fissure) sealants, and diet counseling. The CDC has reported on these issues in "Preventing Dental Caries with Community Programs" (2006) and "Recommendations for Using Fluoride to Prevent and Control Dental Caries in the United States" (2001) (see CD-ROM). Discussion covers community promotions for use of fluoride, sealants, and diet counseling.

- See Chapters 6, General and Oral Pathology: fluorosis; 7, Nutrition: diet counseling; 11, Clinical Treatment: caries classification and charting, patient-use fluoride products and toxicity, enamel sealants, oral microbials.

A. Community fluoride promotions:

1. Primary preventive oral care services to reduce or prevent dental caries.

2. Measured use of fluoride modalities is particularly appropriate during time of anterior tooth enamel development (i.e., age <6 years).

3. Community water fluoridation:

    a. **Artificial fluoridated water** is the addition of fluoride compounds to the community water supply; amount is maintained at an optimum level to decrease caries without causing fluorosis.

    b. CDC and PHS recommend OPTIMUM concentration of fluoride in community water supply to be 0.7 to 1.2 ppm (depending on average maximum daily air temperature):

        (1) If rate is 1 ppm, necessary to consume 1 L of water in order to take in 1 mg of fluoride; highly improbable a person will receive more than the tolerable upper limit from consuming optimally fluoridated water alone.

        (2) Individuals in hotter climates are likely to drink MORE water and thus receive MORE fluoride, so amounts are adjusted for warmer air temperatures.

        (3) Example of addition of fluoride to a community water supply (where temperature is not a consideration): a town naturally has 0.25 ppm concentration of fluoride, the community added 0.75 ppm to make community water supply achieve an optimum concentration of fluoride at 1 ppm.

    c. Environmental Protection Agency (EPA), which is responsible for the safety and quality of drinking water in the United States, sets maximum concentration of fluoride in community water supply at 4 ppm (and secondary limit [i.e., nonenforceable] guideline at 2 ppm).

        (1) If the water supply has **natural fluoridated water** over 2 to 4 ppm, the water supply undergoes **defluoridation** (partial) so the water is at optimum concentration of fluoride to prevent serious side effects.

        (2) Community water supply becomes naturally fluoridated as ground water that is fluoridated by water flowing over rocks and soil containing fluoride.

        (3) Example of defluoridation (partial) to remove fluoride: a rural town naturally has 4 ppm in their community water supply; the community removes 3 ppm to achieve an optimum concentration of fluoride at 1 ppm.

    d. Serves as a model health promotion intervention, since it is socially equitable.

(1) Effectively prevents dental caries in communities with varying disease prevalence; children in communities with water fluoridation experienced 29% fewer cavities.

(2) At present, 67% of individuals on public water supply, MORE than 170 million people receiving community water fluoridation.

(3) Water fluoridation is NOT expensive to administer; very inexpensive, with costs ranging from $0.12 to $1.16 per individual per year; every dollar spent on community water fluoridation saves from $7 to $42 in treatment costs depending on the size of the community; savings are greatest in large communities.

(4) At least 60% of U.S. population on public water supply has received fluoridated water since 1990, translating to savings in dental treatment costs of over $25.7 billion in past decade.

   (a) However, LACK of fluoridation in other 30% of communities may disproportionately affect poor and minority children.

e. Bottled water: some contain optimum concentrations (1.0 ppm); MOST contain <0.3 ppm, if being used to replace tap water, may NOT be receiving benefit of fluoride in community water supply; FDA regulations ONLY required to be listed if added during processing.

4. School water fluoridation: NOT as successful as community water fluoridation, so phased out.

a. Used MAINLY in rural areas, where students attend school together or in adjacent buildings with the same stand alone, separate from community water supply.

b. Since children are at school only part of each day, recommended level was 4.5 times the optimum concentration for community water supply; however, could result in *higher* than recommended concentrations, although NO lasting effects on children noted.

5. Fluoride supplementation: prescribed by supervising dentist or physician because of low levels of fluoride in community water supply (controversial method of prevention) (Table 17-1).

a. For optimum benefits, use of dietary fluoride supplements SHOULD begin when 6 months old and be *continued* daily until 16 years old.

b. Evidence for using to control dental caries is *mixed*; taken by pregnant (or lactating) women, provides NO benefit for offspring.

c. In form of tablets and lozenges, liquids (including fluoride-vitamin preparations); MOST contain sodium fluoride (NaF) as active ingredient.

d. Manufactured with 1.0 mg, 0.5 mg, or 0.25 mg fluoride; to maximize topical effect of fluoride, tablets or lozenges intended to be chewed or sucked for 1 to 2 minutes before being swallowed; for infants, supplements are available as a liquid (with dropper).

e. For infants and children aged <6 years, BOTH benefit of dental caries prevention and risk for *mild* enamel fluorosis for developing, unerupted teeth are possible; although primary teeth of children aged 1 to 6 years would benefit from fluoride's posteruptive action, and some preeruptive benefit for developing permanent teeth could exist, fluoride supplements could also INCREASE the risk for enamel fluorosis at this age.

f. MUST not have prescription larger than 120 mg of fluoride at one time to prevent accidental toxicity; NO storage of large quantities in the home.

g. However, lozenges for elderly or medically compromised, especially those who have limitations with toothbrushing, may be effective for topical use.

h. Example of fluoride supplementation (controversial): a 4-year-old child lives in a community that naturally has 0.4 ppm in community water supply, could receive daily fluoride supplement of 0.25 mg until 16 years old.

Table 17-1 Fluoride supplementation dosage schedule*

Age	Fluoride ion level in drinking water (ppm)[†]		
	<0.3 ppm	0.3-0.6 ppm	>0.6 ppm
Birth–6 months	None	None	None
6 months–3 years	0.25 mg/day[‡]	None	None
3-6 years	0.50 mg/day	0.25 mg/day	None
6-16 years	1.00 mg/day	0.50 mg/day	None

*Approved by the American Dental Association, American Academy of Pediatrics, and American Academy of Pediatric Dentistry, 1994 (only if needed, controversial).
[†]1.0 ppm = 1 mg/liter
[‡]2.2 mg NaS = 1 mg fluoride ion.

6. School-based fluoride mouthrinses: NOT as successful as community water fluoridation, so phased out.
   a. Rinsing (swishing) with diluted formulations of NaF, stannous (SnF_2), or acidulated phosphate (APF) fluoride daily or weekly; rinsing with a 10-mL solution for 1 minute provides topical effect.
   b. Programs done during the 1980s had 3 million children enrolled; little success noted in caries reduction, especially when children were also exposed to fluoridated water; involved teachers and other nondental personnel and consent was difficult to achieve; risk of swallowing was pronounced in younger groups.
7. Community fluoride varnishes: successful program but MUST involve trained healthcare professionals.
   a. Holds high concentration of fluoride on teeth for many hours; MOST effective method of fluoride application for primary caries.
   b. Has ease of application, nonoffensive taste; smaller amounts required than gel or foam application.
   c. BEST if incorporated for the very young such as WIC programs, Head Start, or well-child checkups.
B. Community-based enamel sealant promotions: successful program but MUST involve trained dental professionals.
   1. School-based programs have 60% fewer new decayed pit and fissure surfaces in posteriors for up to 2 to 5 years after a single application; among children, 90% of caries is in pits and fissures.
   2. School-based sealant programs provide sealants to children UNLIKELY to receive them otherwise (e.g., children in low-income households); children of racial and ethnic minority groups have *twice* as much untreated caries in permanent teeth, but receive only about *half* as many dental sealants.
   3. However, although 29 states reported dental sealant programs serving 193,000 children, number represents ONLY about 3% of poor children who could receive sealants.
C. Diet counseling in community programs:
   1. Avenue for helping to control dental caries in patients with high sugar consumption, high rates of caries, or salivary flow problems:
      a. All schoolchildren.
      b. Children, adolescents, and adults with high rates of caries.
      c. Medically compromised patients.
      d. Patients with decreased salivary flow or salivary gland hypofunction (xerostomia).
   2. Characteristics of diet counseling:
      a. Assesses cariogenic food intake by means of a diet diary.
      b. Identifies cariogenic foods and makes recommendations for alternative food choices without significantly changing the diet.
      c. Allows patient and/or guardian to play role in alternative food selections; also allows consideration of likes and dislikes.
      d. Success is dependent on four elements:
         (1) Motivation and cooperation of the patient.
         (2) Establishment of a professional rapport.
         (3) Consideration and fulfillment of the patient's individual needs.
         (4) Completion of a follow-up assessment and evaluation.

COMMUNITY HEALTH STUDY

Scenario: A dental hygienist is conducting a dental needs assessment on 12-year-old children in a small community. Most of these children have not had regular dental care for several years. Clinical findings indicate that most of the children have moderate marginal inflammation and dental biofilm. In addition, decay is present on many occlusal surfaces and along the gingival margin in some of the children. Survey results show that a large number of these children frequently consume candy and sugared sodas and that their homecare is poor (average child brushes with a fluoride toothpaste once daily and flosses sporadically). Community water supply is fluoridated at 1 ppm in their moderate climate.

1. Identify two indices that would be most appropriate for assessing the children's oral condition and for use as motivational tools.
2. Should these children receive fluoride supplementation in the form of tablets?
3. What is the optimum concentration level for fluoride in a community water supply?
4. Describe two other dental and oral public healthcare measures that might be recommended.

1. The DMFS (decayed, missing, filled surfaces) index would be appropriate for identifying specific caries activity and restorative needs and has greater sensitivity than the DMFT (decayed, missing, filled teeth) index. In addition, for both the children and their parents, may be used as visual tool to identify patterns of caries and areas that need concentration. O'Leary plaque index would be appropriate for identifying the dental biofilm present and providing the children with opportunity to see exactly which surfaces have dental biofilm. This index also gives the patient an effective visual display of areas that require attention (e.g., dental biofilm along margins, which can be removed by brushing, and/or in interproximal areas, which must be removed by flossing).

2. No, since they are receiving for the most part benefits from an optimum concentration level of fluoride in the community water supply.

3. CDC and PHS recommend optimum fluoride concentration of 0.7 to 1.2 ppm, depending on average maximum daily air temperature; individuals in hotter climates are likely to drink more water and thus receive more fluoride. EPA, which is responsible for the safety and quality of drinking water in the United States, sets maximum allowable limit for fluoride concentration in community water supply at 4 ppm (and secondary limit [i.e., nonenforceable] guideline at 2 ppm).

4. Two dental and oral public health measures to recommend for these children are enamel sealants (occlusal caries reduction) and some form of topical fluoride application (smooth surface caries reduction). Because most of these children have several areas of occlusal caries, sealants are recommended for the occlusal surfaces that remain caries free. Topical fluoride (such as that furnished by varnish) is recommended to strengthen the outer layer of enamel and to protect and decrease areas of decalcification along the margins. Use of topical fluoride in combination with enamel sealant placement will help to decrease both smooth surface and pit and fissure caries activity. Varnish has some advantages such as ease of application, nonoffensive taste, and smaller amounts required than with gel or foam application.

Prevention and Control of Periodontal Disease

Prevention and control of periodontal disease have traditionally focused on the mechanical removal of dental biofilm and calculus deposits. Process is accomplished by supragingival dental biofilm removal, daily toothbrushing and flossing, use of mouthrinses, regular supragingival and subgingival removal of deposits by a dental hygienist and/or dentist, and use of chemotherapeutic agents. Future treatment may increase the patient's host immune response, identify susceptibility and risk for periodontal disease, and focus on the elimination of specific bacteria.

Prevention and Control of Oral Cancer

Dental professional must conduct thorough head and neck examinations of patients and become familiar with the prevalence of oral cancer, characteristics, and risk factors. Dental professionals should identify, document, and refer patients with suspicious lesions.

DEVELOPING COMMUNITY ORAL HEALTH PROGRAMS

Developing community oral health programs involves determining a problem, assessment, planning, implementation, and evaluation. In addition, developers must possess the skills and knowledge of communication and educational principles necessary to develop and practice the teaching and presentation of oral health education programs.

Assessment of Public Health Problem

Public health problem is a condition or situation that is widespread or has potential to cause morbidity and mortality. Public health problem is one that is perceived by public, government, or public health authority as an existing problem. **Population assessment** is an organized, systematic approach to identifying a group with a health need, in this case an oral health need. An assessment defines the oral health problem, identifies the extent and severity of the problem, and assists in development of a community profile. Then the data are collected in several ways such as survey questionnaire, clinical examination, or personal communication.

Developing a Community (Population) Profile

A **community profile** is developed by gathering comprehensive facts about a particular community regarding income, education, size, location, disease, health, and other characteristics.

A. Community profiles are developed from population characteristics that are determined by studying the following information:
   1. Number of individuals in a population; geographical distribution of the population.
   2. Growth rate of the population, density of the population, urbanization vs. rural areas.
   3. Ethnicity of the population, socioeconomic status of the population, nutritional status of the population.
   4. Types of housing available and standard of living (number of upper, middle, lower class).
   5. Public services and utility types, general health status.
B. Dental disease profiles indicate patterns and distributions of disease, evaluated by the following:
   1. Clinical examination.
   2. Review of patient dental records.
   3. National health surveys.
C. Dental program profiles include assessment of:
   1. Histories and types of currently existing programs.
      a. Preventive.
      b. Treatment oriented.
      c. Educational.
      d. Research.
   2. Individual or organization responsible for each program.
   3. Success of the programs.
   4. Community's acceptance of the programs.
D. Policy- and decision-making profiles include information on:
   1. Occupations of financial leaders.
   2. Community's policy makers.

3. Community's organizational structure.
4. Oral health attitudes of community leaders.
E. Community resources profile includes assessment of:
1. Funding:
   a. Availability of state and local funding for oral care, third-party coverage.
   b. Availability of federal funding, number of private funds through endowments and foundations.
2. Facilities:
   a. Location of the closest major medical center; specialty services available at local medical center.
   b. Number, type, and locations of dental facilities; use, accessibility, and provision of available dental services.
   c. Whether OSHA and CDC guidelines are in place at each facility.
   d. Adequacy and efficiency of dental equipment, number of available operatories in each facility.
   e. Number of dental laboratories available.
3. Labor:
   a. Number of active, licensed dentists and dental hygienists, and number of dental assistants and laboratory technicians in the area.
   b. Availability and location of dental and dental hygiene schools in the immediate and surrounding areas.
   c. Number of active nurse aides in the community.
   d. Number of public health nurses, public health dental hygienists, voluntary health agencies, and nutritionists available.
F. Fluoridated water profile includes:
1. Type of drinking water available (well water versus central community water supplies).
2. Fluoride content of water supply and whether or not it is at optimum levels.
3. History of water fluoridation in the community.
4. Attitudes concerning water fluoridation held by the community, dental professionals, decision makers.
5. Existence of fluoridation laws and referendum availability.
6. Fluoride status of the school water supply.
G. Profile of professionally applied fluorides assesses:
1. Fluoride supplement prescription recommendations of community dentists and physicians.
2. Fluoride supplement and rinse programs available in community schools.
3. Status of fluoride administration at health centers and/or hospitals.
4. Toothbrushing program implementation in schools.
5. Use of fluoride dentifrice and frequency of brushing in these programs.
6. Success of all programs.

H. Interpretation of community profile data:
1. After all of the information regarding community profile is gathered, current oral health needs and priorities are established.
2. Program goals and objectives subsequently are developed and are aimed at meeting the specific needs identified.

Planning the Program

Program planning involves developing a lesson plan and defining goals and objectives.
A. Goals: general statements that describe major purpose of program, lecture, course, or unit of instruction.
B. Objectives: specific, precise, and immediate steps to achieving a goal.
C. Lesson plan:
1. Instructional "set":
   a. Introduces content procedures.
   b. Indicates the value and usefulness of information about to be presented.
   c. Motivates and arouses student interest by making it real.
   d. Ascertains the knowledge base of the audience by presenting information that brings the entire audience to the same level; involves administering quiz and discussing material from the last presentation.
   e. States objectives for the presentation.
   f. Establishes the mood and climate.
2. Lecture "body":
   a. Delivers the bulk of the information.
   b. Presents the major points.
   c. Relates information to personal experiences.
   d. Solicits audience participation and uses appropriate humor.
3. The "closure":
   a. Summarizes material presented in the "body."
   b. Provides a sense of cohesiveness, purpose, and accomplishment of stated objectives.
   c. Reviews and summarizes major principles and key points.
   d. Does NOT introduce new material.
   e. Involves taking questions from the audience and giving announcements.
   f. Provides the audience with a sense of achievement; involves thanking group for attention and participation.

Program Implementation

Program implementation is process by which a program is conducted and involves participants, roles, program specifics.
A. Integrates all external variables.
B. Involves teamwork.
C. Includes the operation of the plan.

D. Involves following a list of steps in the exact order in which they should occur.

E. Involves assigning each individual to a specific task.

F. Defines who does what, when, where, and how.

G. Specifies the time allotment for each task and activity.

Program Evaluation

Evaluation of a program involves defining the program purpose and evaluating the plan, the delivery, and the test results.

A. Purpose of evaluation:

1. To assess and determine the health needs of an individual, group, or population; directly determines the content of the health instruction and ensures that the information will be meaningful to the specific group identified.

2. To determine the strengths and weaknesses of the teaching personnel, the teaching strategies, and the organization of the instruction.

3. To assess the desired outcomes of oral health programs and the extent to which program objectives are met, and to determine a range of cognitive and behavioral outcomes.

B. Evaluating the plan:

1. Presenter should be thoroughly familiar with the subject matter; the material should be current and accurate.

2. Information should be appropriate to the level and needs of the audience.

3. Introduction ("set") should be interesting and appropriate, bulk ("body") of the lecture should be organized and logical.

4. Plan for explaining important points fully and thoroughly should be established.

5. Supplementary materials must be as current as possible, technical terms must be defined, transitions from one piece of information to another should be smooth; audiovisual materials should help illustrate and enhance the main points.

6. Points in the program for assessing the audience's understanding of the information presented should be identified.

7. Ending ("closure") should be effective and include NO new material.

8. Lecture notes should be easy to read; information presented should allow students to reach the stated instructional objectives.

C. Evaluating the delivery:

1. Can be accomplished by reviewing a videotape of the presentation and gathering feedback from the audience and peers.

2. All parts of the presentation must be assessed, including content, organization, and style.

3. Following items should be evaluated:

a. Clarity of speech, enthusiasm, body and facial expression, positive response to audience questions, maintenance of eye contact.

b. Smooth implementation of audiovisual materials, appropriate physical movement when communicating, organization of presentation, comfortable and appropriate atmosphere.

c. Allotment of appropriate time for entire presentation, minimal use of notes, provision of transitions and summaries.

D. Evaluating test results:

1. Instructional objectives serve as a guide for the lecture; exams and quizzes are developed to correlate with stated objectives.

2. Exams and quizzes subsequently can be used for evaluation; SHOULD accurately reflect the effectiveness of instruction; student feedback can provide information for the revision of future lessons.

COMMUNITY HEALTH STUDY

Scenario: A dental hygienist prepared an oral health education program regarding smokeless tobacco for a sixth-grade class. One of the objectives of the program was as follows: "After the lecture and videotape, 'Big Dipper,' the student will list and describe three ingredients in a can of chew." The major points of the lecture were presented. The dental hygienist related specific information in the content to personal experiences with patients.

1. Describe the "condition element" of the instructional objective.

2. Identify how the dental hygienist can best evaluate the learning of the sixth-grade class.

3. During the lecture the dental hygienist presented the major points and related specific information to personal experiences. Which part of the lecture was being delivered?

4. In which population group noted is oral cancer prevalent?

1. "After the lecture and videotape" best describes condition element of the instructional objective. Gives the stipulation of the objective, "the student" refers to the audience; "will describe and list" is a behavior required of the student; and "three ingredients" describes the degree element, or how many the student must be able to list in order to pass.

2. Dental hygienist can best evaluate the learning of the sixth-grade class through testing.

3. Presenting the major points of the lecture and relating specific information to personal experiences occurs in the body of the lecture. Other components

of the lecture format include the set, during which materials are introduced, and the closure, during which information is summarized and NO new material is presented.

4. Oral cancer is MOST prevalent among male and female tobacco users.

RESEARCH METHODS IN COMMUNITY DENTISTRY

Research can be defined as a continual search for truth by means of the scientific method. Research in community dentistry is categorized as biomedical research, which encompasses basic laboratory and clinical research, behavioral science, research regarding educational techniques, and administrative and evaluative research of community dental programs.

A. Biomedical clinical and experimental research typically involve clinical trials:
  1. Involve the use and application of epidemiology and basic laboratory research.
  2. Used to evaluate specific dental AND dental hygiene techniques and therapeutic agents.
    a. Investigational new drug (IND) number:
      (1) Must be obtained before assessing and evaluating a drug that has NOT been tested on a human population.
      (2) Obtained from Food and Drug Administration (FDA).
  3. Requires review by **Institutional Review Board** (IRB).
    a. Committee that reviews proposed research protocols involving human subjects for the protection, safety, and privacy of participants.
    b. Committee must include the following:
      (1) Minimum of five members, male and female members.
      (2) Professional representation by at least one nonscientific professional and at least one consumer or lay individual NOT directly involved with the institution.
  4. Three categories of research:
    a. **True experimental research:**
      (1) Involves random selection; all subjects in the sample have an independent and equal chance of being selected; all elements are selected at random (e.g., numbers are drawn from a hat and replaced before each consecutive drawing).
      (2) Involves random assignment; population subjects are assigned to each group at random.
    b. **Quasi-experimental research:**
      (1) Does NOT involve random selection; the subjects are selected as groups.
      (2) Involves random assignment.
    c. **Single-subject research:** studies that outline only one or a few subjects who may have a special problem or disorder rarely described in the literature.
    d. Important components:
      (1) **Reliability:** measure of accuracy of the research methods (e.g., whether the test, instrument, inventory, or questionnaire gives the same results each time so it is reproducible).
        (a) **Inter-rater reliability:** measure of reliability among two or more evaluators over time; calibration conducted periodically during the study to check concurrence among examiners.
        (b) **Intra-rater reliability:** measure of the reliability of one evaluator over time; calibration of individual examiners conducted throughout study to ensure that diagnostic technique does NOT change.
      (2) **Calibration:** method of unifying examiners in the diagnostic technique; accomplished by having examiners engage in trial runs on several sample cases and comparing findings of and between examiners; process repeated until all examiners concur; should be checked and recalibrated during study.
      (3) **Validity:** measure of accuracy of the research methods (e.g., does the test, instrument, inventory, or questionnaire measure what it intended to measure?).

B. Educational and behavioral research:
  1. Assesses and evaluates application of an educational or behavioral technique in dentistry or dental hygiene to individual or group.
  2. Focuses on knowledge, attitudes, behaviors regarding oral health and disease.
  3. Typically involves studies of short duration; typically involves smaller populations than experimental studies.

C. Administrative and evaluative research:
  1. Used for program evaluation in community dentistry:
    a. Assesses program's operation, effectiveness, and need for improvements.
    b. Determines how a newest innovation has been accepted and used in professional dental community (e.g., placement of sealants over incipient decay).
  2. Often involves questionnaire surveys:
    a. **Survey instrument:** set of specifically designed questions that are carefully planned and tested in terms of context, structure, appearance.
      (1) Used to gain knowledge from particular population regarding information useful to researcher.

(2) Number of subjects depends on the complexity of the study.

(3) Goals of the study should be well defined; ability to evaluate differences among groups should be tested.

(4) Survey question types:

(a) Dichotomous response involves yes/no *or* true/false questions.

(b) Multiple choice involves list of possible answers.

(c) Quantifiable number response, answers involve specific number (e.g., number of days per week, month, or year).

(d) Written response involves subjective answers to questions (difficult to interpret).

(e) Likert scale MOST often used to elicit feelings and NOT mere facts.

3. Pretesting:

a. Involves testing survey instrument on a small group of individuals who are not part of, but have characteristics similar to, the study sample.

b. Assists in gathering information and comments regarding questionnaire itself.

c. Allows errors, inconsistencies, misunderstandings, length to be commented on and corrected before the study takes place.

COMMUNITY HEALTH STUDY

Scenario: The activities coordinator of a senior citizens' center in a rural community asked the dental hygiene program director to present a 1-hour dental program. Eighty-eight senior citizens attend the local senior center. The program director decided to survey the attendees to determine their dental concerns and possible needs before developing the program. Twelve dental hygiene students volunteered to gather the information. An eight-item survey was developed that requested information regarding age, the number of remaining natural teeth, whether dentures are worn, whether the senior citizen has difficulty eating, swallowing, or speaking, perceived cause of any difficulties, and perceived needs. Eighty-one seniors were surveyed. Table 17-2 summarizes the results.

1. What is the mean number of teeth for seniors 65 to 69 years of age? 70 to 74 years of age? 75 to 79 years of age?

2. Based on the results of the survey, which one of these statements could be made: (a) These senior citizens have fewer teeth than the general population; (b) Most of these senior citizens wear dentures; (c) These senior citizens have more bad breath than other groups; or (d) The senior citizens between the ages of 70 and 74 are more likely to suffer a stroke.

3. Based on the results of the survey, what should be the emphasis of the 1-hour dental presentation for senior citizens?

4. What recommendations would help the senior citizens who are having difficulty swallowing?

1. Mean number of teeth remaining in seniors between ages of 65 and 69 is 16, between ages of 70 and 74 is 13, and between ages of 75 and 79 is 5.

2. According to results of the survey, most of these senior citizens wear dentures. General population data are not available for comparison to determine whether these senior citizens have fewer teeth or more bad breath than others. No information is provided that allows assumptions regarding likelihood of strokes in this group.

3. Based on the results of survey, emphasis of the 1-hour dental presentation should be on loose dentures. Two of the three groups had perceived needs involving loose dentures. Third group indicated that denture sores were problematic and may be related to loose dentures.

Table 17-2 Senior citizen survey results for community health study

Item	Age 65-69 (46 persons)	Age 70-74 (33 respondents)	Age 75-79 (2 respondents)
Average number of remaining teeth	16	13	5
Wear dentures	78%	87%	100%
Difficulty swallowing	52%	67%	50%
Difficulty speaking	23%	28%	50%
Difficulty eating	44%	33%	100%
Cause of difficulty	Dry mouth, loose dentures	Dry mouth, loose dentures, stroke	Dry mouth
Perceived needs	Loose dentures, bad breath, yellow teeth	Cleaning dentures, loose dentures, toothpaste selection, yellow teeth	Preventing denture sores, bad breath

4. Because many seniors felt that dry mouth contributes to difficulty, they need the following recommendations: sipping water, oral lubricants, air humidification, chewing sugar-free gum and candy. Referral to a physician recommended if moistening therapies do not help problem.

Government-Conducted Community Dental Research

Much of the money spent on community dental research is provided by NIDCR; research is funded according to its current priorities.

A. Intramural research: conducted within a facility by in-house researchers employed by that facility (e.g., NIDCR).

B. Extramural research:
   1. Agreement between the federal government and an outside institution to conduct identified research.
   2. Two types of extramural research:
      a. Grants:
         (1) Research money awarded to individual or institution to conduct research protocol.
         (2) Protocol has been developed and defined by individual or institution requesting money.
      b. Contracts:
         (1) Research money awarded to individual or institution to conduct research protocol.
         (2) Differs from grant in that the protocol has been defined by the federal government, NOT by the researcher.
         (3) Researchers do NOT develop their own protocols; they consent to conduct research that already has been defined by the federal government.
   3. Announcement and application of grants and contracts; two types:
      a. Requests for application (RFAs):
         (1) Federal government announces a general area of research priority.
         (2) Researchers who desire to apply submit a grant with a protocol that addresses the priority area.
         (3) Researchers may define and develop their own goals and protocols for conducting the research
      b. Requests for proposal (RFPs):
         (1) Federal government develops a detailed definition of the research goals and protocol.
         (2) Researchers and institutions interested in the defined protocol are invited to apply through a contract.
         (3) Interested researchers must describe methods for meeting the specific protocol terms.

COMMUNITY HEALTH STUDY

Scenario: Omar University has just been awarded funds to conduct research in an elementary school setting that targets fifth- and sixth-grade children. The dental hygiene professors at the university developed the research design and submitted a plan regarding the research and education they would provide. The target elementary school was located in a nonfluoridated, rural community. After examining the data collection, researchers found that the incidence of caries, dental biofilm, and gingivitis was high. The researchers planned intervention that includes oral health education and sealant placement and not a school fluoridation program.

1. What type of extramural research and approval, funding, and announcement process did Omar University use to obtain funding?
2. What primary limitation is involved in the implementation of a school water fluoridation program?
3. After the oral health education program has been implemented, how can the presenters best evaluate whether the desired outcomes of the program were accomplished?
4. Explain why many dental public health education programs are conducted in the elementary school setting.

1. Extramural research and approval, funding, and announcement process that Omar University used to obtain funding involved a grant and request for application (RFA). Grants are awarded to individuals and institutions who develop their own protocol for a specific research area. Money is applied for through an RFA.
2. Primary limitation of a school water fluoridation program is that the children are already 5 to 6 years of age when fluoridation begins, which decreases the beneficial effects on their teeth. However, fluoride level of water is adjusted to 4.5 ppm for school fluoridation, which may lead to higher than recommended concentrations. Involving teachers and other nontrained personnel and getting permission are also disadvantages. At least the children would not swallow the rinse, which younger children may do.
3. Best way for the presenters to evaluate whether the desired outcomes have been accomplished is by evaluating the extent to which the objectives were met. One must compare the objectives to the actual content delivered.
4. Many oral health education programs are conducted in school settings because the information can be delivered to large groups of students at once. Use of school typically is the most time- and cost-effective approach, and a school is often selected because of location and availability.

Review Questions

1 Placing an amalgam restoration after removing caries from the tooth surface is an example of
   A. health promotion.
   B. primary prevention.
   C. secondary prevention.
   D. tertiary prevention.

2 The number of individuals in a given population who received dental care services during a specific time period refers to
   A. demand.
   B. need.
   C. use.
   D. normative need.

3 Which of the following statements is NOT correct?
   A. More women than men use dental services.
   B. As an individual's socioeconomic status (SES) rises, his or her use of dental services increases.
   C. Caucasians use dental services more often than African Americans or Hispanic Americans.
   D. Individuals with poor general health are more likely to use dental services.

4 Which factor below is interrelated with all of the factors that influence the use of dental care services?
   A. Age
   B. Ethnicity
   C. Gender
   D. Socioeconomic status

5 Which of the following is a contract between the patient, the dental office, and the insurance company?
   A. Fee for service
   B. Indemnity plan
   C. Third-party plan
   D. Capitation plan

6 Which statement below BEST describes the term "reasonable fee"?
   A. The actual fee charged by the provider for a rendered service
   B. The most frequently charged fee for a particular service
   C. A minimum fee set by the dental insurance company or plan
   D. A charged fee that exceeds the fee set by an insurance company

7 An insurance plan that gives a fixed, monthly payment to a dentist provider, whether or NOT an individual assigned to that dentist receives care, is BEST described by which of the following terms?
   A. Third-party plan
   B. Indemnity plan
   C. Capitation plan
   D. Delta Dental Plan

8 Which of the following statements correctly describes direct reimbursement?
   A. An insurance company directly reimburses an individual for a fee paid to a provider.
   B. An employer directly reimburses an employee for dental services paid for out of his or her pocket.
   C. A fixed, monthly fee is paid to a providing dentist.
   D. An actual fee exceeds the fee set by an insurance company.

9 In 2008, 250 cases of squamous cell carcinoma were reported among a group of 10,000 18-year-olds examined in Fort Rock, Arizona. This is an example of
   A. rate.
   B. incidence.
   C. prevalence.
   D. morbidity.
   E. mortality.

10 Which of the following epidemiological indices would be BEST for evaluating caries in a group of adults between the ages of 70 and 85 who experience gingival recession, inflammation, and bleeding?
   A. DMFT
   B. DMFS
   C. UTN
   D. RCI

11 Joe Black presents with generalized, moderate marginal dental biofilm, inflammation, and bleeding. He indicates that he brushes once a day and flosses when food is caught between his teeth. Which of the following indices would be BEST for monitoring Joe's oral hygiene performance, indicating specific areas of need, and helping Joe with his oral care at home?
   A. OHI-S
   B. PHP
   C. GI
   D. O'Leary plaque index

12 Which of the following indices uses the selection of six teeth to compare dental biofilm removal performance at each subsequent visit and helps move a patient toward better oral health?
   A. OHI-S
   B. PHP
   C. GI
   D. Russell's periodontal index (PI)

13 Which of the following indices contains BOTH a debris index and a calculus index, which are summed for a single score?
   A. OHI-S
   B. PHP
   C. GI
   D. PI

14 The ideal epidemiological index for evaluating specific oral disease is one in which
   A. elaborate mechanisms are used to evaluate all aspects of the disease.
   B. simple indices, which are easily understood and explained, are used.
   C. the index is not reproducible.
   D. all possible factors are recorded.

15 After the gingival health of Tom Cook, a 43-year-old businessman, is evaluated, his teeth are divided into facial, lingual, distal, and mesial areas and the tissue is assessed for color, contour, bleeding, and ulceration. Which of the following indices is being used?
   A. O'Leary plaque index
   B. PHP
   C. PI
   D. Ramfjord's periodontal disease index (PDI)
   E. GI

16 Which of the following indices evaluates attachment loss and the progressive stages of periodontal disease?
   A. PI
   B. PDI
   C. CPITN
   D. GI

17 A public health dental hygienist has been asked to assess the periodontal status and treatment needs of the older adult patients in an assisted living community. To collect this information, the dental hygienist would use which of the following indices?
   A. PI
   B. PDI
   C. CPITN
   D. GI

18 One of the following is an INCORRECT statement about water fluoridation. Which one is INCORRECT?
   A. Has been shown to be effective against decay
   B. Requires no individual effort
   C. Is relatively expensive to administer
   D. Is a safe measure against caries

19 Enamel sealant placement is
   A. recommended for children and young adults living in fluoridated or nonfluoridated communities.
   B. recommended for all age groups in fluoridated and non-fluoridated communities.
   C. recommended for all age groups in nonfluoridated communities only.
   D. limited in its use and is applied only by a dentist.
   E. limited in its use because of low rates of retention and efficacy.

20 Roselyn, a 16-year-old, presents with several carious lesions on occlusal surfaces. She lives in a community with 0.7 ppm of fluoride in the drinking water. Which of the following would be the BEST oral health measure for preventing further decay?
   A. Enamel sealants
   B. Fluoride mouthrinse
   C. Diet counseling
   D. Fluoride supplements

21 All of the following are necessary for successful diet counseling, EXCEPT one. Which one is the EXCEPTION?
   A. Evaluation and counseling regarding food consumption are conducted in the same manner with all patients.
   B. Patients exhibit cooperation and motivation.
   C. Rapport has been established between the oral health professional and the patient.
   D. Reevaluation and assessment have been completed.

22 When research is conducted in a university setting, a project must receive which of the following before research is allowed to start?
   A. IND
   B. IRB approval
   C. Informed consent
   D. FDA approval

23 The IRB is responsible primarily for
   A. approving research on human subjects.
   B. practically applying research.
   C. regulating administrative procedures.
   D. approving and improving the operation of a program.

24 The University of Troy has proposed a study to evaluate the effects of a new antigingivitis drug, which has NOT been tested in a human population. To conduct this study, researchers must FIRST obtain
   A. approval from the IRB.
   B. an IND number.
   C. FDA approval.
   D. informed consent.

25 Which type of clinical trial research exhibits properties of both random assignment and random selection?
   A. True experimental
   B. Quasi-experimental
   C. Single-subject
   D. Questionnaire survey

26 After the implementation of an early childhood caries (ECC) program for low-income mothers, data were collected to determine the program's effectiveness. This study is an example of
   A. clinical trial research.
   B. administrative and evaluative research.
   C. educational and behavioral research.
   D. experimental research.

27 A dental hygienist wishes to assess the current skill level of a group of school nurses regarding the administration of a fluoride mouthrinse program in the local elementary schools. Which of the following is the suggested method for collecting data regarding the skill level of these nurses?
   A. Interview
   B. Written questionnaire
   C. Interviews with the school principals
   D. Direct observation

28 When conducting a questionnaire survey, it is important to
   A. have respondents include their names on returned questionnaires.
   B. use questions that require a written response of feelings.
   C. identify specific populations who possess information that is useful to the survey.
   D. send the questionnaire to as many individuals as possible.

29 Foster University recently was awarded money to conduct research concerning the geriatric population. The professors at Foster developed the research design and submitted a plan to address the oral health needs of the geriatric population in their state. Which type of extramural research and approval, funding, and announcement process did Foster University undergo to receive this money?
   A. Grant, RFA
   B. Grant, RFP
   C. Contract, RFA
   D. Contract, RFP

30 All of the following are characteristics of informed consent given during a research project, EXCEPT one. Which one is the EXCEPTION?
   A. Each subject is guaranteed confidentiality.
   B. Subjects are penalized for withdrawal.
   C. An explanation of the purpose of the research is given.
   D. An explanation of procedures and treatments is given.

31 Information regarding the growth rate, geographical distribution, ethnicity, and socioeconomic status of a population refers to which component of the community profile?
A. Community resources
B. Population characteristics
C. Dental disease
D. Policies and decision making

32 In the community resources component of the community profile, which of the following terms BEST describes the use, accessibility, and provision of available dental services?
A. Labor
B. Funds
C. Facilities
D. Fluorides

33 A student is providing a lecture on smokeless tobacco. She presents the major principles and key points of her lecture. Which part of the lecture (program) is the student delivering?
A. The set
B. The body
C. The closure
D. The introduction

34 A public health dental hygienist has designed an educational program on early childhood caries for expectant parents. Information regarding the audience's current knowledge of the disease is gathered by means of a quiz administered at the beginning of the presentation. The administration of the quiz occurs during which part of the program?
A. The set
B. The body
C. The closure
D. The introduction

35 Two students are reviewing a videotape of their presentation. These students are evaluating the
A. plan.
B. delivery.
C. learning.
D. plan and the delivery.
E. plan, the delivery, and the learning.

36 It is MOST advantageous to conduct evaluation during which part of oral health education?
A. The plan
B. The delivery
C. The learning
D. The plan and the delivery
E. The plan, the delivery, and the learning

37 How can a program presenter BEST evaluate the desired outcome of his or her oral health education program?
A. By evaluating the extent to which the objectives were met
B. By evaluating the teaching strategies used
C. By evaluating the organization of the instruction
D. By evaluating the format and style of the presenter

38 One of the following is NOT a criterion for determining whether a particular disease constitutes a public health problem. Which one is the EXCEPTION?
A. The knowledge of how to alleviate the problem is not being applied.
B. The disease is widespread throughout the community.
C. The disease cannot be prevented by any means.
D. The disease can be cured easily.

39 Which teeth are known as the Ramfjord teeth?
A. #2, #6, #12, #19, #25, and #31
B. #2, #8, #13, #18, #26, and #29
C. #3, #9, #12, #19, #25, and #28
D. #3, #10, #13, #17, #24, and #30

40 Which of the following was developed by the Office of Economic Opportunity and provides services to low-income preschool children?
A. Medicaid
B. Medicare
C. Head Start
D. Maternal and Child Health Services

41 Which of the following BEST describes dental services rendered through the Indian Health Service?
A. Are provided by dentists and auxiliaries who are employed by the federal government
B. Are provided by dentists and auxiliaries and are financed by the patient or through other means
C. Are provided by dentists and auxiliaries who are not government employees
D. Are provided by dentists and auxiliaries who are in a group practice with a health maintenance organization

42 Troy, Colorado, is a rural mountain town of approximately 400 people. The town has inadequate dental services, and the closest town with comprehensive dental services is 180 miles away. The federal government sends commissioned and civil service dental professionals to the area to meet the dental needs of this community. This service is provided by:
A. Maternal and Child Health services
B. National Health Services Corps
C. State Health Agency services
D. Medicaid services

43 Which government program includes an early periodic screening, diagnosis, and treatment component?
A. Medicaid
B. Head Start
C. Medicare
D. Maternal and Child Health Services

44 Which of the following was the primary goal of the health maintenance organizations (HMOs)?
A. To provide a range of healthcare services to participants
B. To help lower the costs of healthcare
C. To increase competition for patients
D. To enable patients to have a wider choice of providers

45 A contract between several practitioners and an insurer to provide healthcare services for lower-than-average fees is referred to as a(n)
A. health maintenance organization (HMO).
B. capitation plan.
C. group practice.
D. preferred provider organization (PPO).

46 The rate of occurrence of a new disease in a population during a given period is referred to as its
A. incidence.
B. prevalence.
C. patterns.
D. severity.

47 All of the following statements are true, EXCEPT one. Which one is the EXCEPTION?

A. The prevalence of periodontal disease does not increase with age.

B. Blacks consistently demonstrate a higher incidence of periodontal disease than whites.

C. Periodontal disease is inversely related to levels of education.

D. The prevalence of periodontal disease is higher in rural than in urban areas.

48 Which of the following is a method of unifying examiners in the diagnostic technique?

A. Calibration

B. Reliability

C. Validity

D. Pretesting

49 The Plaque Assessment Scoring System (PASS) evaluates

A. supragingival dental biofilm.

B. fissure dental biofilm.

C. subgingival dental biofilm.

D. both supragingival and subgingival dental biofilm.

50 What is the MOST appropriate index to use to measure progressive stages of periodontal disease and amount of clinical attachment loss?

A. DFTS

B. PI

C. deft

D. dmfs

E. PDI

Answer Key and Rationales

1 (C) Placing an amalgam is a *secondary* prevention technique, designed to terminate a disease (e.g., caries) and restore tissues to near normal function (e.g., amalgam restoration). *Primary* prevention prevents, reverses, or arrests disease before treatment is needed such as with the use of fluoride and enamel sealants in regard to caries. *Tertiary* prevention replaces lost tissues and rehabilitates to near normal function such as the delivery of a denture when teeth are lost so as to still allow a person to eat and speak. Health promotion refers to individual's health-related behavior change.

2 (C) Use of dental services is defined as proportion of a population who receive dental care services within a given period. Demand is a combination of perceiving need and seeking services. Need is identification of an oral disease, and normative need is amount of oral care needed to keep a community healthy.

3 (D) The statement that "individuals with poor general health are MORE likely to use dental services" is false. Those who do NOT seek routine, preventive care for general health are NOT likely to seek care for oral health. Others are TRUE.

4 (D) Socioeconomic status (SES), measure of BOTH income and education, is interrelated with all of the other factors that affect individual's use of dental services. Other factors (age, ethnicity, and gender) are NOT interrelated with regard to effect on individual's use of dental services.

5 (C) Third-party payment plans are insurance contract between dental office, patient, and insurance company. Fee-for-service is a two-party plan whereby patient pays an out-of-pocket fee to provider. Indemnity plans operate in the same way as traditional insurance. Capitation plans refer to contracts between dentists and insurance companies to provide services to patients.

6 (A) Reasonable fees are actual fees charged by dental provider, modified according to each patient's individual need. These fees may or may NOT exceed dentist's usual fee and/or customary fee allowed by insurance company. MOST frequently charged fee is the usual fee. Customary fee is maximum benefit payable under particular plan.

7 (C) Capitation plan is defined as fixed monthly payment based on the number of patients assigned to the dentist. Insurance company takes into account that some patients will seek significant amount of care and others will NOT seek any care. Third-party plan is a contract between dental office, patient, and insurance company. Indemnity plans are traditional insurance plans with submittal and reimbursement, and Delta Dental provides dental care contracts through a customary fee structure.

8 (B) Direct reimbursement occurs when an employer agrees to pay a portion of an employee's dental services. The employee seeks care and pays the dentist directly, and the employer reimburses the employee for those services. When insurance company directly reimburses individual, this is through an indemnity plan. Capitation refers to fixed monthly fee that is paid to providing dentist. Actual fee charged by the dentist or provider can exceed the fee set by the insurance company and is referred to as customary; however, patient typically pays difference.

9 (D) Prevalence is term that describes 250 cases of squamous cell carcinoma in a group of 10,000 18-year-olds in 2008. Prevalence is defined as the total number of cases of disease in a given population at a specific time. Rate refers to a ratio of actual to possible cases. Incidence is number of new cases of a disease. Morbidity refers to disease, and mortality refers to death; BOTH are typically described as rates.

10 (D) Root caries index evaluates BOTH the risk and the extent of root caries in areas exposed by gingival recession and would be the BEST index for a group of adults between the ages of 70 and 85 who exhibit recession, inflammation, and bleeding. DMFT and

DMFS indices evaluate decayed, missing, and filled teeth and surfaces, respectively. The UTN index divides the mean number of decayed teeth by the mean number of decayed and filled teeth to determine the percentage of teeth that need treatment. The DMFT, DMFS, and UTN indices do NOT address root caries.

11 (D) O'Leary plaque index would be the BEST selection for monitoring Joe's oral hygiene performance by indicating the location of dental biofilm. It would enable him to visualize areas that need concentration and areas of thorough dental biofilm removal. The OHI-S evaluates BOTH debris and calculus and is used MAINLY on large populations. The GI evaluates gingivitis, and the PHP evaluates dental biofilm on six selected teeth.

12 (B) The PHP index evaluates dental biofilm on six selected teeth, gives specific information about a patient's dental biofilm removal ability, and can also be used during subsequent visits to demonstrate improvement over time. The OHI-S evaluates BOTH debris and calculus for large populations. The GI evaluates gingivitis, and Russell's PI assesses the progressive stages of periodontal disease and attachment loss.

13 (A) The OHI-S contains BOTH debris and calculus components and examines the facial surfaces of teeth #3, #8, #14, and 24 and the lingual surfaces of teeth #19 and #30 (see rationale for question 12).

14 (B) Ideal index is reliable, reproducible, valid, easily understood, and easily explained. Elaborate mechanisms that evaluate several factors are MORE difficult to understand and reproduce. Indices should be able to be replicated easily, and only necessary factors should be recorded for the study.

15 (E) The GI is used MAINLY to evaluate gingivitis by assessing tissue for bleeding, color, contour, and ulceration. The O'Leary PI ONLY records the location of dental biofilm. The PHP assesses soft and hard debris and deposits. Russell's PI assesses periodontal disease and attachment loss, and Ramfjord's index evaluates gingival dental biofilm, probing depths, and calculus.

16 (A) Russell's PI is used MAINLY to evaluate the progressive stages of periodontal disease and attachment loss in major populations. Scores range from 0 to 8 in severity. Ramfjord's PDI evaluates gingival dental biofilm, probing depths, and calculus. The CPITN evaluates pockets, bleeding, and dental biofilm in six sextants and is also used MAINLY to identify the treatment needs of specific groups. The GI evaluates gingivitis.

17 (C) The CPITN would be MOST appropriate for older adult patients in the assisted living community. It was developed by the World Health Organization to assess pocketing, bleeding, dental biofilm retention.

This information is used to determine specific periodontal treatment needs of a given population. Other indices are NOT designed to determine the specific needs of a population.

18 (C) Water fluoridation is NOT expensive to administer; very inexpensive, ranging in cost from \$0.12 to \$1.16 per individual per year. The other statements are TRUE.

19 (A) Enamel sealants are recommended for children and young adults in fluoridated and nonfluoridated communities. They can be applied by dentists and dental hygienists or assistants (depending on state practice acts) and have excellent retention and efficacy against decay.

20 (C) Diet counseling is indicated when a patient has a high rate of caries but is still taking the appropriate amount of fluoride. The age of the patient (16) indicates the possible consumption of highly cariogenic foods. Enamal (pit and fissure) sealants are NOT indicated for carious lesions. She is receiving the CORRECT amount of fluoride from the water supply; therefore supplementation is NOT indicated.

21 (A) Success requires that patients be evaluated and counseled according to their specific needs and NOT in the same manner as other patients. Recommendations SHOULD be different for each patient. When successful counseling takes place, patients exhibit cooperation and motivation, especially when rapport has been established. Reevaluation and assessment also must take place after the patient implements new recommendations.

22 (B) IRB approval is necessary before any research is conducted on human subjects. An IND number is obtained before evaluating new drugs never tested on human populations. Informed consent occurs after IRB approval and refers to obtaining the consent of the patient enrolled in a research study. FDA approval is required to market a new drug after research has been conducted.

23 (A) Primary responsibility of the IRB is to review and approve research on human subjects in order to protect their privacy and safety.

24 (B) University of Troy must obtain an IND number through the FDA if the drug being evaluated has NOT been tested in a human population. The IRB reviews proposed research on human subjects to protect their safety and privacy. Patients MUST give their informed consent to participate in a study.

25 (A) True experimental research includes BOTH random selection and random assignment; quasi-experimental research does NOT involve random selection. Single-subject studies are conducted on one or a few subjects who exhibit a rare or specific condition. Questionnaire surveys refer to research through written or oral response.

26 (B) Collection of data to determine a program's effectiveness BEST describes administrative and evaluative research, which evaluates the operation and effectiveness of and the need for improvement in an oral health education program. Clinical trials evaluate techniques and therapeutic interventions. Education and behavioral research assess behavioral education techniques and focus on knowledge, attitudes, and behaviors. Experimental research involves clinical trials and experiments.

27 (D) Direct observation would be the BEST method for learning about the school nurses' skill level in fluoride administration. It would enable the researcher to identify any inconsistencies and/or needs for improvement. Interviewing would provide ONLY self-reported information, whereas a written questionnaire would limit actual implementation techniques, and interviewing the principals would NOT gather information from the individuals directly involved.

28 (C) Questionnaire surveys SHOULD be sent to subjects who possess specific information that the researcher wants to capture. Having the individuals write their names would violate confidentiality, response of feelings is difficult to interpret, and sending the questionnaires to as many individuals as possible would elicit unwanted information.

29 (A) Grant is awarded to researchers to conduct research protocol that has been defined by party receiving the award. Grants are applied for through a request for application (RFA), in which a plan for meeting the priority area is submitted. Contract is awarded to individual or institution, and protocol already is defined by government agency awarding the money, applied for through an RFP (request for proposal).

30 (B) Subjects are NOT penalized for withdrawing from a study; rather, all subjects are guaranteed the ability to withdraw at any time without prejudice or repercussion. Confidentiality is kept throughout the study. Purpose of the research and its procedures and treatments are fully explained to each participant.

31 (B) Population characteristics of a community profile include the number of individuals in the population and their geographical distribution, growth rate, population density, urban vs. rural areas, ethnicity, SES, nutrition and diet, types of housing availability, standard of living, public services, utilities, and general health status. Community resources include funds, facilities, and labor available for use in the community. Dental disease tracks the patterns and distribution of disease. Policy making and decision making outline the community's organizational structure and the oral health attitudes of its leaders.

32 (C) Facilities describe the use, accessibility, and provision of dental services, including the location of the closest major medical center in a community,

the specialty services available, the number, type, and location of dental facilities, the number of operatories and laboratories available, and the adequacy of equipment. Labor describes the number of active dental and other healthcare workers. Funds encompass all available monetary resources, and fluorides refer to BOTH water fluoridation and professionally applied fluorides in the community.

33 (B) The "body" portion of a presentation provides the major points and key principles. The "set" introduces content and establishes mood. The "closure" summarizes the body and does NOT provide new material. "Introductions" are similar to the set.

34 (A) Instructional set of a presentation introduces the content or procedure to be discussed, describes usefulness of the information, motivates the student and arouses the student's interest, can be used to assess the audience's knowledge base by administering a quiz or reviewing previous material, states the objectives, and establishes a mood for the presentation.

35 (B) Evaluating delivery of one's presentation can be accomplished by reviewing a videotape and/or gathering feedback from the audience and peers. Students' learning can be evaluated through testing, and the plan is evaluated by comparison with the stated objectives.

36 (E) Evaluation should take place during all steps of developing an oral health education program.

37 (A) The outcome of a program can be evaluated by comparing the objectives with the outcome and assessing the degree to which each objective was met. Evaluating teaching strategies gives information on the delivery and plan, the organization, and the presentation format and style.

38 (C) Public health problem must meet the following criteria: (a) disease is widespread, (b) disease can be prevented, alleviated, or cured; (c) knowledge of how to alleviate problem is NOT being applied.

39 (C) Ramfjord teeth are teeth #3, #9, #12, #19, #25, and #28, MOSTLY used in clinical trial research as representative sample of the entire dentition.

40 (C) Head Start was developed by Office of Economic Opportunity as result of the Economic Opportunity Act. Primary purpose was to provide social services and health education to low-income preschool children so that they would be able to enter school on an equal ground with higher income peers.

41 (A) Dental services rendered by the Indian Health Service are provided by dentists and auxiliaries who are employed by the PHS. These providers are commissioned officers of the Dental Service Corps. Others do not fit this description.

42 (B) National Health Services Corps is a federal health labor deployment program. It provides commissioned officers and civil service individuals of the

PHS to areas where there are inadequate health services because of shortages. The federal government provides Maternal and Child Health Services for women of childbearing age with low incomes and for children under 21 years of age. State health agencies provide services locally in each state, and Medicaid provides healthcare to those under 21 years of age who are in a "needy" group.

43 (A) Medicaid administers early periodic screening, diagnosis, and treatment program. Medicaid services are provided to specific needy people. Head Start is a federally funded program distributed by the Office of Economic Opportunity to provide educational and social services to low-income preschool children. Medicare offers health insurance to individuals 65 years of age and older. Maternal and Child Health Services provide health services for women of childbearing age and for children under 21 years of age.

44 (B) HMOs were developed MAINLY to help lower the costs of healthcare. Range of services, competition, and a choice of providers are available without an HMO.

45 (D) A PPO is a contract between several practitioners and an insurer to provide healthcare services for lower-than-average fees. Participants in HMOs pay a fixed fee for healthcare and choose physicians within their HMO. Capitation plan pays a fixed fee to a provider to deliver care to participants who are assigned for care. Group practice refers to a group of several healthcare professionals who provide services together.

46 (A) Incidence refers to the rate of occurrence of a new disease in a population during a given period of time. Prevalence refers to the number of persons affected by a disease at a specific point in time. Patterns are formed when data are repeated over time. Severity refers to the extent of a disease.

47 (A) Although aging does NOT preordain periodontal disease, studies have shown that the prevalence of periodontal disease increases directly with age, MOST likely because of repeated exposures to bacterial infection over a lifetime.

48 (A) Calibration is a method of unifying examiners in the diagnostic technique.

49 (C) PASS index evaluates subgingival dental biofilm, unlike the O'Leary plaque index, which only evaluates supragingival dental biofilm.

50 (B) Russell's periodontal index (PI) assesses progressive stages of periodontal disease and amount of attachment loss; used MAINLY for major population groups.

CHAPTER 18

Ethics and Jurisprudence

ETHICS IN DENTISTRY AND RELATIVISM ▬▬

The study of ethics in dental hygiene involves the understanding of concepts of **ethics, morals, mores. Relativism** in ethics involves issues of behavior and belief. What is judged right varies among individuals, situations, cultures. Ethical theories form the basis of principles and rules.

- See CD-ROM for Chapter Terms and WebLinks.

A. Relativism:
  1. Cultural relativism: defines moral rightness and wrongness based on cultural beliefs (common or social morality).
  2. Descriptive relativism: people from different cultures have different views regarding morals.
  3. Normative relativism: ultimately, ALL ethical judgments are arbitrary and not justifiable.
  4. Personal relativism: individual determines what is right or wrong according to personal standards of goodness and NOT according to cultural influences.

B. Ethical theories:
  1. Utilitarian theory: encompasses "the greatest good for the greatest number" or **universality;** addresses consequences:
    a. Also known as Mills' "greatest happiness" theory.
      (1) Act: doing the right act will result in the best consequences.
      (2) Rule: actions are right or wrong based on their consequences.
    b. Value: depends on whether something is determined to be good or harmful.
  2. Deontological theory: focuses on the action, rule, or practice of an act rather than on the consequences; involves performing the right action regardless of the consequences (Kantian theory).
  3. **Virtue** theory: focuses on judging traits of character as good or bad; promotes good choices.

Ethical Principles

Ethical principles are the laws or doctrines of ethics (see CD-ROM for ADHA Code of Ethics).

A. **Autonomy:** everyone has the right to hold and act on personal values and beliefs such as the right to privacy, freedom of choice, and accepting responsibility for one's actions as long as harm is NOT inflicted on others.

B. **Nonmaleficence:** action is wrong if harm is inflicted on others (e.g., staying current with advances in dental hygiene and dentistry and taking CE courses).

C. **Beneficence:** action is moral if it is good and helps a person or enhances the welfare of person.
  1. Rules:
    a. Avoid inflicting harm (principle of nonmaleficence).
    b. Prevent or remove harm.
    c. Promote good and do well.
  2. Problems in dentistry related to beneficence:
    a. Balancing good against harm for the patient.
    b. Conflicts between patients and healthcare providers as to what is a good treatment record result.
    c. Influence of a third party (e.g., caretaker, insurance carrier) on what treatment can be done.
    d. Conflicts that occur when patients refuse or disagree with treatment.
  3. Paternalism: acting as a parent would on behalf of a child, including overriding an autonomous decision for the good of a patient.

D. **Justice:** treating individuals fairly; involves giving patients their due or what is owed to them ("golden rule"). Example: production goals should not affect the treatment we offer a patient.
  1. Distributive justice applies to the proper and fair allocation of many aspects of society (e.g., political rights such as voting privileges, rights of women and minorities).
  2. Formal principle of justice or equality means that "equals must be treated equally, unequals treated unequally."
  3. Theories of distribution:
    a. Utilitarian theory: combines the principles of beneficence and nonmaleficence; aims to maximize good and minimize bad.
    b. Libertarian theory: offers healthcare based on respecting autonomy; need is NOT a factor; giving healthcare charitably based on patient's wishes.
    c. Egalitarian theory: emphasizes equality; based on the idea that everything is for everyone.
  4. Example of violation of justice: dentist uses a specific lab for HMO patients and another for private pay patients to save overall costs.

E. **Veracity:** obligation to speak the truth and disclose information that is necessary for the patient to make sound treatment decisions.

F. **Fidelity:**
   1. Moral obligation to keep promises and other commitments.
   2. Duty on confidentiality: MUST keep confidential the information provided by the patient.

Ethical Dilemma and Decision Making

An **ethical dilemma** occurs when two or more ethical principles are morally justifiable but only one is acted on. The outcome of such a situation varies according to the principle that is chosen. **Ethical decision** making involves several steps of analysis. Person responsible for the decision may need to make a **moral evaluation** of those involved, based on **altruism.** Patient is the autonomous person, and practitioner's value system should NOT come into play; patient's values are what is important.

With moral evaluation of **publicity,** the person publicly states his or her evaluation and on what it is based, while **ultimacy** is a judgment based on a moral evaluation that has no higher standard, based on **societal trust.** Example of societal trust is maintaining patient confidentiality and being concerned for the patient instead of one's self-interest.

A. Identify the problem.

B. Relevant facts must be gathered; decision making before receiving information should be avoided.

C. **Values** must be identified, and for the dental professional these involve **core values;** we must put the patient first without discrimination, which will help to ensure optimal care for the patient and to maintain competency:
   1. Acknowledging the **rights** of the patient.
   2. Granting patient autonomy; allowing patient to participate in decision making regarding treatment; allowing patient right to consent to or refuse treatment.
   3. Avoiding harm to others according to principle of nonmaleficence.
   4. Having respect for the dental profession.
   5. Being true to oneself; following one's conscience.
   6. Following the law.
   7. Generating options and reviewing available options.
   8. Choosing an option and justifying it.

D. Things that SHOULD be taken into consideration:
   1. Rights of the individuals involved.
   2. Duties of the professional involved.
   3. Core values that apply.
   4. Benefits of the care provided or offered.
   5. Realistic alternatives.
   6. Patient knowledge.
   7. Financial or legal factors.
   8. Need for outside consultation.

DENTAL LIABILITY, JURISPRUDENCE, AND TYPES OF LAW

Understanding types of law and methods of avoiding lawsuits or dental liability is vitally important in the practice of dental hygiene. **Jurisprudence** is the philosophy of law. Civil law, which includes contract law and tort law, and criminal law are the two major types of law.

• See CD-ROM for Chapter Terms and WebLinks.

A. Civil law:
   1. Involves crime against a person; concerned with actions that cause harm to an individual.
   2. Individual files suit with a private attorney; response to damages is typically measured in terms of money.

B. Contract law (form of civil law):
   1. Involves a breach of contract; involves the breaking of a contract by either party (healthcare provider or patient) or failing to keep one's part of the contract.
   2. Examples: provider does not provide care that was discussed and agreed to, patient does not pay, or services take too long to complete.

C. Tort law (form of civil law): involves a civil wrong or injury to another person.
   1. Technical assault or battery is a wrongful act that is NOT consented to; includes performing a procedure that patient has NOT been agreed to have done. Examples: placing sealants or performing fluoride treatment on a minor without consent of parent or guardian.
   2. Maligning a patient involves saying or writing something that may damage the patient's reputation; includes slander (verbal) and libel (written).
   3. **Negligence** (often considered synonymous with malpractice) is carelessness, without the intent to harm a patient; it occurs when the appropriate standard of care is NOT met and some damage results. Example: dentist knowingly permits a hazard to exist in the office, and consequently patient is injured.
      a. Liability for negligence requires the existence of:
         (1) Healthcare provider undertaking care of the patient; a duty to the patient results.
         (2) Healthcare provider breaching a duty owed to the patient.
         (3) Evidence of damage or harm to the patient.
         (4) Harm or damage to the patient being related to the breach of duty.
   4. Grounds for malpractice: MOST lawsuits involve failure to diagnose and treat periodontal disease.
      a. Failure to sterilize: sterilization practices should be in accordance with recommendations of the Centers for Disease Control and Prevention (CDC) and the American Dental Association (ADA).

b. Failure to obtain or produce adequate radiographs; this may involve:
   (1) Failure to obtain radiograph when radiograph is indicated.
   (2) Unskillful use or improper processing of radiograph, which jeopardizes diagnosis.
   (3) Refusal by the patient; if a patient refuses to have a radiograph, a written release form should be signed by the patient; a refusal MUST be noted in the patient's chart; radiographs are used for diagnosis and therefore must remain a part of a patient's record.
c. Failure to refer: patient SHOULD be referred to a specialist when "average" dentist knows that procedure is complex.
d. Causing trauma: slipping of an instrument alone does NOT constitute negligence; however, making a statement that may indicate that an error was made by the healthcare provider (e.g., "I should have had a fulcrum") is known as admission against interest: a statement, spoken or written, that may prove the opposite of what the person contends in court.
e. Failure to inform: patient must be informed before he or she can give consent.

D. Criminal law: pertains to actions that constitute a wrong against society.
E. State officials respond to such actions, which on conviction are punishable by death, imprisonment, fine, or removal from office.
F. Examples: practicing profession of dental hygiene or dentistry without a license.

PROFESSIONAL PRACTICE STUDY ▰▰▰▰▰▰

Scenario: The dental hygienist is completing an oral prophylaxis on a new patient. While she is retrieving a posterior scaler from her tray, the instrument slips from her hand and lands on her patient's head. The instrument tip embeds in the scalp tissues. The hygienist carefully removes the instrument, cleanses the wound with antibacterial soap, applies pressure to stop the bleeding, and apologizes for the injury. The patient remains calm and says, "Don't worry about it." The hygienist documents the incident in the patient's record.

1. Is this an incidence of negligence? Why or why not?
2. Did the dental hygienist handle the situation appropriately?
3. What types of information regarding the incident should the dental hygienist include in the patient's record?

1. Not incidence of negligence because there is no indication that accident was caused by particular action, such as not using a fulcrum. If the hygienist had indicated to patient that there was a particular cause for incident

(admission against interest), a case could be made for negligence, which is grounds for malpractice.
2. No one wishes to injure a patient; however, accidents do occur. The hygienist showed concern for her patient by taking immediate care of the wound. She handled the situation well. There is evidence that concern and care on part of clinician can greatly reduce incidences of litigation by patients.
3. Patient's record should include date and time of incident, detailed description of what occurred, hygienist's actions, patient's actions and reactions. The clinician should obtain the patient's signature that patient was informed and note on the record that patient agreed that everything was all right.

Prudent Dental Care

Measures that are used to help avoid legal action include reasonably prudent or sensible practitioner, admissions against interest, *res ipsa loquitur,* proper documentation. Informed consent is discussed next.

A. Be aware that the reasonably prudent practitioner measure is used by law to determine whether provider has exercised reasonable care.
B. Avoid admissions against interest, or making a statement that serves to defeat your own interest; such admissions are legally admissible in court.
   1. Admission of negligence by employee occurs when the healthcare provider admits to improper conduct.
   2. *Res gestae* means "part of the action" and refers to a statement made during the time of the negligent act.
C. Avoid *res ipsa loquitur* or "a matter that speaks for itself," referring to an injury that is directly related to an instance of negligence (e.g., healthcare provider fails to take a medical history or renders services while intoxicated).
D. Prove contributory negligence: that patient has contributed to harmful result.
E. Identify another proximate cause; reveal that harm to patient may have resulted from another incident.
F. Keep accurate and complete patient records, single MOST important factor in the defense of MOST malpractice cases; record information in indelible ink; if an error is made in a patient's chart, mark one line through the statement and place your initials next to the area (do NOT erase, black-out, or use correction fluid).
   1. Medical history should be current, include patient's signature, and be reviewed at each visit.
   2. Diagnosis should be recorded (including dental hygiene diagnosis).
   3. Treatment plan(s) should include ALL options given to patient. Note that all benefits, risks, and alternatives (RB&A) were explained to patient verbally and in writing, and have the patient sign the chart stating that he or she understands the treatment and risks.

4. Record of treatment should include date(s) of treatment, procedure(s) performed, drugs used and/or administered; record should also indicate canceled and broken appointments.
5. Copies of all correspondence regarding patients should be kept, together with receipts of registered mail.
   a. Radiographs should be:
      (1) Processed properly to avoid deterioration with age.
      (2) Carefully labeled with patient's name, date taken, and dentist's name.
      (3) Taken properly so that they are diagnostically acceptable.
      (4) Retained for minimum length of time required by statute of limitations in a state.
6. Letters to patients (correspondence) should be carefully worded to ensure understanding and minimize chance for libel.
G. Transfer of records:
   1. For inactive patient, records are typically kept for length of time required by the statute of limitations and/or state dental practice act.
   2. For active patients, records are kept by dentist unless requested by another dentist.
   3. Steps for requesting transfer of records:
      a. Always keep on record the letter(s) requesting records.
      b. Send copies of records by way of registered mail; request a receipt.
      c. Request that records be returned to the office after their use.
H. Insurance claims include records only of performed procedures; falsifying information is fraudulent and may result in a legal action.
I. Statute of limitations is the legal time span in which a lawsuit (civil) for a wrong must be filed.
   1. Malpractice suit, in most states, must be initiated within 2 years of time that the wrongful act was committed.
   2. Limitation for filing a breach of contract suit typically is 6 years; recommended that records be retained for minimum of 10 years.
J. Liability insurance should be carried by each licensed professional.
   1. Professional reliability: every professional has a responsibility to provide high-quality dental care.
   2. *Respondeat superior:* employer is often named in a suit in which an employee caused harm to a patient.

PROFESSIONAL PRACTICE STUDY ▬▬▬▬

Scenario: A dentist after 33 years of the practice of dentistry receives a letter from an attorney stating that one of his patients has contracted infectious endocarditis (IE) from a routine oral prophylaxis appointment 6 months ago. The dentist reviews the patient's medical history from the last visit and finds no indication on the record of any medical problems, including IE or conditions that involve its risk. The record of treatment indicates that the patient had generalized moderate chronic periodontitis, with moderate subgingival calculus, and that homecare instruction was given because of excess calculus, the condition of the patient's tissue, and excess bleeding. The chart also indicates that the patient was scheduled to have tooth #31 extracted by an oral surgeon the day after the oral prophylaxis appointment.

1. What suit will the attorney most likely file against the dentist?
2. Is this suit processed under civil or criminal law?
3. Is the dentist and/or dental hygienist liable for this suit?
4. What can the dentist do to help prove that the patient may not have contracted IE from the visit to the dentist's office?

1. Negligence or malpractice; negligence implies care lessness without intent of harming a patient
2. Negligence is categorized under tort law, which is a branch of civil law (actions causing harm to individual).
3. There are four factors that must be present before dentist and/or dental hygienist is liable for negligence: (1) healthcare provider must have undertaken the care of patient; (2) healthcare provider must have breached a duty that was owed to patient; (3) harm or damage to patient must be proved; and (4) harm must be related to breach of duty. If any one of these four factors is missing, ruling will be in favor of dentist or dental hygienist.
4. Two considerations may be used to spare the dentist from judgment. First, dentist may try to prove contributory negligence. Patient may have knowingly failed to inform dentist or note on the medical history that the patient had a heart condition (such as an artificial valve replacement) or history of IE that poses risk for IE with dental treatment. The patient also may have contributed to the negligence by not taking the antibiotic premedication that the physician prescribed. Second, the dentist may try to prove proximate cause. Cause of patient's IE may have been the visit to oral surgeon because the tooth extraction may have necessitated antibiotic premedication. For these reasons the dental team must make sure that patient's medical history is updated regularly and any medical consultations followed through. Moreover, all records must be complete.

Informed Consent

Informed consent (in a contractual relationship) means that a patient has given a healthcare provider permission to perform certain procedure(s) and that the patient understands any risks involved in the treatment.

A. To give consent and avoid breach of contract, patient must understand the following:
  1. Nature of his or her condition.
  2. Treatment proposed.
  3. Any risks involved or chances of failure.
  4. Possible results of NOT treating the condition.
  5. Any alternative procedures that may be necessary.
B. To validate consent, the following requirements must be met:
  1. Consent must be informed.
  2. Consent must be given for specific treatment(s).
  3. Individual giving consent must be legally competent.
  4. Treatments consented to must be legal.
  5. Consent must NOT have been obtained through deceit or fraud.
C. Types of consent and refusal:
  1. **Implied consent:** implied by the actions of the patient (e.g., a patient comes to the office for an examination and consultation; therefore consent is established by the actions of provider).
     a. Quasi consent is a type of implied consent.
     b. Patient is in danger of injury or death and is unable to give consent; emergency treatment is given.
  2. **Expressed consent:** informed consent that is given verbally or in writing (provides the MOST protection).
  3. **Parental or guardian consent:** required when a minor or an individual who is NOT mentally competent to give consent needs treatment; usually provided by a parent or other legal caretaker, preferably in writing.
  4. Written and verbal mandatory consent MUST be given for the following situations:
     a. Administration of new drugs.
     b. Use of a patient's photograph (must be recognizable).
     c. Administration of general anesthesia.
     d. Treatment that will take longer than 1 year to complete.
     e. Treatment of children in a public program.
  5. **Informed refusal** against dental advice occurs when patient declines treatment after treatment plan is presented and has been advised of the risks associated with refusing a recommended procedure.

Federal Government Provisions

Many federal government provisions involve the dental practice. The *Health Insurance Portability and Accountability Act* (HIPAA) was enacted by U.S. Congress; Title II of HIPAA, *Administrative Simplification* (AS) provisions. Note that use of Medical Safety Data Sheets (MSDS) is a concern of the Occupational and Safety Health Administration (OSHA), NOT HIPAA.
A. HIPAA with AS provisions requires establishment of national standards for electronic healthcare transactions and national identifiers for providers, health insurance plans, employers.
  1. The AS provisions also address security and privacy of health data.
  2. Standards are meant to improve efficiency and effectiveness of U.S. healthcare system by encouraging widespread use of electronic data interchange within U.S. healthcare system.
B. *Privacy Rule* was added to establish regulations for use and disclosure of *Protected Health Information* (PHI).
  1. General information:
     a. PHI is any information about health status, provision of healthcare, or payment for healthcare that can be linked to an individual. Includes any part of patient's medical record or payment history.
     b. Covered entities must disclose PHI to individual within 30 days upon request. They must also disclose PHI when required to do so by law, such as reporting suspected abuse to state agencies.
     c. Covered entity may disclose PHI to facilitate treatment, payment, or healthcare operations or if the covered entity has obtained authorization from the individual. However, when covered entity discloses any PHI, must make a reasonable effort to disclose only minimum necessary information required to achieve its purpose.
  2. *Dental setting* implementation:
     a. Thus HIPAA requires the covered entity to designate a privacy officer who understands how the privacy rules affect the dental office and patient care.
        (1) This individual is familiar with the requirements and makes certain that policies and procedures have been implemented and training has been conducted.
        (2) In many dental offices, office manager or front desk coordinator serves as privacy officer.
     b. PHI includes any information that is created or received by dental office as it relates to patient's care.
        (1) Includes radiographs, images (both intraoral and photographic), and traditional dental record.
        (2) Also includes oral discussion of patient care that may be overhead by other parties.
     c. Dental office should create a notice of privacy policy that informs patients how their information will be used and disclosed.
        (1) The privacy rules require covered entities to have written, site-specific privacy procedures detailing how staff members may have access to PHI and how PHI is used and disclosed.

(2) In addition to the practice's team members, business associates have access to PHI; business associates are defined as third parties, including consultants, billing and collection agencies, attorneys, software trainers, and hardware technicians; privacy rules address how to deal with business associates to ensure the privacy of PHI.

(3) Dental office needs to make a good faith effort to obtain each patient's acknowledgment of receipt of notice of privacy practices.

  (a) May be a separate form or incorporated within the office's consent forms. NOT to be confused with the patient's consent to use or disclose PHI, which may be required in some states.

  (b) It is highly recommended, when dealing with any media materials that contain PHI, to obtain a special authorization that details how the PHI will be used and for how long.

(4) According to federal law and most state laws, patient has a legal right to the information contained in the dental record; HIPAA gives patients the right to examine and obtain a copy of their records, access needs to be made within 30 days of the request, and offices may charge patients for the cost of duplicating and sending the records.

(5) Patients have the right to file a complaint if they feel their privacy rights have been violated; this complaint is filed directly with the provider or the U.S. Department of Health and Human Services Office for Civil Rights; therefore information on how to file a complaint should be included with the notice of privacy policy.

(6) Dental offices must provide training for their team and maintain documentation of the training; employees should be familiar with practice's privacy policies and procedures and be aware of the disciplinary actions that will be taken if employee fails to follow these procedures.

C. *Security Rule* complements *Privacy Rule,* deals specifically with *Electronic Protected Health Information* (EPHI).

  1. Lays out three types of security safeguards required for compliance: administrative, physical, technical.

    a. For each of these types, the Security Rule identifies various security standards, and for each standard it names both required and addressable implementation specifications.

    b. Required specifications must be adopted and administered as dictated by the rule.

    c. Addressable specifications are more flexible. Individual covered entities can evaluate their own situation and determine the best way to implement addressable specifications.

D. HIPAA has also standardized the use of *Health Care Financing Administration's Health Care Procedural Coding System,* which contains codes for dental services that were created by American Dental Association and published as current dental terminology; first digit, "0," was replaced by a "D"; refer to "Current Dental Terminology, CDT 2007-2008" for the current version of the *Code on Dental Procedures and Nomenclature* ("the Code").

E. *National Health Information Infrastructure Act,* established through the Department of Health and Human Services, mandates electronic medical records (EMRs); ensures that patient health records are capable of being sent electronically anywhere in the country with the patient's agreement, as well as being safely stored electronically.

PROFESSIONAL PRACTICE STUDY

Scenario: A 47-year-old patient in a general dental practice has a thorough periodontal evaluation that reveals generalized severe chronic periodontitis. The dental hygienist explains treatment options to the patient and asks whether there are further questions. A series of four appointments is scheduled. The patient completes the series of appointments and agrees to return in 6 weeks for a reevaluation of treatment. The supervising dentist wants to place images of the patient, before and after the treatment, in his reception room for other patients to see.

1. Did the patient give consent for her treatment? If so, what type of consent did she give?
2. The dental hygienist asks the patient to allow the case to be used as a teaching tool in the practice, which would involve both extraoral and intraoral photographs of both the face and mouth and full-mouth series of radiographs. What type of consent is required before photographs are taken?
3. If, after thorough treatment of the periodontal condition, further loss of alveolar bone is detected, what should be done?
4. What does the supervising dentist need to consider when using the patient's images in his reception room?

1. The patient gave consent for treatment when it was agreed to schedule appointments and then agreed to return for reevaluation. This type of consent is called implied consent.
2. Written, mandatory consent is required in situations in which new drugs are used, recognizable photographs of

a patient are used, general anesthetics are administered, or treatment takes longer than 1 year to complete.

3. If the treatment performed is unsuccessful (as evidenced by further progression of the disease), the general dentist should refer patient to an appropriate specialist, which in this case would be a periodontist.

4. The images of the patient would be considered protected health information (PHI) under the Health Insurance Portability and Accountability Act (HIPAA). It is recommended that the dentist obtain special authorization for use of these images from the patient.

Legal Responsibilities and Duties

Legal responsibilities in the dental practice setting include the duties of the healthcare provider and the patient. Duties are the obligations that one person owes another.

A. Duties of the healthcare provider:
   1. Hold licensure; the healthcare provider must have a valid professional license to practice.
   2. Protect and respect the personal and property rights of the patient; includes respecting patient's right to the ownership of dentures, even if patient has NOT paid for them.
      a. Healthcare provider should AVOID asking patients personal questions.
      b. Patient has right to confidentiality; photographs of patients cannot be displayed and/or published without written permission from patient.
      c. Any discussion in the office between the healthcare provider and patient is considered privileged communication.
      d. There are two exceptions to privileged communication:
         (1) Abuse.
         (2) Communicable diseases.
   3. Provide only care that is necessary and to which the patient has agreed.
   4. Exercise reasonable skill, care, and judgment.
      a. Reasonable skill involves not ONLY having knowledge but the ability to use such knowledge.
      b. Reasonable care relates to how skill is used; the healthcare provider should use the degree of care that a reasonably prudent practitioner would use under similar circumstances.
      c. Reasonable judgment involves making the best decision(s) possible regarding the procedures performed.
   5. Do NOT abandon the patient after individual becomes a patient of record.
      a. Abandonment is desertion; involves failure to provide services and needs to be agreed on by healthcare provider and patient; applies to practitioner who is NOT available.

   b. Withdrawal from a contract:
      (1) Written letter of intent to withdraw is sent to patient by certified or registered mail (with return receipt).
      (2) Contains a statement of care that must be completed.
      (3) Suggests to patient how care can be obtained.
      (4) States that emergency care will be provided for 30 days and all treatment in progress will be completed.
   6. Use standard materials, techniques, and drugs; any experimental procedures, techniques, or drugs used for treatment require the patient's informed consent.
   7. Charge reasonable fees; charge is reasonable when customary and ordinary for service in the same or a similar community.
   8. Keep the patient informed of the progress of treatment; give adequate and understandable instructions to patient so they can be followed.
   9. Achieve reasonable results; healthcare provider has a legal duty to provide standard care but does NOT have to obtain perfect results.
   10. Arrange for care during any temporary absence; if a healthcare provider is unavailable to treat patient, competent care must be available (e.g., a dentist who goes on vacation arranges to have someone available for emergency care); failure to do so may result in abandonment.
   11. Refer the patient to a specialist when patient's needs CANNOT be met; referral should be made when a case is particularly difficult or beyond the dentist's capabilities.
   12. Complete care within a reasonable amount of time; if the completion of treatment exceeds 1 year, patient must give written consent.
B. Duties of the patient:
   1. Pay reasonable fees; fees should be paid within a reasonable period of time.
   2. Cooperate during treatment; involves following instructions given by healthcare provider and keeping appointments.

Government Regulations and Dental Practice Act

Dental profession is regulated by government regulations of state dental practice acts. Dental practice act defines the practice of the dental profession, including dental hygiene, and indicates how an individual may be granted a license to practice within a given state. Practice acts vary from state to state. NO one should provide treatment that their Dental Statute Act does not allow.

A. Purpose of dental practice act:
   1. Protects the public from incompetent practitioners and ensures they will receive a minimum standard of care.

2. Prohibits individuals from practicing in the profession before meeting specific qualifications.

3. Gives authority to state boards of dentistry to issue or deny licensure.

4. Empowers state boards of dentistry to suspend or revoke licenses.

B. Violations of the dental practice act:

1. Are crimes against society; involve any acts in violation of dental practice act of a particular state.

2. Subject individual to professional discipline if convicted.

3. Include illegal acts that do NOT necessarily result in physical harm (e.g., dental hygienist performs an oral prophylaxis before receiving licensure).

4. Examples of infractions:

   a. Sex offenses against patients or employees.

   b. Illegal prescription of narcotics.

   c. Delegation of tasks to one who is NOT qualified.

   d. Poor documentation or improper documentation.

   e. Insurance fraud.

   f. Tax evasion.

C. State board of dentistry:

1. Members are appointed or elected and may include dentists, dental hygienists (in most states), and consumers (in many states).

2. Duties:

   a. Administering the written word of state's practice act.

   b. Issuing and revoking licenses.

   c. Investigating complaints and taking disciplinary action when necessary.

   d. Measuring the competence of graduates by way of state board examinations.

PROFESSIONAL PRACTICE STUDY ▬▬▬▬▬

Scenario: A recent graduate from a dental hygiene program has completed all requirements for licensure. The state board of dentistry will meet in 6 weeks to issue new licenses. A local dentist has just hired the new graduate and would like him to begin practicing immediately as a dental hygienist.

1. What government regulation defines the requirements that an individual must meet to practice dental hygiene in a given state?

2. What is the state board of dentistry, and what are their duties?

3. Can the dental hygiene graduate begin practicing before obtaining his professional license if he has met the requirements for licensure?

1. Dental practice act is the government regulation that includes a definition for the practice of dental hygiene and how an individual can be granted a license to practice in the state.

2. State board of dentistry is a group of appointed or elected members (dentists, dental hygienists, and/or consumers) who administer the practice act, make rules on the administrative act, issue and revoke licenses, investigate complaints, take disciplinary action, and measure competence of graduates through state boards.

3. The hygiene graduate would violate the dental practice act, a crime against society, if he began practicing his profession without a license. If he were convicted of such a violation, he would be subject to professional discipline.

Review Questions

1 What is the study of conduct, which is based on right and wrong issues, known as?

A. Morals

B. Mores

C. Ethics

D. Values

2 The moral evaluation that because it is acceptable for one individual to act a particular way, it is therefore acceptable for others to act in the same way is referred to as

A. publicity.

B. ultimacy.

C. neutrality.

D. universality.

3 An individual who focuses on which actions are right is known as a(n)

A. action utilitarian.

B. value utilitarian.

C. consequential utilitarian.

D. deontologist.

E. "golden rule" keeper.

4 What is treating others fairly and living by the "golden rule" known as?

A. Justice

B. Nonmaleficence

C. Beneficence

D. Paternalism

5 A healthcare provider is responsible for speaking the truth and giving adequate information to allow sound decisions regarding treatment. This is referred to as

A. fidelity.

B. reparation.

C. gratitude.

D. veracity.

6 When an ethical decision must be made, all of the following steps are recommended, EXCEPT one. Which one is the EXCEPTION?

A. Granting patient autonomy

B. Following an employer's directive

C. Avoiding harm

D. Respecting the profession

7 When a dental hygienist does NOT perform a procedure included in the contract with a patient, that is referred to as
A. technical battery.
B. breach of contract.
C. malpractice.
D. negligence.

8 Saying or writing something that may damage a patient's reputation is
A. breach of contract.
B. technical assault.
C. maligning.
D. negligence.

9 Malpractice is one type of
A. tort law.
B. breach of contract.
C. criminal law.
D. technical battery.

10 When an individual commits a wrongful act against society, it is considered an offense of
A. tort law.
B. civil law.
C. contract law.
D. criminal law.

11 Failure on the part of the patient to follow instructions given by the dentist during and after treatment is an example of
A. contributory negligence.
B. *respondeat superior.*
C. *res gestae.*
D. admission against interest.

12 All of the following are CORRECT regarding patient records, EXCEPT one. Which one is the EXCEPTION?
A. Are kept for 1 year
B. Include diagnoses
C. Are recorded in ink
D. Include treatment plans

13 What is the principle that makes the dentist responsible for injuries caused by employees?
A. Admission against interest
B. *Respondeat superior*
C. *Res gestae*
D. Professional reliability

14 A contract initiated by the actions of the parties concerned, in absence of a legally binding contract, is a(n)
A. parental contract.
B. expressed contract.
C. written contract.
D. implied contract.

15 Information acquired about a patient during the course of treatment is considered privileged communication, even in a court of law. EXCEPTIONS to this rule are made when patients exhibit signs or symptoms of (1) alcoholism; (2) child abuse; (3) illegal drug use; (4) communicable disease.
A. 1 and 2
B. 2 and 3
C. 1 and 3
D. 2 and 4
E. 3 and 4

16 When a dentist is NOT available to a patient at any time during treatment, it may be considered an act of
A. withdrawal.
B. abandonment.
C. neglect.
D. technical assault.

17 A patient should give written consent to continue dental treatment if the treatment extends beyond
A. 3 months.
B. 6 months.
C. 1 year.
D. 2 years.

18 Who handles the violations of legal principles?
A. State board of dentistry
B. American Dental Association
C. State practice act
D. American Dental Hygienists' Association

19 Treatment plan(s) should include all options given to the patient. All risks are explained to the patient orally and in writing, and the patient signs the chart stating that he or she understands the treatment and risks.
A. Both statements are true.
B. Both statements are false.
C. The first statement is true, the second is false.
D. The first statement is false, the second is true.

20 According to HIPAA, patients have the right to file a complaint if they feel their privacy rights have been violated; this complaint is filed directly with the provider or with the
A. state board of dentistry.
B. American Dental Association and American Dental Hygienists' Association.
C. U.S. Department of Health and Human Services Office for Civil Rights.
D. attorney general of the state.

Answer Key and Rationales

1 **(C)** Ethics deals with issues of right and wrong regarding conduct and character. Mores are customs of a group. Morals are standards of thought or specific judgments that are typically, but not always, based on strong religious beliefs. Values are beliefs and attitudes that are often established by individual's upbringing or religious affiliation.

2 **(D)** Universality stresses that if it is good for individual to act a certain way, it must be acceptable for others to act in same way. With moral evaluation of publicity, one publicly states his or her evaluation and on what it is based. Neutralism (altruism) is based on how an evaluation is best for someone else, and ultimacy is a judgment based on a moral evaluation that has no higher standard.

3 **(A)** An action utilitarian deals with the actions of what is right and is responsible for the consequences of those actions. A value utilitarian focuses on what counts as a good or harm. A consequential utilitarian decides that an action is either right or wrong based on the consequences of the action. A deontologist focuses on the action of an act without worrying about its consequences. The "golden rule" refers to treating individuals fairly; involves giving patients their due or what is owed to them, that is, justice.

4 (A) Treating others fairly and giving them their just due is known as justice. Nonmaleficence is identifying an action as wrong if harm is inflicted on an individual. Beneficence defines an action as moral if it is good and helps a person. Paternalism involves acting as a parent would, including overriding a decision for the good of an individual.

5 (D) Veracity claims that a healthcare provider has an obligation to speak the truth and keep the patient abreast of all information that is needed to make sound decisions during treatment. Fidelity stresses the duty to maintain confidentiality. Reparation is the act of making amends to an individual who was harmed, and gratitude is the act of showing respect to someone who has helped you.

6 (B) When making an ethical decision, it is important to evaluate own values. Granting a patient's autonomy is a necessary part of the process. Patient can be active in determining his or her treatment and can participate in the decision making regarding the treatment plan. Avoiding harm to others is vital. Healthcare provider should have a conscience and a respect for the profession. Employer's direction may NOT offer the appropriate guidelines for making a decision.

7 (B) Breach of contract involves the breaking of a contract (an agreement) by either party involved. Technical battery is an act performed that was NOT agreed on by the patient. Malpractice, often considered synonymous with negligence, is a form of carelessness that brings harm to a patient. Act that results in harm to the patient does NOT have to be intentional.

8 (C) Maligning an individual involves saying or writing something that can damage that individual's reputation. Slander involves saying something that can destroy an individual's reputation, and libel involves writing something that yields the same result.

9 (A) Malpractice is a civil wrong that is handled under tort law. It involves an injury to a patient that occurs without intent to harm the patient. Such injuries typically are a result of carelessness. Criminal law involves wrongs against society. In such cases the state takes action against the healthcare provider.

10 (D) A criminal law pertains to a criminal action that is a wrong against society (e.g., individual practicing dental hygiene without a license). Tort and contract laws are examples of civil law; lawsuits are filed with a private attorney, and damages typically are measured monetarily.

11 (A) Contributory negligence describes a patient's contribution to the harm. Example: a patient has periodontal problems and is advised to follow a 3-month periodontal maintenance program. However, patient has failed to keep his appointments for the past 2 years. When he finally does keep the appointment, his condition has become worse. Because the broken appointments were recorded in the patient's chart, the dentist can claim that the patient contributed to the negligence. *Respondeat superior* indicates that the dentist is responsible for the wrongful actions of his or her employees. *Res gestae* is a statement that an individual makes during a negligent act and that can be used against him or her in a lawsuit. Admission against interest is a statement made at any time that goes against the legal interest of the person making the statement.

12 (A) Patient records should be kept on file for the length of the statute of limitations within a state. They should always be neatly recorded in ink and SHOULD include a complete record of the diagnosis, treatment plans, updated medical history, correspondence, radiographs, record of treatment.

13 (B) *Respondeat superior* is the principle that makes the dentist responsible for a wrongful action by an employee that caused harm to a patient. Admission against interest is a statement that a person makes, orally or in writing, that may prove to be the opposite of what that person is contending in court; statement can be used in a lawsuit. Professional reliability states that every professional has the responsibility to provide good dental care to patients.

14 (D) An implied contract is established by certain actions on the part of the healthcare provider or patient. An expressed contract is informed consent given in writing or orally. Parental or guardian consent is given when the patient is a minor or is mentally incompetent to give consent. Written consent provides the MOST protection for the patient and is a form of expressed consent.

15 (D) Privileged communication grants the patient autonomy. What the patient confides in the office MUST remain confidential. However, there are two exceptions. When suspected abuse or communicable disease has NOT been reported, proper authorities must be contacted.

16 (B) Abandonment is the result of desertion. Healthcare provider fails to provide services that the two parties had agreed on to be done. If the dentist is on vacation, provision must be made for the period of absence. Withdrawal is the act of terminating treatment before it is completed. Neglect is failure to meet the appropriate standard of care, and technical assault is a wrongful act that has NOT been agreed on.

17 (C) Treatment should be completed within 1 year of its initiation. If it extends beyond that time, the patient should give written consent.

18 (A) State board of dentistry members are appointed or elected and are responsible for administering the written law of a state, or its practice act. They also are responsible for issuing and revoking licenses and investigating any complaints submitted to them. The American Dental Association and the American Dental Hygienists' Association do NOT administer any legal actions. State practice act defines the practice of the dental profession and provides guidelines regarding licensure within the state.

19 (A) Both statements are true. Treatment plan(s) SHOULD include all options given to patient; all risks are explained to patient orally and in writing, and patient signs the chart stating that he or she understands the treatment and risks.

20 (C) According to HIPAA, patients have the right to file a complaint if they feel their privacy rights have been violated; this complaint is filed directly with the provider or with the U.S. Department of Health and Human Services Office for Civil Rights; therefore information on how to file a complaint SHOULD be included with the notice of privacy policy.

Index

Note: Page numbers followed by f indicate illustrations; t, tables; and b, boxed material.